Clinical
Periodontology

8th Edition

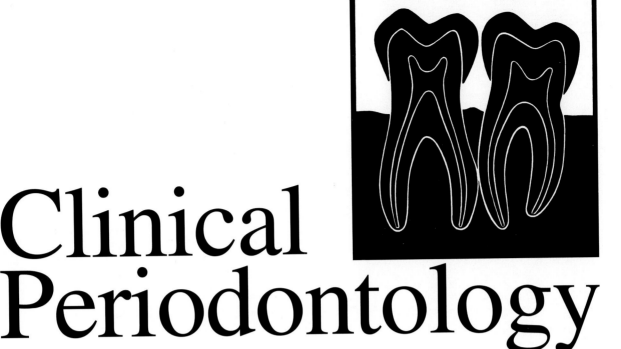

Clinical Periodontology

8th Edition

FERMIN A. CARRANZA, JR., DR. ODONT.
Research Professor of Periodontology and
   Professor Emeritus
School of Dentistry
University of California, Los Angeles
Los Angeles, California

MICHAEL G. NEWMAN, D.D.S.
Adjunct Professor of Periodontology
School of Dentistry
University of California, Los Angeles
Los Angeles, California

W.B. SAUNDERS COMPANY
A Division of Harcourt Brace & Company
Philadelphia   London   Toronto   Montreal   Sydney   Tokyo

W.B. SAUNDERS COMPANY
A Divison of Harcourt Brace & Company

The Curtis Center
Independence Square West
Philadelphia, Pennsylvania   19106

Library of Congress Cataloging-in-Publication Data

Clinical periodontology.—8th ed./[edited by] Fermin A. Carranza, Jr.,
Michael G. Newman.
    p.   cm.
Rev. ed. of: Glickman's clinical periodontology. 7th ed./Fermin A.
Carranza, Jr. 1990.
Includes bibliographical references and index.

ISBN 0-7216-6728-7

1. Periodontics.   I. Carranza, Fermin A.   II. Newman, Michael G.
    III. Glickman, Irving.   Glickman's clinical periodontology.
[DNLM: 1. Periodontal Diseases.   WU 240 C641 1996]
RK361.G58   1996   617.6'32—dc20
DNLM/DLC
                                                    94-37666

Clinical periodontology, 8th edition   ISBN 0-7216-6728-7

Printed in the United States of America

Last digit is the print number: 9   8   7   6   5

Contributors

DONALD F. ADAMS, D.D.S., M.S.
Professor and Chairman, Department of Periodontology, Oregon Health Sciences University, School of Dentistry; Clinical Professor, Department of Surgery, Oregon Health Sciences University Hospital, Portland, Oregon.
Slowly Progressive Periodontitis; Rapidly Progressive Periodontitis, Necrotizing Ulcerative Periodontitis, and Refractory Periodontitis; Treatment of Aggressive Forms of Periodontitis: Refractory, Rapidly Progressive, Necrotizing Ulcerative, and Juvenile.

GEORGE W. BERNARD, D.D.S., PH.D.
Professor and Chair, Section of Oral Biology, School of Dentistry, University of California, Los Angeles, Los Angeles, California.
Biologic Aspects of Dental Implants.

JAIME BULKACZ, DR. ODONT., PH.D.
Lecturer in Periodontics and Oral Biology, University of California, Los Angeles, Los Angeles, California; Staff Member, Northridge Hospital Medical Center, Northridge, California.
Defense Mechanisms of the Gingiva.

FERMIN A. CARRANZA, JR., DR. ODONT.
Research Professor of Periodontology and Professor Emeritus, School of Dentistry, University of California, Los Angeles, Los Angeles, California.
Introduction: The Historical Background of Periodontology; The Gingiva; The Tooth-Supporting Structures; Aging and the Periodontium; Classification of Diseases of the Periodontium; Defense Mechanisms of the Gingiva; Dental Calculus; The Role of Iatrogenic and Other Local Factors; Influence of Systemic Diseases on the Periodontium; Gingival Inflammation; Clinical Features of Gingivitis; Gingival Enlargement; Acute Gingival Infections; Gingival Diseases in Childhood; The Periodontal Pocket; Bone Loss and Patterns of Bone Destruction; Periodontal Response to External Forces; Slowly Progressive Periodontitis; Rapidly Progressive Periodontitis, Necrotizing Ulcerative Periodontitis, and Refractory Periodontitis; Prepubertal and Juvenile Periodontitis; Clinical Diagnosis; Radiographic and Other Aids in the Diagnosis of Periodontal Disease; Determination of the Prognosis;

The Treatment Plan; Rationale for Periodontal Treatment; Treatment of Acute Gingival Disease; Treatment of the Periodontal Abscess; Treatment of Uncomplicated Chronic Gingivitis; Treatment of Aggressive Forms of Periodontitis: Refractory, Rapidly Progressive, Necrotizing Ulcerative, and Juvenile; Orthodontic Considerations in Periodontal Therapy; The Surgical Phase of Therapy; General Principles of Periodontal Surgery; Surgical Anatomy of the Periodontium and Related Structures; Gingival Curettage; The Gingivectomy Technique; The Periodontal Flap; The Flap Technique for Pocket Therapy; Resective Osseous Surgery; Reconstructive Osseous Surgery; Treatment of Furcation Involvement and Combined Periodontal-Endodontic Therapy; Mucogingival Surgery; Treatment of Gingival Enlargement; Biologic Aspects of Dental Implants; Preparation of the Periodontium for Restorative Dentistry.

EDMUND CATALDO, D.D.S., M.S.
Professor of Oral Pathology, Tufts University, School of Dental Medicine; Chief, Oral Pathology, New England Medical Center, Boston, Massachusetts.
AIDS and the Periodontium; Periodontal Management of HIV-Infected Patients.

SEBASTIAN G. CIANCIO, D.D.S., PH.D.
Professor and Chair, Department of Periodontics, School of Dental Medicine, State University of New York at Buffalo, Buffalo, New York.
Antimicrobial and Other Chemotherapeutic Agents in Periodontal Therapy.

SUSAN KINDER HAAKE, D.M.D., PH.D.
Assistant Professor of Periodontics, School of Dentistry, University of California, Los Angeles, Los Angeles, California.
Periodontal Microbiology; Host–Bacteria Interactions in Periodontal Diseases.

THOMAS J. HAN, D.D.S., M.S.
Adjunct Associate Professor of Periodontics, University of California, Los Angeles, Los Angeles, California.
Surgical Aspects of Dental Implants.

v

MARIA E. ITOIZ, Dr. Odont.
Professor and Chair, Oral Pathology Department, Faculty of Dentistry, University of Buenos Aires, Buenos Aires, Argentina.
The Gingiva

DAVID L. JOLKOVSKY, D.D.S., M.S.
Lecturer, Section of Periodontics, School of Dentistry, University of California, Los Angeles, Los Angeles, California.
Antimicrobial and Other Chemotherapeutic Agents in Periodontal Therapy.

SASCHA A. JOVANOVIC, D.D.S., M.S.
Adjunct Assistant Professor of Periodontics, School of Dentistry, University of California, Los Angeles, Los Angeles, California.
Biologic Aspects of Dental Implants; Clinical Aspects of Dental Implants; Diagnosis and Treatment of Peri-implant Disease.

VANESSA MARINHO, D.D.S.
Postdoctoral Student, University of Southern California, School of Dentistry, Department of Periodontics, Los Angeles, California.
Treatment of Aggressive Forms of Periodontitis: Refractory, Rapidly Progressive, Necrotizing Ulcerative, and Juvenile.

MICHAEL K. McGUIRE, D.D.S.
Assistant Clinical Professor of Periodontics, University of Texas Dental Branch, Houston, Texas, and University of Texas Health Science Center, San Antonio, Texas.
Periodontal-Restorative Interrelationships.

ROBERT L. MERIN, D.D.S.
Lecturer in Periodontics, School of Dentistry, University of California, Los Angeles, Los Angeles, California.
Supportive Periodontal Treatment; Results of Periodontal Treatment.

KENNETH T. MIYASAKI, D.D.S, Ph.D.
Associate Professor of Oral Biology, School of Dentistry, University of California, Los Angeles, Los Angeles, California.
Altered Leukocyte Function and Periodontal Disease.

NEAL C. MURPHY, D.D.S., M.S.
Lecturer in Periodontics and Orthodontics, University of California, Los Angeles, Los Angeles, California.
Orthodontic Considerations in Periodontal Therapy.

MICHAEL G. NEWMAN, D.D.S.
Adjunct Professor of Periodontology, School of Dentistry, University of California, Los Angeles, Los Angeles, California.
Host Response: Basic Concepts; Host–Bacteria Interactions in Periodontal Diseases; Advanced Diagnostic Techniques; Slowly Progressive Periodontitis; Rapidly Progressive Periodontitis, Necrotizing Ulcerative Periodontitis, and Refractory Periodontitis; Treatment of Aggressive Forms of Periodontitis: Refractory, Rapidly Progressive, Necrotizing Ulcerative, and Juvenile.

RUSSELL C. NISENGARD, D.D.S., Ph.D.
Distinguished Teaching Professor of Periodontology and Associate Dean for Research and Advanced Education, School of Dental Medicine, and Professor of Microbiology, School of Medicine, State University of New York at Buffalo; Attending Dentist, Buffalo General Hospital and VA Hospital, Buffalo, New York.
Host Response: Basic Concepts; Host–Bacteria Interactions in Periodontal Diseases.

JOAN OTOMO-CORGEL, D.D.S., M.P.H.
Adjunct Assistant Professor of Periodontics, School of Dentistry, University of California, Los Angeles; Director of Research/Faculty, VAMC West Los Angeles Periodontics Residency; Faculty, Rancho Los Amigos Hospital, Los Angeles, California.
Periodontal Treatment of Medically Compromised Patients; Periodontal Treatment of Geriatric Patients.

ANNA M. PATTISON, R.D.H., M.S.
Associate Professor, Department of Dental Hygiene, School of Dentistry, University of Southern California, Los Angeles, Los Angeles, California.
The Periodontal Instrumentarium; Principles of Periodontal Instrumentation; Instrumentation in Different Areas of the Mouth.

GORDON L. PATTISON, D.D.S.
Lecturer in Periodontics, School of Dentistry, University of California, Los Angeles, Los Angeles, California.
The Periodontal Instrumentarium; Principles of Periodontal Instrumentation; Instrumentation in Different Areas of the Mouth.

DOROTHY A. PERRY, R.D.H., Ph.D.
Assistant Professor and Chair, Division of Dental Hygiene and Preventive Dentistry, School of Dentistry, University of California, San Francisco, San Francisco, California.
Plaque Control.

JOHN W. RAPLEY, D.D.S.
Director, Graduate Periodontics, School of Dentistry, University of Missouri at Kansas City, Kansas City, Missouri.
Gingival Inflammation.

TERRY D. REES, D.D.S., M.S.D.
Professor and Chair, Department of Periodontics, Baylor College of Dentistry, Dallas, Texas.
AIDS and the Periodontium; Periodontal Management for HIV-Infected Patients.

MARIANO SANZ, M.D., D.D.S.
Professor of Periodontics, Universidad Complutense de Madrid, Madrid, Spain.
Host Response: Basic Concepts; Host–Bacteria Interactions in Periodontal Diseases; Advanced Diagnostic Techniques.

MAX O. SCHMID, D.M.D.

Former Associate Professor of Periodontics, School of Dentistry, University of California, Los Angeles, Los Angeles, California; Private practice, Aarau, Switzerland.
Preparation of the Tooth Surface; Plaque Control.

DONALD A. SELIGMAN, D.D.S.

Adjunct Assistant Professor, Section of Orofacial Pain and Occlusion, School of Dentistry, University of California, Los Angeles, Los Angeles, California.
Dental Occlusion; Coronoplasty in Periodontal Therapy.

DENNIS A. SHANELEC, D.D.S.

Private practice in periodontics, Santa Barbara, California.
Recent Advances in Surgical Technology.

GERALD SHKLAR, D.D.S., M.S.

Charles A. Brackett Professor of Oral Pathology, Harvard University School of Dental Medicine; Lecturer in Oral Pathology, Tufts University School of Dental Medicine; Senior Clinical Investigator, Forsyth Dental Center; Consultant in Oral Pathology, Brigham and Women's Hospital, Children's Hospital Medical Center, and Massachusetts General Hospital, Boston, Massachusetts.
Introduction: The Historical Background of Periodontology; Desquamative Gingivitis and Oral Mucous Membrane Diseases.

THOMAS N. SIMS, D.D.S.

Lecturer in Periodontics, University of California, Los Angeles, Los Angeles, California.
Resective Osseous Surgery.

WILLIAM K. SOLBERG, D.D.S., M.S.D.

Professor, School of Dentistry, University of California, Los Angeles; Attending Dentist, University of California Los Angeles Hospitals; Co-Director, Pain Management Center, School of Dentistry, University of California, Los Angeles, Los Angeles, California.
Dental Occlusion; Coronoplasty in Periodontal Therapy.

VLADIMIR W. SPOLSKY, D.M.D., M.P.H.

Associate Professor of Public Health Dentistry and Associate Director of the Clinical Research Center, University of California, Los Angeles, Los Angeles, California.
Epidemiology of Gingival and Periodontal Disease.

HENRY H. TAKEI, D.D.S., M.S.

Clinical Professor of Periodontology, School of Dentistry, University of California, Los Angeles, Los Angeles, California.
The Periodontal Instrumentarium; The Periodontal Flap; The Flap Technique for Pocket Therapy; Treatment of Furcation Involvement and Combined Periodontal-Endodontic Therapy; Mucogingival Surgery; Preparation of the Periodontium for Restorative Dentistry.

LEONARD S. TIBBETTS, D.D.S.

Private practice in periodontics, Arlington, Texas.
Recent Advances in Surgical Technology.

ANGELA M. UBIOS, Dr. Odont.

Professor and Chair, Department of Histology and Embryology, Faculty of Dentistry, University of Buenos Aires, Buenos Aires, Argentina.
The Tooth-Supporting Structures.

Preface

This is a textbook for practitioners of general dentistry and students preparing to become general practitioners. It is predicated on the premise that the periodontal care of the public is primarily the concern of the general dentist, and that the general dentist cannot disregard his or her responsibility to provide periodontal care for all patients. The extremely high incidence of periodontal problems in the population makes it impossible for the small number of specialists in periodontics to cope with them; in addition, the close relationship between periodontal and restorative dental therapies makes it very important for the general dentist to have a thorough knowledge of periodontics. A well-trained group of periodontists who specialize in the diagnosis and treatment of severe or unusual problems should serve only to supplement the general dental care available to our population.

In our experience, in order to manage periodontal problems, dental students and dentists need most to understand the clinical phenomena in terms of underlying tissue changes and comprehend the biologic nature of the periodontal responses. Once this aspect is mastered, most treatment techniques can be mastered with the degree of skill possessed by every qualified general dentist.

A great amount of information regarding the nature of periodontal disease and its treatment has resulted from the efforts of clinicians and researchers. A considerable portion of this information is applicable to the practice of dentistry. It is the purpose of this textbook to present knowledge regarding periodontal problems and their possible solutions in such a manner that they can be incorporated into the practice of dentistry.

This edition incorporates all the major advances that have taken place in periodontics in recent years. The entire book has been brought up to date, extensive portions have been rewritten, and new chapters added. It remains, however, a standard textbook with exhaustive coverage of past and present basic and clinical developments in periodontics and related fields.

FERMIN A. CARRANZA, JR. AND MICHAEL G. NEWMAN

Acknowledgments

The first four editions of *Clinical Periodontology,* which is currently in its eighth edition, were published in 1953, 1958, 1964, and 1972 under the authorship of Dr. Irving Glickman. Dr. Glickman, who died on October 2nd, 1972, at the age of 58, was Professor and Chairman of the Department of Periodontics at Tufts University School of Dental Medicine in Boston, Massachusetts. He was a prominent researcher and superb teacher, whose profound knowledge, clear judgment, and dynamic personality made him a leader in the progress of periodontology for a quarter of a century.

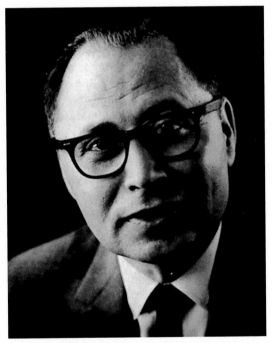

Irving Glickman (1914–1972)

Dr. Glickman was also a gifted speaker and a brilliant writer, and his concepts shaped periodontal thinking for many years. His style of writing and many of his original illustrations, and more importantly many of his ideas in periodontics and his periodontal philosophy of dental practice, can still be found in many areas of this book.

The next three editions (1979, 1984, and 1990) were edited by Dr. Fermin Alberto Carranza, Jr., once a student and then a collaborator of Dr. Glickman's, later Professor and Chairman of Periodontics, and now Professor Emeritus at the School of Dentistry, University of California, Los Angeles. For this eighth edition Dr. Carranza has been joined by Dr. Michael Gary Newman, Adjunct Professor of Periodontics at the University of California, Los Angeles.

In the 43 years that have elapsed since the first edition of this book was published, periodontology has made tremendous progress. The analysis of periodontal tissues and of the mechanisms and causes of their involvement in various pathologic processes has gone beyond histology and physiology into cellular and molecular research. Therapeutic goals and techniques, based on the improved biologic foundation and multiple technologic advances, have surpassed the goal of attaining periodontal health and adequate function. Today, reconstruction of lost structures, replacement of teeth by implants, and achievement of aesthetic results are integral parts of clinical periodontology. All this development and growth has resulted in revisions of, additions to, and modifications in the book's content and organization throughout the editions and has required the inclusion of numerous experts in the various fields into which our discipline has entered.

We would like to express our gratitude to all those who have contributed their knowledge and expertise to the previous editions of this book, but whose names no longer appear as authors or coauthors of chapters:

Drs. Juan J. Carraro, Louis A. Cohn, John E. Flocken, E. Barrie Kenney, Vojislav Lekovic, Francis McCarthy, Philip McCarthy, F. Reinaldo Saglie, and *Alfred Weinstock.*

Many of their concepts and the spirit of their valuable contributions are still evident in this book.

For this edition, we have again been fortunate to obtain the valuable help of a group of scientists with remarkable expertise and knowledge in different clinical and research areas of periodontics.

We are grateful to the following colleagues who contributed previously unpublished information or illustrations:

Enrique Albano, Robert Azzi, E.I. Ball, Ronald L. Barbanell, B. Oscar Barletta, Michael Barnett, Burton E. Becker, William Becker, Sol Bernick, Jean-Pierre Bernimoulin, Raúl G. Caffesse, John J. Cane, Anand P. Chaudhry, Charles Cobb, Edward S. Cohen, Jean-Jacques Elbaz, L. Roy Eversole, Robert M. Frank, Steven Garrett, Charles Gibbs, Max Goodson, Barton Gratt, Ann Haffajee, Thomas J. Han, Stanley C. Holt, Joseph Hsiou, John I. Ingle, Jules Klingsberg, Perry Klokkevold, Stephen Kwan, Stephen D. Levine, Jan Lindhe, Max Listgarten, I. Logan, Frank Lucatorto, Harry Lundeen, Agusti Marfany, Maury Massler, Irving Meyer, Philip R. Melnick, David F. Mitchell, Silvia Oreamuno, Charles A. Palioca, Benjamin Patur, R. Earl Robinson, Max O. Schmid, Nils J. Selliseth, Knut A. Selvig, Z. Skobe, Sigmund S. Socransky, John Sottosanti, B.O.A. Thomas, Carlo Tinti, Sam Toll, Ralph P. Vandersloot, Spencer N. Woolfe, and *Kim D. Zussman.*

We wish to gratefully acknowledge the valuable help of colleagues who read various chapters and offered valuable advice and constructive criticism:

Drs. Rómulo L. Cabrini, Andrew D. Dixon, Karl Donath, Gary Greenstein, and *Thomas R. Wilson.*

We are grateful to the following companies that have shared information and/or illustrations with us:

Thos. B. Hartzell, Hu-Friedy, Interpore International (IMZ), Procter & Gamble, The Straumann Company, and *3i/Implant Innovations, Inc.*

We are indebted to *Ms. Irena Petravicius* and *Mr. Patrick Masson* for their excellent artwork and their untiring efforts to follow our ideas; to *Mr. Richard Friske, Ms. B.J. Coburn,* and *Mr. Reed Hutchinsons* for their photographic expertise; and to *Ms. Marsha Hood* for her invaluable administrative and secretarial help.

Our thanks to the W.B. Saunders Co., and particularly to *Mr. Ray Kersey* and *Mr. Lawrence McGrew,* Senior Medical Editors, as well as to *Ms. Linda R. Garber, Ms. Kendall W. Sterling,* and *Ms. Amy Norwitz.* Their expertise and their detailed attention to every word and every concept have contributed greatly to improving the quality of the book.

Last but not least, we wish to acknowledge the constant support of our families, who have always been so tolerant and understanding.

FERMIN A. CARRANZA, JR. AND MICHAEL G. NEWMAN

Contents

Color Plates

INTRODUCTION

The Historical Background of Periodontology

GERALD SHKLAR and FERMIN A. CARRANZA, JR.

Gingival and periodontal diseases, in their various forms, have afflicted humans since the dawn of history, and studies in paleopathology have indicated that destructive periodontal disease, as evidenced by bone loss, affected early humans in such diverse cultures as ancient Egypt and early pre-Columbian America.[48] The earliest historical records dealing with medical topics reveal an awareness of periodontal disease and the need for treating it. Almost all of the early writings that have been preserved have sections or chapters dealing with oral diseases, and periodontal problems take up a significant amount of space in these writings. The relationship of calculus to periodontal disease was often considered, and underlying systemic disease was often postulated as a cause of periodontal disorders. However, methodical, carefully reasoned, therapeutic discussions did not exist until the Arabic surgical treatises of the Middle Ages; and modern treatment, with illustrated texts and sophisticated instrumentation, did not develop until the time of Pierre Fauchard.

EARLY CIVILIZATIONS

Oral hygiene was practiced by the Sumerians of 3000 BC, and elaborately decorated gold toothpicks found in the excavations at Ur in Mesopotamia suggest an interest in cleanliness of the mouth. The Babylonians and Assyrians, like the earlier Sumerians, apparently suffered from periodontal problems, and a clay tablet of the period tells of treatment by gingival massage combined with various herbal medications.[25]

Periodontal disease was the most common of all diseases evidenced in the embalmed bodies of the ancient Egyptians. It is thus not surprising that the problem received attention in medical and surgical writings of the time. The *Ebers papyrus* contains many references to gingival disease and offers a number of prescriptions for strengthening the teeth and gums. These remedies were made from various plants and minerals and were applied to the gums in the form of a paste with honey, vegetable gum, or residue of beer as a vehicle.[14]

Among the various medical papyri that have been preserved, the most sophisticated, in terms of modern medical practice, is the *Edwin Smith surgical papyrus.*[7] This remnant of a larger work presents 48 cases and discusses diagnosis, prognosis, and appropriate therapy. Mandibular fractures and mandibular dislocations are considered, but periodontal problems are not mentioned as diseases requiring surgical therapy.

The medical works of ancient India devote a significant amount of space to oral and periodontal problems. In the *Susruta Samhita,* there are numerous descriptions of severe periodontal disease with loose teeth and purulent discharge from the gingiva.[51] In a later treatise, the *Charaka Samhita,* toothbrushing and oral hygiene are stressed: "The stick for brushing the teeth should be either astringent or pungent or bitter. One of its ends should be chewed in the form of a brush. It should be used twice a day, taking care that the gums not be injured."[11]

Ancient Chinese medical works also discussed periodontal disease. In the oldest book, written by Huang-Ti about 2500 BC, there is a chapter devoted to dental and gingival diseases. Oral diseases were divided into three types: Fong Ya, or inflammatory conditions; Ya Kon, or diseases of the soft investing tissues of the teeth; and Chong Ya, or dental caries.[12]

Gingival inflammations, periodontal abscesses, and gingival ulcerations are described in accurate detail. One gingival condition is described as follows: "The gingivae are pale or violet red, hard and lumpy, sometimes bleeding: the toothache is continuous." Herbal remedies ("Zn-hine-tong") are mentioned for the treatment of these conditions. The Chinese were among the earliest people to use the "chew stick" as a toothpick and toothbrush to clean the teeth and massage the gingival tissues.

The importance of oral hygiene was recognized by the early Hebrews. Many pathologic conditions of the teeth and their surrounding structures are described in the Talmudic writings. Artifacts of the Phoenician civilization include a specimen of wire splinting, apparently constructed to stabilize teeth loosened by periodontal disease.[25]

GREECE

With the development of Greek culture and science came one of the golden ages of Western civilization. The Greeks attained preeminence in almost every field or discipline they attempted. Architecture, painting, sculpture, pottery, poetry, drama, philosophy, and history reached a degree of perfection rarely surpassed in succeeding ages. This was the age of Homer, Plato, and Aristotle; of Euripides, Aeschylus, and Sophocles; of Herodotus and Xenophon; of Phidias and Praxiteles. Modern science also had its birth in Greece, and medicine developed in terms of diagnostic approach and technical skill. Greek medicine continued into the succeeding Roman civilization and the early Byzantine Age.

Among the ancient Greeks, Hippocrates of Cos (460–377 BC) was the father of modern medicine, the first to institute a systematic examination of the patient's pulse, temperature, respiration, excreta, sputum, and pulse.[9,36] He discussed the function and eruption of the teeth and also the etiology of periodontal disease. He believed that inflammation of the gums could be caused by accumulations of pituita or calculus, with gingival hemorrhage occurring in cases of persistent splenic maladies; one splenic malady was described as follows: "The belly becomes swollen, the spleen enlarged and hard, the patient suffers from acute pain. The gums are detached from the teeth and smell bad."[28]

ROME

The Etruscans, long before 735 BC, were adept in the art of constructing artificial dentures, but there is no evidence that they were aware of the existence of periodontal disease or its treatment.

Among the Romans, Aulus Cornelius Celsus (25 BC–50 AD) referred to diseases that affect the soft parts of the mouth and their treatment as follows: "If the gums separate from the teeth, it is beneficial to chew unripe pears and apples and keep their juices in the mouth." He described looseness of the teeth caused by the weakness of their roots or by flaccidity of the gums and noted that in these cases it is necessary to touch the gums lightly with a red-hot iron and then smear them with honey.[10] The Romans were very interested in oral hygiene. Celsus believed that stains on the teeth should be removed and the teeth then rubbed with a dentifrice. The use of the toothbrush is mentioned in the writings of many of the Roman poets. Gingival massage was an integral part of oral hygiene.

Paul of Aegina (625–690 AD) differentiated between epulis, a fleshy excrescence of gums in the area of a tooth, and parulis, which he described as an abscess of the gums. He wrote that tartar incrustations must be removed with either scrapers or a small file, and that the teeth should be carefully cleaned after the last meal of the day.[43]

THE MIDDLE AGES

The decline and eventual fall of the Roman Empire that plunged Europe into an age of darkness was accompanied by the rise of Islam and the golden age of Arabic science and medicine. The astonishing attainments of Islamic medicine provided for the rise of European medicine in the late Middle Ages and Renaissance. In the early medical schools of Salerno and Montpellier, the available texts were primarily the renowned Arabic treatises, in adequate (but far from accurate) Latin translations.

Much of medieval and Renaissance stomatology and dentistry was derived directly from Arabic writings, particularly the treatises of Ibn Sina (Avicenna) and Abu'l-Qasim (Albucasis). The Arabic treatises derived much of their information from Greek medical treatises, but many refinements and novel approaches were added, particularly in surgical specialties.[49] Many of the Greek medical classics translated into Arabic in Baghdad during the Abbassid Caliphate were eventually retranslated into Latin after the destruction and virtual disappearance of scholarship in Europe during the Dark Ages. Baghdad, along with Córdoba, Spain, enjoyed both intellectual and medical eminence; these two cities represented the greatness of the Eastern and Western Caliphates, respectively.

Hunayn ibn-Ishaq (809–873) and his associates translated into Arabic the original Greek texts of Galen, Oribasius, Paul of Aegina, Dioscorides, and the Hippocratic corpus, as well as the philosophy of Plato and Aristotle and the mathematics of Archimedes. Abu Bakr Muhammed ibn Zakariya al Razi (Rhazes) (841–926) wrote an encyclopedic work on medicine and surgery in 25 books. He was also physician-in-chief at the great Baghdad hospital and taught medicine in terms of clinical cases. Ali ibn Abbas al Majousi (Haly Abbas) (930–994) described many dermatologic diseases and recommended such surgical advances as the suturing of blood vessels prior to the removal of tumors. He also wrote extensively on dental subjects.

Ibn Sina (Avicenna) (980–1037), born in Persia, was possibly the greatest of the Arabic physicians. His *Canon,* a comprehensive treatise on medicine, is probably the most famous medical text of all time and was in continuous use for almost 600 years. Avicenna used an extensive materia medica for oral and periodontal diseases and rarely resorted to surgery. Headings in the *Canon* on gingival disease include "Bleeding Gums," "Fissures of the Gums," "Ulcers of the Gums," "Separation of the Gums," "Recession of the Gums," "Looseness of the Gums," and "Epulis."[4]

Abu'l-Qasim (836–1013) was the preeminent physician and surgeon of the Western Caliphate at Córdoba. His contributions to dentistry and periodontology were among his outstanding achievements. He had a clear understanding of the major etiologic role of calculus deposits and described in detail the technique of scaling the teeth, using a sophisticated set of instruments that he developed. He also wrote in detail on the extraction of teeth, on splinting loose teeth with gold wire, and on filing gross occlusal abnormalities. The fame of his treatise spread through the Arab world and beyond. It was translated into Latin by Gerard of Cremona in the 12th century and greatly influenced the surgeons Guglielmo Saliceti (1201–1277) and Guy de Chauliac (c. 1300–1368)[44] in the 13th and 14th centuries and Fabricius of Aquapendente (1537–1619) in the 16th century. Abu'l-Qasim described as follows how to remove calculus from teeth:[1]

Occasionally there is deposited in the inner and outer surfaces of the teeth or between the gums, large and rough ugly concretion: the teeth take on a black, yellow or green color following which the gums are altered and the teeth become unsightly.

To treat this disease, seat the patient in front of you, placing the head in your lap. Scale [scrape] the teeth and molars that present the concretions or the gritty deposits until nothing remains. Scrape also throughout where the teeth are black, yellow, green or otherwise colored, until they [the calculus deposits] are gone. It is possible that one scaling will suffice. If not, begin a second, third or fourth time, until your purpose is completely attained.

You should know that the scaling of teeth is done with instruments of various shapes according to the use that is required for them. The scalers that one uses for scaling the inner surfaces of the teeth are different than those employed for the scaling of the exterior surfaces, and those that are used to scale the interdental surfaces. Here is an assortment of scalers all of which you have at your disposition (Fig. 1).

In Japan in 984, a book by Yasuyori Tanba, entitled *I-Shin-Po,* which means *Essential Method of Medicine,* was published.[17a] *I-Shin-Po* consisted of 30 volumes, and in volume 5 the treatment of diseases of the mouth, teeth, throat,

and nose was described. The author wrote that the teeth receive their nutrition from the bone marrow, and tooth mobility is caused by malnutrition.

RENAISSANCE

During the Renaissance, with the rebirth of classical scholarship and the development of scientific thought and medical knowledge in addition to the flowering of art, music, and literature, there were significant contributions to anatomy and surgery.

Andreas Vesalius (1514–1564), born in Brussels, taught at the University of Padua in the Venetian Republic, where he performed human dissections and wrote a magnificent book on anatomy, with excellent illustrations throughout, which were drawn by a student of Titian's.[52] Bartholomaeus Eustachius (1520–1574), of Rome, was another outstanding anatomist and wrote a small book on dentistry, *Libellus de Dentibus,* in 30 chapters. He described the firmness of the teeth in the jaws as follows: "There exists besides a very strong ligament, principally attached to the roots by which these later are tightly connected with the alveoli. . . . The gums also contribute to their firmness." Eustachius compares this with the joining of the skin to the fingernails.[15]

Ambroise Paré (1509–1590), head surgeon at the Hotel Dieu in Paris, was the outstanding surgeon of the Renaissance, and his contributions to dental surgery were substantial. He developed many oral surgical procedures in detail, including gingivectomy for hyperplastic gingival tissues.[42] He also understood the etiologic significance of calculus and had a set of scalers to remove the hard deposits on the teeth. Paré wrote in French rather than in Latin, and therefore his works could be widely read and understood.

The first book written in a common language (German) and specifically devoted to dental practice, entitled *Artzney Buchlein or Zene Artzney*[3] (Fig. 2), was published in Leipzig in 1530; 15 separate editions were published between that time and 1576. The author of this book remains unknown in spite of considerable historic research attempting to discover his identity.[8] The book was essentially a compendium of previous writings on oral and dental diseases and their management. Three chapters are devoted specifically to periodontal problems. In Chapter 7, entitled "Concerning Yellow and Black Teeth," the author describes "tartar . . . a white, yellow and black slime that settles on the lower part of the teeth and over the gums." The author also suggests scraping black teeth and the use of toothpastes or powders to rub against the teeth. "Recipes" for several pastes and powders are offered.

In Chapter 9, "Of Loose Teeth," there is a description of periodontitis "which happens either through negligence or weakness or disease of the gums, or through the separation of those substances that hold the teeth in their places which happens when humors from the head drop down upon the gums or roots of the teeth and loosen them by their noxious action." Thus, a crude concept is presented of both systemic and local factors in the etiology of periodontal disease. The presence of local infective agents, or "worms," is also mentioned. A variety of ointments, often astringent in nature, are suggested, and it is recommended that loose

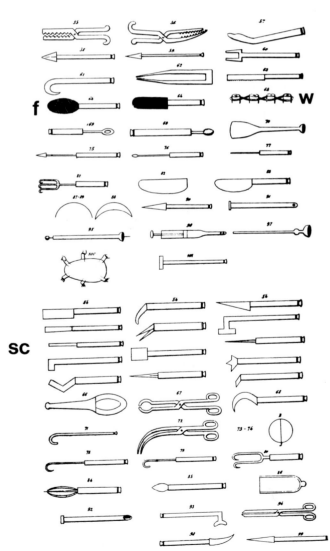

FIGURE 1. Illustration of Abu'l-Qasim's periodontal instruments, showing scalers *(sc),* files *(f),* and the wiring of loose teeth *(w).*

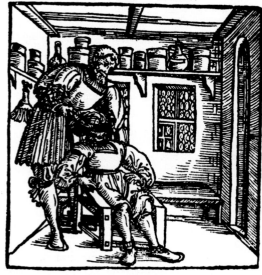

FIGURE 2. Frontispiece of *Artzney Buchlein* (1530).

teeth be bound to sound ones with silk or gold thread. Cauterizing the gingiva with a hot iron is mentioned, but "this burning is dangerous and needs an expensive skilled master." In Chapter 11, "Ulceration, Bad Smell and Decay of the Gums," the management of necrotizing gingivitis with medicines containing vinegar and alum is discussed.

The Italian physician, mathematician, and philosopher Girolamo Cardano (1501–1576) seems to have been the first to differentiate types of periodontal disease. In a publication dated 1562, he mentions one type of disease that occurs with advancing age and leads to progressive loosening and loss of teeth and a second very aggressive type that occurs in younger patients.[27] It was not until late in the 20th century that this classification was rediscovered and became widely accepted!

Anton van Leeuwenhoek (1632–1723) of Delft, Holland, contributed more to the development of modern biologic science than any classically trained scholar of his age. A layman with an inquisitive mind and a hobby of grinding lenses, he developed the microscope and used it to discover microorganisms, cellular structure, blood cells, sperm, and various other microscopic structures, including the tubular structure of dentin.[13] Using material from his gingival tissues, van Leeuwenhoek first described oral bacterial flora, and his drawings offered a reasonably good presentation of oral spirochetes and bacilli (Fig. 3). "I didn't clean my teeth (on purpose) for three days and then took the material

that had lodged in small amounts on the gums above my front teeth. . . . I found a few living animalcules." He described a great amount of bacteria in a man who had never cleaned his mouth.[34]

18TH CENTURY

Modern dentistry essentially developed in 18th century Europe, particularly France and England. Pierre Fauchard, born in Brittany in 1678, is rightly regarded as the father of the profession as we know it. Although he was self-educated in dentistry, he was able to develop a systematic approach to dental practice based on the knowledge of his age. Fauchard significantly improved the instruments and the technical skills required for dental treatment, and his book, *The Surgeon Dentist,* published in 1728 (Fig. 4), gave respectability to the profession and developed a wide appreciation for the technical and surgical skills of the dental practitioner.[16] Fauchard became the leading dentist in Paris and died in 1761 after a long life of service and achievement.

Fauchard's book not only transformed dental practice, but also served to educate the succeeding generation of dentists, some of whom emigrated to America and practiced in the early years of the Republic. Some of George Washington's dentures were made with springs similar to those in the design illustrated by Fauchard. All aspects of dental practice are presented in his book (i.e., restorative dentistry, prosthodontics, oral surgery, periodontics, and orthodontics). Preventive dentistry is described in Chapter 4 ("The Regimen and Care Required for the Preservation of the Teeth") and in Chapter 5 ("How to Keep the Teeth White and Strengthen the Gums"). Fauchard wrote that confections and sweets destroy the teeth by sticking to their surfaces and producing an acid. He described in detail his periodontal instruments (Fig. 5) and the scaling technique to "detach hard matter or tartar from the teeth."

John Hunter (1728–1793), the most distinguished anatomist, surgeon, and pathologist of 18th century England, wrote an excellent treatise on dentistry entitled *The Natural History of the Human Teeth.*[30] He offered remarkably clear

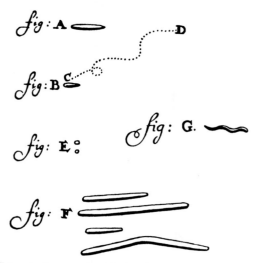

FIGURE 3. van Leeuwenhoek's drawing of oral spirochetes, bacilli, and other microorganisms.

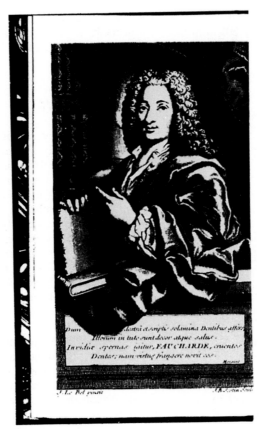

FIGURE 4. Frontispiece of *The Surgeon Dentist* of Fauchard (1746).

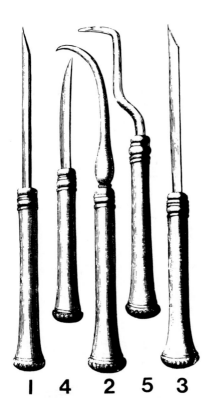

FIGURE 5. The five types of instruments used by Fauchard for detaching tartar from the teeth: 1, chisel; 2, parrot beak; 3, graver; 4, convex blade; 5, Z-shaped hook.

illustrations of the anatomy of the teeth and their supporting structures. He also described the features of periodontal diseases and enunciated the concept of active and passive eruption of teeth.

A contemporary of Hunter, Thomas Berdmore (1740–1785), was considered to be the outstanding dentist in England and was known as "Dentist to His Majesty." He published the *Treatise in the Disorders and Deformities of the Teeth and Gums* in 1770, with several chapters devoted to periodontal problems.[6] In Chapter 7, "Of Tartar of the Teeth, and the Recess of the Gums, and Toothache Occasioned by Tartarous Concretions Long Neglected," Berdmore offered detailed descriptions of instrumentation for tartar removal but stressed prevention. He also used surgery when necessary to remove hyperplastic gingival tissue once the tartar was removed, "for without this, the gums will not closely embrace a tooth which has been made smaller at the collar by the removal of its tartar."

The first qualified American dentists were trained in England or France.[54] Robert Woffendale (1742–1828) was trained in London by Thomas Berdmore, who was dentist to King George III. Woffendale wrote one of the early dental books in America. In an advertisement in the *New York Weekly Journal* of 1766, he "begs Leave to inform the Public that he performs all Operations upon the Teeth, Gums, Sockets and Palate." Similar advertisements were placed by many contemporary dentists. John Baker (1732?–1796) was one of George Washington's dentists and had a very successful career. He imparted his dental knowledge to Paul Revere, Isaac Greenwood, and Josiah Flagg. In an advertisement in the *New York Weekly Journal* of 1768, Baker tells the public that he ". . . cures the scurvy in the gums, be it ever so bad; first cleans and scales the teeth from that corrosive tartarous gritty substance, which hinders the gums from growing, infects the breath and is one of the principle causes of scurvy, and, if not timely prevented, eats away the gums so that many people's teeth fall out fresh. . . . His dentifrice with proper directions for preserving the teeth and gums is to be had at his lodgings."

19TH CENTURY

Leonard Koecker (1785–1850) was a German-born dentist who practiced in Baltimore. In a paper in 1821, in the *Philadelphia Journal of Medicine and Physical Sciences,* he described inflammatory changes in the gingiva and the presence of calculus on teeth, leading to their looseness and exfoliation.[33] He mentioned the careful removal of tartar and the need for oral hygiene by the patient, which he recommended to be performed in the morning and after every meal, using an astringent powder and a toothbrush, placing "the bristles. . . . into the spaces of the teeth." He also discouraged splinting because it loosened firm teeth and recommended that treatment of caries be postponed until after the gum treatment is completed and that placement of artificial teeth be avoided. Koecker was an early advocate of the odontogenic focal infection theory and recommended the extraction of all severely involved teeth and roots, including all unopposed molars, to prevent systemic infections.[33]

The term *pyorrhea alveolaris* was used for the first time by Alphonse Toirac (1791–1863) in 1823, although some authors dispute this.[29] It was introduced in the United States by F. H. Rehwinkel, a German physician who emigrated to the United States and attended the Baltimore College of Dental Surgery.[27]

In the mid-19th century, John W. Riggs (1811–1885) (Fig. 6) was the leading authority on periodontal disease and its treatment in the United States, to the point that periodontitis, or alveolar pyorrhea, was known as "Riggs' disease." He was born in Seymour, CT, on October 25, 1811, and graduated from the Baltimore College of Dental Surgery in 1854. He practiced in Hartford, where he died on November 11, 1885. Riggs seems to have been the first individual to limit his practice to periodontics and therefore can be considered the first specialist in this field. Riggs was an associate of Horace Wells in Hartford, and he performed the first surgical operation under anesthesia, extracting a tooth of Dr. Wells' under nitrous oxide in 1844.

Riggs described his treatment of periodontal disease to an audience at the Connecticut Valley Dental Society at Northampton, MA, in June 1867.[35] His publications, however, are very few; in a paper published in 1876 in the *Pennsylvania Journal of Dental Science,*[46] Riggs strongly advocated cleanliness of the mouth, as he believed that "the teeth themselves, with their accumulated accretions and roughened surfaces. . . . are the exciting cause of the disease"; he strongly opposed surgery, which at the time consisted of resection of the gums.

Riggs and his disciples had great influence in the dental profession. They were the proponents of the so-called conservative approach to periodontal therapy, developing the concept of oral prophylaxis and prevention. Among his fol-

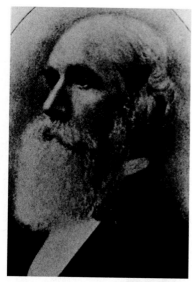

FIGURE 6. John W. Riggs (1811–1885). (From Hoffman-Axthelm W. History of Dentistry. Chicago, Quintessence Books, 1981.)

lowers were L. Taylor, D. D. Smith, R. B. Adair, and W. J. Younger.[27] Many papers by followers and contemporaries of Riggs described clinical features and treatment of periodontal disease, the latter based mostly on hygienic measures.[36,45] William J. Younger (1838–1920) considered periodontal disease a local infection and was the first to discuss, in 1893, the possibility of "reattachment." In 1902, Younger reported on a case in which he grafted gingival tissue "from behind the third molar" to an extensive area of recession in an upper cuspid of the same patient. He first treated the root of the cuspid with lactic acid and then fixed the gum graft with "fine cambric needles," and he claims the operation to have been a success.[2]

In the late 19th century, studies by Rudolph Virchow (1821–1902), Julius Cohnheim (1839–1884), Elie Metchnikoff (1845–1916), and others had started to shed light on the microscopic changes occurring in inflammation. This resulted in an understanding of the pathogenesis of periodontal disease, based on histopathologic studies. N. N. Znamensky, in Moscow, understood the complex interaction of local and systemic factors in the etiology of periodontal disease[61] (Fig. 7), and his observations and concepts were summarized in 1902 in a classic paper, "Alveolar Pyorrhoea—Its Pathological Anatomy and Its Radical Treatment," in which he describes the presence in inflamed gingivae of a cellular infiltrate that extends deeper as the disease progresses, causing bone resorption associated to multinucleated cells (osteoclasts) and Howship's lacunae. Znamensky treated pyorrhea with removal of calculus and deep curettage of the pockets, using cocaine anesthesia.

The first individual to identify bacteria as the cause of periodontal disease appears to have been the German dentist Adolph Witzel (1847–1906),[21,58] who taught at the University of Jena, but the first true oral microbiologist was Willoughby D. Miller (1853–1907), who was born in Ohio and received training in basic sciences at the University of Michigan and dental training at the Pennsylvania Dental College. He emigrated to Germany, where he worked in Robert Koch's microbiology laboratory and embarked on a research career that introduced modern bacteriology princi-

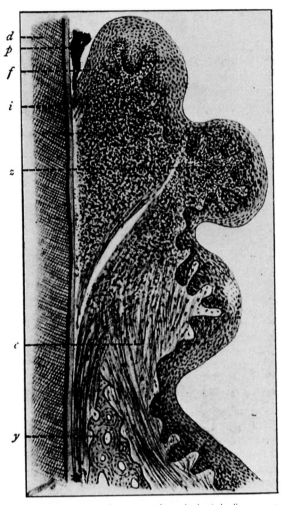

d
p
f
i
z
c
y

FIGURE 7. Microscopic features of periodontal disease as presented by Znamensky.

ples to dentistry. His greatest accomplishments were in caries research, where he developed the chemicoparasitic theory of caries. In his classic book *The Microorganisms of the Human Mouth,* published in 1890, he described the features of periodontal disease and considered the role of predisposing factors, irritational factors, and bacteria in the etiology of pyorrhea alveolaris. He believed that the disease was not caused by a specific bacterium but by a complex array of various bacteria normally present in the oral cavity. This constitutes what was later known as the nonspecific plaque hypothesis that went unchallenged for seven decades.[21]

Miller did not, however, recognize bacterial plaque. This was left to J. Leon Williams (1852–1932), an American dentist who practiced in London, England, and who in 1897 described a gelatinous accumulation of bacteria adherent to the enamel surface in relation to caries;[57] and to G. V. Black (1836–1915), who in 1899 coined the term *gelatinous microbic plaque.*

J. H. Vincent (1862–1950) was a French physician working at the Pasteur Institute in Paris; in 1896 and 1898 he described the spirillum and fusiform bacilli associated with what later became known as Vincent's angina, and in 1904 he described these organisms in acute ulceronecrotic gingivitis.[21,53]

Salomon Robicsek (1845–1928), born in Hungary, obtained his medical degree and practiced dentistry in Vienna. He developed a surgical technique consisting of a scalloped continuous gingivectomy excision exposing the marginal bone for subsequent curettage and remodeling.[50] The first description, in 1901, of a possible role of trauma from occlusion and bruxism in periodontal disease is generally attributed to the Austrian dentist Moritz Karolyi (1865–1945),[32] who also recommended its correction by grinding occlusal surfaces and preparation of bite plates.

20TH CENTURY

In the first third of the 20th century, periodontics flourished in Central Europe, with two major centers of excellence: Vienna and Berlin.

Vienna. The Viennese school developed the basic histopathologic concepts on which modern periodontics was built. The major representative from this group was Bernhard Gottlieb (1885–1950) (Fig. 8), who published extensive microscopic studies of periodontal disease performed on human autopsy specimens. His major contributions appeared in the German literature in the 1920s and described the attachment of the gingival epithelium to the tooth,[22] the histopathology of inflammatory and degenerative periodontal disease,[17,23] the biology of the cementum, active and passive tooth eruption, and traumatic occlusion. Gottlieb also carried out histologic studies on animal periodontal tissues in the laboratory of Julius Tandler. Reviews of Gottlieb's studies appeared in English in 1921 in *The Dental Cosmos* and in 1927 in the *Journal of the American*

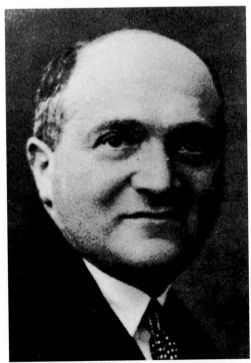

FIGURE 8. Bernhard Gottlieb (1885–1950). (From Gold SI. Periodontics. The past. Part II. J Clin Periodontol *12:*171, 1985. © 1985, Munksgaard International Publishers Ltd, Copenhagen, Denmark.)

Dental Association. A book published in 1938 by Gottlieb and Orban, *Biology and Pathology of the Tooth and Its Supporting Mechanism,* presented in English a complete review of the concepts developed by Gottlieb and his coworkers in Vienna.[24]

A younger contemporary of Gottlieb's in Vienna was Balint J. Orban (1899–1960) (Fig. 9), who carried out extensive histologic studies on periodontal tissues that serve as the basis for much of current therapy. Other members of the Viennese school were Rudolph Kronfeld (1901–1940), Joseph P. Weinmann (1889–1960), and Harry Sicher (1889–1974). All of these scientists emigrated to the United States in the 1930s and contributed greatly to the progress of American dentistry.

Berlin. The Berlin group consisted mostly of clinical scientists who developed and refined the surgical approach to periodontal therapy. Prominent in this group were Oskar Weski and Robert Neumann.

Weski (1879–1952) (Fig. 10) carried out pioneering studies correlating radiographic and histopathologic changes in periodontal disease.[55] He also conceptualized the periodontium as formed by cementum, gingiva, periodontal ligament, and bone and gave it the name *paradentium,* which was later changed (owing to etymologic reasons) to *parodontium,* a term still used in Europe. The contributions of Alfred Kantorowicz (1880–1962), Karl Haupl (1893–1960), and others to the histopathology of the periodontal tissues also deserve mention.

Neumann (1882–1958) (Fig. 11) published a book entitled *Die Alveolarpyorrhoe und Ihre Behandlung* in 1912,[38] with new editions published in 1915, 1920, and 1924. He described the principles of periodontal flap surgery, including osseous recontouring, as it is currently known[18] (Fig. 12). Other clinicians who described flap surgery at the beginning of the century were Leonard Widman, of Sweden (1871–1956),[56] and A. Cieszynski, of Poland. A bitter controversy developed among Widman, Cieszynski, and Neumann in the 1920s over the priority in the description of the periodontal flap.[40]

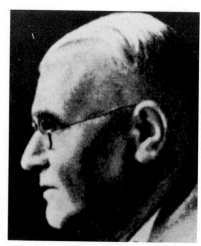

FIGURE 10. Oskar Weski (1879–1952). (From Hoffman-Axthelm W. History of Dentistry. Chicago, Quintessence Books, 1981.)

United States and Other Countries. In the United States, periodontal surgery developed in the first decades of the century with important contributions by A. Zentler,[60] J. Zemsky,[59] G. V. Black, O. Kirkland, A. W. Ward, A. B. Crane, H. Kaplan, and others. Early in the 20th century, surgical techniques were developed for the coverage of denuded roots (W. J. Younger, 1902[2]; A. W. Harlan, 1906[5,26]; and P. Rosenthal, 1912).[47] However, these techniques did not attain wide usage.

The nonsurgical approach was championed by Isadore Hirschfeld (1882–1965), of New York, who wrote classic papers on oral hygiene and local factors. In 1913, the first school for dental hygienists was created by Alfred Fones (1869–1938), in Bridgeport, CT.

In other countries, H. K. Box (Canada); M. Roy and R. Vincent (France); R. Jaccard and A.-J. Held (Switzerland); F. A. Carranza, Sr., and R. Erausquin (Argentina); W. W. James, A. Counsell, and E. W. Fish (Great Britain); and A. Leng (Chile) are well known for their important contribu-

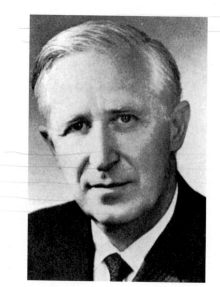

FIGURE 9. Balint J. Orban (1899–1960). (From J Periodontol 31:266, 1960.)

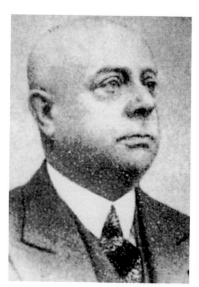

FIGURE 11. Robert Neumann (1882–1958). (Courtesy of Dr. Steven I. Gold.)

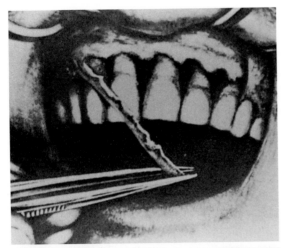

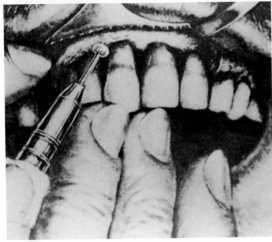

FIGURE 12. Surgical procedure advocated by Robert Neumann in the early part of the 20th century. *Top,* After raising a mucoperiosteal flap, its edge is trimmed with scissors, leaving a scalloped outline. *Bottom,* Osseous recontouring with burs. (From Gold SI. Robert Neumann—a pioneer in periodontal flap surgery, J Periodontol *53:*456, 1982.)

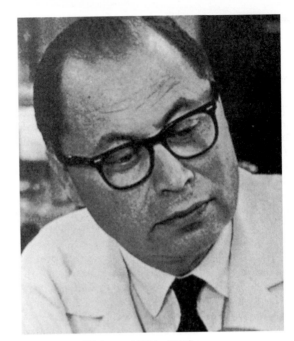

FIGURE 13. Irving Glickman (1914–1972).

tions. Probably the most comprehensive book on periodontics published in the first half of the 20th century was *El Paradencio, Su Patologia y Tratamiento,* by the Uruguayan F. M. Pucci, which appeared in 1939.

After World War II. The United States and Scandinavia took a leading role in basic and clinical periodontal research from the 1950s on, with major advances in the fields of experimental pathology, microbiology, and immunology. Animal models of periodontal disease were developed and the role of local and systemic factors studied by many investigators. Irving Glickman (1914–1972) (Fig. 13) was a leading researcher in this period. Among other scientists who contributed to the knowledge of the experimental pathology of the periodontal tissues were Herman Becks (1897–1962), Paul Boyle (1901–1980), Henry Goldman (1911–1991), Balint Orban (1899–1960), Sigurd Ramfjord (1911–), Isaac Schour (1900–1964), Joseph Weinmann (1889–1960), and Helmut Zander (1912–1991). In the clinical area, many authors expanded this knowledge, including Frank Beube (1904–1995), Samuel Charles Miller (1902–1957), Timothy O'Leary (1921–1991), John Prichard (1907–1990), Saul Schluger (1908–1990), and Sidney Sorrin (1900–1978).

The leading figure of the Scandinavian group was Jens Waerhaug (1907–1980) (Fig. 14), of Oslo, Norway, whose dissertation, *The Gingival Pocket,* published in 1952, opened a new era in the understanding of the biology of the periodontium. Prominent members of the Scandinavian school include Harald Löe, Jan Lindhe, and Jan Egelberg.

At present the role of microorganisms and the immuno-

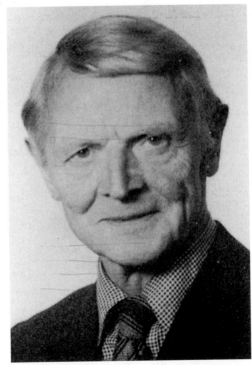

FIGURE 14. Jens Waerhaug (1907–1980). (From J Clin Periodontol *7:*534, 1980. © 1980, Munksgaard International Publishers Ltd, Copenhagen, Denmark.)

logic response are the center of attention of many research groups. Investigators such as Robert Genco, Max Listgarten, Walter Loesche, Roy Page, Jorgen Slots, Sigmund Socransky, and many others are carrying the torch into the future. The pages of this book document their contributions.

Several workshops and international conferences have summarized the existing knowledge on the biologic and clinical aspects of periodontology. Worthy of mention are those conducted in 1951, 1966, 1977, and 1989 that were cosponsored and published by the American Academy of Periodontology.

The American Academy of Periodontology, founded in 1914 by two women periodontists, Grace Rogers Spalding (1881–1953) and Gillette Hayden (1880–1929), has become the leader in organized periodontics. Its monthly scientific publication, *The Journal of Periodontology*, presents all the advances in this discipline. Other scientific periodontal journals are the *Journal of Periodontal Research,* the *Journal of Clinical Periodontology, Periodontology 2000,* and the *International Journal of Periodontics and Restorative Dentistry.* In other languages, the *Journal de Parodontologie* (France) and the *Journal of the Japanese Association of Periodontology* (Japan) deserve mention.

Periodontal education in the United States has also grown in the second half of the 20th century, and most dental schools have separate and independent units for teaching and research in this discipline. Periodontics was recognized as a specialty of dentistry by the American Dental Association in 1947. The first university-based programs for the training of specialists in periodontics were begun in several universities (Columbia, Michigan, Tufts) in the late 1940s; these 1-year programs expanded to 2-year programs about 10 years later. There are currently more than 50 periodontal graduate programs based in universities and hospitals; all of these are 3-year programs.

REFERENCES

1. Albucasis. La Chirurgie. Translated by Lucien LeClere. Paris, Baillière, 1861.
2. American Dental Club of Paris. Meetings of December 1902 and January and March 1903. Dent Cosmos 46:39, 1904.
3. Artzney Buchlein. Leipzig, Michael Blum, 1530. English translation in Dent Cosmos, 29:1, 1887.
4. Avicenna. Liber Canonis. Venice, 1507. Reprinted, Hildesheim, Georg Olms, 1964.
5. Baer PN, Benjamin SD. Gingival grafts; a historical note. J Periodontol 52:206, 1981.
6. Berdmore T. A Treatise on the Disorders and Deformities of the Teeth and Gums. London, B White, 1786.
7. Breasted JH. The Edwin Smith Surgical Papyrus. Chicago, University of Chicago Press, 1930.
8. Budjuhn K. The 1920 German commentary based on original sources regarding the history of the oldest printed book in dentistry. English translation by HE Cooper. In The Classics of Dentistry Library. Zene Artzney, Birmingham, AL, 1981.
9. Castiglione A. History of Medicine. 2nd ed. New York, AA Knopf, 1941.
10. Celsus A. De Medicina. Translated by WG Spencer, London, Heinemann, 1935–1938.
11. Charaka Samhita. Edited, translated, and published by AC Kaviratna, Calcutta, 1892–1905.
12. Dabry P. La Medicine chez les Chinois. Paris, Plon, 1863.
13. Dobell C. Anatomy van Leeuwenhoek and His "Little Animals." New York, Harcourt, 1932. Reprinted, New York, Dover Publications, 1960.
14. Ebbel B. The Papyrus Ebers. Copenhagen, Levin and Munksgaard, 1937.
15. Eustachius B. Libellus de Dentibus. Venice, 1563. Reprinted in facsimile, Vienna, Urban and Schwarzenberg, 1951.
16. Fauchard P. Le Chirurgien Dentiste, ou Traite des Dents. Paris, J Maruiette, 1728. Reprinted in facsimile, Paris, Prélat, 1961. (An English translation by Lillian Lindsay appeared in 1946, published by Butterworth and Company, London.)
17. Fleischmann L, Gottlieb B. Beitrage zur Histologie und Pathogenese der Alveolarpyorrhoe. Z Stomatol 2:44, 1920.
17a. Funakoshi M. Personal communication, 1993.
18. Gold SI. Robert Neumann—a pioneer in periodontal flap surgery. J Periodontol 53:456, 1982.
19. Gold SI. Periodontics. The past. Part I. Early sources. J Clin Periodontol 12:79, 1985.
20. Gold SI. Periodontics. The past. Part II. The development of modern periodontics. J Clin Periodontol 12:171, 1985.
21. Gold SI. Periodontics. The past. Part III. Microbiology. J Clin Periodontol 12:257, 1985.
22. Gottlieb B. Der Epithelansatz am Zahne. Dtsch Monatschr Zahn 39:142, 1921.
23. Gottlieb B. Die diffuse Atrophie der Alveolarknochen. Z Stomatol 21:195, 1923.
24. Gottlieb B, Orban B. Biology and Pathology of the Tooth and Its Supporting Mechanism. Translated and edited by M Diamond, New York, Macmillan, 1938.
25. Guerini V. History of Dentistry. Philadelphia, Lea & Febiger, 1909.
26. Harlan AW. Restoration of gum tissue on the labial aspect of teeth. D Cosmos 48:927, 1906.
27. Held A-J. Periodontology. From its origins up to 1980: A survey. Birkhäuser, Boston, 1989.
28. Hippocrates. Works. Edited and translated by WHS Jones and ET Withington. London, Heinemann, 1923–1931.
29. Hoffman-Axthelm W. History of Dentistry. Chicago, Quintessence Publishing, 1981.
30. Hunter J. The Natural History of the Human Teeth. London, J Johnson, 1771. Reprinted as Treatise in the natural history and diseases of the human teeth. In Bell T, ed. Collected Works. London, Longman Rees, 1835.
31. Jastrow N. The medicine of the Babylonians and Assyrians. Proc Soc Med London 7:109, 1914.
32. Karolyi M. Beobachtungen über Pyorrhea Alveolaris. Vjschr Zahnheilk 17:279, 1901.
33. Koecker A. An essay on the devastation of the gums and the alveolar processes. Philadelphia J Med Phys Sci 2:282, 1821.
34. Leeuwenhoek A van. Arcana Naturae. Delphis Bartavorum, 1695. Reprinted in facsimile, Brussels, Culture et Civilization, 1966.
35. MacManus C. The makers of dentistry. Dent Cosmos 44:1105, 1902.
36. Major RHL. A History of Medicine. Springfield, IL, Charles C Thomas, 1954.
37. Mills GA. Some of the phases of Riggs' disease (so-called). Dent Cosmos 19:185,254,347, 1877.
38. Neumann R. Die Alveolarpyorrhoe und ihre Behandlung. Berlin, Meusser, 1912.
39. Neumann R. Die Radikal-Chirurgische Behandlung der Alveolarpyorrhoe. Vjschr Zahnheilk 37:113, 1921.
40. Neumann R. Erwiderung zu Widmans auffassungen über die Prioritatsfrage betreffs der radikalchirurgischen Behandlung der sogenannten Alveolarpyorrhoe. Vjschr Zahnheilk 39:170, 1923.
41. Nicaise E. La Grande Chirurgie de Guy de Chauliac. Paris, Alean, 1890.
42. Paré A. Oeuvres Completes. Edited by JF Malgaigne, Paris, Baillière, 1840–1841.
43. Paul of Aegina. The Seven Books. Translated by F Adams, London, Sydenham Society, 1844–1847.
44. Pifteau P. Chirurgie de Guillaume de Salicet: Traduition et Commentaire. Toulouse, France, St Cyprien, 1989.
45. Rawls AO. Pyorrhea alveolaris. D Cosmos 27:265, 1885.
46. Riggs JW. Suppurative inflammation of the gums and absorption of the gums and alveolar process. Pa J Dent Sci 3:99, 1876. Reprinted in Arch Clin Oral Pathol 2:423, 1938.
47. Rosenthal P. Recovering the exposed necks of teeth by autoplasty. Dent Cosmos 54:377, 1912.
48. Ruffer MA. Studies in the Paleopathology of Egypt. Chicago, University of Chicago Press, 1921.
49. Shklar G. Stomatology and dentistry in the golden age of Arabian medicine. Bull Hist Dent 17:17, 1969.
50. Stern IB, Everett FG, Robicsek K. S Robicsek—a pioneer in the surgical treatment of periodontal disease. J Periodontol 36:265, 1965.
51. Susruta Samhita. Edited, translated, and published by KKL Bhishagratna, Calcutta, 1907–1916.
52. Vesalius S. De Humanis Corporis Fabrica, Basle, 1542. Reproduced in facsimile, Brussels, Culture et Civilisation, 1966.
53. Vincent JH. Recherche sur l'etiologie de la stomatitis ulceromembraneuse primitive. Arch Int Laryngol 17:355, 1904.
54. Weinberger BW. An Introduction to the History of Dentistry. St Louis, CV Mosby, 1948.
55. Weski O. Roentgenographische-anatomische Studien auf dem Gebiete der Kieferpathologie. Vjrsch Zahnh 37:1, 1921.
56. Widman L. Surgical treatment of pyorrhea alveolaris. J Periodontol 42:571, 1971.
57. Williams JL. A contribution to the study of pathology of enamel. Dent Cosmos 39:169,269,353, 1897.
58. Witzel A. The treatment of pyorrhea alveolaris or infectious alveolitis. Br J Dent Sci 25:153,209,257, 1882.
59. Zemsky J. Surgical treatment of periodontal disease with the author's open view operation for advanced cases of dental periclasia. Dent Cosmos 68:465, 1926.
60. Zentler A. Suppurative gingivitis with alveolar involvement. A new surgical procedure. JAMA 71:1530, 1918.
61. Znamensky NN. Alveolar pyorrhoea—its pathological anatomy and its radical treatment. J Br Dent Assoc 23:585, 1902.

Section One

The Normal Periodontium

The periodontium consists of the investing and supporting tissues of the tooth (gingiva, periodontal ligament, cementum, alveolar bone). The cementum is considered a part of the periodontium because, along with the bone, it serves as the support for the fibers of the periodontal ligament. The periodontium is subject to morphologic and functional variations, as well as changes associated with age. This section deals with the normal features of the tissues of the periodontium, knowledge of which is necessary for an understanding of periodontal diseases.

The soft and hard tissues surrounding dental implants have many features similar to and some important differences from the periodontal tissues. These features and differences are dealt with in Chapter 62.

1

The Gingiva

MARIA E. ITOIZ and FERMIN A. CARRANZA, Jr.

Normal Clinical Features
Marginal Gingiva
Attached Gingiva
Interdental Gingiva
Normal Microscopic Features
Gingival Epithelium
Gingival Connective Tissue

Correlation of Normal Clinical and Microscopic Features
Color
Size
Contour
Shape
Consistency
Surface Texture
Position

The oral mucosa consists of three zones: the gingiva and the covering of the hard palate, termed the *masticatory mucosa;* the dorsum of the tongue, covered by *specialized mucosa;* and the oral mucous membrane lining the remainder of the oral cavity. *The gingiva is the part of the oral mucosa that covers the alveolar processes of the jaws and surrounds the necks of the teeth.*

NORMAL CLINICAL FEATURES

The gingiva is divided anatomically into marginal, attached, and interdental areas.

marginal
attached
interdental

Marginal Gingiva

The marginal, or unattached, gingiva is the terminal edge or border of the gingiva surrounding the teeth like a collar (Figs. 1–1 and 1–2). In about 50% of cases, it is demarcated from the adjacent attached gingiva by a shallow linear depression, the *free gingival groove.*[3] Usually about 1 mm wide, the marginal gingiva forms the soft tissue wall of the gingival sulcus. It can be separated from the tooth surface with a periodontal probe.

Gingival Sulcus

The gingival sulcus is the shallow crevice or space around the tooth bounded by the surface of the tooth on one side and the epithelium lining the free margin of the gingiva on the other. It is V shaped and barely permits the entrance of a periodontal probe. The clinical determination of the depth of the gingival sulcus is an important diagnostic parameter. Under absolutely normal or ideal conditions, the depth of the gingival sulcus is 0 or about 0.[42,87] These strict conditions of normalcy can be produced experimentally only in germ-free animals[5] or after intense, prolonged plaque control.[8,23]

In clinically healthy gingiva in humans, a sulcus of some depth can be found. The depth of this sulcus, as determined in histologic sections, has been reported as 1.8 mm, with variations of from 0 to 6 mm[77]; other studies have reported depths of 1.5 mm[118] and 0.69 mm.[40] The clinical maneuver used to determine the depth of the sulcus is the introduction of a metallic instrument—the periodontal probe—and the estimation of the distance it penetrates. The histologic depth of a sulcus need not be and is not exactly equal to the depth of penetration of the probe. The so-called probing depth of a clinically normal gingival sulcus in humans is 2 to 3 mm (see Chapter 28).

Attached Gingiva

The attached gingiva is continuous with the marginal gingiva. It is firm, resilient, and tightly bound to the underlying periosteum of alveolar bone. The facial aspect of the attached gingiva extends to the relatively loose and movable alveolar mucosa, from which it is demarcated by the *mucogingival junction* (see Fig. 1–2).

The *width of the attached gingiva* is another important clinical parameter. It is the distance between the mucogingival junction and the projection on the external surface of the bottom of the gingival sulcus or the periodontal pocket. It should not be confused with the width of the keratinized gingiva, because the latter also includes the marginal gingiva (see Fig. 1–2).

The width of the attached gingiva on the facial aspect differs in different areas of the mouth.[16] It is generally greatest in the incisor region (3.5 to 4.5 mm in the maxilla and 3.3 to 3.9 mm in the mandible) and less in the posterior segments, with the least width in the first premolar area (1.9 mm in the maxilla and 1.8 mm in the mandible)[3] (Fig. 1–3).

The mucogingival junction remains stationary throughout adult life[1]; therefore, changes in the width of the attached gingiva are due to modifications in the position of its coro-

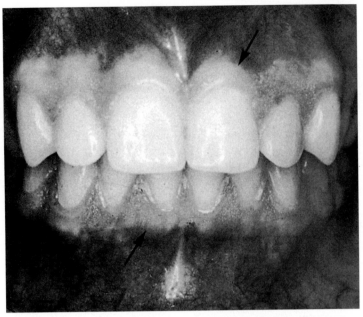

FIGURE 1–1. Normal gingiva in a young adult. Note the demarcation (mucogingival line) *(arrows)* between the attached gingiva and the darker alveolar mucosa.

nal end. The width of the attached gingiva increases with age[4] and in supraerupted teeth.[2] On the lingual aspect of the mandible, the attached gingiva terminates at the junction with the lingual alveolar mucosa, which is continuous with the mucous membrane lining the floor of the mouth. The palatal surface of the attached gingiva in the maxilla blends imperceptibly with the equally firm, resilient palatal mucosa.

Interdental Gingiva

The interdental gingiva occupies the gingival embrasure, which is the interproximal space beneath the area of tooth contact. The interdental gingiva can be pyramidal or have a "col" shape. In the former, there is one papilla with its tip immediately beneath the contact point; the latter shape presents a depression that connects a facial and a lingual papilla and conforms to the shape of the interproximal contact[29] (Figs. 1–4 and 1–5).

The shape of the gingiva in a given interdental space depends on the contact point between the two adjoining teeth and the presence or absence of some degree of recession. Figure 1–6 depicts the variations in normal interdental gingiva.

The facial and lingual surfaces are tapered toward the interproximal contact area, and the mesial and distal surfaces are slightly concave. The lateral borders and tip of the interdental papillae are formed by a continuation of the marginal gingiva from the adjacent teeth. The intervening portion consists of attached gingiva (Fig. 1–7).

If a diastema is present, the gingiva is firmly bound over

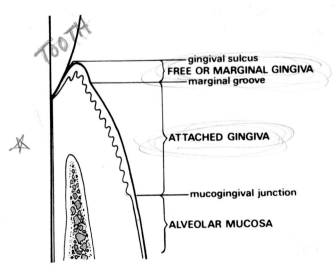

FIGURE 1–2. Diagram showing anatomic landmarks of the gingiva.

- gingival sulcus
- **FREE OR MARGINAL GINGIVA**
- marginal groove
- **ATTACHED GINGIVA**
- mucogingival junction
- **ALVEOLAR MUCOSA**

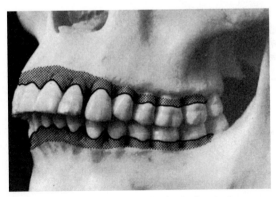

FIGURE 1–3. Mean width of attached gingiva in human permanent dentition.

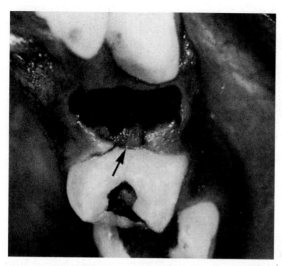

FIGURE 1–4. Site of extraction showing the facial and palatal interdental papillae and the intervening col *(arrow).*

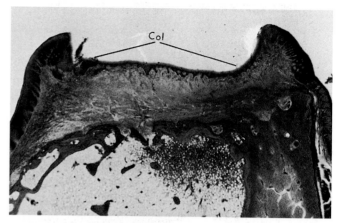

FIGURE 1–5. Faciolingual section (monkey) showing the col between the facial and lingual interdental papillae. The col is covered with nonkeratinized stratified squamous epithelium.

the interdental bone and forms a smooth, rounded surface without interdental papillae (Fig. 1–8).

NORMAL MICROSCOPIC FEATURES*

The gingiva consists of a central core of connective tissue covered by stratified squamous epithelium. These two tissues will be considered separately.

Gingival Epithelium

General Aspects of Gingival Epithelium Biology

Although the gingival epithelium constitutes a continuous lining of stratified squamous epithelium, three different areas can be defined from the morphologic and functional points of view: the oral or outer epithelium, the sulcular epithelium, and the junctional epithelium.

The principal cell type of the gingival epithelium, as well as of other stratified squamous epithelia, is the *keratinocyte.* Other cells found in the epithelium are the clear cells or nonkeratinocytes, which include the Langerhans cells, the Merkel cells, and the melanocytes.

The main function of the gingival epithelium is to protect the deep structures while allowing a selective interchange with the oral environment. This is achieved by proliferation and differentiation of the keratinocyte.

Proliferation of keratinocytes takes place by mitosis in the basal layer and, less frequently, in the suprabasal layers, where a small proportion of cells remain as a proliferative compartment while a larger number begin to migrate to the surface.

Differentiation involves the process of keratinization, which consists of a sequence of biochemical and morphologic events that occur in the cell as it migrates from the basal layer (Fig. 1–9). The main morphologic change is a progressive flattening of the cell, with an increasing prevalence of tonofilaments and intercellular junctions coupled to the production of keratohyaline granules and the disappearance of the nucleus. (See the discussion by Schroeder[87] for further details.)

A complete keratinization process leads to the production of an *orthokeratinized* superficial horny layer similar to that of the skin, with no nuclei in the stratum corneum and a well-defined stratum granulosum (Fig. 1–10). Only some areas of the outer gingival epithelium are orthokeratinized;

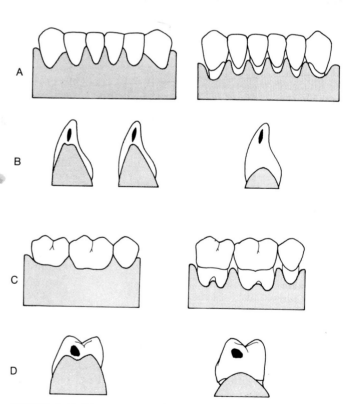

FIGURE 1–6. Diagram comparing anatomic variations of the interdental col in the normal gingiva *(left)* and after gingival recession *(right).* A and B, Mandibular anterior segment, facial and buccolingual views, respectively. C and D, Mandibular posterior region, facial and buccolingual views, respectively. Tooth contact points are shown in B and D.

---

* A detailed description of periodontal histology with an exhaustive literature review can be found in the book *The Periodontium,* by H. E. Schroeder, published by Springer-Verlag in 1986.

Wed., May 12th - TEST! - Ch. 1 & 2

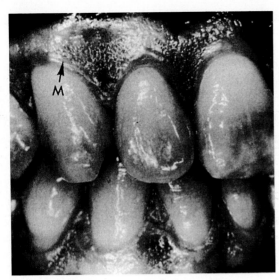

FIGURE 1–7. Interdental papillae with the central portion formed by attached gingiva. The shape of the papillae varies according to the dimension of the gingival embrasure. M, marginal gingiva.

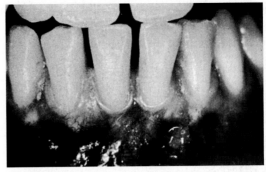

FIGURE 1–8. Absence of interdental papillae and col where proximal tooth contact is missing.

the other gingival areas are covered by parakeratinized or nonkeratinized epithelium,[20] considered to be at intermediate stages of keratinization. These areas can progress to maturity or dedifferentiate under different physiologic or pathologic conditions.

In *parakeratinized epithelia* the stratum corneum retains pyknotic nuclei, and the keratohyalin granules are dis-

persed, not giving rise to a stratum granulosum. The *nonkeratinized epithelium* (although cytokeratins are the major component, as in all epithelia) has neither granulosum nor corneum strata, and superficial cells have viable nuclei.

Immunohistochemistry, gel electrophoresis, and immunoblot techniques have made it possible to identify the characteristic pattern of cytokeratins in each epithelial type. The keratin proteins are composed of different polypeptide subunits characterized by their isoelectric point and their molecular weight. They have been numbered in a sequence contrary to their molecular weight. Generally, basal cells start synthesizing lower molecular weight keratins (such as K19, 40 kd) and express other higher molecular weight keratins as they migrate to the surface. K1 keratin polypep-

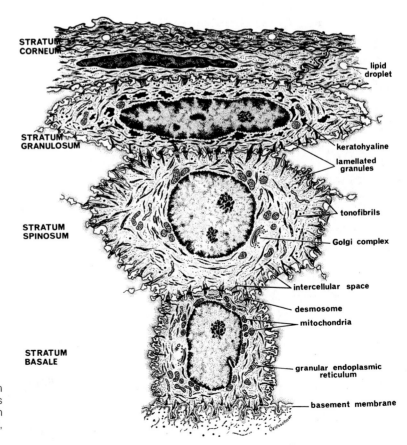

FIGURE 1–9. Diagram showing representative cells from the various layers of stratified squamous epithelium as seen by electron microscopy. (From Weinstock A. In Ham AW, ed. Histology. 7th ed. Philadelphia, JB Lippincott, 1974.)

STRATUM CORNEUM

STRATUM GRANULOSUM

STRATUM SPINOSUM

STRATUM BASALE

lipid droplet

keratohyaline

lamellated granules

tonofibrils

Golgi complex

intercellular space

desmosome

mitochondria

granular endoplasmic reticulum

basement membrane

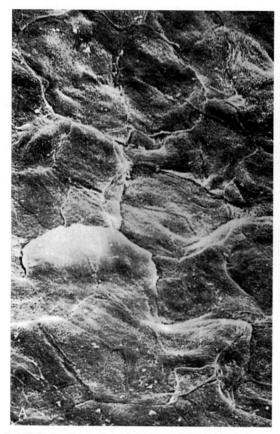
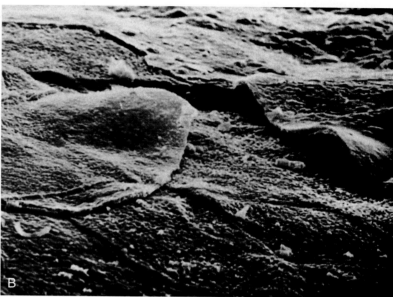

FIGURE 1–10. *A,* Scanning electron micrograph of keratinized gingiva showing the flattened keratinocytes and their boundaries on the surface of the gingiva. ×1000. *B,* Scanning electron micrograph of the gingival margin at the edge of the gingival sulcus showing a close-up view of several keratinocytes about to be exfoliated. ×3000. (From Kaplan GB, Pameijer CH, Ruben MP. Scanning electron microscopy of sulcular and junctional epithelia correlated with histology (Part I). J Periodontol *48:*446, 1977.)

tide of 68 kd is the main component of the stratum corneum.[27]

Other proteins unrelated to keratins are synthesized during the maturation process. The most extensively studied are *keratolinin* and *involucrin,* which are precursors of a chemically resistant structure (the envelope) located below the cell membrane, and *filaggrin,* whose precursors are packed into the keratohyalin granules. In the sudden transition to the horny layer, the keratohyalin granules disappear and give rise to filaggrin, which forms the matrix of the most differentiated epithelial cell, the *corneocyte.*

Thus, in the fully differentiated state, the corneocytes are mainly formed by bundles of keratin tonofilaments embedded in an amorphous matrix of filaggrin and surrounded by a resistant envelope under the cell membrane. The immunohistochemical patterns of the different keratin types—envelope proteins and filaggrin—change under normal or pathologic stimuli, modifying the keratinization process.[50–52]

Electron microscopy reveals that keratinocytes are interconnected by structures on the cell periphery called *desmosomes.*[60] These desmosomes have a typical structure consisting of two dense attachment plaques into which tonofibrils insert, and an intermediate, electron-dense line in the extracellular compartment. Tonofilaments, which are the morphologic expression of the cytoskeleton of keratin proteins, radiate in brush-like fashion from the attachment plaques into the cytoplasm of the cells. The space between the cells shows cytoplasmic projections resembling microvilli that extend into the intercellular space and often interdigitate.

Less frequently observed forms of epithelial cell connections are tight junctions (zonae occludens) where the membranes of the adjoining cells are believed to be fused.[107,116,119] There is evidence suggesting that these structures allow ions and small molecules to pass from one cell to another.

Cytoplasmic organelle concentration varies among different epithelial strata. Mitochondria are more numerous in deeper strata and decrease toward the surface. Accordingly, histochemical demonstration of succinic dehydrogenase, nicotinamide-adenine dinucleotide, cytochrome oxidase, and other mitochondrial enzymes revealed a more active tricarboxylic cycle in basal and parabasal cells, where the proximity of the blood supply facilitates energy production via aerobic glycolysis.

Conversely, enzymes of the pentose shunt (an alternative pathway of glycolysis), such as glucose-6-phosphatase, increase their activity toward the surface. This pathway produces a larger amount of intermediate products for the production of RNA, which in turn can be used for the synthesis of keratinization proteins. This histochemical pattern is in accordance with the increased volume and amount of tonofilaments observed in cells reaching the surface.[35,36,48,80]

The uppermost cells of the stratum spinosum contain numerous dense granules known as *keratinosomes* or *Odland bodies,* which are modified lysosomes. They contain a large amount of acid phosphatase, an enzyme involved in the destruction of organelle membranes; this destruction occurs suddenly between the granulosum and corneum strata and during the intercellular cementation of cornified cells. Thus, acid phosphatase activity is closely related to the degree of keratinization.[18,46,113]

Nonkeratinocyte cells are present in gingival epithelium as in other malpighian epithelia. *Melanocytes* are dendritic cells located in the basal and spinous layers of the gingival epithelium. They synthesize melanin in organelles called *premelanosomes* or *melanosomes*[30,86,100] (Fig. 1–11). These contain tyrosinase, which hydroxylates tyrosine to dihydroxyphenylalanine (dopa), which in turn is progressively converted to melanin. Melanin granules are phagocytosed and contained within other cells of the epithelium and connective tissue, called *melanophages* or *melanophores.*

Langerhans cells are dendritic cells located among keratinocytes at all suprabasal levels (Fig. 1–12). They belong to the mononuclear phagocyte system (reticuloendothelial system) as modified monocytes derived from the bone marrow. They have an important role in the immune reaction as antigen-presenting cells for lymphocytes. They contain specific granules (Birbeck's granules) and marked adenosine triphosphatase activity. They are found in oral epithelium of normal gingiva and in smaller amounts in the sulcular epithelium; they are probably absent from the junctional epithelium of normal gingiva. (For a review on Langerhans cells, see the article by Bouchard.[15])

Merkel cells are located in the deeper layers of the epithelium, harbor nerve endings, and are connected to adjacent cells by desmosomes. They have been identified as tactile perceptors.[74]

The epithelium is joined to the underlying connective tissue by a *basal lamina* 300 to 400 Å thick, which lies approximately 400 Å beneath the epithelial basal layer.[58,91,101] The basal lamina consists of lamina lucida and lamina densa. Hemidesmosomes of the basal epithelial cells abut the lamina lucida, which is composed mainly of the glyco-

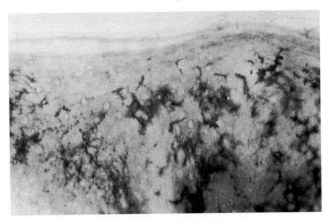

FIGURE 1–12. Human gingival epithelium, oral aspect. Immunoperoxidase technique showing Langerhans cells.

protein laminin. The lamina densa is composed of type IV collagen. The basal lamina, clearly distinguishable at the ultrastructural level, is connected to a reticular condensation of the underlying connective tissue fibrils (mainly collagen type IV) by the anchoring fibrils.[73,81,104] The complex of basal lamina and fibrils is the periodic acid–Schiff (PAS)–positive and argyrophilic line observed at the optical level[93,105] (Fig. 1–13). The basal lamina is permeable to fluids but acts as a barrier to particulate matter.

Structural and Metabolic Characteristics of the Gingival Epithelium

Oral or Outer Epithelium

The oral or outer epithelium covers the crest and outer surface of the marginal gingiva and the surface of the attached gingiva. It is keratinized (Fig. 1–14) or parakeratinized or presents various combinations of these conditions. The prevalent surface, however, is parakeratinized.[13,114]

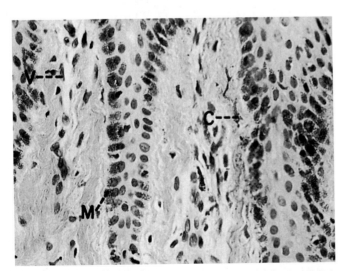

FIGURE 1–11. Pigmented gingiva, showing melanocytes (M) in the basal epithelial layer and melanophores (C) in the connective tissue. Also shown is a capillary (V) in the papillary connective tissue.

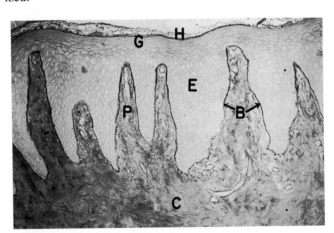

FIGURE 1–13. Normal human gingiva stained with the periodic acid–Schiff (PAS) histochemical method. The basement membrane (B) is seen between the epithelium (E) and the underlying connective tissue (C). In the epithelium, there is glycoprotein material between the cells and in the cell membrane of the superficial hornified (H) and underlying granular (G) layers. The connective tissue presents a diffuse amorphous ground substance and collagen fibers. The blood vessel walls stand out clearly in the papillary projections of the connective tissue (P).

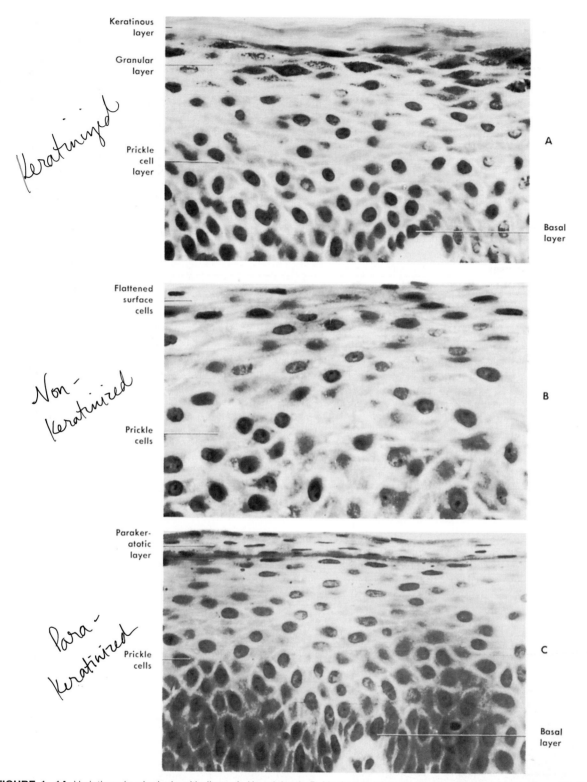

FIGURE 1-14. Variations in gingival epithelium. *A*, Keratinized. *B*, Nonkeratinized. *C*, Parakeratinized. (From Stern IB. Oral mucous membrane. In Bhaskar SN, ed. Orban's Oral Histology and Embryology. 8th ed. St Louis, CV Mosby, 1976.)

The degree of gingival keratinization diminishes with age and the onset of menopause[79] but is not necessarily related to the different phases of the menstrual cycle.[53] Keratinization of the oral mucosa varies in different areas in the following order: palate (most keratinized), gingiva, tongue, and cheek (least keratinized).[70]

Keratins K1 and K2 and K10–K12, which are specific to epidermal differentiation, are immunohistochemically expressed with high intensity in orthokeratinized areas and with less intensity in parakeratinized areas. K6 and K16, characteristic of highly proliferative epithelia, and K5 and K14, stratification-specific cytokeratins, are also present.

Parakeratinized areas express K19, which is usually absent from orthokeratinized normal epithelia.[14,85]

In keeping with complete or almost complete maturation, histoenzyme reactions for acid phosphatase and pentose-shunt enzymes are very strong.[19,48]

Glycogen can accumulate intracellularly when it is not completely degraded by any of the glycolytic pathways. Thus, its concentration in normal gingiva is inversely related to the degree of keratinization[92,114] and inflammation.[31,109,112]

Sulcular Epithelium

The sulcular epithelium lines the gingival sulcus (Fig. 1–15). It is a thin, nonkeratinized, stratified squamous epithelium without rete pegs and extends from the coronal limit of the junctional epithelium to the crest of the gingival margin (Fig. 1–16). It usually shows numerous cells with hydropic degeneration.[13]

As other nonkeratinized epithelia, it lacks granulosum and corneum strata and K1, K2, and K10–K12 cytokeratins but contains K4 and K13, the so-called esophageal type cytokeratins. It also expresses K19 and normally does not contain Merkel cells.

Histochemical studies of enzymes have consistently revealed a lower degree of activity than in the outer epithelium, particularly in the case of enzymes related to keratinization. Glucose-6-phosphate dehydrogenase expressed a faint and homogeneous reaction in all strata, unlike the increasing gradient toward the surface observed in cornified epithelia.[48] Acid phosphatase staining is negative,[18] although lysosomes have been described in exfoliated cells.

In spite of these morphologic and chemical characteristics, the sulcular epithelium has the potential to keratinize if (1) it is reflected and exposed to the oral cavity[17,21] or (2) the bacterial flora of the sulcus is totally eliminated.[22] Conversely, the outer epithelium loses its keratinization when it is placed in contact with the tooth.[22] These findings suggest that local irritation of the sulcus prevents sulcular keratinization.

The sulcular epithelium is extremely important, because it may act as a semipermeable membrane through which injurious bacterial products pass into the gingiva and through which tissue fluid from the gingiva seeps into the sulcus.[106]

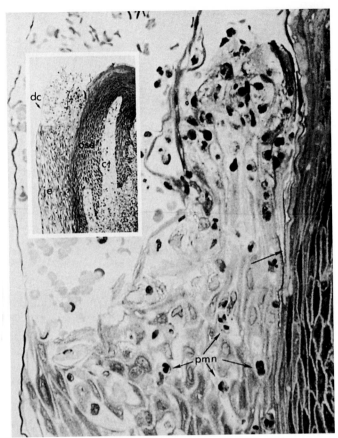

FIGURE 1–16. An Epon-embedded human biopsy specimen showing a relatively normal gingival sulcus. The soft tissue wall of the gingival sulcus is made up of the oral sulcular epithelium (ose) and its underlying connective tissue (ct), whereas the base of the gingival sulcus is formed by the sloughing surface of the junctional epithelium (je). The enamel space is delineated by a dense cuticular structure (dc). There is a relatively sharp line of demarcation between the junctional epithelium and the oral sulcular epithelium *(arrow)*, and several polymorphonuclear leukocytes (pmn) can be seen traversing the junctional epithelium. The sulcus contains red blood cells resulting from the hemorrhage occurring at the time of biopsy. × 391; inset × 55. (From Schluger S, Youdelis R, Page RC. Periodontal Disease. Philadelphia, Lea & Febiger, 1977.)

Junctional Epithelium

The junctional epithelium consists of a collar-like band of stratified squamous nonkeratinizing epithelium. It is three to four layers thick in early life, but the number of layers increases with age to 10 or even 20; these cells can be grouped in two strata: basal and suprabasal. The length of the junctional epithelium ranges from 0.25 to 1.35 mm (Fig. 1–17).

Cell layers not juxtaposed to the tooth exhibit numerous free ribosomes and prominent membrane-bound structures such as Golgi complexes, lysosome-like bodies, and cytoplasmic vacuoles, presumably phagocytic. Similar morphologic findings have been described in the gingiva of germ-free rats. Polymorphonuclear neutrophil leukocytes are found routinely in the junctional epithelium of both conventional and germ-free rats.[120]

The different keratin polypeptides of junctional epithelium have a particular immunochemical pattern. Junctional epithelium expresses K19 (which is absent from keratinized epithelia) and the stratification-specific cytokeratins K5 and

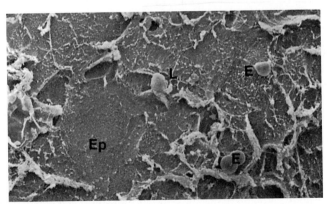

FIGURE 1–15. Scanning electron microscopic view of the epithelial surface facing the tooth in a normal human gingival sulcus. The epithelium (Ep) shows desquamating cells, some scattered erythrocytes (E), and a few emerging leukocytes (L). × 1000.

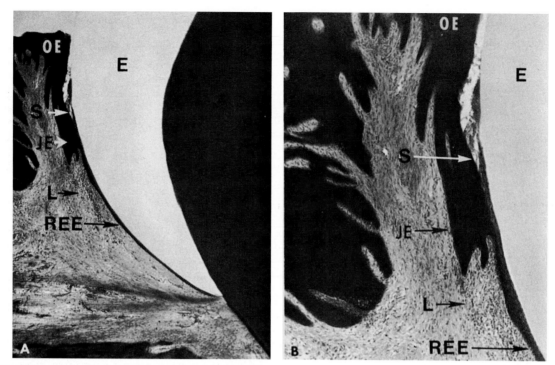

FIGURE 1–17. Gingival sulcus in an erupting monkey tooth. *A,* The gingival sulcus (S), the enamel (E), and the junctional epithelium (JE). Note the oral epithelium (OE), the reduced enamel epithelium (REE), and the leukocytic infiltration (L). *B,* High-power section showing the base of the sulcus (S), the enamel (E), and the junctional epithelium (JE). Leukocytic infiltration (L), which is usually present in clinically normal gingiva, is shown beneath the base of the sulcus. Tissues within the sulcus are artifact and debris.

K14.[85] Morgan et al.[71] reported that reactions to demonstrate K4 or K13 reveal a sudden change between sulcular and junctional epithelium, with the junctional area being the only stratified nonkeratinized epithelium in the oral cavity that does not synthesize these specific polypeptides. Another particular behavior is the lack of expression of K6 and K16 (proliferation-specific keratins), although the turnover of the cells is very high.

Similar to sulcular epithelium, junctional epithelium exhibits less glycolytic enzyme activity than outer epithelium and lacks acid phosphatase activity.[18,48]

The junctional epithelium is attached to the tooth surface (epithelial attachment) by means of an internal basal lamina and to the gingival connective tissue by an external basal lamina that has the same structure as other epithelial–connective tissue attachments elsewhere in the body.[66]

The internal basal lamina consists of a lamina densa (adjacent to the enamel) and a lamina lucida to which hemidesmosomes are attached (Fig. 1–18). Organic strands from the enamel appear to extend into the lamina densa.[103] The junctional epithelium attaches to afibrillar cementum when it is present on the crown (usually restricted to an area within 1 mm of the cemento-enamel junction)[90] (see Fig. 1–18) and to root cementum in a similar manner.

Histochemical evidence for the presence of neutral polysaccharides in the zone of the epithelial attachment has been reported.[108] Data have also shown that the basal lamina of the junctional epithelium resembles that of endothelial and epithelial cells in its laminin content, but the junctional epithelium differs in its internal basal lamina, which has no type IV collagen.[55,84] These findings indicate that the cells of the junctional epithelium are involved in the pro-

duction of laminin and play a key role in the adhesion mechanism.

The attachment of the junctional epithelium to the tooth is reinforced by the gingival fibers, which brace the marginal gingiva against the tooth surface. For this reason, the junctional epithelium and the gingival fibers are considered to be a functional unit, referred to as the *dentogingival unit.*

Development of the Gingival Sulcus

After enamel formation is complete, the enamel is covered with reduced enamel epithelium, which is attached to the tooth by a basal lamina and hemidesmosomes.[62,102] When the tooth penetrates the oral mucosa, the reduced enamel epithelium unites with the oral epithelium and transforms itself into the junctional epithelium. As the tooth erupts, this united epithelium condenses along the crown, and the ameloblasts, which form the inner layer of the reduced enamel epithelium (see Fig. 1–17), gradually become squamous epithelial cells. The transformation of the reduced enamel epithelium into junctional epithelium proceeds in an apical direction, without interrupting the attachment to the tooth; according to Schroeder and Listgarten, this process takes between 1 and 2 years.[90]

The junctional epithelium is a continually self-renewing structure, with mitotic activity occurring in all cell layers.[62,102] The regenerating epithelial cells move toward the tooth surface and along it in a coronal direction to the gingival sulcus, where they are shed[11] (Fig. 1–19). The migrating daughter cells provide a continuous attachment to the tooth surface. The strength of the epithelial attachment to the tooth has not been measured.

The gingival sulcus is formed when the tooth erupts into

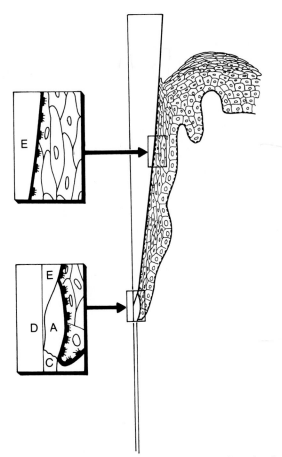

FIGURE 1–18. Diagram of the dentogingival junction showing the junctional epithelium adhering to the tooth surface. At upper left, an enlarged view of epithelial cells showing hemidesmosomes in those cells along the enamel surface (E). Intervening between the epithelial cells and the enamel are the basal lamina and dental cuticle, respectively; both of these structures are represented by the single thick line along the enamel. At lower left, an enlarged view of the cemento-enamel junction shows a small area of afibrillar cementum (A). C, Cementum; D, dentin.

the oral cavity. At that time, the junctional epithelium and reduced enamel epithelium together form a broad band that is attached to the tooth surface from near the tip of the crown to the cemento-enamel junction.

The gingival sulcus is the shallow, V-shaped space or groove between the tooth and gingiva that encircles the newly erupted tip of the crown. In the fully erupted tooth, only the junctional epithelium persists. *The sulcus consists of the shallow space that is coronal to the attachment of the junctional epithelium and is bounded by the tooth on one side and the sulcular epithelium on the other. The coronal extent of the gingival sulcus is the gingival margin.*

Renewal of Gingival Epithelium

The oral epithelium undergoes continuous renewal. Its thickness is maintained by a balance between new cell formation in the basal and spinous layers and the shedding of old cells at the surface. The mitotic activity exhibits a 24-hour periodicity, with highest and lowest rates occurring in the morning and evening, respectively.[110] The mitotic rate is higher in nonkeratinized areas and is increased in gingivitis, without significant sex differences. Opinions differ as to

whether the mitotic rate is increased[66,69] or decreased[10] with age.

The mitotic rate in experimental animals varies in different areas of the oral epithelium in the following descending order: buccal mucosa, hard palate, sulcular epithelium, junctional epithelium, outer surface of the marginal gingiva, and attached gingiva.[6,44,65,110] The turnover times for different areas of the oral epithelium in experimental animals have been reported as follows: palate, tongue, and cheek, 5 to 6 days; gingiva, 10 to 12 days, with the same or more time required with age; and junctional epithelium, 1 to 6 days.[11,98]

Cuticular Structures on the Tooth

The term *cuticle* is used to describe a thin, acellular structure with a homogeneous matrix, sometimes enclosed within clearly demarcated linear borders.

Listgarten has classified cuticular structures into acquired coatings and coatings of developmental origin.[64] *Acquired coatings* include those of exogenous origin, such as saliva, bacteria, calculus, and surface stains. They are discussed in Chapters 6 and 11. *Coatings of developmental origin* are those normally formed as part of tooth development. They include the reduced enamel epithelium, the coronal cementum, and the dental cuticle.

After enamel formation is completed, the ameloblastic epithelium becomes reduced to one or two layers of cells

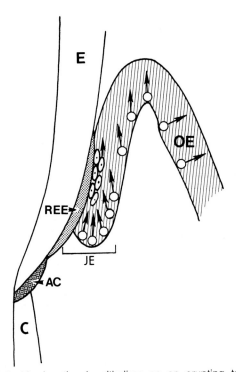

FIGURE 1–19. Junctional epithelium on an erupting tooth. The junctional epithelium (JE) is formed by the joining of the oral epithelium (OE) and the reduced enamel epithelium (REE). Afibrillar cementum (AC), sometimes formed on enamel after degeneration of the reduced enamel epithelium, is shown. The *arrows* indicate the coronal movement of the regenerating epithelial cells, which multiply more rapidly in the junctional epithelium than in the oral epithelium. A similar cell turnover pattern exists in the fully erupted tooth. C, Root cementum; E, enamel. (From Listgarten MA. J Can Dent Assoc *36:*70, 1970.)

that remain attached to the enamel surface by hemidesmosomes and a basal lamina. This *reduced enamel epithelium* consists of postsecretory ameloblasts and cells from the stratum intermedium of the enamel organ.

In some animal species, the reduced enamel epithelium disappears entirely very rapidly, thereby placing the enamel surface in contact with the connective tissue. Connective tissue cells then deposit a thin layer of cementum, known as *coronal cementum,* on the enamel. In humans, thin patches of afibrillar cementum may sometimes be seen in the cervical half of the crown.

Electron microscopy has shown a *dental cuticle* consisting of a layer of homogeneous organic material of variable thickness (approximately 0.25 μm) overlying the enamel surface. It is nonmineralized and is not always present. In some instances near the cemento-enamel junction, it is deposited over a layer of afibrillar cementum, which in turn overlies enamel. The cuticle may or may not be present between the junctional epithelium and the tooth. Ultrastructural histochemical studies have shown the dental cuticle to be proteinaceous,[56] and it may be an accumulation of tissue fluid components.[39,88]

Gingival Fluid (Sulcular Fluid)

The gingival sulcus contains a fluid that seeps into it from the gingival connective tissue through the thin sulcular epithelium. The gingival fluid is believed to (1) cleanse material from the sulcus, (2) contain plasma proteins that may improve adhesion of the epithelium to the tooth, (3) possess antimicrobial properties, and (4) exert antibody activity in defense of the gingiva.

The gingival fluid and its significance in health and disease are discussed in detail in Chapter 7.

Gingival Connective Tissue

The connective tissue of the gingiva is known as the *lamina propria* and consists of two layers: a *papillary layer* subjacent to the epithelium that consists of papillary projections between the epithelial rete pegs, and a *reticular layer* contiguous with the periosteum of the alveolar bone.

Connective tissue has a cellular and an intercellular compartment. Collagen type I forms the bulk of the lamina propria and provides tensile strength to the gingival tissue. Type IV collagen (argyrophilic reticulum fibers) bundles branch between the collagen type I bundles and are continuous with those of the basement membrane and blood vessel walls.[66]

The elastic fiber system is composed of oxytalan, elaunin, and elastin fibers distributed among collagen fibers.[26] The intercellular matrix also contains proteoglycans (mainly hyaluronic acid and chondroitin sulfate) and glycoproteins (mainly fibronectin). Glycoproteins account for the faint PAS-positive reaction of the ground substance.[36] Fibronectin binds fibroblasts to the fibers and to many other components of the intercellular component.

Gingival Collagen Fibers

The connective tissue of the marginal gingiva is densely collagenous, containing a prominent system of collagen fiber bundles called the *gingival fibers* that consist of type I collagen.[81] The gingival fibers have three functions:

1. To brace the marginal gingiva firmly against the tooth.
2. To provide the rigidity necessary to withstand the forces of mastication without being deflected away from the tooth surface.
3. To unite the free marginal gingiva with the cementum of the root and the adjacent attached gingiva.

The gingival fibers are arranged in three groups: gingivodental, circular, and transseptal.[7,57]

Gingivodental Group. The gingivodental fibers are the fibers of the facial, lingual, and interproximal surfaces. They are embedded in the cementum just beneath the epithelium at the base of the gingival sulcus. On the facial and lingual surfaces, they project from the cementum in fan-like conformation toward the crest and outer surface of the marginal gingiva and terminate short of the epithelium (Figs. 1–20 and 1–21). They also extend external to the periosteum of the facial and lingual alveolar bone and terminate in the attached gingiva or blend with the periosteum of the bone. Interproximally, the gingivodental fibers extend toward the crest of the interdental gingiva.

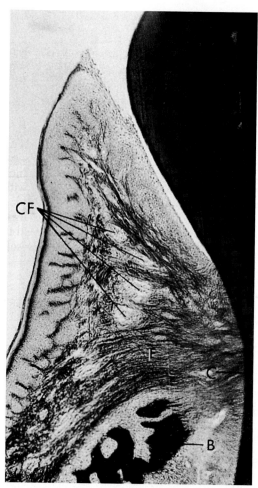

FIGURE 1–20. Faciolingual section of marginal gingiva, showing gingival fibers (F) extending from the cementum (C) to the crest of the gingiva, to the outer gingival surface, and external to the periosteum of the bone (B). Circular fibers (CF) are shown in cross section between the other groups. (Courtesy of Dr. Sol Bernick.)

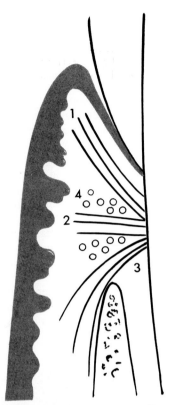

FIGURE 1–21. Diagram of the gingivodental fibers extending from the cementum to the crest of the gingiva (1), to the outer surface (2), and external to the periosteum of the labial plate (3). Circular fibers (4) are shown in cross section.

Circular Group. Circular fibers course through the connective tissue of the marginal and interdental gingivae and encircle the tooth in a ring-like fashion.

Transseptal Group. Located interproximally, the transseptal fibers form horizontal bundles that extend between the cementum of approximating teeth into which they are embedded. They lie in the area between the epithelium at the base of the gingival sulcus and the crest of the interdental bone and are sometimes classified with the principal fibers of the periodontal ligament.

Page and coworkers[78] have also described (1) a group of *semicircular fibers* that attach at the proximal surface of a tooth, immediately below the cemento-enamel junction, and go around the facial or lingual marginal gingiva of the tooth and attach on the other proximal surface of the same tooth and (2) a group of *transgingival fibers* that attach in the proximal surface of one tooth, traverse the interdental space diagonally, go around the facial or lingual surface of the adjacent tooth, then again traverse the interdental space diagonally, and attach in the proximal surface of the next tooth.

Connective Tissue Cellular Compartment

The preponderant cellular element in the gingival connective tissue is the *fibroblast*. Numerous fibroblasts are found between the fiber bundles. As in connective tissue elsewhere in the body, fibroblasts synthesize collagen and elastic fibers, as well as the glycoproteins and glycosamino-

glycans of the amorphous intercellular substance. Fibroblasts also regulate collagen degradation.

Mast cells, which are distributed throughout the body, are numerous in the connective tissue of the oral mucosa and the gingiva.[24,96,97,117] *Fixed macrophages* and *histiocytes* are present in the gingival connective tissue as components of the mononuclear phagocyte system (reticuloendothelial system) and derived from blood monocytes. *Adipose cells* and *eosinophils*, although scarce, are also present in the lamina propria.

In clinically normal gingiva, *small foci of plasma cells and lymphocytes* are found in the connective tissue near the base of the sulcus. Neutrophils can be seen in relatively high numbers in both the gingival connective tissue and the sulcus. These inflammatory cells are usually present in small amounts in clinically normal gingiva. Their presence is believed to be related to the penetration of antigenic substances from the oral cavity via the sulcular and junctional epithelia (Fig. 1–22) (see Chapters 7 and 8). They are not present, however, if gingival normalcy is judged by very strict clinical criteria.[76] Therefore, *in spite of the frequency of their occurrence, the inflammatory infiltrate cells are not a normal component of the gingival tissue.*

Blood Supply, Lymphatics, and Nerves

Vascularization patterns can be visualized in tissue sections by means of the histoenzymatic reactions for alkaline phosphatase and adenosine triphosphatase owing to the great activity of these enzymes in endothelial cells.[25,121] In experimental animals, the injection and posterior demonstration of peroxidase allow blood vessel identification and permeability studies.[95] The PAS reaction also outlines vascular walls by a positive line in their basal membrane.[93] Endothelial cells also express 5-nucleotidase activity.[47] Scanning electron microscopy can be used after injection of plastic into the vessels, via the carotid artery, followed by corrosion of the soft tissues to visualize.

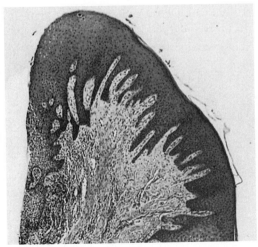

FIGURE 1–22. Section of clinically normal gingiva, showing inflammation, which is almost always present near the base of the sulcus. Keratin strands are visible on the outer surface, where they have been displaced as a result of artifact.

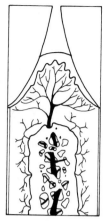
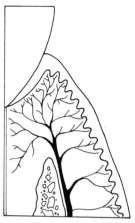

FIGURE 1–23. Diagrammatic representation of an arteriole penetrating the interdental alveolar bone to supply the interdental tissues *(left)* and a supraperiosteal arteriole overlying the facial alveolar bone, sending branches to the surrounding tissue *(right).*

There are three sources of blood supply to the gingiva:

1. *Supraperiosteal arterioles* along the facial and lingual surfaces of the alveolar bone, from which capillaries extend along the sulcular epithelium and between the rete pegs of the external gingival surface.[34,45] Occasional branches of the arterioles pass through the alveolar bone to the periodontal ligament or run over the crest of the alveolar bone (Fig. 1–23).

2. *Vessels of the periodontal ligament,* which extend into the gingiva and anastomose with capillaries in the sulcus area.

or (intraosseous) artery

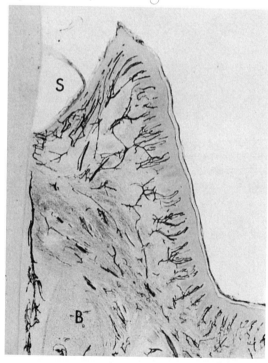

FIGURE 1–24. Blood supply and peripheral circulation of the gingiva. Tissues perfused with India ink. Note the capillary plexus parallel to the sulcus (S) and the capillary loops in the outer papillary layer. Note also the supraperiosteal vessels external to the bone (B) that supply the gingiva and a periodontal ligament vessel anastomosing with the sulcus plexus (see also Fig. 2–5). (Courtesy of Dr. Sol Bernick.)

3. *Arterioles that emerge from the crest of the interdental septa*[37] and extend parallel to the crest of the bone to anastomose with vessels of the periodontal ligament, with capillaries in the gingival crevicular areas, and with vessels that run over the alveolar crest.

Beneath the epithelium on the outer gingival surface, capillaries extend into the papillary connective tissue between the epithelial rete pegs in the form of terminal hairpin loops with efferent and afferent branches, spirals, and varices[25,45] (Figs. 1–24 and 1–25). The loops are sometimes linked by cross-communications,[38] and there are also flattened capillaries that serve as reserve vessels when the circulation is increased in response to irritation.[41]

Along the sulcular epithelium, capillaries are arranged in a flat, anastomosing plexus that extends parallel to the enamel from the base of the sulcus to the gingival margin.[25] In the col area, there is a mixed pattern of anastomosing capillaries and loops.

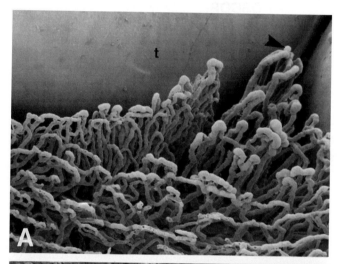
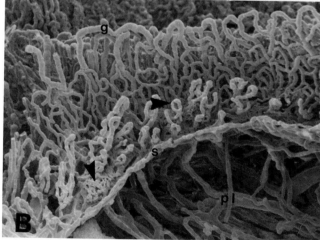

FIGURE 1–25. Scanning electron microscopic view of gingival tissues of rat molar palatal gingiva after vascular perfusion of plastic and corrosion of soft tissue. *A,* Oral view of gingival capillaries. ×180. *Arrowhead,* interdental papilla; t, tooth. *B,* View from the tooth side. Note the vessels of the plexus next to the sulcular and the junctional epithelium. The *arrowheads* point to vessels in the sulcus area with mild inflammatory changes. ×150. g, Crest of marginal gingiva; pl, periodontal ligament vessels; s, bottom of gingival sulcus. (Courtesy of Dr. N. J. Selliseth and Dr. K. Selvig, University of Bergen, Norway.)

The *lymphatic drainage of the gingiva* brings in the lymphatics of the connective tissue papillae. It progresses into the collecting network external to the periosteum of the alveolar process and then to the regional lymph nodes (particularly the submaxillary group). In addition, lymphatics just beneath the junctional epithelium extend into the periodontal ligament and accompany the blood vessels.

Gingival innervation is derived from fibers arising from nerves in the periodontal ligament and from the labial, buccal, and palatal nerves.[12] The following nerve structures are present in connective tissue: a meshwork of terminal argyrophilic fibers, some of which extend into the epithelium; Meissner-type tactile corpuscles; Krause-type end bulbs, which are temperature receptors; and encapsulated spindles.[9]

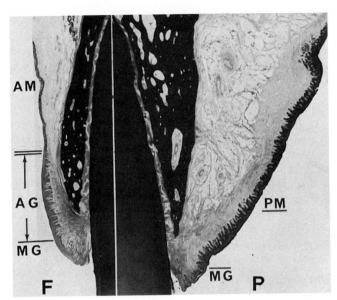

FIGURE 1–26. Oral mucosa, facial and palatal surfaces. The facial surface (F) shows the marginal gingiva (MG), attached gingiva (AG), and alveolar mucosa (AM). The double line (=) marks the mucogingival junction. Note the differences in the epithelium and connective tissue in the attached gingiva and alveolar mucosa. The palatal surface (P) shows the marginal gingiva (MG) and thick, keratinized palatal mucosa (PM).

CORRELATION OF NORMAL CLINICAL AND MICROSCOPIC FEATURES

To understand the normal clinical features of the gingiva, the clinician must be able to interpret them in terms of the microscopic structures they represent.

Color

The color of the attached and marginal gingivae is generally described as coral pink and is produced by the vascular supply, the thickness and degree of keratinization of the epithelium, and the presence of pigment-containing cells. The color varies among persons and appears to be correlated with the cutaneous pigmentation. It is lighter in blond individuals with a fair complexion than in dark-complexioned brunettes (Plate I).

The attached gingiva is demarcated from the adjacent alveolar mucosa on the buccal aspect by a clearly defined mucogingival line. The alveolar mucosa is red, smooth, and shiny rather than pink and stippled. Comparison of the microscopic structure of the attached gingiva with that of the alveolar mucosa affords an explanation for the difference in appearance. The epithelium of the alveolar mucosa is thinner, nonkeratinized, and contains no rete pegs (Fig. 1–26). The connective tissue of the alveolar mucosa is loosely arranged, and the blood vessels are more numerous.

Physiologic Pigmentation (Melanin)

Melanin, a non–hemoglobin-derived brown pigment, is responsible for the normal pigmentation of the skin, gingiva, and remainder of the oral mucous membrane. It is present in all normal individuals, although often not in sufficient quantities to be detected clinically, but it is absent or severely diminished in albinos. Melanin pigmentation in the oral cavity is prominent in blacks (see Plate I).

According to Dummett,[33] the distribution of oral pigmentation in blacks is as follows: gingiva, 60%; hard palate, 61%; mucous membrane, 22%; and tongue, 15%. *Gingival pigmentation occurs as a diffuse, deep purplish discoloration or as irregularly shaped brown and light brown patches. It may appear in the gingiva as early as 3 hours after birth and often is the only evidence of pigmentation.*[33]

Size

The size of the gingiva corresponds to the sum total of the bulk of cellular and intercellular elements and their vascular supply. Alteration in size is a common feature of gingival disease.

Contour

The contour or shape of the gingiva varies considerably and depends on the shape of the teeth and their alignment in the arch, the location and size of the area of proximal contact, and the dimensions of the facial and lingual gingival embrasures. The marginal gingiva envelops the teeth in collar-like fashion and follows a scalloped outline on the facial and lingual surfaces. It forms a straight line along teeth with relatively flat surfaces. On teeth with pronounced mesiodistal convexity (e.g., maxillary canines) or teeth in labial version, the normal arcuate contour is accentuated, and the gingiva is located farther apically. On teeth in lingual version, the gingiva is horizontal and thickened (Fig. 1–27).

Shape

The shape of the interdental gingiva is governed by the contour of the proximal tooth surfaces and the location and shape of gingival embrasures. When the proximal surfaces of the crowns are relatively flat faciolingually, the roots are close together, the interdental bone is thin mesiodistally, and the gingival embrasures and interdental gingiva are narrow mesiodistally. Conversely, with proximal surfaces that flare away from the area of contact, the mesiodistal diameter of the interdental gingiva is broad (Fig. 1–28). The height of the interdental gingiva varies with the location of the proximal contact.

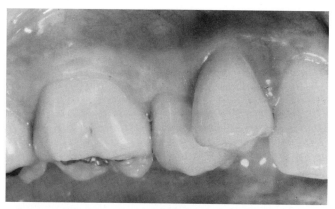

FIGURE 1–27. Thickened, shelf-like contour of the gingiva on a tooth in lingual version aggravated by local irritation caused by plaque accumulation.

Consistency

The gingiva is firm and resilient and, with the exception of the movable free margin, tightly bound to the underlying bone. The collagenous nature of the lamina propria and its contiguity with the mucoperiosteum of the alveolar bone determine the firm consistency of the attached gingiva. The gingival fibers contribute to the firmness of the gingival margin.

Surface Texture

The gingiva presents a textured surface like that of an orange peel and is referred to as being stippled; Stippling is best viewed by drying the gingiva (see Plate I). *The attached gingiva is stippled; the marginal gingiva is not.* The central portion of the interdental papillae is usually stippled, but the marginal borders are smooth. The pattern and

extent of stippling vary from person to person and in different areas of the same mouth.[43,82] It is less prominent on lingual than on facial surfaces and may be absent in some persons.

Stippling varies with age. It is absent in infancy, appears in some children at about 5 years of age, increases until adulthood, and frequently begins to disappear in old age.

Microscopically, stippling is produced by alternate rounded protuberances and depressions in the gingival surface. The papillary layer of the connective tissue projects into the elevations, and both the elevated and the depressed areas are covered by stratified squamous epithelium (Fig. 1–29). The degree of keratinization and the prominence of stippling appear to be related.

Scanning electron microscopy has shown considerable variation in shape but a relatively constant depth; at low magnification a rippled surface is seen, interrupted by irregular depressions 50 μm in diameter. At higher magnification, cell micropits are seen.[28]

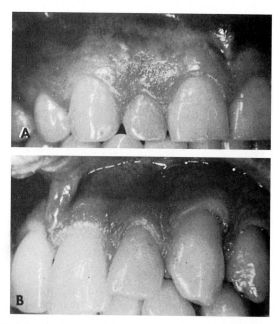

FIGURE 1–28. Shape of interdental gingival papillae correlated with the shape of teeth and embrasures. *A,* Broad interdental papillae. *B,* Narrow interdental papillae.

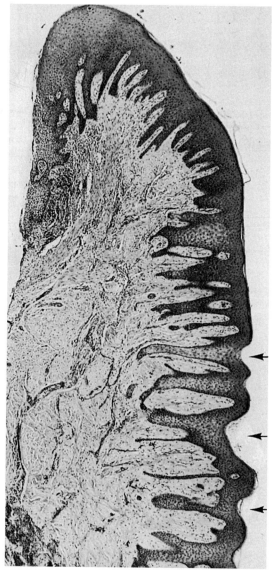

FIGURE 1–29. Gingival biopsy from the same patient as in Figure 1–7, demonstrating alternating elevations and depressions *(arrows)* in the attached gingiva, creating a stippled appearance.

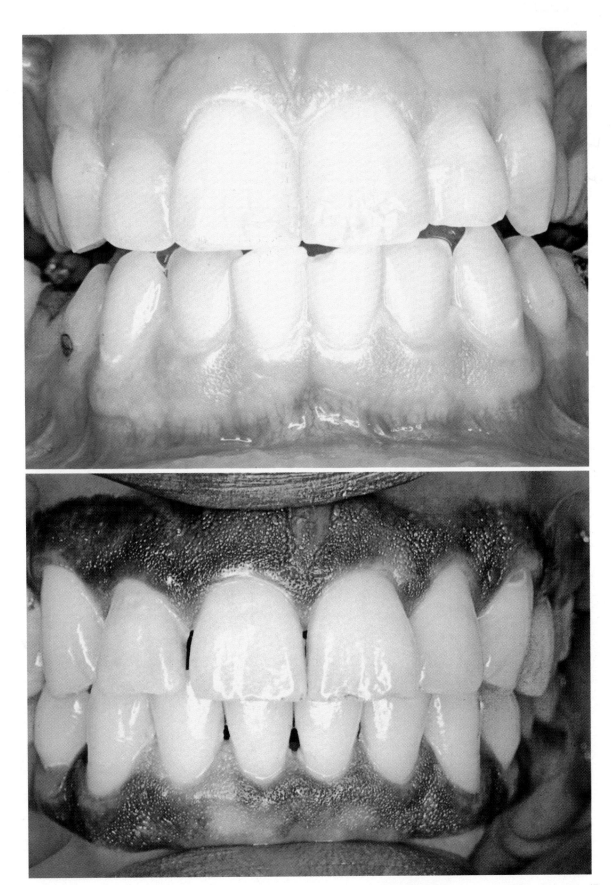

PLATE I. *Top,* Clinically normal gingiva in a young adult. *Bottom,* Heavily pigmented (melanotic) gingiva in a middle-aged adult. (From Glickman I, Smulow JB. Periodontal Disease: Clinical. Radiographic, and Histopathologic Features. Philadelphia, WB Saunders, 1974.)

Attrition = normal wearing away of teeth (chewing) (active)

The Gingiva

27

Stippling is a form of adaptive specialization or reinforcement for function. It is a feature of healthy gingiva, and reduction or loss of stippling is a common sign of gingival disease. When the gingiva is restored to health with treatment, the stippled appearance returns.

The surface texture of the gingiva is also related to the presence and degree of epithelial keratinization. Keratinization is considered to be a protective adaptation to function. It increases when the gingiva is stimulated by toothbrushing. However, research on free gingival grafts (see Chapter 59) has shown that when connective tissue is transplanted from a keratinized area to a nonkeratinized area, it becomes covered by a keratinized epithelium.[54] This finding suggests a connective tissue–based genetic determination of the type of epithelial surface.

Position

The position of the gingiva refers to the level at which the gingival margin is attached to the tooth. When the tooth erupts into the oral cavity, the margin and sulcus are at the tip of the crown; as eruption progresses, they are seen closer to the root. During this eruption process, as described earlier, the junctional epithelium, oral epithelium, and reduced enamel epithelium undergo extensive alterations and remodeling, while at the same time maintaining the shallow physiologic depth of the sulcus. Without this remodeling of the epithelia, an abnormal anatomic relationship between the gingiva and the tooth would result.

Continuous Tooth Eruption

According to the concept of continuous eruption,[42] eruption does not cease when teeth meet their functional antagonists but continues throughout life. It consists of an active and a passive phase. *Active eruption* is the movement of the teeth in the direction of the occlusal plane, whereas *passive eruption* is the exposure of the teeth by apical migration of the gingiva.

This concept distinguishes between the *anatomic crown* (the portion of the tooth covered by enamel) and the *anatomic root* (the portion of the tooth covered by cementum), and between the *clinical crown* (the part of the tooth that has been denuded of its gingiva and projects into the oral cavity) and the clinical root (that portion of the tooth covered by periodontal tissues). When the teeth reach their functional antagonists, the gingival sulcus and junctional epithelium are still on the enamel, and the clinical crown is approximately two thirds of the anatomic crown.

Active and passive eruption were believed by Gottlieb to proceed together. Active eruption is coordinated with attrition. The teeth erupt to compensate for tooth substance worn away by attrition. Attrition reduces the clinical crown and prevents it from becoming disproportionately long in relation to the clinical root, thus avoiding excessive leverage on the periodontal tissues. Ideally, the rate of active eruption keeps pace with tooth wear, preserving the vertical dimension of the dentition.

As the teeth erupt, cementum is deposited at the apices and furcations of the roots, and bone is formed along the fundus of the alveolus and at the crest of the alveolar bone.

In this way, part of the tooth substance lost by attrition is replaced by lengthening of the root, and socket depth is maintained to support the root.

Passive eruption is divided into four stages (Fig. 1–30). Although this was originally thought to be a normal physiologic process, it is currently considered a pathologic process.

1. *Stage one:* The teeth reach the line of occlusion. The junctional epithelium and base of the gingival sulcus are on the enamel.
2. *Stage two:* The junctional epithelium proliferates so that part is on the cementum and part is on the enamel. The base of the sulcus is still on the enamel.
3. *Stage three:* The entire junctional epithelium is on the cementum, and the base of the sulcus is at the cemento-enamel junction. As the junctional epithelium proliferates from the crown onto the root, it remains at the cemento-enamel junction no longer than at any other area of the tooth.
4. *Stage four:* The junctional epithelium has proliferated farther on the cementum. The base of the sulcus is on the cementum, a portion of which is exposed. Proliferation of the junctional epithelium onto the root is accompanied by degeneration of gingival and periodontal ligament fibers and their detachment from the tooth. The cause of this degeneration is not understood. At present, however, it is believed to be the result of chronic inflammation and, therefore, a pathologic process.

As noted previously, apposition of bone accompanies active eruption. The distance between the apical end of the junctional epithelium and the crest of the alveolus remains constant throughout continuous tooth eruption (1.07 mm).[40]

Exposure of the tooth by the apical migration of the gingiva is called *gingival recession,* or *atrophy.* According to the concept of continuous eruption, the gingival sulcus may be located on the crown, cemento-enamel junction, or root, depending on the age of the patient and the stage of eruption. Therefore, some root exposure with age is considered normal and is referred to as *physiologic recession.* As mentioned previously, this concept is not accepted at present. Excessive exposure is termed *pathologic recession* (see Chapter 17).

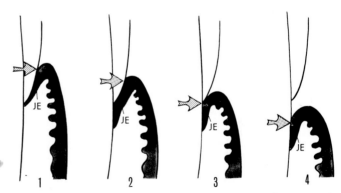

FIGURE 1–30. Diagrammatic representation of the four steps in passive eruption according to Gottlieb and Orban.[42] 1, The base of the gingival sulcus (*arrow*) and the junctional epithelium (JE) are on the enamel. 2, The base of the gingival sulcus (*arrow*) is on the enamel, and part of the junctional epithelium is on the root. 3, The base of the gingival sulcus (*arrow*) is at the cemento-enamel line, and the entire junctional epithelium is on the root. 4, The base of the gingival sulcus (*arrow*) and the junctional epithelium are on the root.

REFERENCES

1. Ainamo A. Influence of age on the location of the maxillary mucogingival junction. J Periodont Res *13*:189, 1978.
2. Ainamo A, Ainamo J. The width of attached gingiva on supraerupted teeth. J Periodont Res *13*:194, 1978.
3. Ainamo J, Löe H. Anatomical characteristics of gingiva. A clinical and microscopic study of the free and attached gingiva. J Periodontol *37*:5, 1966.
4. Ainamo J, Talari A. The increase with age of the width of attached gingiva. J Periodont Res *11*:182, 1976.
5. Amstad-Jossi M, Schroeder HE. Age related alterations of periodontal structures around the cemento-enamel junction and of the gingival connective tissue composition in germfree rats. J Periodont Res *13*:76, 1978.
6. Anderson GS, Stern I. The proliferation and migration of the attachment epithelium on the cemental surface of the rat incisor. Periodontics *4*:115, 1966.
7. Arnim SS, Hagerman DA. The connective tissue fibers of the marginal gingiva. J Am Dent Assoc *47*:271, 1953.
8. Attstrom RM, Graf de Beer M, Schroeder HE. Clinical and histologic characteristics of normal gingiva in dogs. J Periodont Res *10*:115, 1975.
9. Avery JK, Rapp R. Pain conduction in human dental tissues. Dent Clin North Am *July*:489, 1959.
10. Barakat MH, Toto PD, Choukas NC. Aging and cell renewal of oral epithelium. J Periodontol *40*:599, 1969.
11. Beagrie GS, Skougaard MR. Observations on the life cycle of the gingival epithelial cells of mice as revealed by autoradiography. Acta Odontol Scand *20*:15, 1962.
12. Bernick S. Innervation of the teeth and periodontium. Dent Clin North Am *July*:503, 1959.
13. Biolcati EL, Carranza FA Jr, Cabrini RL. Variaciones y alteraciones de la queratinizacion en encias humanas clinicamente sanas. Rev Asoc Odontol Argent *41*:446, 1953.
14. Bosch FX, Ouyahoun JP, Bader BL, et al. Extensive changes in cytokeratin expression patterns in pathologically affected human gingiva. Arch VB Cell Pathol *58*:59, 1989.
15. Bouchard P. La cellule de Langerhans: Un role immunitaire pour l'epithelium gingivale. J Parodontol *6*:249, 1987.
16. Bowers GM. A study of the width of the attached gingiva. J Periodontol *34*:210, 1963.
17. Bral MM, Stahl SS. Keratinizing potential of human crevicular epithelium. J Periodontol *48*:381, 1977.
18. Cabrini RL, Carranza FA Jr. Histochemical distribution of acid phosphatase in human gingiva. J Periodontol *29*:34, 1958.
19. Cabrini RL, Carranza FA Jr. Histology of periodontal tissues. A review of the literature. Int Dent J *16*:476, 1966.
20. Cabrini R, Cabrini RL, Carranza FA Jr. Estudio histologico de la queratinizacion del epitelio gingival y de la adherencia epitelial. Rev Asoc Odontol Argent *41*:212, 1953.
21. Caffesse RG, Karring T, Nasjleti CE. Keratinizing potential of sulcular epithelium. J Periodontol *48*:140, 1977.
22. Caffesse RG, Nasjleti CE, Castelli WA. The role of the sulcular environment in controlling epithelial keratinization. J Periodontol *50*:1, 1979.
23. Caffesse RG, Kornman KS, Nasjleti CE. The effect of intensive antibacterial therapy on the sulcular environment in monkeys. II. Inflammation, mitotic activity and keratinization of the sulcular epithelium. J Periodontol *5*:155, 1980.
24. Carranza FA Jr, Cabrini RL. Mast cells in human gingiva. Oral Surg *8*:1093, 1955.
25. Carranza FA Jr, Itoiz ME, Cabrini RL, Dotto CA. A study of periodontal vascularization in different laboratory animals. J Periodont Res *1*:120, 1966.
26. Chavier C. Elastic fibers of healthy human gingiva. J Periodontol *9*:29, 1990.
27. Clausen H, Moe D, Buschard K, Dabelsteen E. Keratin proteins in human oral mucosa. J Oral Pathol *15*:36, 1986.
28. Cleaton-Jones P, Buskin SA, Volchansky A. Surface ultrastructure of human gingiva. J Periodont Res *13*:367, 1978.
29. Cohen B. Morphological factors in the pathogenesis of periodontal disease. Br Dent J *107*:31, 1959.
30. Cohen L. ATPase and dopa oxidase activity in human gingival epithelium. Arch Oral Biol *12*:1241, 1967.
31. Dewar MR. Observations on the composition and metabolism of normal and inflamed gingivae. J Periodontol *26*:29, 1955.
32. DiFranco CF, Toto PD, Rowden G, Gargiulo AW. Identification of Langerhans cells in human gingival epithelium. J Periodontol *56*:48, 1985.
33. Dummett CO. Physiologic pigmentation of the oral and cutaneous tissues in the Negro. J Dent Res *25*:422, 1946.
34. Egelberg J. The topography and permeability of blood vessels at the dentogingival junction in dogs. J Periodont Res *2*(suppl 1), 1967.
35. Eichel B, Shahrik HA, Lisanti VF. Cytochemical demonstration and metabolic significance of reduced diphosphopyridinenucleotide and triphosphopyridinenucleotide reductases in human gingiva. J Dent Res *43*:92, 1964.
36. Engel MB. Water-soluble mucoproteins of the gingiva. J Dent Res *32*:779, 1953.
37. Folke LEA, Stallard RE. Periodontal microcirculation as revealed by plastic microspheres. J Periodont Res *2*:53, 1967.
38. Forsslund G. Structure and function of capillary system in the gingiva in man. Development of stereophotogrammetric method and its application for study of the subepithelial blood vessels in vivo. Acta Odontol Scand *17*(suppl 26):9, 1959.
39. Frank RM, Cimasoni G. Ultrastructure de l'epithelium cliniquement normal du sillon et de la jonction gingivo-dentaire. Z Zellforsch *109*:356, 1970.
40. Gargiulo AW, Wentz FM, Orban B. Dimensions and relations of the dentogingival junction in humans. J Periodontol *32*:261, 1961.
41. Glickman I, Johannessen L. Biomicroscopic (slitlamp) evaluation of the normal gingiva of the albino rat. J Am Dent Assoc *41*:521, 1950.
42. Gottlieb B, Orban B. Active and passive eruption of the teeth. J Dent Res *13*:214, 1933.
43. Greene AH. A study of the characteristics of stippling and its relation to gingival health. J Periodontol *33*:176, 1962.
44. Hansen ER. Mitotic activity of the gingival epithelium in colchicinized rats. Odont T *74*:229, 1966.
45. Hansson BO, Lindhe J, Branemark PI. Microvascular topography and function in clinically healthy and chronically inflamed dentogingival tissues. A vital microscopic study in dogs. Periodontics *6*:265, 1968.
46. Itoiz ME, Carranza FA Jr, Cabrini RL. Histotopographic distribution of alkaline and acid phosphatase in periodontal tissues of laboratory animals. J Periodontol *35*:470, 1964.
47. Itoiz ME, Carranza FA Jr, Cabrini RL. Histotopographic study of esterase and 5-nucleotidase in periodontal tissues of laboratory animals. J Periodontol *38*:130, 1967.
48. Itoiz ME, Carranza FA Jr, Gimenez I, Cabrini RL. Microspectrophotometric analysis of succinic dehydrogenase and glucose-6-phosphate dehydrogenase in human oral epithelium. J Periodont Res *7*:14, 1972.
49. Itoiz ME, Carranza FA Jr, Neira V, Cabrini RL. Fine structural localization of thiamine pyrophosphatase in normal human gingiva. J Periodontol *45*:579, 1974.
50. Itoiz ME, Lanfranchi HE, Gimenez-Conti IB, Conti CJ. Immunohistochemical demonstration of keratins in oral mucosa lesions. Acta Odont Lat-Am *1*:47, 1984.
51. Itoiz ME, Conti CJ, Lanfranchi HE, et al. Immunohistochemical detection of filaggrin in preneoplastic and neoplastic lesions of the human oral mucosa. J Oral Pathol *15*:205, 1986.
52. Itoiz ME, Conti CJ, Gimenez-Conti IB, et al. Immunodetection of involucrin in lesions of the oral mucosa. J Oral Pathol *15*:205, 1986.
53. Iusem R. A cytological study of the cornification of the oral mucosa in women. Oral Surg *3*:1516, 1950.
54. Karring T, Lang NP, Löe H. The role of gingival connective tissue in determining epithelial differentiation. J Periodont Res *10*:1, 1975.
55. Kobayashi K, Rose GG. Ultrastructural histochemistry of the dentoepithelial junction. II. Colloidal thorium and ruthenium red. J Periodont Res *13*:164, 1978.
56. Kobayashi K, Rose GG. Ultrastructural histochemistry of the dentoepithelial junction. III. Chloramine T-silver methenamine. J Periodont Res *14*:123, 1979.
57. Kronfeld R. Histopathology of the Teeth and Their Surrounding Structures. Philadelphia, Lea & Febiger, 1939.
58. Kurahashi Y, Takuma S. Electron microscopy of human gingival epithelium. Bull Tokyo Dent Col *3*:29, 1962.
59. Lange D, Camelleri GE. Cytochemical demonstration of lysosomes in the exfoliated epithelial cells of the gingival cuff. J Dent Res *46*:625, 1967.
60. Listgarten MA. The ultrastructure of human gingival epithelium. Am J Anat *114*:49, 1964.
61. Listgarten MA. Electron microscopic study of the gingivodental junction of man. Am J Anat *119*:147, 1966.
62. Listgarten MA. Phase contrast and electron microscopic study of the junction between reduced enamel epithelium and enamel in unerupted human teeth. Arch Oral Biol *11*:999, 1966.
63. Listgarten M. Changing concepts about the dentogingival junction. J Can Dent Assoc *36*:70, 1970.
64. Listgarten MA. Structure and surface coatings on teeth. A review. J Periodontol *47*:139, 1976.
65. Löe H, Karring T. Mitotic activity and renewal time of the gingival epithelium of young and old rats. J Periodont Res *4*(suppl):18, 1969.
66. Löe H, Karring T. A quantitative analysis of the epithelium–connective tissue interface in relation to assessments of the mitotic index. J Dent Res *48*:634, 1969.
67. McHugh WD. Keratinization of gingival epithelium in laboratory animals. J Periodontol *35*:338, 1964.
68. McHugh WD, Zander HA. Cell division in the periodontium of developing and erupted teeth. Dent Pract *15*:451, 1965.
69. Meyer J, Marwah AS, Weinmann JP. Mitotic rate of gingival epithelium in two age groups. J Invest Dermatol *27*:237, 1956.
70. Miller SC, Soberman A, Stahl S. A study of the cornification of the oral mucosa of young male adults. J Dent Res *30*:4, 1951.
71. Morgan PR, Leigh IM, Purkis PE, et al. Site variation in keratin expression in human oral epithelia. An immunocytochemical study of individual keratins. Epithelia *1*:31, 1987.
72. Mori M, Kishiro A. Histochemical observation of aminopeptidase activity in the normal and inflamed oral epithelium. J Osaka Univ Dent School *1*:39, 1961.
73. Moss ML. Phylogeny and comparative anatomy of oral ectodermal ectomesenchymal inductive interactions. J Dent Res *48*:732, 1969.

74. Ness KH, Morton TH, Dale BA. Identification of Merker cells in oral epithelium using antikeratin and antineuroendocrine monoclonal antibodies. J Dent Res 66:1154, 1987.
75. Newcomb GM, Powell RN. Human gingival Langerhans cells in health and disease. J Periodont Res 21:640, 1986.
76. Oliver RC, Holm-Pedersen P, Löe H. The correlation between clinical scoring, exudate measurements and microscopic evaluation of inflammation in the gingiva. J Periodontol 40:201, 1969.
77. Orban B, Kohler J. Die physiologische Zahn-fleischtasche, Epithelansatz und Epitheltiefenwucherung. Z Stomatol 22:353, 1924.
78. Page RC, Ammons WF, Schectman LR, Dillingham LA. Collagen fibre bundles of the normal marginal gingiva in the marmoset. Arch Oral Biol 19:1039, 1972.
79. Papic M, Glickman I. Keratinization of the human gingiva in the menstrual cycle and menopause. Oral Surg 3:504, 1950.
80. Person P, Felton J, Fine A. Biochemical and histochemical studies of aerobic oxidative metabolism of oral tissues. III. Specific metabolic activities of enzymatically separated gingival epithelium and connective tissue components. J Dent Res 44:91, 1965.
81. Romanos GE, Bernimoulin J-P. Das Kollagen als Basiselement des Parodonts: Immunohistochemische Aspekte beim Menschen und bei Tieren. Parodontologie 4:363, 1990.
82. Rosenberg H, Massler MJ. Gingival stippling in young adult males. J Periodontol 38:473, 1967.
83. Saglie R, Sabag N, Mery C. Ultrastructure of the normal human epithelial attachment. J Periodontol 50:544, 1979.
84. Sawada T, Yamamoto T, Yanagisawa T, et al. Electron immunochemistry of laminin and type IV collagen in the junctional epithelium of rat molar gingiva. J Periodont Res 25:372, 1990.
85. Sawaf MH, Ouyahoun JP, Forest N. Cytokeratin profiles in oral epithelia: A review and new classification. J Biol Buccale 19:187, 1991.
86. Schroeder HE. Melanin containing organelles in cells of the human gingiva. J Periodont Res 4:1, 1969.
87. Schroeder HE. Differentiation of Human Oral Stratified Epithelia. New York, S Karger, 1981.
88. Schroeder HE. The Periodontium. Berlin, Springer-Verlag, 1986.
89. Schroeder HE, Amstad-Jossi M. Type and variability of the stratum corneum in normal and diseased human oral stratified epithelia. J Biol Buccale 12:101, 1984.
90. Schroeder HE, Listgarten MA. Fine structure of the developing epithelial attachment of human teeth. Monographs in Developmental Biology. Vol. 2. 1971.
91. Schroeder HE, Theilade J. Electron microscopy of normal human gingival epithelium. J Periodont Res 1:95, 1966.
92. Schultz-Haudt SD, From S. Dynamics of periodontal tissues. I. The epithelium. Odont T 69:431, 1961.
93. Schultz-Haudt SD, Paus S, Assev S. Periodic acid–Schiff reactive components of human gingiva. J Dent Res 40:141, 1961.
94. Schweitzer G. Lymph vessels of the gingiva and teeth. Arch Mik Anat Ent 69:807, 1907.
95. Schwint AE, Itoiz ME, Cabrini RL. A quantitative histochemical technique for the study of vascularization using horseradish peroxidase. Histochem J 16:907, 1984.
96. Shapiro S, Ulmansky M, Scheuer M. Mast cell population in gingiva affected by chronic destructive periodontal disease. J Periodontol 40:276, 1969.
97. Shelton L, Hall W. Human gingival mast cells. J Periodont Res 3:214, 1968.
98. Skougaard MR, Beagrie GS. The renewal of gingival epithelium in marmosets (Callithrix jacchus) as determined through autoradiography with thymidine-H3. Acta Ondontol Scand 20:467, 1962.
99. Soni NN, Silberkweit M, Hayes RL. Pattern of mitotic activity and cell densities in human gingival epithelium. J Periodontol 36:15, 1965.
100. Squier CA, Waterhouse LP. The ultrastructure of the melanocyte in human gingival epithelium. J Dent Res 46:112, 1967.
101. Stern IB. Electron microscopic observations of oral epithelium. I. Basal cells and the basement membrane. Periodontics 3:224, 1965.
102. Stern IB. The fine structure of the ameloblast-enamel junction in rat incisors, epithelial attachment and cuticular membrane. In 5th International Congress for Electron Microscopy, Vol 2, 1966, p 6.
103. Stern IB. Further electron microscopic observations of the epithelial attachment. 45th General Meeting of the International Association for Dental Research Abstracts, 1967, p 118.
104. Susi F. Histochemical, autoradiographic and electron microscopic studies of keratinization in oral mucosa. PhD thesis, Tufts University, 1967.
105. Swift JA, Saxton CA. The ultrastructural location of the periodate Schiff reactive basement membrane of the dermoepidermal junctions of human scalp and monkey gingiva. J Ultrastruct Res 17:23, 1967.
106. Thilander H. Permeability of the gingival pocket epithelium. Int Dent J 14:416, 1964.
107. Thilander H, Bloom GD. Cell contacts in oral epithelia. J Periodont Res 3:96, 1968.
108. Thonard JC, Scherp HW. Histochemical demonstration of acid mucopolysaccharides in human gingival epithelial intercellular spaces. Arch Oral Biol 7:125, 1962.
109. Trott JR. An investigation into the glycogen content of the gingivae. Dent Pract 7:234, 1957.
110. Trott JR, Gorenstein SL. Mitotic rates in the oral and gingival epithelium of the rat. Arch Oral Biol 8:425, 1963.
111. Turesky S, Crowley J, Glickman I. A histochemical study of protein-bound sulfhydryl and disulfide groups in normal and inflamed human gingiva. J Dent Res 36:225, 1957.
112. Turesky S, Glickman I, Litwin T. A histochemical evaluation of normal and inflamed human gingivae. J Dent Res 30:792, 1951.
113. Waterhouse JP. The gingival part of the human periodontium. Its ultrastructure and the distribution in it of acid phosphatase in relation to cell attachment and the lysosome concept. Dent Prac 15:409, 1965.
114. Weinmann JP, Meyer J. Types of keratinization in the human gingiva. J Invest Dermatol 32:87, 1959.
115. Weinstock A. Secretory function of postsecretory ameloblasts as shown by electron microscope radioautography. J Dent Res 50:82, 1972.
116. Weinstock A, Albright JT. Electron microscopic observations on specialized structures in the epithelium of the normal human palate. J Dent Res 45(suppl):79, 1966.
117. Weinstock A, Albright JT. The fine structure of mast cells in normal human gingiva. J Ultrastruct Res 17:245, 1967.
118. Weski O. Die chronische marginales Entzündungen des Alveolar-fortsatzes mit besonderer Berücksichtigung der Alveolarpyorrhoe. Vierteljahrsschr Zahnheilk 38:1, 1922.
119. Wilgram GF, Weinstock A. Advances in genetic dermatology: Acantholysis, hyperkeratosis, and dyskeratosis. Arch Dermatol 94:456, 1966.
120. Yamasaki A, Nikai H, Niltani K, Ijuhin N. Ultrastructure of the junctional epithelium of germfree rat gingiva. J Periodontol 50:641, 1979.
121. Zander HA. The distribution of phosphatase in gingival tissue. J Dent Res 20:347, 1941.

2

The Tooth-Supporting Structures

FERMIN A. CARRANZA, JR. and ANGELA M. UBIOS

[handwritten: Gingivitis turns into periodontitis when it involves bone. (bone loss)]

[handwritten: The stronger the fibers, the lower the Roman numeral #.]

[handwritten: Periodontium]

The attachment apparatus of the tooth is composed of the periodontal ligament, the cementum, and the alveolar bone. The structure of these tissues will be considered first, followed by a description of their development, vascularization, innervation, and functions.*

PERIODONTAL LIGAMENT

The periodontal ligament is the connective tissue that surrounds the root and connects it with the bone. It is continuous with the connective tissue of the gingiva and communicates with the marrow spaces through vascular channels in the bone.

Periodontal Fibers

The most important elements of the periodontal ligament are the *principal fibers,* which are collagenous, are arranged in bundles, and follow a wavy course when viewed in longitudinal sections (Fig. 2–1). Terminal portions of the principal fibers that insert into cementum and bone are termed *Sharpey's fibers* (Fig. 2–2). The principal fiber bundles consist of individual fibers that form a continuous anastomosing network between tooth and bone.[8,21]

Collagen is a protein composed of different amino acids, the most important of which are glycine, proline, hydroxylysine, and hydroxyproline.[17] The amount of collagen in a tissue can be determined by its hydroxyproline content.

Collagen biosynthesis occurs inside the fibroblasts to form tropocollagen molecules. These aggregate into microfibrils that are packed together to form fibrils. Collagen fibrils have a transverse striation with a characteristic periodicity of 64 nm; this striation is caused by the overlapping arrangement of the tropocollagen molecules. In collagen types I and III these fibrils associate to form fibers, and in collagen type I the fibers associate to form bundles (Fig. 2–3).[70] *[handwritten: Collagen regenerates fast]*

Collagen is synthesized by fibroblasts, chondroblasts, osteoblasts, odontoblasts, and other cells. There are several types of collagen, all distinguishable by their chemical composition, distribution, function, and morphology.[58] The principal fibers are composed mainly of collagen type I,[91] whereas reticular fibers are collagen type III. Collagen type IV is found in the basal lamina.[89,90]

The molecular configuration of collagen fibers confers to them a tensile strength greater than that of steel. Consequently, collagen imparts a unique combination of flexibility and strength to the tissues where it lies.[58]

The principal fibers of the periodontal ligament are arranged in six groups: transseptal, alveolar crest, horizontal, oblique, apical, and interradicular (Fig. 2–4):

1. *Transseptal Group.* Transseptal fibers extend interproximally over the alveolar crest and are embedded in the cementum of adjacent teeth (Fig. 2–5). They are a remarkably constant finding and are reconstructed even after destruction of the alveolar bone has occurred in periodontal disease.

2. *Alveolar Crest Group.* Alveolar crest fibers extend obliquely from the cementum just beneath the junctional epithelium to the alveolar crest (Fig. 2–6). They prevent the extrusion of the tooth[19] and resist lateral tooth movements. Their incision does not significantly increase tooth mobility.[37]

3. *Horizontal Group.* Horizontal fibers extend at right angles to the long axis of the tooth from the cementum to the alveolar bone.

4. *Oblique Group.* Oblique fibers, the largest group in the periodontal ligament, extend from the cementum in a coronal direction obliquely to the bone (Fig. 2–7). They bear the brunt of vertical masticatory stresses and transform them into tension on the alveolar bone.

---

* For a more complete analysis, the reader is referred to Berkovitz BKB, Moxham BJ, Newman HN, eds. The Periodontal Ligament in Health and Disease. London, Pergamon Press, 1982; and Schroeder HE. The Periodontium. Berlin, Springer-Verlag, 1986.

Perivstat stops collagenase → which is what destroys structures

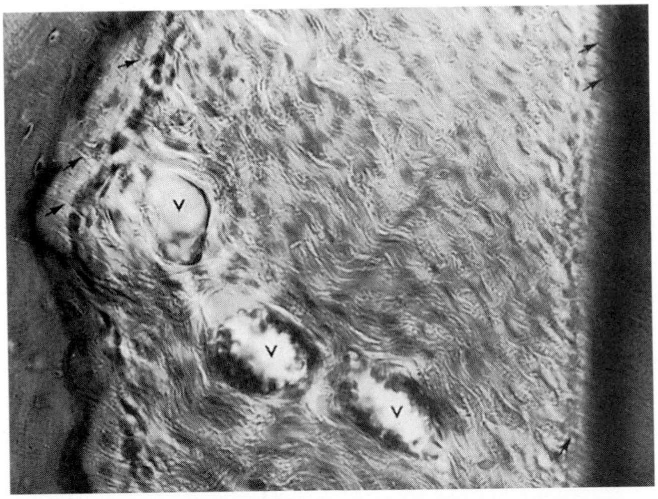

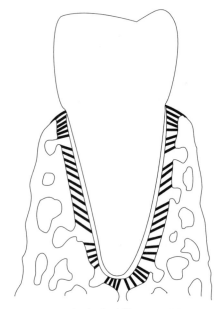

FIGURE 2-1. Principal fibers of the periodontal ligament follow a wavy course when sectioned longitudinally. The formative function of the periodontal ligament is illustrated by the newly formed osteoid and osteoblasts along a previously resorbed bone surface *(left)* and the cementoid and cementoblasts *(right)*. Note the fibers embedded in the forming calcified tissues *(arrows)*. V, Vascular channels.

5. *Apical Group.* The apical fibers radiate from the cementum to the bone at the fundus of the socket. They do not occur on incompletely formed roots.
6. *Interradicular Fibers.* These fibers fan out from the cementum to the tooth in the furcation areas of multirooted teeth.

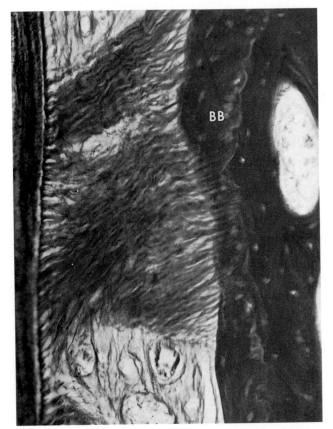

FIGURE 2-2. Collagen fibers embedded in the cementum *(left)* and bone *(right)* (silver stain). Note Sharpey's fibers within the bundle bone (BB) overlying lamellar bone.

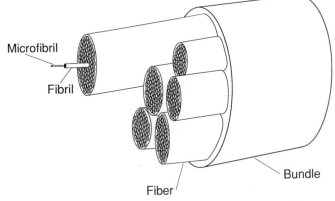

FIGURE 2-3. Collagen microfibrils, fibrils, fibers, and bundles.

Other well-formed fiber bundles interdigitate at right angles or splay around and between regularly arranged fiber bundles. Less regularly arranged collagen fibers are found in the interstitial connective tissue between the principal fiber groups; this tissue contains the blood vessels, lymphatics, and nerves.

Although the periodontal ligament does not contain mature elastin, two immature forms are found: oxytalan and eluanin. The so-called oxytalan fibers[32,41] run parallel to the root surface in a vertical direction and bend to attach to cementum[32] in the cervical third of the root. They are thought to regulate vascular flow.[31] An elastic meshwork has been described in the periodontal ligament[54] as being composed of many elastin lamellae with peripheral oxytalan fibers and eluanin fibers.

The principal fibers are remodeled by the periodontal ligament cells to adapt to physiologic needs[101,116] and in response to different stimuli.[108]

In addition to these fiber types, Shackleford has described small collagen fibers in association with the larger principal collagen fibers. These fibers run in all directions, forming a plexus that has been termed the *indifferent fiber plexus.*[97]

Many different fibers!

FIGURE 2-4. Diagram of principal fiber groups.

Gingivodental group: coronal, horizontal, & apical

32

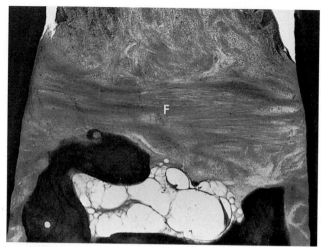

FIGURE 2–5. Transseptal fibers (F) at the crest of the interdental bone.

Cellular Elements

Four types of cells have been identified in the periodontal ligament: connective tissue cells, epithelial rest cells, defense cells, and cells associated with neurovascular elements.[7]

Connective tissue cells include fibroblasts, cementoblasts, and osteoblasts. Fibroblasts are the most common cells in the periodontal ligament and appear as ovoid or elongated cells oriented along the principal fibers and exhibiting pseudopodia-like processes (Fig. 2–8).[87] These cells synthesize collagen and have also been shown to possess the capacity to phagocytose "old" collagen fibers and degrade them[101] by enzyme hydrolysis. Thus, collagen turnover appears to be regulated by fibroblasts.

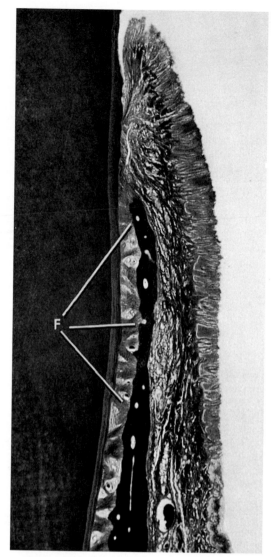

FIGURE 2–7. Principal fiber bundles (F) of the periodontal ligament on the facial surface of a mandibular premolar (silver stain).

Hassell and Stanek[46] have demonstrated that phenotypically distinct and functionally different subpopulations of fibroblasts exist in the adult periodontal ligament, although these subpopulations look identical at both light and electron microscopic levels. Different subpopulations may have different functions, such as secretion of collagen of different types or production of collagenase.

Osteoblasts and cementoblasts, as well as osteoclasts and odontoclasts, are also seen in the cemental and osseous surfaces of the periodontal ligament.

The *epithelial rests of Malassez* form a latticework in the periodontal ligament and appear as either isolated clusters of cells or interlacing strands (Fig. 2–9), depending on the plane in which the microscopic section is cut. Continuity with the junctional epithelium in experimental animals has been suggested.[43] The epithelial rests are considered to be remnants of Hertwig's root sheath, which disintegrates during root development.

Epithelial rests are distributed close to the cementum throughout the periodontal ligament of most teeth and are

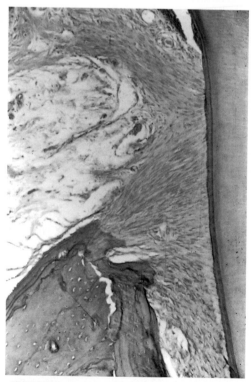

FIGURE 2–6. Alveolar crest fibers in rat molar.

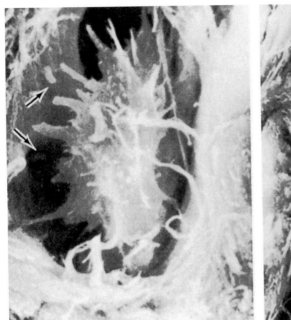
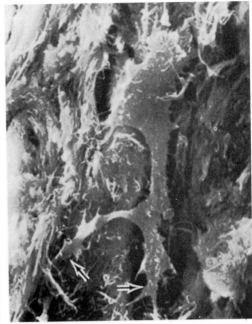

FIGURE 2–8. *Left,* Stellate cell with abundant cellular processes and enclosed in a lacunar structure formed by primary collagen fibers of the periodontal ligament. Broken cell processes *(arrows)* are probably dehydration artifacts. ×8157. *Right,* Large (60-μm-long) fibroblast-like periodontal ligament cell with multiple cellular processes and pseudopodia-like structures *(arrows)*. ×3062. (From Roberts WE, Chamberlain JG. Scanning electron microscope view of the cellular elements of rat periodontal ligament. Arch Oral Biol *23*:587, 1978. © 1978 with kind permission from Elsevier Science Ltd, The Boulevard, Langford Lane, Kidlington OX5 1GB, UK.)

most numerous in the apical areas[83] and cervical areas.[110,111] They diminish in number with age[99] by degenerating and disappearing or by undergoing calcification to become cementicles. They are surrounded by a periodic acid–Schiff (PAS)–positive, argyrophilic, fibrillar, sometimes hyaline capsule, from which they are separated by a distinct basal lamina. Epithelial rests proliferate when stimulated[102,105,107] and participate in the formation of periapical cysts and lateral root cysts.

The *defense cells* include macrophages, mast cells, and eosinophils. These, as well those *cells associated with neurovascular elements*, are similar to those in other connective tissues.

Ground Substance

The periodontal ligament also contains a large proportion of ground substance filling the spaces between fibers and

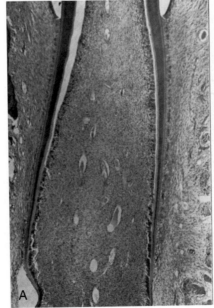
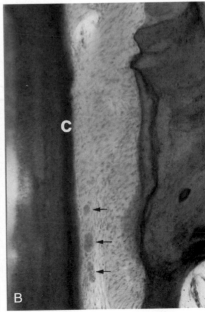

FIGURE 2–9. Epithelial rests of Malassez. *A,* Erupting tooth in a cat. Fragmentation of Hertwig's epithelial root sheath giving rise to epithelial rests located along, and close to, the root surface. *B,* Human periodontal ligament with rosette-shaped epithelial rests *(arrows)* lying close to the cementum (C).

cells. It consists of two main components: *glycosaminogly-cans* such as hyaluronic acid and proteoglycans, and *glyco-proteins* such as fibronectin and laminin. It also has a high water content (70%).

The periodontal ligament may also contain calcified masses called *cementicles,* which are adherent to or detached from the root surfaces (Fig. 2–10). Cementicles may develop from calcified epithelial rests; around small spicules of cementum or alveolar bone traumatically displaced into the periodontal ligament; from calcified Sharpey's fibers; and from calcified, thrombosed vessels within the periodontal ligament.[69]

Functions of the Periodontal Ligament

The functions of the periodontal ligament are physical, formative and remodeling, nutritional, and sensory.

Physical Function

The physical functions of the periodontal ligament entail (1) provision of a soft tissue "casing" to protect the vessels and nerves from injury by mechanical forces, (2) transmission of occlusal forces to the bone, (3) attachment of the teeth to the bone, (4) maintenance of the gingival tissues in their proper relationship to the teeth, and (5) resistance to the impact of occlusal forces (shock absorption).

Resistance to the Impact of Occlusal Forces (Shock Absorption). Three theories relative to the mechanism of tooth support have been considered: the tensional theory, the viscoelastic system theory, and the thixotropic theory.

The *tensional theory* of tooth support ascribes to the principal fibers of the periodontal ligament the major responsibility in supporting the tooth and transmitting forces to the bone. When a force is applied to the crown, the principal fibers first unfold and straighten and then transmit

forces to the alveolar bone, causing an elastic deformation of the bony socket; finally, when the alveolar bone has reached its limit, the load is transmitted to the basal bone. Many investigators find this theory insufficient to explain available experimental evidence.

The *viscoelastic system theory* considers the displacement of the tooth to be largely controlled by fluid movements, with fibers having only a secondary role.[10,16] When forces are transmitted to the tooth, the extracellular fluid passes from the periodontal ligament into the marrow spaces of bone through foramina in the cortical layer. These perforations of the lamina dura link the periodontal ligament with the cancellous portion of the alveolar bone and are more abundant in the cervical third than in the middle and apical thirds (Fig. 2–11).

After the depletion of tissue fluids, the fiber bundles absorb the slack and tighten. This leads to blood vessel stenosis; arterial back-pressure causes ballooning of the vessels and passage of blood ultrafiltrates into the tissues, thereby replenishing the tissue fluids.[10]

The *thixotropic theory*[59] claims that the periodontal ligament has the rheologic behavior of a thixotropic gel (i.e., the property of becoming fluid when shaken or stirred and then becoming semisolid again). The physiologic response of the periodontal ligament may be explained by changes in the viscosity of the biologic system. According to Schroeder,[94] the presence of organized collagen fibers makes this theory untenable.

Transmission of Occlusal Forces to the Bone. The arrangement of the principal fibers is similar to a suspension bridge or a hammock. When an axial force is applied to a tooth, there is a tendency toward displacement of the root into the alveolus. The oblique fibers alter their wavy, untensed pattern, assume their full length, and sustain the major part of the axial force. When a horizontal or tipping force is applied, there are two phases of tooth movement. The first is within the confines of the periodontal ligament, and the second produces a displacement of the facial and lingual bony plates.[26] The tooth rotates about an axis that may change as the force is increased.

The apical portion of the root moves in a direction opposite to the coronal portion. In areas of tension, the principal fiber bundles are taut rather than wavy. In areas of pressure, the fibers are compressed, the tooth is displaced, and

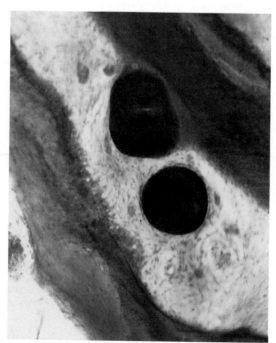
FIGURE 2–10. Cementicles in the periodontal ligament, one lying free and the other adherent to the tooth surface.

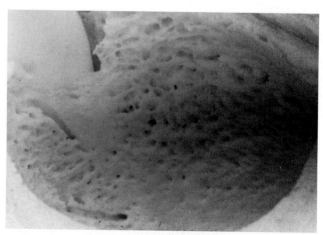
FIGURE 2–11. Foramina perforating the lamina dura (dog jaw).

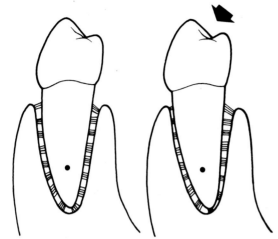

FIGURE 2–12. *Right,* distribution of faciolingual forces *(arrow)* around the axis of rotation *(black circle on root)* in a mandibular premolar. The periodontal ligament fibers are compressed in areas of pressure and tension. *Left,* The same tooth in a resting state.

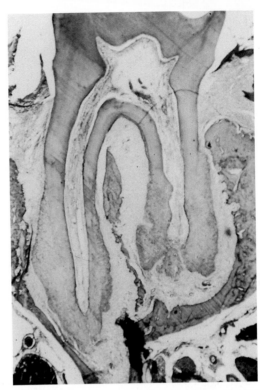

FIGURE 2–13. Microscopic view of rat molar subjected to occluso-horizontal forces. Note the widened and narrowed areas of the periodontal ligament. The axis of rotation is in the interradicular space.

there is a corresponding distortion of bone in the direction of root movement.[80]

In single-rooted teeth, the axis of rotation is located in the area between the apical third and the middle third of the root (Fig. 2–12). The root apex[72] and the coronal half of the clinical root have been suggested as other locations of the axis of rotation. The periodontal ligament, which is shaped like an hourglass, is narrowest in the region of the axis of rotation[24,62] (Table 2–1). In multirooted teeth, the axis of rotation is located in the bone between the roots (Fig. 2–13). In compliance with the physiologic mesial migration of the teeth, the periodontal ligament is thinner on the mesial root surface than on the distal surface (Figs. 2–14 and 2–15).

Formative and Remodeling Function

Cells of the periodontal ligament participate in the formation and resorption of cementum and bone, which occur in physiologic tooth movement; in the accommodation of the periodontium to occlusal forces; and in the repair of injuries. Variations in cellular enzyme activity[34–36] are correlated with the remodeling process.

Cartilage formation in the periodontal ligament, although unusual, may represent a metaplastic phenomenon in the repair of this ligament after injury[4] or result from some toxins such as uranium.

The periodontal ligament is constantly undergoing remodeling. Old cells and fibers are broken down and replaced by new ones, and mitotic activity can be observed in the fibroblasts and endothelial cells.[71] Fibroblasts form the collagen fibers and may also develop into osteoblasts and cementoblasts. Therefore, the rate of formation and the differentiation of fibroblasts affect the rate of formation of collagen, cementum, and bone.

Radioautographic studies with radioactive thymidine, proline, and glycine indicate a very high turnover rate of collagen in the periodontal ligament. The rate of collagen

Table 2–1. THICKNESS OF PERIODONTAL LIGAMENT OF 172 TEETH FROM 15 HUMAN JAWS

	Average of Alveolar Crest (mm)	Average of Mid-root (mm)	Average of Apex (mm)	Average of Tooth (mm)
Ages 11–16 83 teeth from 4 jaws	0.23	0.17	0.24	0.21
Ages 32–50 36 teeth from 5 jaws	0.20	0.14	0.19	0.18
Ages 51–67 35 teeth from 5 jaws	0.17	0.12	0.16	0.15
Age 24 (1 case) 18 teeth from 1 jaw	0.16	0.09	0.15	0.13

From Coolidge ED. The thickness of the human periodontal membrane. J Am Dent Assoc *24*:1260, 1937. Reprinted by permission of ADA Publishing Co., Inc.

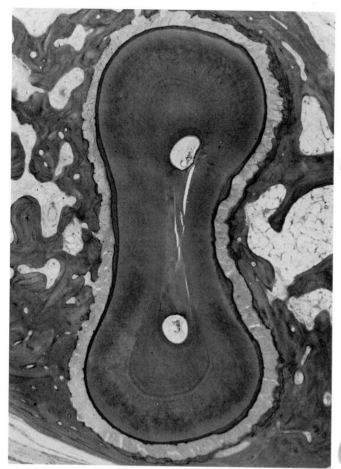

FIGURE 2–14. Physiologic mesial migration. Horizontal section through the molar root. The periodontal ligament is thinner on the side toward which the tooth is migrating (mesial surface, *left*) than on the distal surface *(right)*. The distal fibers are taut.

synthesis, as established in the rat molar, is twice as fast as that in the gingiva and four times as fast as that in the skin.[100] There is also a rapid turnover of sulfated glycosaminoglycans in the cells and amorphous ground substance of the periodontal ligament.[5]

It should be noted that most of these studies have been performed in rodents, and information on primates and humans is scarce.[94]

Nutritional and Sensory Functions

The periodontal ligament supplies nutrients to the cementum, bone, and gingiva by way of the blood vessels and provides lymphatic drainage (see later discussion).

The periodontal ligament is abundantly supplied with sensory nerve fibers capable of transmitting tactile, pressure, and pain sensations by the trigeminal pathways.[3,9] Nerve bundles pass into the periodontal ligament from the periapical area and through channels from the alveolar bone that follow the course of the blood vessels. They divide into single myelinized fibers, which ultimately lose their myelin sheaths and end in one of four types of neural termination: free endings, which have a tree-like configuration; Ruffini-like corpuscles, located primarily in the apical area; coiled forms, found mainly in the midroot region; and spindle-like endings, which are surrounded by a fibrous capsule and located mainly in the apex.[31,66]

CEMENTUM

Types of Cementum

Cementum is the calcified mesenchymal tissue that forms the outer covering of the anatomic root. There are two

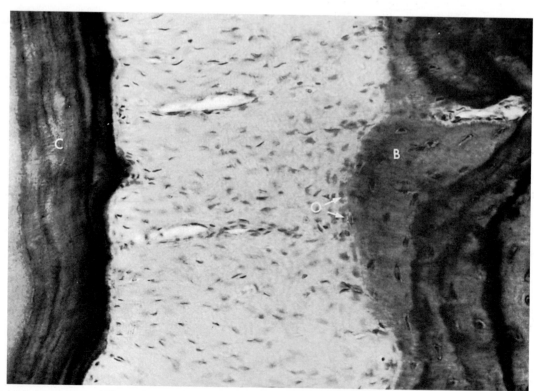

FIGURE 2–15. High-power view of Figure 2–14. Distal surface, showing cementum (C), periodontal ligament, and bone. The tooth is migrating mesially (toward the left). Note the osteoblasts (O) and new bone formation (B) *(right)*.

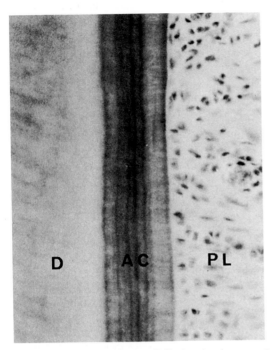

FIGURE 2–16. Acellular cementum (AC) showing incremental lines running parallel to the long axis of the tooth. These lines represent the appositional growth of cementum. Note the thin, light lines running into the cementum perpendicular to the surface; these represent Sharpey's fibers of the periodontal ligament (PL). D, Dentin. ×300.

main types of root cementum: acellular (primary) and cellular (secondary).[42] Both consist of a calcified interfibrillar matrix and collagen fibrils.

There are two sources of collagen fibers in cementum: Sharpey's (extrinsic) fibers, which are the embedded portion of the principal fibers of the periodontal ligament[88] and are formed by the fibroblasts; and fibers that belong to the cementum matrix per se (intrinsic) and are produced by the cementoblasts.[95] Cementoblasts also form the noncollagenous components of the interfibrillar ground substance, such as proteoglycans, glycoproteins, and phosphoproteins. *Acellular cementum* is the first to be formed and covers approximately the cervical third or half of the root; it does not contain cells (Fig. 2–16). This cementum is formed before the tooth reaches the occlusal plane, and its thickness ranges from 30 to 230 μm.[94] Sharpey's fibers make up most of the structure of acellular cementum, which has a principal role in supporting the tooth. Most of the fibers are inserted at approximately right angles into the root surface and penetrate deep into the cementum, but others enter from several different directions. Their size, number, and distribution increase with function.[52] Sharpey's fibers are completely calcified, with the mineral crystals oriented parallel to the fibrils, as they are in dentin and bone, except in a 10- to 50-μm-wide zone near the cementodentinal junction, where they are only partially calcified. The peripheral portions of Sharpey's fibers in actively mineralizing cementum tend to be more calcified than the interior regions, according to evidence obtained by scanning electron microscopy.[56] Acellular cementum also contains other collagen fibrils that are calcified and irregularly arranged or parallel to the surface.[96]

Cellular cementum, formed after the tooth reaches the occlusal plane, is more irregular and contains cells (cementocytes) in individual spaces (lacunae) that communicate with each other through a system of anastomosing canaliculi (Fig. 2–17). Cellular cementum is less calcified than the acellular type.[53] Sharpey's fibers occupy a smaller portion of cellular cementum and are separated by other fibers that are arranged either parallel to the root surface or at random. Sharpey's fibers may be completely calcified or partially calcified or have a central, uncalcified core surrounded by a calcified border.[56,95]

Both acellular and cellular cementum are arranged in lamellae separated by incremental lines parallel to the long axis of the root (see Figs. 2–16 and 2–17). These lines represent rest periods in cementum formation and are more mineralized than the adjacent cementum.[91] In addition, loss of the cervical part of the reduced enamel epithelium at the time of tooth eruption may place portions of mature enamel in contact with the connective tissue, which will then deposit over it an acellular afibrillar type of cementum.[64]

Based on these findings, Schroeder[94] has classified cementum as follows:

Acellular afibrillar cementum (AAC) contains neither cells nor extrinsic or intrinsic collagen fibers, apart from a mineralized ground substance. It is a product of cementoblasts and in humans is found in coronal cementum.

Acellular extrinsic fiber cementum (AEFC) is composed almost entirely of densely packed bundles of Sharpey's fibers and lacks cells. It is a product of fibroblasts and cementoblasts and in humans is found in the cervical third of roots but may extend further apically.

Cellular mixed stratified cementum (CMSC) is composed of extrinsic (Sharpey's) and intrinsic fibers and contains

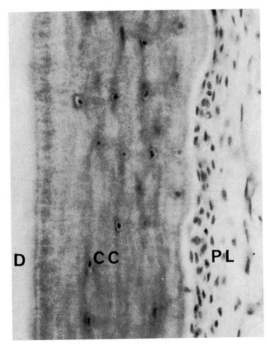

FIGURE 2–17. Cellular cementum (CC) showing cementocytes lying within lacunae. Cellular cementum is thicker than acellular cementum (cf. Fig. 2–16). There is also evidence of incremental lines, but they are less distinct than in acellular cementum. The cells adjacent to the surface of the cementum in the periodontal ligament (PL) space are cementoblasts. D, Dentin. ×300.

cells. It is a coproduct of fibroblasts and cementoblasts, and in humans it appears primarily in the apical third of the roots and the apices and in furcation areas.

Cellular intrinsic fiber cementum (CIFC) contains cells but no collagen fibers. It is formed by cementoblasts, and in humans it fills resorption lacunae.

Intermediate cementum is an ill-defined zone near the cemento-dentinal junction of certain teeth that appears to contain cellular remnants of Hertwig's sheath embedded in calcified ground substance.[28,63]

The inorganic content of cementum (hydroxyapatite; $Ca_{10}[PO_4]_6[OH]_2$) is 45% to 50%, which is less than that of bone (65%), enamel (97%), or dentin (70%).[118] Opinions differ about whether the microhardness increases[73] or decreases with age,[113] and no relationship has been established between aging and the mineral content of cementum.

Permeability of Cementum

In very young animals, both cellular and acellular cementum are very permeable and permit the diffusion of dyes from the pulp and from the external root surface. In cellular cementum, the canaliculi in some areas are contiguous with the dentinal tubuli. With age, the permeability of cementum diminishes.[13]

Cemento-enamel Junction

The cementum at and immediately subjacent to the cemento-enamel junction is of particular clinical importance in root scaling procedures.[84] Three types of relationships involving the cementum may exist at the cemento-enamel junction.[39,74] In about 60% to 65% of cases cementum overlaps the enamel (Fig. 2–18); in about 30% there is an edge-to-edge butt joint; and in 5% to 10% the cementum and enamel fail to meet. In the last instance, gingival recession may be accompanied by an accentuated sensitivity because the dentin is exposed.

Thickness of Cementum

Cementum deposition is a continuous process that proceeds at varying rates throughout life. Cementum formation is most rapid in the apical regions, where it compensates

for tooth eruption, which itself compensates for attrition. The thickness of cementum on the coronal half of the root varies from 16 to 60 μm, or about the thickness of a hair. It attains its greatest thickness (up to 150 to 200 μm) in the apical third and in the bifurcation and trifurcation areas[76]; it is thicker in distal surfaces than in mesial surfaces, probably because of functional stimulation from mesial drift over time.[25] Between the ages of 11 and 70, the average thickness of the cementum increases threefold, with the greatest increase in the apical region. Average thicknesses of 95 μm at age 20 and 215 μm at age 60 have been reported.[117]

The term *hypercementosis* (cementum hyperplasia) refers to a prominent thickening of the cementum. It may be localized to one tooth or affect the entire dentition. Because of considerable physiologic variation in the thickness of cementum among different teeth in the same person and also among different persons, it is sometimes difficult to distinguish between hypercementosis and physiologic thickening of cementum.

Hypercementosis occurs as a generalized thickening of the cementum, with nodular enlargement of the apical third of the root. It also appears in the form of spike-like excrescences (cemental spikes) created by either the coalescence of cementicles that adhere to the root or the calcification of periodontal fibers at the sites of insertion into the cementum.[63]

The etiology of hypercementosis varies and is not completely understood. The spike-like type of hypercementosis generally results from excessive tension from orthodontic appliances or from occlusal forces. The generalized type occurs in a variety of circumstances. In teeth without antagonists, hypercementosis is interpreted as an effort to keep pace with excessive tooth eruption. In teeth subject to low-grade periapical irritation arising from pulp disease, it is considered to be compensation for the destroyed fibrous attachment to the tooth. The cementum is deposited adjacent to the inflamed periapical tissue. Hypercementosis of the entire dentition may occur in patients with Paget's disease.[93]

Cementum Resorption and Repair

The cementum of erupted as well as unerupted teeth is subject to resorption. The resorptive changes may be of microscopic proportion or sufficiently extensive to present a radiographically detectable alteration in the root contour. Cementum resorption is extremely common. In one microscopic study, it occurred in 236 of 261 teeth (90.5%).[49] The average number of resorption areas per tooth was 3.5. Of the 922 areas of resorption, 708 (76.8%) were located in the apical third of the root, 177 (19.2%) in the middle third, and 37 (4.0%) in the gingival third. Seventy percent of all resorption areas were confined to the cementum without involving the dentin.

Cementum resorption may be due to local or systemic causes or may occur without apparent etiology (i.e., idiopathic). Among the local conditions in which it occurs are trauma from occlusion[77] (Fig. 2–19); orthodontic movement[48,60,75,92]; pressure from malaligned erupting teeth, cysts, and tumors[61]; teeth without functional antagonists; embedded teeth; replanted and transplanted teeth[1,55]; periapical disease; and periodontal disease. Among the sys-

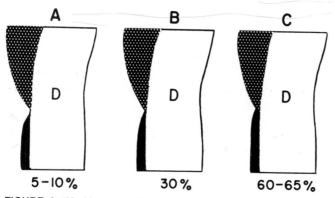

FIGURE 2–18. Normal variations in tooth morphology at the cemento-enamel junction. *A*, Space between enamel and cementum with dentin (D) exposed. *B*, End-to-end relationship of enamel and cementum. *C*, Cementum overlapping the enamel.

5–10%   30%   60–65%

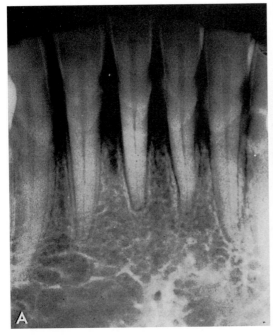

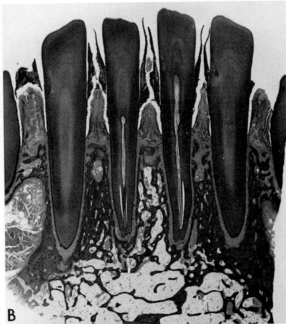

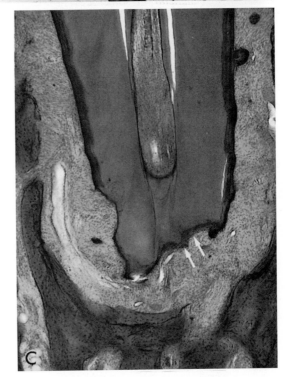

In organic portion of cementum & bone, 90% is PROTEIN.

In ligaments (gingival & perio), 70-80% is protein.

FIGURE 2–19. Cemental resorption associated with excessive occlusal forces. *A,* Radiograph of mandibular anterior teeth. Note the thickening of the periodontal ligament space and lamina dura, with blunting of the apices of the central incisors. *B,* Low-power histologic section of the mandibular anterior teeth. *C,* Higher power micrograph of the left central incisor shortened by resorption of cementum and dentin. Note partial repair of the eroded areas *(arrows)* and cementicle at upper right.

temic conditions mentioned as predisposing to or inducing cemental resorption are calcium deficiency,[57] hypothyroidism,[6] hereditary fibrous osteodystrophy,[106] and Paget's disease.[93]

⊗ Boards ↑

Cementum resorption appears microscopically as bay-like concavities in the root surface (Fig. 2–20). Multinucleated giant cells and large mononuclear macrophages are generally found adjacent to cementum undergoing active resorption (Fig. 2–21). Several sites of resorption may coalesce to

form a large area of destruction. The resorptive process may extend into the underlying dentin and even into the pulp, but it is usually painless.

Cementum resorption is not necessarily continuous and may alternate with periods of repair and the deposition of new cementum. The newly formed cementum is demarcated from the root by a deeply staining irregular line, termed a *reversal line,* which delineates the border of the previous resorption (Fig. 2–22). Embedded fibers of the periodontal ligament re-establish a functional relationship in the new cementum. Cementum repair requires the presence of viable connective tissue. If epithelium

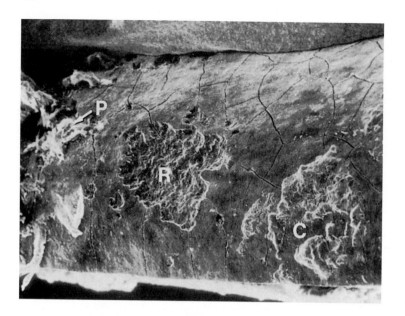

FIGURE 2–20. Scanning electron micrograph of root exposed by periodontal disease showing large resorption bay (R). Remnants of the periodontal ligament (P) and calculus (C) are visible. Cracking of the tooth surface occurs as a result of the preparation technique. × 160. (Courtesy of Dr. John Sottosanti.)

proliferates into an area of resorption, repair will not take place. Cementum repair can occur in devitalized as well as in vital teeth.

Ankylosis. Fusion of the cementum and alveolar bone with obliteration of the periodontal ligament is termed *ankylosis*. Ankylosis occurs in teeth with cemental resorption, which suggests that it may represent a form of abnormal repair. Ankylosis may also develop after chronic peri-

apical inflammation, tooth replantation, and occlusal trauma and around embedded teeth.

Ankylosis results in resorption of the root and its gradual replacement by bone tissue. For this reason, reimplanted teeth that ankylose will lose their roots after a period of 4 to 5 years and exfoliate.

When titanium implants are placed in the jaw, healing results in bone formed in direct apposition to the implant without any intervening connective tissue. This may be interpreted as a form of ankylosis. Because resorption of the metallic implant cannot occur, the implant remains indefi-

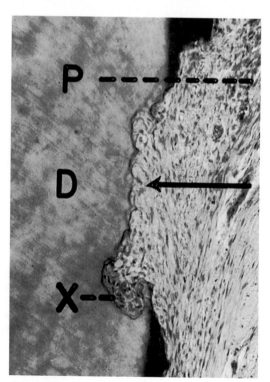

FIGURE 2–21. Resorption of cementum and dentin. A multinuclear osteoclast is seen at X. The direction of resorption is indicated by the arrow. Note the scalloped resorption front in the dentin (D). The cementum is the darkly stained band at upper and lower right. P, Periodontal ligament.

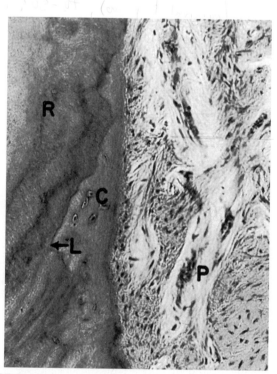

FIGURE 2–22. Section showing repair of previously resorbed root. The defect is filled in with cellular cementum (C), which is separated from the older cementum (R) by an irregular line (L) that indicates the pre-existent outline of the resorbed root. P, Periodontal ligament.

nitely "ankylosed" to the bone. Also, because apical proliferation of the epithelium along the root, a key element of pocket formation, is not possible owing to the ankylosis, a true periodontal pocket will not form.

ALVEOLAR PROCESS

The *alveolar process* is the portion of the maxilla and mandible that forms and supports the tooth sockets (alveoli). It forms when the tooth erupts to provide the osseous attachment to the forming periodontal ligament; it disappears gradually after the tooth is lost.

The alveolar process consists of (1) an external plate of cortical bone formed by haversian bone and compacted bone lamellae; (2) the inner socket wall of thin, compact bone called the *alveolar bone proper* (also known as the *cribriform plate* or *lamina dura*) and also formed by bundle bone; and (3) cancellous trabeculae, between these two compact layers, which act as supporting alveolar bone. The *interdental septum* consists of cancellous supporting bone enclosed within a compact border (Fig. 2–23).

The alveolar process is divisible into separate areas on an anatomic basis, but it functions as a unit, with all parts interrelated in the support of the teeth. Occlusal forces that are transmitted from the periodontal ligament to the inner wall of the alveolus are supported by the cancellous trabeculae, which in turn are buttressed by the labial and lingual cortical plates.

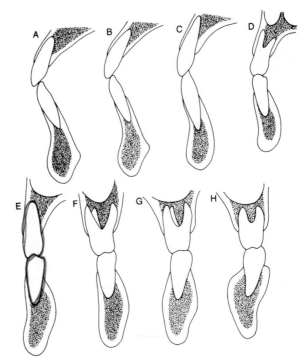

FIGURE 2–24. Relative proportions of cancellous bone and compact bone in a longitudinal faciolingual section of central incisors *(A)*, lateral incisors *(B)*, canines *(C)*, first premolars *(D)*, second premolars *(E)*, first molars *(F)*, second molars *(G)*, and third molars *(H)*.

Figures 2–24 and 2–25 show the relative proportions of cancellous bone and compact bone that form the alveolar process. Most of the facial and lingual portions of the sockets are formed by compact bone alone; cancellous bone surrounds the lamina dura in apical, apicolingual, and interradicular areas.

Cells and Intercellular Matrix

Alveolar bone is formed during fetal growth by intramembranous ossification and consists of a calcified matrix with osteocytes enclosed within spaces called *lacunae*. The osteocytes extend processes into canaliculi that radiate from the lacunae. The canaliculi form an anastomosing sys-

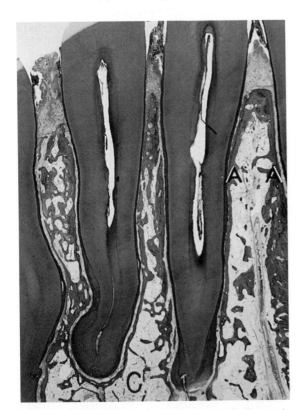

FIGURE 2–23. Mesiodistal section through mandibular canine and premolars showing interdental bony septa. The dense bony plates (A) represent the alveolar bone proper (cribriform plates) and are supported by cancellous bony trabeculae (C). Note the vertical blood vessels within a nutrient canal in the interdental septum at the right.

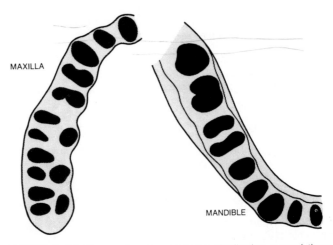

FIGURE 2–25. Shape of roots and bone distribution around them in a transverse section of maxilla and mandible at mid-root level.

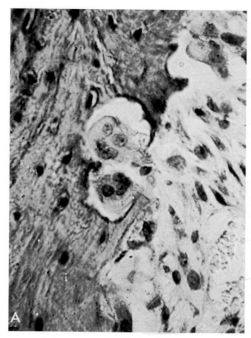
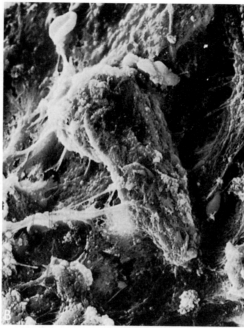

FIGURE 2-26. Rat alveolar bone. *A*, Histologic view of two multinucleated osteoclasts in a Howship lacuna. *B*, Scanning electron microscopic view of osteoclast on bone surface.

tem through the intercellular matrix of the bone, which brings oxygen and nutrients to the osteocytes via the blood and removes metabolic waste products. Blood vessels branch extensively and travel through the periosteum. The endosteum lies adjacent to the marrow vasculature. Bone growth occurs by apposition of an organic matrix that is deposited by osteoblasts.

Bone consists of two thirds inorganic matter and one third organic matrix. The inorganic matter is composed principally of the minerals calcium and phosphate, along with hydroxyl, carbonates, citrate, and trace amounts of other ions,[40] such as sodium, magnesium, and fluorine. The mineral salts are in the form of hydroxyapatite crystals of ultramicroscopic size and constitute approximately 65% to 70% of the bone structure.

The organic matrix[27] consists mainly (90%) of collagen type I,[70] with small amounts of noncollagenous proteins, such as osteocalcin, osteonectin, bone morphogenetic protein, phosphoproteins, and proteoglycans.[82] The apatite crystals are generally aligned with their long axes parallel to the long axes of collagen fibers and appear to be deposited on and within the collagen fibers. In this fashion, bone matrix is able to withstand the heavy mechanical stresses applied to it during function.

Although the alveolar bone tissue is constantly changing in its internal organization, it retains approximately the same form from childhood through adult life. Bone deposition by osteoblasts is balanced by resorption by osteoclasts during tissue remodeling and renewal.

The bone matrix that is laid down by osteoblasts is not mineralized and is referred to as *osteoid*. While new osteoid is being deposited, the older osteoid located below the surface becomes mineralized as the mineralization front advances.

Bone resorption is a complex process morphologically related to the appearance of eroded bone surfaces (Howship's lacunae) and large, multinucleated cells (osteoclasts) (Fig. 2-26). When osteoclasts are active, as opposed to resting, they possess an elaborately developed ruffled bor-

der from which hydrolytic enzymes are believed to be secreted.[109] These enzymes digest the organic portion of bone. The activity of osteoclasts and the morphology of the ruffled border can be modified and regulated by hormones such as parathormone and calcitonin. Osteoclasts originate

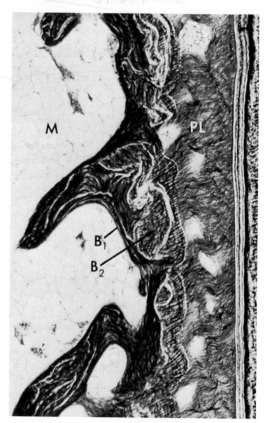

FIGURE 2-27. Deep penetration of Sharpey's fibers into bundle bone. The darkly stained bone (B$_1$) is lamellar bone. Bundle bone (B$_2$) takes up less stain and shows numerous white lines running more or less parallel to each other; these lines correspond to Sharpey's fibers. M, Fatty marrow; PL, periodontal ligament.

from hematopoietic tissue[20,45,67] and are formed by the fusion of mononuclear cells of asynchronous populations.[79,108] Small mononucleated cells have also been described as bone-resorbing cells.[112]

Another mechanism of bone resorption that has been described consists of the creation of an acidic environment on the bone surface, leading to the dissolution of the mineral component of bone. This event can be produced by different conditions, among them a proton pump through the cell membrane of the osteoclast,[12] bone tumors, or local pressure.[65]

Socket Wall

thicker
You find it where there is tension

The socket wall consists of dense, lamellated bone, some of which is arranged in haversian systems, and bundle bone. *Bundle bone* is the term given to bone adjacent to the periodontal ligament that contains a great number of Sharpey's fibers (Fig. 2–27).[114] It is characterized by thin lamellae arranged in layers parallel to the root, with intervening appositional lines (Fig. 2–28). Some Sharpey's

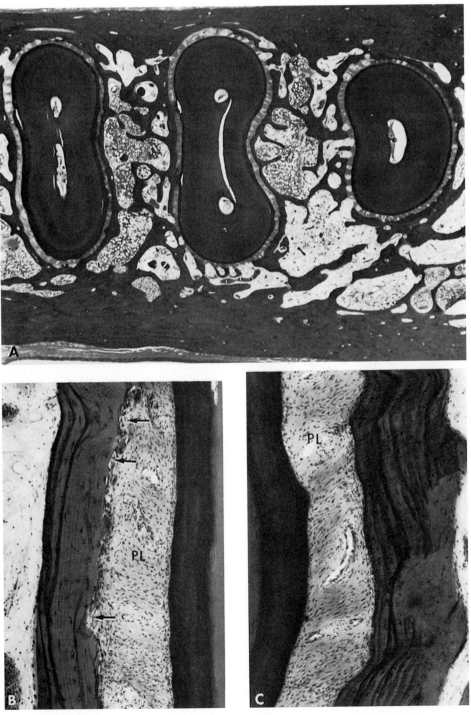

FIGURE 2–28. Bundle bone associated with physiologic mesial migration of the teeth. *A,* Horizontal section through molar roots in the process of mesial migration *(left,* mesial; *right,* distal). *B,* Mesial root surface showing osteoclasis of bone *(arrows). C,* Distal root surface showing bundle bone that has been partially replaced with dense bone on the marrow side. PL, Periodontal ligament.

fibers are completely calcified, but most contain an uncalcified central core within a calcified outer layer.[95] Bundle bone is not unique to the jaws; it occurs throughout the skeletal system wherever ligaments and muscles are attached.

The cancellous portion of the alveolar bone consists of trabeculae that enclose irregularly shaped marrow spaces lined with a layer of thin, flattened endosteal cells. There is wide variation in the trabecular pattern of cancellous bone,[78] which is affected by occlusal forces. The matrix of the cancellous trabeculae consists of irregularly arranged lamellae separated by deeply staining incremental and resorption lines indicative of previous bone activity, with an occasional haversian system.

Cancellous bone is found predominantly in the interradicular and interdental spaces and in limited amounts facially or lingually, except in the palate. In the adult human there is more cancellous bone in the maxilla than in the mandible.[94]

Bone Marrow

In the embryo and newborn, the cavities of all bones are occupied by red hematopoietic marrow. The red marrow gradually undergoes a physiologic change to the fatty or yellow inactive type of marrow. In the adult, the marrow of the jaw is normally of the latter type, and red marrow is found only in the ribs, sternum, vertebrae, skull, and humerus. However, foci of red bone marrow are occasionally seen in the jaws, often accompanied by resorption of bony trabeculae.[14] Common locations are the maxillary tuberosity (Fig. 2–29) and the maxillary and mandibular molar and premolar areas, which may be visible radiographically as zones of radiolucency.

Periosteum and Endosteum

All bone surfaces are covered by layers of differentiated osteogenic connective tissue. The tissue covering the outer surface of bone is termed *periosteum*, whereas the tissue lining the internal bone cavities is called *endosteum*.

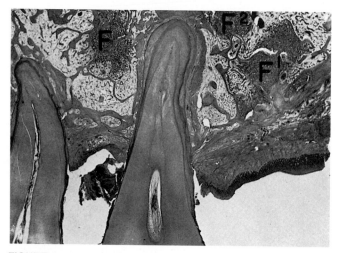

FIGURE 2–29. Mesiodistal section in the molar area of the maxilla of a 59-year-old male, showing foci of hematopoiesis in the marrow (F, F[1], F[2]).

The periosteum consists of an inner layer composed of cells that have the potential to differentiate into osteoblasts and an outer layer that is rich in blood vessels and nerves and is composed of collagen fibers and fibroblasts. Bundles of periosteal collagen fibers penetrate the bone, binding the periosteum to the bone. The endosteum is composed of a single layer of osteoprogenitor cells and a small amount of connective tissue.

Interdental Septum

The interdental septum consists of cancellous bone bordered by the socket walls of approximating teeth and the facial and lingual cortical plates (Fig. 2–30). If the interdental space is narrow, the septum may consist of only lamina dura. For example, the space between mandibular second premolars and first molars consists of lamina dura and cancellous bone in 85% of the cases and of only lamina dura in the remaining 15%.[47] If roots are too close together, an irregular "window" can appear in the bone between adjacent roots (Fig. 2–31). Between maxillary molars, the septum consists of lamina dura and cancellous bone in 66.6% of cases, is composed of only lamina dura in 20.8% of cases, and has a fenestration in 12.5% of cases.[47] Determining root proximity radiographically is important (see Chapter 29). The mesiodistal angulation of the crest of the interdental septum usually parallels a line drawn between the cemento-enamel junctions of the approximating teeth.[86] The distance between the crest of the alveolar bone and the cemento-enamel junction in young adults varies between 0.75 and 1.49 mm (average, 1.08 mm).[33] This distance increases with age to an average of 2.81 mm.[33] However, this phenomenon may not be as much a function of age as of periodontal disease.

The mesiodistal and faciolingual dimensions and shape of the interdental septum are governed by the size and convexity of the crowns of the two approximating teeth, as well as by the position of the teeth in the jaw and their degree of eruption.[86]

Osseous Topography

The bone contour normally conforms to the prominence of the roots, with intervening vertical depressions that taper toward the margin (Fig. 2–32). Alveolar bone anatomy varies from patient to patient and has important clinical implications. The height and thickness of the facial and lingual bony plates are affected by the alignment of the teeth, by the angulation of the root to the bone, and by occlusal forces.

On teeth in labial version, the margin of the labial bone is located farther apically than on teeth in proper alignment. The bone margin is thinned to a knife edge and presents an accentuated arc in the direction of the apex. On teeth in lingual version, the facial bony plate is thicker than normal. The margin is blunt and rounded and horizontal rather than arcuate. The effect of the root-to-bone angulation on the height of alveolar bone is most noticeable on the palatal roots of maxillary molars. The bone margin is located farther apically on the roots, which form relatively acute angles with the palatal bone.[51] The cervical portion of the alveolar plate is sometimes considerably thickened on

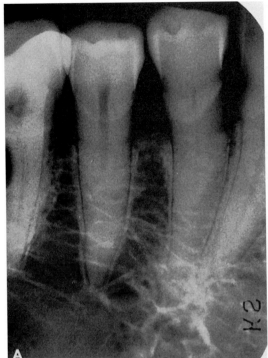
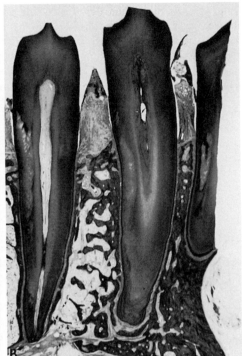
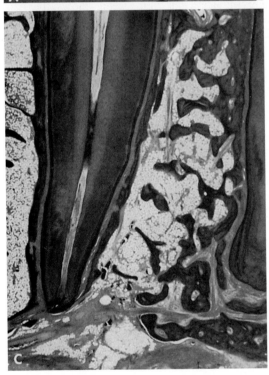

FIGURE 2–30. Interdental septa. *A,* Mandibular premolar area. Note the prominent lamina dura. *B,* Interdental septa between the canine *(right)* and premolars. The central cancellous portion is bordered by the dense bony cribriform plates of the socket. (This forms the lamina dura around the teeth in the radiograph.) *C,* Interdental septum between the premolars, showing central cancellous bone and dense cribriform plate around the roots.

the facial surface, apparently as reinforcement against occlusal forces (Fig. 2–33).

Fenestrations and Dehiscences

Isolated areas in which the root is denuded of bone and the root surface is covered only by periosteum and overlying gingiva are termed *fenestrations.* In these instances the marginal bone is intact. When the denuded areas extend through the marginal bone, the defect is called a *dehiscence*

(Fig. 2–34). Such defects occur on approximately 20% of the teeth; they occur more often on the facial bone than on the lingual, are more common on anterior teeth than on posterior teeth, and are frequently bilateral. There is microscopic evidence of lacunar resorption at the margins. The cause of these defects is not clear. Prominent root contours, malposition, and labial protrusion of the root combined with a thin bony plate are predisposing factors.[29] Fenestration and dehiscence are important, because they may complicate the outcome of periodontal surgery.

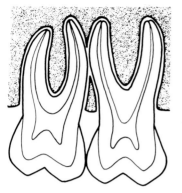
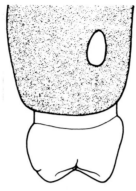

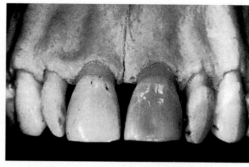

FIGURE 2–32. Normal bone contour conforms to the prominence of the roots.

FIGURE 2–31. Boneless "window" between adjoining close roots of molars.

Remodeling of Alveolar Bone

In contrast to its apparent rigidity, alveolar bone is the least stable of the periodontal tissues, because its structure is in a constant state of flux. A considerable amount of internal remodeling takes place by means of resorption and formation, which are regulated by local and systemic influences. Local influences include functional requirements on the tooth as well as age-related changes in bone cells. Systemic influences are probably hormonal (parathyroid hormone, calcitonin, and others).

Remodeling of alveolar bone affects its height, contour, and density and is manifested in three areas: adjacent to the periodontal ligament, in relation to the periosteum of the facial and lingual plates, and along the endosteal surface of the marrow spaces.

DEVELOPMENT OF THE ATTACHMENT APPARATUS

After the crown has formed, the stratum intermedium and the stellate reticulum of the enamel organ disappear. The outer and the inner epithelia of the enamel organ remain and form the so-called reduced enamel epithelium. The apical portion of this constitutes Hertwig's epithelial root sheath, which will continue to grow apically and determines the shape of the root. Prior to the beginning of root formation, the root sheath bends horizontally at the future cemento-enamel junction, narrowing the cervical opening and forming what is known as the *epithelial diaphragm.* After dentin formation starts, Hertwig's root sheath breaks up and partially disappears; the remaining cells form the epithelial clusters or strands known as epithelial rests of Malassez (see Fig. 2–9A). In multirooted teeth, the epithelial diaphragm grows in such a way that tongue-like extensions develop horizontally, leaving spaces for each of the future roots to form.

The rupture of Hertwig's root sheath allows the mesenchymal cells of the dental follicle to contact the dentin, where they start forming a continuous layer of cementoblasts that begin depositing a meshwork of irregularly arranged collagen fibrils sparsely distributed in an irregularly arranged ground substance or matrix called *precementum* or *cementoid.* This is followed by a phase of matrix maturation, which subsequently mineralizes to form cementum. Cementoblasts, initially separated from the cementum by uncalcified cementoid, sometimes become enclosed within the matrix and become trapped. Once enclosed, they are referred to as *cementocytes,* and they remain viable in a fashion similar to osteocytes.

The enamel organ—including, as it develops, the epithelial root sheath—is surrounded by a layer of connective tissue known as the *dental sac.* The zone immediately in contact with the dental organ and continuous with the ectomesenchyme of the dental papilla is called the *dental follicle*[102–104] and consists of undifferentiated fibroblasts. As the crown approaches the oral mucosa during tooth eruption, these fibroblasts become active and start producing

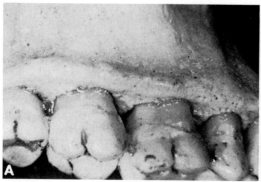
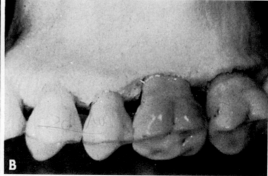

FIGURE 2–33. Variation in the cervical portion of the buccal alveolar plate. *A,* Shelf-like conformation. *B,* Comparatively thin buccal plate.

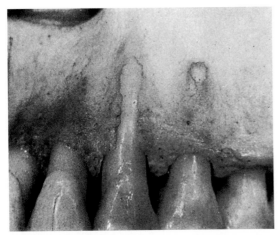

FIGURE 2–34. Dehiscence on the canine and fenestration of the first premolar.

collagen fibrils. These initially lack orientation, but they soon acquire an orientation oblique to the tooth. The first collagen bundles then appear in the region immediately apical to the cemento-enamel junction and give rise to the gingivodental fiber groups. As tooth eruption progresses, additional oblique fibers appear and become attached to the newly formed cementum and bone. The transseptal and alveolar crest fibers develop when the tooth merges into the oral cavity. Alveolar bone deposition occurs simultaneously with periodontal ligament organization.[103]

Studies on the squirrel monkey[44] have shown that during eruption, cemental fibers appear first, followed by Sharpey's fibers emerging from bone. Sharpey's fibers are fewer in number and are more widely spaced than those emerging from the cementum. At a later stage, alveolar fibers extend into the middle zone to join the lengthening cemental fibers and attain their classic orientation, thickness, and strength when occlusal function is established.

Early investigators had suggested that the individual fibers, rather than being continuous, consisted of two separate parts spliced together midway between cementum and bone in a zone called the *intermediate plexus.* The plexus has been reported in the periodontal ligament of continuously growing incisors but not in the posterior teeth of rodents[50,68,119] and in actively erupting human and monkey teeth,[44] but not after they reach occlusal contact. Rearrangement of the fiber ends in the plexus is supposed to accommodate tooth eruption without necessitating the embedding of new fibers into tooth and bone.[68] The existence of such a plexus, however, has not been confirmed by radioautographic data and other studies and is considered to be a microscopic artifact.[94]

Physiologic Migration of the Teeth

Tooth movement does not end when active eruption is completed and the tooth is in functional occlusion. With time and wear, the proximal contact areas of the teeth are flattened and the teeth tend to move mesially. This is referred to as *physiologic mesial migration.* By age 40, it results in a reduction of about 0.5 cm in the length of the dental arch from the midline to the third molars. Alveolar bone is reconstructed in compliance with the physiologic mesial migration of the teeth. Bone resorption is increased in areas of pressure along the mesial surfaces of the teeth, and new layers of bundle bone are formed in areas of tension on the distal surfaces (Fig. 2–35; see also Fig. 2–28).

Occlusal Forces and the Periodontium

The periodontium exists for the purpose of supporting teeth during function and depends on the stimulation it receives from function for the preservation of its structure. Therefore, there is a constant and sensitive balance between occlusal forces and the periodontal structures.

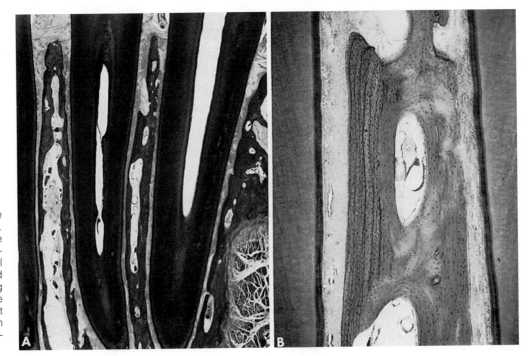

FIGURE 2–35. Bone response to physiologic mesial migration. *A,* Interdental septa between the canine *(left)* and first and second premolars. *B,* Interdental septum between the first and second premolars, showing lamellae of newly apposed bone opposite the distal of the first premolar *(left)* and resorption opposite the mesial of the second premolar *(right).*

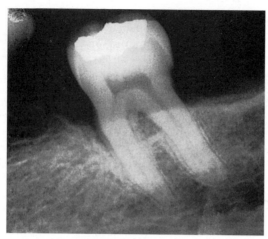

FIGURE 2–36. Bony trabeculae realigned perpendicular to the mesial root of tilted molar.

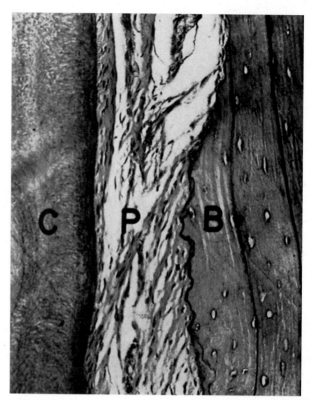

FIGURE 2–37. Atrophic periodontal ligament (P) of a tooth devoid of function. Note the scalloped edge of the alveolar bone (B), indicating that resorption has occurred. C, Cementum.

Alveolar bone undergoes constant physiologic remodeling in response to occlusal forces. Bone is removed from areas where it is no longer needed and is added to areas where new needs arise. The socket wall reflects the responsiveness of alveolar bone to occlusal forces. Osteoblasts and newly formed osteoid line the socket in areas of tension; osteoclasts and bone resorption occur in areas of pressure. Occlusal forces also influence the number, density, and alignment of cancellous trabeculae. The bony trabeculae are aligned in the path of the tensile and compressive stresses to provide maximal resistance to the occlusal force with a minimum of bone substance (Fig. 2–36).[38,98] When occlusal forces are increased, the cancellous bony trabeculae increase in number and thickness, and bone may be added to the external surface of the labial and lingual plates.

The periodontal ligament also depends on stimulation provided by occlusal function to preserve its structure. Within physiologic limits, the periodontal ligament can accommodate increased function with an increase in width (Table 2–2), a thickening of its fiber bundles, and an increase in diameter and number of Sharpey's fibers. Forces that exceed the adaptive capacity of the periodontium produce injury called *trauma from occlusion*. This condition is described in Chapter 24.

When occlusal forces are reduced, the number and thickness of the trabeculae are reduced.[23,60] The periodontal ligament also atrophies, appearing thinned, and the fibers are reduced in number and density, disoriented,[2,85] and ulti-

mately arranged parallel to the root surface (Fig. 2–37). This is termed *disuse* or *afunctional atrophy*. In this condition, the cementum is either unaffected[23] or thickened, and the distance from the cemento-enamel junction to the alveolar crest is increased.[81]

VASCULARIZATION OF THE SUPPORTING STRUCTURES

The blood supply to the supporting structures of the tooth is derived from the inferior and superior alveolar arteries to the mandible and maxilla, respectively, and reaches the periodontal ligament from three sources: apical vessels, penetrating vessels from the alveolar bone, and anastomosing vessels from the gingiva.[22] The apical vessels give off branches supplying the apical region of the periodontal ligament before entering the dental pulp. The transalveolar vessels are branches of the intraseptal vessels

Table 2–2. COMPARISON OF PERIODONTAL WIDTH OF FUNCTIONING AND FUNCTIONLESS TEETH IN A 38-YEAR-OLD MAN

	Heavy Function: Left Upper 2nd Bicuspid	Light Function: Left Lower 1st Bicuspid	Functionless: Left Upper 3rd Molar
Average width of periodonal space at entrance of alveolus	0.35 mm	0.14 mm	0.10 mm
Average width of periodontal space at middle of alveolus	0.28 mm	0.10 mm	0.06 mm
Average width of periodontal space at fundus of alveolus	0.30 mm	0.12 mm	0.06 mm

From Kronfeld R. Histologic study of the influence of function on the human periodontal membrane. J Am Dent Assoc *18*:1242, 1931. Reprinted by permission of ADA Publishing Co., Inc.

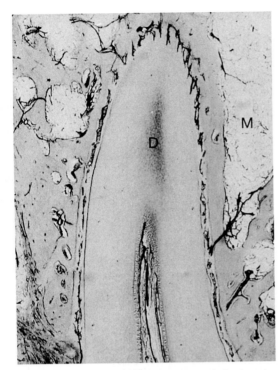

FIGURE 2–38. Vascular supply of monkey periodontium (perfused with India ink). Note the longitudinal vessels in the periodontal ligament and alveolar arteries passing through channels between the bone marrow (M) and periodontal ligament. D, Dentin. (Courtesy of Dr. Sol Bernick.)

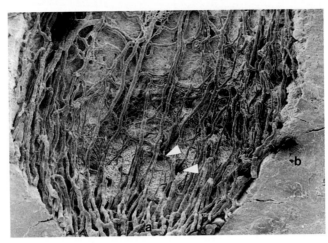

FIGURE 2–39. Vascular supply to the periodontal ligament in rat molar, as viewed by scanning electron microscopy after perfusion with plastic and tissue corrosion. Middle and apical areas of the periodontal ligament are shown with longitudinal blood vessels from apex *(below)* to gingiva *(above)*, perforating vessels entering the bone (b), and many transverse connections *(arrowheads)*. Apical vessels (a) form a cap that connects with the pulpal vessels. (Courtesy of Dr. N. J. Selliseth and Dr. K. Selvig, University of Bergen, Norway.)

that perforate the lamina dura and enter into the ligament. The intraseptal vessels continue on to vascularize the gingiva; these gingival vessels in turn anastomose with the periodontal ligament vessels of the cervical region.[30]

The vessels within the periodontal ligament are contained in interstitial spaces of loose connective tissue between the principal fibers and are connected in a net-like plexus that runs longitudinally and closer to the bone than to the cementum[18] (Figs. 2–38 and 2–39). The blood supply increases from the incisors to the molars; is greatest in the gingival third of single-rooted teeth, less in the apical third, and least in the middle; is equal in the apical and middle thirds of multirooted teeth; is slightly greater on the mesial and distal surfaces than on the facial and lingual; and is greater on the mesial surfaces of mandibular molars than on the distal.[11]

The vascular supply to the bone enters the interdental septa via nutrient canals together with veins, nerves, and lymphatics. Dental arterioles, also branching off the alveolar arteries, send tributaries through the periodontal ligament, and some small branches enter the marrow spaces of the bone via the perforations in the cribriform plate. Small vessels emanating from the facial and lingual compact bone also enter the marrow and spongy bone.

Venous Drainage

The venous drainage of the periodontal ligament accompanies the arterial supply. Venules receive the blood via the abundant capillary network; there are also arteriovenous anastomoses that bypass the capillaries. These are more frequent in apical and interradicular regions, and their significance is unknown.

Lymphatics

Lymphatics supplement the venous drainage system. Those draining the region just beneath the junctional epithelium pass into the periodontal ligament and accompany the blood vessels into the periapical region.[15] From there they pass through the alveolar bone to the inferior dental canal in the mandible or the infraorbital canal in the maxilla and then to the submaxillary lymph nodes.

Acknowledgment
The authors are grateful to Dr. R.L. Cabrini for his constructive critical analysis of this chapter.

REFERENCES

1. Agnew RG, Fong CC. Histologic studies on experimental transplantation of teeth. Oral Surg *9:*18, 1956.
2. Anneroth G, Ericsson SG. An experimental histological study of monkey teeth without antagonist. Odont Revy *18:*345, 1967.
3. Avery JK, Rapp R. Pain conduction in human dental tissues. Dent Clin North Am July 1959, p. 489.
4. Bauer WH. Effect of a faultily constructed partial denture on a tooth and its supporting tissue, with special reference to formation of fibrocartilage in the periodontal membrane as a result of disturbed healing caused by abnormal stresses. Am J Orthod Oral Surg *27:*640, 1941.
5. Baumhammers A, Stallard R. S35 sulfate utilization and turnover by connective tissues of the periodontium. J Periodont Res *3:*187, 1968.
6. Becks H. Root resorptions and their relation to pathologic bone formation. Int J Orthod Oral Surg *22:*445, 1936.
7. Berkovitz BKB, Shore RC. Cells of the periodontal ligament. In Berkovitz BKB, Moxham BJ, Newman HE, eds. The Periodontal Ligament in Health and Disease. London, Pergamon Press, 1982.
8. Berkovitz BKB. The structure of the periodontal ligament: an update. Eur J Orthod *12:*51, 1990.
9. Bernick S. Innervation of the teeth and periodontium. Dent Clin North Am 503, 1959.
10. Bien SM. Hydrodynamic damping of tooth movement. J Dent Res *45:*907, 1966.
11. Birn H. The vascular supply of the periodontal membrane. J Periodont Res *1:*51, 1966.
12. Blair HC, Teitelbaum SC, Ghiselli R, Gluck S. Osteoclastic bone resorption by a polarized vacuolar proton pump. Science *245:*855, 1989.

13. Blayney JR, Wasserman F, Groetzinger G, DeWitt TF. Further studies on mineral metabolism of human teeth by the use of radioactive isotopes. J Dent Res 29:559, 1941.

14. Box HK. Bone resorption in red marrow hyperplasia in human jaws. Bulletin 21, Canadian Dental Research Foundation, 1936.

15. Box KF. Evidence of lymphatics in the periodontium. J Can Dent Assoc 15:8, 1949.

16. Boyle PE. Tooth suspension. A comparative study of the paradental tissues of man and of the guinea pig. J Dent Res 17:37, 1938.

17. Carneiro J, Fava de Moraes F. Radioautographic visualization of collagen metabolism in the periodontal tissues of the mouse. Arch Oral Biol 10:833, 1955.

18. Carranza FA Jr, Itoiz ME, Cabrini RL, Dotto CA. A study of periodontal vascularization in different laboratory animals. J Periodont Res 1:120, 1966.

19. Carranza FA Sr, Carranza FA Jr. The management of the alveolar bone in the treatment of the periodontal pocket. J Periodontol 27:29, 1956.

20. Chambers TJ. The cellular basis of bone resorption. Clin Orthop 251:283, 1980.

21. Ciancio SC, Neiders ME, Hazen SP. The principal fibers of the periodontal ligament. Periodontics 5:76, 1967.

22. Cohen L. Further studies into the vascular architecture of the mandible. J Dent Res 39:936, 1960.

23. Cohn SA. Disease atrophy of the periodontium in mice. Arch Oral Biol 10:909, 1965.

24. Coolidge ED. The thickness of the human periodontal membrane. J Am Dent Assoc 24:1260, 1937.

25. Dastmalchi R, Polson A, Bouwsma O, Proskin H. Cementum thickness and mesial drift. J Clin Periodontol 17:709, 1990.

26. Davies WI, Picton DC. Dimensional changes in the periodontal membrane of monkey's teeth with horizontal thrusts. J Dent Res 46:114, 1967.

27. Eastoe JE. The organic matrix of bone. In Bourne GH, ed. The Biochemistry and Physiology of Bone. New York, Academic Press, 1956, p 81.

28. El Mostehy MR, Stallard RE. Intermediate cementum. J Periodont Res 3:24, 1968.

29. Elliot JR, Bowers GM. Alveolar dehiscence and fenestration. Periodontics 1:245, 1963.

30. Folke LEA, Stallard RE. Periodontal microcirculation as revealed by plastic microspheres. J Periodont Res 2:53, 1967.

31. Freeman E. The periodontium. In Ten Cate R, ed. Oral Histology. 4th ed. St Louis, CV Mosby, 1994.

32. Fullmer HM, Sheetz JH, Narkates AJ. Oxytalan connective tissue fibers: a review. J Oral Pathol 3:291, 1974.

33. Gargiulo AW, Wentz FM, Orban B. Dimensions and relations of the dentogingival junction in humans. J Periodontol 32:261, 1961.

34. Gibson W, Fullmer H. Histochemistry of the periodontal ligament. I. The dehydrogenases. Periodontics 4:63, 1966.

35. Gibson W, Fullmer H. Histochemistry of the periodontal ligament. II. The phosphatases. Periodontics 5:226, 1967.

36. Gibson W, Fullmer H. Histochemistry of the periodontal ligament. III. The esterases. Periodontics 6:71, 1968.

37. Gillespie BR, Chasens AF, Brownstein CN, Alfano MC. The relationship between the mobility of human teeth and their supracrestal fiber support. J Periodontol 50:120, 1979.

38. Glickman I, Roeber FW, Brion M, Pameijer JHN. Photoelastic analysis of internal stresses in the periodontium created by occlusal forces. J Periodontol 41:30, 1970.

39. Glimcher MJ, Friberg U, Levine P. The identification and characterization of a calcified layer of coronal cementum in erupted bovine teeth. J Ultrastruct Res 10:76, 1964.

40. Glimcher MJ. The nature of the mineral component of bone and the mechanism of calcification. In Avioli LV, Krane SM, eds. Metabolic Bone Disease and Clinical Related Disorders. Philadelphia, WB Saunders, 1990, pp 42–68.

41. Goggins JF. The distribution of oxytalan connective tissue fibers in periodontal ligaments of deciduous teeth. Periodontics 4:182, 1966.

42. Gottlieb B. Biology of the cementum. J Periodontol 17:7, 1942.

43. Grant D, Bernick S. A possible continuity between epithelial rests and epithelial attachment in miniature swine. J Periodontol 40:87, 1969.

44. Grant D, Bernick S. The formation of the periodontal ligament. J Periodontol 43:17, 1972.

45. Hagel-Bradway S, Dziak R. Regulation of bone cell metabolism. J Oral Pathol Med 18:344, 1989.

46. Hassell TM, Stanek EJ. Evidence that healthy human gingiva contains functionally heterogenous fibroblast subpopulations. Arch Oral Biol 28:617, 1983.

47. Heins PJ, Wieder SM. A histologic study of the width and nature of inter-radicular spaces of human adult premolars and molars. J Dent Res 65:948, 1986.

48. Hemley S. The incidence of root resorption of vital permanent teeth. J Dent Res 20:133, 1941.

49. Henry JL, Weinmann JP. The pattern of resorption and repair of human cementum. J Am Dent Assoc 42:271, 1951.

50. Hindle MC. Quantitative differences in periodontal membrane fibers. J Dent Res 43:953, 1964.

51. Hirschfeld I. A study of skulls in the American Museum of Natural History in relation to periodontal disease. J Dent Res 5:241, 1923.

52. Inoue M, Akiyoshi M. Histologic investigation on Sharpey's fibers in cementum of teeth in abnormal function. J Dent Res 41:503, 1962.

53. Ishikawa J, Yamamoto H, Ito K, Masuda M. Microradiographic study of cementum and alveolar bone. J Dent Res 43:936, 1964.

54. Johnson RB, Pylypas SP. A re-evaluation of the distribution of the elastic meshwork within the periodontal ligament of the mouse. J Periodont Res 27:239, 1992.

55. Jones ML, Alfred MJ, Hardy P. Tooth resorption in the two-stage transplantation technique. Br J Orthodont 10:157, 1983.

56. Jones SJ, Boyde A. A study of human root cementum surfaces as prepared for and examined in the scanning electron microscope. Z Zellforsch 130:318, 1972.

57. Jones MR, Simonton FV. Mineral metabolism in relation to alveolar atrophy in dogs. J Am Dent Assoc 15:881, 1928.

58. Junqueira LC, Carneiro J, Kelley RO. Basic Histology. 6th ed. Norwalk, CT, Appleton & Lange, 1989.

59. Kardos TB, Simpson LD. A theoretical consideration of the periodontal membrane as a collagenous thixotropic system and its relationship to tooth eruption. J Periodont Res 14:444, 1979.

60. Kellner E. Histologic findings on teeth without antagonists. Z Stomatol 26:271, 1928.

61. Kronfeld R. Biology of the cementum. J Am Dent Assoc 25:1451, 1938.

62. Kronfeld R. Histologic study of the influence of function on the human periodontal membrane. J Am Dent Assoc 18:1242, 1931.

63. Lester K. The incorporation of epithelial cells by cementum. J Ultrastruct Res 27:63, 1969.

64. Listgarten MA. A light and electron microscopic study of coronal cementogenesis. Arch Oral Biol 13:93, 1968.

65. Lopez Otero R, Parodi RJ, Ubios AM, et al. Histologic and histometric study of bone resorption after tooth movement in rats. J Periodont Res 8:327, 1973.

66. Maeda T, Kannari K, Sato O, Iwanaga T. Nerve terminals in human periodontal ligament as demonstrated by immunohistochemistry for neurofilament protein (NFP) and S-100 protein. Arch Histol Cytol 53:259, 1990.

67. Marks CS, Jr. The origin of osteoclasts: Evidence, clinical implications and investigative challenges of an extra-skeletal source. J Pathol 12:226, 1983.

68. Melcher AH. Remodelling of the periodontal ligament during eruption of the rat incisor. Arch Oral Biol 12:1649, 1967.

69. Mikola OJ, Bauer WH. Cementicles and fragments of cementum in the periodontal membrane. Oral Surg 2:1063, 1949.

70. Miller EJ. A review of biochemical studies on the genetically distinct collagens of the skeletal system. Clin Orthop 92:260, 1973.

71. Mühlemann HR, Zander HA, Halberg F. Mitotic activity in the periodontal tissues of the rat molar. J Dent Res 33:459, 1954.

72. Mühlemann HR. The determination of tooth rotation centers. Oral Surg 7:392, 1954.

73. Nihei I. A study of the hardness of human teeth. J Osaka Univ Dent Soc 4:1, 1959.

74. Noyes FB, Schour I, Noyes HJ. A Textbook of Dental Histology and Embryology. 5th ed. Philadelphia, Lea & Febiger, 1938, p 113.

75. Oppenheim A. Human tissue response to orthodontic intervention of short and long duration. Am J Orthodont Oral Surg 28:263, 1942.

76. Orban B. Oral Histology and Embryology. 2nd ed. St. Louis, CV Mosby, 1944, p 161.

77. Orban B. Tissue changes in traumatic occlusion. J Am Dent Assoc 15:2090, 1928.

78. Parfitt GJ. An investigation of the normal variations in alveolar bone trabeculation. Oral Surg 15:1453, 1962.

79. Parodi RJ, Ubios AM, Mayo J, Cabrini RL. Total body irradiation effects on the bone resorption mechanism in rats subjected to orthodontic movement. J Oral Pathol 2:1, 1973.

80. Picton DC, Davies WI. Dimensional changes in the periodontal membrane of monkeys (Macaca irus) due to horizontal thrusts applied to the teeth. Arch Oral Biol 12:1635, 1967.

81. Pihlstrom BL, Ramfjord SP. Periodontal effects of nonfunction in monkeys. J Periodontol 42:748, 1971.

82. Raisz LG, Rodan GA. Cellular basis for bone turnover. In Avioli LV, Krane SM, eds. Metabolic Bone Disease and Clinical Related Disorders. Philadelphia, WB Saunders, 1990, pp 1–41.

83. Reeve CM, Wentz FJ. The prevalence, morphology and distribution of epithelial rests in the human periodontal ligament. Oral Surg 15:785, 1962.

84. Riffle AB. Cementoenamel junction. J Periodontol 23:41, 1952.

85. Rippin JW. Collagen turnover in the periodontal ligament under normal and altered functional forces. II. Adult rat molars. J Periodont Res 13:149, 1978.

86. Ritchey B, Orban B. The crests of the interdental alveolar septa. J Periodontol 24:75, 1953.

87. Roberts WE, Chamberlain JG. Scanning electron microscopy of the cellular elements of rat periodontal ligament. Arch Oral Biol 23:587, 1978.

88. Romaniuk K. Some observations of the fine structure of human cementum. J Dent Res 46:152, 1967.

89. Romanos GE, Schroter-Kermani C, Bernimoulin J-P. Das Kollagen als Basiselement des Parodonts: Immunohistochemische Aspekte beim Menschen und bei Tieren. Parodontologie 1:47, 1991.

90. Romanos GE, Schroter-Kermani C, Hinz N, Bernimoulin J-P. Immunohistochemical distribution of the collagen types IV, V and VI and glycoprotein laminin in the healthy rat, marmoset (Callithrix jacchus) and human gingiva. Matrix 11:125, 1991.

91. Romanos GE, Schroter-Kermani C, Hinz N, et al. Immunohistochemical localization of collagenous components in healthy periodontal tissues of the rat and

marmoset *(Callithrix jacchus)*. I. Distribution of collagens type I and III. J Periodont Res *27:*101, 1992.

92. Rudolph CE. An evaluation of root resorption occurring during orthodontic therapy. J Dent Res *19:*367, 1940.
93. Rushton MA. Dental tissues in osteitis deformans. Guys Hosp Rep *88:*163, 1938.
94. Schroeder HE. The Periodontium. Berlin, Springer-Verlag, 1986.
95. Selvig KA. The fine structure of human cementum. Acta Odontol Scand *23:*423, 1965.
96. Sequeira P, Domenicucci C, Wasi S, Sodek J. Specific immunohistochemical localization of osteonectin and collagen types I and III in fetal and adult porcine dental tissues. J Histochem Cytochem *33:*531, 1985.
97. Shackleford JM. The indifferent fiber plexus and its relationship to principal fibers of the periodontium. Am J Anat *131:*427, 1971.
98. Sicher H, DuBrul EL. Oral Anatomy. 6th ed. St. Louis, CV Mosby, 1975.
99. Simpson HE. The degeneration of the rests of Malassez with age as observed by the apoxestic technique. J Periodontol *36:*288, 1965.
100. Sodek J. A comparison of the rates of synthesis and turnover of collagen and non-collagen proteins in adult rat periodontal tissues and skin using a microassay. Arch Oral Biol *22:*655, 1977.
101. Ten Cate AR, Deporter DA. The degradative role of the fibroblast in the remodelling and turnover of collagen in soft connective tissue. Anat Rec *182:*1, 1975.
102. Ten Cate AR, Mills C, Solomon G. The development of the periodontium. A transplantation and autoradiographic study. Anat Rec *170:*365, 1971.
103. Ten Cate AR. Formation of supporting bone in association with periodontal ligament organization in the mouse. Arch Oral Biol *20:*137, 1975.
104. Ten Cate AR. The development of the periodontium. In Melcher AH, Bowen WH, eds. Biology of the Periodontium. New York, Academic Press, 1969.
105. Ten Cate AR. The histochemical demonstration of specific oxidative enzymes and glycogen in the epithelial cell of Malassez. Arch Oral Biol *10:*207, 1965.
106. Thoma KH, Sosman MC, Bennett GA. An unusual case of hereditary fibrous osteodystrophy (fragilitas ossium) with replacement of dentine by osteocementum. Am J Orthodont Oral Surg *29:*1, 1943.
107. Trowbridge HO, Shibata F. Mitotic activity in epithelial rests of Malassez. Periodontics *5:*109, 1967.
108. Ubios AM, Cabrini RL. Tritiated thymidine uptake in periodontal tissues subjected to orthodontic movement. J Dent Res *50:*1160, 1971.
109. Vaes G. Cellular biology and biochemical mechanism of bone resorption. Clin Orthop *231:*239, 1988.
110. Valderhaug JP, Nylen MU. Function of epithelial rests as suggested by their ultrastructure. J Periodont Res *1:*69, 1966.
111. Valderhaug JP, Zander H. Relationship of epithelial rests of Malassez to other periodontal structures. Periodontics *5:*254, 1967.
112. Vilmarin H. Characteristics of growing bone surfaces. Scand J Dent Res *87:*65, 1979.
113. Warren EB, Hansen NM, Swartz ML, Phillips RW. Effects of periodontal disease and of calculus solvents on microhardness of cementum. J Periodontol *35:*505, 1964.
114. Weinmann JP, Sicher H. Bone and Bones. Fundamentals of Bone Biology. 2nd ed. St. Louis, CV Mosby, 1955.
115. Yamamoto H, et al. Microradiographic and histopathological study of the cementum. Bull Tokyo Dent Univ *9:*141, 1962.
116. Yamamoto T, Wakita M. Bundle formation of principal fibers in rat molars. J Periodont Res *27:*20, 1992.
117. Zander HA, Hurzeler B. Continuous cementum apposition. J Dent Res *37:*1035, 1958.
118. Zipkin J. The inorganic composition of bones and teeth. In Schraer H, ed. Biological Calcification. New York, Appleton-Century-Crofts, 1970.
119. Zwarych PD, Quigley MB. The intermediate plexus of the periodontal ligament: History and further observations. J Dent Res *44:*383, 1965.

3

Aging and the Periodontium

FERMIN A. CARRANZA, JR.

General Effects of Aging
Aging-Related Changes in the Periodontium
Gingiva and Other Areas of the Oral Mucosa
Periodontal Ligament
Alveolar Bone and Cementum

Tooth–Periodontium Relationships
Masticatory Efficiency
Aging and the Cumulative Effects of Oral Disease

Disease of the periodontium occurs in childhood, adolescence, and early adulthood, but the prevalence of periodontal disease and the tissue destruction and tooth loss it causes increase with age. Many tissue changes occur with aging, some of which may affect the diseases of the periodontium. In fact, it is sometimes difficult to differentiate between physiologic aging and the cumulative effects of disease.

Aging is a slowing of natural function, a disintegration of the balanced control and organization that characterize the young adult.[29] It is a process of physiologic and morphologic disintegration, unlike infancy, childhood, and adolescence, which are typified by processes of integration and coordination. However, it is often difficult to separate age-related changes from those induced by disease or by pharmacotherapeutic agents used for their treatment.

Aging is described in detail in texts devoted to the subject. Some general age-related changes and alterations in the periodontium are considered here. For further reading on the oral and periodontal aspects of aging, the book *Geriatric Dentistry: A Textbook of Oral Gerontology,* by Holm-Pedersen and Löe,[18] is recommended.

GENERAL EFFECTS OF AGING

Aging is manifested to different degrees and in different manners in various tissues and organs, but in all tissues it includes general features[46,50] such as tissue desiccation, reduced elasticity, diminished reparative capacity, and altered cell permeability.

In the skin, the dermis and epidermis are thinned, keratinization is diminished,[21] the blood supply is decreased, and the nerve endings show degeneration. Capillaries appear to become more fragile with age, which may result in development of large hematomas after minor traumas. Tissue elasticity is reduced with aging,[23] and there is degeneration of the elastic tissue fibers of the corium. The atrophic skin changes are less marked in females and may be reversed in local areas by application of estrogen.

Bone undergoes osteoporosis with aging. The bone is rarified, trabeculae are reduced in number, the cortical plates are thinned, vascularity is reduced, lacunar resorption is more prominent, and susceptibility to fracture is increased. Generalized osteoporosis occurs in aged females more commonly than in aged males and has been associated with sex hormone dysfunction.[22] With age, water content of bone is reduced, the mineral crystals are increased in size, and collagen fibrils are thickened.[17]

AGING-RELATED CHANGES IN THE PERIODONTIUM

Gingiva and Other Areas of the Oral Mucosa

The following changes in the gingiva have been identified with aging: diminished keratinization, in both men and women[38]; a reduced[15] or an unchanged[40] amount of stippling; increased width of attached gingiva,[2] with constant location of the mucogingival junction throughout adult life[1]; decreased connective tissue cellularity; a greater amount of intercellular substances[56]; and reduced oxygen consumption, a measure of metabolic activity.[55] An increase[11,33,34] or no change[42] in the mitotic index of gingival epithelium in aged humans has been reported.

Thinning of the oral epithelium[45] or no change in width[30] has also been reported to occur with age. The keratinizing potential of the hard palate epithelium does not change with age.[35] An increased keratinization of lip and cheek mucosa with age has been reported[45]; however, this might be related to smoking.[35] Other changes noted in the oral mucosa include atrophy of the connective tissue with loss of elasticity,[43] a decrease in the number of protein-bound hexoses and mucoproteins,[7] and an increase in the number of mast cells.[8]

Although different opinions have been expressed, studies indicate that there is no reduction in salivary gland performance as a result of aging.[6]

Periodontal Ligament

In the periodontal ligament, aging results in a greater number of elastic fibers[16]; decreases in vascularity, mitotic activity,[51] fibroplasia,[20,28] and the number of collagen fibers[13,44] and mucopolysaccharides[39,47,52]; and increases in arteriosclerotic changes.[13] Both an increase[24] and a decrease[10] in width of the ligament have been described in aging. A reduction in width may be accounted for by a lower functional demand owing to the decrease in strength of the masticatory musculature. An increase in width may be due to the availability of fewer teeth to support the entire functional load. The decreased width may also result

from encroachment on the ligament by continuous deposition of cementum and bone.[26]

Alveolar Bone and Cementum

Changes in alveolar bone with aging are similar to those occurring in the remainder of the skeletal system. These include osteoporosis,[3,27] decreased vascularity, and a reduction in metabolic rate and healing capacity.[50] Bone resorption may be increased[32] or decreased,[12] and the density of bone may increase or decrease, depending on its location in the body and the animal species.[25,32]

There is greater irregularity in the surfaces of both the cementum and the alveolar bone facing the periodontal ligament with advancing age.[13,19] A continuous increase in the amount of cementum also occurs with age.[19,59] The total width of cementum at age 76 is three times that at age 11.[59]

Tooth–Periodontium Relationships

The most obvious change in the teeth with aging is a loss of tooth substance caused by attrition. Occlusal wear reduces cusp height and inclination (Fig. 3–1), with a resultant increase in the food table area and loss of sluiceways. The degree of attrition is influenced by the musculature, the consistency of the food, the tooth hardness, occupational factors, and habits such as grinding (bruxism) and clenching.[26,41]

The rate of attrition may be coordinated with other aging-related changes such as continuous tooth eruption and gingival recession (Fig. 3–2). As the tooth erupts, cementum is usually deposited in the apical region of the root. The reduction in bone height that occurs with aging is not necessarily related to occlusal wear.[5] If bone support is reduced, the clinical crown tends to become disproportionately long and exerts excessive leverage on the bone. By reducing the clinical crown length, attrition appears to preserve the balance between the tooth and its bony support.

Wear of teeth also occurs on the proximal surfaces, accompanied by mesial migration of the teeth.[36] Proximal wear reduces the anteroposterior length of the dental arch by approximately 0.5 cm by age 40.[58] Anteroposterior narrowing from proximal wear is greater in teeth that taper toward the cervical aspect, such as the incisors.[58] Progressive attrition and proximal wear result in a reduced

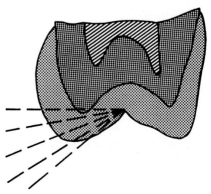

FIGURE 3–1. Diminution in cuspal inclination with increasing age.

FIGURE 3–2. Tooth–periodontium relationships at different ages. *A,* Age 12. The gingiva is located on the enamel, and the clinical crown is shorter than the anatomic crown. *B,* Age 25. The gingiva is attached close to the cemento-enamel junction. *C,* Age 50. Slight occlusal wear and slight recession. *D,* Age 72. Moderate attrition and slight to moderate recession. These variations may be due not to an aging process but to the cumulative effect of injurious factors.

maxillary–mandibular overjet in the molar area and an edge-to-edge bite anteriorly.

Masticatory Efficiency

Slight atrophy of the buccal musculature has been described as a physiologic feature of aging. However, reduction in masticatory efficiency in aged individuals is more likely to be the result of unreplaced missing teeth, loose teeth, poorly fitting dentures, or an unwillingness to wear dentures. Reduced masticatory efficiency leads to poor chewing habits and the possibility of associated digestive disturbances. Aged persons select foods requiring less chewing effort when masticatory efficiency is impaired.

Avitaminosis is relatively common in aged persons, but the extent to which it results from impaired masticatory efficiency has not been established. Most nutrient requirements of older persons are similar to those of younger people, but some nutrients are especially important. An adequate intake of vitamins, calcium, iron, and potassium is particularly important to geriatric patients, and dietary supplementation may be advisable. A diet high in fiber and vitamins and comparatively low in fat may also be beneficial.[18]

AGING AND THE CUMULATIVE EFFECTS OF ORAL DISEASE

With time, chronic disease can produce many oral changes, and it is difficult to determine how much physiologic aging contributes to the total picture. However, changes such as gingival recession, tooth attrition, and reduction in bone height in the elderly result from disease and factors in the oral environment and not from physiologic aging[4] (Figs. 3–3 through 3–5).

Plaque accumulation starts as soon as teeth erupt. However, the experimental gingivitis model has shown that inflammation develops more rapidly in older individuals than in children.[18] This may occur in part because areas of recession in older individuals may favor plaque accumulation; it may also be due to a reduction in immune response with aging.[9]

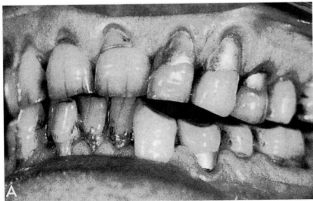
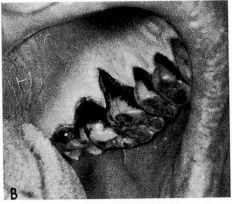

FIGURE 3–3. *A,* Attrition of the teeth and gingival recession in a 65-year-old man. Note the elliptical contour of the tooth wear associated with biting the stem of a pipe while smoking. *B,* Lingual view showing accentuated recession on the first molar.

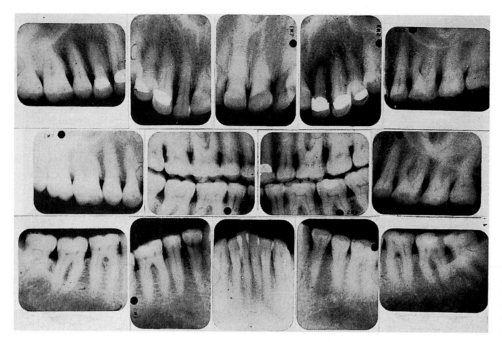

FIGURE 3-4. Radiographs of the patient shown in Figure 3-3. Aside from a few localized areas of bone loss, there is little evidence of reduced bone height, which is considered by some investigators to be a physiologic feature of aging.

Studies on experimental gingivitis in young and old individuals with high and low susceptibility to periodontal destruction have shown that susceptibility to disease can overshadow the effect of age.[53,54,57] Inflammation develops more rapidly and wound healing proceeds more slowly in old than in young individuals with the same susceptibility to periodontal disease. But when susceptible young individuals are compared to nonsusceptible old individuals, inflammation develops in the former more rapidly and more intensely than in the latter, thereby overshadowing the effect of age.

Senescence of the immune system has been considered to enhance susceptibility to diseases associated with abnormalities in T-cell function; these include viral and fungal (but not bacterial) infections.[37]

Rapidly destructive forms of periodontal disease occur in young patients and are usually associated with deficient leukocyte function. Elderly individuals have a slowly progressive form of the disease that does not result from impaired leukocyte function or host defense mechanisms.

The clinical management of geriatric patients is discussed in Chapter 35.

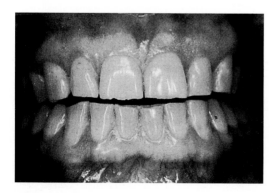

FIGURE 3-5. Bruxing habit and marked attrition in a 25-year-old woman.

REFERENCES

1. Ainamo A. Influence of age on the location of the maxillary mucogingival junction. J Periodont Res *13*:189, 1978.
2. Ainamo J, Talari A. The increase with age of the width of attached gingiva. J Periodont Res *11*:182, 1976.
3. Atkinson PJ, Woodhead C. Changes in human mandibular structure with age. Arch Oral Biol *13*:1453, 1968.
4. Baer PN, Bernick S. Age changes in the periodontium of the mouse. Oral Surg *10*:430, 1957.
5. Baer PN, Kakehashi S, Littleton NW, et al. Alveolar bone loss and occlusal wear. Periodontics *1*:91, 1963.
6. Baum BJ. Age changes in salivary glands and salivary secretion. In Holm-Pedersen P, Löe H, eds. Geriatric Dentistry. Copenhagen, Munksgaard, 1986.
7. Burzynski NJ. Relationship between age and palatal tissue and gingival tissue in the guinea pig. J Dent Res *46*:539, 1967.
8. Carranza FA Jr, Cabrini RL. Age variations in the number of mast cells in oral mucosa and skin of albino rats. J Dent Res *38*:631, 1959.
9. Church H, Dolby AE. The effect of age on the cellular immune response to dentogingival plaque extract. J Periodont Res *13*:120, 1978.
10. Coolidge E. The thickness of the periodontal membrane. J Am Dent Assoc *24*:1200, 1937.
11. Gargiulo AW, Wentz FM, Orban B. Mitotic activity of human oral epithelium exposed to 20% hydrogen peroxide. Oral Surg *14*:474, 1961.
12. Gilmore N, Glickman I. Some age changes in the periodontium of the albino mouse. J Dent Res *38*:1195, 1959.
13. Grant D, Bernick S. Arteriosclerosis in periodontal vessels of aging humans. J Periodontol *41*:170, 1970.
14. Grant D, Bernick S. The periodontium of aging humans. J Periodontol *43*:660, 1972.
15. Greene AJ. Study of the characteristics of stippling and its relation to gingival health. J Periodontol *33*:176, 1962.
16. Haim G, Baumgartel R. Alterations in the periodontal ligament due to age. Dtsch Zahnaerztl Z *23*:340, 1968.
17. Hall DA. The Aging of Connective Tissue. London, Academic Press, 1976.
18. Holm-Pedersen P, Löe H, eds. Geriatric Dentistry: A Textbook of Oral Gerontology. Copenhagen, Munksgaard, 1986.
19. Ive JC, Shapiro PA, Ivey JL. Age related changes in the periodontium of pigtail monkeys. J Periodont Res *15*:420, 1980.
20. Jensen JL, Toto PD. Radioactive labeling index of the periodontal ligament in aging rats. J Dent Res *47*:149, 1968.
21. Joseph NR, Molimard R, Bourliere F. Aging of skin. I. Titration curves of human epidermis in relation to age. Gerontologia *1*:18, 1957.
22. Kesson CM, Morris N, McCutcheon A. Generalized osteoporosis in old age. Ann Rheum Dis *6*:146, 1947.
23. Kirk E, Kvorning SA. Quantitative measurements of the elastic properties of the skin and subcutaneous tissue in young and old individuals. J Gerontol *4*:273, 1949.
24. Klein A. Systemic investigations concerning the thickness of the periodontal membrane. Z Stomatol *26*:417, 1928.
25. Klingsberg J, Butcher EO. Comparative histology of age changes in oral tissues of rat, hamster and monkey. J Dent Res *39*:158, 1960.

26. Kronfeld R. Structure, function, and pathology of the human periodontal membrane. NY J Dent *6:*112, 1936.
27. Kronfeld R. Biology of cementum. J Am Dent Assoc *25:*1451, 1938.
28. Lavelle CLB. The effect of age on the proliferative activity of the periodontal membrane of the rat incisor. J Periodont Res *3:*48, 1968.
29. Little CC. Growth and individuality. In Muller HS, Little CC, Snyder LH. Genetics, Medicine and Man. Ithaca, NY, Cornell University Press, 1947, p 104.
30. Löe H, Karring T. The three-dimensional morphology of the epithelium–connective tissue interface of the gingiva as related to age and sex. Scand J Dent Res *79:*315, 1971.
31. Lopez Otero R, Carranza FA Jr, Cabrini RL. Histometric study of age changes in interradicular bone of Wistar rats. J Periodont Res *2:*40, 1967.
32. Manson JD, Lucas RB. A microradiographic study of age changes in the human mandible. Arch Oral Biol *7:*761, 1962.
33. Marwah AS, Weinmann JP, Meyer J. Effect of chronic inflammation on the epithelial turnover of human gingiva. Arch Pathol *69:*147, 1960.
34. Meyer J, Marwah AS, Weinmann JP. Mitotic rate of gingival epithelium in two age groups. J Invest Dermatol *27:*237, 1956.
35. Mosadomi A, Shklar G, Loftus DR, Chauncey HH. Effects of tobacco smoking and age on the keratinization of palatal mucosa. A cytological study. Oral Surg *40:*413, 1970.
36. Murphy TR. Reduction of the dental arch by approximal attrition. Br Dent J *116:*483, 1964.
37. Page RC. Periodontal diseases in the elderly: A critical evaluation of current information. Gerodontology *3:*63, 1984.
38. Papic M, Glickman I. Keratinization of the human gingiva in the menstrual cycle and menopause. Oral Surg *3:*504, 1950.
39. Paunio K. The age change of acid mucopolysaccharides in the periodontal membrane of man. J Periodont Res suppl *4:*27, 1969.
40. Riethe P. Surface changes in the attached gingiva in young and old people. Dtsch Zahnaerztl Z *9:*1028, 1965.
41. Robinson HBG. Some clinical aspects of intraoral age change. Geriatrics *2:*9, 1947.
42. Ryan EJ, Toto PD, Gargiulo AW. Aging in human attached gingival epithelium. J Dent Res *53:*74, 1974.
43. Schei O, Waerhaug J, Lovdal A, Arno A. Alveolar bone loss as related to oral hygiene and age. J Periodontol *30:*7, 1959.
44. Severson JA, Moffett BC, Kokich V, Selipsky H. A histologic study of age changes in the adult human periodontal joint (ligament). J Periodontol *49:*189, 1987.
45. Shklar G. The effects of aging upon oral mucosa. J Invest Dermatol *47:*115, 1966.
46. Simms HS, Stolman A. Changes in human tissue electrolytes in senescence. Science *86:*269, 1937.
47. Skougaard MR, Levy BM, Simpson J. Collagen metabolism in skin and periodontal membrane of the marmoset. J Periodont Res suppl *4:*28, 1969.
48. Soni NN. Quantitative study of bone activity in alveolar and femoral bone of the guinea pig. J Dent Res *47:*584, 1968.
50. Thomas BOA. Gerodontology. The study of changes in oral tissue associated with aging. J Am Dent Assoc *33:*207, 1946.
51. Toto PD, Borg M. Effect of age changes on the premitotic index in the periodontium of mice. J Dent Res *47:*70, 1968.
52. Toto PD, Jensen J, Sawinski J. Sulfate uptake and cell kinetics in teeth and bone of aging mice. Periodontics *5:*292, 1967.
53. van der Velde V. Effect of age on the periodontium. J Clin Periodontol *11:*281, 1984.
54. van der Velde V, Abbas F, Hart AM. Experimental gingivitis in relation to susceptibility to periodontal disease. I. Clinical observations. J Clin Periodontol *12:*61, 1985.
55. Volpe AR, Manhold JH, Manhold BS. Effect of age and other factors upon normal gingival tissue respiration. J Dent Res *41:*1060, 1962.
56. Wentz FW, Maier AW, Orban B. Age changes and sex differences in the clinically normal gingiva. J Periodontol *23:*13, 1952.
57. Winkel, ES, Abbas F, van der Velde V, et al: Experimental gingivitis in relation to age in individuals not susceptible to periodontal destruction. J Clin Periodontol *14:*499, 1987.
58. Wood HE. Causal factors in shortening tooth series with age. J Dent Res *17:*1, 1938.
59. Zander H, Hurzeler B. Continuous cementum apposition. J Dent Res *37:*1035, 1958.

Section Two

Classification and Epidemiology of Periodontal Diseases

4

Classification of Diseases of the Periodontium

FERMIN A. CARRANZA, JR.

Gingival Diseases
Types of Gingival Disease
Diseases of the Tooth-Supporting Structures
Classification

Disease classifications are useful for the purposes of diagnosis, prognosis, and treatment planning. Different classifications of periodontal diseases have been used over the years and have been replaced as new knowledge has improved our understanding of the etiology and pathology of the diseases of the periodontium.

The term *periodontal disease* has been given different meanings and is used rather ambiguously. It is used in a general sense to encompass all diseases of the periodontium in much the same way as the terms *liver disease* and *kidney disease* are used. It may be considered synonymous with *periodontopathia,* although this term is not in current usage.

Traditionally, periodontal diseases have been divided into two major categories: gingival diseases and periodontal diseases. The former includes diseases that attack only the gingiva, whereas the latter includes diseases that involve the supporting structures of the tooth.

GINGIVAL DISEASES

Gingivitis (inflammation of the gingiva) is the most common form of gingival disease. Inflammation is almost always present in all forms of gingival disease, because bacterial plaque, which causes inflammation, and irritating factors, which favor plaque accumulation, are often present in the gingival environment.

This has led to the tendency to designate all forms of gingival disease as gingivitis, as if inflammation were the only disease process involved. However, pathologic processes not caused by local irritation, such as atrophy, hyperplasia, and neoplasia, also occur in the gingiva. The presence of inflammation does not necessarily make all cases of gingivitis the same, and it is often necessary to differentiate between inflammation and other pathologic processes that may be present in the gingival disease.

The role of inflammation in gingival diseases varies in three ways:

1. Inflammation may be the primary and only pathologic change. This is by far the most prevalent type of gingival disease.
2. Inflammation may be a secondary feature, superimposed on systemically caused gingival disease. For example, inflam-

mation commonly complicates gingival hyperplasia caused by the systemic administration of phenytoin.
3. Inflammation may be the precipitating factor responsible for clinical changes in patients with systemic conditions that of themselves do not produce clinically detectable gingival disease. Gingivitis in pregnancy is an example.

Types of Gingival Disease

The most common type of gingival disease is the simple inflammatory involvement caused by bacterial plaque attached to the tooth surface. This type of gingivitis, called *chronic marginal gingivitis* or *simple gingivitis,* may remain stationary for indefinite periods of time or may proceed to destroy the supporting structures (i.e., periodontitis). The reasons for these different behaviors are not clearly understood.

In addition, the gingiva can be involved in other diseases, often but not always related to chronic inflammatory problems. Classification of these diseases is difficult, and its usefulness doubtful. These other types of gingival disease include the following:

1. Acute necrotizing ulcerative gingivitis (see Chapter 19), as well as the gingival changes seen in acquired immunodeficiency syndrome (AIDS) patients (see Chapter 15).
2. Acute herpetic gingivostomatitis (see Chapter 19) and other viral, bacterial, or fungal diseases (see Chapter 20).
3. Allergic gingivitis (see Chapter 20).
4. Skin diseases that also involve the gingival tissues, inducing characteristic types of gingival disease, such as that seen in lichen planus, pemphigus, erythema multiforme, and other dermatoses. These are described in detail in Chapter 20.
5. Gingivitis that is initiated by bacterial plaque, but in which the tissue response is modified by systemic factors. Such is the case with nutritional deficiencies (see Chapter 14), endocrine diseases such as diabetes, and conditions such as pregnancy, puberty (see Chapter 14), and hematologic and immunologic problems (see Chapters 10 and 14).
6. Gingival enlargement, in which the gingival response to a variety of pathogenic agents results in an increase in volume. Included in this group are drug-associated changes such as those induced by phenytoin, cyclosporine, and other drugs (see Chapter 18).
7. Different benign and malignant tumors may appear in the gingiva either as primary tumors or as metastases (see Chapter 18).

DISEASES OF THE TOOTH-SUPPORTING STRUCTURES

There are several different diseases that involve the tooth-supporting tissues. Many older classifications considered them in terms of the pathologic changes they produced (e.g., inflammatory, degenerative, or neoplastic). Although there are degenerative and neoplastic periodontal diseases, the most common disease by far is initiated by plaque accumulation in the gingivodental area and is basically inflammatory in character. Initially it is confined to the gingiva and is called *chronic marginal gingivitis.* Later the supporting structures become involved, and the disease is termed *periodontitis.* There is a continuum of changes from marginal gingivitis to periodontitis, and the term *periodontal disease* has been used generically to refer to the entire process and more specifically to refer to periodontitis. The term *chronic destructive periodontitis,* however, is a more accurate designation for this disease.

The periodontal tissues can also be involved by other nosologic entities unrelated to plaque; many of these fall into the degenerative or neoplastic categories. These diseases frequently involve other organs or systems and are considered periodontal manifestations of systemic diseases; these may have their initiation in the gingival tissues, in the underlying supporting structures, or both.

Classification

The classification given in Table 4–1 includes all forms of chronic destructive periodontitis and attempts to provide a useful tool for the analysis and diagnosis of clinical cases. It does not include the purely gingival diseases. As background information, other relevant classifications proposed for the clinical management of chronic destructive periodontitis are presented in Table 4–2.

Periodontitis

Periodontitis is the most common type of periodontal disease and results from extension of the inflammatory process initiated in the gingiva to the supporting periodontal tissues (see Chapter 23). Synonyms not in current use include schmutz pyorrhea (Gottlieb), paradentitis (Weski, Beck), paradentosis, periodontoclasia, pericementitis, parodontitis, alveolar pyorrhea, alveoloclasia, Riggs' disease, and chronic suppurative periodontitis.

Periodontitis has been classified according to the rate of progression (slowly progressive and rapidly progressive) and according to the age at onset (adult periodontitis and early-onset periodontitis). Other forms are necrotizing ulcerative periodontitis and refractory periodontitis.

Slowly Progressive Periodontitis

Chronic inflammation of the gingiva, pocket formation, and bone loss usually accompany slowly progressive periodontitis (SPP). Tooth mobility and pathologic migration appear in advanced cases. Although SPP can be preceded by long-standing chronic gingivitis, its destructive features are usually seen at age 35 or beyond.

SPP is caused by dental plaque; immunologic defects have not been found. The accumulation of plaque can be facilitated by a large variety of local irritants such as calculus, faulty restorations, and food impaction.

The disease is either generalized or affects many teeth; the severity of lesions can vary in different sites but is usually correlated with the amount of plaque (see Chapter 25).

Rapidly Progressive Periodontitis

Rapidly progressive periodontitis (RPP) can occur at an early age (before the end of puberty) or during the adult years. The adult onset forms of RPP can be associated with a lack of clinical inflammation or with marked inflammatory changes. RPP is associated with scantier amounts of plaque and calculus but results in deep pocket formation and rapid bone loss (see Chapter 26).

Early onset RPP includes advanced destructive lesions in children and adolescents. The two major forms are prepubertal and juvenile periodontitis. Prepubertal periodontitis appears before the age of puberty and is a very rapidly destructive disease. It is associated with immunologic or other systemic problems, such as Papillon-Lefèvre syndrome, hypophosphatasia, agranulocytosis, Down syndrome, and others (see Chapter 27).

Juvenile periodontitis is seen during puberty; previous terms for the condition include *periodontosis, precocious advanced alveolar atrophy, juvenile atrophy, juvenile paradentosis, juvenile parodontopathia,* and *localized juvenile periodontitis.* It is characterized by deep angular lesions localized in the first molars and incisors and occurs in otherwise healthy adolescents (see Chapter 27).

Necrotizing Ulcerative Periodontitis

Necrotizing ulcerative periodontitis follows repeated long-term episodes of acute necrotizing ulcerative gingivitis and exhibits deep interdental osseous craters, usually in localized areas, although it can be fairly generalized (see Chapter 19). This type of periodontitis is also seen in patients with AIDS (see Chapters 15 and 26).

Refractory Periodontitis

These are cases that, for unknown reasons, fail to respond to adequate treatment (see Chapter 26).

Table 4–1. CLASSIFICATION OF CHRONIC DESTRUCTIVE PERIODONTITIS

I. Periodontitis
   A. Slowly progressive periodontitis
   B. Rapidly progressive periodontitis
      1. Adult onset periodontitis
      2. Early onset periodontitis
         a. Prepubertal periodontitis
         b. Juvenile periodontitis
   C. Necrotizing ulcerative periodontitis
   D. Refractory periodontitis
II. Trauma from occlusion*
III. Periodontal atrophy*
IV. Periodontal manifestations of systemic diseases

---

* Both trauma from occlusion and periodontal atrophy, in their pure forms, are accommodation phenomena to changes in the environment. They are *not* actually "diseases," but are included for the sake of completeness and convenience for the clinician.

DEFINITIONS: *adolescence:* the period of life beginning with the appearance of secondary sex characteristics and terminating with the cessation of somatic growth (roughly from 11 to 19 years of age); *adult:* having attained full growth or maturity; *juvenile:* pertaining to youth or childhood; *puberty:* the period during which secondary sex characteristics begin to develop and the capability of sexual reproduction is attained.

Table 4–2. CURRENT CLASSIFICATIONS OF PERIODONTAL DISEASE*

Page and Schroeder, 1982[3]

Prepubertal periodontitis
  Generalized
  Localized
Juvenile periodontitis
Rapidly progressing periodontitis
Adult type periodontitis

Grant, Stern, and Listgarten, 1988[2]

Bacterially induced diseases
  Gingivitis
  Periodontitis
    Adult type
    Postjuvenile
    Early onset
      Juvenile
        Localized
        Generalized
  Acute necrotizing ulcerative gingivitis
  Acute abscess
  Pericoronitis
Functionally induced diseases
  Traumatic occlusion
  Disuse atrophy
Trauma
  Habits, accidents

Suzuki, 1988[5]

Adult periodontitis
Rapidly progressing periodontitis
  Type A
  Type B
Juvenile periodontitis
Postjuvenile periodontitis
Prepubertal periodontitis

World Workshop in Clinical Periodontics, 1989[6]

Adult periodontitis
Early onset periodontitis
  Prepubertal
    Generalized or localized
  Juvenile
    Generalized or localized
  Rapidly progressive periodontitis
Periodontitis associated with systemic diseases
  Down syndrome
  Diabetes type I
  Papillon-Lefèvre syndrome

AIDS
  Other diseases
Necrotizing ulcerative periodontitis
Refractory periodontitis

Genco, 1990[1]

Periodontitis in adults
Periodontitis in juveniles
  Localized form
  Generalized form
Periodontitis with systemic involvement
  Primary neutrophil disorders
  Secondary or associated neutrophil impairment
  Other systemic diseases
Miscellaneous conditions

Ranney, 1993[4]

Gingivitis
  Gingivitis, plaque bacterial
    Nonaggravated
    Systemically aggravated by sex hormones, drugs, systemic
      disease
  Necrotizing ulcerative gingivitis
    Systemic determinants unknown
    Related to HIV
  Gingivitis, nonplaque
    Associated with skin disease; allergic; infectious
Periodontitis
  Adult periodontitis
    Nonaggravated
    Systemically aggravated (neutropenias, leukemias, lazy leuko-
      cyte syndrome, AIDS, diabetes mellitus, Crohn's disease,
      Addison's disease)
  Early-onset periodontitis
    Localized early-onset periodontitis
      Neutrophil abnormality
    Generalized early-onset periodontitis
      Neutrophil abnormality; immunodeficient
    Early-onset periodontitis related to systemic disease
      Leukocyte adhesion deficiency, hypophosphatasia, Papillon-
      Lefèvre syndrome, neutropenias, leukemias, Chédiak-
      Higashi syndrome, AIDS, diabetes mellitus type I, trisomy
      21, histiocytosis X, Ehlers-Danlos syndrome (type VIII)
    Early-onset periodontitis, systemic determinants unknown
  Necrotizing ulcerative periodontitis
    Systemic determinants unknown
    Related to HIV
    Related to nutrition
  Periodontal abscess

* Note that some of these classifications (Grant et al, Ranney) include gingival and periodontal diseases, whereas others, including the one used in this book, classify only periodontal diseases.

Trauma From Occlusion

Because gingival inflammation is very common, trauma from occlusion seldom occurs without it. When it is the sole pathologic process, trauma from occlusion presents two predominant clinical features: increased tooth mobility and widening of the periodontal space, particularly in the gingival region of the root. These changes are adaptation phenomena to increased function. Trauma from occlusion does not produce gingival inflammation or the formation of periodontal pockets (see Chapter 24).

Periodontal Atrophy

Atrophy is a decrease in the size of a tissue or organ or of its cellular elements after it has attained its normal ma-

ture size. Generalized reduction in the height of the periodontium results in gingival recession and may or may not be associated with overt inflammation. Periodontal atrophy occurs as a result of repeated traumatic insults such as aggressive toothbrushing, frenum pull, and other causes. Because its incidence increases with age, it has been termed *physiologic* or *senile atrophy.* However, it is not a result of aging but of the cumulative effect of repeated injuries to the periodontium.

Periodontal Manifestations of Systemic Diseases

A partial list of systemic diseases involving the periodontal tissues is presented in Table 4–3. A considerable over-

Table 4–3. SOME SYSTEMIC DISEASES INVOLVING THE PERIODONTAL TISSUES

1. Necrotizing ulcerative periodontitis
   a. AIDS-associated
   b. Non-AIDS associated
2. Disorders of neutrophil function
   a. Agranulocytosis
   b. Cyclic neutropenia
   c. Chédiak-Higashi syndrome
   d. Other diseases
3. Hematologic diseases
   a. Leukemia
   b. Anemias
   c. Histiocytosis X
4. Metabolic diseases
   a. Gaucher's disease
   b. Niemann-Pick disease
5. Connective tissue disorders
   a. Ehlers-Danlos syndrome
   b. Wegener's granulomatosis
   c. Sarcoidosis
6. Bone diseases
   a. Hypophosphatasia
   b. Paget's disease
7. Neoplastic diseases
   a. Benign tumors
   b. Malignant tumors

lap may be found between diseases listed here and disorders that predispose to or aggravate periodontitis. For example, some of these diseases may play a role in different types of early onset periodontitis and probably in rapidly progressive and refractory periodontitis. Necrotizing ulcerative periodontitis may be considered to belong in this list because of the key systemic component of its etiology. However, it is also included in the classification of periodontitis because traditionally it has been considered a type of periodontitis. Other diseases in the list, such as neoplasias, are totally unrelated to chronic destructive periodontitis.

REFERENCES

1. Genco RJ. Classification and clinical and radiographic features of periodontal disease. In Genco RJ, Goldman HM, Cohen DW, eds. Contemporary Periodontics. St. Louis, CV Mosby, 1990.
2. Grant DA, Stern IB, Listgarten MA. Periodontics. 6th ed. St Louis, CV Mosby, 1988.
3. Page RC, Schroeder HE. Periodontitis in Man and Other Animals. Basel, S Karger, 1982.
4. Ranney RR: Classification of periodontal diseases, Periodontology 2000 2:13, 1993.
5. Suzuki J. Diagnosis and classification of the periodontal diseases. Dent Clin North Am *32*:195, 1988.
6. World Workshop in Clinical Periodontics. Report of Section on Periodontal Diagnosis and Diagnostic Aids. Princeton, NJ, July 23–27, 1989.

5

Epidemiology of Gingival and Periodontal Disease

VLADIMIR W. SPOLSKY

Indices Used to Study Periodontal Problems
Indices Used to Assess Gingival Inflammation
Indices Used to Measure Periodontal Destruction
Indices Used to Measure Plaque Accumulation
Indices Used to Measure Calculus
Indices Used to Assess Treatment Needs
Reliability of Dental Indices
Descriptive Epidemiology of Gingival and Periodontal Disease
Prevalence of Gingivitis

Prevalence of Periodontitis
Prevalence of Juvenile Periodontitis
Risk Factors Affecting the Prevalence and Severity of Gingivitis and Periodontitis
Etiologic Risk Factors for Gingival and Periodontal Disease
Distribution of Disease in Different Areas of the Mouth
The Relationship Between Periodontal Disease and Dental Caries

Epidemiologic surveys conducted throughout the world point to the almost universal distribution of caries and periodontal disease.[131] Progress in the study of the epidemiology of periodontal diseases has been slower than that in the study of dental caries because of several important factors that do not exist in the study of dental caries. The pathologic changes of dental caries involve hard, calcified tissues, whereas periodontal disease involves soft and

hard tissues. Unlike dental caries, periodontal disease does not lend itself easily to objective measurement, because the signs of periodontal pathologic alteration involve color changes in the soft tissues, swelling, bleeding, and bone changes that are reflected in crevice depth changes or pathologic pockets, as well as loss of tooth function because of tooth mobility. Therefore, examining the teeth for the signs of dental caries is far easier than evaluting the pathologic variables used to define periodontal diseases.

Dental epidemiology is the study of the pattern (distribution) and dynamics of dental diseases in a human population. "Pattern" implies that certain people are affected by a disease and that the association between the disease and the affected population can be described by variables such as age, sex, racial or ethnic group, occupation, social characteristics, place of residence, susceptibility, and exposure to specific agents. The term *dynamics* refers to a temporal pattern (distribution) and is concerned with trends, cyclic patterns, and the time that elapses between the exposure to inciting factors and the onset of the specific disease.[138] Russell[132] defined dental epidemiology as "not so much the study of disease as a process as it is a study of the condition of the people in whom the disease occurs."

The purpose or objective of epidemiology is to increase understanding of the disease process (i.e., to identify the risk factors or determinants of disease), thereby leading to the development of methods of control and prevention. In addition, epidemiology attempts to discover populations at high and low risk, to define the specific problem under investigation, and to determine trends in disease patterns. The design, conduct, and interpretation of clinical trials of preventive and curative measures are also within its purview.[138] Ainamo[5] has astutely described the significance of epidemiologic research to the understanding of periodontal disease. Epidemiologic research has clarified the prevalence of periodontal disease, provided new insights on its pathogenesis through controlled clinical trials, and focused attention on assessing treatment needs for improving the periodontal health of the public.

One of the most valuable techniques employed in dental epidemiology is the epidemiologic index. *Epidemiologic indices* are attempts to quantitate clinical conditions on a graduated scale, thereby facilitating comparison among populations examined by the same criteria and methods. Unlike the absolute or definitive diagnosis that can be made of disease in a solitary patient, an epidemiologic index (which is a numerical value) estimates only the relative prevalence or occurrence of the clinical condition. (*Prevalence* is the proportion of persons affected by a disease at a specific point in time, as determined by a cross-sectional survey. *Incidence* is defined as the rate of occurrence of new disease in a population during a given interval of time.) In general, indices are actually underestimates of the true clinical condition. A good epidemiologic index must be easy to use, permit the examination of many people in a short period of time, define clinical conditions objectively, be highly reproducible in assessing a clinical condition when used by one or more examiners, be amenable to statistical analysis, and be strongly related numerically to the clinical stages of the specific disease under investigation. Calibration or standardization in reference to the use of an index's criteria by an examiner or examiners is imperative to ensure the reliability of the data.[132]

In general, there are two types of dental indices. The first type of index measures the number or proportion of people in a population with or without a specific condition at a specific point in time or interval of time. The second type of dental index measures the number of people affected and the severity of the specific condition at a specific time or interval of time.[132] More explicitly, the second type of index not only helps to identify the person in the population affected with a specific condition, but also assesses the condition under study on a graduated scale. Most of the indices described in this chapter are of the second type.

INDICES USED TO STUDY PERIODONTAL PROBLEMS

Although there are many indices for recording and quantitating the entities that make up periodontal disease, space limitations permit the inclusion only of indices that historically have contributed to the understanding of periodontal diseases or are currently in frequent use. Two excellent comprehensive reviews of indices not covered in this chapter are available elsewhere.[42,45] A scholarly overview of epidemiologic research in periodontal disease is provided by Ainamo.[5] The indices that are discussed in this chapter can, for the purposes of convenience and reason, be divided according to the following measured variables:

1. The degree of inflammation of the gingival tissues
2. The degree of periodontal destruction
3. The amount of plaque accumulated
4. The amount of calculus present

In addition, indices developed to assess treatment needs will be discussed.

Indices Used to Assess Gingival Inflammation

Papillary-Marginal-Attachment Index. Originally the Papillary-Marginal-Attachment (PMA) Index[144] was used to count the number of gingival units affected with gingivitis.[143,144] This approach was predicated on the belief that the number of units affected correlated with the degree or severity of gingival inflammation. The facial surface of the gingiva around a tooth was divided into three gingival scoring units: the mesial dental papilla (P), the gingival margin (M), and the attached gingiva (A). The presence or absence of inflammation on each gingival unit was recorded as 1 or 0, respectively. The P, M, and A numerical values for all teeth were totaled separately and then added together to express the PMA Index score per person. Although all of the facial tissues surrounding all of the teeth could be assessed in this manner, usually only the maxillary and mandibular incisors, the canines, and the premolars were examined. The developers of this index eventually added a severity component for assessing gingivitis; the papillary units (P) were scored on a scale of 0 to 5, and the marginal (M) and attached (A) gingivae were scored on a scale of 0 to 3.[101]

The value of this index lies in its broad application to epidemiologic surveys and clinical trials and in its capacity for use in individual patients. The criteria for and approach to assessing gingival inflammation developed by Schour and Massler[144] served as the basis for many other indices. Examples of indices that are based on modifications of the PMA Index are those developed by Mühlemann and Mazor,[106] Lobene,[87] and Suomi and Barbano.[157] Excellent reviews of indices of gingivitis have been presented by Ciancio[43] and Fischman.[55]

Periodontal Index. The Periodontal Index (PI)[127] was intended to estimate the extent of deeper periodontal disease than the PMA Index could measure by determining the presence or absence of gingival inflammation and its severity, pocket formation, and masticatory function. The criteria given in Table 5–1 are used to assess all of the gingival tissue circumscribing each tooth (i.e., all of the tissue circumscribing a tooth is considered a scoring or gingival unit). Because the PI measures both reversible and irreversible aspects of periodontal disease, it is an epidemiologic index with a true biologic gradient.[132] A PI score for an individual is determined by adding all of the tooth scores and dividing by the number of teeth examined. Because only a mouth mirror and no calibrated probes or radiographs are used when performing a PI examination, the results tend to underestimate the true level of periodontal disease, especially early bone loss, in a population.[150] The number of periodontal pockets without obvious supragingival calculus is also underestimated in the PI.

The PI is important, because more data have been assembled using it than using any other index of periodontal disease. Thus, much of what is known about the distribution of periodontal disease in the United States and throughout the world resulted from using this index. The PI also was used in the Ten-State Nutrition Survey,[160] the National Health Survey (NHS),[78] the National Health and Nutrition Examination Survey (NHANES I),[76] and the Hispanic Health and Nutrition Examination Survey (HHANES).[71] The NHS and NHANES 1 (NHANES 2 is currently in progress) were the largest health surveys ever conducted in the United States.

Gingivitis Component of the Periodontal Disease Index. The Periodontal Disease Index (PDI)[123] is similar to the PI in that both are used to measure the presence and severity of periodontal disease. The PDI does so by combining the assessments of gingivitis and gingival sulcus depth on six selected teeth (teeth #3, 9, 12, 19, 25, and 28). This group of teeth, frequently referred to as the *Ramfjord teeth,* have been tested as reliable indicators for the various regions of the mouth. Calculus and plaque are also examined to assist in formulating a comprehensive assessment of periodontal status and are described in the following discussions.

The criteria used to assess the tissue circumscribing the Ramfjord teeth combine elements of the PMA Index and the PI and appear in Table 5–2. A numerical score for the gingival status component of the PDI (i.e., the Gingivitis Index score per person) (see following section) is obtained

---

Table 5–1. THE PERIODONTAL INDEX[127]

Score	Criteria and Scoring for Field Studies	Additional Radiographic Criteria Followed in the Clinical Test
0	*Negative.* There is neither overt inflammation in the investing tissues nor loss of function owing to destruction of supporting tissues.	Radiographic appearance is essentially normal.
1	*Mild GIngivitis.* There is an overt area of inflammation in the free gingivae, but this area does not circumscribe the tooth.	
2	*Gingivitis.* Inflammation completely circumscribes the tooth, but there is no apparent break in the epithelial attachment.	
4	(Used when radiographs are available.)	There is early, notch-like resorption of the alveolar crest.
6	*Gingivitis with pocket formation.* The epithelial attachment has been broken, and there is a pocket (not merely a deepened gingival crevice as a result of swelling in free gingivae). There is no interference with normal masticatory function; the tooth is firm and has not drifted.	There is horizontal bone loss involving the entire alveolar crest, up to half of the length of the tooth root.
8	*Advanced destruction with loss of masticatory function.* The tooth may be loose, may have drifted, may sound dull on percussion with a metallic instrument, or may be depressible in its socket.	There is advanced bone loss involving more than one half of the length of the tooth root or a definite infrabony pocket with widening of the periodontal ligament. There may be root resorption or rarefraction at the apex.

RULE: When in doubt, assign the lesser scores.

$$\text{Periodontal index score per person} = \frac{\text{Sum of individual scores}}{\text{Number of teeth present}}$$

Clinical Condition	Group Pi Scores	Stage of Disease
Clinically normal supportive tissues	0 to 0.2	
Simple gingivitis	0.3 to 0.9	
Beginning destructive periodontal disease	0.7 to 1.9	Reversible
Established destructive periodontal disease	1.6 to 5.0	
Terminal disease	3.8 to 8.0	Irreversible

Modified from Russell AL. The periodontal index. J Periodontol *38*:585, 1967.

Table 5-2. CRITERIA FOR SEVERAL COMPONENTS OF THE PERIODONTAL DISEASE INDEX[123]

Gingival status (Gingivitis index)

0 = Absence of signs of inflammation
1 = Mild to moderate inflammatory gingival changes, not extending around the tooth
2 = Mild to moderately severe gingivitis extending all around the tooth
3 = Severe gingivitis characterized by marked redness, swelling, tendency to bleed, and ulceration[124]

Crevicular Measurements

A. If the gingival margin is on the enamel, measure from the gum margin to the cemento-enamel junction and record the measurement. If the epithelial attachment is on the crown and the cemento-enamel junction cannot be felt by the probe, record the depth of the gingival sulcus on the crown. Then record the distance from the gingival margin to the bottom of the pocket if the probe can be moved apically to the cemento-enamel junction without resistance or pain. The distance from the cemento-enamel junction to the bottom of the pocket can then be found by subtracting the first from the second measurement.
B. If the gingival margin is on the cementum, record the distance from the cemento-enamel junction to the gingival margin as a minus value. Then record the distance from the cemento-enamel junction to the bottom of the gingival sulcus as a plus value. Both loss of attachment and actual sulcus depth can easily be assessed from the scores.[124]

Periodontal Disease Index (PDI) Criteria for Surveys

If the gingival sulcus in none of the measured areas extended apically to the cemento-enamel junction, the recorded score for gingivitis is the PDI score for that tooth. If the gingival sulcus in any of the two measured areas extended apically to the cemento-enamel junction but not more than 3 mm (including 3 mm in any area), the tooth is assigned a PDI score of 4. The score for gingivitis is then disregarded in the PDI score for that tooth. If the gingival sulcus in either of the two recorded areas of the tooth extends apically to from 3 to 6 mm (including 6 mm) in relation to the cemento-enamel junction, the tooth is assigned a PDI score of 5 (again, the gingivitis score is disregarded). Whenever the gingival sulcus extends more than 6 mm apically to the cemento-enamel junction in any of the measured areas of the tooth, the score of 6 is assigned as the PDI score for that tooth (again disregarding the gingivitis score).[124]

Shick-Ash Modification[151] of Plaque Criteria

0 = Absence pf dental plaque
1 = Dental plaque in the interproximal area or at the gingival margin covering less than one third of the gingival half of the facial or lingual surface of the tooth
2 = Dental plaque covering more than one third but less than two thirds of the gingival half of the facial or lingual surface of the tooth
3 = Dental plaque covering two thirds or more of the gingival half of the facial or gingival surface of the tooth

Calculus Criteria

0 = Absence of calculus
1 = Supragingival calculus extending only slightly below the free gingival margin (not more than 1 mm)
2 = Moderate amount of supragingival and subgingival calculus or subgingival calculus alone
3 = An abundance of supragingival and subgingival calculus[124]

---

by adding the values for all of the gingival units and dividing by the number of teeth present.[124] The PDI has been used in epidemiologic surveys, longitudinal studies of periodontal disease, and clinical trials of therapeutic or preventive procedures.[62]

Gingival Index. The Gingival Index (GI)[93] was developed solely for the purpose of assessing the severity of gingivitis and its location in four possible areas. The tissues surrounding each tooth are divided into four gingival scoring units: the distofacial papilla, the facial margin, the mesiofacial papilla, and the entire lingual gingival margin. To minimize examiner variability in scoring, the lingual surface is not subdivided, because it will most likely be viewed indirectly with a mouth mirror. A blunt instrument, such as a periodontal pocket probe, is used to assess the bleeding potential of the tissues. Each of the four gingival units is assessed according to the criteria shown in Table 5-3.

Totaling the scores around each tooth yields the GI score for the area. If the scores around each tooth are totaled and divided by four, the GI score for the tooth is obtained. To-

taling all of the scores per tooth and dividing by the number of teeth examined provides the GI score per person. The GI may also be used to evaluate a segment of the mouth or a group of teeth.[89]

The numerical scores of the GI are associated with varying degrees of clinical gingivitis as follows:

GINGIVAL SCORES	DEGREE OF GINGIVITIS
0.1–1.0	Mild
1.1–2.0	Moderate
2.1–3.0	Severe

The index can be used to determine the prevalence and severity of gingivitis in both epidemiologic surveys and in an individual. This latter attribute has contributed to making the GI the index of choice in controlled clinical trials of preventive or therapeutic agents.[62]

Lobene and associates[88] created the modified GI (MGI) by eliminating the bleeding criterion, making the MGI a noninvasive index. By redefining the criteria for mild and moderate inflammation, the MGI increases sensitivity in the

Table 5–3. CRITERIA FOR THE GINGIVAL INDEX,[93] THE PLAQUE INDEX,[152] AND THE MODIFIED GINGIVAL INDEX[88]

Gingival Index (GI)

0 = Normal gingiva
1 = Mild inflammation, slight change in color, slight edema; *no bleeding on palpation*
2 = Moderate inflammation, redness, edema, and glazing; *bleeding on probing**
3 = Severe inflammation, marked redness and edema, ulcerations; *tendency to spontaneous bleeding*[89]

Plaque Index (PI)

0 = No plaque in the gingival area
1 = A film of plaque adhering to the free gingival margin and adjacent area of the tooth. The plaque may be recognized only by running a probe across the tooth surface
2 = Moderate accumulation of soft deposits within the gingival pocket and on the gingival margin and/or adjacent tooth surface that can be seen by the naked eye
3 = Abundance of soft matter within the gingival pocket and/or on the gingival margin and adjacent tooth surface[89]

Modified Gingival Index (MGI)

0 = Absence of inflammation
1 = Mild inflammation; slight change in color, little change in texture of any portion of the marginal or papillary gingival unit
2 = Mild inflammation; criteria as above but involving the entire marginal or papillary gingival unit
3 = Moderate inflammation; glazing, redness, edema, and/or hypertrophy of the marginal or papillary gingival unit
4 = Severe inflammation; marked redness, edema, and/or hypertrophy of the marginal or papillary gingival unit, spontaneous bleeding, congestion, or ulceration

* A periodontal probe is drawn horizontally along the soft tissue wall of the entrance to the gingival sulcus.

lower portion of the scoring scale. The criteria for the MGI are given in Table 5–3.

Indices of Gingival Bleeding. Two indices that combine clinical estimates of inflammation and bleeding have been described. The Sulcus Bleeding Index (SBI) of Mühlemann and Mazor[106] uses bleeding on gentle probing as the first criterion for indicating gingival inflammation. In 1971, Mühlemann and Son[107] added an additional category to the original criteria, resulting in a 0 to 5 scale for assessing inflammation or sulcular bleeding.

Several years later Mühlemann[105] assessed sulcus bleeding on probing at the interdental papilla. This Papillary Bleeding Index (PBI) used a scale of 0 to 4. A timing component was added to the PBI by Barnett and colleagues[16] in an effort to make the PBI more sensitive than the GI in assessing gingival changes.

All of Mühlemann's indices are predicated on an understanding of sulcular bleeding as a precursor of gingival inflammation and as the first sign of inflammation. The GI of Löe and Silness,[93] however, uses the presence of a slight color change and the absence of bleeding when a blunt instrument is used to palpate the soft tissue wall at the gingival margin to indicate initial gingival inflammation. Although the correlation between the two variables (inflammation and bleeding) is not perfect, the histologic evidence for associating inflammation with the GI criteria is stronger than that for associating gingival fluid flow and the SBI. From the epidemiologic viewpoint, it is better to measure single elements than to measure a combination of several. The MGI[88] illustrates how the signs of inflammation and bleeding in the GI were separated.

Several other indices are worthy of mention. The Bleeding Points Index[86] was developed to assess a patient's oral hygiene performance. It determines the presence or absence of gingival bleeding interproximally and on the facial and lingual surfaces of each tooth. A periodontal probe is drawn horizontally through the gingival crevice of a quadrant, and the gingiva is examined for bleeding after 30 seconds.

The Gingival Bleeding Index[39] also assesses the presence or absence of gingival bleeding, but only at the interproximal spaces and using unwaxed dental floss. The floss is thought to assess a larger area more quickly than a periodontal probe, and it can be used by both the professional and the patient when the latter is instructed to perform self-evaluation in a control program.

The Interdental Bleeding Index,[40] also referred to as the Eastman Interdental Bleeding Index, utilizes a triangle-shaped toothpick made of soft, pliable wood to stimulate the interproximal gingival tissue. The presence or absence of bleeding with a specific stimulus permits the dentist and, perhaps more important, the patient to monitor interproximal gingival health. The interproximal cleaner is inserted horizontally between the teeth from the facial surface, depressing the interproximal papilla by up to 2 mm. The wooden cleaner is inserted and removed four times, and the presence or absence of bleeding within 15 seconds is noted. The Interdental Bleeding Index score is determined by dividing the number of bleeding sites by the number of sites evaluated.

The Gingival Bleeding Index (GBI) of Ainamo and Bay[7] was developed as an easy and suitable way for the practitioner to assess a patient's progress in plaque control. The presence or absence of gingival bleeding is determined by gentle probing of the gingival crevice with a periodontal probe. The appearance of bleeding within 10 seconds indicates a positive score, which is expressed as a percentage of the total number of gingival margins examined.

Gingival Index Used by the National Institute of Dental Research. The dichotomous criteria used by the National Institute of Dental Research (NIDR) to assess gingi-

Table 5–4. CRITERIA USED BY THE NIDR TO ASSESS GINGIVAL INFLAMMATION AND CALCULUS[103]

Gingival Inflammation (Bleeding Index)

0 = No bleeding present
1 = Bleeding results after probe is placed in gingival sulcus up to 2 mm and drawn along the inner surface of the gingival sulcus.

Calculus Assessment (Calculus Index)

0 = Calculus is absent
1 = Supragingival calculus,* but no subgingival calculus is present
2 = Supragingival and subgingival calculus, or subgingival calculus only is present

* Supragingival calculus includes calculus located on the exposed crown and root of the tooth and extending to 1 mm below the free gingival margin.

val inflammation (Table 5–4) are the presence or absence of bleeding. Two sites per tooth (mesial-buccal interproximal and mid-buccal on all teeth *excluding* the molars; and mesial-buccal interproximal and mid-buccal of the mesial root of molars) on one half of the maxillary arch and the contralateral half of the mandibular arch are assessed after excess moisture is dried with air. The decision of starting at either the right or left half on the maxillary arch is decided randomly. The NIDR probe (a periodontal probe that is graduated in 2-mm increments, with alternating increments colored in yellow) is gently inserted up to 2 mm into the gingival sulcus at the midpoint of the buccal and then drawn gently into the mesial-buccal interproximal area. After all the sites in both halves of the arches are probed (i.e., the gingival sulcus is palpated), the bleeding sites are counted. This number is divided by the total number of sites assessed and then multiplied by 100 to yield the percentage of sites with gingival bleeding.

In conclusion, the use of gingival bleeding indices is desirable, because bleeding is a more objective indicator than early gingival color changes and provides evidence of recent plaque exposure.[86] In general, the indices that utilize palpation or interproximal cleaning aids are more suitable for the diagnosis of gingivitis and evaluation of a patient's progress in plaque control than are indices that utilize apical probing (i.e., probing to the bottom of the gingival sulcus or pocket). (Palpation refers to the gentle touching of the surface gingival tissue with the blunt end of a periodontal probe and/or the gentle sweeping of the probe in a horizontal direction along the inner surface of the gingival sulcus *without* apical pressure.) The indices that utilize apical probing, however, are more suitable for diagnosing periodontitis and for assessing the effects of subgingival pocket therapy.

Indices Used to Measure Periodontal Destruction

The destruction of bone is still the most important criterion for assessing the severity of periodontal disease.[121] Some of the approaches to measuring bone loss that are discussed are gingival crevice measurements, radiographic evaluations of bone loss, and assessments of gingival recession and tooth mobility.

Gingival Sulcus Measurement Component of the PDI. The technique developed by Ramfjord[124] for determining gingival sulcus depth with a calibrated periodontal probe involves measuring the distance from the cemento-enamel junction to the free gingival margin and the distance from the free gingival margin to the bottom of the gingival sulcus or pocket. The difference between the two measurements yields the clinical attachment level. This is considered the most important clinical measurement (i.e., the "gold standard") in determining the status of the periodontium. Ramfjord's technique is considered useful in epidemiologic surveys, longitudinal studies of periodontal disease, and clinical trials of preventive and therapeutic agents.[125]

The first measurement in this two-step process may be used in assessing gingival loss (recession) or gain. It is considered more accurate and reliable in clinical trials than the Gingival Recession Index used in epidemiologic surveys.[125]

The criteria developed by Ramfjord for making sulcus depth determinations are shown in Table 5–2. The Ramfjord criteria are most applicable to longitudinal studies of periodontal disease and clinical trials of preventive or therapeutic agents. Either the six teeth used by Ramfjord (teeth #3, 9, 12, 19, 25, and 28) or other teeth appropriate to the objective of the study may be assessed. Quadrants of teeth or all teeth should be considered in longitudinal studies.

In an epidemiologic survey (e.g., a cross-sectional survey) in which the purpose is to determine the prevalence of total periodontal disease, only the six index teeth should be used. The set of criteria for a cross-sectional survey is the PDI (see Table 5–2). The PDI score for the individual is obtained by totaling the scores of the teeth and dividing by the number of teeth examined (a maximum of six).[124]

Extent and Severity Index. The Extent and Severity Index (ESI)[38] was developed because of a lack of satisfaction with previous indices of periodontal disease and because of the emergence of a newer conceptual model of periodontal disease pathogenesis developed by Socransky and associates.[153] The older model, the PI, was based on the concept of periodontal disease as a slowly progressing, continuous disease process; it dealt with gingivitis as part of the biologic gradient that extended from health to advanced periodontal disease. In the newer model, periodontal disease is viewed as a chronic process with intermittent periods of activity and remission that affects individual teeth and sites around teeth at different rates within the same mouth. Unlike the PI, which uses a mouth mirror only, the ESI uses a periodontal probe (the NIDR periodontal probe) to determine attachment levels.

The ESI score is a bivariate statistic. It expresses the percentage of sites that exhibit disease (E for Extent) and measures mean attachment loss in millimeters (S for Severity). Hence the ESI = (E,S). Disease is defined arbitrarily as any site with more than 1 mm of attachment loss. Unlike the PI, which examines the tissues surrounding all teeth present, the ESI is based on probe measurements (at the mesio-buccal interproximal and mid-buccal locations on all teeth *excluding* molars and at the mesio-buccal interproximal and mid-buccal of the mesial root of molars) at 14 sites in half of the maxillary arch and at 14 sites in the contralateral mandibular arch. The decision to start at either the right or left half of the maxillary arch is made randomly. Attachment level measurements are made using the criteria of Ramfjord[124] (see Table 5–2). Carlos and coworkers[38] found that interexaminer agreement on site scores was within 1 mm more than 95% of the time. Unlike the PI or PDI, the ESI describes the distribution (extent) of disease.[38] Currently, the NIDR diagnostic criterion includes the methodology of the ESI but has modified the definition of disease to be more than 3 mm of attachment loss.

Radiographic Approaches to Measuring Bone Loss. In general, the use of radiographs in the study of the epidemiology of periodontal disease would appear to overcome some of the criticisms of the more subjective clinical measurements. Radiographs present a permanent objective record of interdental bone levels; in longitudinal studies they may ensure less variability than poorly standardized evaluations by dental examiners, and they offer the only method available for making crown and root measurements. Their disadvantages are that they are not useful in the buccal or lingual assessment of bone level, they do not provide adequate information on soft tissue attachment, and their value may be lost if improper angulation is used.[50] Furthermore, obtaining radiographs of survey participants, without the intent of providing treatment if needed, is unethical.

Only a few indices have been specifically designed to evaluate the radiographic assessment of periodontal disease, but other, more precise techniques for making reasonably accurate measurements from radiographs have been developed.

Of historical interest are indices developed by Dunning and Leach[48] (the Gingival–Bone Count Index), which records the gingival condition on a scale of 0 to 3 and the level of the crest of the alveolar bone, and a similar index by Sheiham and Striffler.[150] The strength of each of these radiographic indices is in epidemiologic surveys in which evaluation time is limited because of large study populations.

The Periodontitis Severity Index (PSI)[2] assesses the presence or absence of periodontitis as the product of clinical inflammation (CIS) and interproximal bone loss (BLS) determined radiographically using a modified Schei ruler.[142] Because of the need for periapical radiographs, the PSI is limited to longitudinal studies and lacks validation.

Indices Used to Measure Plaque Accumulation

In general, most of the indices used to measure plaque accumulation utilize a numerical scale to measure the extent of the surface area of a tooth covered by plaque. For these purposes, plaque is defined as a soft, nonmineralized tooth deposit, which includes debris and materia alba.

Plaque Component of the PDI. The first index that attempted to use a numerical scale to assess the extent of plaque covering the surface area of a tooth was developed by Ramfjord.[124] The plaque component of the PDI is used on the six teeth selected by Ramfjord[124] (teeth #3, 9, 12, 19, 25, and 28) after staining with Bismarck brown solution. The criteria measure the presence and extent of plaque on a scale of 0 to 3, looking specifically at all interproximal facial and lingual surfaces of the index teeth. The criteria are suitable for longitudinal studies of periodontal disease.[124] Even though the plaque component is not a part of the PDI score, it is helpful in a total assessment of periodontal status.

Shick and Ash[151] modified the original criteria of Ramfjord[124] by excluding consideration of the interproximal areas of the teeth and "restricting the scoring of plaque to the gingival half"[125] of the facial and lingual surfaces of the index teeth. The criteria for the Shick-Ash modification of the Ramfjord plaque criteria are shown in Table 5–2.

The plaque score per person is obtained by totaling all of the individual tooth scores and dividing by the number of teeth examined. These modified plaque criteria are suitable for clinical trials of preventive or therapeutic agents.

Simplified Oral Hygiene Index. Greene and Vermillion[66] developed the Oral Hygiene Index (OHI) in 1960 and later simplified it to include only six tooth surfaces that were representative of all anterior and posterior segments of the mouth. This modification was called the Simplified OHI (OHI-S).[67] The OHI-S measures the surface area of the tooth that is covered by debris and calculus. The imprecise term *debris* was used because it was not practical to distinguish among plaque, debris, and materia alba. In addition, the practicality of determining the weight and thickness of the soft deposits prompted the assumption that the dirtier the mouth is, the greater is the tooth surface area covered by debris. This assumption also implied a time factor, because the longer oral hygiene practices are neglected, the greater the likelihood that the surface area of the tooth will be covered by debris.

The OHI-S consists of two components: a Simplified Debris Index (DI-S) and a Simplified Calculus Index (CI-S). Each component is assessed on a scale of 0 to 3. Only a mouth mirror and a shepherd's crook or sickle type dental explorer, and no disclosing agent, are used for the examination. The six tooth surfaces examined in the OHI-S are the facial surfaces of teeth #3, 8, 14, and 24 and the lingual surfaces of teeth #19 and 30. Each tooth surface is divided horizontally into gingival, middle, and incisal thirds. For the DI-S, a dental explorer is placed on the incisal third of the tooth and moved toward the gingival third according to the criteria in Table 5–5. The DI-S score per person is obtained by totaling the debris score per tooth surface and dividing by the number of surfaces examined.

The CI-S assessment is performed by gently placing a dental explorer into the distal gingival crevice and drawing it subgingivally from the distal contact area to the mesial contact area (one half of a tooth's circumference is considered a scoring unit). The criteria for scoring the calculus component of the OHI-S are given in Table 5–5. The CI-S

Table 5–5. CRITERIA FOR SCORING THE ORAL DEBRIS (DI-S) AND CALCULUS (CI-S) COMPONENTS OF THE SIMPLIFIED ORAL HYGIENE INDEX (OHI-S)[67]

Oral Debris Index (DI-S)

0 = No debris or stain present
1 = Soft debris covering not more than one third of the tooth surface or the presence of extrinsic stains without other debris, regardless of surface area covered
2 = Soft debris covering more than one third but not more than two thirds of the exposed tooth surface
3 = Soft debris covering more than two thirds of the exposed tooth surface

Calculus Index (CI-S)

0 = No calculus present
1 = Supragingival calculus covering not more than one third of the exposed tooth surface
2 = Supragingival calculus covering more than one third but not more than two thirds of the exposed tooth surface or the presence of individual flecks of subgingival calculus around the cervical portion of the tooth, or both
3 = Supragingival calculus covering more than two thirds of the exposed tooth surface or a continuous heavy band of subgingival calculus around the cervical portion of the tooth, or both

score per person is obtained by totaling the calculus scores per tooth surface and dividing by the number of surfaces examined. The OHI-S score per person is the total of the DI-S and CI-S scores per person.

The clinical levels of oral cleanliness for debris that can be associated with group DI-S scores are as follows:[65]

Good	0.0–0.6
Fair	0.7–1.8
Poor	1.9–3.0

The clinical levels of oral hygiene that can be associated with group OHI-S scores are as follows:[65]

Good	0.0–1.2
Fair	1.3–3.0
Poor	3.1–6.0

The importance of the OHI-S is that, like the PI of Russell,[127] it has been used extensively throughout the world and has contributed greatly to the understanding of periodontal disease. It was also used in the Ten-State Nutrition Survey,[160] NHS,[79] NHANES I,[76] and HHANES.[71] The high degree of correlation ($r = 0.82$)[146] between the OHI-S and the PI makes it possible, if one of the two scores is known, to calculate the other score with regression analysis.[64] The major strength of the OHI-S is its use in epidemiologic surveys and in evaluation of dental health education programs (longitudinal studies). It can also evaluate an individual's level of oral cleanliness and can, to a more limited extent, be used in clinical trials. The index is easy to use because the criteria are objective, the examination may be performed quickly, and a high level of reproducibility is possible with a minimum of training sessions.[65]

Turesky-Gilmore-Glickman[161] Modification of the Quigley-Hein[122] Plaque Index. In 1962 Quigley and Hein[122] reported a plaque measurement that focused on the gingival third of the tooth surface. They examined only the facial surfaces of the anterior teeth, using a basic fuchsin mouthwash as a disclosing agent and a numerical scoring system of 0 to 5. Turesky and colleagues[161] strengthened the objectivity of the Quigley-Hein criteria by redefining the scores of the gingival third area. The Turesky-Gilmore-Glickman modification of the Quigley-Hein criteria appears in Table 5–6. Plaque was assessed on the facial and lingual surfaces of all of the teeth after using a disclosing agent. A plaque score per person was obtained by totaling all of the plaque scores and dividing by the number of surfaces examined. This system of scoring plaque is relatively easy to use because of the objective definitions of each numerical score. The strength of this plaque index is its application to longitudinal studies and clinical trials of preventive and therapeutic agents. The Turesky-Gilmore-Glickman modification of the Quigley-Hein criteria is considered one of the two indices of choice when assessing plaque in clinical trials.[54]

Plaque Index. The Plaque Index (PII)[152] is unique among the indices described so far because it ignores the coronal extent of plaque on the tooth surface area and assesses only the thickness of plaque at the gingival area of the tooth. Because it was developed as a component to parallel the GI of Löe and Silness,[93] it examines the same scoring units of the teeth: distofacial, facial, mesiofacial,

Table 5–6. TURESKY-GILMORE-GLICKMAN[161] MODIFICATION OF THE QUIGLEY-HEIN[122] PLAQUE INDEX

0 = No plaque
1 = Separate flecks of plaque at the cervical margin of the tooth
2 = A thin, continuous band of plaque (up to 1 mm) at the cervical margin
3 = A band of plaque wider than 1 mm but covering less than one third of the crown
4 = Plaque covering at least one third but less than two thirds of the crown
5 = Plaque covering two thirds or more of the crown[97]

and lingual surfaces. A mouth mirror and a dental explorer are used after air drying of the teeth to assess plaque. Unlike most indices, the PlI does not exclude or substitute for teeth with gingival restorations or crowns. Either all or only selected teeth may be used in the PlI. The criteria for the PlI of Silness and Löe are given in Table 5–3.

The PlI score for the area is obtained by totaling the four plaque scores per tooth. If the sum of the PlI scores per tooth is divided by four, the PlI score for the tooth is obtained. The PlI score per person is obtained by adding the PlI scores per tooth and dividing by the number of teeth examined. The PlI may be obtained for a segment of the mouth or a group of teeth in a similar manner.

The strength of the PlI is in its application to longitudinal studies and clinical trials. In spite of the studies that have been conducted to ensure the reliability of PlI data, the assessment of plaque thickness is so subjective that obtaining valid data requires highly trained and experienced examiners.[97,98]

Other Plaque Indices. The Modified Navy Plaque Index[49] records the presence or absence of plaque with a score of 1 or 0, respectively, on nine areas of each tooth surface of the six index teeth used by Ramfjord.[124] Like the Patient Hygiene Performance (PHP) Index of Podshadley and Haley,[120] the Modified Navy Plaque Index is of value in assessing health education programs and the ability of individuals to perform oral hygiene practices. A variation of the Modified Navy Plaque Index is the Distal Mesial Plaque Index (DMPI), which places more emphasis on the gingival and interproximal areas of a tooth.[56] Plaque is one of the two factors measured in the Irritants Index,[110,112] which is a component of the Gingival Periodontal Index (GPI) of O'Leary and associates.[112] The presence and coronal extent of plaque are scored on a scale of 0 to 3. Other factors that contribute to the Irritants Index are supragingival and subgingival calculus and subgingival irritants, such as overhanging or deficient restorations.

PHP Index. The PHP Index[120] was the first index developed for the sole purpose of assessing an individual's performance in removing debris after toothbrushing instruction. It records the presence or absence of debris as 1 or 0, respectively, using the six surfaces of the six OHI-S teeth. The PHP Index is more sensitive than the OHI-S because it divides each tooth surface into five areas: three longitudinal thirds, with the middle third subdivided horizontally into thirds. Scoring is preceded by the use of a disclosing agent. The index is easy to use because its criteria are dichotomous and it can be performed quickly. Its value lies chiefly in its application to individual patient education.

Two other indices with a similar purpose that also use dichotomous criteria are the Plaque Control Record[111] and the plaque portion of the Bleeding Points Index.[86]

Bjorby and Löe[23] developed a Retention Index that not only examined supragingival and subgingival calculus, but also grossly assessed dental caries and the quality of the margins of restorations. Collectively, all of these variables were scored on a numerical scale of 0 to 3.[89]

Indices Used to Measure Calculus

In general, the indices used to assess calculus may be conveniently divided into those that are most appropriate to epidemiologic surveys; those that are appropriate to longitudinal studies, with an examination every 3 to 6 months; and those that are used in short-term clinical studies, usually no longer than 6 weeks.

Calculus Component of the Simplified Oral Hygiene Index. The Simplified Calculus Index (CI-S)[67] component of the OHI-S was previously discussed with indices used to measure plaque accumulation because it is less separable from the combined scoring system than are any of the other indices that include several component measures. The value of the CI-S component is its application to epidemiologic surveys and longitudinal studies of periodontal disease.[65] Table 5–5 presents the specific criteria of the OHI-S used to assess calculus.

Calculus Component of the Periodontal Disease Index. The calculus component of the PDI[123] assesses the presence and extent of calculus on the facial and lingual surfaces of Ramfjord's six index teeth (i.e., teeth #3, 9, 12, 19, 25, and 28) on a numerical scale of 0 to 3. A mouth mirror and a dental explorer and/or a periodontal probe are used in the examination. The criteria for assigning a score to each tooth surface for the calculus component of the PDI are given in Table 5–2.

The calculus scores per tooth are totaled and then divided by the number of teeth examined to yield the calculus score per person. Like the CI-S of the OHI-S, the calculus component of the PDI has a high degree of examiner reproducibility, can be performed quickly, and has its best application in epidemiologic surveys and longitudinal studies.[124]

Probe Method of Calculus Assessment. The Probe Method of Calculus Assessment[163] was developed for longitudinal studies of the quantity of supragingival calculus formed. A periodontal probe graduated in millimeter divisions is used to measure the deposits of calculus on the lingual surfaces of the six mandibular anterior teeth. The Probe Method of Calculus Assessment has been shown to possess a high degree of inter- and intraexaminer reproducibility. However, extensive training under an experienced investigator is required to master it.[162]

Calculus Surface Index. The Calculus Surface Index (CSI)[53] is one of two indices that are used in short-term (e.g., less than 6 weeks) clinical trials of calculus-inhibiting agents. The objective of this type of study is to determine rapidly whether a specific agent has any effect on reducing or preventing supragingival or subgingival calculus. The CSI assesses the presence or absence of supragingival and/or subgingival calculus on the four mandibular incisors. The index has also been applied to the six mandibular anterior teeth. The presence or absence of calculus is determined by visual examination or by tactile examination using a mouth mirror and a sickle type dental explorer.

A companion index to the CSI is the Calculus Surface Severity Index (CSSI).[53] The CSSI measures the quantity of calculus present on the surfaces examined for the CSI.

Marginal Line Calculus Index. A second index that is frequently used in short-term clinical trials of anticalculus agents is the Marginal Line Calculus Index (MLCI).[108] This index was developed to assess the accumulation of supragingival calculus on the gingival third of the tooth or, more specifically, supragingival calculus along the margin of the gingiva.

Calculus Index Used by NIDR. The NIDR uses a three-point ordinal scale for the assessment of calculus (see Table 5–4). Unlike the NIDR gingival assessment, the Calculus Index[103] assigns only one score per tooth, after examining both the mid-buccal and mesial-buccal interproximal sites, on one half of the maxillary and one half of the contralateral mandibular arch. As in the gingival assessment, the decision to start at either the right or left half of the maxillary arch is made randomly. Both sites are examined for the presence and extent of calculus (with either the NIDR periodontal probe or a no. 17 dental explorer) after all of the teeth in one half of an arch are air dried. The Calculus Index score is obtained by dividing the score for each tooth by the number of teeth examined.

Indices Used to Assess Treatment Needs

Interpretations of the indices described in this section are to be viewed with caution because of the difficulty that exists concerning the estimation of treatment needs. Without knowing the response of the periodontal tissues to phase 1 or initial therapy, any estimate of treatment needs may be subject to over- or underestimation of what is clinically prudent.

GPI. The GPI[112] is a modification of the PDI of Ramfjord[123] for the purpose of screening persons to determine who needs periodontal treatment. The GPI assesses three components of periodontal disease: gingival status; periodontal status (crevice depth); and, collectively, materia alba, calculus, and overhanging restorations. The latter triad is independently called the Irritation Index. Only the criteria for the gingival status component are described.

The maxillary and mandibular arches are each divided into three segments: the six anterior teeth, the left posterior teeth, and the right posterior teeth. The primary objective in using the index is to determine the tooth or surrounding tissues with the severest condition within each of the six segments. Each segment is assessed for each of the three components of periodontal disease described previously. The specific criteria for the gingival status component of the GPI are as follows:

  0 = tissue tightly adapted to the teeth; firm consistency with physiologic architecture.
  1 = slight to moderate inflammation, as indicated by changes in color and consistency, involving one or more teeth in the same segment but not completely surrounding any one tooth.
  2 = the above changes either singly or combined completely encircling one or more teeth in a segment.
  3 = marked inflammation, as indicated by loss of surface

continuity (ulceration), spontaneous hemorrhage, loss of faciolingual continuity or any interdental papilla, marked deviation from normal contour (such as gross thickening or enlargement covering more than one third of the anatomic crown), recession, and clefts.

The area with the highest score determines the gingival score for the entire segment, and the gingival status for the mouth is obtained by dividing the sum of the gingival scores by the number of segments.

The GPI has been used extensively in military populations. Unlike the traditional indices used in epidemiology (which attempt primarily to assess the status of a specific disease condition, with only the crudest suggestion of determining treatment needs), the GPI was developed for the specific purpose of detecting periodontal disease early so that treatment may be instituted promptly.[110]

Periodontal Treatment Need System. The next index to evolve with the purpose of assessing treatment needs was the Periodontal Treatment Need System (PTNS),[19] which has been used with interesting results.[20,62] It attempts to place individuals into one of four classes based on treatment procedures relative to time requirements. It considers the presence or absence of gingivitis and plaque and the presence of pockets 5 mm or deeper in each quadrant of the mouth, as shown in Table 5–7.

Community Periodontal Index of Treatment Needs. In 1977, the World Health Organization (WHO) appointed an expert committee to review the methods available to assess periodontal status and treatment needs.[166] The index that resulted after extensive field testing by investigators from the WHO and the International Dental Federation (FDI) was called the *Community Periodontal Index of Treatment Needs* (CPITN).[6] The CPITN was "primarily designed to assess periodontal treatment needs rather than periodontal status."[6] Combining elements of the GPI and PTNS, the CPITN assesses the presence or absence of gingival bleeding on gentle probing; the presence or absence of supragingival or subgingival calculus; and the presence or absence of periodontal pockets, subdivided into shallow and deep. A specially designed periodontal probe with a 0.5-mm ball tip and gradations corresponding to shallow and deep pockets was developed to probe for bleeding and calculus and to determine pocket depth. In epidemiologic surveys, 10 index teeth are examined, but only the worst finding from the index teeth is recorded per sextant of teeth. In determining the treatment needs of individual patients, only the worst finding from all of the teeth in a sextant is recorded, resulting in six scores. The CPITN criteria for determining periodontal status and the corresponding treatment needs ap-

Table 5–7. CRITERIA FOR THE PERIODONTAL TREATMENT NEED SYSTEM (PTNS) CLASSIFICATION

PTNS Classification	Unit	Plaque	Calculus and/or Overhangs	Inflammation	Pocket Depth
Class O	Mouth	No	No	No	Not considered
Class A	Mouth	Yes	No	Yes	≤ 5 mm
Class B	Quadrant	Yes	Yes	Yes	< 5 mm
Class C	Quadrant	Yes	Yes	Yes	> 5 mm

Adapted from A system to classify the need for periodontal treatment, by Johansen JR, Gjermo P, Bellini HT, from Acta Odontol Scand, 1973 *31*:297, by permission of Scandinavian University Press.

Table 5–8. CRITERIA FOR THE COMMUNITY PERIODONTAL INDEX OF TREATMENT NEEDS

Periodontal Status[166]	Treatment Needs[6]
0 = Healthy periodontium	0 = No treatment needed
1 = Bleeding observed, directly or by using mouth mirror, after sensing	I = Oral hygiene needs improvement
2 = Calculus felt during probing, but the entire black area* of the probe is visible	II = I + professional scaling
3 = Pocket 4 or 5 mm (gingival margin is situated on black area* of probe)	II = I + professional scaling
4 = Pocket > 6 mm (black area* of probe *not* visible)	III = I + II + complex treatment†

* Portion of probe between 3.5 and 5.5 mm.
† Complex treatment may require scaling and root planing under local anesthesia, with or without surgical exposure for access.

pear in Table 5–8. Each subject or sextant of teeth is classified according to one of the treatment needs.

The value of the CPITN is that it permits rapid examination of a population to determine periodontal treatment needs. However, a lot of effort is expended and a great deal of useful information is lost when only the worst score per sextant is recorded. Gaengler and colleagues[61] found that the CPITN underestimated the number of pockets larger than 6 mm in older age groups and overestimated the need for scaling in younger age groups. The American Academy of Periodontology (AAP) has proposed the use of the CPITN for individual patients as a periodontal screening and recording (PSR) tool for general practitioners.

RELIABILITY OF DENTAL INDICES

In the context of epidemiologic indices, the term *reliability* means the ability of a dental index to measure a condition in the same subject repeatedly and obtain the same score results each time. The definition implies that reliability is a matter of degree, because all measurements are subject to error (method and observer) or variability. Replicate (repeat) examinations by one examiner will assess intraexaminer variability, whereas duplicate examinations by two or more examiners will assess interexaminer variability. The most obvious implications of unreliable measures are that prevalence estimates (from surveys) become questionable when comparisons are made between groups and that measurements from longitudinal studies may no longer reveal the likelihood of differences between treatment and control groups. Reliability is considered a more general term than reproducibility or repeatability, the latter of which is usually restricted to repeat examination data.[126]

The literature describing the reliability of the indices used in measuring periodontal disease and oral hygiene status, in contrast to similar literature about dental caries, is sparse. Clemmer and Barbano[44] described several statistical techniques used in assessing intra- and interexaminer reproducibility of periodontal scores. They discussed the proportion of agreement (similarity or "alikeness" on each unit scored), the paired *t* test, the analysis of variance (ANOVA), and the correlation coefficient. The last three tests measure the alikeness of the average score per person.

The κ statistic may be applied to quantitative data (e.g., attachment level measurements and intraclass correlation coefficients) and to qualitative data (e.g., dichotomous criteria).[58,59] The κ statistic corrects "the observed proportion

of agreement for the proportion of agreement to be expected by chance alone."[59] Fleiss[57] described the interpretation of κ statistics as: excellent agreement beyond chance when κs are >0.75; fair to good agreement for κs between 0.40 and 0.75; and poor agreement for κs <0.40. Reports suggest that even when studies are conducted well, κ statistics may not always meet these high criteria. The reasons for this variance are (1) the condition under observation may result in different levels of agreement by chance; (2) the examination process may influence or be influenced by the severity of the clinical condition under observation; (3) the time interval between the first and second examinations (e.g., the examination process may influence the clinical condition if the time between observations is too short, or the clinical condition may change if the time between observations is too long); and (4) the physical environment (i.e., office or field conditions) in which the examination is conducted may influence the outcome of duplicate examinations.[82]

To ensure the reliability of periodontal indices, all studies should incorporate measures of reliability into the study design. Because there is no agreement as to the best statistical method for describing reliability, several methods should be used.

DESCRIPTIVE EPIDEMIOLOGY OF GINGIVAL AND PERIODONTAL DISEASE

Prevalence of Gingivitis*

A review of prevalence data from surveys in the United States conducted between 1960 and 1985 (Table 5–9) illustrates the difficulty in stating a precise prevalence for gingivitis and, to a lesser extent, interpreting trend changes. Although it is tempting to say that the prevalence figures for gingivitis in Table 5–9 suggest a decrease in gingivitis when compared with figures from earlier surveys, changes in examination criteria, sampling techniques, and age-specific grouping of data make true comparisons impossible and trend changes speculative. In general, the prevalence and severity of gingivitis increase with age (Table 5–10), beginning at approximately 5 years of age,[160] reaching their highest point in puberty,[22] and then gradually decreasing but remaining relatively high throughout life.[76] Hence, the highest prevalence of gingivitis occurs during puberty.

* The reader is referred to an excellent review on the epidemiology of gingivitis by Stamm.[154]

Table 5–9. PREVALENCE* OF GINGIVITIS AND PERIODONTITIS IN ADULTS 18
TO 80[†] YEARS OF AGE IN U.S. SURVEYS, 1960 TO 1985

Condition	NHES[78] (1960–1962)[†]	NHANES1[76] (1971–1974)[‡]	HRSA-DHOP[25,31] (1981)[§]	NIDR[103] (1985)[∥]
No disease	26.1	45.4	14.8	42.1 (30.0)
Gingivitis	48.5	20.7	49.2	43.6 (46.9)
Periodontitis	25.4[¶]	33.9[¶]	36.0[#]	14.3 (22.2)[#]
Total with disease	73.9	54.6	85.2	57.9 (69.1)

* Percentages may not total 100 because of rounding.
[†] Persons age 18–79 yrs
[‡] Persons age 18–74 yrs
[§] Persons age 19–65[+] yrs
[∥] Persons age 18–64[+] yrs and 65–80[+] yrs
[¶] Periodontal disease with one or more pockets
[#] One or more pockets ≥ 4 mm
HRSA-DHOP = Health Resources & Services Administration–Dental Health Outcomes related to dental Prepayment

Data from NHANES I suggest that there was a dramatic decrease in the prevalence of gingivitis in the early 1970s: for children 6 to 11 years of age (see Table 5–10), from 38% to 13.6%; for adolescents 12 to 17 years, from 62% to 32.2%; and for adults 18 to 74 years (see Table 5–9), from 48.5% to 20.7%.[76]

Almost a decade later (see Table 5–10), Ismail and colleagues[71] found a higher percentage of gingivitis (80%) in children 6 to 17 years of age in HHANES. Using an index of gingival bleeding instead of the PI, Wolfe and Carlos[165] found that 70.6% of 14- to 19-year-old Navajo Indians had gingivitis.

The prevalence of gingivitis (defined as at least one bleeding site) in employed adults 18 to 64 years of age in the NIDR survey (see Table 5–9) was 43.6% (with 5.8% of sites with bleeding); in senior adults (65 to 80 years of age and older), the prevalence of gingivitis was 46.9% (with 10.3% of sites with bleeding).[103]

Speculation about the causes of the dramatic decrease in gingivitis (see Table 5–9) from the NHES (1960–1962) to the NHANES I (1971–1974) included many variables (e.g., oral hygiene, fluoride intake, diet, preventive care, lifestyle, and antibiotic intake).[115] A concomitant decrease in oral hygiene scores from the same surveys, in conjunction with an increase in preventive services, provided some basis for ex-

plaining a decrease in gingivitis prevalence. The decrease may be partially attributed to a departure from the criteria originally applied by the examiners, even though both surveys employed the PI. This is especially true in the lower end of the PI scale that classifies the presence or absence of gingivitis and its severity. Although some decrease in prevalence may have occurred between the two surveys, the magnitude of the decrease prompts caution in interpreting the data.

Prevalence of Periodontitis*

On a worldwide basis, the United States ranks relatively low in the magnitude and prevalence of periodontitis. Table 5–11 shows mean PI scores by various population groups throughout the world. Compared with that in South America and the Asian countries, the severity of periodontal disease in people in the United States is relatively low.[131] Evidence for the belief that the prevalence of severe periodontitis is greater in underdeveloped countries than industrialized countries, however, is currently not as clear-cut as once thought.[118,119,149]

---

* The reader is referred to an insightful description of periodontal disease over time by Löe and associates.[91]

Table 5–10. PREVALENCE OF GINGIVITIS* FOR PERSONS 6 TO 65[+] YEARS
OF AGE IN U.S. SURVEYS, 1960 TO 1987

Survey (Year)	Age (yr)				
	6–11	12–17	18–44	45–64	65[+]
NHES (1960–1962)[78]	—	—	51.8	43.7	40.1[†]
NHES (1963–1965)[77]	37.9	—	—	—	—
NHES (1966–1970)[137]	—	62.1	—	—	—
NHANES1 (1971–1974)[76]	13.6	32.2	28.6	17.0	13.5
HRSA-DHOP (1981)[25,31]	—	—	53.9	44.2	36.3
HHANES (1982–1983)[71]	78.4	81.3	—	—	—
NIDR (1985)[103]	—	—	44.8	41.1	46.9[‡]
NIDR (1986–1987)[22]	—	58.8[§]	—	—	—

* Gingival inflammation without pockets
[†] Persons age 65–79 yrs
[‡] Persons age 65–80[+] yrs
[§] Persons age 14–17 yrs
HRSA-DHOP = Health Resources & Services Administration–Dental Health Outcomes related to dental Prepayment

Table 5–11. AVERAGE PERIODONTAL INDEX
SCORES IN CIVILIANS (BOTH SEXES)
40 TO 49 YEARS OF AGE SURVEYED BY
EXAMINERS OF THE NIDR

Population Group	Average Periodontal Index Score
Baltimore, MD (whites)	1.03
Colorado Springs, CO	1.04*
Alaska (primitive Eskimos)	1.17†
Ecuador	1.85
Ethiopia	1.86
Baltimore, MD (blacks)	1.99
Uganda	2.50‡
Vietnam (Vietnamese)	2.18
Colombia	2.21
Alaska (urban Eskimos)	2.31†
Chile	2.74
Lebanon (Lebanese)	2.98
Thailand	3.30
Lebanon (Palestinian refugees)	3.52
Burma	3.58
Jordan (Jordanian civilians)	3.96
Vietnam (Hill tribesmen)	3.97
Trinidad	4.21
Jordan (Palestinian refugees)	4.41

* Ages 40 to 44 only
† Males only
‡ Persons over 40 only
Modified from Russell AL. The periodontal index. J Periodontol *38*:585, 1967.

Table 5–9 summarizes the relative magnitude of periodontal disease from 1960 to 1985 as measured by the largest surveys conducted in the United States: two National Center for Health Statistics (NCHS) surveys, the NHES[78] and the NHANES I[76]; the Health Resources and Services Administration survey on the Dental Health Outcomes related to dental Prepayment (HRSA-DHOP)[25,31]; and the NIDR survey of the oral health of U.S. adults.[103] The NCHS surveys shared a common examination criterion (PI) that was applied to all teeth present and a sampling design (a national probability sample of households) that was representative of the noninstitutionalized civilian population. The HRSA-DHOP survey (based on a multistage probability sample of households) used the gingivitis criteria of the PI and a calibrated periodontal probe to determine moderate and severe pockets. The NIDR survey measured attachment level, pocket depths, gingival bleeding on palpation at two sites per tooth, and supragingival and subgingival calculus at one site per tooth on one maxillary quadrant and one mandibular quadrant. Instead of selecting households for its sample, the NIDR survey selected business establishments (adults 18 to 64 years of age or older) and multipurpose senior centers (senior adults 65 to 80 years of age and older). The shortcoming of the NIDR sampling method is that it excluded certain groups, such as senior adults not visiting senior centers, self-employed workers, unpaid family workers, agricultural and mining workers, college and graduate students, and the unemployed.[37] The measurements selected by the NIDR are consistent with current understanding of gingival and periodontal pathogenesis and are therefore appropriate. However, they are still underestimates of the true conditions because they are based on only two examination sites per tooth (instead of the usual six sites examined for probing depth), only half of the mouth is examined, and the sample is different. The definition of periodontitis, or the point at which health becomes disease, confounds an accurate prevalence value. Because of the fundamental differences between the NCHS, HRSA, and NIDR surveys, it is impossible to make direct comparisons between the surveys, and even indirect comparisons should be viewed with caution. The NIDR data are presented because they are the most current information available and because of the changes in measurement of periodontal disease that they exemplify.

In the oldest of the surveys (NHES[78]; see Table 5–9), one of four adults (25.4%) had destructive periodontal disease (one or more pockets).[78] Approximately 10 years later, the NHANES I data suggested that one of three adults (33.9%) had destructive periodontal disease.[76] There was a decrease in overall disease prevalence, which was attributed to a decrease in gingivitis (see preceding discussion). The prevalence of destructive disease, however, appeared slightly higher. The HRSA-DHOP survey also suggested that approximately one of three adults (36%) had one or more pockets greater than 4 mm.[25,31] Using the same criteria as the HRSA, the NIDR data showed that among employed adults (18 to 64 years), one of seven (14.3%) had destructive periodontal disease. Even though the prevalence of destructive disease appears low (14.3%), the percentage of adults in the NIDR sample who had dental insurance was 57.9% (31.6% for those 65 years of age and older). These percentages of dentally insured adults are significantly higher than those during the 1960s and 1970s.[60] If the percentage of adults with destructive periodontal disease is 14.3% in a sample that is heavily weighted with employed people who have dental insurance, then the prevalence of destructive disease would very likely be higher in a probability sample in which the proportion of dentally insured adults is lower. The percentage of sites (i.e., the distribution of sites) with pockets greater than 4 mm was 10.9% among employed adults. Among senior adults (65 to 80 years of age), one of five (22.2%) had destructive disease, and for senior adults the percentage of sites with pockets greater than 4 mm was 13.7%.[103]

The prevalence of edentulous adults over the span of these three surveys gradually diminished from 18.8%[73] to 14.7%[69] to 4.2% in employed adults (41.1% in senior adults) by 1985.[103] This decreasing trend in the prevalence of edentulous adults illustrates that more persons are retaining a greater number of their teeth throughout their lifetimes. However, as the proportion of older persons increases, more teeth will be at risk to periodontal disease. The fact that fewer teeth were being extracted suggests that the periodontal status of adults was improving over the span of these three surveys. One interesting observation from the NHES (1960–1962) was that adults who had teeth in only one arch had more severe periodontal disease than persons with some teeth in both arches.[78] The converse of this should be that the severity of periodontal disease may decrease as the trend to longer tooth retention increases among more persons. However, even if the severity of periodontal disease decreases in the future, the prevalence may remain relatively constant or even increase. The NIDR data should be thought of as a baseline until a second survey using the same criteria and sample design is conducted.

Prevalence of Juvenile Periodontitis

Before the NIDR survey of children,[33] two radiographic studies of 16-year-old adolescents and one clinicoradiographic study of 15- to 19-year-old persons showed a prevalence of 0.1%.[85,139,140,141] The first two studies surveyed whites only, but the third study included other ethnic groups and reported the following prevalence rates: whites, 0.02%; Afro-Caribbeans, 0.8%; and Asians, 0.2%. Earlier studies do not differentiate juvenile periodontitis from other periodontal diseases.

Using loss of periodontal attachment to classify adolescents (14 to 17 years of age), the NIDR survey of children found that 0.53% had localized juvenile periodontitis (LJP), 0.13% had generalized juvenile periodontitis (GJP), and 1.61% had incidental loss of attachment (at least one tooth with 3 or more mm of attachment loss).[92] The teeth most severely affected, in descending order, were the first molars, second molars, and incisors.

The age group that appears to be most affected by juvenile periodontitis consists of those between puberty and approximately 30 years of age.[74,134] In general, blacks were more likely to have LJP and GJP than whites. Males were more likely to have GJP than females. Black males were more likely to have LJP than black females, whereas white females were more likely to have LJP than white males. The estimated incidence for GJP and LJP is 1.5 cases per 1000 person-years at risk.[92] For further discussion of this disease, see Chapter 27.

RISK FACTORS AFFECTING THE PREVALENCE AND SEVERITY OF GINGIVITIS AND PERIODONTITIS

Age. The prevalence of periodontal disease increases directly with increasing age.[131] This is not to imply that aging causes an increase in the prevalence, extent, and severity of periodontal disease, because cross-sectional descriptive data can only suggest associations between variables and cannot prove cause-and-effect relationships. The progression and accumulative effects of periodontal disease are more severe in older adults. Both cross-sectional and longitudinal data support the diminishing importance of age as a risk factor.[1,91] Figure 5–1 shows the distribution of periodontal disease using the gold standard of attachment loss to illustrate this pattern. Specifically, Figure 5–1 shows the prevalence (percentage of persons) and extent (mean number of sites) of loss of attachment (LA) ≥3 mm in adults according to age. The percentage of persons with LA ≥3 mm starts at approximately 16% in the 18- to 24-year-old age group and gradually rises to 83% in the 55- to 64-year-old age group. The combined percentage for the entire age range (18 to 64 years) is 44%. The extent or average number of sites (LA ≥ 3 mm) for the same age-specific groups starts at four and increases to 10, with an overall average of eight sites for the 18- to 64-year-old age group. If other variables, such as one or more pockets or pockets ≥4 mm, were used to examine prevalence, the pattern would be the same.

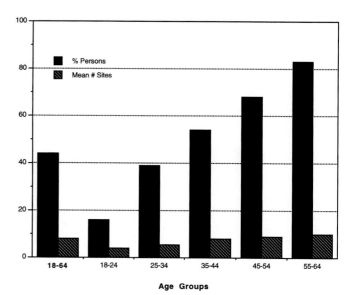

FIGURE 5–1. Prevalence and extent of attachment loss by age. Data are from NIDR survey of employed adults (18–64 years), 1985.[114] Loss of attachment (LA) was defined as ≥3 mm. The solid bars refer to the percentage of persons with LA ≥ 3 mm (prevalence), and the hashed bars refer to the mean number of sites with LA ≥ 3 mm (extent).

In the NIDR survey of adults, the prevalence of pockets >4 mm among employed adults was approximately 6% at 20 years of age and 13% at 35 years and among senior adults was 22% at 70 years of age.[103] Similar patterns were observed in previous surveys.[76–78,136]

This pattern of disease with pockets closely parallels that of the reduction in bone height that occurs with increasing age.[100] Although destructive periodontal disease is primarily a disease of adults, its onset during puberty has been observed with greater frequency in countries other than the United States.[129,136]

The severity of periodontal disease, as indicated by mean attachment loss in millimeters, increases directly with age (Fig. 5–2). Among employed adults, mean attachment loss started at 1.2 mm in the 18- to 24-year-old age group and increased gradually to 3.6 mm in the 75- to 80 +-year-old senior group.[103] Mean PI scores in previous surveys, showed a similar pattern.[73,76,78]

Sex. In general, males consistently have a higher prevalence and severity of periodontal disease than females. In earlier surveys the difference between males and females was slight before 20 years of age.[76,77,136] A comparison of periodontal disease severity (mean attachment loss) by sex (Fig. 5–3) in the NIDR survey reveals that males consistently experience more severe periodontal disease than females and average approximately 10% higher attachment loss in millimeters than females from 18 to 80 + years of age.[103] A similar pattern was observed in earlier surveys.[73,78]

In the NIDR survey,[103] mean pocket depth (4.3 mm) was comparable for employed males and females. Females, however, had slightly fewer sites (9.8%) with pockets ≥4 mm than males (11.5%). A similar pattern existed for attachment loss (mean, 2.5 mm). Again, females had fewer sites with attachment loss (25.0%) when compared with males (30.9%).

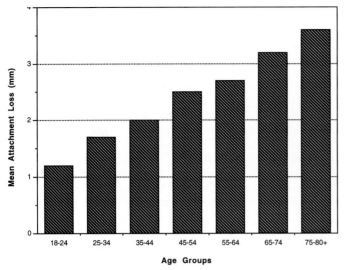

FIGURE 5-2. Severity of periodontal disease by age. Data for mean attachment loss (mm) from the NIDR 1985 survey for employed adults (18–64 years) and seniors (65–80+ years). Severity of disease is reflected in mean attachment loss.[103]

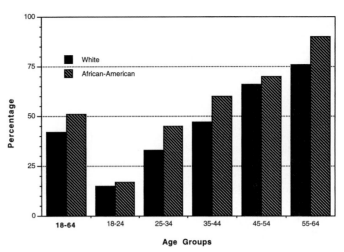

FIGURE 5-4. Comparison of periodontal disease prevalence of attachment loss by racial-ethnic group and age. Data are from 1985 NIDR survey of employed adults (18–64 years).[114] Prevalence is indicated by the percentage of persons with LA ≥ 3 mm.

Race. When the prevalence of periodontal disease (percentage of persons with loss of attachment ≥3 mm) is compared by racial and ethnic group, blacks consistently have a higher prevalence than whites in the NIDR survey.[18,78,103,114] Starting in the 18- to 24-year-old age group (Fig. 5–4), the prevalence was 15% and 17% for whites and blacks, respectively; this increased to 76% and 90%, respectively, for the 55- to 64-year-old age group. When the extent of LA (average number of sites with LA ≥3 mm) was compared between whites and blacks, the two groups were almost identical. Crude comparisons of either prevalence or severity between whites and blacks have shown similar differences, varying in magnitude, in previous surveys.[76,160] The real test of this comparison, which illustrates an important underlying epidemiologic principle, is to compare whites and blacks of similar education and income. Although these comparisons were not presented in the NIDR report, previous surveys have made these com-

parisons and have shown that racial and ethnic risk factors do not contribute to increased periodontal disease susceptibility.[78]

In the southwestern HHANES survey (1982–1983), the prevalence of periodontal disease with pockets among Hispanics ranged from 3.6% (18 to 24 years old) to 51.6% (65 to 74 years old) for those below poverty status, and from 0.9% (18 to 24 years old) to 48.2% (65 to 74 years old) for those above poverty status.[72] Among Hispanic children and youths (5 to 17 years of age), there was a high prevalence of gingivitis (76.9%) and a low prevalence of periodontal pockets (0.2%).[71] In the Ten-State Nutrition Survey, the severity of periodontal disease among Hispanics appeared to be higher than that among both whites and blacks, but because of disproportionate differences in the number of persons examined, a definitive statement on disease severity cannot be made.[160]

Education. Figure 5–5 illustrates an important associa-

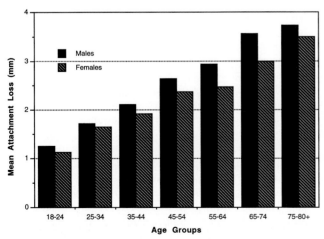

FIGURE 5-3. Severity of periodontal disease by sex and age. Data for mean attachment loss (mm) from NIDR 1985 survey for employed adults (18–64 years) and seniors (65–80+ years). Severity of disease is reflected in mean attachment loss.[103]

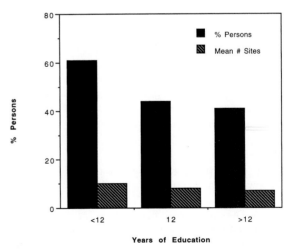

FIGURE 5-5. Prevalence and extent of attachment loss by years of education. Data are from 1985 NIDR survey of employed adults, 18 to 64 years of age.[114] Loss of attachment (LA) was defined as ≥3 mm. Prevalence is indicated by the percentage of persons with LA ≥ 3 mm, and extent by the mean number of sites with LA ≥ 3 mm.

tion relative to periodontal disease.[114] Periodontal disease is inversely related to increasing levels of education. Specifically, Figure 5–5 shows that the prevalence and extent of LA ≥3 mm is inversely related to increasing levels of education (i.e., <12 years, 12 years, or >12 years). The magnitude of the decrease in prevalence (from 61% to 41%) and extent (from a mean of 10 sites to a mean of seven sites) is approximately 30%. A similar pattern was observed in employed adults with pockets ≥4 mm. The prevalence of persons with pockets ≥4 mm decreased from 26% (<12 years of education) to 11% (>12 years); and the extent (mean number of sites) decreased from five (<12 years of education) to four (>12 years).

This inverse relationship was observed in other surveys[70,78,129] and by Burt and associates[35] on analysis of the NHANES I data.* In a survey of adults who were predominantly Hispanic living in New Mexico, Ismail and colleagues[72a] found an inverse relationship between educational levels and periodontal pockets greater than 4 mm.

It is not surprising that the relationship between periodontal disease and occupation, which is so closely tied to education in the United States, is similar to that between periodontal disease and education.

Income. The association between periodontal disease and income is similar to that between periodontal disease and education,[35,78] with periodontal disease inversely related to increasing levels of income. This was shown previously[78] and to a lesser degree in the NIDR survey of adults.[114] When the prevalence and extent of LA (≥3 mm) were examined by income levels (<$20,000; $20,000 to $39,999; and >$40,000), the prevalence decreased almost 19% as income increased from less than $20,000 to greater than $40,000. However, the extent of LA (mean number of sites) did not decrease with increasing income.

Place of Residence. In general, the prevalence and severity of periodontal disease are slightly higher in rural areas than in urban areas.[78]

Geographic Area. In the United States there have been no significant regional differences in the prevalence and severity of periodontal disease for adults in the NHES[78] (6672 persons, 18 to 79 years of age) and in the NHANES I[76] (13,645 persons, 18 to 74 years of age). Children (7109, 6 to 11 years of age)[77] and youths (6768, 12 to 17 years of age)[136] living in the South, however, did have slightly higher PI scores than their counterparts living in the Midwest and West. Slight but insignificant differences were observed in the regional findings of the NIDR survey of adults. Employed males in the Southwest, Northeast, and Pacific regions had a higher prevalence of LA (85% to 87%) than in the Midwest (72%).[32]

ETIOLOGIC RISK FACTORS FOR GINGIVAL AND PERIODONTAL DISEASE

Oral Hygiene. The strong positive association that exists between poor oral hygiene and gingival and periodontal

---

* Education, income, residence, and geographic area were not analyzed as a function of disease levels in the original publications by the NCHS on the NHANES I.

disease[64,67,79,95,158] makes poor oral hygiene the primary etiologic agent. On the basis of observations of periodontal disease in the United States and throughout the world, Russell stated, ". . . active (gingival and periodontal) disease is rarely found in the absence of oral debris (plaque) or calculus."[133] One vivid example that puts in perspective the importance of oral hygiene relative to demographic variables (detailed in the preceding discussion) is a multiple correlation analysis of the combined effects of age, sex, and oral hygiene (OHI-S scores) to PI scores in 752 South Vietnamese persons older than 15 years of age.[135] The coefficient of multiple correlation was $r = 0.82$, which, under the above conditions, means that statistically 67% (two thirds) of the variance was attributed to oral hygiene and approximately 31% (one third) was attributed to age. As previously noted, the second most significant correlate associated with at least one periodontal pocket >6 mm was the number of teeth with plaque.[72a]

In the NHES, a comparison of the partial correlation coefficients of oral hygiene (OHI-S), age, education level of the head of the household, and family income with PI scores showed that oral hygiene was the best predictor of the prevalence and severity of periodontal disease.[136,137] The first analytical analysis of the NHANES I data showed a strong, statistically significant inverse relationship between the frequency of brushing and the level of periodontal disease.[34] In an analysis of the NHANES I of adults 24 to 74 years of age, Burt and coworkers[35] concluded that even when gingivitis and periodontal pocketing (based on PI scores) increased with increasing age, tooth loss was not inevitable as long as good oral hygiene existed. They hypothesized that OHI-S scores in the range of 0.3 to 0.6 with Simplified Calculus Index scores of 0.1 to 0.2 were compatible with a dentition free of periodontal disease. Slightly higher scores (OHI-S = 0.7 to 1.3; CI-S = 0.3 to 0.6), which are associated with low to moderately severe periodontal disease, were still compatible with tooth retention. Hence, statistically as well as clinically, *bacterial plaque is a primary etiologic factor of periodontal disease.*

A slight clarification of the importance of oral hygiene as a risk factor is possible because of the chronic disease model of periodontal disease (i.e., disease activity followed by remission and tissue repair with many cycles of varying length)[63] and the findings of the natural history of periodontal disease by Löe and associates.[90,91] Even when poor oral hygiene exists, not all individuals experience periodontal disease. Only those who are highly susceptible succumb to the risks presented by poor oral hygiene. *Therefore, poor oral hygiene is an important risk factor in highly susceptible individuals and is of less importance in individuals with strong host resistance.*

Nutrition. The nutrients that have been specifically associated with the periodontal tissues are vitamins A, B complex, C, and D and calcium and phosphorus (see Chapter 14). Deficiencies in each of these nutrients and their effects on the periodontium have been clearly demonstrated in appropriately designed animal studies. The evidence for association of deficiencies in these nutrients with periodontal disease in humans, however, has been less than convincing.[147]

In a series of nutrition surveys conducted under the auspices of the Interdepartmental Committee on Nutrition for National Defense (ICNND),[130] designed specifically to determine associations between nutrient levels and disease, the strongest residual associations between periodontal disease and nutritional deficiencies were expressed in partial correlations (holding the effects of age, debris, and calculus constant) of −0.11 for vitamin A and −0.19 for hematocrit levels.[131] The partial correlation coefficient (−0.11) for the vitamin A deficiency accounts for approximately 1% of the variance in the PI scores; the strongest partial correlation coefficient (−0.19) accounts for less than 4% of the variance in the PI scores.

Little or no effect could be attributed to levels of serum ascorbic acid, serum carotene, total serum protein, urinary thiamine, riboflavin, and N'-methylnicotinamide and hemoglobin concentration. A vitamin A deficiency and a subnormal hematocrit level were found in a South Vietnamese population, but neither of these deficiencies was found to be associated with periodontal disease in subsequent ICNND surveys.[135] In the Ten-State Nutrition Survey,[160] the simple correlation coefficient (−0.03) for PI scores and plasma vitamin A deficiency accounted for 0.1% of the variance in PI scores. All of these correlation coefficients are weak associations at best. The ICNND surveys found no consistent correlation between nutrition and periodontal disease. However, they concluded that despite the independence of the nutritive state of the individual adult and his or her periodontal condition, there is a trend toward a higher prevalence and severity of periodontal disease in adults in areas[81] where protein calorie malnutrition and vitamin A deficiency are common in children.[130] *Therefore, nutrition is a secondary factor in the etiology of periodontal disease.*

Fluorides. No definitive statement can be made concerning the prevalence and severity of gingival or periodontal disease in cities with optimal or high levels of fluoride in the drinking water. Some investigators reported that optimal levels of fluoride do not have any effect on the gingival tissues,[52,104,109] but other researchers reported a lower prevalence and severity of gingivitis and periodontal disease in optimally fluoridated areas.[13,51,128] In a comparison of adults who were continuous residents of two communities with water supplies containing 3.5 ppm and 0.7 ppm fluoride, respectively, no differences were observed between the residents in the distribution of pocket depth and in the mean number of tooth sites with pockets.[72a]

Adverse Habits. Tobacco smoking[11,12,156] and betel nut chewing[15] have been associated with increased periodontal disease.[46] Although this association is not unequivocal, it seems reasonable that any habit that increases irritation of the gingival tissues or lowers their resistance would be a predisposing or secondary factor in initiating periodontal disease (see Chapter 12). In Burt et al.'s analysis of the NHANES I data, adults with the highest levels of periodontal disease were also among the group of smokers. Adults with the lowest levels of periodontal disease were found among the group who never smoked.[34]

Professional Dental Care. The incidence and severity of periodontal disorders are lower in individuals who receive regular dental care.[28,96,158,164] The prevalence and severity of disease increase with dental neglect (see Chapter 68).

DISTRIBUTION OF DISEASE IN DIFFERENT AREAS OF THE MOUTH

The strong association previously described between plaque and calculus and periodontal disease in its initial stages may be explained by the dynamics of plaque and gingivitis formation over time. Figure 5–6 shows the rate of plaque and gingivitis formation observed by Löe and associates[94] in their classic study of experimental gingivitis. It can be seen that when brushing is omitted from oral hygiene cleansing procedures, the formation of plaque and the development of gingivitis are closely parallel. In the study both increased with time, reaching a maximum at 15 to 21 days, when all subjects experienced a maximum of gingivitis. Reinstitution of toothbrushing not only demonstrated the reversible nature of gingival inflammation, but also showed a concomitant decrease in plaque and gingivitis formation.

Dividing the mouth into interproximal, buccal, and lingual areas by upper and lower arches (Table 5–12), Löe and associates[94] showed that the interproximal area was the area most severely affected by gingivitis, followed by the buccal and lingual surfaces. Dividing each of the areas into upper and lower arches revealed that gingivitis was more severe in the upper arch than in the lower arch for the interproximal and buccal areas, and was more severe in the lower arch than in the upper arch in the lingual area.[94]

Suomi and Barbano[157] examined the severity of gingivitis by facial and lingual surfaces for three areas of the mouth (Fig. 5–7) and found the same general pattern observed by Löe and associates.[94] For facial surfaces the areas most severely affected by gingivitis, in descending order, were the upper first and second molars, the lower anteriors, the upper anteriors, the upper premolars, the lower first and second molars, and the lower premolars. For lingual surfaces

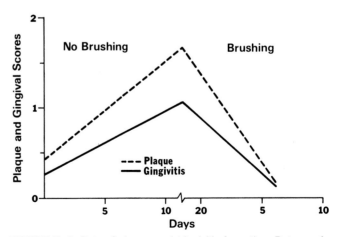

FIGURE 5–6. Rate of plaque and gingivitis formation. Data are for 12 young Scandinavian adults, averaging 23 years of age. The Gingival Index and the Plaque Index were used for the clinical assessments. (Adapted from Löe H, Theilade E, Jensen SB. Experimental gingivitis in man. *J Periodontol 36:*177, 1965.)

Table 5–12. SEVERITY OF GINGIVITIS FOR THREE DIFFERENT AREAS BY ARCH*

Area	Arch	Mean Gingival Index Score
Interproximal	Upper > lower	1.44 > 1.20
Buccal	Upper > lower	1.23 > 1.13
Lingual	Lower > upper	0.89 > 0.46

* Adapted from Löe H, Theilade E, Jensen SB. Experimental gingivitis in man. J Periodontol *36*:177, 1965.

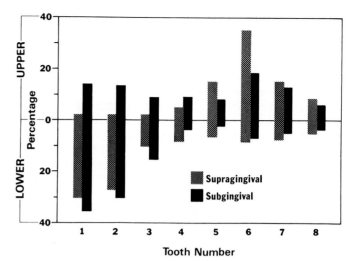

FIGURE 5–8. Intraoral prevalence of calculus by individual teeth. The percentage of supragingival and subgingival calculus is presented by tooth and arch. Tooth numbers are as defined in Figure 5–7; 8, third molar. (Adapted from Schroeder HE. Formation and Inhibition of Dental Calculus. Vienna, H. Huber Publishers, 1969.)

the areas most severely affected by gingivitis, in descending order, were the lower first and second molars, the lower premolars, the lower anteriors, the upper first and second molars, the upper premolars, and the upper anteriors. This intraoral pattern of gingivitis was similar to that observed by Marshall-Day,[99] with the exception of the facial surfaces of the upper anteriors, which he found to be the most severely affected by gingivitis. Several investigators[3,21,157] observed a slightly higher tendency toward gingivitis on the right half of the arch than on the left half. This may be because of the difficulty that right-handed persons have in brushing the right half of the mouth.

The intraoral pattern of supragingival and subgingival calculus by individual teeth appears in Figure 5–8. For supragingival calculus, the upper first molars had the most calculus, followed by the lower centrals and laterals; the upper anteriors (centrals, laterals, and canines) had the least calculus. For subgingival calculus, the lower centrals and laterals had the most calculus, followed by the upper first molars; the upper anteriors (centrals, laterals, and canines) and the upper second molars had intermediate amounts of calculus; and the lower first and second premolars and the lower third molars had the least calculus. When measurements of supragingival and subgingival calculus were combined, the lower centrals and laterals and the upper first molars had the most calculus; the upper second premolars and the upper second molars had intermediate amounts of

calculus; and the lower second premolars and the lower third molars had the least calculus.[116,145]

In general, the severity of bone loss follows the intraoral pattern of subgingival calculus and the intraoral pattern of calculus when supragingival and subgingival calculus are combined. The incisor and molar areas are more severely involved than the canine and premolar areas,[100,142] with the least bone loss occurring in the lower canine and premolar region. Bone loss in the maxilla is generally more severe than that in the mandible,[17] except for the anterior region, where the situation is reversed.[100,164] In addition, the severity of bone loss is greater interproximally than it is facially and lingually.

The upper and lower limits of the various patterns of plaque, gingivitis, calculus, and bone loss together produce the intraoral pattern of periodontal disease in individual teeth presented in Figure 5–9. Measurement of all of these

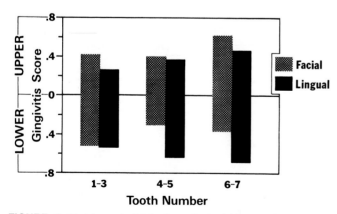

FIGURE 5–7. Intraoral distribution of gingivitis severity by tooth surface and area of mouth. Data are for 400 males 15 to 34 years of age. The Dental Health Center Index (DHCI) was used to assess gingivitis by marginal and papillary units for all teeth. Tooth numbers are defined as follows: 1, central incisor; 2, lateral incisor; 3, canine; 4, first premolar; 5, second premolar; 6, first molar; 7, second molar. (Adapted from Suomi JD, Barbano JP. Patterns of gingivitis. J Periodontol *39*:71, 1968.)

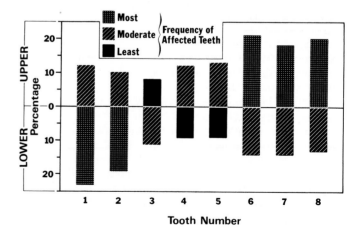

FIGURE 5–9. Intraoral prevalence of periodontal disease by individual teeth. The percentages of teeth affected by periodontal disease are classified as most, moderate, and least. Data are for industrial workers 40 to 44 years of age, with men and women combined. Tooth numbers are defined in Figures 5–7 and 5–8. (Adapted from Bossert WA, Marks HH. J Am Dent Assoc *52*:429, 1956 by permission of ADA Publishing Co., Inc.)

variables shows that the teeth that are most severely affected by periodontal disease are the lower centrals and laterals and the upper molars (first, second, and third). The teeth that are moderately affected by periodontal disease are the lower first molars (first, second, and third); the upper centrals, laterals, and premolars (first and second); and the lower canines. Finally, the teeth that are least affected by periodontal disease are the lower premolars (first and second) and the upper canines.

THE RELATIONSHIP BETWEEN PERIODONTAL DISEASE AND DENTAL CARIES

Even though numerous investigators have attempted to determine the relationship between the occurrence of periodontal disease and dental caries, no clear-cut positive or negative relationship has been established.[80] Some investigators consider these antagonistic processes, with the presence of one precluding the occurrence of the other.[30,80] Several statistical studies suggest a positive correlation between caries and gingival disease,[24,148] but this has not been substantiated.[164] Although both have dental plaque as their chief etiologic factor, caries and periodontal disease appear to be two independent processes.[34,164]

The final result of either untreated dental caries or advanced periodontal disease is the loss of teeth. Hence, comparing the percentages of teeth extracted as a result of caries and of periodontal disease provides one outcome measure for examining the relationship between the two processes. An excellent review of periodontal disease and tooth loss has been presented by Oliver and Brown.[113]

Although no data were gathered on reasons for tooth extraction during the NHES (1960–1962), information on this topic was obtained during the NHANES I (1971–1974) and was presented as averages for age-specific groups. For the overall survey (ages 1 to 74 years), more teeth were recommended for extraction as a result of periodontal disease (6.7 per person) than as a result of dental caries (0.7 per person) or all other reasons (3.2 per person).[76]

A subtle but important point must be clarified when summarizing the literature from the United States that describes the reasons for extractions. Starting with the first study by Brekhus in 1926,[29] every study[9,10,47,68,84] except one[117] showed that the overall proportion of teeth extracted for dental caries was always greater than the proportion extracted for periodontal disease. When the number of extractions was compared by age, however, periodontal disease was the primary cause of extractions in certain older age-specific groups. However, a study by Chauncey and associates[41] failed to support this age-specific relationship. Studies conducted outside of the United States[4,8,27,36,75,83,155] have observed a pattern similar to that seen in the United States, in spite of cultural and geographic differences.

One major problem in almost all of the studies cited is the definition and application of the reasons for extraction. Retrospective studies must reconstruct the reasons for tooth removal from dental records, and prospective studies must deal with examiner variability in applying the definitions over time. The subjective nature of clinical judgment and the dentist's ability to prevent extractions seriously compromise any study that attempts to examine tooth mortality according to reason for extraction.

It is clear that many factors, such as oral hygiene, socioeconomic status, fluoride exposure, and professional treatment philosophies, have influenced the reasons for extraction. The secular decline in dental caries, continued exposure to fluorides, greater preventive orientation of the general population and the dental profession, and improved socioeconomic status can contribute collectively to an overall decrease in tooth loss for any reason and for all ages in the future.

REFERENCES

1. Abdellatif HM, Burt BA. An epidemiological investigation into the relative importance of age and oral hygiene status as determinants of periodontitis. J Dent Res 66:13, 1987.
2. Adams RA, Nystrom GP. A periodontitis severity index. J Periodontol 57:176, 1986.
3. Addy M, Griffiths D, Dummer P, et al. The distribution of plaque and gingivitis and the influence of toothbrushing hand in a group of South Wales 11–12 year old children. J Clin Periodontol 14:564, 1987.
4. Agerholm DM, Sidi AD. Reasons given for extraction of permanent teeth by general dental practitioners in England and Wales. Br Dent J 164:345, 1988.
5. Ainamo J. Significance of epidemiologic research in the understanding of periodontal disease. Scand J Dent Res 100:39, 1992.
6. Ainamo J, Barmes D, Beagrie G, et al. Development of the World Health Organization (WHO) Community Periodontal Index of Treatment Needs (CPITN). Int Dent J 32:281, 1982.
7. Ainamo J, Bay I. Problems and proposals for recording gingivitis and plaque. Int Dent J 25:229, 1975.
8. Ainamo J, Sarkki L, Kuhalampi ML, et al. The frequency of periodontal extractions in Finland. Community Dent Health 1:165, 1984.
9. Allen EF. Statistical study of the primary causes of extraction. J Dent Res 23:453, 1944.
10. Andrews G, Krogh HW. Permanent tooth mortality. Dent Progress, 1:130, 1961.
11. Arno A, Schei O, Lovdal A, Waerhaug J. Alveolar bone loss as a function of tobacco consumption. Acta Odontol Scand 17:3, 1959.
12. Arno A, Waerhaug J, Lovdal A, Schei O. Incidence of gingivitis as related to sex, occupation, tobacco consumption, toothbrushing and age. Oral Surg 11:587, 1958.
13. Ast DB, Schlesinger ER. The conclusion of a ten-year study of fluoridation. Am J Public Health 46:265, 1956.
14. Baer PN. The case for periodontosis as a clinical entity. J Periodontol 42:516, 1971.
15. Balendra W. The effect of betel chewing on the dental and oral tissues and its possible relationship to buccal carcinoma. Br Dent J 87:83, 1949.
16. Barnett M, Ciancio S, Mather M. The modified Papillary Bleeding Index: Comparison with Gingival Index during the resolution of gingivitis. J Prev Dent 6:135, 1980.
17. Beagrie GS, James GA. The association of posterior tooth irregularity and periodontal disease. Br Dent J 113:239, 1962.
18. Beck JD, Löe H. Epidemiological principles in studying periodontal diseases. Periodontology 2000 2:34, 1993.
19. Bellini HT. A System to Determine the Periodontal Therapeutic Needs of a Population. Oslo, Universitetsforlagets Trykningssentral, 1973.
20. Bellini HT, Gjermo P. Application of the Periodontal Treatment Need System (PTNS) in a group of Norwegian industrial employees. Community Dent Oral Epidemiol 1:22, 1973.
21. Beube FE, Schwartz M, Thompson RH. A comparison of effectiveness in plaque removal of an electric toothbrush and a conventional hand toothbrush. Periodontics 2:71, 1964.
22. Bhat M. Periodontal health of 14–17-year-old US schoolchildren. J Public Health Dent 51:5, 1991.
23. Bjorby A, Löe H. The relative significance of different local factors in the initiation and development of periodontal inflammation. Abstract. J Periodont Res 2:76, 1967.
24. Black GV. Something of the etiology and early pathology of the diseases of the periodontal membrane with suggestions as to treatment. Dent Cosmos 55:1219, 1913.
25. Bonito A, Iannachione V, Jones S, Stuart C. A study of dental health outcomes related to prepayment. Final report. Part I, DHEW contract No. HRA 231-76-0093. Research Triangle Park, NC: Research Triangle Institute, 1984.
26. Bossert WA, Marks HH. Prevalence and characteristics of periodontal disease of 12,800 persons under periodic dental observation. J Am Dent Assoc 52:429, 1956.
27. Bouma J, Schaub RM, van de-Poel AC. Relative importance of periodontal disease for full mouth extractions in the Netherlands. Community Dent Oral Epidemiol 15:41, 1987.

28. Brandtzaeg P, Jamison HC. The effect of controlled cleansing of the teeth on periodontal health and oral hygiene in Norwegian army recruits. J Periodontol *35:*308, 1964.
29. Brekhus PJ. Dental disease and its relation to the loss of human teeth. J Am Dent Assoc *16:*2237, 1929.
30. Broderick FW. Antagonism between dental caries and pyorrhea. Am Dent Surg *49:*103, 1929.
31. Brown LJ, Oliver RC, Löe H. Periodontal disease in the U.S. in 1981: Prevalence, severity, extent, and role in tooth mortality. J Periodontol *60:*368, 1989.
32. Brunelle JA, Miller-Chisholm AJ, Löe H. Oral health of United States adults regional findings: 1985–1986. NIH publication no. 88-2869. Bethesda, MD: U.S. Department of Health and Human Services, May, 1988.
33. Brunelle JA. Dental health of United States children. The National Survey of Dental Caries in U.S. School Children: 1986–1987. National and regional findings. NIH publication no. 89-2247. Bethesda, MD: U.S. Department of Health and Human Services, September, 1989.
34. Burt BA, Eklund SA, Landis JR, et al. Diet and dental health, a study of relationships. Hyattsville, MD, U.S. Public Health Service, U.S. Department of Health and Human Services, Publication no. (PHS) 82-1675, series 11, no. 225. National Center for Health Statistics, 1982.
35. Burt BA, Ismail AI, Eklund SA. Periodontal disease, tooth loss, and oral hygiene among older Americans. Community Dent Oral Epidemiol *13:*93, 1985.
36. Cahen PM, Frank RM, Turlot JC. A survey of the reasons for dental extractions in France. J Dent Res *64:*1087, 1985.
37. Capilouto ML, Douglass CW. Trends in the prevalence and severity of periodontal diseases in the United States: Is it a public health problem? J Public Health Dent *48:*245, 1988.
38. Carlos JP, Wolfe MD, Kingman A. The Extent and Severity Index: A simple method for use in epidemiologic studies of periodontal disease. J Clin Periodontol *13:*500, 1986.
39. Carter HG, Barnes GP. The Gingival Bleeding Index. J Periodontol *45:*801, 1974.
40. Caton JG, Polson AM. The Interdental Bleeding Index: A simplified procedure for monitoring gingival health. Comp Cont Educ Dent *6:*88, 1985.
41. Chauncey HH, Glass RL, Alman JE, Feller RF. Dental caries: The primary cause of tooth extraction in a sample of U.S. male adults. Abstract no. 9. Caries Res *21:*161, 1987.
42. Chilton NW, ed. International Conference on Clinical Trials of Agents Used in the Prevention/Treatment of Periodontal Diseases. J Periodont Res suppl 14:7, 1974.
43. Ciancio SG. Current status of indices of gingivitis. J Clin Periodontol *13:*375, 1986.
44. Clemmer BA, Barbano JP. Reproducibility of periodontal score in clinical trials. J Periodont Res Suppl 14:118, 1974.
45. Cohen DW, Ship II, eds. Clinical methods in periodontal diseases, based on a conference held on May 20–23, 1967. J Periodontol *38:*580, 1967.
46. Davies GN. Social customs and habits and their effect on oral disease. J Dent Res *42:*209, 1963.
47. Davis CH. Relative causes of tooth mortality. A pilot study. J Public Health Dent *22:*85, 1961.
48. Dunning JM, Leach LB. Gingival bone count: A method for epidemiological study of periodontal disease. J Dent Res *39:*506, 1960.
49. Elliott JR, Bowers GM, Clemmen BA, Rovelstad GH. Evaluation of an oral physiotherapy center in the reduction of bacterial plaque and periodontal disease. J Periodontol *43:*221, 1972.
50. Emslie RD. Formal discussion. Design of studies or clinical trials to evaluate the effectiveness of agents or procedures for the prevention, or treatment, of loss of the periodontium. J Periodont Res suppl 14:78, 1974.
51. Englander HR, Kesel RG, Gupta OP. Effect of natural fluoride on the periodontal health of adults. Am J Public Health *53:*1233, 1963.
52. Englander HR, White CL. Periodontal and oral hygiene status of teenagers in optimum and fluoride-deficient cities. J Am Dent Assoc *68:*173, 1964.
53. Ennever J, Sturzenberger CP, Radlike AW. Calculus Surface Index for scoring clinical calculus studies. J Periodontol *32:*54, 1961.
54. Fischman SL. Current status of indices of plaque. J Clin Periodontol *13:*371, 1986.
55. Fischman SL. Clinical index systems used to assess the efficacy of mouth rinses on plaque and gingivitis. J Clin Periodontol *15:*506, 1988.
56. Fischman SL, Cancro LP, Pretara-Spanedda P, Jacobs D. Distal Mesial Plaque Index: A technique for assessing dental plaque about the gingiva. Dent Hygiene *61:*404, 1986.
57. Fleiss JL. Statistical Methods for Rates and Proportions. 2nd ed. New York, John Wiley, 1981.
58. Fleiss JL. The Design and Analysis of Clinical Experiments. New York, John Wiley, 1986.
59. Fleiss JL, Fischman SL, Chilton NW, Park MH. Reliability of discrete measurements in caries trials. Caries Res *13:*23, 1979.
60. Frankel JM, Boffa J. Prepaid Dental Care—A Technical Assistant Manual. 3rd ed. Atlanta, Marketing Associates, 1974.
61. Gaengler P, Goebel G, Kurbad A, Kosa W. Assessment of periodontal disease and dental caries in a population survey using the CPITN, GPM/T and DMF/T indices. Community Dent Oral Epidemiol *16:*236, 1988.
62. Gjermo P. Formal discussion. Indices for the measurement of gingival inflammation in clinical studies of oral hygiene and periodontal disease. J Periodont Res suppl 14:61, 1974.
63. Goodson JM, Tanner ACM, Haffajee AD, et al. Patterns of progression and regression of advanced destructive periodontal disease. J Clin Periodontol *9:*472, 1982.
64. Greene JC. Oral hygiene and periodontal disease. Am J Public Health *53:*913, 1963.
65. Greene JC. The Oral Hygiene Index: Development and uses. J Periodontol *38:*625, 1967.
66. Greene JC, Vermillion JR. Oral Hygiene Index: A method for classifying oral hygiene status. J Am Dent Assoc *61:*172, 1960.
67. Greene JC, Vermillion JR. The Simplified Oral Hygiene Index. J Am Dent Assoc *68:*7, 1964.
68. Grewe JM, Gorlin RJ, Meskin LH. Human tooth mortality: A clinical-statistical study. J Am Dent Assoc *72:*106, 1966.
69. Harvey C, Kelly JE. Decayed, missing, and filled teeth among persons 1–74 years, United States. Publication no. (PHS) 81-1673, series 11, no. 223. Hyattsville, MD, U.S. Public Health Service, U.S. Department of Health and Human Services, National Center for Health Statistics, 1981.
70. Horton JE, Sumnicht RW. Relationships of educational levels to periodontal disease and oral hygiene with variables of age and geographic regions. J Periodontol *38:*335, 1967.
71. Ismail AL, Burt BA, Brunelle JA. Prevalence of dental caries and periodontal disease in Mexican American children aged 5 to 17 years: Results from southwestern HHANES, 1982–1983. Am J Public Health *77:*967, 1987.
72. Ismail AL, Burt BA, Brunelle JA. Prevalence of tooth loss, dental caries, and periodontal disease in Mexican American adults: Results from the southwestern HHANES. J Dent Res *66:*1183, 1987.
72a. Ismail AI, Eklund AS, Burt BA, Calderone JJ. Prevalences of deep periodontal pockets in New Mexico adults aged 27 to 74 years. J Public Health Dent *46:*199, 1986.
73. Johnson ES, Kelly JE, Van Kirk LE. Selected dental findings in adults by age, race and sex, United States 1960–1962. Publication no. 1000, series 11, no. 7. Washington, DC, U.S. Department of Health, Education, and Welfare, National Center for Health Statistics, 1965.
74. Kaslick RS, Chasens A. Periodontosis with periodontitis: A study involving young adult males. I. Review of the literature and incidence in a military population. Oral Surg *25:*305, 1968.
75. Kay EJ, Blinkhorn AS. The reasons underlying the extraction of teeth in Scotland. Br Dent J *160:*287, 1986.
76. Kelly JE, Harvey CR. Basic dental examination findings of persons 1–74 years, United States 1971–1974. Publication no. (PHS) 79-1662, series 11, no. 214. Hyattsville, MD, U.S. Public Health Service, U.S. Department of Health, Education, and Welfare, National Center for Health Statistics, 1979.
77. Kelly JE, Sanchez MJ. Periodontal disease and oral hygiene among children, United States. Publication no. (HSM) 72-1060, series 11, no. 117. Washington, DC, U.S. Public Health Service, U.S. Department of Health, Education, and Welfare, National Center for Health Statistics, 1972.
78. Kelly JE, Van Kirk LE. Periodontal disease in adults, United States 1960–1962. Publication no. 1000, series 11, no. 12. Washington, DC, U.S. Public Health Service, U.S. Department of Health, Education, and Welfare, National Center for Health Statistics, 1966.
79. Kelly JE, Van Kirk LE, Garst CC. Oral hygiene in adults, United States 1960–1962. Publication no. 1000, series 11, no. 16. Washington, DC, U.S. Public Health Service, U.S. Department of Health, Education, and Welfare, National Center for Health Statistics, 1966.
80. Kesel RG. Are dental caries and periodontal disease incompatible? J Periodontol *21:*30, 1950.
81. King JD. Dental disease in the Isle of Lewis. Medical Research Council, Special report series, no. 241. London, His Majesty's Stationery Office, 1940.
82. Kingman A, Löe H, Ånerud Å, Boysen H. Errors in measuring parameters associated with periodontal disease and disease. J Periodontol *62:*477, 1991.
83. Klock KS, Haugejorden O. Primary reasons for extraction of teeth in Norway: Changes from 1968 to 1988. Community Dent Oral Epidemiol *19:*336, 1991.
84. Krogh HW. Permanent tooth mortality: A clinical study of causes of loss. J Am Dent Assoc *57:*670, 1958.
85. Kronauer E, Borsa G, Lang NP. Prevalence of incipient juvenile periodontitis at age 16 years in Switzerland. J Clin Periodontol *13:*103, 1986.
86. Lenox JA, Kopczyk RA. A clinical system for scoring a patient's oral hygiene performance. J Am Dent Assoc *86:*849, 1973.
87. Lobene RR. The effect of an automatic toothbrush on gingival health. J Periodontol *35:*137, 1964.
88. Lobene R, Weatherford T, Ross W, et al. A modified gingival index for use in clinical trials. Clin Prev Dent *8:*3, 1986.
89. Löe H. The Gingival Index, the Plaque Index and the Retention Index systems. J Periodontol *38:*610, 1967.
90. Löe H, Ånerud Å, Boysen H, Smith M. The natural history of periodontal disease in man: The rate of periodontal destruction before 40 years of age. J Periodontol *49:*607, 1978.
91. Löe H, Ånerud Å, Boysen H, Morrison E. The natural history of periodontal disease in man: Rapid, moderate, and no loss of attachment in Sri Lankan laborers 14 to 46 years of age. J Clin Periodontol *13:*431, 1986.
92. Löe H, Brown LJ. Early onset periodontitis in the United States of America. J Periodontol *62:*608, 1991.
93. Löe H, Silness J. Periodontal disease in pregnancy. Acta Odontol Scand *21:*533, 1963.

94. Löe H, Theilade E, Jensen SB. Experimental gingivitis in man. J Periodontol *36:*177, 1965.

95. Lovdal A, Arno A, Schei O, Waerhaug J. Combined effect of subgingival scaling and controlled oral hygiene on the incidence of gingivitis. Acta Odontol Scand *19:*537, 1961.

96. Lovdal A, Arno A, Waerhaug J. Incidence of clinical manifestations of periodontal disease in light of oral hygiene and calculus formation. J Am Dent Assoc *56:*21, 1958.

97. Mandel ID. Indices for measurement of soft accumulations in clinical studies of oral hygiene and periodontal disease. J Periodont Res Suppl 14:7, 1974.

98. Mandel ID. Indices for measurement of soft accumulations in clinical studies of oral hygiene and periodontal disease (continued). J Periodont Res Suppl 14:106, 1974.

99. Marshall-Day CD. The epidemiology of periodontal disease. J Periodontol *22:*13, 1951.

100. Marshall-Day CD, Shourie KL. A roentgenographic study of periodontal disease in India. J Am Dent Assoc *39:*572, 1949.

101. Massler M. The P-M-A Index for the assessment of gingivitis. J Periodontol *38:*592, 1967.

102. Massler M, Schour I, Chopra B. Occurrence of gingivitis in suburban Chicago school children. J Periodontol *21:*146, 1950.

103. Miller AJ, Brunelle JA, Carlos JP, et al. Oral health of United States adults. NIDR publication no. (NIH) 87-2868. Bethesda, MD, U.S. Public Health Service, U.S. Department of Health and Human Services, 1987.

104. Moore RM, Muhler JC, McDonald RE. A study of the effect of water fluoride content and socioeconomic status on the occurrence of gingivitis in school children. J Dent Res *43:*782, 1964.

105. Mühlemann HR. Psychological and chemical mediators of gingival health. J Prev Dent *4:*6, 1977.

106. Mühlemann HR, Mazor ZS. Gingivitis in Zurich school children. Helv Odontol Acta *2:*3, 1958.

107. Mühlemann HR, Son S. Gingival sulcus bleeding—a leading symptom in initial gingivitis. Helv Odontol Acta *15:*107, 1971.

108. Mühlemann HR, Villa P. The Marginal Line Calculus Index. Helv Odontol Acta *11:*175, 1967.

109. Murray JJ. Gingivitis in 15-year-old children from high fluoride and low fluoride areas. Arch Oral Biol *14:*951, 1969.

110. O'Leary TJ. The periodontal screening examination. J Periodontol *38:*617, 1967.

111. O'Leary TJ, Drake RB, Naylor JE. The plaque control record. J Periodontol *43:*38, 1972.

112. O'Leary TJ, Gibson WA, Shannon IL, et al. A screening examination for detection of gingival and periodontal breakdown and local irritants. Periodontics *1:*167, 1963.

113. Oliver RC, Brown LJ. Periodontal diseases and tooth loss. Periodontology 2000 *2:*117, 1993.

114. Oliver RC, Brown LJ, Löe H. Variations in the prevalence and extent of periodontitis. J Am Dent Assoc *122:*43, 1991.

115. Page RC. Oral health status in the United States: Prevalence of inflammatory periodontal diseases. J Dent Educ *49:*354, 1985.

116. Parfitt GJ. A survey of the oral health of Navajo Indian children. Arch Oral Biol *1:*193, 1959.

117. Pelton WJ, Pennell EH, Druzina A. Tooth morbidity experience of adults. J Am Dent Assoc *49:*439, 1954.

118. Pilot T, Barmes DE, Leclercq MH, et al. Periodontal conditions in adolescents, 15–19 years of age: An overview of CPITN data in the WHO Global Oral Data Bank. Community Dent Oral Epidemiol *15:*336, 1987.

119. Pilot T, Barmes DE, Leclercq MH, et al. Periodontal conditions in adults, 35–44 years of age: An overview of CPITN data in the WHO Global Oral Data Bank. Community Dent Oral Epidemiol *14:*310, 1986.

120. Podshadley AG, Haley JV. A method for evaluating patient hygiene performance by observation of selected tooth surfaces. Public Health Rep *83:*259, 1968.

121. Proceedings of the Workshop on Quantitative Evaluation of Periodontal Diseases by Physical Measurement Techniques. J Dent Res *58:*547, 1979.

122. Quigley G, Hein J. Comparative cleansing efficiency of manual and power brushing. J Am Dent Assoc *65:*26, 1962.

123. Ramfjord SP. Indices for prevalence and incidence of periodontal disease. J Periodontol *30:*51, 1959.

124. Ramfjord SP. The Periodontal Disease Index (PDI). J Periodontol *38:*602, 1967.

125. Ramfjord SP. Design of studies or clinical trials to evaluate the effectiveness of agents or procedures for the prevention, or treatment, of loss of the periodontium. J Periodont Res suppl 14:78, 1974.

126. Rugg-Gunn AJ, Holloway PJ. Methods of measuring the reliability of caries prevalence and incremental data. Community Dent Oral Epidemiol *2:*287, 1974.

127. Russell AL. A system of classification and scoring for prevalence surveys of periodontal disease. J Dent Res *35:*350, 1956.

128. Russell AL. Fluoride, domestic water and periodontal disease. Am J Public Health *47:*688, 1957.

129. Russell AL. A social factor associated with the severity of periodontal disease. J Dent Res *36:*922, 1957.

130. Russell AL. International nutrition surveys: A summary of preliminary dental findings. J Dent Res *42:*233, 1963.

131. Russell AL. Epidemiology of periodontal disease. Int Dent J *17:*282, 1967.

132. Russell AL. Epidemiology and the rational bases of dental public health and dental practice. In Young WO, Striffler DF, eds. The Dentist, His Practice, and His Community. 2nd ed. Philadelphia, WB Saunders, 1969, pp 35–57.

133. Russell AL. The epidemiology of dental caries and periodontal diseases. In Young WO, Striffler DF, eds. The Dentist, His Practice, and His Community. 2nd ed. Philadelphia, WB Saunders, 1969, pp 73–86.

134. Russell AL. The prevalence of periodontal disease in different populations during the circumpubertal period. J Periodontol *42:*508, 1971.

135. Russell AL, Leatherwood EC, Consolazio CF, Van Reen R. Periodontal disease and nutrition in South Vietnam. J Dent Res *44:*775, 1965.

136. Sanchez MJ. Periodontal disease among youths 12–17 years, United States. Publication no. (HRA) 74-1623, series 11, no. 141. Washington, DC, U.S. Public Health Service, U.S. Department of Health, Education, and Welfare, National Center for Health Statistics, 1974.

137. Sanchez MJ. Oral hygiene among youths 12–17 years, United States. Publication no. (HRA) 76-1633, series 11, no. 151, Washington, DC, U.S.P.H.S., U.S. Department of Health, Education, and Welfare, National Center for Health Statistics, 1975.

138. Sartwell PE, ed. Maxcy-Rosenau Preventive Medicine and Public Health. 10th ed. New York, Appleton-Century-Crofts, 1973, p 1.

139. Saxby L. Juvenile periodontitis: An epidemiologic study in the West Midlands of the United Kingdom. J Clin Periodontol *14:*594, 1987.

140. Saxen L. Juvenile periodontitis. J Clin Periodontol *7:*1, 1980.

141. Saxen L. Prevalence of juvenile periodontitis in Finland. J Clin Periodontol *7:*177, 1980.

142. Schei O, Waerhaug J, Lovdal A, Arno A. Alveolar bone loss as related to oral hygiene and age. J Periodontol *30:*7, 1959.

143. Schour I, Massler M. Gingival disease in postwar Italy (1945). I. Prevalence of gingivitis in various age groups. J Am Dent Assoc *35:*475, 1947.

144. Schour I, Massler M. Survey of gingival disease using the PMA Index. J Dent Res *27:*733, 1948.

145. Schroeder HE. Formation and Inhibition of Dental Calculus. Berne, H Huber Publishers, 1969, p 66.

146. Shapiro S, Pollack BR, Gallant D. A special population available for periodontal research. Part II. A correlation and association analysis between oral hygiene and periodontal disease. J Periodontol *42:*161, 1971.

147. Shaw JH, Sweeney EA. Nutrition in relation to dental medicine. In Goodhart RS, Shils ME, eds. Modern Nutrition in Health and Disease. Philadelphia, Lea & Febiger, 1973, p 756.

148. Shay H, Smart GA. The association of local factors with gingivitis. Br Dent J *78:*135, 1945.

149. Sheiham A. The epidemiology of periodontal disease. In Kieser JB, ed. Periodontics: A Practical Approach. London, Wright, 1990, pp 40–45.

150. Sheiham A, Striffler DF. A comparison of four epidemiological methods of assessing periodontal disease. J Periodont Res *5:*155, 1970.

151. Shick RA, Ash MM. Evaluation of the vertical method of toothbrushing. J Periodontol *32:*346, 1961.

152. Silness P, Löe H. Periodontal disease in pregnancy. Acta Odontol Scand *22:*121, 1964.

153. Socransky SS, Haffajee AD, Goodson JM, Lindhe J. New concepts of destructive periodontal disease. J Clin Periodontol *11:*21, 1984.

154. Stamm JW. Epidemiology of gingivitis. J Clin Periodontol *13:*360, 1986.

155. Stephens RG, Kogon SL, Jarvis AM. A study of the reasons for tooth extraction in a Canadian population sample. J Can Dent Assoc *57:*501, 1991.

156. Summers C, Oberman A. Association of oral disease with twelve selected variables. I. Periodontal disease. J Dent Res *47:*457, 1968.

157. Suomi JD, Barbano JP. Patterns of gingivitis. J Periodontol *39:*71, 1968.

158. Suomi JD, Greene JC, Vermillion JR, et al. The effect of controlled oral hygiene procedures on the progression of periodontal disease in adults: Results after third and final year. J Periodontol *42:*152, 1971.

159. Suomi JD, Smith LW, McClendon BJ. Marginal gingivitis during a sixteen week period. J Periodontol *42:*268, 1971.

160. Ten-State Nutrition Survey 1968–1970. Publication no. (HSM) 72-8131. Vol. 3. Washington, DC, Health Services and Mental Health Administration, U.S. Department of Health, Education, and Welfare; Atlanta, Centers for Disease Control, 1972, pp 111, 126–131.

161. Turesky S, Gilmore ND, Glickman I. Reduced plaque formation by the chloromethyl analogue of victamine C. J Periodontol *41:*41, 1970.

162. Volpe AR. Indices for the measurement of hard deposits in clinical studies of oral hygiene and periodontal disease. J Periodont Res suppl 14:31, 1974.

163. Volpe AR, Manhold JH, Hazen SP. In vivo calculus assessment: A method and its reproducibility. J Periodontol *36:*292, 1965.

164. White CL, Russell AL. Some relations between dental caries experience and active periodontal disease in two thousand adults. NY J Dent *32:*211, 1962.

165. Wolfe MD, Carlos JP. Periodontal disease in adolescents: Epidemiologic findings in Navajo Indians. Community Dent Oral Epidemiol *15:*33, 1987.

166. World Health Organization. Oral Health Surveys: Basic Methods. 3rd ed. Geneva, WHO, 1987.

Section Three

Etiology of Periodontal Diseases

6

Periodontal Microbiology

SUSAN KINDER HAAKE

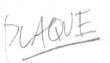

Periodontal disease comprises a group of inflammatory conditions of the supporting tissues of the teeth that are caused by bacteria. Our understanding of the etiology of periodontal diseases has undergone major advances in recent decades.[102] In the mid-1900s it was believed that all bacterial species found in dental plaque were equally capable of causing disease and that periodontitis was the result of cumulative exposure to dental plaque. The association of specific bacterial species with disease came about in the early 1960s, when microscopic examination of plaque revealed that different bacterial morphotypes were found in periodontally healthy versus periodontally diseased sites. Then in the 1960s and 1970s, technical improvements in the procedures used to isolate, cultivate, and identify periodontal microorganisms resulted in refinements in bacterial taxonomy (Table 6–1) and clarification of the specific groups of microorganisms present with diseases of the periodontium.

The identification of bacterial pathogens in periodontal diseases has been difficult because of a number of factors.[102] The periodontal microbiota is a complex community of microorganisms, many of which are still difficult or impossible to isolate in the laboratory. Currently it is apparent that multiple species function as pathogens, and that species that function as pathogens in one site may also be present in low numbers in healthy sites. Furthermore, the interpretation of microbiologic data is greatly influenced by the clinical classification of disease status. Misclassification, or grouping together of different disease states, in some cases has obscured microbiologic associations. In addition, the chronic nature of periodontal disease has complicated the search for bacterial pathogens. It was previously thought that periodontal diseases progressed at a slow but steady rate. However, epidemiologic studies have established that the disease progresses at different rates, with episodes of rapid tissue destruction alternating with periods of remission. Identification of the microorganisms found during the different phases of the disease process is technically challenging.

Despite the difficulties inherent in characterizing the microbiology of periodontal diseases, a small group of pathogens is recognized owing to their association with disease. The properties of these microorganisms that enable them to function as pathogens in the periodontal environment are currently under investigation and promise to provide much information about the basic mechanisms involved in the disease process. Technologic advances in the field of immunologic, enzymatic, and recombinant DNA probes have improved the ability to detect specific bacteria and their products, which may serve as markers of ongoing disease or predictors of future disease. Some of these technologies have led to commercial products that are currently available for use in clinical therapy. However, while considerable advances have been made toward understanding the bacterial etiology of periodontal diseases, a complete answer to the question of what causes periodontal diseases is not known.

DENTAL PLAQUE: A HOST-ASSOCIATED BIOFILM

Dental plaque is a host-associated biofilm. This is important, as the biofilm environment is often advantageous for a microorganism and may have significant effects on the properties of bacteria that exist there. For example, the susceptibility of bacteria to antimicrobial agents may be significantly reduced by the biofilm structure itself.[15]

The biofilm community is initially formed through bacterial interactions with the tooth, and then through physical and physiologic interactions among different species within the microbial mass. Furthermore, the bacteria found in the plaque biofilm are also strongly influenced by external environmental factors that may be host mediated. Periodontal health can be considered to be a state of balance in which the bacterial population coexists with the host, and no irreparable damage occurs to either the bacteria or the host tissues. Disruption of this balance causes alterations in both

Table 6-1. RECLASSIFICATIONS OF PERIODONTAL BACTERIA

Previous Classifications	New Classification
Bacteroides gingivalis	*Porphyromonas gingivalis*
Bacteroides endodontalis	*Porphyromonas endodontalis*
Bacteroides intermedius	*Prevotella intermedia*
Bacteroides melaninogenicus	*Prevotella melaninogenica*
Bacteroides denticola	*Prevotella denticola*
Bacteroides loescheii	*Prevotella loescheii*
Wolinella recta	*Campylobacter rectus*
Wolinella curva	*Campylobacter curvus*

Based on Shah HN, Collins MD. Proposal for reclassification of *Bacteroides asaccharolyticus, Bacteroides gingivalis,* and *Bacteroides endodontalis* in a new genus, *Porphyromonas*. Int J Sys Bacteriol 38:128, 1988; *Prevotella*, a new genus to include *Bacteroides melaninogenicus* and related species formally classified in the genus *Bacteroides*. Int J Sys Bacteriol 40:205, 1990; and Vandamme P, Falsen E, Rossau R, et al. Revision of *Campylobacter, Helicobacter,* and *Wolinella* taxonomy: Emendation of generic descriptions and proposal of *Arcobacter* gen. nov. Int J Sys Bacteriol 41:88, 1991.

the host and biofilm bacteria and results ultimately in the destruction of the connective tissues of the periodontium.

Structure and Composition of Dental Plaque

Dental plaque can be defined as the soft deposits that form the biofilm adhering to the tooth surface or other hard surfaces in the oral cavity, including removable and fixed restorations.[3] Plaque is differentiated from other deposits that may be found on the tooth surface such as materia alba and calculus (Plate II). *Materia alba* refers to soft accumulations of bacteria and tissue cells that lack the organized structure of dental plaque and are easily displaced with a water spray. *Calculus* is a hard deposit that forms by mineralization of dental plaque and is generally covered by a layer of unmineralized plaque.

Dental plaque is broadly classified as supragingival or subgingival based on its position on the tooth surface. *Supragingival plaque* is found at or above the gingival margin; the supragingival plaque that is in direct contact with the gingival margin is referred to as *marginal plaque.*

Subgingival plaque is found below the gingival margin, between the tooth and the gingival sulcular tissue. Morphologic studies[1,9,52,55,74,76,88,89] indicate a differentiation of tooth-associated and tissue-associated regions of subgingival plaque, and in certain cases bacteria are found within the host tissues (see later discussion of invasion). The different regions of plaque are significant to different processes associated with diseases of the teeth and periodontium. For example, marginal plaque is of prime importance in the development of gingivitis. Supragingival plaque and tooth-associated subgingival plaque are critical in calculus formation and root caries, whereas tissue-associated subgingival plaque is important in the soft tissue destruction characteristic of different forms of periodontitis.

Dental plaque is composed primarily of microorganisms. One gram of plaque (wet weight) contains approximately 2×10^{11} bacteria.[101] Because 1 gm of pure streptococcal cells packed by centrifugation contains 2.3×10^{11} bacteria, bacteria account for almost all of the plaque weight.[101] It has been estimated that more than 325 different bacterial species may be found in plaque[71] (Fig. 6-1). Nonbacterial microorganisms that are found in plaque include *Mycoplasma* species, yeasts, protozoa, and viruses. The microorganisms exist within an intercellular matrix that also contains a few host cells, such as epithelial cells, macrophages, and leukocytes (Fig. 6-2).

The intercellular matrix, estimated to account for 20% to 30% of the plaque mass, consists of organic and inorganic materials derived from saliva, gingival crevicular fluid, and bacterial products. Organic constituents of the matrix include polysaccharides, proteins, glycoproteins, and lipid material. Glycoproteins from saliva are an important component of the pellicle that initially coats a clean tooth surface (see later discussion), but they also become incorporated into the developing plaque biofilm. Polysaccharides produced by bacteria, of which dextran is the predominant form, contribute to the organic portion of the matrix. Albumin, probably originating from crevicular fluid, has been identified as a component of plaque matrix. The lipid material consists of debris from the membranes of disrupted bacterial and host cells and possibly food debris.

The inorganic component of plaque is primarily calcium and phosphorus, with trace amounts of other minerals such as sodium, potassium, and fluoride. The source of inorganic constituents of supragingival plaque is primarily saliva; as the mineral content increases, the plaque mass becomes calcified to form calculus. Calculus is frequently found in areas of the dentition adjacent to salivary ducts (e.g., the lingual surface of the mandibular anteriors and the buccal surface of the maxillary first molars), reflecting the high concentration of minerals available from saliva in those regions.

The inorganic component of subgingival plaque is derived from crevicular fluid, which is a serum transudate. Calcification of subgingival plaque also results in calculus formation. Subgingival calculus is typically dark green or dark brown, probably reflecting the presence of subgingival matrix components distinct from those of supragingival calculus (e.g., blood products associated with subgingival hemorrhage). The fluoride component of plaque is largely derived from external sources such as fluoridated toothpastes and rinses. Fluoride is used therapeutically to aid in remineralization of tooth structure, prevention of demineralization of tooth structure, and inhibition of the growth of many plaque microorganisms.[85]

The intercellular matrix forms a hydrated gel in which the embedded bacteria exist and proliferate. This gel-like matrix is a primary characteristic of biofilms. The matrix confers specialized properties on bacteria that exist within the biofilm, in contrast to free-floating bacteria. For example, the biofilm gel functions as a barrier. Substances produced by bacteria within the biofilm are retained and essentially concentrated, which fosters metabolic interactions among the different bacteria (see later discussion of physiologic properties). In addition, the matrix is thought to protect resident bacteria from potentially harmful substances such as antimicrobial agents, which may be unable to diffuse through the matrix to reach the bacterial cells.

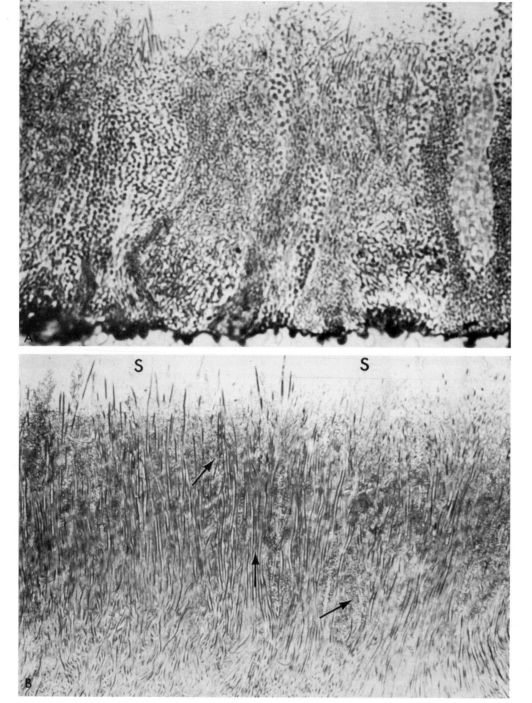

FIGURE 6–1. *A,* One-day-old plaque. Microcolonies of plaque bacteria extend perpendicularly away from tooth surfaces. (From Listgarten M. Development of dental plaque on epoxy resin crowns in man. A light and electron microscopic study. J Periodontol *46:*10, 1975.) *B,* Developed supragingival plaque showing overall filamentous nature and microcolonies *(arrows)* extending perpendicularly away from tooth surface. Saliva–plaque interface shown (S). (Courtesy of Dr. Max Listgarten.)

Formation of Dental Plaque

Dental plaque may be readily visualized on teeth after 1 to 2 days with no oral hygiene measures. Plaque is white, grayish, or yellow and has a globular appearance. Movement of tissues and food materials over the teeth results in mechanical removal of plaque; such removal is particularly effective on the coronal two thirds of the tooth surface. Thus, plaque is typically observed on the gingival third of the tooth surface, where it accumulates without disruption by the movement of food and tissues over the tooth surface during mastication. Plaque deposits also form preferentially in cracks, pits, and fissures in the tooth structure; under overhanging restorations; and around malaligned teeth.

The location and rate of plaque formation vary among individuals, and determining factors include oral hygiene, as well as host factors such as diet or salivary composition and flow rate.[64]

Small amounts of plaque that are not discernible on the tooth surface may be detected by running a periodontal probe or explorer along the gingival third of the tooth. Another common method of detecting small amounts of plaque is the use of disclosing solutions (see Plate II). Interproximal plaque formation is less evident visually but may also be monitored with an explorer or probe.

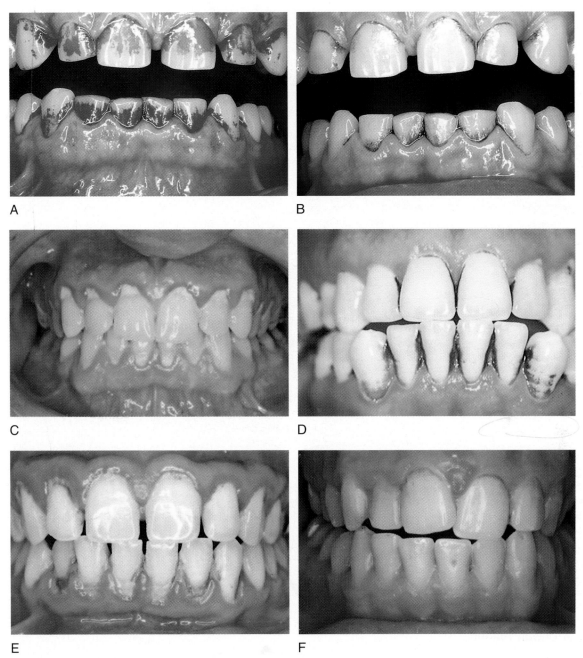

PLATE II. *A,* Disclosed supragingival plaque covering one half to two thirds of the clinical crowns. *B,* Same patient as in *A.* Supragingival plaque disclosed with an oxidation-reduction dye that indicates reduced (anaerobic) areas of plaque. The supragingival anaerobic areas (purple stain) are located interproximally and along the gingival margin. (*A* and *B* courtesy of Dr. S. Socransky.) *C,* Materia alba generalized throughout the mouth, with heaviest accumulation near the gingiva. Note the gingivitis present. *D,* Teeth stained by several weeks of mouth rinses with alexidine. This stain can be easily removed. *E,* Supragingival calculus in a patient with gingival inflammation. *F,* Green stain on anterior teeth. Note the inflamed, enlarged interdental papilla between the maxillary central incisors.

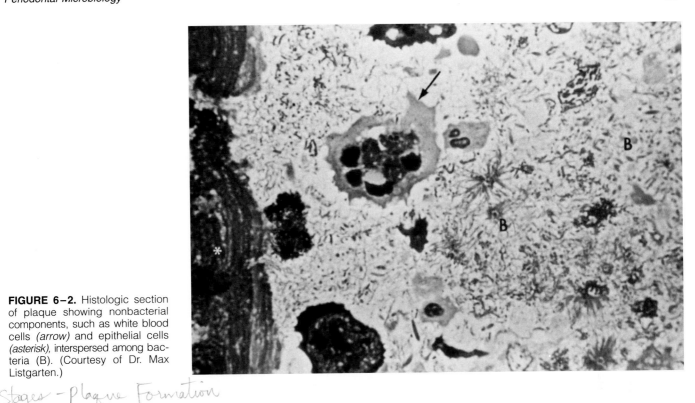

FIGURE 6–2. Histologic section of plaque showing nonbacterial components, such as white blood cells *(arrow)* and epithelial cells *(asterisk),* interspersed among bacteria (B). (Courtesy of Dr. Max Listgarten.)

3 Stages – Plague Formation

In the absence of oral hygiene measures, plaque will continue to accumulate until a balance is reached between the forces of plaque removal and those of plaque formation. The formation of dental plaque at the microscopic level represents a highly ordered and predictable ecologic succession.

The process of plaque formation can be divided into three phases: the formation of the pellicle coating on the tooth surface, initial colonization by bacteria, and secondary colonization and plaque maturation.

① **Formation of the Dental Pellicle.** Formation of the dental pellicle on the tooth surface is the initial phase of plaque development. All surfaces of the oral cavity, including all tissue surfaces as well as surfaces of teeth and fixed and removable restorations, are coated with a glycoprotein pellicle. This pellicle is derived from components of saliva and crevicular fluid, as well as from bacterial and host tissue cell products and debris.

The specific components of pellicles on different surfaces vary in composition. Studies of early (2-hour) enamel pellicle reveal that its amino acid composition differs from that of saliva,[91] indicating that the pellicle forms by *selective adsorption of the environmental macromolecules.* The mechanisms involved in enamel pellicle formation include electrostatic, van der Waals, and hydrophobic forces. The hydroxyapatite surface has a predominance of negatively charged phosphate groups that interact directly or indirectly with positively charged components of salivary and crevicular fluid macromolecules.[84]

Pellicles function as a protective barrier, providing lubrication for the surfaces and preventing tissue dessication. However, they also provide a substrate to which bacteria in the environment attach. Because the epithelial tissue cells are continually sloughed, the bacterial population on the tissue surfaces is continually disrupted. In contrast, pellicle on the nonshedding hard surfaces provides a substrate on which bacteria progressively accumulate to form dental plaque.

② **Initial Colonization of the Tooth Surface.** Within a few hours bacteria are found on the dental pellicle. The initial bacteria colonizing the pellicle-coated tooth surface are predominantly gram-positive facultative microorganisms such as *Actinomyces viscosus* and *Streptococcus sanguis.* These initial colonizers adhere to the pellicle[22,24,68] through specific molecules, termed *adhesins,* on the bacterial surface that interact with receptors in the dental pellicle. For example, cells of *A. viscosus* possess fibrous protein structures called *fimbriae* that extend from the bacterial cell surface. Protein adhesins on these fimbriae specifically bind to proline-rich proteins that are found in dental pellicle,[68] resulting in the attachment of the bacterial cell to the pellicle-coated tooth surface.

The plaque mass then matures through the growth of attached species, as well as the colonization and growth of additional species. *In this ecologic succession of the biofilm, there is a transition from the early aerobic environment characterized by gram-positive facultative species to a highly oxygen-deprived environment in which gram-negative anaerobic microorganisms predominate.*

③ **Secondary Colonization and Plaque Maturation.** Secondary colonizers are the microorganisms that do not initially colonize clean tooth surfaces, including *Prevotella intermedia, Prevotella loescheii, Capnocytophaga* species, *Fusobacterium nucleatum,* and *Porphyromonas gingivalis.*[42] These microorganisms adhere to cells of bacteria already in the plaque mass. Extensive laboratory studies have documented the ability of different species and genera of plaque microorganisms to adhere to one another, a process known as *coaggregation.* This process occurs primarily through the highly specific stereochemical interaction of protein and carbohydrate molecules located on the bacterial cell surfaces,[40,42] in addition to the less specific interactions result-

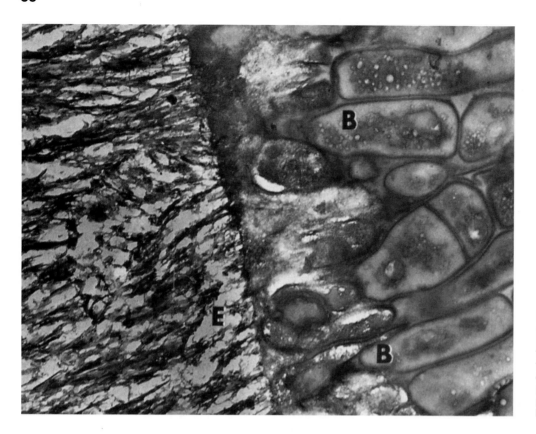

FIGURE 6–3. Plaque formed directly on enamel surface. Electron micrograph of decalcified, noncarious enamel surface showing remnants of enamel matrix (E) and gram-positive bacteria (B) in attached plaque. (Courtesy of Dr. R. M. Frank and Dr. A. Brendel.)

ing from hydrophobic, electrostatic, and van der Waals forces.[17,25]

The significance of coaggregation in oral colonization has been documented in animal model studies.[66] Well-characterized interactions of secondary colonizers with early colonizers include the coaggregation of *F. nucleatum* with *S. sanguis*,[37] *P. loescheii* with *A. viscosus*,[115,116] and *Capnocytophaga ochracea* with *A. viscosus*.[114] Most studies of coaggregation have focused on interactions between different gram-positive species and between gram-positive and gram-negative species. In the latter stages of plaque formation, coaggregation between different gram-negative species is likely to predominate. An example of this type of interaction is the coaggregation of *F. nucleatum* with *P. gingivalis*.[38,39,41]

Structural and Physiologic Properties of Dental Plaque

A high degree of specificity is found in the interactions between bacteria in dental plaque as demonstrated by the studies of coaggregation. This is further evident from light and electron microscopic studies of the structure of dental plaque formed in vivo.[52]

Supragingival plaque typically demonstrates a stratified organization of the bacterial morphotypes. Gram-positive cocci and short rods predominate at the tooth surface (Fig. 6–3), whereas gram-negative rods and filaments (see Fig. 6–1), as well as spirochetes, predominate in the outer surface of the mature plaque mass. Highly specific cell-to-cell interactions are also evident from the "corncob" structures[54] that are often observed (Fig. 6–4). "Corncob" formations have been observed between rod-shaped bacterial cells

(e.g., *Bacterionema matruchotii* or *F. nucleatum*) that form the inner core of the structure, and coccal cells (e.g., streptococci or *P. gingivalis*) that attach along the surface of the rod-shaped cell.[40,46,75]

The environmental parameters of the subgingival region differ from those of the supragingival region. The gingival crevice or pocket is bathed by the flow of crevicular fluid, which contains many substances that the bacteria may use as nutrients (see later discussion). Host inflammatory cells and mediators are likely to have considerable influence on the establishment and growth of bacteria in this region. Morphologic and microbiologic studies of subgingival plaque reveal distinctions between the tooth-associated and

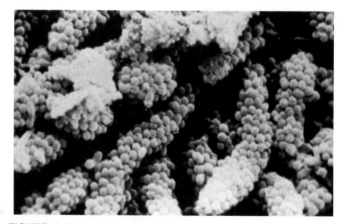

FIGURE 6–4. Long-standing supragingival plaque near the gingival margin demonstrates "corncob" arrangement. A central gram-negative filamentous core supports the outer coccal cells, which are firmly attached by interbacterial adherence or coaggregation.

tissue-associated regions of subgingival plaque (Figs. 6-5 and 6-6).

The tooth-associated (attached) plaque (Figs. 6-7 and 6-8) is characterized by gram-positive rods and cocci, including bacteria such as *Streptococcus mitis, S. sanguis, A. viscosus, Actinomyces naeslundii,* and *Eubacterium* species. *The apical border of the plaque mass is separated from the junctional epithelium by a layer of host leukocytes, and the bacteria of this apical tooth-associated region show an increased concentration of gram-negative rods.* The portion of plaque adjacent to the tissue surfaces (Figs. 6-9 and 6-10) is more loosely organized than the very dense tooth-associated region. It contains primarily gram-negative rods and cocci, as well as large numbers of filaments, flagellated rods, and spirochetes. Host tissue cells (e.g., white blood cells and epithelial cells) may also be found in this region. Cultural studies of tissue-associated plaque indicate a predominance of species such as *P. gingivalis, P. intermedia,* and *C. ochracea.*[19] Bacteria found in tissue-associated plaque (e.g., *P. gingivalis*) have also been found in host tissues.[87] Thus, the physical proximity of these bacteria to the host tissues in the plaque mass may be important in the process of tissue invasion (see later discussion).

The transition from gram-positive to gram-negative microorganisms observed in the structure of dental plaque is paralleled by a physiologic transition in the developing plaque. The early colonizers (e.g., streptococci and *Actinomyces*) utilize oxygen and lower the reduction-oxidation potential of the environment, which then favors the growth of anaerobic species.[112] Gram-positive species utilize sugars as an energy source and saliva as a carbon source. The bacteria that predominate in mature plaque are anaerobic, asaccharolytic, and use amino acids and small peptides as energy sources.[61]

Laboratory studies have demonstrated many physiologic interactions among the different bacteria found in dental plaque (Fig. 6-11). Lactate and formate are by-products of the metabolism of streptococci and *Actinomyces* and may be utilized in the metabolism of other plaque microorganisms. The growth of *P. gingivalis* is enhanced by metabolic by-products produced by other microorganisms, such as succinate from *C. ochracea* and protoheme from *Campylobacter rectus.*[32,33,65]

The host also functions as an important source of nutrients. For example, the bacterial enzymes that degrade host proteins result in the release of ammonia, which may be used by bacteria as a nitrogen source.[8] Hemin iron from the breakdown of host hemoglobin may be important in the metabolism of *P. gingivalis.*[4] Increases in steroid hormones are associated with significant increases in the proportions of *P. intermedia* found in subgingival plaque.[44] Thus, physiologic interactions occur both between different microorganisms in plaque and between the host and plaque microorganisms. These nutritional interdependencies are probably critical to the growth and survival of microorganisms in dental plaque and may partly explain the highly specific structural interactions observed among bacteria in plaque.

ASSOCIATION OF PLAQUE MICROORGANISMS WITH PERIODONTAL DISEASES

Microbial Specificity of Periodontal Diseases

In the mid-1900s periodontal disease was believed to result from an accumulation of plaque over time in conjunction with a diminished host response and increased host susceptibility with age. This thinking was supported by epidemiologic studies that correlated both age and the amount of plaque with evidence of periodontitis.[63,86,92] Periodontal disease was clearly associated with plaque, and it was thought that all plaque was alike and equally capable of causing disease.

Several observations, however, contradicted these conclusions. First, some individuals with considerable amounts of plaque and calculus, as well as gingivitis, never developed destructive periodontitis. Furthermore, individuals who did present with periodontitis demonstrated considerable site specificity in the pattern of disease. Some sites were unaffected, while advanced disease was found in adjacent sites. In the presence of a uniform host response, these findings were inconsistent with the concept that all plaque was equally pathogenic. Recognition of the differences in

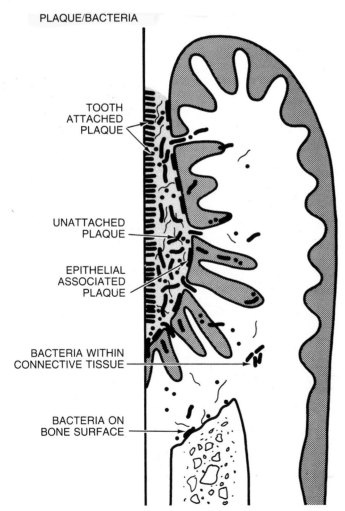

PLAQUE/BACTERIA

TOOTH ATTACHED PLAQUE

UNATTACHED PLAQUE

EPITHELIAL ASSOCIATED PLAQUE

BACTERIA WITHIN CONNECTIVE TISSUE

BACTERIA ON BONE SURFACE

FIGURE 6-5. Diagram depicting the plaque/bacteria association with tooth surface and periodontal tissues.

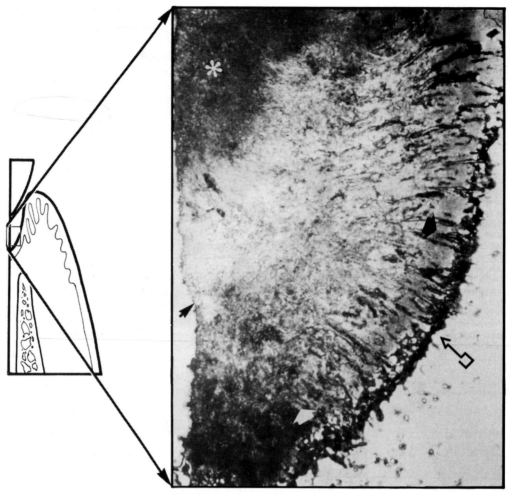

FIGURE 6–6. *Left,* Diagrammatic representation of the histologic structure of subgingival plaque. *Right,* Histologic section of subgingival plaque. *Arrow with box,* Sulcular epithelium. *White arrow,* Predominantly gram-negative unattached zone. *Black arrow,* Tooth surface. *Asterisk,* Predominantly gram-positive attached zone. (From Listgarten M. Development of dental plaque on epoxy resin crowns in man. A light and electron microscopic study. J Periodontol *46:*10, 1975.)

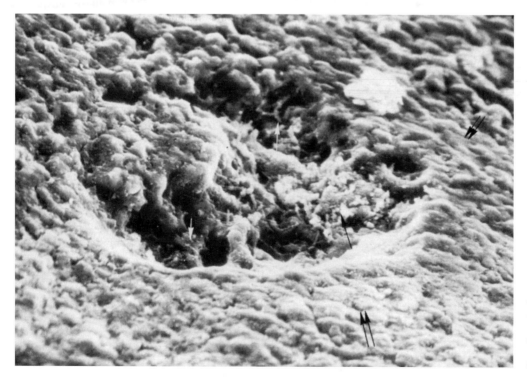

FIGURE 6–7. Minute lesion on surface of root (resorption cavity) previously covered by attached plaque. Note microorganisms *(single arrows)* within resorption cavity. Cemental mounds can easily be identified *(double arrows).* (Courtesy of Dr. J. Sottosanti.)

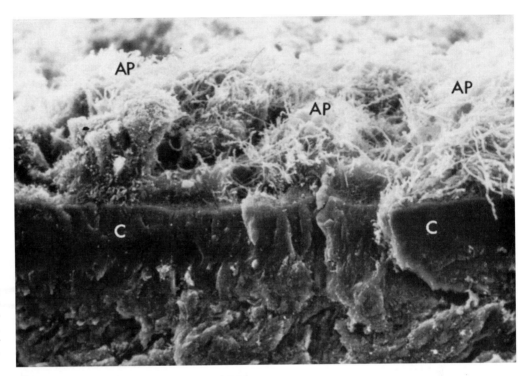

FIGURE 6-8. Scanning electron photomicrograph of cross section of cementum (C) with attached subgingival plaque (AP). Area shown is within a periodontal pocket. (Courtesy of Dr. J. Sottosanti.)

plaque at sites of different clinical status (i.e., disease versus health)[58,97,101] led to a renewed search for specific pathogens in periodontal diseases and a conceptual transition from the nonspecific to the specific plaque hypothesis.

Nonspecific Plaque Hypothesis

The nonspecific and specific plaque hypotheses were delineated in 1976 by Walter Loesche, a researcher at the University of Michigan. The nonspecific plaque hypothesis maintains that periodontal disease results from the "elaboration of noxious products by the entire plaque flora."[60] According to this thinking, when only small amounts of

plaque are present, the noxious products are neutralized by the host. Similarly, large amounts of plaque would produce large amounts of noxious products, which would essentially overwhelm the host's defenses. Inherent in the nonspecific plaque hypothesis is the concept that control of periodontal disease depends on control of the amount of plaque accumulation. Treatment of periodontitis by debridement (nonsurgical or surgical) and oral hygiene measures focuses on the removal of plaque and its products and is founded in the nonspecific plaque hypothesis. Thus, although the nonspecific plaque hypothesis has been discarded in favor of the specific plaque hypothesis, much clinical treatment is still based on the nonspecific plaque hypothesis.

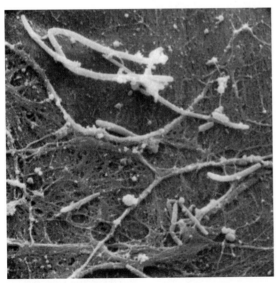

FIGURE 6-9. Scanning electron micrograph of cocci and filaments associated with surface of pocket epithelium in a case of marginal gingivitis. ×3000.

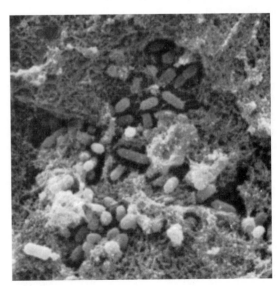

FIGURE 6-10. Scanning electron micrograph of frontal view of pocket wall showing short rods on epithelial surface. ×10,000.

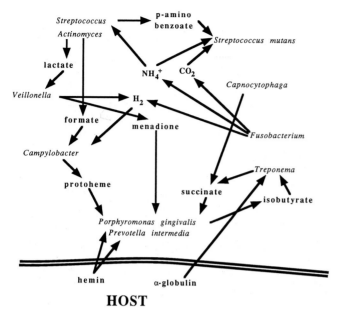

FIGURE 6–11. Schematic illustration of metabolic interactions among different bacterial species found in plaque, as well as between the host and plaque bacteria. These interactions are likely to be important to the survival of bacteria in the periodontal environment. (Based on Grenier,[30] Loesche,[61] Walden and Hentges,[112] and Carlsson.[8])

Specific Plaque Hypothesis

The specific plaque hypothesis states that only certain plaque is pathogenic, and its pathogenicity depends on the presence of or increase in specific microorganisms.[60] This concept predicts that plaque harboring specific bacterial pathogens results in periodontal disease, because these organisms produce substances that mediate the destruction of host tissues.

At about the same time that Loesche proposed the specific plaque hypothesis, major advances were made in techniques used to isolate and identify periodontal microorganisms. These included improvements in procedures to sample subgingival plaque, in handling samples to prevent killing the bacteria, and in the media used to grow the bacteria in the laboratory.[102] The result was a tremendous increase in the ability to isolate periodontal microorganisms and considerable refinement in bacterial taxonomy. Acceptance of the specific plaque hypothesis was spurred by the recognition of *Actinobacillus actinomycetemcomitans* as a pathogen in localized juvenile periodontitis.[77,97] A series of association studies was begun that focused on identifying specific periodontal pathogens by examining the microbiota associated with states of health and disease in cross-sectional and longitudinal studies.

Microorganisms Associated With Specific Periodontal Diseases

The microbiota associated with periodontal health and disease has been studied with a wide variety of techniques for sampling and cultivation of bacteria, as well as different classifications of disease status.[8,20,62,71,77,101,107,119] These variables make direct comparisons of such studies difficult. However, comparisons do reveal the general characteristics of the microbial populations found in the presence of different clinical states and implicate a discrete group of bacteria that function as periodontal pathogens.

Early studies that used appropriate microbiologic procedures clearly demonstrated that the number and proportions of different subgingival bacterial groups varied in periodontal health when compared with the disease state.[53,97,101] The total number of bacteria, determined by microscopic counts per gram of plaque, are twice as high in periodontally diseased sites than in healthy sites.[101] Because considerably more plaque is found at diseased sites, this suggests that the total bacterial load is much greater than that at healthy sites.

The differences between periodontal health and disease are also evident when the morphotypes of the bacteria from healthy and diseased sites are examined. There are fewer coccal cells and more motile rods and spirochetes in diseased sites than in healthy sites (Fig. 6–12).[53] The bacteria cultivated from periodontally healthy sites[97] consist predominantly of gram-positive facultative rods and cocci (approximately 75%). The recovery of this group of microorganisms is decreased proportionally in gingivitis (44%) and periodontitis (10% to 13%). These decreases are accompanied by increases in the proportions of gram-negative rods from 13% in health to 40% in gingivitis, 65% in localized juvenile periodontitis, and 74% in advanced periodontitis (Fig. 6–13).

The specific bacterial species associated with the different states of disease and health based on studies in human populations are discussed in the following sections. The classification of periodontal diseases has evolved considerably,[81] so for the purposes of this discussion, broad categories of disease are used.

Periodontal Health. The recovery of microorganisms from periodontally healthy sites is meager when compared

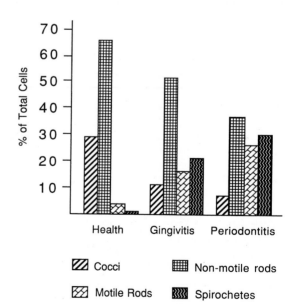

FIGURE 6–12. Bacterial morphotypes in the subgingival microbiota associated with periodontal health and disease based on direct microscopic examination. (Adapted from Slots J, Rams TE. Microbiology of periodontal disease. In Slots J, Taubman MA, eds. Contemporary Oral Microbiology and Immunology. St Louis, CV Mosby, 1992.)

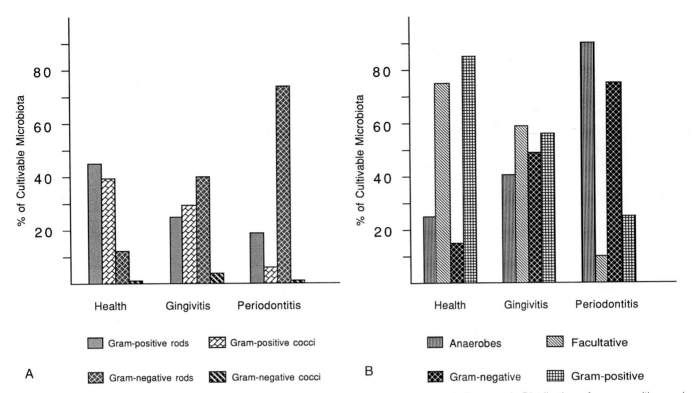

FIGURE 6-13. Cultivable subgingival microbiota associated with periodontal health and disease. *A,* Distribution of gram-positive and gram-negative rods and cocci. *B,* Distribution of anaerobic, facultative, gram-positive and gram-negative species. (Adapted from Slots J, Rams TE. Microbiology of periodontal disease. In Slots J, Taubman MA, eds. Contemporary Oral Microbiology and Immunology. St Louis, CV Mosby, 1992.)

with that from diseased sites. The bacteria associated with periodontal health are primarily gram-positive facultative species and members of the genera *Streptococcus* and *Actinomyces* (e.g., *S. sanguis, S. mitis, A. viscosus,* and *A. naeslundii*). Small proportions of gram-negative species are also found, most frequently *P. intermedia, F. nucleatum,* and *Capnocytophaga, Neisseria,* and *Veillonella* spp. Microscopic studies indicate that a few spirochetes and motile rods may also be found.

Certain bacterial species have been proposed to be protective or beneficial to the host, including *S. sanguis, Veillonella parvula,* and *C. ochracea.* They are typically found in high numbers at periodontal sites that do not demonstrate attachment loss (inactive sites), but in low numbers at sites where active periodontal destruction occurs.[21,102] These species probably function in preventing the colonization or proliferation of pathogenic microorganisms. One example of a mechanism by which this may occur is the production of H_2O_2 by *S. sanguis;* H_2O_2 is known to be lethal to cells of *Actinobacillus actinomycetemcomitans.*[102] Clinical studies have shown that sites with high levels of *C. ochracea* and *S. sanguis* are associated with a greater gain of attachment level after therapy,[102] further supporting this concept. A better understanding of plaque ecology and the interactions between bacteria and their products in plaque will undoubtedly reveal many other examples.

Gingivitis. The development of gingivitis has been extensively studied in a model system referred to as *experimental gingivitis* and initially described by Löe and coworkers.[58,109] Periodontal health is first established in human subjects by cleaning and rigorous oral hygiene mea-

sures, followed by abstinence from oral hygiene for 21 days. After 8 hours without oral hygiene, bacteria may be found at concentrations of 10^3 to 10^4 per square millimeter of tooth surface and will increase in number by a factor of 100 to 1000 in the next 24-hour period.[104] A healthy periodontium will develop gingivitis within 3 to 4 days.

The initial microbiota of experimental gingivitis consists of gram-positive rods, gram-positive cocci, and gram-negative cocci. The transition to gingivitis is evident by inflammatory changes observed in the gingival tissues and is accompanied first by the appearance of gram-negative rods and filaments (Fig. 6–14), then by spirochetal and motile microorganisms.[109]

The bacteria found in *chronic gingivitis* consist of roughly equal proportions of gram-positive (56%) and gram-negative (44%) species, as well as facultative (59%) and anaerobic (41%) microorganisms (see Fig. 6–13).[97] The gram-positive species are primarily *S. sanguis, S. mitis, A. viscosus, A. naeslundii,* and *Peptostreptococcus micros.* The gram-negative microorganisms are predominantly *F. nucleatum, P. intermedia, V. parvula,* and *Haemophilus* and *Campylobacter* spp.[97]

Pregnancy gingivitis is an acute inflammation of the gingival tissues associated with pregnancy. This condition is accompanied by increases in steroid hormones in crevicular fluid and dramatic increases in the levels of *P. intermedia,* which use the steroids as growth factors.[44]

Acute necrotizing ulcerative gingivitis (ANUG) is an acute inflammation of the gingiva characterized by tissue necrosis of the gingival margin and interdental papillae. Clinically the condition is often associated with stress or

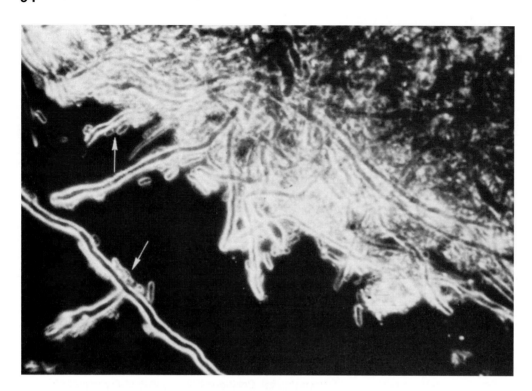

FIGURE 6–14. Darkfield photomicrograph demonstrating the filamentous nature of plaque associated with gingivitis. Note attachment of smaller bacteria to filaments *(arrows).*

human immunodeficiency virus (HIV) infection. It is accompanied by malodor, pain, and possibly systemic symptoms, including lymphadenopathy, fever, and malaise. Microbiologic studies indicate that high levels of *P. intermedia* and spirochetes are found in ANUG lesions. Spirochetes are found to penetrate necrotic tissue as well as apparently unaffected connective tissue.[51,56]

Studies of gingivitis support the conclusion that disease development is associated with characteristic alterations in the microbial composition of dental plaque and are not due simply to an accumulation of plaque. Gingivitis is generally believed to precede the development of chronic periodontitis; however, many individuals demonstrate long-standing gingivitis that never advances to destruction of the periodontal attachment.[6,57]

Adult Periodontitis. The hallmark of periodontitis is the loss of connective tissue attachment to the tooth. Numerous forms of periodontal disease are found in adult populations; these forms are characterized by different rates of progression (Fig. 6–15) and different responses to therapy. Studies in which untreated populations were examined over long time intervals indicate disease progression at mean rates ranging from 0.05 to 0.3 mm of attachment loss per year ("gradual model").[6] When populations are examined over short time intervals, individual sites demonstrated short phases of attachment destruction interposed by periods of no disease activity ("burst model").[29] It is unclear from current studies whether the gradual or burst model of disease progression, or some other model, is correct.[6]

Microbiologic examinations of adult periodontitis have been carried out in both cross-sectional and longitudinal studies; the latter have been conducted both with and without treatment. These studies support the concept that adult periodontitis is associated with specific bacterial agents.

Microscopic examination of plaque from sites with periodontitis have consistently revealed elevated proportions of spirochetes (see Fig. 6–12).[53,62] Cultivation of plaque microorganisms from sites of adult periodontitis reveals high percentages of anaerobic (90%) gram-negative (75%) species (see Fig. 6–13).[96,97]

In *chronic adult periodontitis* the microorganisms most often cultivated at high levels include *P. gingivalis, Bacteroides forsythus, P. intermedia, C. rectus, Eikenella corrodens, F. nucleatum, A. actinomycetemcomitans,* and *Treponema* and *Eubacterium* spp.[62,71,96,97,102,103,107] When periodontally active sites (i.e., with recent attachment loss) were examined in comparison with inactive sites (i.e., with no recent attachment loss), *C. rectus, P. gingivalis, P. intermedia, F. nucleatum,* and *B. forsythus* were found to be elevated in the active sites.[20] Furthermore, detectable levels of *P. gingivalis, P. intermedia, B. forsythus, C. rectus,* and *A. actinomycetemcomitans* are associated with disease progression,[20,117] and elimination of specific bacterial pathogens with therapy is associated with an improved clinical response.[13,98]

Rapidly Progressive Periodontitis. Epidemiologic data indicate that between 7% and 15% of the populations studied experienced severe or rapidly progressing periodontitis.[14] Microbiologic studies indicate an association between this disease and elevated levels of *P. gingivalis, P. intermedia, A. actinomycetemcomitans, E. corrodens, C. rectus,* and *Bacteroides* capillus.[73,108] It may be significant in aggressive forms of adult periodontitis that both *P. gingivalis* and *A. actinomycetemcomitans* have been shown to invade host tissue cells.[9,10,87]

Juvenile Periodontitis. Several forms of periodontitis are characterized by rapid and severe attachment loss occurring in individuals at or prior to puberty. They are al-

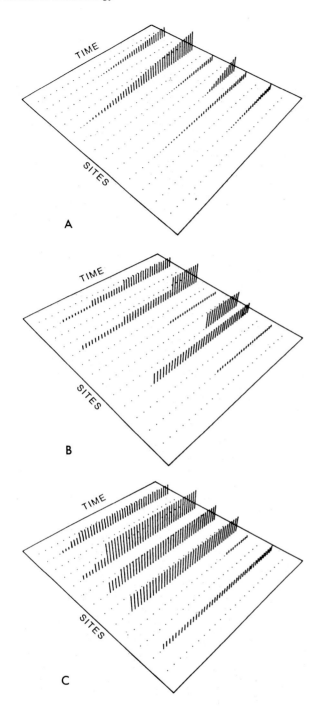

FIGURE 6-15. Diagrammatic representation of different possible modes of progression of chronic destructive periodontal disease. Sites on the x-axis are plotted against time on the y-axis, and activity is shown on the z-axis. A, Some sites show progressive loss of attachment over time, whereas others show no destruction. The time of onset and the extent of destruction vary from site to site. B, Random burst model. Activity occurs at random at any site. Some sites show no activity, whereas others show one or several bursts of activity. The cumulative extent of destruction varies from site to site. C, Asynchronous multiple burst model. Several sites show bursts of activity over a finite period, followed by prolonged periods of inactivity. Occasional bursts may occur infrequently at certain sites at later periods. Other sites show no periodontal disease activity at any time. The difference from the model shown in B is that here the majority of destructive disease activity takes place within a few years of the individual's life. (Courtesy of Drs. S. Socransky, A. Haffajee, M. Goodson, and J. Lindhe.)

most uniformly seen in individuals who demonstrate a systemic defect in immune regulation. Juvenile periodontitis (also called *localized juvenile periodontitis* [LJP]) (see Chapter 27) develops around the time of puberty, is observed in females more often than in males, and typically affects the permanent molars and incisors. Most affected individuals demonstrate defective neutrophil function.

The microbiota associated with juvenile periodontitis is predominantly composed of gram-negative, capnophilic, and anaerobic rods.[77-79,97] Microbiologic studies indicate that almost all LJP sites harbor *A. actinomycetemcomitans,* which may make up as much as 90% of the total cultivable microbiota.[45,71] Other organisms found in significant levels include *P. gingivalis, E. corrodens, C. rectus, F. nucleatum, B. capillus, Eubacterium brachy,* and *Capnocytophaga* spp. and spirochetes.[45,71,72] It is generally accepted that *A. actinomycetemcomitans* is the primary etiologic agent in most, but not all, cases of LJP (see later discussion of virulence factors).[43,102] Studies of therapy indicate that both mechanical debridement and systemic antibiotic treatment are necessary to control the levels of *A. actinomycetemcomitans* in LJP.[45,82,83] The failure of mechanical therapy alone may relate to the ability of this organism to invade host tissues.[9,10,87]

Prepubertal Periodontitis. Prepubertal periodontitis is a rare form of the disease that affects the primary dentition (see Chapter 27). The microorganisms associated with localized forms of the disease include *P. gingivalis, P. intermedia, A. actinomycetemcomitans,* and *F. nucleatum.*[80] Most afflicted individuals also demonstrate profound immunologic abnormalities, and identification of the periodontal condition may be one of the first signs of systemic disease.

Conclusions From Studies of the Association of Microorganisms With Periodontal Diseases

Studies examining the microbiota associated with periodontal diseases versus the healthy state indicate that a discrete number of microorganisms appear to function as pathogens in the disease process. Association is important but is only one aspect of demonstrating an etiologic role for a particular bacterium (see later discussion). The periodontal microbiota is a very complex ecologic system with many structural and physiologic interactions among the resident bacteria and between the bacteria and the host. It is clearly possible that levels of a particular species may be elevated as a result of environmental changes produced by the disease process and may not be a causative agent. For example, in studies on the development of gingivitis in humans at the time of puberty, it was found that only the proportions of *Capnocytophaga* species increased prior to the development of gingivitis, and *P. intermedia* was recovered only after the onset of gingivitis.[70] This suggests a causative role for the *Capnocytophaga* species and that environmental changes associated with disease then favor the emergence of species such as *P. intermedia.* Thus, the association studies represent a first step in critically identifying pathogens in periodontal diseases.

CRITERIA FOR IDENTIFICATION OF PERIODONTAL PATHOGENS

In the 1870s Robert Koch developed the criteria by which a microorganism can be judged to be a causative agent in human infections. These criteria, known as *Koch's postulates,* stipulate that the causative agent must

1. Be routinely isolated from diseased individuals;
2. Be grown in pure culture in the laboratory;
3. Produce a similar disease when inoculated into susceptible laboratory animals; and
4. Be recovered from lesions in a diseased laboratory animal.

These criteria remain the basis for elucidating infectious agents. For example, *Streptococcus mutans* has been shown to fulfill Koch's postulates as an etiologic agent of dental caries. However, difficulties exist in the application of these postulates to other types of diseases, including periodontitis. Three primary problems are the inability to culture all the organisms that have been associated with disease (e.g., many of the oral spirochetes), the difficulties inherent in defining and culturing sites of active disease, and the lack of a good animal model system for the study of periodontitis.[102]

In response to the difficulties inherent in the application of Koch's postulates, Sigmund Socransky, a researcher at the Forsyth Dental Center in Boston, proposed criteria by which periodontal microorganisms may be judged to be potential pathogens.[102] According to these criteria, a potential pathogen must

1. Be associated with disease, as evident by increases in the number of organisms at diseased sites;
2. Be eliminated or decreased in sites that demonstrate clinical resolution of disease with treatment;
3. Demonstrate a host response, in the form of an alteration in the host cellular or humoral immune response;
4. Be capable of causing disease in experimental animal models; and
5. Demonstrate virulence factors responsible for enabling the microorganism to cause destruction of the periodontal tissues.

Data supporting the role of two microorganisms as periodontal pathogens, based on these criteria, are presented in Table 6–2. The association and elimination criteria are discussed in detail in the preceding sections, the host response is dealt with in Chapters 8 and 9, and the discussion below focuses on virulence factors of putative pathogens.

VIRULENCE FACTORS OF PERIODONTAL PATHOGENS

The properties that enable a bacterium to cause disease are termed *virulence factors,* and considerable research is currently focused on defining the virulence factors of periodontal pathogens. From a simplistic viewpoint, to function as a pathogen, a bacterium must colonize the appropriate host tissue site and then cause destruction of the host tissues. In periodontitis, the initial step in the disease process is the colonization of the periodontal tissues by pathogenic species. Entry of the bacterium itself (invasion) or of bacterial products into the periodontal tissues may be essential in the disease process. Furthermore, inherent in successful colonization of host tissues is the ability of the bacterium to evade host defense mechanisms aimed at eliminating the bacterium from the periodontal environment.

The process of tissue destruction results from the elaboration of bacterial substances that directly or indirectly cause degradation of the periodontal tissues. Thus, virulence properties can be broadly categorized into two groups: factors that enable a bacterial species to colonize and invade host tissues, and factors that enable a bacterial species to directly or indirectly cause host tissue damage.

Colonization and Invasion of Periodontal Tissues

Bacterial Adherence in the Periodontal Environment. The gingival sulcus and periodontal pocket are bathed in gingival crevicular fluid, which flows from the base of the pocket outward. Bacterial species that colonize this region must attach to available surfaces to avoid displacement by the fluid flow. Therefore, adherence represents a virulence factor for periodontal pathogens.

The surfaces available for attachment include the tooth or root, the tissues, and the pre-existing plaque mass. Nu-

Table 6–2 EVIDENCE SUPPORTING A ROLE FOR *A. ACTINOMYCETEMCOMITANS* AND *P. GINGIVALIS* AS PATHOGENS IN PERIODONTAL DISEASES: SOCRANSKY'S CRITERIA

Criterion	*A. actinomycetemcomitans*	*P. gingivalis*
Association	Increased in LJP lesions Increased in some periodontitis lesions Detected in the tissues of LJP lesions	Increased in periodontitis lesions Found associated with crevicular epithelium
Elimination	Suppressed or eliminated in successful therapy Found in recurrent lesions	Suppressed or eliminated in successful therapy Found in recurrent lesions
Host response	Increased serum and local antibody levels in LJP	Increased systemic and local antibody levels in periodontitis
Animal studies	Capable of inducing disease in gnotobiotic rats	Found to be important in experimental mixed infections and in periodontitis in the cynomolgus monkey
Virulence factors	Host tissue cell invasion, leukotoxin, collagenase, endotoxin (LPS), epitheliotoxin, fibroblast inhibiting factor, bone resorption–inducing factor	Host tissue cell adherence and invasion, collagenase, trypsin-like enzyme, fibrinolysin, phospholipase A, phosphatases, endotoxin (LPS), H_2S, NH_3, fatty acids, factors that affect PMN function

Adapted from Socransky SS, Haffajee AD. The bacterial etiology of destructive periodontal disease: Current concepts. J Periodontol *63*:322, 1992.

Table 6-3 SELECTED BACTERIAL ADHESINS AND TARGET SUBSTRATES

Probable Attachment Surface	Substrate	Bacterial Species	Bacterial Adhesin	Substrate Receptor
Tooth	Saliva-coated mineralized surfaces	*A. viscosus*	Fimbriae	Saliva-treated hydroxyapatite
		A. viscosus	Fimbriae	Proline-rich proteins
	Saliva-coated surfaces	*S. mitis*	70-, 90-kd protein	Sialic acid residues
		F. nucleatum	300- to 330-kd outer membrane protein	Galactosyl residue
Tissue	Epithelial cells	*P. gingivalis*	Fimbriae	Galactosyl residues
		A. viscosus, A. naeslundii	Fimbriae	Galactosyl residues
	Fibroblasts	*T. denticola*	Surface protein	Galactosyl or mannose residues
	Polymorphonuclear leukocytes	*A. viscosus, A. naeslundii*	Fimbriae	Galactosyl residues
		F. nucleatum	Protein	Galactosyl residues
	Connective tissue components	*P. gingivalis*	Membrane protein	Fibrinogen/Fibronectin
		P. intermedia	Membrane protein	Fibrinogen
Pre-existing plaque mass	*S. sanguis*	*A. viscosus*	Fimbriae	Repeating heptasaccharide on polysaccharide
	S. sanguis *A. naeslundii* *A. israelii*	*C. ochracea*	Heat-sensitive protein	Rhamnose, fucose, or *N*-acetylneuraminic acid residue
	S. sanguis *A. israelii*	*P. loescheii*	75- 45-kd fimbrial proteins	Galactosyl residues
	P. gingivalis	*F. nucleatum*	Outer membrane protein	Galactosyl residue

Adapted from Socransky SS, Haffajee AD. Microbiol mechanisms in the pathogenesis of destructive periodontal diseases: A critical assessment. J Periodontal Res *26*:195, 1991; Lantz MS, Allen RD, Bounelis P, et al. *Bacteroides gingivalis* and *Bacteroides intermedius* recognize different sites on human fibrinogen. J Bacteriol *172*:716, 1990; and Lantz MS, Allen RD, Duck LW, et al. Identification of *Porphyromonas gingivalis* components that mediate its interactions with fibronectin. J Bacteriol *173*:4263, 1991.

merous interactions between periodontal bacteria and these surfaces have been characterized, and in some cases the molecules responsible for mediating these highly specific interactions have been determined (Table 6-3). Bacteria that initially colonize the periodontal environment most likely attach to the pellicle- or saliva-coated tooth surface. A relevant example is the adherence of *A. viscosus* through fimbria on the bacterial surface to proline-rich proteins found on saliva-coated tooth surfaces.[68]

Bacterial attachment to pre-existing plaque is studied by examining the adherence between different bacterial strains (coaggregation). One of the best characterized interactions is the adherence of *A. viscosus* through surface fimbriae to a polysaccharide receptor on cells of *S. sanguis*.[67] These types of interactions are thought to be of primary importance in colonization of the periodontal environment. In addition, the adherence of bacteria to host tissues is likely to play a role in colonization and may be a critical step in the process of bacterial invasion. Thus, the ability of *P. gingivalis* to attach to other bacteria,[38,39,41] to epithelial cells,[16] and to the connective tissue components fibrinogen and fibronectin[48,49] are all likely to be important in the virulence of this organism.

Host Tissue Invasion. The presence of bacteria in host tissues in patients with ANUG has been recognized for years, based on histologic studies.[51,56] Investigations carried out largely in the 1980s demonstrated the presence of bacteria in periodontal tissues in gingivitis,[23] advanced chronic adult periodontitis,[26,89] and juvenile periodontitis.[9,10,12,28,87] Both gram-positive and gram-negative bacteria, including cocci, rods, filaments, and spirochetes, have been observed in gingival connective tissue and in proximity to alveolar bone. Bacteria may enter host tissues through ulcerations in the epithelium of the gingival sulcus or pocket, and microorganisms have been observed in intercellular spaces of the gingival tissues (Figs. 6-16 to 6-19). Another means of tissue invasion may involve the direct penetration of bacteria into host epithelial or connective tissue cells. Laboratory investigations have demonstrated the ability of *A. actinomycetemcomitans*,[69,105] *P. gingivalis* (Fig. 6-20),[18,90]

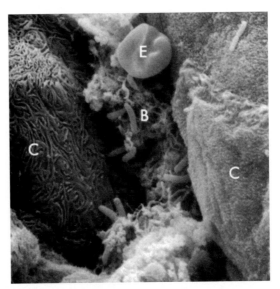

FIGURE 6-16. Scanning electron micrograph of epithelial intercellular spaces containing bacterial plaque (B) enmeshed in a fibrin-like material. C, epithelial cells; E, erythrocyte. The cells to the left show signs of necrosis. ×4000.

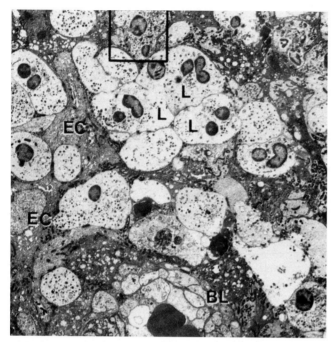

FIGURE 6–17. Interface between pocket epithelium and connective tissue separated by the basement lamina (BL). Abundant bacteria can be seen in the intercellular spaces. Numerous infiltrating polymorphonuclear leukocytes (L) are seen between epithelial cells (EC). Some of the leukocytes show engulfed bacteria. ×3908.

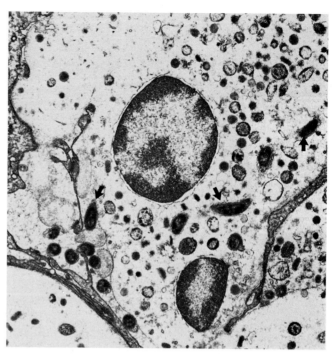

FIGURE 6–18. Higher magnification of the polymorphonuclear leukocyte in square in Figure 6–17 with engulfed bacteria *(arrows)*; ×15,000.

and *Treponema denticola*[113] to directly invade host tissue cells.

The clinical significance of bacterial invasion is not clear. Bacterial species that have been identified as capable of tissue invasion are strongly associated with diseased sites, and the ability to invade has been proposed as a key factor distinguishing pathogenic from nonpathogenic gram-negative species.[59] Certainly localization of bacteria to the tissues provides an ideal position from which the organism

can effectively deliver toxic molecules and enzymes to the host tissue cells, and this may be the significance of invasion as a virulence factor. Indeed, some investigators have speculated that the "bursts of disease activity" observed in periodontitis may be related to phases of bacterial invasion of the tissues.[87] An additional possibility is that bacteria in the tissues may enable persistence of that species in the periodontal pocket by providing a reservoir for recolonization. Consistent with this hypothesis is the observation that

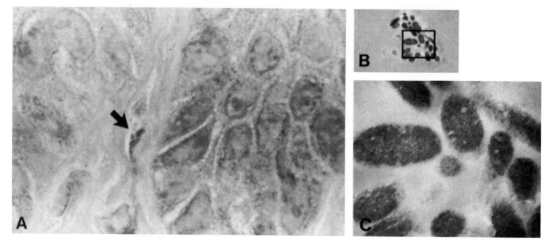

FIGURE 6–19. *A,* Gingival tissue of a patient with localized juvenile periodontitis showing granular positive (dark gray) staining in the connective tissue for *Actinobacillus actinomycetemcomitans (arrow).* Formalin paraffin section, peroxidaseantiperoxidase method, anti-*Actinobacillus actinomycetemcomitans,* counterstained with hematoxylin. ×1200. *B,* Electron micrograph of the same paraffin section showing the area indicated by the arrow in part *A,* which was re-embedded in plastic (modified "pop-off" technique). ×40,000. *C,* Higher magnification of the rectangle in part *B* showing the short coccobacillary rod with approximately the size and shape of *A. actinomycetemcomitans.* ×80,000.

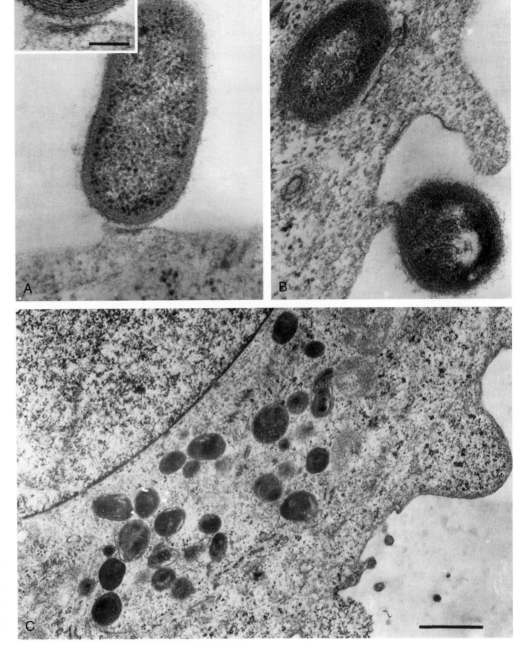

FIGURE 6–20. High-magnification electron photomicrographs of the interaction of *Porphyromonas gingivalis* strain W50 with the epithelial cell, HEp-2. *A, P. gingivalis* is attached to the HEp-2 plasma membrane by its tip. *Insert:* Note the electron-dense region juxtaposed to the site of interaction, possibly an early stage of clatherin pit formation. *B, P. gingivalis* is seen in transverse section attached to a microvillus extension. An internalized *P. gingivalis* is also apparent in the cell section. *C,* Numerous *P. gingivalis* W50 cells are seen in the HEp-2 cytoplasm. (Courtesy of Dr. Stanley C. Holt.)

mechanical debridement alone is insufficient, and that systemic antibiotics in combination with surgical therapy are required to eliminate *A. actinomycetemcomitans* from lesions in patients with LJP.[11,45]

Bacterial Evasion of Host Defense Mechanisms. For bacteria to survive in the periodontal environment, they must neutralize or evade the host mechanisms involved in bacterial clearance and killing. Adherence and invasion of bacteria are representative strategies by which microorganisms accomplish this task. The ability to adhere allows bacteria to avoid displacement by host secretions, and eukaryotic cell invasion disrupts the natural barriers formed by host tissue cells. There are numerous other mechanisms by which periodontal bacteria neutralize or evade host de-

fenses; selected examples are presented in Table 6–4. For example, immunoglobulins might function to facilitate phagocytosis of the bacteria by opsonization or to block adherence by binding to the bacterial cell surface and restricting access to bacterial adhesins. The production of immunoglobulin-degrading proteases by specific microorganisms may counteract these host defenses. Similarly, bacteria produce substances that suppress the activity of or kill polymorphonuclear leukocytes and lymphocytes that are normally involved in host defenses. An example of this is the production by *A. actinomycetemcomitans* of a leukotoxin that may be important in the virulence of this microorganism in LJP and possibly in chronic adult periodontitis (see Tables 6–2 and 6–4).

Table 6-4 SELECTED BACTERIAL PROPERTIES INVOLVED IN EVASION OF HOST DEFENSE MECHANISMS

Host Defense Mechanism	Bacterial Species	Bacterial Property	Biologic Effect
Specific antibody	*P. gingivalis* *P. intermedia* *P. melaninogenica* *Capnocytophaga sp.*	IgA and IgG degrading proteases	Degradation of specific antibody
Polymorphonuclear leukocytes	*A. actinomycetemcomitans* *P. gingivalis* *P. gingivalis* *T. denticola*	Leukotoxin Capsule Inhibition of superoxide production Inhibition of superoxide production	Inhibition of PNM function Inhibition of phagocytosis Decreased bacterial killing Decreased bacterial killing
Lymphocytes	*A. actinomycetemcomitans* *A. actinomycetemcomitans* *A. actinomycetemcomitans* *P. intermedia*	Leukotoxin Leukotoxin Suppression	Killing of mature B and T cells Nonlethal suppression of activity Decreased immune response
	P. intermedia	Suppression	Decreased response to antigens and mitogens
	T. denticola *A. actinomycetemcomitans*		

Adapted from Socransky SS, Haffejee AD. Microbial mechanisms in the pathogenesis of destructive periodontal diseases: A critical assessment. J Periodontal Res *26*:195, 1991.

Mechanisms of Host Tissue Damage

Much research on virulence factors has focused on the properties of bacteria related to the destruction of host tissues. These bacterial properties can be broadly categorized as those resulting directly in degradation of host tissues and those that cause the release of biologically active substances from host tissue cells.

Some bacterial products inhibit the growth or alter the metabolism of host tissue cells; these include a number of metabolic by-products such as ammonia; volatile sulfur compounds; and fatty acids, peptides, and indole.[95,110] An important class of molecules in tissue destruction is the variety of enzymes produced by periodontal microorganisms (Table 6-5). These enzymes appear to be capable of degrading essentially all the host tissue and intercellular matrix molecules.[2,7,27,31,34,35,47,49,100,118] In particular, *P. gingivalis* produces a wide range of proteases, including a trypsin-like enzyme, enzymes that degrade collagen, fibronectin, and immunoglobulins. Bacterial enzymes may facilitate tissue destruction and invasion of the bacteria into host tissues. However, the exact role of bacterially derived proteases in the disease process has not been determined, as similar enzymes in the periodontal environment may originate from host tissue cells.

The host immune system involves a complex network of interactions between cells and regulatory molecules. Bacterial products may perturb the system, resulting in tissue destruction (Table 6-6). A well-characterized interaction involves the release of interleukin-1, tumor necrosis factor, and prostaglandins from macrophages and monocytes exposed to bacterial endotoxin (lipopolysaccharide).[5,36] These host-derived cytokines have the potential to stimulate bone resorption and to activate or inhibit other host immune cells. There are many examples of this type of interaction. The bacterial modulation of the host immune system is dealt with in detail in Chapter 9.

Table 6-5. BACTERIAL ENZYMES CAPABLE OF DEGRADING HOST TISSUES

Bacterial Enzyme	Species
Collagenase	*P. gingivalis* *A. actinomycetemcomitans*
Trypsin-like enzyme	*P. gingivalis* *A. actinomycetemcomitans* *T. denticola*
Keratinase	*P. gingivalis* *T. denticola*
Arylsulfatase	*C. rectus*
Neuraminidase	*P. gingivalis* *B. forsythus* *P. melaninogenica*
Fibronectin-degrading enzyme	*P. gingivalis* *P. intermedia*
Phospholipase A	*P. intermedia* *P. melaninogenica*

Adapted from Socransky SS, Haffejee AD. Microbial mechanisms in the pathogenesis of destructive periodontal diseases: A critical assessment. J Periodontal Res *26*:195, 1991; and Loesche WJ. Bacterial mediators in periodontal disease. Clin Infect Dis *16*(suppl 4):S203, 1993.

FUTURE ADVANCES IN PERIODONTAL MICROBIOLOGY

Several scientific advances will have a direct impact on future advances in the understanding of periodontal microbiology. First, the development and utilization of DNA probes for identification of specific microorganisms represent a significant advantage in time and cost compared with the cultivation of bacterial samples. The use of DNA probes in clinical studies will allow for analysis of larger populations and at a greater number of time points.

Second, studies of the virulence factors of periodontal pathogens have documented many mechanisms by which the infecting bacteria may cause disease. To determine

Table 6-6. EXAMPLES OF BACTERIA AND THEIR PRODUCTS THAT CAUSE BIOLOGICAL EFFECTS ON HOST CELLS

Biological Effect	Bacterial Species	Bacterial Components Involved
Release of interleukin-1 from monocytes	*P. gingivalis* *A. actinomycetemcomitans*	LPS or bacterial suspensions
Release of interleukin-1 from monocytes or macrophages	*C. rectus* *F. nucleatum* *A. actinomycetemcomitans*	LPS
Release of prostaglandins from monocytes or macrophages	*P. gingivalis* *P. intermedia* *C. rectus* *A. actinomycetemcomitans*	LPS
Release of tumor necrosis factor from monocytes	*P. gingivalis* *A. actinomycetemcomitans*	LPS or bacterial suspensions
Release of thymocyte-activating factor from fibroblasts	*P. gingivalis*	Fimbriae
B cell activation and mitogenicity; macrophage stimulation	*F. nucleatum*	Outer membrane protein (porin)
Activation of natural killer cells	*A. actinomycetemcomitans*	LPS
Release of collagenase from osteoblast-like cells	*P. gingivalis*	LPS
Stimulation of bone resorption	*P. gingivalis* *A. actinomycetemcomitans*	LPS Capsular material

Adapted from Socransky SS, Haffajee AD. Microbial mechanisms in the pathogenesis of destructive periodontal diseases: A critical assessment. J Periodontal Res *26:*195. 1991.

which factors are actually functioning in the disease process, it will be essential to isolate mutant strains that are defective only in the property in question. Molecular genetic approaches will allow this to be accomplished. The mutant strain then must be compared with the wild type (i.e., the type possessing the virulence factor) in experimental animal models to assess the effect of loss of the putative virulence factor.

Tremendous advances in the molecular biology of periodontal microorganisms have been made, and this area represents a very active field of current research. Clarification of the role of specific virulence factors in periodontal disease may ultimately lead to strategies (e.g., vaccines or therapeutic agents) to prevent or arrest the disease process.

REFERENCES

1. Berthold P, Lai CH, Listgarten MA. Immunoelectron microscopic studies of *Actinomyces viscosus.* J Periodont Res *17:*26, 1982.
2. Birkedal-Hansen H, Taylor RE, Zambon JJ, et al. Characterization of collagenolytic activity from strains of *Bacteroides gingivalis.* J Periodont Res *23:*258, 1988.
3. Bowen W. Nature of plaque. Oral Sci Rev *9:*3, 1976.
4. Bramanti TE, Holt SC. Roles of porphyrins and host iron transport proteins in regulation of growth of *Porphyromonas gingivalis* W50. J Bacteriol *173:*7330, 1991.
5. Bramanti TE, Wong GG, Weintraub ST, Holt SC. Chemical characterization and biologic properties of lipopolysaccharide from *Bacteroides gingivalis* strains W50, W83, and ATCC 33277. Oral Microbiol Immunol *4:*183, 1989.
6. Brown LJ, Löe H. Prevalence, extent, severity and progression of periodontal disease. Periodontol 2000 *2:*57, 1993.
7. Bulkacz J, Schuster GS, Singh B, Scott DF. Phospholipase A activity of extracellular products from *Bacteroides melaninogenicus* on epithelial tissue cultures. J Periodont Res *20:*146, 1985.
8. Carlsson J. Microbiology of plaque associated periodontal disease. In Linde J, ed. Textbook of Clinical Periodontology. Copenhagen, Munksgaard International Publishers, 1983.
9. Carranza FA Jr, Saglie R, Newman MG, Valentin P. Scanning and transmission electron microscopic study of tissue-invading microorganisms in localized juvenile periodontitis. J Periodontol *54:*598, 1983.
10. Christersson LA, Alibini A, Zambon JJ, et al. Tissue localization of *Actinobacillus actinomycetemcomitans* in human periodontitis. I. Light, immunofluorescence and electron microscopic studies. J Periodontol *58:*529, 1987.
11. Christersson LA, Slots J, Rosling B, Genco RJ. Microbiological and clinical effects of *Actinobacillus actinomycetemcomitans* in localized juvenile periodontitis. J Clin Periodontol *12:*465, 1985.
12. Christersson LA, Slots J, Rosling B, Genco RJ. Transmission and colonization of *Actinobacillus actinomycetemcomitans* in localized juvenile periodontitis. J Periodontol *56:*127, 1985.
13. Christersson LA, Zambon JJ, Genco RJ. Dental bacterial plaques. Nature and role in periodontal disease. J Clin Periodontol *18:*441, 1991.
14. Clark WB, Löe H. Mechanisms of initiation and progression of periodontal disease. Periodontol 2000 *2:*72, 1993.
15. Costerton JW, Cheng K, Geesey GG, et al. Bacterial biofilms in nature and disease. Annu Rev Microbiol *41:*435, 1987.
16. Dickinson DP, Kubiniec MA, Yoshimura F, Genco RJ. Molecular cloning and sequencing of the gene encoding the fimbrial subunit protein of *Bacteroides gingivalis.* J Bacteriol *170:*1658, 1988.
17. Doyle RJ, Rosenberg M, Drake D. Hydrophobicity of oral bacteria. In Doyle RJ, Rosenberg M, ed. Microbial Cell Surface Hydrophobicity. Washington DC, American Society for Microbiology, 1990.
18. Duncan MJ, Nakao S, Skobe Z, Xie H. Interactions of *Porphyromonas gingivalis* with epithelial cells. Infect Immun *61:*2260, 1993.
19. Dzink JL, Gibbons RJ, Childs WC III, Socransky SS. The predominant cultivable microbiota of crevicular epithelial cells. Oral Microbiol Immunol *4:*1, 1989.
20. Dzink JL, Socransky SS, Haffajee AD. The predominant cultivable microbiota of active and inactive lesions of destructive periodontal diseases. J Clin Periodontol *15:*316, 1988.
21. Dzink JL, Tanner ACR, Haffajee AD, Socransky SS. Gram negative species associated with active destructive periodontal lesions. J Clin Periodontol *12:*648, 1985.
22. Fachon-Kalweit S, Elder BL, Fives-Taylor P. Antibodies that bind to fimbriae block adhesion of *Streptococcus sanguis* to saliva-coated hydroxyapatite. Infect Immun *48:*617, 1985.
23. Fillery ED, Pekovic DD. Identification of microorganisms in immunopathological mechanisms on human gingivitis. J Dent Res *61:*253, 1982.
24. Fives-Taylor PM, Thompson DW. Surface properties of *Streptococcus sanguis* FW213 mutants nonadherent to saliva-coated hydroxyapatite. Infect Immun *47:*752, 1985.
25. Fletcher M. The physiological activity of bacteria attached to solid surfaces. Adv Microbiol Physiol *32:*53, 1991.
26. Frank RM. Bacterial penetration in the apical wall of advanced human periodontitis. J Periodont Res *15:*563, 1980.
27. Fujimura S, Nakamura T. Isolation and characterization of a protease from *Bacteroides gingivalis.* Infect Immun *55:*716, 1987.
28. Gillett R, Johnson NW. Bacterial invasion of the periodontium in a case of juvenile periodontitis. J Clin Periodontol *9:*93, 1982.
29. Goodson JM, Tanner ACR, Haffajee AD, et al. Patterns of progression and regression of advanced destructive periodontal disease. J Clin Periodontol *9:*472, 1982.
30. Grenier D. Nutritional interaction between two suspected periodontopathogens, *Treponema denticola* and *Porphyromonas gingivalis.* Infect Immun *60:*5298, 1992.
31. Grenier D, Chao G, McBride BC. Characterization of sodium dodecyl sulfate-stable *Bacteroides gingivalis* proteases by polyacrylamide gel electrophoresis. Infect Immun *57:*95, 1989.
32. Grenier D, Mayrand D. Etudes d'infections mixtes anaerobies comportant *Bacteroides gingivalis.* Can J Microbiol *29:*612, 1983.

33. Grenier D, Mayrand D. Nutritional relationships between oral bacteria. Infect Immun *53:*616, 1986.

34. Grenier D, McBride BC. Isolation of a membrane-associated *Bacteroides gingivalis* glycylprolyl protease. Infect Immun *55:*3131, 1987.

35. Grenier D, McBride BC. Surface location of a *Bacteroides gingivalis* glycylprolyl protease. Infect Immun *57:*3265, 1989.

36. Hanazawa S, Nakada K, Ohmori Y, et al. Functional role of interleukin 1 in periodontal disease: Induction of interleukin 1 production by *Bacteroides gingivalis* lipopolysaccharide in peritoneal macrophages from C3H/HeN and C3H/HeJ mice. Infect Immun *50:*262, 1985.

37. Kaufman J, DiRienzo JM. Isolation of a corncob (coaggregation) receptor polypeptide from *Fusobacterium nucleatum.* Infect Immun *57:*331, 1989.

38. Kinder SA, Holt SC. Carbohydrate receptor on *Porphyromonas gingivalis* T22 mediating coaggregation with *Fusobacterium nucleatum* T18. J Dent Res *70:*275, 1991.

39. Kinder SA, Holt SC. Characterization of coaggregation between *Bacteroides gingivalis* T22 and *Fusobacterium nucleatum* T18. Infect Immun *57:*3425, 1989.

40. Kolenbrander PE. Surface recognition among oral bacteria: Multigeneric coaggregations and their mediators. Crit Rev Microbiol *17:*137, 1989.

41. Kolenbrander PE, Andersen RN. Inhibition of coaggregation between *Fusobacterium nucleatum* and *Porphyromonas (Bacteroides) gingivalis* by lactose and related sugars. Infect Immun *57:*3204, 1989.

42. Kolenbrander PE, London J. Adhere today, here tomorrow: Oral bacterial adherence. J Bacteriol *175:*3247, 1993.

43. Kornman KS, Löe H. The role of local factors in the etiology of periodontal diseases. Periodontol 2000 *2:*83, 1993.

44. Kornman KS, Loesche WJ. Effects of estradiol and progesterone on *Bacteroides melaninogenicus* and *Bacteroides gingivalis.* Infect Immun *35:*256, 1982.

45. Kornman KS, Robertson PB. Clinical and microbiological evaluation of therapy for juvenile periodontitis. J Periodontol *56:*443, 1985.

46. Lancy P, DiRienzo JM, Appelbaum B, et al. Corncob formation between *Fusobacterium nucleatum* and *Streptococcus sanguis.* Infect Immun *40:*303, 1983.

47. Lantz MS, Allen RD, Bounelis P, et al. *Bacteroides gingivalis* and *Bacteroides intermedius* recognize different sites on human fibrinogen. J Bacteriol *172:*716, 1990.

48. Lantz MS, Allen RD, Duck LW, et al. Identification of *Porphyromonas gingivalis* components that mediate its interactions with fibronectin. J Bacteriol *173:*4263, 1991.

49. Lantz MS, Rowland RW, Switalski LM, Hook M. Interactions of *Bacteroides gingivalis* with fibrinogen. Infect Immun *54:*654, 1986.

50. Lindhe J, Slots J. Juvenile periodontitis (periodontosis). In Lindhe J, ed. Textbook of Clinical Periodontology. Copenhagen, Munksgaard, 1983.

51. Listgarten MA. Electron microscopic observations on the bacterial flora of acute necrotizing ulcerative gingivitis. J Periodontol *36:*328, 1965.

52. Listgarten MA. Structure of the microbial flora associated with periodontal health and disease in man. J Periodontol *47:*1, 1976.

53. Listgarten MA, Hellden L. Relative distribution of bacteria at clinically healthy and periodontally diseased sites in humans. J Clin Periodontol *5:*115, 1978.

54. Listgarten MA, Mayo H, Amsterdam M. Ultrastructure of the attachment device between coccal and filamentous microorganisms in "corn cob" formations in dental plaque. Arch Oral Biol *18:*651, 1973.

55. Listgarten MA, Mayo HE, Tremblay R. Development of dental plaque on epoxy resin crowns in man. A light and electron microscopic study. J Periodontol *46:*10, 1975.

56. Listgarten MA, Socransky SS. Ultrastructural characteristics of a spirochete in lesions of acute necrotizing ulcerative gingivostomatitis (Vincent's infection). Arch Oral Biol *9:*95, 1964.

57. Löe H. Periodontal diseases: A brief historical perspective. Periodontol 2000 *2:*7, 1993.

58. Löe H, Theilade E, Jensen SB. Experimental gingivitis in man. J Periodontol *36:*177, 1965.

59. Loesche WJ. Bacterial mediators in periodontal disease. Clin Infect Dis *16*(suppl 4):S203, 1993.

60. Loesche WJ. Chemotherapy of dental plaque infections. Oral Sci Rev *9:*65, 1976.

61. Loesche WJ. Importance of nutrition in gingival crevice microbial ecology. Periodontics *6:*245, 1968.

62. Loesche WJ, Syed SA, Schmidt E, Morrison EC. Bacterial profiles of subgingival plaques in periodontitis. J Periodontol *56:*447, 1985.

63. Lovdal A, Arno A, Waerhaug J. Evidence of clinical manifestations of periodontal disease in light of oral hygiene and calculus formation. J Am Dent Assoc *56:*21, 1958.

64. Manganiello AD, Socransky SS, Smith C, et al. Attempts to increase viable count recovery of human supragingival dental plaque. J Periodont Res *12:*107, 1977.

65. Mayrand D, McBride BC. Ecological relationships of bacteria involved in a simple mixed anaerobic infection. Infect Immun *27:*44, 1980.

66. McBride BC, van der Hoeven JS. Role of interbacterial adherence in colonization of the oral cavities of gnotobiotic rats infected with *Streptococcus mutans* and *Veillonella alcalescens.* Infect Immun *33:*467, 1981.

67. McIntire FC. Structure of a new hexasaccharide from the coaggregation polysaccharide of *Streptococcus sanguis* 34. Carbo Res *166:*133, 1987.

68. Mergenhagen SE, Sandberg AL, Chassy BM, et al. Molecular basis of bacterial adhesion in the oral cavity. Rev Infect Dis *9:*S467, 1987.

69. Meyer DH, Sreenivasan PK, Fives-Taylor PM. Evidence for invasion of a human oral cell line by *Actinobacillus actinomycetemcomitans.* Infect Immun *59:*2719, 1991.

70. Mombelli A, Lang NP, Burgin WB, Gusberti FA. Microbial changes associated with the development of puberty gingivitis. J Periodont Res *25:*331, 1990.

71. Moore WEC. Microbiology of periodontal disease. J Periodont Res *22:*335, 1987.

72. Moore WEC, Holdeman LV, Cato EP, et al. Comparative bacteriology of juvenile periodontitis. Infect Immun *48:*507, 1985.

73. Moore WEC, Holdeman LV, Smibert RM, et al. Bacteriology of severe periodontitis in young adult humans. Infect Immun *38:*1137, 1982.

74. Mosques T, Listgarten MA, Phillips RW. Effect of scaling and root planning on the composition of the human subgingival microbial flora. J Periodont Res *15:*144, 1980.

75. Mouton C, Reynolds HS, Genco RJ. Characterization of tufted streptococci isolated from the "corn cob" configuration of human dental plaque. Infect Immun *27:*235, 1980.

76. Newman HN. The approximal apical border of plaque on children's teeth. I. Morphology, structure and cell content. J Periodontol *50:*561, 1979.

77. Newman MG, Socransky SS. Predominant cultivable microbiota in periodontosis. J Periodont Res *14:*1, 1977.

78. Newman MG, Socransky SS, Listgarten MA. Relationship of microorganisms to the etiology of periodontosis. J Dent Res *53:*290, 1974.

79. Newman MG, Socransky SS, Savitt ED, et al. Studies of the microbiology of periodontosis. J Periodontol *47:*373, 1976.

80. Page RC, Schroeder H. Periodontitis in Man and Other Animals. Basel, Karger, 1982.

81. Ranney RR. Classification of periodontal diseases. Periodontol 2000 *2:*13, 1993.

82. Renvert S, Wikstrom M, Dahlen G, et al. On the inability of root debridement and periodontal surgery to eliminate *Actinobacillus actinomycetemcomitans* from periodontal pockets. J Clin Periodontol *17:*351, 1990.

83. Renvert S, Wikstrom M, Dahlen S, et al. Effect of root debridement on the elimination of *Actinobacillus actinomycetemcomitans* and *Bacteroides gingivalis* from periodontal pockets. J Clin Periodontol *17:*345, 1990.

84. Rolla G. Pellicle formation. In Lazzari EP, ed. Handbook of Experimental Aspects of Oral Biochemistry. Boca Raton, FL, CRC Press, 1983.

85. Rolla G, Ogaard B, Cruz RA. Topical application of fluorides on teeth. New concepts of mechanisms of interaction. J Clin Periodontol *20:*105, 1993.

86. Russel AL. Epidemiology of periodontal disease. Int Dent J *17:*282, 1967.

87. Saglie FR, Marfany A, Camargo P. Intragingival occurrence of *Actinobacillus actinomycetemcomitans* and *Bacteroides gingivalis* in sections of gingival tissue in localized juvenile periodontitis. J Periodontol *59:*259, 1988.

88. Saglie R, Carranza FA Jr, Newman MG, et al. Identification of tissue-invading bacteria in human periodontal disease. J Periodont Res *17:*452, 1982.

89. Saglie R, Carranza FA Jr, Newman MG, Pattison GA. Bacterial invasion of gingiva in advanced periodontitis in humans. J Periodontol *53:*217, 1982.

90. Sandros J, Papapanou P, Dahlen G. *Porphyromonas gingivalis* invades oral epithelial cells in vitro. J Periodont Res *28:*219, 1993.

91. Scannapieco FA, Levine MJ. Saliva and dental pellicles. In Genco RJ, Goldman HM, Cohen DW, eds. Contemporary Periodontics. St Louis, CV Mosby, 1990.

92. Schei O, Waerhaug J, Lovdal A, Aron A. Alveolar bone loss as related to oral hygiene and age. J Periodontol *30:*7, 1959.

93. Shah HN, Collins MD. *Prevotella*, a new genus to include *Bacteroides melaninogenicus* and related species formally classified in the genus *Bacteroides.* Int J Sys Bacteriol *40:*205, 1990.

94. Shah HN, Collins MD. Proposal for reclassification of *Bacteroides asaccharolyticus, Bacteroides gingivalis,* and *Bacteroides endodontalis* in a new genus, *Porphyromonas.* Int J Sys Bacteriol *38:*128, 1988.

95. Singer RE, Buckner BA. Butyrate and propionate: Important components of toxic dental plaque extracts. Infect Immun *32:*458, 1981.

96. Slots J. The predominant cultivable microflora of advanced periodontitis. Scand J Dent Res *85:*114, 1977.

97. Slots J. Subgingival microflora and periodontal disease. J Clin Periodontol *6:*351, 1979.

98. Slots J, Listgarten MA. *Bacteroides gingivalis, Bacteroides intermedius* and *Actinobacillus actinomycetemcomitans* in human periodontal diseases. J Clin Periodontol *15:*85, 1988.

99. Slots J, Rams TE. Microbiology of periodontal disease. In Slots J, Taubman MA, eds. Contemporary Oral Microbiology and Immunology. St Louis, CV Mosby, 1992.

100. Smalley JW, Birss AJ, Shuttleworth CA. The degradation of type I collagen and human plasma fibronectin by the trypsin-like enzyme and extracellular membrane vesicles of *Bacteroides gingivalis* W50. Arch Oral Biol *33:*323, 1988.

101. Socransky SS, Gibbons RJ, Dale AC, et al. The microbiota of the gingival crevice area of man. I. Total microscopic and viable counts of specific microorganisms. Arch Oral Biol *8:*275, 1953.

102. Socransky SS, Haffajee AD. The bacterial etiology of destructive periodontal disease: Current concepts. J Periodontol *63:*322, 1992.

103. Socransky SS, Haffajee AD. Microbial mechanisms in the pathogenesis of destructive periodontal diseases: A critical assessment. J Periodont Res *26:*195, 1991.

104. Socransky SS, Manganiello AD, Propas D, et al. Bacteriological studies of developing supragingival dental plaque. J Periodont Res *12:*90, 1977.
105. Sreevnivasan PK, Meyer DH, Fives-Taylor PM. Requirements for invasion of epithelial cells by *Actinobacillus actinomycetemcomitans.* Infect Immun *61:*1239, 1993.
106. Takada H, Tomohiko O, Yoshimura F, et al. Immunobiological activities of a porin fraction isolated from *Fusobacterium nucleatum* ATCC 10953. Infect Immun *56:*855, 1988.
107. Tanner ACR, Haffer C, Bratthall GT, et al. A study of the bacteria associated with advancing periodontitis in man. J Clin Periodontol *6:*278, 1979.
108. Tanner ACR, Socransky SS, Goodson JM. Microbiota of periodontal pockets loosing crestal alveolar bone. J Periodont Res *19:*279, 1984.
109. Theilade E, Wright WH, Jensen SB, Löe H. Experimental gingivitis in man. II. A longitudinal clinical and bacteriological investigation. J Periodont Res *1:*1, 1966.
110. van Steenbergen TJM, van der Mispel LMS, de Graff J. Effects of ammonia and volatile fatty acids produced by oral bacteria on tissue culture cells. J Dent Res *65:*909, 1986.
111. Vandamme P, Falsen E, Rossau R, et al. Revision of *Campylobacter, Helicobacter,* and *Wolinella* taxonomy: Emendation of generic descriptions and proposal of *Arcobacter* gen. nov. Int J Sys Bacteriol *41:*88, 1991.
112. Walden WC, Hentges DC. Differential effects of oxygen and oxidation-reduction potential on the multiplication of three species of anaerobic bacteria. Appl Microbiol *30:*781, 1975.
113. Wang B, Holt SC. Interaction of *Treponema denticola* with HEp-2 cells. J Dent Res *72:*324, 1993.
114. Weiss EI, Eli I, Shenitzki B, Smorodinsky N. Identification of the rhamnose-sensitive adhesin of *Capnocytophaga ochracea* ATCC 33596. Arch Oral Biol *35:*127, 1990.
115. Weiss EI, London J, Kolenbrander PE, et al. Characterization of monoclonal antibodies to fimbria-associated adhesins of *Bacteroides loescheii* PK1295. Infect Immun *56:*219, 1988.
116. Weiss EI, London J, Kolenbrander PE, et al. Localization and enumeration of fimbria-associated adhesins of *Bacteroides loescheii.* J Bacteriol *170:*1123, 1988.
117. Wennstrom JL, Dahlen G, Svensson J, Nyman S. *Actinobacillus actinomycetemcomitans, Bacteroides gingivalis* and *Bacteroides intermedius:* Predictors of attachment loss? Oral Microbiol Immunol *2:*158, 1987.
118. Wikstrom M, Linde A. Ability of oral bacteria to degrade fibronectin. Infect Immun *51:*707, 1986.
119. Zambon JJ, Reynolds HS, Slots J. Black-pigmented *Bacteroides* spp. in the human oral cavity. Infect Immun *32:*198, 1981.

7

Defense Mechanisms of the Gingiva

FERMIN A. CARRANZA, JR. and JAIME BULKACZ

Sulcular Fluid
Methods of Collection
Permeability of Junctional and Sulcular Epithelia
Amount
Composition
Cellular and Humoral Activity in GCF
Clinical Significance
Drugs in the Sulcular Fluid

Leukocytes in the Dentogingival Area
Saliva
Antibacterial Factors
Salivary Antibodies
Salivary Buffers and Coagulation Factors
Leukocytes
Role in Periodontal Pathology

The gingival tissue is constantly subjected to mechanical and bacterial aggressions. Resistance to these actions is provided by the saliva, the epithelial surface, and the initial stages of the inflammatory response. The role of the epithelium, through its degree of keratinization and turnover rate, were considered in Chapter 1. The permeability of the junctional and sulcular epithelia and the role of sulcular fluid, leukocytes, and saliva will be described here.

SULCULAR FLUID

The presence of sulcular fluid* or gingival crevicular fluid (GCF) has been known since the 19th century, but its composition and possible role in oral defense mechanisms were elucidated by the pioneering work of Waerhaug[128] and Brill and Krasse[14] in the 1950s. The latter investigators introduced filter paper into the gingival sulci of dogs that had previously been injected intramuscularly with fluorescein; within 3 minutes the fluorescent material was recovered on the paper strips. This indicated a passage of fluid from the blood stream through the tissues and exiting via the gingival sulcus.

In subsequent studies Brill[11,12] confirmed the presence of GCF in humans and considered it a transudate. However, others[74,129] demonstrated that GCF is an inflammatory exudate, not a continuous transudate. In a strictly normal gingiva, little or no fluid can be collected.

More recently, interest in the development of tests for the detection or prediction of periodontal disease has resulted in numerous research papers dealing with the components, origin, and function of GCF.

_____
* For background information the reader is referred to the comprehensive reviews by Cimasoni.[20,21]

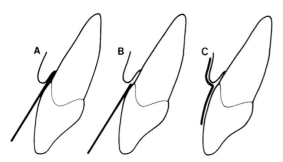

FIGURE 7–1. Placement of filter strip in gingival sulcus for collection of fluid. *A,* Intrasulcular method. *B* and *C,* Extrasulcular methods.

Methods of Collection

The most difficult hurdle to overcome when collecting gingival fluid is the scarcity of material that can be obtained from the sulcus. Numerous collection methods have been tried.[10,13,59,63,64,74,76,104,124,125] These methods include the use of absorbing paper strips, twisted threads placed around and into the sulcus, micropipettes, and intracrevicular washings.

The absorbing paper strips are placed within the sulcus (intrasulcular method) or at its entrance (extrasulcular method) (Fig. 7–1). The placement of the filter paper strip in relation to the sulcus or pocket is important. The Brill technique places it into the pocket until resistance is encountered (see Fig. 7–1A). This method introduces a degree of irritation of the sulcular epithelium that can, by itself, trigger the oozing of fluid.

To minimize this irritation, Löe and Holm-Pedersen[74] placed the filter paper strip just at the entrance of the pocket or over the pocket entrance (see Fig. 7–1B,C). In this way fluid seeping out is picked up by the strip, but the sulcular epithelium will not be in contact with the paper.

Preweighed twisted threads were used by Weinstein et al.[129] The threads were placed in the gingival crevice around the tooth, and the amount of fluid collected was estimated by weighing the sample thread.

The use of micropipettes permits the absorption of fluid by capillarity. Capillary tubes of standardized length and diameter are placed in the pocket, and their content is later centrifuged and analyzed.[10,12,13]

Crevicular washings can be used to study crevicular fluid from clinically normal gingiva. One method uses an appliance consisting of a hard acrylic plate covering the maxilla with soft borders and a groove following the gingival margins, connected to four collection tubes. The washings are obtained by rinsing the crevicular areas from one side to the other, using a peristaltic pump.[21]

A modification of the method uses two injection needles fitted one within the other such that during sampling the inside, or ejection, needle is at the bottom of the pocket and the outside, or collecting, one is at the gingival margin. The collection needle is drained into a sample tube by continuous suction.[104]

Permeability of Junctional and Sulcular Epithelia

The initial studies by Brill and Krasse[14] with fluorescein were later confirmed with substances such as India ink[97]

and saccharated iron oxide.[21] Substances that have been shown to penetrate the sulcular epithelium include albumin,[96,125] endotoxin,[95,100,101,109] thymidine,[49] histamine,[28] phenytoin,[120] and horseradish peroxidase.[80,81] These findings indicate permeability to substances with a molecular weight of up to 1 million.[110]

The mechanisms of penetration through an intact epithelium were reviewed by Squier and Johnson.[119] Intercellular movement of molecules and ions along intercellular spaces appears to be a possible mechanism. Substances taking this route do not traverse the cell membranes.

Amount

The amount of fluid collected on a paper strip can be evaluated in a variety of ways. The wetted area can be made more visible by staining with ninhydrin; it is then measured planimetrically on an enlarged photograph or with the help of a magnifying glass or a microscope.

An electronic method has been devised for measuring the fluid collected on a "blotter" (Periopaper), employing an electronic transducer (Periotron, Harco Electronics, Winnipeg, Manitoba, Canada) (Fig. 7–2). The wetness of the paper strip affects the flow of an electronic current and gives a digital read-out. A comparison of the ninhydrin-staining method and the electronic method performed in vitro revealed no significant differences between the two techniques.[122]

The amount of fluid collected is extremely small. Measurements performed by Cimasoni[21] showed that a strip of paper 1.5 mm wide inserted 1 mm within the gingival sulcus of a slightly inflamed gingiva absorbs about 0.1 mg of fluid in 3 minutes. Challacombe[19] used an isotope dilution method to measure the amount of gingival fluid present in a particular space at any given time. His calculations in human volunteers with a mean gingival index of less than 1 showed that the mean crevicular fluid volume in proximal spaces from molar teeth ranged from 0.43 to 1.56 μl.

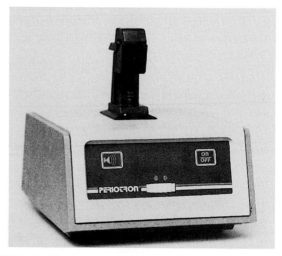

FIGURE 7–2. Electronic machine for measuring the amount of fluid collected on filter paper.

Composition

The components of sulcular fluid can be characterized according to individual proteins,[76,87,106] specific antibodies and antigens,[35,94] and enzymes of several specificities.[15] The gingival fluid contains cellular elements.[28,31,131]

Many research efforts have attempted to use gingival fluid components to detect or diagnose active disease or to predict patients at risk for periodontal disease.[2] So far, more than 40 compounds found in GCF have been analyzed,[91] but their origin is not known with certainty. These compounds can be host derived or produced by the bacteria in the gingival crevice, but their source can be hard to elucidate. Examples of this are β-glucuronidase, a lysosomal enzyme, and lactic acid dehydrogenase, a cytoplasmic enzyme; the source for collagenases can be fibroblasts or polymorphonuclear neutrophils (PMNs),[89] or collagenases can be secreted by bacteria.[35] Phospholipases are lysosomal enzymes but are also produced by microorganisms.[15] The

majority of GCF elements detected thus far have been enzymes, but there are nonenzymatic substances as well (Table 7–1).

Cellular Elements. Cellular elements found in the gingival fluid include bacteria, desquamated epithelial cells, and leukocytes (PMNs, lymphocytes, and monocytes), which migrate through the sulcular epithelium.[28,31]

Electrolytes. Potassium, sodium, and calcium have been studied in gingival fluid. Most studies have shown a positive correlation of calcium and sodium concentrations and the sodium-to-potassium ratio with inflammation.[56-58,63] (For further information, see references 12 and 13 in Table 7–2.)

Organic Compounds. Both carbohydrates and proteins have been investigated. Glucose hexosamine and hexuronic acid are two of the compounds found in gingival fluid.[47] Blood glucose levels do not correlate with gingival fluid glucose levels; glucose concentration in gingival fluid is three to four times greater than that in serum.[47] This is in-

Table 7–1. ENZYMES AND OTHER COMPOUNDS REPORTED IN GCF

Compound	References	Compound	References
Acid phosphatase	19	Endopeptidases	
Alkaline phosphatase	11	Cathepsin D	12
α_1-Antitrypsin	1	Cathepsin B/L	6
α_2-Macroglobulins	1	Cathepsin G	5,6
Aryl sulfatase	15	Elastase	5,6
Aspartate aminotransferase	4	Plasminogen activator	8
β-Glucuronidase	2,15	Collagenase	7
Chondroitin sulfatase	21	Tryptase–like	6
Citric acid	17	Trypsin–like	6
Cytokines	13,14,16	Dipeptidyl peptidase IV–like	6
Interleukin-1α		Elastase-α_1 proteinase inhibitor	9
Interleukin-1β		Exopeptidases	18
IgA, IgG, IgG4, IgM		Fibrin	20
Cystatins	10	Fibronectin	20
		Glycosidases	3

1. Adonogianaki E, Mooney J, Kinane DF. The ability of acute gingival crevicular fluid phase proteins to distinguish gingivitis and periodontitis sites. J. Clin Periodontol *19:*98, 1992.
2. Bang J, Cimasoni G, Held A. Beta glucuronidase correlated with inflammation in the exudate from human gingiva. Arch Oral Biol *15:*445, 1970.
3. Beighton D, Radford JR, Naylor MN. Glycosidase activity in gingival crevicular fluid in subjects with adult periodontitis or gingivitis. Arch Oral Biol *37:*43, 1992.
4. Chambers DA, Imrey PB, Cohen AL, et al. A longitudinal study of aspartate aminotransferase in human gingival crevicular fluid. J Periodont Res *26:*65, 1991.
5. Cimasoni G. Crevicular fluid updated. In Myers H, ed. Monographs in Oral Science. Vol. 12. Basel, S Karger, 1983.
6. Eley BM, Cox SW. Cathepsin B/L-, elastase-, tryptase-, trypsin-, and dipeptidyl peptidase IV-like activities in gingival crevicular fluid: A comparison of levels before and after periodontal surgery in chronic periodontitis. J Periodontol *63:*412, 1992.
7. Fullmer HM, Gibson WA. Collagenolytic activity in gingiva in man. Nature *209:*728, 1966.
8. Gustaffson GT, Nilsson IM. Fibrinolytic activity in fluid from gingival crevice. Proc Soc Exp Biol Med *106:*277, 133.
9. Huynk C, Roch-Arveiller M, Meyer J, Giroud JP. Gingival crevicular fluid of patients with gingivitis or periodontal disease: Evaluation of elastase-alpha 1 proteinase inhibitor complexes. J Clin Periodontol *19:*187, 1992.
10. Ichimaru E, Imura K, Hara Y, et al. Cystatin activity in gingival crevicular fluid from periodontal disease patients, measured by a new quantitative analysis method. J Periodont Res *27:*119, 1992.
11. Ishikawa I, Cimasoni G. Alkaline phosphatase in human gingival fluid and its relation to periodontitis. Arch Oral Biol *15:*1401, 1970.
12. Ishikawa I, Cimasoni G, Ahmad-Zadeh C. Possible roles of lysosomal enzymes in the pathogenesis of periodontitis: A study in cathepsin D in human gingival fluid. Arch Oral Biol *17:*111, 1972.
13. Kabashima H, Maeda K, Iwamoto Y, et al. Partial characterization of an interleukin-1-like factor in human gingival crevicular fluid from patients with chronic inflammatory periodontal disease. Infect Immun *58:*2621, 1990.
14. Kinane DF, Winstanley FP, Adonogianak E, Moughal NA. Bioassay of interleukin-1 (IL-1) in human crevicular fluid during experimental gingivitis. Arch Oral Biol *37:*153, 1992.
15. Lamster IB, Vogel RI, Hartley LJ, et al. Lactate dehydrogenase, beta-glucuronidase, and arylsulfatase activity in gingival crevicular fluid associated with experimental gingivitis in man. J Periodontol *56:*139, 1985.
16. Life JS, Johnson NW, Powell JR, et al. Interleukin-1 beta (IL-1β) levels in gingival crevicular fluid from adults without previous evidence of destructive periodontitis. A cross sectional study. J Clin Periodontol *19:*53, 1992.
17. Miyajima K, Ohmo Y, Iwata T, et al. The lactic acid and citric acid content in the gingival fluid of orthodontic patients. Aichi-Gakuin Dent Sci *4:*75, 1991.
18. Smalley J, Birss AJ, Kay HM, et al. The distribution of trypsin-like enzyme activity in cultures of a virulent and an avirulent strain of *Bacteroides gingivalis* W50. Oral Microbiol Immunol *4:*178, 1989.
19. Sueda T, Cimasoni G, Held AJ. High levels of acid phosphatase in human crevicular fluid. Arch Oral Biol *12:*1205, 1967.
20. Talonopoika J. Characterization of fibrin(ogen) fragments in gingival crevicular fluid. Scand J Periodont Res *99:*40, 1991.
21. Tipler LS, Emberg G. Glycosaminoglycan depolymerizing enzymes from oral microorganisms. Arch Oral Biol *30:*391, 1985.

Table 7-2. COMPOUNDS AND ENZYMES OF POSSIBLE BACTERIAL ORIGIN DETECTED IN GCF

Product	Reference	Product	Reference
Acid phosphatase	17,18	Glucosidases	17
Alkaline phosphatase	10	Hemolysin	8
Aminopeptidases	15	Hyaluronidase	21
β-Lactamase	17,18	Iminopeptidases	2
Chondroitin sulfatase	22	Immunoglobulinases	12,14,20
Chymotrypsin-like	23	Lysophospholipase	3,4
Collagenase	11,13,15	Phospholipase A	3
Dipeptidyl aminopeptidase IV-like	1	Phospholipase C	5,6
Deoxyribonuclease	17	Prostaglandin-like	7
Fibrinolysin	9,16	Trypsin-like enzyme	17,19

1. Abiko Y, Hayakawa M, Murai, S, Takiguchi H. Glycylpropyl dipeptidyl amino-peptidase from *Bacteroides gingivalis*. J Dent Res *64*:106, 1985.
2. Brandtzaeg P, Mann WA. A comparative study of the lysozyme activity of human gingival pocket fluid, serum and saliva. Acta Odont Scand *29*:441, 1964.
3. Bulkacz J. Enzymatic activities in gingival fluid with special emphasis on phospholipases. J Western Soc Periodont *36*:145, 1986.
4. Bulkacz J, Erbland JF, MacGregor J. Phospholipase activity in supernatants from cultures of *Bacteroides melaninogenicus*. Biochim Biophys Acta *664*:148, 1981.
5. Bulkacz J, Erbland JF, Sutter VL. Phospholipase activity of *Propionibacterium acnes*. Abstract no. 996. J Dent Res *61*:289, 1982.
6. Bulkacz J, Garnick J, Barclay JE. Detection of phospholipase activity in crevicular fluid. Abstract no. 1187. J Dent Res *60*:606, 1981.
7. Bulkacz J, Grenett H. Synthesis of prostaglandin-like substances by oral gram negative rods. Abstract no. 421. J Dent Res *60*:415, 1981.
8. Chu, L, Bramanti TE, Holt SC, Ebersole JL. Hemolytic activity in the periodontopathogen *Porphyromonas gingivalis*: Kinetics of enzyme formation and localization. Infect Immun *59*:1932, 1991.
9. Eley BM, Cox SW. Cathepsin B/L-, elastase-, tryptase-, trypsin-, and dipeptidyl peptidase IV-like activities in gingival crevicular fluid: A comparison of levels before and after periodontal surgery in chronic periodontitis. J Periodontol *63*:412, 1992.
10. Franker CK, McGee M, Rezzo T. Alkaline phosphatase activity in a strain of *Bacterionema matruchotti*. J Dent Res *58*:1705, 1979.
11. Gibbons RJ, MacDonald JB. Degradation of collagenous substrates by *Bacteroides melaninogenicus*. J. Bacteriol *81*:614, 1964.
12. Gregory RL, Kim DE, Kindel JC, et al. Immunoglobulin degrading enzymes in localized juvenile periodontitis. J Periodont Res *27*:176, 1992.
13. Grenier D, Mayrand D. Selected characteristics of pathogenic and non-pathogenic strains of *Bacteroides gingivalis*. J Clin Microbiol *25*:738, 1987.
14. Killian M. Degradation of immunoglobulins A1, A2, and G by suspected principal periodontal pathogens. Infect Immun *34*:757, 1981.
15. Makinen KK, Syed SA, Loesche WJ, Makinen PL. Proteolytic profile of *Treponema vincentii* ATCC 35580 with special reference to collagenolytic and arginine aminopeptidase activity. Oral Microbiol Immunol *3*:121, 1988.
16. Nitzan D, Sperry JF, Wilkins TD. Fibrinolytic activity of oral anaerobic bacteria. Arch Oral Biol *23*:465, 1978.
17. Slots J. Enzymatic characterization of some oral and non-oral gram-negative bacteria with the API ZYM system. J Clin Microbiol *14*:288, 1981.
18. Slots J, Dahlen G. Subgingival microorganisms and bacterial virulence factors in periodontitis. Scand J Dent Res *93*:119, 1985.
19. Smalley J, Birss AJ, Kay HM, et al. The distribution of trypsin-like enzyme activity in cultures of a virulent and an avirulent strain of *Bacteroides gingivalis* W 50. Oral Microbiol Immunol *4*:178, 1989.
20. Sundqvist GK, Carlsson J, Herrman B, Tranvik A. Degradation of human immunoglobulins G and M and complement factors C3 and C5 by black-pigmented *Bacteroides*. J Med Microbiol *1*:85, 1985.
21. Tynelius-Brathall G. Hyaluronidase activity in gingival crevicular fluid and in peritoneal exudate leukocytes in dogs. J Periodont Res *7*:307, 1972.
22. Vito VJ. Degradation of basement membrane collagen by proteinases from human gingiva, leukocytes and bacterial plaque. J Periodont *54*:740, 1983.
23. Vito VJ, Grenier D, Chan ECS, McBride BC. Isolation of a chymotrypsin-like enzyme from *Treponema denticola*. Infect Immun *56*:2717, 1988.

terpreted not only as a result of metabolic activity of adjacent tissues, but also as a function of the local microbial flora.

The total protein content of gingival fluid is much less than that of serum.[13,14] No significant correlations have been found between the concentration of proteins in the gingival fluid and the severity of gingivitis, pocket depth, or extent of bone loss.[7]

Metabolic and bacterial products identified in gingival fluid include lactic acid,[48] urea,[42] hydroxyproline,[93] endotoxins,[114,115] cytotoxic substances, hydrogen sulphide,[118] and antibacterial factors.[27] Many enzymes have also been identified (see Tables 7-1 and 7-2).

The methodology utilized for the analysis of GCF components is as varied as the diversity of those components. A few examples will suffice: fluorometry for the detection of metalloproteases[28]; Elisa tests to detect enzyme levels and interleukin 1-beta[69]; radio-immunoassays to detect cyclooxygenase derivatives[88] and procollagen III[123]; timidazole detected by high-pressure liquid chromatography (HPLC)[68]; acute phase proteins detected by direct and indirect immunodots[113]; and others.

Cellular and Humoral Activity in GCF

Monitoring periodontal disease is a complicated task, because there are very few noninvasive procedures that can follow the initiation and progress of the disease. Analysis of GCF constituents in health and disease may be extremely useful because of GCF's simplicity and the fact that it can be obtained with noninvasive methods.

Analysis of GCF has identified cell and humoral responses in both healthy individuals and those with periodontal disease.[66] The cellular immune response includes the appearance in GCF of cytokines (see Table 7-1), but there is no clear evidence of a relationship between them and disease. However, interleukin-1α and -1β are known to increase the binding of PMNs and monocytes to endothelial cells, stimulate the production of prostaglandin (PGE_2) and release of lysosomal enzymes, and stimulate bone resorption.[69] There is also preliminary evidence of the presence of interferon-γ in GCF,[66] which may have a protective role in periodontal disease because of its ability to inhibit the bone resorption activity of interleukin-1β.[44]

Because the amount of fluid recoverable from gingival crevices is small, only the use of very sensitive immunoassays permits the analysis of the specificity of antibodies.[27] A study comparing antibodies in different crevices with serum antibodies directed at specific microorganisms did not provide any conclusive evidence about the significance of the antibody presence in GCF in periodontal disease.[66]

Even though the role of antibodies in the gingival defense mechanisms is hard to ascertain, there is a consensus indicating that (1) in a patient with periodontal disease, a reduction in antibody response is detrimental, and (2) an antibody response plays a protective role in periodontal disease.[65]

Clinical Significance

As mentioned previously, gingival fluid is an inflammatory exudate.[74] Its presence in clinically normal sulci can be explained by the fact that gingiva that appears clinically normal invariably exhibits inflammation when examined microscopically.

The amount of gingival fluid is greater when inflammation is present[34,111] and is sometimes proportional to the severity of inflammation.[90] Gingival fluid production is not increased by trauma from occlusion[79] but is increased by mastication of coarse foods, toothbrushing and gingival massage, ovulation,[71] hormonal contraceptives,[72] and smoking.[82] Other factors that influence the amount of gingival fluid are circadian periodicity and periodontal therapy.

Circadian Periodicity. There is a gradual increase in gingival fluid amount from 6:00 A.M. to 10:00 P.M. and a decrease afterward.[9]

Sex Hormones. Female sex hormones increase the gingival fluid flow, probably because they enhance vascular permeability.[69] Pregnancy, ovulation,[68] and hormonal contraceptives[70] all increase gingival fluid production.

Mechanical Stimulation. Chewing[12] and vigorous gingival brushing stimulate the oozing of gingival fluid. Even the minor stimuli represented by intrasulcular placement of paper strips increases the production of fluid.

Smoking. Smoking produces an immediate transient but marked increase in gingival fluid flow.[82]

Periodontal Therapy. There is an increase in gingival fluid production during the healing period after periodontal surgery.[3]

Drugs in the Sulcular Fluid

Drugs that are excreted through the gingival fluid may be used advantageously in periodontal therapy. Bader and Goldhaber[6] demonstrated in dogs that tetracyclines are excreted through the gingival fluid; this finding triggered extensive research.[43] Metronidazole is another antibiotic that has been detected in human gingival fluid[32] (see Chapter 44).

LEUKOCYTES IN THE DENTOGINGIVAL AREA

Leukocytes have been found in clinically healthy gingival sulci in humans and experimental animals. The leukocytes found are predominantly neutrophils. They appear in small numbers extravascularly in the connective tissue adjacent to the bottom of the sulcus; from there they travel across the epithelium[18,45] to the gingival sulcus, where they are expelled (Figs. 7–3 and 7–4).

Leukocytes are present in sulci even when histologic sections of adjacent tissue are free of inflammatory infiltrate. Differential counts of leukocytes from clinically healthy human gingival sulci have shown 91.2% to 91.5% PMNs and 8.5% to 8.8% mononuclear cells.[117,131]

Mononuclear cells were identified as 58% B lymphocytes, 24% T lymphocytes, and 18% mononuclear phagocytes. The ratio of T lymphocytes to B lymphocytes was found to be reversed from the normal ratio of about 3:1 found in peripheral blood to about 1:3 in crevicular fluid.[131]

Leukocytes are attracted by different plaque bacteria[54,130] but can also be found in the dentogingival region of germ-free adult animals.[75,103] Leukocytes were reported in the gingival sulcus in nonmechanically irritated (resting) healthy gingiva, indicating that their migration may be independent of an increase in vascular permeability.[5,124] The majority of these cells are viable and have been found to have phagocytic and killing capacity.[62,92,98] Therefore, they constitute a major protective mechanism against the extension of plaque into the gingival sulcus.

Leukocytes are also found in saliva (see following discussion). The main port of entry of leukocytes into the oral cavity is the gingival sulcus.[107]

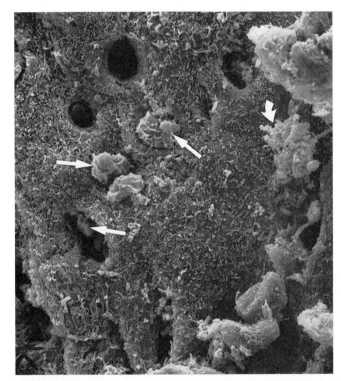

FIGURE 7–3. Scanning electron microscope view of periodontal pocket wall. Several leukocytes are emerging *(straight arrows),* some partially covered by bacteria *(curved arrow).* Empty holes correspond to tunnels through which leukocytes have emerged.

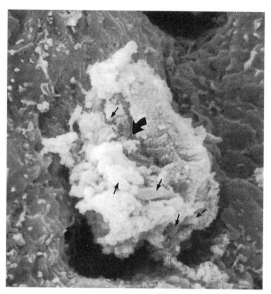

FIGURE 7-4. Scanning electron microscope view at higher magnification than Figure 7-3. A leukocyte emerging from the pocket wall is covered with bacteria *(small arrows)*. The *large curved arrow* points to a phagosomal vacuole through which bacteria are being engulfed.

SALIVA

Salivary secretions are protective in nature because they maintain the oral tissues in a physiologic state (Table 7-3). Saliva exerts a major influence on plaque by mechanically cleansing the exposed oral surfaces, by buffering acids produced by bacteria, and by controlling bacterial activity.

Antibacterial Factors

Saliva contains numerous inorganic and organic factors that influence bacteria and their products in the oral environment. Inorganic factors include ions and gases, bicarbonate, sodium, potassium, phosphates, calcium, fluorides, ammonium, and carbon dioxide. Organic factors include lysozyme, lactoferrin, myeloperoxidase, lactoperoxidase, and agglutinins such as glycoproteins, mucins, β_2-macroglobulins, fibronectins,[123] and antibodies.

Lysozyme is a hydrolytic enzyme that cleaves the linkage between structural components of the glycopeptide muramic acid–containing region of the cell wall of certain bacteria in vitro. Lysozyme works on both gram-negative

and gram-positive organisms[50]; *Veillonella* species and *Actinobacillus actinomycetemcomitans* are some of their targets. It probably repels certain transient bacterial invaders of the mouth.[53]

The lactoperoxidase-thiocyanate system in saliva has been shown to be bactericidal to some strains of *Lactobacillus* and *Streptococcus*[84,102] by preventing the accumulation of lysine and glutamic acid, both of which are essential for bacterial growth. Another antibacterial finding includes lactoferrin, which is effective against *Actinobacillus* species.[55]

Myeloperoxidase, an enzyme similar to salivary peroxidase, is released by leukocytes and is bactericidal for *Actinobacillus*[83] but has the added effect of inhibiting the attachment of *Actinomyces* strains to hydroxyapatite.[16]

Salivary Antibodies

Saliva, like sulcular fluid, contains antibodies that are reactive with indigenous oral bacterial species. Although immunoglobulins G (IgG) and M (IgM) are present, the preponderant immunoglobulin found in saliva is immunoglobulin A (IgA), whereas IgG is more prevalent in sulcular fluid.[121] Major and minor salivary glands contribute with all the secretory IgA (sIgA) and lesser amounts of IgG and IgM. The crevicular fluid contributes with most of the IgG complement components and cells that, in conjunction with IgG or IgM, inactivate or opsonize bacteria.

Salivary antibodies appear to be synthesized locally, for they react with strains of bacteria indigenous to the mouth but not with organisms characteristic of the intestinal tract.[36,38] Many bacteria found in saliva have been shown to be coated with IgA, and the bacterial deposits on teeth contain both IgA and IgG in quantities greater than 1% of their dry weight.[37] It has been shown that IgA antibodies present in parotid saliva can inhibit the attachment of oral *Streptococcus* species to epithelial cells.[33,128] Gibbons and coworkers[36-38] suggested that antibodies in secretions may impair the ability of bacteria to attach to mucosal or dental surfaces.

The enzymes normally found in the saliva are derived from the salivary glands, bacteria, leukocytes, oral tissues, and ingested substances; the major enzyme is parotid amylase. Certain salivary enzymes have been reported in increased concentrations in periodontal disease; these are hyaluronidase and lipase,[17] β-gluronidase and chondroitin sulfatase,[41] amino acid decarboxylases,[41] catalase, peroxidase, and collagenase.[60]

Table 7-3. ROLE OF SALIVA IN ORAL HEALTH

Function	Salivary Components	Probable Mechanism
Lubrication	Glycoproteins, mucoids	Coating similar to gastric mucin
Physical protection	Glycoproteins, mucoids	Coating similar to gastric mucin
Cleansing	Physical flow	Clearance of debris and bacteria
Buffering	Bicarbonate and phosphate	Antacids
Tooth integrity maintenance	Minerals	Maturation, remineralization
	Glycoprotein pellicle	Mechanical protection
Antibacterial action	IgA	Control of bacterial colonization
	Lysozyme	Breaks bacterial cell walls
	Lactoperoxidase	Oxidation of susceptible bacteria

Proteolytic enzymes in the saliva are generated by both the host and oral bacteria. These enzymes have been recognized as contributors to the initiation and progression of periodontal disease.[49,78] To combat these enzymes, saliva contains antiproteases that inhibit cysteine proteases such as cathepsins[51] and antileucoproteases that inhibit elastase.[89] Another antiprotease identified as a tissue inhibitor of matrix metalloproteinase (TIMP) has been shown to inhibit the activity of collagen-degrading enzymes.[26]

High-molecular-weight mucinous glycoproteins in saliva bind specifically to many plaque-forming bacteria. The glycoprotein–bacteria interactions facilitate bacterial accumulation on the exposed tooth surface.[33,36–38,130] The specificity of these interactions has been demonstrated. The interbacterial matrix of human plaque appears to contain polymers similar to salivary glycoproteins that may aid in maintaining the integrity of plaque. In addition, these glycoproteins selectively adsorb to the hydroxyapatite to make up part of the acquired pellicle. Other salivary glycoproteins inhibit the sorption of some bacteria to the tooth surface and to epithelial cells of the oral mucosa. This activity appears to be associated with the glycoproteins that possess blood group reactivity.[1,33,36,38,128] Another effect of mucin is the deletion of bacterial cells from the oral cavity by aggregation with mucin-rich films.

Glycoproteins and a glycolipid present on mammalian cell surfaces appear to serve as receptors for the attachment of some viruses and bacteria. Thus, the close similarity between glycoproteins of salivary secretions and components of the epithelial cell surface suggests that the secretions can competitively inhibit antigen sorption and therefore may limit pathologic alterations.

Salivary Buffers and Coagulation Factors

The maintenance of physiologic hydrogen ion concentration (pH) at the mucosal epithelial cell surface and the tooth surface is an important function of salivary buffers. Their primary effect has been studied in relationship to dental caries. In saliva the most important salivary buffer is the bicarbonate–carbonic acid system.[77]

Saliva also contains coagulation factors (factors VIII, IX, and X; plasma thromboplastin antecedent [PTA]; and the Hageman factor) that hasten blood coagulation and protect wounds from bacterial invasion.[67] The presence of an active fibrinolytic enzyme has also been suggested.

Leukocytes

In addition to desquamated epithelial cells, the saliva contains all forms of leukocytes, of which the principal cells are *polymorphonuclear leukocytes*. The number of leukocytes varies from person to person and at different times of the day and is increased in gingivitis. Leukocytes reach the oral cavity by migrating through the lining of the gingival sulcus. Living polymorphonuclear leukocytes in saliva are sometimes referred to as *orogranulocytes,* and their rate of migration into the oral cavity is termed the *orogranulocytic migratory rate*. Some investigators think that the rate of migration is correlated with the severity of gingival inflammation and is therefore a reliable index for assessing gingivitis.[117]

Role in Periodontal Pathology

Saliva exerts a major influence on plaque initiation, maturation, and metabolism. Calculus formation, periodontal disease, and caries are also influenced by salivary flow and composition. The removal of the salivary glands in experimental animals significantly increases the incidence of dental caries[39] and periodontal disease[46] and delays wound healing.[112]

In humans, an increase in inflammatory gingival diseases, dental caries, and rapid tooth destruction associated with cervical or cemental caries is partially a consequence of decreased salivary gland secretion (xerostomia). Xerostomia may result from a variety of factors, among them sialolithiasis, sarcoidosis, Sjogren's syndrome, Mikulicz's disease, irradiation, and surgical removal of the salivary glands (see Chapter 35).

REFERENCES

1. Adinolfi M, Mollison PL, Polley MJ, Rose JM. A blood group antibodies. J Exp Med *123:*951, 1966.
2. Armitage G. Diagnostic tests for periodontal diseases. Curr Opinion Dent *2:*53, 1992.
3. Arnold R, Lunstad, G, Bissada, N, Stallard R. Alterations in crevicular fluid flow during healing following gingival surgery. J Periodont Res *1:*303, 1966.
4. Attstrom R. Presence of leukocytes in the crevices of healthy and clinically inflamed gingiva. J Periodontol *5:*42, 1970.
5. Attstrom R, Egelberg J. Emigration of blood neutrophils and monocytes into the gingival crevices. J Periodont Res *5:*48, 1970.
6. Bader HJ, Goldhaber P. The passage of intravenously administered tetracycline in the gingival sulcus of dogs. J Oral Ther *2:*324, 1966.
7. Bang J, Cimasoni G. Total protein in human crevicular fluid. J Dent Res *50:*1683, 1971.
8. Birkedal-Hansen H, Taylor RE, Zambon JJ, et al. Characterization of collagenolytic activity from strains of *Bacteroides gingivalis*. J Periodont Res *23:*258, 1988.
9. Bissada NF, Schaffer EM, Haus E. Circadian periodicity of human crevicular fluid. J Periodontol *38:*36, 1967.
10. Bjorn HL, Koch G, Lindhe J. Evaluation of gingival fluid measurements. Odont Rev *16:*300, 1965.
11. Brill N. The gingival pocket fluid. Studies of its occurrence, composition and effect. Acta Odont Scand *20*(suppl 32):159, 1969.
12. Brill N. Effect of chewing on flow of tissue fluid into gingival pockets. Acta Odontol Scand *17:*277, 1959.
13. Brill N, Bronnestam R. Immunoelectrophoretic study of tissue fluid from gingival pockets. Acta Odontol Scand *18:*95, 1960.
14. Brill N, Krasse B. The passage of tissue fluid into the clinically healthy gingival pocket. Acta Odontol Scand *11:*223, 1958.
15. Bulkacz J. Enzymatic activities in gingival fluid with special emphasis on phospholipases. J Western Soc Periodont *36:*145, 1986.
16. Camargo PM de, Miyasaki KT, Wolinsky LE. Host modulation of adherence: The effect of human neutrophil myeloperoxidase on the attachment of *Actinomyces viscosus* and *naeslundii* to saliva coated hydroxyapatite. J Periodont Res *23:*334, 1988.
17. Carlsson J, Egelberg J. Local effect of diet on plaque formation and development of gingivitis in dogs. II. Effect of high carbohydrate versus high protein/fat diets. Odont Rev *16:*42, 1965.
18. Cattoni M. Lymphocytes in the epithelium of healthy gingiva. J Dent Res *30:*627, 1951.
19. Challacombe SJ. Passage of serum immunoglobulin into the oral cavity. In Lehner, T, Cimasoni, G, eds. Borderland Between Caries and Periodontal Disease. Vol II. London, Academic Press, 1980, p 55.
20. Cimasoni G. The crevicular fluid. In Myers, H., ed. Monographs in Oral Science. Vol 3. Basel, S Karger, 1974.
21. Cimasoni G. Crevicular fluid updated. In Myers H, ed. Monographs in Oral Science. Vol. 12. Basel, S Karger, 1983.
22. Cobb CM, Brown LR. The effects of exudate from the periodontal pocket on cell culture. Periodontics *5:*5, 1967.
23. Dawes C. The chemistry and physiology of saliva. In Shaw JH, Sweeney EA, Cappuccino CC, Meller SM, eds. Textbook of Oral Biology. Philadelphia, WB Saunders, 1978.
24. Dawes C, Jenkins GM, Tonge CH. The nomenclature of the integuments of the enamel surface of teeth. Br Dent J *115:*65, 1963.
25. Dinarello CA. Interleukin-1 and its biologically related cytokines. In Cohen S, ed. Lymphokines and the Immune Response. Boca Raton, FL, CRC Press, 1990.

26. Drouin L, Overall CM, Sodek J. Identification of matrix metallo-endoproteinase inhibitor (TIMP) in human parotid and submandibular saliva: Partial purification and characterization. J Periodont Res 23:370, 1988.

27. Ebersole JL, Taubman MA, Smith DJ. Gingival crevicular fluid antibody to oral microorganisms. II. Distribution and specificity of local antibody responses. J Periodont Res 20:349, 1985.

28. Egelberg J. Cellular elements in gingival pocket fluid. Acta Odontol Scand 21:283, 1963.

29. Egelberg J. Gingival exudate measurements for evaluation of inflammatory changes of the gingiva. Odont Rev 15:381, 1964.

30. Egelberg J. Permeability of the dentogingival vessels. II. Clinically healthy gingiva. J Periodont Res 1:276, 1966.

31. Egelberg J, Attstrom R. Presence of leukocytes within crevices of healthy and inflamed gingiva and their immigration from the blood. J Periodont Res (suppl 4):23, 1969.

32. Eisenberg L, Suchow R, Coles RS, Deasy MJ. The effects of metronidazole administration on clinical and microbiologic parameters of periodontal disease. Clin Prevent Dent 13:28, 1991.

33. Ellen RP, Gibbons RJ. Protein associated adherence of *Streptococcus pyogenes* to epithelial surfaces: Prerequisite for virulence. Infect Immun 5:826, 1972.

34. Garnick JJ, Pearson R, Harrell D. The evaluation of the Periotron. J Periodontol 50:424, 1979.

35. Genco RJ, Zambon JJ, Murray PA. Serum and gingival fluid antibodies as an adjunct in the diagnosis of *Actinobacillus actinomycetemcomitans*–associated periodontal disease. J Periodontol 56:41, 1985.

36. Gibbons RJ, van Houte J. Selective bacterial adherence to oral epithelial surfaces and its role as an ecological determinant. Infect Immun 3:567, 1971.

37. Gibbons RJ, van Houte J. On the formation of dental plaques. J Periodontol 44:347, 1973.

38. Gibbons RJ, van Houte J, Liljemark WF. Some parameters that effect the adherence of *S. salivarius* to oral epithelial surfaces. J Dent Res 51:424, 1972.

39. Gilda JE, Keyes PH. Increased dental caries activity in the Syrian hamster following desalivation. Proc Soc Exp Biol Med 66:28, 1947.

40. Glas JE, Krasse B. Biophysical studies on dental calculus from germ-free and conventional rats. Acta Odontol Scand 20:127, 1962.

41. Gochman N, Meyer RK, Blackwell RQ, Fosdick LS. The aminoacid decarboxylase of salivary sediment. J Dent Res 38:998, 1959.

42. Golub LM, Borden SM, Kleinberg K. Urea content of gingival crevicular fluid and its relation to periodontal disease in humans. J Periodont Res 6:243, 1971.

43. Gordon JM, Walker CB, Goodson JM, Socransky SS. Sensitive assay for measuring tetracycline levels in gingival crevice fluid. Antimicrob Agents Chemother 17:193, 1980.

44. Gowan M, Mundy GR. Actions of recombinant interleukin 1, interleukin 2 and interferon-gamma on bone resorption. In vitro. J Immunol 136:2478, 1986.

45. Grant DA, Orban BJ. Leukocytes in the epithelial attachment. J Periodontol 31:87, 1960.

46. Gupta OH, Blechman H, Stahl SS. The effects of desalivation on periodontal tissues of the Syrian hamster. Oral Surg 13:470, 1960.

47. Hara K, Löe H. Carbohydrate components of the gingival exudate. J Periodont Res 4:202, 1969.

48. Hasegawa K. Biochemical study of gingival fluid. Lactic acid in gingival fluid. Bull Tokyo Med Dent Univ 14:359, 1967.

49. Holt SC, Bramanti TE. Factors in virulence expression and their role on periodontal disease pathogenesis. Crit Rev Oral Biol Med 2:177, 1991.

50. Iacono VC, Bolot PR, Mackay JB, et al. Lytic sensitivity of *Actinobacillus actinomycetemcomitans* to lysozyme. Infect Immun 40:773, 1983.

51. Isemura S, Ando K, Nakashizoka T, Hayakawa T. Cystatin S: A cystein-proteinase inhibitor of human saliva. J Biochem 96:1311, 1984.

52. Jensen RL, Folke LEA. The passage of exogenous tritiated thymidine into gingival tissues. J Periodontol 45:786, 1974.

53. Jolles P, Petit JF. Purification and analysis of human saliva lysozyme. Nature 200:168, 1963.

54. Kahnberg KE, Lindhe J, Helden J. Initial gingivitis induced by topical application of plaque extract. A histometric study in dogs with normal gingiva. J Periodont Res 11:218, 1976.

55. Kalmar JP, Arnold RP. Killing of *Actinobacillus actinomycetemcomitans* by human lactoferrin. Infect Immun 56:2552, 1988.

56. Kaslick RS, Mandel ID, Chasens AI, et al. Concentration of inorganic ions in gingival fluid. J Dent Res 49:887, 1970.

57. Kaslick RS, Chasens AI, Mandel ID, et al. Quantitative analysis of sodium, potassium and calcium in gingival fluid from gingiva in varying degrees of inflammation. J Periodontol 41:93, 1970.

58. Kaslick RS, Chasens AI, Mandel ID, et al. Sodium, potassium and calcium in gingival fluid. A study of the relationship of the ions to one another, to circadian rhythms, gingival bleeding, purulence, and to conservative periodontal therapy. J Periodontol 41:442, 1970.

59. Kaslik RS, Chasens AI, Weinstein O, Waldman R. Ultramicromethods for the collection of gingival fluid and quantitative analysis of its sodium content. J Dent Res 47:1192, 1986.

60. King JD. Experimental investigation of periodontal disease in the ferret and in man, with special reference to calculus formation. Dent Pract 4:157, 1954.

61. Kiroshita JJ, Muhlemann HR. Effect of sodium ortho and pyrophosphate on supragingival calculus. Helv Odontol Acta 10:46, 1966.

62. Kowolik MJ, Raeburn JA. Functional integrity of gingival crevicular neutrophil polymorphonuclear leukocytes as demonstrated by nitroblue tetrazolium reduction. J Periodont Res 15:483, 1980.

63. Krasse B, Egelberg J. The relative proportions of sodium, potassium and calcium in gingival-free pocket fluid. Acta Odontol Scand 20:143, 1962.

64. Krekeler G. Quantitative determination of the gingival sulcus fluid by means of microcapillaries. Dtsch Zahnaertzl Z 30:544, 1975.

65. Lamster IB, Celenti R, Ebersole J. The relationship of serum IgG antibody titers to periodontal pathogens to indicators of the host response in gingival crevicular fluid. J Clin Periodontol 17:419, 1990.

66. Lamster IB, Novak MJ. Host mediators in gingival crevicular fluid: Implications for the pathogenesis of periodontal disease. Crit Rev Oral Biol Med 3:31, 1992.

67. Leung SW, Jensen AT. Factors controlling the deposition of calculus. Int Dent J 8:613, 1958.

68. Liew V, Mack G, Tseng P, et al. Single-dose concentrations of timidazole in gingival crevicular fluid, serum and gingival tissue in adults with periodontitis. J Dent Res 70:910, 1991.

69. Life JS, Johnson NW, Powell JR, et al. Interleukin-1 beta (IL-1β) levels in gingival crevicular fluid from adults without previous evidence of destructive periodontitis. A cross sectional study. J Clin Periodontol 19:53, 1992.

70. Lindhe J, Attstrom R. Gingival exudation during the menstrual cycle. J Periodont Res 2:194, 1967.

71. Lindhe J, Attstrom R, Bjorn AL. Influence of sex hormones on gingival exudate of gingivitis-free female dogs. J Periodont Res 3:273, 1968.

72. Lindhe J, Bjorn AL. Influence of hormonal contraceptives on the gingiva of women. J Periodont Res 2:1, 1967.

73. Lisanti VF. Hydrolytic enzymes in periodontal tissues. Ann NY Acad Sci 85:461, 1960.

74. Löe H, Holm-Pedersen P. Absence and presence of fluid from normal and inflamed gingiva. Periodontics 3:171, 1965.

75. Magnusson B. Mucosal changes at erupting molars in germ-free rats. J Periodont Res 4:181, 1969.

76. Marcus ER, Jooste CP, Driver HS, Hatting J. The quantification of individual proteins in crevicular gingival fluid. J Periodont Res 20:444, 1985.

77. Mandel I. Relation of saliva and plaque to caries. J Dent Res 53(suppl):246, 1974.

78. Mandel ID. Markers of periodontal disease susceptibility and activity derived from saliva. In Johnson NW, ed. Risk Markers of Oral Diseases. Vol 3. New York, Cambridge University Press, 1991, p 228.

79. Martin LP, Noble WH. Gingival fluid in relation to tooth mobility and occlusal interferences. J Periodontol 45:444, 1974.

80. McDougall WA. Pathways of penetration and effects of horseradish peroxidase in rat molar gingiva. Arch Oral Biol 15:621, 1970.

81. McDougall WA. The effect of topical antigen on the gingiva of sensitized rabbits. J Periodont Res 9:153, 1974.

82. McLaughlin WS, Lovat FM, Macgregor IDM, Kelly PJ. The immediate effects of smoking on gingival fluid flow. J Clin Periodontol 20:448, 1993.

83. Miyasaki KT, Wilson ME, Genco RJ. Killing of *Actinobacillus actinomycetemcomitans* by the human peroxide chloride system. Infect Immun 53:161, 1986.

84. Muhlemann HR, Schroeder H. Dynamics of supragingival calculus formation. Adv Oral Biol 1:175, 1964.

85. Nagao M. Influence of prosthetic appliances upon the flow of crevicular tissue fluid. I. Relation between crevicular tissue fluid and prosthetic appliances. Bull Tokyo Med Dent Univ 14:241, 1967.

86. Nakamura M, Slots J. Salivary enzymes: Origin and relationship to periodontal disease. J Periodont Res 18:559, 1983.

87. Novaes AB Jr, Ruben MP, Kramer GM. Proteins of the gingival exudate: A review and discussion of the literature. J Western Soc Periodontol 27:12, 1979.

88. Offenbacher S, Williams RC, Jeffcoat MK, et al. Effects of NAIDS on beagle crevicular cyclo-oxyegnase metabolites and periodontal bone loss. J Periodont Res 27:207, 1992.

89. Ohlsson M, Rosengreen M, Tegner H, Ohlsson K. Quantification of granulocyte elastase inhibitor in human mixed saliva and in pure parotid secretion. Phys Chem 364:1323, 1983.

90. Orban JE, Stallard RE. Gingival crevicular fluid: A reliable predictor of gingival health? J Periodontol 40:231, 1969.

91. Page RC. Host response tests designed for diagnosing periodontal disease. J Periodontol 63:356, 1992.

92. Passo SA, Tsai CC, McArthur WP, et al. Interaction of inflammatory cells and oral microorganisms. IX. The bacterial effect of human PMN leukocytes on isolated plaque microorganisms. J Periodont Res 15:470, 1980.

93. Paunio K. On the hydroxyproline-containing components in the gingival exudate. J Periodont Res 6:115, 1971.

94. Pollock JJ, Andors L, Gulumoglu A. Direct measurement of hepatitis B virus antibody and antigen markers in gingival crevicular fluid. Oral Surg, Oral Med, Oral Pathol 57:499, 1984.

95. Ranney RR, Montgomery EH. Vascular leakage resulting from topical application of endotoxin to the gingiva of the beagle dog. Arch Oral Biol 18:963, 1973.

96. Ranney RR, Zander HA. Allergic periodontal disease in sensitized squirrel monkeys. J Periodontol 41:12, 1970.

97. Ratcliff P. Permeability of healthy gingival epithelium by microscopically observable particles. J Periodontol 37:291, 1966.

98. Renggli HH. Phagocytosis and killing by crevicular neutrophils. *In* Lehner T,

ed. The Borderland Between Caries and Periodontal Disease. New York, Grune & Stratton, 1977.

99. Renggli HH, Regolatti B. Intracrevicular sampling of leukocytes using plastic strips. Helv Odont Acta *16:*93, 1972.

100. Rizzo AA. Absorption of bacterial endotoxin into rabbit gingival pocket tissue. Periodontics *6:*65, 1968.

101. Rizzo AA. Histologic and immunologic evaluation of antigen penetration with oral tissues after topical application. Periodontics *41:*210, 1970.

102. Rosebury R, Karshan M. Salivary Calculus: Dental Science and Dental Art. Philadelphia, Lea & Febiger, 1938.

103. Rovin S, Costich ER, Gordon HA. The influence of bacteria and irritation in the initiation of periodontal disease in germfree and conventional rats. J Periodont Res *1:*193, 1966.

104. Salonen JI, Paunio KU. An intracrevicular washing method for collection of intracrevicular contents. Scand J Dent Res *99:*406, 1991.

105. Sandalli P, Wade AB. Alterations in crevicular fluid flow during healing following gingivectomy and flap procedures. J Periodont Res *4:*314, 1969.

106. Sano K, Nakao M, Shiba A, Kobayashi K. An ultra-micro assay for proteins in biological fluids other than blood using a combination of agarose gel isoelectric focusing and silver staining. Clin Chim Acta *137:*115, 1984.

107. Schiott CR, Löe H. The origin and variation in the number of leukocytes in the human saliva. J Periodont Res (suppl 4):24, 1969.

108. Schultz-Haudt S, Bibby BG, Bruce MA. Tissue destructive products of gingival bacteria from nonspecific gingivitis. J Dent Res *33:*624, 1954.

109. Schwartz J, Stinson FL, Parker RB. The passage of tritiated bacterial endotoxin across intact gingival crevicular epithelium. J Periodontol *43:*270, 1972.

110. Selvig K. Structure and metabolism of the normal periodontium. Position paper. International Conference on Research in the Biology of Periodontal Disease, Chicago, IL, June 12–15, 1977.

111. Shapiro L, Goldman H, Bloom A. Sulcular exudate flow in gingival inflammation. J Periodontol *50:*301, 1979.

112. Shen LS, Ghavamzadeh G, Shklar G. Gingival healing in sialadenectomized rats. J Periodontol *50:*533, 1979.

113. Sibraa PD, Reinhardt AA, Dyer JK, DuBois LM. Acute-phase protein detection and quantification in gingival crevicular fluid by direct and indirect immuno-dot. J Clin Periodont *18:*101, 1991.

114. Simon B, Goldman HM, Ruben MP, et al. The role of endotoxin in periodontal disease. II. Correlation of the amount of endotoxin in human gingival exudate with the clinical degree of inflammation. J Periodontol *42:*81, 1970.

115. Simon B, Goldman HM, Ruben MP, et al. The role of endotoxin in periodontal disease. III. Correlation of the amount of endotoxin with the histologic degree of inflammation. J Periodontol *42:*210, 1971.

116. Skapski H, Lehner T. A crevicular washing method for investigating immune components of crevicular fluid in man. J Periodont Res *11:*19, 1976.

117. Skougaard MR, Bay I, Kilnkhammer JM. Correlation between gingivitis and orogranuloyctic migratory rate. J Dent Res *48:*716, 1994.

118. Solis Gaffar MC, Rustogi KN, Gaffar A. Hydrogen sulfide production from gingival crevicular fluid. J Periodontol *51:*603, 1980.

119. Squier CA, Johnson NW. Permeability of oral mucosa. Br Med Bull *31:*169, 1975.

120. Steinberg AD, Steinberg J, Allen P, et al. The effect of alteration in the sulcular environment upon the movement of 14C-diphenylhydantoin through rabbit sulcular tissues. J Periodont Res *11:*47, 1976.

121. Sueda T, Bang J, Cimasoni G. Collection of gingival fluid for quantitative analysis. J Dent Res *48:*159, 1969.

122. Suppipat W, Suppipat N. Evaluation of an electronic device for gingival fluid quantitation. J Periodontol *48:*388, 1977.

123. Talonopoika JT, Hamalainen MM. Collagen III aminoterminal propeptide in gingival crevicular fluid before and after periodontal disease. Scand J Dent Res *100:*107, 1992.

124. Theilade J, Egelberg J, Attstrom R. Vascular permeability to colloidal carbon in clinically inflamed gingiva. J Periodont Res *6:*100, 1971.

125. Tolo K. Transport across stratified nonkeratinized epithelium. J Periodont Res *6:*237, 1971.

126. Tomasi TB, Bienenstock J. Secretory immunoglobulins. Adv Immunol *9:*1, 1968.

127. Vogel JJ, Amdur BH. Inorganic pyrophosphate in parotid saliva. Arch Oral Biol *12:*159, 1967.

128. Waerhaug J. The gingival pocket. Anatomy, pathology deepening and elimination. Odont Tidskaift *60*(suppl 1):1, 1952.

129. Weinstein E, Mandel ID, Salkind A, et al. Studies of gingival fluid. Periodontics *5:*161, 1967.

130. Williams RW, Gibbons RG. Inhibition of bacterial adherence by secretory immunoglobulin A: A mechanism of antigen disposal. Science *177:*697, 1972.

131. Wilton JMA, Renggli HH, Lehner T. The isolation and identification of mononuclear cells from the gingival crevice in man. J Periodont Res *11:*243, 1976.

132. Winkelhoff AJ van, Steenberger TJM van, de Graaff J. The role of black-pigmented *Bacteroides* in human oral infections. J Clin Periodontol *15:*145, 1988.

8

Host Response: Basic Concepts

RUSSELL C. NISENGARD, MICHAEL G. NEWMAN, and MARIANO SANZ

Inflammatory Cell Response
Mast Cells
Neutrophils
Macrophages
Lymphocytes
Plasma Cells
Antibody
Biologic Properties of Immunoglobulins
Complement

Immune Mechanisms
Anaphylaxis (Type I)
Cytotoxic Reactions (Type II)
Immune Complex (Arthus) Reactions (Type III)
Cell-Mediated Immunity or Delayed Hypersensitivity
 (Type IV)
Cytokines
Classification
Assays

It is recognized that host responses play a role in most forms of periodontal disease. *In gingivitis, periodontitis, and juvenile periodontitis, the development of the disease depends on the interaction between the resident microbiota and the host response. In other types of periodontal disease, such as desquamative gingivitis, the lesions frequently result from a host response.*

This chapter briefly reviews the basis of the immunologic and inflammatory responses as they may relate to the etiology and pathogenesis of periodontal diseases.

INFLAMMATORY CELL RESPONSE

In response to specific stimuli, inflammatory cells chemotactically migrate and concentrate in localized areas where they phagocytize bacteria and bacterial components or remove damaged tissue. Some of these, such as T and B lymphocytes, divide and increase in number by blastogenesis. Others release vasoactive products, and still others produce substances such as plasma cells and macrophages that cause or assist in the lysis of other host cells or the destruction of alveolar bone.[3] The cells involved are mast cells, neutrophils (polymorphonuclear leukocytes), macrophages, lymphocytes, and plasma cells.

Mast Cells

Mast cells are important because of their cytoplasmic granules, which contain histamine, slow-reacting substance of anaphylaxis (SRS-A), heparin, eosinophil chemotactic factor of anaphylaxis, and bradykinin, all of which are released into the gingival tissues.[3] Degranulation of mast cells occurs during nonimmunologic and immunologic immediate hypersensitivity reactions of the anaphylactic type, when antigens react with surface-bound immunoglobulin E (IgE) antibody. In addition, a mast cell interleukin has been shown to enhance collagenase activity,[44] and heparin (contained in other granules) may augment bone resorption[30] by potentiating the effect of parathyroid hormone.

Neutrophils

Neutrophils (polymorphonuclear leukocytes) are important in the host defense against injury and infection and are thought to play an important role in periodontal disease (see Chapter 10). These cells are found in all inflammatory lesions, particularly in the more acute lesions, where they concentrate at sites of injury, chemically attracted to the area through the process of chemotaxis. The neutrophils then engulf (phagocytosis) and subsequently kill and digest most microorganisms and neutralize other noxious substances. Phagocytosis is enhanced immunologically by the presence of C3b surface receptors. These receptors bind complexes of bacteria (antigen)–antibody–complement through C3b, a fragment of the third component of complement formed by immune complexes.

Neutrophils may also cause tissue destruction. Their granules contain substances capable of killing, digesting, and neutralizing microorganisms and/or their products.[15,17,42,43] Their granules also contain lysozyme, acid hydrolase, myeloperoxidase, collagenase I and III, cathepsin D, cathepsin G, elastase, and lactoferrin. It is important to note that the localized tissue damage in the Arthus reaction (see below) depends on the presence of neutrophils.

Leukocyte abnormalities, including chemotactic defects, deficiencies in adhesion, inability to mount a necessary respiratory burst, and lack of specific granules, can lead to more severe periodontal disease.[30]

Macrophages

Macrophages play a direct, important function in cell-mediated immunity (see later discussion). These large, highly phagocytic cells are part of the scavenger reticuloendothelial system; their phagocytic activity is enhanced by surface receptors for the Fc portion of immunoglobulin G (IgG), which provides increased contact of antigens with the macrophage following antigen–antibody interaction. They participate with T lymphocytes in aiding the response of B lymphocytes to many immunogens.[7,14] It is thought that the macrophage "processes" the antigen for the B lymphocyte. In inflammatory lesions, macrophages are formed by differentiation of monocytes that are carried to the lesion by the blood. These cells act nonspecifically with antigens, which provide them with the capability of destroying a diverse, antigenically unrelated group of bacteria.[19]

Mononuclear cells are attracted to sites of inflammation by lymphokines (soluble substances released by lymphocytes) such as interferon-γ (IFN-γ) and complement factors (e.g., C5a). They are then retained at these sites by other lymphokines. The ability of the macrophages to ingest, kill, and digest microorganisms is dependent on interaction with other leukocytes, elements of the immune system in general, and complement. The efficiency of bacterial phagocytosis by the macrophages is enhanced by the reaction of the antibody with the antigen and subsequent complement activation.

Macrophages are also important because they secrete Interleukin-1 (IL-1), IL-6, IL-8, IL-10, tumor necrosis factor-γ (TNF-γ), insulin-like growth factors, IFN-α and γ, and other stimulatory, inhibitory and growth factors; they also produce prostaglandins,[25] cyclic adenosine monophosphate (cAMP), and collagenase[9,30,31,45] in response to stimulation by bacterial endotoxin, immune complexes, or lymphokines. Macrophage collagenase may play a significant role in collagen destruction in diseased periodontal tissues.

Lymphocytes

Lymphocytes include three types of cells: (1) T lymphocytes, or T cells, which are derived from the thymus and play a role in cell-mediated immunity; (2) B lymphocytes, or B cells, which are derived from liver, spleen, and bone marrow, are the precursors for plasma cells, and play a role in humoral immunity; and (3) natural killer (NK) and killer (K) cells.[19,33]

The T cells are recognized to be composed of several subsets that modulate the humoral response.[19] These include helper-inducer T cells (T_H cells) (CD4 positive), which aid in the cellular response of B cells to differentiate into plasma cells and produce antibodies and suppressor-cytotoxic T cells (T_S cells) (CD8 positive), which stimulate cytotoxic and microbicidal activity of immune cells. The T_H cells release IL-2 and IFN-g, while the T_S cells release IL-4 and IL-5. T_H cells have been further subdivided into three subsets (T_H1, T_H2, and T_H0) distinguished by their cytokine production profiles. In adult periodontitis, T_H cells increase and T_S cells decrease with increased gingival inflammation.[22]

The B cells are identifiable by their cell surface immunoglobulin, usually immunoglobulin M (IgM) or D (IgD). However, some B cells express IgG, IgA, or IgE. These surface immunoglobulins serve as receptors for antigen. The NK cells are recognized by their absence of T-cell receptors (TCRs) and surface immunoglobulin.[19,33]

The interaction between antigens and macrophages,

Table 8-1. POSSIBLE ROLE OF ANTIBODIES IN INFLAMMATORY DISEASE

Reaction or Process†	Effects
Complement activation by Ag-Ab complexes	Protective early changes in inflammation
Phagocytosis of Ag-Ab complexes by PMNs with release of lysosomes	Destructive
Enhanced lymphocyte stimulation by Ag-Ab complexes	Release of lymphokines with protective and destructive effects
Blocking of lymphocytes by free antibody or by Ag-Ab complexes	Suppression of cell-mediated immune reactions
Neutralization of bacterial allergens, toxins, or histolytic enzymes	Protective
Enhanced opsonization or bacteriolysis of plaque bacteria	Protective

Ag-Ab complexes, Antigen–antibody complexes; PMNs, polymorphonuclear leukocytes.
Adapted from Genco RJ, Mashimo PA, Krygier G, Ellison SA: Antibody mediated effects on the periodontium. J Periodontol 45:336, 1974

known as antigen processing, leads to the activation of NK cells.[27]

Plasma Cells

Plasma cells are the terminal cells in the progression from B cells. They contain abundant cytoplasmic RNA, which is characteristic of a cell actively producing protein. Plasma cells occur in germinal centers and in tissues, where they produce immunoglobulins and antibodies, the effector cells for systemic and local humoral immunity, respectively.

ANTIBODY

The host responds to oral bacteria and their products by plasma cell production of immunoglobulins or antibodies. Prior to this, antigen-presenting cells such as macrophages present processed antigen fragments to T cells via the major histocompatibility complex (MHC) on its surface. After the physical interaction of the T cells with the B cells, the latter respond to T-cell–dependent antigens with plasma cell differentiation and antibody production.[27] The possible role of antibodies in inflammation is summarized in Table 8-1.

Antibodies, which are glycoproteins, are found in blood, tissue fluids, and secretions and are the effectors of humoral immunity.[13] They are highly specific and sensitive. All classes and subsets of immunoglobulins have similar structural organizations, but they differ according to their biologic properties, carbohydrate content, weight, and amino acid sequences. Every antibody molecule has a variable region, which, because of its unique amino acid sequence and tertiary structure of its antibody-combining site, allows it to react highly specifically with a particular antigen.

Human immunoglobulin is divided into five classes on the basis of structural differences. These differences are responsible for the variability in biologic effects (Table 8-2). The five classes are IgG, IgM, IgA, IgE, and IgD. Four subclasses of IgG have been identified (IgG1, IgG2, IgG3, and IgG4), as have two subclasses of IgA (IgA1 and IgA2) and two subclasses of IgM (IgM1 and IgM2). Immunoglobulin molecules are composed of either two κ or two λ light (small) chains and one of five types of heavy (large) polypeptide chains. The class is determined by the type of heavy chain. Each class of immunoglobulin has similar sets of light chains but antigenically distinct sets of heavy chains. A given immunoglobulin molecule has identical heavy chains and identical κ or λ light chains.

The basic immunologic structure appears Y shaped. The tail of the Y contains the ends of two heavy chains and is referred to as the *Fc fragment*. It is in this region that complement binding takes place. The remaining area of the Y-shaped molecule is composed of the light chains and the remainder of the heavy chains. This is the *Fab* or *antibody-binding site*. The number of binding sites is called the *valence* of the molecule. IgG has a valence of 2; secretory IgA containing two monomeric units of IgA has a valence of 4; and IgM containing five monomeric units has a valence of up to 10.

Antibody molecules can be divided into three antigenic determinants or epitopes: isotypic, allotypic, and idiotypic. These determinants are located on discrete regions of the antibody molecule. The isotypic determinant is at the Fc or

Table 8-2. PROPERTIES OF IMMUNOGLOBULINS

	IgG				IgA		IgM	IgD	IgE
	1	2	3	4	1	2			
Serum concentration (mg/ml)	Total IgG: 12				Total IgA: 2		1.2	0.03	0.00004
Complement fixation									
Classic pathway	+	±	+	–	–	–	+	–	–
Alternative pathway	+	+	+	?	+	+	+	–	+
Placental transfer	+	+	+	+	–	–	–	–	–
Reaginic activity	–	–	–	–	–	–	–	–	+
Antibacterial lysis	+	+	+	+	+	+	+	?	?
On B-lymphocyte surface	–	–	–	–	–	–	+	+	–

From Nisengard RJ. The role of immunology in periodontal disease. J Periodontol 48:505,1977.

constant regions of the heavy and light chains, defines the class and subclass of the antibody, and is common to a species.

The allotypic determinants, found on both heavy and light chains at both the Fc and Fab regions of the antibody molecule, may vary from person to person within a species. At present, the γ chain has been identified to have 25 allotypes called Gm markers.

The idiotypic determinant is at the Fab or variable region of the antibody molecule. Multiple idiotypes may be found on an antibody.[19]

Biologic Properties of Immunoglobulins

IgG. IgG, consisting of IgG1, IgG2, IgG3, and IgG4, is the most abundant of the serum immunoglobulins and is distributed equally between the blood and the extravascular fluids. Its major role is to neutralize bacterial toxins by binding to organisms, thereby enhancing their phagocytosis. Although IgG concentration in serum is high, its concentration in secretions is low. IgG constitutes 80% of the total serum immunoglobulin, passes the placental barrier, and provides newborns with the humoral immunity of the mother.[13]

IgM. Antibodies of the IgM class are the first to be formed after challenge with most antigens, but they are usually present in much lower concentrations than IgG. The levels of IgM during the later stages of an infection generally decrease and become negligible in comparison with those of IgG, which usually remain elevated for extended periods. This early synthesis suggests an important role for IgM in the early stages of infection. IgM is also the most efficient activator of the complement system. IgM molecules are composed of five monomeric subunits (each similar to those in the IgG molecule) joined by disulfide bonds to a J chain and, through the Fc region, have a correspondingly larger number of sites for interaction with antigen.

IgE. IgE (reaginic antibody) is present in human serum at about 1/125,000 the level of IgG. Despite the low concentration, this class of antibody is responsible for acute allergic reactions. The cells that produce IgE are abundant in the mucosa of the oral, respiratory, and intestinal tracts. Because of this, IgE is also found in exocrine secretions. Higher concentrations of these antibodies are found in patients with asthma, hay fever, and drug and food allergies. This class of antibodies has an affinity for cell surfaces, which is mediated by an attachment site on their Fc fragment. In humans, IgE is homocytotropic or attaches to mast cells and basophilic leukocytes. Antigen reaction with two IgE molecules previously attached to mast cells or basophils leads to the release of histamine and other pharmacologically active substances.

IgD. IgD is an immunoglobulin that is found at extremely low levels in serum. IgD binds to a receptor on the surface of B lymphocytes. It may play an important role in triggering B-cell stimulation by antigen, thus initiating the immune response.

IgA. IgA occurs in a variety of polymeric forms of the basic immunoglobulin molecule, from monomer to trimer and even higher forms. IgA is the principal immunoglobulin in exocrine secretions (i.e., saliva, milk, respiratory secretions, intestinal mucin, and tears). It is present at one fifth the concentration of IgG in human serum. The cells that produce IgA are concentrated in the subepithelial tissue of the exocrine glands and respond to locally occurring antigens. Serum IgA is mostly monomer, whereas secretory IgA is a dimer, containing a secretory piece and a J chain that binds IgA molecules through disulfide bonds. Gingival tissue and crevicular fluid contain serum IgA rather than secretory IgA.

Properties of secretory IgA antibodies make them unique and influence their function on mucosal surfaces. Secretory IgA is more resistant to digestion by proteolytic enzymes than are other immunoglobulins. It has been suggested that the secretory component of a polypeptide chain attached to the Fc portion of secretory IgA stabilizes this portion of the molecule, facilitating its transport across the glandular epithelium. It is also possible that the J chain, the fourth type of polypeptide chain associated with secretory IgA, may function in making secretory IgA more resistant to proteolysis. The valence of the secretory IgA molecules generally found in saliva is 4.[10]

There has been wide interest in the protective effects of secretory antibodies against bacterial and viral diseases on mucosal surfaces. IgA, unlike IgG and IgM, does not activate complement by the classic pathway, which begins with fixation of complement to the Fc portion of the immunoglobulin molecule. An alternative pathway of complement activation has been described; it involves the later complement components, C3 through C9, but not C1, C4, or C2 (see following discussion of complement). This alternative pathway can be activated by aggregated immunoglobulin, including IgA.

Adhesion of bacteria to tissue surfaces may be prevented or reduced by secretory antibodies.[12] This mechanism of protection is thought to be active in bacterial diseases (e.g., cholera) and dental caries and possibly in the early phase of periodontal disease, in which bacterial adhesion and colonization of mucosal or dental tissues are necessary steps in the pathogenesis[10] (see Chapter 6). An antibacterial role of secretory IgA in established periodontal lesions is doubtful, because saliva probably does not penetrate into the depths of the lesion.

COMPLEMENT

An important consequence of antigen–antibody interaction is the activation of complement (Fig. 8–1). Complement consists of at least 11 proteins and glycoproteins that make up approximately 10% of the proteins in the normal sera of humans and other vertebrates.[19] These proteins are not immunoglobulins, and their concentration is not affected by immunization. They are synthesized in the liver, the small intestine, the macrophages, and other mononuclear cells.[13] Complement reacts with antibody–antigen complexes when the antibodies are of the IgG and IgM classes and exerts its primary biologic effects on cell membranes, causing lysis and functional alteration that can promote phagocytosis. Of primary importance is its effect on mast cells. In these cells, degranulation by complement causes the release of histamine and other biologically active substances that increase the permeability of small blood vessels. Migration of polymorphonuclear neutrophils

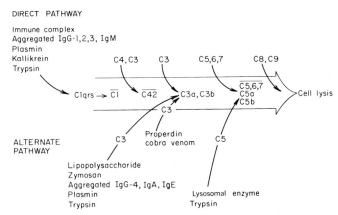

DIRECT PATHWAY

FIGURE 8–1. Schematic diagram of the complement sequence. Direct (classic) and alternate pathways in the activation of complement components. (From Page R. Pathogenic mechanisms. In Schluger S, Yuodelis RA, Page RC. Periodontal Disease. Philadelphia, Lea & Febiger, 1977.)

(PMNs), increased phagocytic activity by leukocytes and macrophages, hemolysis, and bacteriolysis also take place. Red blood cell lysis (hemolysis) as a consequence of complement activation when antibody has reacted with the red blood cell has been analyzed in greatest detail because it is simple to measure. This provides the basis for the complement fixation assay, an important laboratory procedure for detecting and measuring many different kinds of antigens and antibodies and their effect on the complement system.

The reaction sequence in the activation of the complement system has a cascading type pathway similar to that of the blood coagulation system (see Fig. 8–1). After one component of the complement system is bound by the Fc portion of the antibody in the antibody–antigen complex, the other components of the complement system react in an ordered sequence. In general, each activated complement component cleaves the next reacting member of the series into fragments, until the cascade has been completed. Some of the smaller fragments formed during cleavage have phlogistic activity—that is, they cause inflammatory tissue changes[19] (Table 8–3). These include increased vascular permeability and the attraction of PMNs. Other biologic activities of complement fixation are shown in Table 8–3.

Table 8–3. BIOLOGIC EFFECTS OF COMPLEMENT

Activity	Complement Components
Cytolytic and cytotoxic damage to cells	C1–9
Chemotactic activity for leukocytes	C3a, C5a, C567
Histamine release from mast cells	C3a, C5a
Increased vascular permeability	C3a, C5a
Kinin activity	C2, C3a
Lysosomal enzyme release from leukocytes	C5a
Promotion of phagocytosis	C3, C5
Enhancement of blood clotting	C6
Promotion of clot lysis	C3, C4
Inactivation of bacterial lipopolysaccharides from endotoxin	C5, C6

From Nisengard RJ. The role of immunology in periodontal disease. J Periodontol 48:505, 1977.

The classic pathway is activated by a reaction of antigen with IgG or IgM antibodies and by aggregated immunoglobulins. The sequence is C1, C4, C2, C3, C5, C6, C7, C8, and C9. C3 is cleaved by the complex C42 into C3b, which binds to the cell membrane, and C3a, which has biologic activity (see Fig. 8–1).

An alternative pathway for complement activation also exists. Aggregated antibodies of the IgG, IgA, and IgE classes, endotoxin, fungi and yeast cell walls, some viruses, parasites, and other substances can initiate the complement sequence by direct activation of the third component of complement (C3) without triggering the beginning of the cascade starting with C1. The alternative pathway begins with cleavage of C3 after the conversion of C3 proactivator. The sequence after C3 activation is identical to that of the classic pathway: C5, C6, C7, C8, C9.

Bacterial antigens such as endotoxins and polysaccharides such as dextran are also activators of the alternative pathway.[29] Dental plaque and pure cultures of bacteria can also activate complement by the alternative pathway in the absence of antibody.[29] On activation of complement by endotoxin, biologically active fragmentation products are released. Complement components that are present in the gingival sulcular fluid have been shown to decrease and therefore are assumed to be activated by some plaque bacteria and bacterial proteases.[37,38] Complement activation by these various pathways could result in mechanisms that destroy the periodontal tissues.[35]

Although most attention has focused on cell lysis as a result of complement activation, the main physiologic effects are the cellular and tissue changes associated with inflammation. When C3 and C5 components are activated by C3a and C5a, they cause degranulation of mast cells along with the liberation of histamine, leading to a marked increase in capillary permeability. This effect can be specifically blocked by antihistamine drugs.

Chemotaxis of PMNs is brought about by the activation of C5 to the C5a component of the complement system.[40] There is some speculation that the C3a component is also involved in this activity. Chemotaxis is neither stimulated by histamine nor blocked by antihistamine drugs and therefore does not appear to be related to the effect of C3 and C5 on histamine release.

In addition to complement chemotactic factors, certain species of bacteria produce peptides of low molecular weight that are also directly chemotactic and do not require complement.[34] These products could contribute to the accumulation of inflammatory cells in the periodontal lesion.

An important effect of complement occurs when antibodies react with invading gram-negative bacteria, leading to complement activation. These bacteria can be lysed by the same complement reaction sequence as occurs in the lysis of red blood cells. It appears that gram-positive bacteria are not susceptible to this lytic action of complement but are nonetheless effective because they are phagocytosed more rapidly after complement activation.

IMMUNE MECHANISMS

Immune mechanisms are usually protective responses by the host to the presence of foreign substances such as bacteria and viruses. They may at the same time cause local tissue destruction by triggering several types of overreaction or hypersensitivity. Tissue damage (immunopathologic change) may occur in a sensitized host with subsequent exposure to the sensitizing antigen. Four types of hypersensitivity reactions have been described:[8] I, II, III, and IV (Fig. 8–2). Type I, II, and III reactions are humoral and are termed *immediate reactions* because they occur in minutes to hours. Type IV reactions are cellular or cell mediated and are termed *delayed reactions* because they occur within days.

Three of these hypersensitivity reactions are of potential importance in periodontal disease.[36] They are anaphylaxis, or immediate hypersensitivity (type I), cytotoxic reactions (type II), and immune complex, or Arthus, reactions (type III). In addition, reactions to transfused blood are involved in immediate hypersensitivity reactions.

Anaphylaxis (Type I)

Two variations in anaphylactic hypersensitivity occur, depending on the route of administration of the antigen. If the antigen is injected locally into the skin, the reaction is called *cutaneous anaphylaxis*. If the antigen is injected intravenously, it is called *systemic* or *generalized anaphy-*

laxis. The basic mechanisms in both types of immediate hypersensitivity are the same.[4]

Although both IgE and IgG antibodies are involved in anaphylaxis, only IgE plays a direct role in its pathogenesis through its ability to sensitize the skin. This sensitizing capability is referred to as *reaginic* and the IgE antibody as *reagin.* IgG antibody combines with antigen in the circulation before it can bind to IgE in mast cells or basophils and prevents sensitization. These IgG antibodies are referred to as *blocking antibodies.* Several major features distinguish these blocking antibodies from reaginic or sensitizing antibodies.

IgE antibodies involved in anaphylactic reactions attach strongly at the Fc portion of the antibody to receptors found on mast cells and basophilic leukocytes, primarily in the skin and other connective tissues such as the gingiva. Experimentally, this binding lasts for several days. These sensitizing IgE antibodies are called *homocytotropic antibodies* because they normally bind in vivo to specific host cells, in this case both mast cells and basophilic leukocytes. In contrast, IgG-blocking antibodies bind only transiently to mast cells of other phylogenetically distinct species and are termed *heterocytotropic antibodies.* Experimentally, this binding usually lasts for only a few hours. An important component in anaphylactic hypersensitivity is that IgE antibodies normally do not fix (activate) complement.

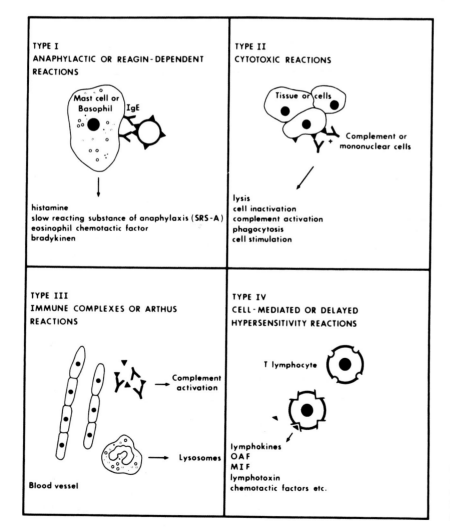

FIGURE 8–2. Immunologic mechanisms of tissue damage. The four types of hypersensitivity reactions described by Gell and Coombs and depicted by Nisengard. (From Nisengard RJ. The role of immunology in periodontal disease. J Periodontol *48*:505, 1977.)

Because plasma cells are known to produce immunoglobulins, the finding of IgE-containing cells in periodontal, bronchial, and other tissues is thought to represent localized synthesis of IgE antibodies.[28] These IgE-containing cells are found primarily in the respiratory and gastrointestinal mucosa and in regional lymph nodes. It has been suggested that IgE formed locally in tissue may then participate in local disease processes.

Mechanisms of Anaphylactic Hypersensitivity. Anaphylaxis occurs when two IgE antibodies that are fixed to a mast cell or basophil react with the sensitizing antigen through the Fab portion of the antibodies (Fig. 8–2). This antibody–antigen reaction causes the release of pharmacologically active substances from the sensitized cells (Table 8–4). These substances cause the response and have the potential to induce tissue damage in periodontal disease.[28]

Of the several active pharmacologic substances released during anaphylaxis, histamine pre-exists in the cells and is promptly released by antibody–antigen complexes. Other pharmacologically active substances, such as the kinins and SRS-A, are produced only *after* the antigen–antibody complexes are formed. An α_2-macroglobulin that blocks the normally found inhibitor for collagenase is also released from challenged sensitized cells, as are prostaglandins and an eosinophil chemotactic factor.

Histamine has been the most extensively studied chemical mediator of immediate hypersensitivity. As mentioned in preceding discussion, it is widely found in mammalian tissues. Mast cells, platelets, and basophilic leukocytes contain this substance. Histamine levels in chronically inflamed gingiva are significantly higher than those in normal gingiva. Some pharmacologic actions of histamine include increased capillary permeability, smooth muscle contraction, stimulation of the exocrine glands, and increased venule dilation and permeability. The biologic effects of histamine can be blocked with antihistamine drugs, but no apparent change in the course of periodontal disease has been demonstrated with these drugs.

Slow-reacting substances of anaphylaxis are acidic lipids that cause a sustained slow contraction of guinea pig ileum. This contraction is not inhibited by antihistamines and occurs even when histamine has been added to the point at which it can no longer cause ileum contraction. In addition to causing contraction of smooth muscle, SRS-A has some permeability-enhancing activity.

Bradykinin, a peptide formed by the enzymatic action of kallikrein on an α_2-globulin of plasma, has a number of pharmacologic activities and is considered a major pharmacologic mediator of anaphylactic hypersensitivity. These biologic activities include smooth muscle contraction, vasodilation, increased capillary permeability, migration of leukocytes, and the stimulation of pain fibers. The action of bradykinin is not inhibited by antihistamine drugs.

Cytotoxic Reactions (Type II)

In cytotoxic (type II) reactions (see Fig. 8–2), antibodies react directly with antigens tightly bound to cells. These antigens may be natural surface components of the cell, such as the cell membrane polysaccharide antigens of red blood cells. A cytotoxic reaction involving these cells may result in hemolysis. Cytotoxic antibodies may also react with antigens associated with tissue cells. These cell-associated antigens include normal cell surface antigens or those derived from bacteria, drugs, or altered tissue components.

Cytotoxic antibodies are of the IgG or the IgM class. These antibodies have the ability to fix complement, although complement fixation is not required for all types of cytotoxic antibody reactions. In addition to inducing cell lysis, cytotoxic antibodies may cause tissue damage by increasing the synthesis and release of lysosomal enzymes by cells (PMNs) coated with antigen. The tissues in the vicinity of these enzymes may then be damaged. Hemolytic transfusion reactions, hemolytic disease of the newborn, and autoallergic hemolytic anemia are examples of cytotoxic reactions induced by these antibody–antigen reactions.[4] Cytotoxic reactions are seen in autoimmune disease in which antibodies react with a patient's own tissue components. This occurs, for example, in pemphigus, in which antibodies react with cell membranes, and in pemphigoid, in which antibodies react with the epithelial basement membrane.[28] To date no evidence suggests an important role for cytotoxic reactions in gingivitis and periodontitis.

Immune Complex (Arthus) Reactions (Type III)

When high levels of antigen to which the host has been sensitized are present and persist without being eliminated, antigen–antibody (IgG and IgM) complexes precipitate in and around small blood vessels and, with subsequent complement activation, cause tissue damage at the site of the local reaction[5,30] (see Fig. 8–2). Inflammation, hemorrhage, and necrosis may occur. Tissue damage appears to be due to the release of lysosomal enzymes from PMNs, mast cell activation, platelet agglutination, microthrombi formation, and neutrophil chemotaxis. This reaction is referred to as an *immune complex,* or *Arthus, reaction* and is usually mediated by IgM or IgG antibodies. These antibodies have the ability to fix complement, which is partially responsible for

---

Table 8–4. PHARMACOLOGICALLY ACTIVE MEDIATORS RELEASED BY HUMAN MAST CELLS

Mediator	Pharmacologic Action
Histamine	Increased capillary permeability
	Smooth muscle contraction
	Stimulation of exocrine glands
	Dilation and increased venule permeability
	Skin response: wheal and erythema
	Bone resorption?
SRS-A	Smooth muscle contraction
	Increased vascular permeability
Bradykinin	Smooth muscle contraction
	Vasodilation
	Increased capillary permeability
	Migration of leukocytes
	Stimulation of pain fibers
α_2-Macroglobulin	Collagenase activation

Adapted from Nisengard RJ. Immediate hypersensitivity and periodontal disease. J Periodontol 45:345, 1972.

the chemotactic attraction of the PMNs crucial to the Arthus reaction (see Fig. 8–1).

Cell-Mediated Immunity or Delayed Hypersensitivity (Type IV)

The phenomenon of delayed hypersensitivity belongs to the class of immune responses known as *cell-mediated immunity*. These reactions are referred to as *type IV reactions* (Fig. 8–3).

Cellular immunity does not involve circulating antibodies but is based on the interaction of antigens with the surface of T lymphocytes. There are actually two populations of lymphocytes (Fig. 8–3). Lymphocytes that can develop into plasma cells that produce antibodies are designated as B cells because they were found to proliferate in the bursa of Fabricius in birds and the bone marrow of mammals. These cells circulate from the blood or the thoracic duct to the lymphatic tissues, the cortical germinal centers of lymph nodes, and the red pulp of the spleen, where they differentiate into plasma cells.[19] These differentiated cells can then produce antibodies. B lymphocytes have been shown to produce biologically active lymphokines[20,30] (see following discussion).

In contrast, the T cells migrate from the bone marrow to the thymus, where they divide and become immunocompetent (Fig. 8–3). From the thymus they migrate to the pericortical areas of lymph nodes and the white pulp of the spleen.[19] The relationship between T and B lymphocytes and cellular and humoral immunity is complex, with frequent interactions between B and T cells.

T lymphocytes or B lymphocytes sensitized to an immunizing antigen can be stimulated to undergo blastogenesis or transformation in vitro and presumably in vivo. This consists of morphologic enlargement and synthesis of proteins, RNA, and DNA and results, ultimately, in mitotic division. This increases the number of immunocompetent lymphoid cells that are specific for a particular antigen. Some oral bacteria, including *Actinomyces* and some strains of *Streptococcus,* produce extracellular substances that inhibit blast transformation of normal peripheral lymphocytes.[18] Similar substances from some bacteria also inhibit fibroblast growth.

CYTOKINES

The complex interactions among lymphocytes, inflammatory cells, and other cellular elements in connective tissue are mediated by a series of low-molecular-weight proteins called *cytokines*. These were originally called *lymphokines* before their production by other cells was recognized.

Cytokines assist in the regulation and development of immune effector cells, cell-to-cell communication, and direct effector functions. Some cytokines exhibit autocrine function, binding to the cell that produced them. Others are panacrine, binding to nearby cells, and still others are endocrine, binding to distant cells. Cytokines may be pleiotrophic, eliciting different biologic activities from different cells. In addition, different cytokines may exhibit similar responses.[19,25]

The accumulation of plasma cells and lymphocytes in the periodontal tissues suggests that cytokines participate in periodontal pathologic changes. Because the number of currently identified cytokines is extensive, only the major ones will be discussed. Originally cytokines were named for their biologic activity. These included macrophage activation factor (MAF), macrophage migration inhibition factor (MIF), leukocyte-derived chemotactic factor (CTX), lymphotoxin (LT), and osteoclast-activating factor (OAF).[26]

More recently the majority of cytokines have been renamed as *interleukins,* referring to their role in communication between leukocytes. Presently 10 interleukins have been identified and are numbered 1 to 10. Other cytokines are still named for their biologic activity (e.g., tumor necrosis factor, transforming growth factor, and interferon).[19]

Classification

IL-1. IL-1 (α and β) is a pleiotrophic cytokine with a variety of activities. It includes OAF[9,25,34] because of its stimulation of osteoclasts and lymphocyte-activating factor (LAF) because of its ability to stimulate proliferation of phytohemagglutination-treated T cells. It is known to also play a role in T_H-cell activation, promotion of B-cell maturation, chemotaxis of neutrophils and macrophages, enhancement of NK cell activity, and other responses. It is secreted by monocytes, macrophages, B cells, fibroblasts, neutrophils, epithelial cells, and many other stimulated cell types. This stimulation results from phagocytosis, complement components (C3a and C5a), and other substances. IL-1 occurs in gingival tissues and crevicular fluid and decreases after periodontal treatment.[6,22,24] It also increases fibroblast procollagen, prostaglandin E_2 (PGE_2), and bone resorption activity.[10]

IL-2. IL-2 (α and β) was originally called *T-cell growth factor* because of its effect on mitogen or antigen-activating

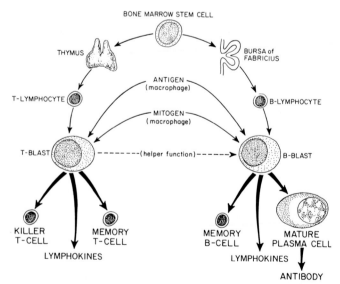

FIGURE 8–3. Schematic diagram illustrating the derivation and response of B and T lymphocytes. Antigen- and mitogen-induced responses result from the presence of macrophages. (From Page R. Pathogenic mechanisms. In Schluger S, Yuodelis RA, Page RC. Periodontal Disease. Philadelphia, Lea & Febiger, 1977.)

T cells (T_H and T_C cells) and is known to play a general role in immune responses.[41] IL-2 also stimulates macrophage functional activity, modulates NK function, and induces NK proliferation.[14,33] It is secreted by T_H cells and NK cells and is increased in periodontal tissues in periodontitis.[24]

IL-3. IL-3 supports the growth and differentiation of hematopoietic cells, including stimulation of mast cell growth and histamine secretion. It is secreted by activated T_H cells and NK cells.[19,33]

IL-4. IL-4 was originally called *T-cell–derived B-cell growth factor* (BCGF-1) because of its activation of B cells and may also be what was previously called *migration inhibition factor* (MIF). It is known to also play a role in the activation, proliferation, and differentiation of B cells; T-cell growth; macrophage function; and growth of mast cells.[19,32] IgE synthesis by B cells is also induced by IL-4. IL-4 is secreted by T_H cells. IL-4 increases in periodontal tissues in periodontitis.[24]

IL-5. IL-5 induces B-cell proliferation and enhances IgA production. Together with IL-4, it also promotes IgE production. It is secreted by T_H cells.

IL-6. IL-6 stimulates plasma cell production of immunoglobulins and, with IL-1, activates T_H production. It is secreted by T_H cells, macrophages, monocytes, fibroblasts, and endothelial cells. IL-6 increases in sites of gingival inflammation and plays a role in bone resorption.[1,22,34]

IL-7. IL-7 induces T-cell proliferation by expressing IL-2 and IL-2 receptors. It is secreted by bone marrow stromal cells.

IL-8. IL-8 is chemotactic for neutrophils and increases their adherence to endothelial cells. It is secreted by macrophages.

IL-9. IL-9, secreted by some T_H cells, induces proliferation of T_H cells in the absence of antigen or antigen-presenting cells and promotes growth of mast cells.

IL-10. IL-10, secreted by T_H cells, is suppressed by T_H cells, IFN-γ production of NK cells that are induced by IL-2. IL-10 inhibits the antigen-presenting capacity of monocytes.[21,27,33]

IFNs. IFNs (α, β, and γ) are a family of three glycoproteins produced by leukocytes, fibroblasts, and T lymphocytes, respectively. They provide antiviral activity, enhance macrophage activity (IFN-γ), T-cell activity, NK-cell activity.[10,33] IFN-γ also plays a role in bone resorption by inhibiting both the proliferation and differentiation of progenitors of osteoclasts.[26]

TNFs. TNF (α and β), produced by macrophages and T_H cells, respectively, cause the necrosis of certain tumors. TNF-α is produced by macrophages after stimulation by gram-negative bacterial components, including lipopolysaccharide (LPS)[30] TNF-β, previously known as *lymphotoxin* (LT), is primarily produced by T_H cells. TNF-α and -β play a role in the activation of osteoclasts and stimulate them to cause bone resorption. TNF-α also aids leukocytes in their ability to adhere to endothelial cells and increases their phagocytosis and chemotaxis. These effects, along with the effect on macrophages leading to macrophage-induced angiogenesis, may play a role in the vascular changes seen in periodontal disease.[30]

In vitro experiments have demonstrated that LT may be cytotoxic for cultures of human gingival fibroblasts.[34] A correlation exists between the degree of periodontal disease of the lymphocyte donor and the amount of LT elaborated by the cells in response to plaque antigens. Thus, there may be some in vivo correlation with the in vitro experiment results.

Cytotoxicity of tissue cells may also be affected by a direct lymphocyte interaction with target cells that contain a specific stimulating antigen on their surface.[4] Although antigen recognition by sensitized lymphocytes is generally quite specific, the cytotoxic effect of the lymphocyte–host cell interaction is generally nonspecific. These lymphocyte interactions suggest that the persistent deposition of plaque antigens into the gingival tissue could favor the generation of LT-producing cells and/or direct lymphocytotoxicity, resulting in the tissue damage seen in periodontal diseases.[28]

Lymphocytes sensitized to plaque antigens undergo morphologic and functional transformation in vitro, which results in a chronic infiltration with lymphocytes and macrophages and the formation of biologically active substances.

The *graft-versus-host reaction* is seen when the lymphocytes are transferred from an immunologically competent donor to an allogeneic immunologically incompetent recipient. These reactions have increasing clinical importance because of therapeutic attempts to transfer normal thymus or bone marrow cells to immunodeficient persons. These transplantation techniques are becoming increasingly common and have been used in patients with genetic defects and in patients with leukemia treated with cytotoxic drugs and whole-body irradiation.[4] Often such patients have concomitant periodontal manifestations of their primary systemic disease (see Chapter 10).

Assays

Originally cytokines were identified by their biologic activities, which led to some confusion because of the overlapping activities of some cytokines. Functional identification has been supplanted as a result of cytokine purification and cloning, which has allowed production of monoclonal antibodies to the cytokines used in specific radioimmunoassays, enzyme-linked immunosorbent assays, and enzyme-linked immunospot assays.[2]

REFERENCES

1. Bartoid PM, Haynes DR. Interleukin-6 production by human gingival fibroblasts. J Periodont Res *26:*339, 1991.
2. Beckman MP, Morrissey PJ. Assays for lymphokines, cytokines and their receptors. Curr Opin Immunol *3:*247, 1991.
3. Benditt EP, Lagunoff D. The mast cell: Its structure and function. Progr Allergy *8:*195, 1964.
4. Brostoff J, Scadding GK, Male D, Roitt IM. Clinical Immunology. Philadelphia, JB Lippincott, 1991.
5. Cochrane CG. Mechanisms involved in the deposition of immune complexes in tissues. J Exp Med *134:*75, 1971.
6. Charon JA, Luger TA, Mergenhagen S, Oppenhein JJ. Increased thymocyte activating factor in human gingival fluid during gingival inflammation. Infect Immun *38:*1190, 1982.
7. Erb P, Feldman M. Role of macrophages in in vitro induction of T-helper cells. Nature *254:*352, 1975.
8. Gell PGH, Coombs RRA, Lachman PJ. Clinical Aspects of Immunology. 3rd ed. Oxford, Blackwell Scientific, 1975.
9. Gemsa D, Steggemann L, Menzel J, et al. Release of cyclic AMP from macrophages by stimulation with prostaglandins. J Immunol *144:*1422, 1975.
10. Genco RJ. Host responses in periodontal tissues: Current concepts. J Periodontol *63:*338, 1992.

11. Genco RJ, Slots J. Host responses in periodontal disease. J Dent Res *63:*441, 1984.

12. Gibbons RJ, Van Houte J. Selective bacterial adherence to oral epithelial surfaces and its role as an ecological determinant. Infect Immun *3:*567, 1971.

13. Goldhaber P. Heparin enhancement of factors stimulating bone resorption in tissue culture. Science *147:*407, 1965.

14. Gordon S, Fraser I, Nath D, et al. Macrophages in tissues and in vitro. Curr Opin Immunol *4:*25, 1992.

15. Hawkins D. Neutrophilic leukocytes in immunologic reactions: Evidence for the selective release of lysosomal constituents. J Immunol *108:*310, 1972.

16. Higerd TB, Vesole DH, Goust J. Inhibitory effects of extracellular products from oral bacteria on human fibroblasts and stimulated lymphocytes. Infect Immun *21:*567, 1978.

17. Ishikawa I, Cimasoni G, Ahmad-Zadeh C. Possible role of lysosomal enzymes in the pathogenesis of periodontitis. A study on cathepsin D in human gingival fluid. Arch Oral Biol *17:*111, 1972.

18. Jayawardine A, Goldner M. Reaginlike activity of serum in human periodontal disease. Infect Immun *15:*665, 1977.

19. Kuby J. Immunology. New York, WH Freeman, 1992.

20. Mackler BF, Altman LC, Wahl S, et al. Blastogenesis and lymphokine synthesis by T and B lymphocytes from patients with periodontal disease. Infect Immun *10:*844, 1974.

21. Malefyt R, Yssel H, Roncarola MG, Spits H, Vries J. Interleukin-10. Curr Opin Immunol *4:*314, 1992.

22. Malberg K, Mölle A, Streuer D, Gängler P. Determination of lymphocyte populations and subpopulations extracted from chronically inflamed periodontal tissues. J Clin Periodontol *19:*155, 1992.

23. Massada MP, Persson P, Kenney JS, et al. Measurement on interleukin-1α and 1β in gingival crevicular fluid. Implications for pathogenesis of periodontal disease. J Periodont Res *25:*156, 1990.

24. McFarlane CG, Meikle MC. Interleukin-2, interleukin-2 receptor and interleukin-4 levels are elevated in the sera of patients with periodontal disease. J Periodont Res *26:*402, 1991.

25. Morley H. Prostaglandins and lymphokines in arthritis. Prostaglandins *8:*315, 1974.

26. Mundy GR. Inflammatory mediators and the destruction of bone. J Periodont Res *26:*213, 1991.

27. Myers CD. Role of B cell antigen processing and presentation in the humoral immune response. FASEB J *5:*2547, 1991.

28. Nisengard RJ. The role of immunology in periodontal disease. J Periodontol *48:*505, 1977.

29. Okuda K, Takazoe I. Activation of complement by dental plaque. J Periodont Res *15:*232, 1980.

30. Page RC. The role of inflammatory mediators in the pathogenesis of periodontal disease. J Periodont Res *26:*230, 1991.

31. Parakkal PF. Involvement of macrophages in collagen resorption. J Cell Biol *41:*345, 1969.

32. Paulnock DM. Macrophage activation by T cells. Curr Opin Immunol *4:*344, 1992.

33. Perussia B. Lymphokine-activated killer cells, natural killer cells and cytokines. Curr Opin Immunol *3:*49, 1991.

34. Ranney RR. Immunologic mechanisms of pathogenesis in periodontal diseases: An assessment. J Periodont Res *26:*243, 1991.

35. Raisz LG, Sandberg AL, Goodson JM, et al. Complement-dependent stimulation of prostaglandin synthesis and bone resorption. Science *185:*789, 1974.

36. Rizzo AA, Mergenhagen SE. Studies on the significance of local hypersensitivity in periodontal disease. Periodontics *3:*271, 1965.

37. Schenkein HA, Genco RJ. Gingival fluid and serum in periodontal diseases. I. Quantitative study of immunoglobulins, complement components and other plasma proteins. J Periodontol *48:*772, 1977.

38. Shillitoe EJ, Lehner T. Immunoglobulins and complement in crevicular fluid, serum and saliva in man. Arch Oral Biol *17:*241, 1972.

39. Snyderman R. Role for endotoxin and complement in periodontal tissue destruction. J Dent Res *51*(suppl 2):356, 1972.

40. Snyderman R, Shin HS, Hausmann MH. A chemotactic factor from mononuclear phagocytes. Proc Soc Exp Biol Med *138:*378, 1971.

41. Swain S. Lymphokines and the immune response: The central role of Interleukin-2. Curr Opin Immunol *3:*304, 1991.

42. Taichman NS, Freedman HL, Uriuhara T. Inflammation and tissue injury. I. The response to intradermal injections of human dentogingival plaque in normal and leukopenic rabbits. Arch Oral Biol *11:*1385, 1966.

43. Taichman NS, Pruzanski W, Ranadive NS. Release of intracellular constituents from rabbit polymorphonuclear leukocytes exposed to soluble and insoluble immune complexes. Int Arch Allergy Appl Immunol *43:*182, 1972.

44. Taylor AC. Collagenolysis in cultured tissue. II. Role of mast cells. J Dent Res *50:*1301, 1971.

45. Terner C. Arthus reaction in the oral cavity of laboratory animals. Periodontics *3:*18, 1965.

9

Host–Bacteria Interactions in Periodontal Diseases

MICHAEL G. NEWMAN, MARIANO SANZ,
RUSSELL C. NISENGARD, and SUSAN KINDER HAAKE

Gingivitis and periodontitis as well as other less common periodontal diseases are chronic bacterial infections. As in other infections, the host–bacteria interactions determine the nature and extent of the resulting disease. *Pathogenic microorganisms may influence the course of the disease process by producing tissue-toxic substances, by directly invading host tissues, and by stimulating a host response.* Bacterial products and bacterial invasion of the tissues are generally harmful to the host, but the host response may be protective or destructive. The varying balance between harmful and beneficial interactions of the pathogenic bacteria and the host accounts for the wide variety of patterns of tissue changes observed in patients.[21]

PERIODONTAL DISEASE AS AN INFECTION

Gingivitis and periodontitis are caused by bacteria that colonize the gingival crevice and attach to tooth surfaces. The pathogenic potential of bacteria within the plaque varies from individual to individual and from gingival site to gingival site. Small amounts of plaque in a healthy person can be tolerated without causing gingival or periodontal disease, probably because of the control exerted by host defense mechanisms. When specific bacteria within the plaque increase to significant numbers and produce virulence factors beyond the individual patient's control threshold, the balance shifts from health to disease. Disease also occurs as a result of a reduction in the host defensive capacity.

The composition of bacterial plaque associated with gingival health differs from that of plaque associated with different periodontal diseases.[45] *In general, gram-negative, facultative, capnophilic or anaerobic microorganisms are the principal bacteria associated with periodontal diseases. Porphyromonas gingivalis, Prevotella intermedia, Actinobacillus actinomycetemcomitans, Fusobacterium nucleatum, Campylobacter rectus, Treponema denticola,* and *Eikenella* species are some of the most common bacteria associated with disease, because of their pathogenic capabilities and their increased numbers in disease.[36,42] Other bacteria found in lower numbers may also be important but have not been investigated to the same extent.

The etiologic relationship of bacteria to different periodontal diseases is based on the following criteria, as proposed by Socransky and colleagues:[45]

1. An organism that is important in a disease process should be commonly found in high numbers at sites of disease and absent or infrequently found at healthy sites.
2. Elimination or suppression of the organism by treatment should have a positive influence.
3. Although many of the host responses are influenced by the immunogenicity of the organism, there should usually be an elevated immune response to the organism. This may be an elevated antibody response or a cellular response.
4. Experimental implantation of the organism into the gingival crevice of an animal should lead to development of at least some of the characteristics of naturally occurring disease (e.g., inflammation, connective tissue destruction, and bone loss).
5. The putative pathogen should possess pathogenic or virulent potential.[45]

MICROBIOLOGY OF PERIODONTAL DISEASE: GENERAL ASPECTS

Often used synonymously with periodontitis, the term *periodontal disease* is currently considered to describe a group of diseases or infections. Each disease is associated with different groups of microorganisms, resulting in clinical signs and symptoms that can be similar or unique.

The mechanisms by which subgingival bacteria contribute to the pathogenesis of periodontal disease are varied. The periodontopathogens possess numerous factors that permit them to damage the periodontium directly or to trigger a pathologic host response indirectly. Table 9–1 lists many of the possible pathogenic mechanisms.

Bacterial Invasion. In early studies of periodontitis, bacteria identified microscopically in gingival tissue were considered artifacts. Bacteria were not thought to invade the periodontium actively but to infiltrate passively after routine, mild gingival trauma such as toothbrushing, chewing hard substances, and subgingival scaling.

In 1965 Listgarten[16] demonstrated with an electron microscope the invasive nature of spirochetes in acute necrotizing ulcerative gingivitis (ANUG). In the 1980s sophisticated techniques, including immunofluorescence and anaerobic culture, as well as electron microscopy, have led to a reconsideration of the role of bacterial invasion of the gingival tissues in periodontal disease.

Bacteria were first identified by transmission electron microscopy within the gingival tissues and close to resorbing bone surfaces in many cases of advanced human periodontitis.[10] Since that finding, bacteria–leukocyte interactions on the surface of pocket epithelium and bacteria between junctional epithelial cells and the epithelium lining the lateral wall of pockets, as well as bacteria within the connective tissue, have been identified.[35] Along with bacterial invasion, alteration in the basement membrane of the pocket epithelium can be observed. In some studies a discontinuous absence of basement membrane antigen can be seen, which suggests basement membrane disruption possibly associated with bacterial invasion.

In localized juvenile periodontitis (LJP), *A. actinomycetemcomitans* has been identified within the gingival connective tissue. The presence of this organism within the tissues appears to make the disease more resistant to treatment and may necessitate the use of antibiotics or other chemotherapeutic agents in refractory LJP cases. Bacterial invasion is discussed in Chapters 6 and 22.

Exotoxins. The production of exotoxins by some plaque microorganisms has been described. *A. actinomycetemcomitans* produces an exotoxin referred to as *leukotoxin* because of its toxic effect on human polymorphonuclear neutrophils (PMNs). The production of leukotoxin may enable *A. actinomycetemcomitans* to evade the host defense of phagocytosis and may be an important property in the virulence of this microorganism.[43]

Cell Constituents. Cell constituents of both gram-positive and gram-negative bacteria may also play a role in periodontal disease. These include endotoxins, bacterial surface components, and capsular components.

The preponderance of gram-negative bacteria within pockets in periodontal disease leads to high concentrations of endotoxin, a constituent of the cell walls of gram-negative bacteria. Endotoxin, or lipo-oligosaccharide (LOS) (previously termed *lipopolysaccharide* [LPS]), is found in the outer membrane of all gram-negative bacteria. LOS is released when the cell dies and disintegrates and may also be released by the bacteria in the form of vesicles, or blebs of membrane derived from viable cells. Endotoxins are highly toxic substances, affecting tissues directly and through activation of host responses.[43] Important in their role in periodontal disease is their ability to (1) produce leukopenia; (2) activate factor XII (or Hageman's factor), which affects the clotting system, leading to intravascular coagulation; (3) activate the complement (C) system by the alternative pathway, which begins with C3 activation and bypasses C1, C4, and C2; (4) lead to a localized Shwartzman phenomenon, with tissue necrosis occurring after two or more exposures to endotoxin; (5) have cytotoxic effects on cells such as fibroblasts; and (6) induce bone resorption in organ culture. Endotoxins penetrate gingival epithelium.

Both gram-positive and gram-negative subgingival bacteria produce a variety of toxic end products that are also capable of tissue destruction. These include fatty and organic acids such as butyric and propionic acids, amines, volatile sulfur compounds, indole, ammonia, and glycans. Peptidoglycan, a cell wall component found in both gram-positive and gram-negative species, may affect a variety of host responses, including complement activation, immunosuppressive activity, stimulation of the reticuloendothelial system, and immunopotentiating properties. Peptidoglycan also appears capable of stimulating bone resorption and stimulating macrophages to produce prostaglandin and collagenases.[54]

Capsular material and slime constituents are found on the outermost surface of many bacterial cells and may play a role in tissue destruction as well as bacterial evasion of host defense mechanisms.[12]

Enzymes. The bacteria found in dental plaque produce a variety of enzymes that undoubtedly contribute to the production of periodontal diseases. Bacterial enzymes that are likely to contribute to the disease process include collagenases, hyaluronidase, gelatinase, aminopeptidases, phospholipases, and alkaline and acid phosphatases.

A central characteristic of periodontal destruction is the degradation of collagen. The primary source of collagenase in the periodontal pocket is probably host tissue cells, but bacterial collagenases may also contribute to collagen degradation. *P. gingivalis* and some strains of *A. actinomycetemcomitans* have been found to produce collagenases.

Bacterial hyaluronidase is capable of altering gingival permeability by allowing apical proliferation of the junctional epithelium along the root surfaces. Hyaluronidase is found in higher concentrations in periodontal pockets than in normal sulci, and a greater number of bacterial isolates that produce hyaluronidase are found in periodontal pockets. In addition, experimental studies have demonstrated that topical application of hyaluronidase on gingival epithelium leads to widening of the intercellular spaces and in-

Table 9–1. PATHOGENIC BACTERIAL MECHANISMS IN PERIODONTAL DISEASE

1. Invasion
2. Production of exotoxins
3. Role of cell constituents (endotoxins, surface components, capsular components, etc.)
4. Production of enzymes
5. Evasion of immunologic host responses

Table 9-2. BACTERIAL FACTORS IMPORTANT IN EVASION OF HOST DEFENSES

Inhibition of PMNs
    Leukotoxin
    Chemotaxis inhibitors
    Decreased phagocytosis and intracellular killing
      Resistance to C-mediated killing
Lymphocyte alterations
Endotoxicity
IgA, IgG proteases
Fibrinolysin
Superoxide dismutase
Catalase

creased permeability. Injection of hyaluronidase into the gingiva causes disruption of gingival connective tissue and apical migration of the gingival epithelium along the cementum, the initial phases of pocket formation.

Evasion of Host Responses. Bacterial factors also help in evasion of host defenses (Table 9-2).[40,43] These factors influence both cellular and humoral immune responses. Polymorphonuclear leukocytes, for example, are influenced by leukotoxins, chemotactic substances, and inhibitors. Immunoglobulins are inactivated or destroyed by proteases.[13,46] The combination of direct bacterial effects on the periodontal tissues and indirect bacterial effects achieved by influencing host defenses determines the response of the periodontium to the periodontopathogens.

IMMUNOLOGY OF PERIODONTAL DISEASE: GENERAL ASPECTS

Host responses play an important role in the pathogenesis of many types of periodontal diseases (Table 9-3) by contributing to the disease process or by modulating the effects of the bacteria.[11,26] Immune responses may be both beneficial (protective) and detrimental (destructive). Several components of the immune system are active in periodontal disease (Table 9-4). The neutrophils, lymphocytes, plasma cells, and macrophages vary in numbers, depending on the disease status of the tissues. Localized and systemic antibodies to the oral bacteria and complement also are of significance.[48] These host variables may influence bacterial colonization, bacterial invasion, tissue destruction, and healing and fibrosis[11] (Table 9-5).

Bacterial Colonization. In periodontal diseases, the major source for immunoglobulins (Ig) and complement is gingival or crevicular fluid, which contains systemically and locally produced antibodies. These antibodies potentially modulate the types and numbers of microorganisms through inhibition of colonization and/or lysis. However, in bacteria-associated periodontal disease, there is an "explosion" in the numbers of subgingival bacteria when compared with the numbers of such bacteria in gingivally healthy patients. This heavy antigen load in an "external" environment may overwhelm the immune system, distorting or obviating any positive protective effects.

Bacterial Invasion. In comparison with the large numbers of bacteria within the gingival crevice or pocket, there are relatively few bacteria beneath the basal lamina of the epithelium. This probably results from the physical barrier provided by the junctional epithelium and from the host protective responses. The gingival tissues are bathed with antibodies to the oral bacteria and complement, which could lead to bacterial lysis. In addition, chemotactic factors could lead to PMN and monocyte infiltration, with bacterial phagocytosis and lysis.

The importance of PMNs and macrophages as phagocytes in defense against periodontopathic microorganisms has become evident. Even in clinically normal gingiva, small numbers of neutrophils are seen in the gingival

Table 9-3. SIGNIFICANT IMMUNE FINDINGS IN PERIODONTAL DISEASES

Disease	Immune Response
ANUG	PMN chemotactic defect Elevated antibody titers to *P. intermedia* and intermediate-sized spirochetes
Pregnancy gingivitis	No significant findings reported
Adult periodontitis	Elevated antibody titer to *P. gingivalis* and other periodontopathogens Occurrence of immune complexes in tissues Immediate hypersensitivity to gingival bacteria Cell-mediated immunity to gingival bacteria
Juvenile periodontitis LJP	PMN chemotactic defect and depressed phagocytosis Elevated antibody levels to *A. actinomycetemcomitans*
GJP	PMN chemotactic defect and depressed phagocytosis Elevated antibody levels to *P. gingivalis*
Prepubertal	PMN and monocyte chemotactic defects
Rapidly progressing periodontitis	Suppressed or enhanced PMN or monocyte chemotaxis Elevated antibody levels to several gram-negative bacteria
Refractory periodontitis	Reduced PMN chemotaxis
Desquamative gingivitis	Diagnostic or characteristic immunopathologic changes in two thirds of cases Autoimmune cause in cases resulting from pemphigus and pemphigoid

Table 9–4. COMPONENTS OF THE IMMUNE SYSTEM AFFECTING PERIODONTAL DISEASE

System	Function
Secretory immune system	Decreases bacterial colonization on surfaces exposed to saliva
Neutrophil, antibody, complement	Bactericidal
Lymphocyte, macrophage, lymphokine	Tissue destruction
Immunoregulatory system	Controls immune responses to bacteria

Data from Genco RJ, Slots J. Host responses in periodontal disease. J Dent Res 63:441, 1984.

Table 9–6. NEUTROPHIL-RELATED PERIODONTAL DISEASE

Neutrophil Disorders Associated With Periodontal Disease

Diabetes mellitus
Papillon-Lefèvre syndrome
Down syndrome
Chédiak-Higashi syndrome
Drug-induced agranulocytosis
Cyclic neutropenia

Periodontal Disease With Neutrophil Disorders

Acute necrotizing ulcerative gingivitis
Localized juvenile periodontitis
Prepubertal periodontitis
Rapidly progressing periodontitis
Refractory periodontitis

crevice. With gingival inflammation, increasing numbers of neutrophils infiltrate within and directly below the dentogingival region. Phagocytes are usually chemotactically attracted to invading bacteria and attach to the bacteria via C3b and other receptors.[37] After phagocytosis, the bacteria are usually lysed. Functional neutrophil or macrophage defects in chemotaxis predispose to periodontal disease. Patients with systemic diseases entailing neutrophil disorders frequently have severe periodontitis, and several periodontal diseases have characteristic chemotactic defects[11] (Table 9–6).

Tissue Destruction. Several bacterial mechanisms could contribute to the pathogenesis of periodontal disease. These include anaphylactic (or reagin-dependent) reactions, cytotoxic reactions, immune complex (or Arthus) reactions, and cell-mediated (or delayed hypersensitivity) reactions (see Chapter 8).

In *anaphylactic reactions,* immunoglobulin E (IgE) produced by plasma cells fixes to or sensitizes mast cells and basophilic leukocytes. Subsequent antigenic exposure leads to antigen–antibody complexes on the cell surface, with the degranulation of mast cells and basophils and the release of mediators, including histamine.

Cytotoxic reactions occur when immunoglobulin G (IgG)

Table 9–5. INFLUENCE OF HOST RESPONSES ON PERIODONTAL DISEASE

Aspect of Disease	Host Factors
Bacterial colonization	Subgingivally, antibody–complement in crevicular fluid inhibits adherence and coaggregation of bacteria and potentially reduces their numbers by lysis
Bacterial invasion	Antibody–complement–mediated lysis reduces bacterial counts
	Neutrophils as a consequence of chemotaxis, phagocytosis, and lysis reduce bacterial counts
Tissue destruction	Antibody-mediated hypersensitivity
	Cell-mediated immune responses
	Activation of tissue factors such as collagenase
Healing and fibrosis	Lymphocytes and macrophage-produced chemotactic factors for fibroblasts; fibroblast-activating factors

and M (IgM) antibodies react with cell or tissue antigens. Consequent complement activation further contributes to the pathogenesis.[39]

In *immune complex reactions,* microprecipitates of antigen with IgG and IgM antibodies occur in tissues in and around blood vessels.[27] Microcomplexes that form in moderate antigen excess activate the complement system, leading to hormonal, vascular, and cytotoxic effects. Associated with the reaction is a leukocytic infiltrate that releases lysozymes, causing further tissue damage.

Cell-mediated reactions occur when sensitized T lymphocytes react with the sensitizing antigen, leading to the lymphocytic release of lymphokines such as osteoclast-activating factor (OAF).[28] Although host mechanisms leading to tissue destruction could be activated in any of the bacteria-associated periodontal diseases, most research has focused on gingivitis and periodontitis.

Healing and Fibrosis. Macrophages influence fibroblast activity. They play a role in healing through their release of fibronectin, which is chemotactic for fibroblasts and other factors that influence fibroblast function and lead to fibroblast activation.[54] Lymphocytes also release lymphokines capable of activating and recruiting fibroblasts.

Immunoregulation appears to play a role in periodontal disease.[39] One important immune mediator is interleukin-1 (IL-1), a cytokine produced by macrophages, B cells, and squamous epithelial cells. IL-1 release is stimulated from these cells by LOSs of periodontopathogens such as *P. gingivalis* and *C. rectus.* IL-1 influences thymocytes, T cells, B cells, and fibroblasts, as well as other cells, and induces the proliferation of thymocytes, T cells, B cells, and fibroblasts. It also enhances the production of lymphokines, including T-cell growth factor (IL-2) and OAF.[38] Furthermore, IL-1 enhances antibody production by B cells and production of collagenase and prostaglandin by fibroblasts. IL-1 is found in greater amounts in gingival fluid at inflamed sites, suggesting that it may play a role in periodontal disease by influencing the host immunologic and inflammatory responses to bacterial antigens and mitogens.

Lymphocytes from chronically inflamed gingival tissues have also been shown to be capable of producing IL-2. However, no relationship has been found between IL-2 and the severity of periodontal disease.

The role of bacteria in modulating the immune response as well as connective tissue function has been demonstrated. Some periodontopathogens chemotactically attract leukocytes, reduce chemotactic ability, elaborate leukotoxins, resist phagocytosis, inhibit their own phagocytic killing, and interfere with fibroblast proliferation.[43] For example, LOSs from gram-negative bacteria activate the complement system by the classic and alternative pathways, inducing PMN chemotaxis. However, soluble bacterial products can also block receptors on leukocytes, thus reducing the chemotactic response. A distinguishing difference between pathogenic and less pathogenic strains of black-pigmented bacilli is that the pathogenic strains are more resistant to phagocytosis. Resistance to PMN killing appears to be due to capsular material, an unknown mechanism dependent on serum and on the ability to split PMN-derived hydrogen peroxide and superoxide dismutase.

The humoral response to subgingival bacteria can be nonspecifically altered by bacterial production of IgG, IgA, IgM, C3, and C5 proteases.[46] Enzymes to some or all of the humoral components are elaborated by black-pigmented bacilli and *Capnocytophaga*.[43] Black-pigmented bacilli completely degrade the immunoglobulins, whereas *Capnocytophaga* splits the immunoglobulin into Fab and Fc fragments, which may still have some biologic activity. This protease activity may inhibit the local host response and allow penetration and spread of bacteria within the tissues.

Subgingival bacteria also affect the humoral immune response by polyclonal B-cell activation.[3] Bacteria nonspecifically induce multiple clones of B lymphocytes to produce immunoglobulins so that B cells stimulated by one microorganism produce antibodies to other microorganisms. The immunoglobulin production by B cells is under the regulatory control of T cells. Extracts of *P. gingivalis, P. intermedia, Prevotella melaninogenica, F. nucleatum, A. actinomycetemcomitans, Actinomyces viscosus, Actinomyces naeslundii,* and *Capnocytophaga ochracea* stimulate polyclonal antibody responses and OAF in cultures of normal human peripheral blood lymphocytes. These bacterial activators may play a role in the pathogenesis of periodontal disease.

Bacterial factors affect lymphocytes and other cellular constituents via suppression, activation, and mitogenicity.[20] A factor from *A. actinomycetemcomitans* selectively activates human suppressor T cells.[43] Sonic extracts of *F. nucleatum* lead to immunosuppression either by altering helper T-cell activity or by directly influencing the effector or responding cell population. *F. nucleatum* also suppresses mitogen activation of peripheral leukocytes. Extracellular polysaccharide from *C. ochracea* exerts immunosuppressive activity through macrophages, possibly with the participation of suppressor T cells.[4]

MICROBIOLOGY AND IMMUNOLOGY IN GINGIVAL HEALTH

Microbiology. The gingival crevice is not sterile, but instead harbors a microbial flora in both health and disease. In healthy sulci from young adults, gram-positive cocci are the major morphotype and compose almost two thirds of the total flora. Filamentous forms, small spirochetes,

fusiforms, and motile rods are also identified.[23] In general, gram-negative species and motile forms are considerably less frequent and occur in smaller numbers. Similar bacterial findings are noted in elderly patients with healthy gingival sulci. However, gram-negative bacteria may be slightly more common in these persons.

Immunology. Except in persons receiving an extensive regimen of professional and home care plaque control, the gingival tissues are usually infiltrated by chronic inflammatory cells, primarily lymphocytes. Leukocytes are also common within the junctional epithelium and in the gingival crevice. This cellular infiltrate is thought to be a direct response to plaque. In extreme periodontal health, in which there is an absence of plaque, the cellular infiltrate is not present.

Serum antibodies to the microbial flora occur usually in low titers, reflecting the minimal antigenic stimulation by plaque during gingival health. Titers to some organisms are higher, which is thought to indicate extragingival antigenic stimulation.

MICROBIOLOGY AND IMMUNOLOGY IN SPECIFIC DISEASES AND CONDITIONS

Gingivitis and Periodontitis

The accumulation of crevicular microorganisms adjacent to the gingiva elicits inflammation within the connective tissue.[31] Initially clinical signs of inflammation, such as redness, may not be seen. However, with time and further plaque accumulation, clinical signs of gingivitis become apparent. *In the early stages of gingivitis, the inflammatory infiltrate is predominantly lymphocytic, with a preponderance of T cells. In advanced gingivitis and periodontitis, plasma cells are the most common inflammatory cells.* Lymphocytes found in periodontitis are usually B cells. T cells constitute less than 6% of the lymphoid population. The helper-to-suppressor T-cell ratio in naturally occurring gingivitis in children and in persons with experimentally induced gingivitis is approximately 2:1. In contrast, the ratio in periodontitis is lower (approximately 1:1). In patients with acquired immunodeficiency syndrome (AIDS), the ratio would be expected to be markedly lower, because the human immunodeficiency virus (HIV) primarily infects the helper T cells. This suggests a local alteration in the immunoregulatory mechanisms. As discussed earlier in this chapter, the pocket microorganisms synthesize an array of products, causing direct tissue damage.

The perpetuation of the periodontal lesion is controlled by both local and systemic factors. Active disease is associated with increased proportions of pathogenic bacteria, changes in the host response, and possibly bacterial invasion of the tissues. The exact triggering mechanisms are not known.

Microbiologic Findings. The role of bacteria in the etiology of gingivitis and periodontitis has been well established.

Epidemiologic Studies. Epidemiologic studies have identified plaque as the primary etiologic factor in both gingivitis and periodontitis (see Chapter 5). In cross-sectional studies, an increasing amount of plaque is associated with increasing severity of periodontal disease. In longitudinal studies of several years' duration, poor plaque control leads to increased severity of periodontal disease, whereas good plaque control prevents such periodontal breakdown.

Antimicrobial Studies. Antimicrobial agents, including antibiotics, disinfectants, and antiseptics, directly affect microorganisms and have minimal, if any, effects on host tissue. The chemical control of microorganisms improves the periodontal status (see Chapter 44).

Oral Hygiene Studies. The classic experimental gingivitis model, in which plaque is allowed to form and is then removed, demonstrates the causal relationship between plaque accumulations and gingivitis (see Chapter 42).

Pathogenicity Studies. Numerous subgingival bacteria can induce aspects of periodontal disease when orally implanted into germ-free and conventional animals or injected subcutaneously.[45] Some of the pathologic changes observed include inflammation, destruction of connective tissue, vasculitis, osteoclastic bone resorption, and apical migration of the junctional epithelium. These responses can often be induced by colonization of pure cultures of a single organism such as *A. actinomycetemcomitans,* which leads to rapid bone loss in a germ-free animal within a few months. Selected "mixed cultures" including black-pigmented bacilli can also induce rapid tissue destruction and periodontitis.[41] Bacterial interactions in the complex subgingival flora and environmental and host factors in the pocket can either inhibit or stimulate bacterial growth.

Scaling and Root Planing Treatment. Clinical experience and an overwhelming number of clinical investigations have demonstrated the efficacy of scaling and root planing in periodontal therapy (see Chapter 41). Thorough

removal of the bacterial deposits quickly and effectively reduces gingival inflammation.

With the accumulation of plaque and the development of gingivitis, there is both a quantitative and a qualitative change in plaque.[36,45] There is a shift in the flora from the gram-positive cocci seen in health to one characterized by increased numbers of filamentous bacteria, gram-negative rods, and spirochetes. In the earlier stages of gingivitis, *Actinomyces* species are common. In long-standing gingivitis, gram-negative bacteria, including *Veillonella* and *Fusobacterium,* increase so that they constitute approximately 25% of the flora.

In periodontitis, there is a continued change in the flora to one increasingly characterized by gram-negative rods.[36] The flora is much more varied and complex than that seen in health or in gingivitis.

Studies have demonstrated qualitative differences in the subgingival flora in active sites, defined on the basis of recent loss of alveolar bone or attachment, compared with inactive sites with no recent bone or attachment loss.[8] Active sites usually have elevated numbers of *P. gingivalis, P. intermedia, A. actinomycetemcomitans,* fusiform *Bacteroides, C. rectus, Eikenella* species, and small spirochetes. Conversely, successfully treated sites have small numbers of *P. gingivalis, P. intermedia,* and *A. actinomycetemcomitans* and increased numbers of *Streptococcus sanguis.*[18,25]

Immunologic Findings. Continued exposure to bacterial antigens in the gingival crevice and within the gingival tissues induces systemic and local host responses.[26] In gingivitis and adult periodontitis, these immune responses have both protective and destructive functions (Fig. 9–1).

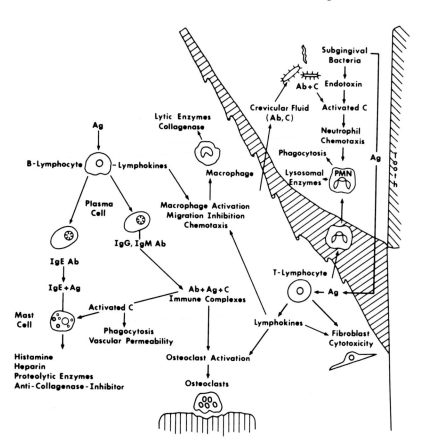

FIGURE 9–1. Immunologic responses in gingivitis and periodontitis. Potential immunopathologic processes that may occur in the course of human gingivitis and periodontitis. (From Nisengard RJ. The role of immunology in periodontal disease. J Periodontol *48:*505, 1977.)

Their relative importance may vary from patient to patient and from site to site.

Protective Functions. There is little evidence of a significant protective immune function, because plaque accumulation inevitably leads to gingivitis. However, crevicular fluid contains immunoglobulins and complement, which constantly bathe and react with the subgingival bacteria.[11] This reactivity may modulate or alter the composition of the subgingival microflora. The bacterial masses could also be reduced via antibody–antigen reactions, with complement activation leading to bacterial cytolysis and phagocytosis. The important role of the neutrophil in control of periodontopathogens is evident in the occurrence of more severe periodontal disease in cases of reduced neutrophil function.

Destructive Functions. The importance of B-cell responses in the pathogenesis of periodontal disease has been demonstrated experimentally in athymic rats devoid of T cells.[49] Athymic rats with preponderantly B cells in their gingival tissues show increased bone loss. In contrast, when T cells preponderate in athymic rats reconstituted by injection of T cells or in normal animals, there is less bone loss. Progressive periodontal disease therefore appears to be associated with B-cell–dominated lesions.

The immunopathologic findings in gingivitis and periodontitis indicate that the gingival tissues contain the necessary elements for humoral responses.[11] IgG-, IgA-, IgM-, and IgE-containing plasma cells are in the inflammatory infiltrate at sites where IgG and IgM predominate. Both local and systemic antibody responses commonly occur to the crevicular microflora. Local production has been demonstrated to *A. actinomycetemcomitans, P. gingivalis, F. nucleatum,* and *C. rectus.*[48] Indirect evidence for a local antibody response is further provided by the finding that many subgingival bacteria are "coated" in vivo with immunoglobulins and complement.[26]

Antibody levels to most periodontopathogens are usually high and often correlate with the severity or type of periodontal disease and bacterial numbers.[11] For example, patients with adult periodontitis usually have high numbers of *P. gingivalis* and significantly elevated antibody levels to this organism compared with subjects with healthy gingiva. Similarly, higher antibody levels also occur in periodontitis patients having higher numbers of *C. ochracea,* some gram-negative anaerobic bacteria, *A. naeslundii, Fusobacterium,* and *Leptotrichia buccalis.* However, the serum antibody levels of some bacteria may be either high or low without regard to the periodontal status.

Dental treatment such as scaling and root planing commonly elicits a humoral response to some but not all subgingival bacteria.[9] The serum antibody response generally peaks 2 to 4 months after scaling and root planing and gradually decreases to the prescaling level within 8 to 12 months. After scaling and root planing, elevated antibody levels occur to black-pigmented bacilli, including *P. gingivalis* and *P. intermedia* as well as *Eikenella corrodens, Campylobacter concisus,* and *A. actinomycetemcomitans.*

Many responses to antigen–antibody interactions are complement dependent. Complement activation is important in bacterial lysis, phagocytosis, bone resorption, chemotaxis, and other biologically significant events. The immunopathologic changes may result from anaphylactic re-

actions, cytotoxic reactions, immune complex reactions, and cell-mediated reactions in the pathogenesis of periodontal disease.[27]

Anaphylactic Reactions. Anaphylactic, or immediate hypersensitivity, reactions occur when IgE fixed to mast cells or basophils reacts with antigens and leads to the release of histamine and other mediators. All of the necessary components for such reactions are associated with periodontitis.[26]

IgE-containing plasma cells occur in the gingival tissues, although they are fewer in number than IgG-, IgA-, or IgM-containing cells. Mast cell numbers increase with progression from gingival health to moderate periodontitis and then decrease. It has been suggested that the decrease is a result of anaphylactic reactions that lead to the degranulation of mast cells. Histamine levels in chronically inflamed gingivae are significantly higher than those in normal tissues, and in vitro challenge of inflamed gingival tissues with anti-IgE leads to histamine release, suggesting that IgE is already fixed to gingival mast cells.

The traditional method of identifying immediate hypersensitivity with skin tests has been applied to studies of periodontal disease. Intradermal skin tests with extracts of *Actinomyces* have revealed both immediate and, less commonly, delayed reactions in humans. There is a significant correlation between the incidence of immediate hypersensitivity to this organism and the severity of periodontal disease. The greatest incidence occurs in periodontitis. Similar immediate skin test responses have been demonstrated to *Bacterionema matruchotii, P. melaninogenica,* and *F. nucleatum.*

Repetitive challenge of the gingival tissues experimentally to induce immediate hypersensitivity reactions in monkeys has evoked an inflammatory response. This response is characterized by a chronic inflammatory infiltrate of plasma cells and lymphocytes, along with connective tissue breakdown. Osteoclastic bone loss is not apparent.

The role of anaphylactic reactions in the pathogenesis of gingivitis and periodontitis has not been definitively shown. Although the potential for this mechanism exists, it is not thought to be a major factor because of the small numbers of IgE-containing cells in the gingival tissues.

Cytotoxic Reactions. Cytotoxic reactions occur when antibodies react with cell or tissue antigens and complement is activated. The antigens can be either host cell constituents or bacterial antigens attached to host cells via receptor sites. An example of cytotoxic reactions is humoral autoimmune disease. *There is no evidence, however, for considering cytotoxic reactions in the pathogenesis of gingivitis and periodontitis.*

Immune Complex Reactions. Immune complex, or Arthus, reactions occur when antigen forms microprecipitates with IgG and/or IgM antibodies in or around blood vessels in tissues. Microcomplexes in moderate antigen excess activate the complement system, leading to hormonal, vascular, and cytotoxic reactions, depending on where the complexes lodge.

The elements for immune complex disease—bacterial antigen, antibodies to the bacteria, and complement for activation—are present in the gingival tissues. The constant shower of bacterial antigens within inflamed gingival tissues, as seen by the occurrence of bacteremias resulting from gingival manipulation and by bacterial invasion, serves both to sensitize and subsequently to challenge the host. These bacterial antigens encounter tissue fluids that contain bacterial antibodies, permitting immune complex formation. Studies with the Raji cell assay showed that immune complexes commonly occur in soluble extracts of human gingival tissue from patients with periodontitis.[27]

Experimental Arthus reactions in monkey gingivae are similar to those in humans with periodontitis. Repetitive reactions can lead to chronic inflammatory infiltrates of macrophages, lymphocytes, and plasma cells, accompanied by collagen breakdown and osteoclastic bone loss.[26]

Cell-Mediated Reactions. Cell-mediated, or delayed hypersensitivity, reactions are dependent on T lymphocytes and release of lymphokines. Numerous studies have demonstrated that peripheral leukocytes from patients with periodontitis blast or proliferate in response to some oral bacteria.

The lymphoproliferative response in the gingival tissues is thought to release potent lymphokines, including OAF. Isolated gingival lymphocytes from nondiseased gingiva produce low levels of the lymphokines, including chemotactic factor, leukocyte migration inhibition factor, and mitogenic factor in response to plaque and specific plaque bacteria. In contrast, lymphocytes from gingivitis and periodontitis tissues produce more lymphokines on challenge with plaque and specific plaque bacteria, suggesting that the lymphocytes are sensitized to the bacterial antigens.[11]

Experimental induction of cell-mediated immunity in the periodontium of monkeys is characterized by massive tissue destruction, including marked bone loss, reduced number of fibroblasts, and collagen breakdown.[26] It has been suggested that the bone loss in cell-mediated immune responses results directly from T-cell effects or enhanced B-cell activation.

Experimental depression of cell-mediated immunity with antithymocyte globulin, however, does not influence development of gingivitis or alter existing gingivitis. In addition, patients receiving immunosuppressive therapy, such as transplant recipient patients, have been evaluated for periodontal status.[29] Most longitudinal studies indicate no difference in the rate of periodontitis between immunosuppressed patients and normal controls. In AIDS patients, reduced numbers of helper T cells may contribute to the frequent occurrence of severe and often acute periodontal disease (see Chapter 15).

The contribution of cell-mediated immunity to the immunopathologic changes of gingivitis and periodontitis is unknown. However, with the relatively low numbers of T cells in the tissue, it is not thought to be a major contributor.

Pregnancy Gingivitis and Hormonally Related Gingivitis

Microbiologic Findings. Bacteriologically, during pregnancy, the changes in hormone levels influence the composition of plaque. There is a shift toward a greater percentage of anaerobic bacteria, particularly *P. intermedia.*[15] It appears that *P. intermedia* can substitute progesterone or estradiol for vitamin K as a growth factor. Steroid hormone concentrations in crevicular fluid may parallel serum concentrations, which dramatically change during pregnancy, puberty, and menstruation and after menopause.

Immunologic Findings. Changes in immune responses to oral flora during pregnancy have not been evaluated.

Periodontitis in Insulin-Dependent Diabetes Mellitus

Microbiologic Findings. In gingivitis associated with insulin-dependent diabetes mellitus (IDDM), the preponderant cultivable organisms include *Actinomyces* (33%), *Streptococcus* (36%), *Veillonella parvula* (12%), and *Fusobacterium* (10%).[19]

The predominant cultivable flora in IDDM-associated periodontitis includes *Capnocytophaga* and anaerobic *Vibrio* spp., which average 24% and 13% of the cultivable flora, respectively. This pattern differs from adult periodontitis, in which *P. gingivalis* is frequently preponderant, and from localized juvenile periodontitis, in which *A. actinomycetemcomitans* is usually preponderant.

Immunologic Findings. As in other aggressive forms of periodontal disease, in IDDM there is frequently a leukocyte chemotactic defect[11] (see Table 9–6). This deficiency is thought to contribute directly to the pathogenesis of the disease.

Periodontal Abscesses

Microbiologic Findings. Early animal studies demonstrated that fulminating, transferable abscesses could be induced by subcutaneous injections of plaque. A limited number of bacteria were necessary for this, and the abscesses were termed *mixed anaerobic infections. P. gingivalis* was found to be an essential component of the bacterial inoculum that resulted in a transferable infection.

Cultural examination of human abscesses reveals a similar microbiota, with gram-negative anaerobic rods preponderant. *P. gingivalis, Fusobacterium* spp., *Capnocytophaga,* and *Vibrio* spp. were the most common gram-negative isolates, making up more than 30% of the total cultivable microbiota.[24]

Localized Juvenile Periodontitis

Microbiologic Findings. Initial anaerobic cultural studies of first molar sites exhibiting localized bone loss in LJP patients revealed a unique bacterial flora consisting of gram-negative anaerobic rods.[25] These organisms were less frequently isolated and were found in significantly lower numbers in healthy subgingival sites in LJP patients and in their non-LJP siblings or other adolescents. These organisms have been subsequently identified as *A. actinomycetemcomitans. A. actinomycetemcomitans* has been implicated in the etiology of LJP as a result of the following findings:[2,43,57]

1. The prevalence of and humoral immune response to this organism are elevated in patients with LJP. *A. actinomycetemcomitans* has been isolated in up to 97% of LJP patients, compared with 21% of adult periodontitis patients and 17% of healthy subjects. Not only is the prevalence of *A. actinomycetemcomitans* six times greater in LJP than in healthy patients, but its proportion of the cultivable subgingival flora

is also elevated. Among the three serotypes, serotype B is the most common, followed by serotype A.

2. The incidence of *A. actinomycetemcomitans* is greater in younger LJP patients than in older LJP patients. If age is considered relative to the duration of the disease, younger patients have more destructive disease developing within a shorter period. This suggests that this organism correlates with disease activity.

3. A large number of *A. actinomycetemcomitans* organisms occur in lesions in LJP patients, but such organisms are absent or occur in low numbers in healthy sites.

4. *A. actinomycetemcomitans* can be identified by electron microscopy, immunofluorescence, and culture from LJP lesions within the gingival connective tissues.

5. The organism is quite virulent, producing a leukotoxin, collagenase, phosphatases, and bone-resorbing factors, as well as other factors important in evasion of host defenses and destruction of periodontal tissues.

6. There is a positive correlation between the elimination of this organism from the subgingival flora and successful clinical treatment of LJP.[44]

The source of *A. actinomycetemcomitans* in LJP patients, as well as of pathogens in other periodontal diseases, is not clear, but it may be derived from the mother, from other family members, or from exogenous sources.[34] An intrafamily transmission of *A. actinomycetemcomitans* has also been suggested by observations that the same biotype and serotype of *A. actinomycetemcomitans* can be isolated in family members of LJP patients, although in smaller numbers.[57] This may be one factor associated with the apparent familial tendency for this disease. Transmission of this organism is difficult to achieve and probably requires extended exposure. Periodontal probes contaminated with *A. actinomycetemcomitans* from LJP lesions during routine examinations can transfer the organism from infected to healthy noninfected sulci.[7] However, the organism does not permanently colonize the healthy sites and is eliminated within a matter of weeks.

Beneficial modes of therapy depend on understanding the ecology of *A. actinomycetemcomitans*. Mechanical methods alone do not predictably eradicate the organism, because it occurs not only in the pocket, but also within the gingival tissues. This intragingival location may permit rapid repopulation of the pocket. Thus, clinical studies suggest a combination of surgery to treat the pocket and antibiotic therapy to suppress the organism as the best therapeutic approach (see Chapter 45).

Immunologic Findings. Studies of LJP were the first to demonstrate the importance of neutrophils in periodontal disease.[11,21,47,52,53] Approximately 75% of patients with LJP exhibit a PMN chemotactic defect and depressed phagocytosis in peripheral blood. The chemotactic defect is a cellular abnormality that is not associated with serum factors or neutrophil ability for random migration, deformation, or adherence. In addition to altered systemic neutrophil function, neutrophil migration into the gingival crevice is slower. The gingival crevicular neutrophils also have grossly altered morphologic appearance and diminished phagocytosis.

The role of the neutrophil chemotactic defect in LJP has been clarified by studying families of patients with LJP.[57] In many cases, brothers and sisters of patients with LJP may also exhibit a chemotactic defect without clinical signs of LJP. This has led to the conclusion that the chemotactic defect is a predisposing factor in LJP. The failure of neu-

trophil chemotactic responsiveness diminishes the host's ability to ward off the effects of periodontopathogens associated with LJP. This reduction in host defenses, coupled with the leukotoxin produced by *A. actinomycetemcomitans* that destroys the reduced numbers of neutrophils that are chemotactically attracted into the gingiva, further complicates the situation.

Associated with the high numbers of *A. actinomycetemcomitans* in LJP are elevated antibody levels to this organism in the serum, the crevicular fluid, and the saliva from LJP patients.[11] Sixty percent to 90% of patients have serum IgG antibodies and, to a lesser extent, IgM, IgA, and IgE antibodies. Although antibody levels in serum and crevicular fluid are usually similar, crevicular fluid antibody levels may exceed serum levels during periods of ongoing attachment loss. This suggests local antibody production within the gingival tissues. As expected, scaling patients with *A. actinomycetemcomitans* introduces bacterial antigens into tissues, leading to a hyperimmune response. Within 2 to 3 months after scaling, IgG serum and salivary antibody levels increase.

Capnocytophaga species are also common inhabitants of the subgingival flora in LJP. In contrast to the response to *A. actinomycetemcomitans,* however, antibody levels to this organism are low. It has been suggested that this is a result of suppressor cell activation or tolerance to the *Capnocytophaga* antigens.

Generalized Juvenile Periodontitis

Microbiologic Findings. The preponderant cultivable microorganisms in generalized juvenile periodontitis (GJP) differ from those found in LJP. *P. gingivalis* is the most common isolate and constitutes 13% to 20% of the total cell counts.[55] Other common isolates include *E. corrodens, P. intermedia, Capnocytophaga,* and *Neisseria. A. actinomycetemcomitans* is present in lower numbers in GJP than in LJP.

Immunologic Findings. Like LJP patients, GJP patients frequently have a neutrophil chemotactic defect and reduced phagocytosis.[55] The chemotactic defect is cellular in nature, but the neutrophils have normal random migration and oxidative metabolic activity. Although the incidence of chemotactic defects is similar but somewhat less in GJP than in LJP, GJP patients are less likely to exhibit decreased phagocytosis. Twenty-nine percent of GJP patients and 62% of LJP patients have decreased phagocytosis compared with healthy controls.

Patients exhibit high IgG antibody titers to *P. gingivalis,* reflecting the high incidence and numbers of this organism in GJP.[50,55] Approximately two thirds of GJP patients have these elevated antibody levels. Antibodies to *A. actinomycetemcomitans* are less frequent in GJP than in LJP; there are low titers to serotypes A and B but unexpectedly high titers to serotype C, approximating the levels in LJP patients.

Rapidly Progressing Periodontitis

Microbiologic Findings. Limited microbiologic examination has been performed on the subgingival flora in pockets from patients with rapidly progressing periodontitis. *P.*

gingivalis, P. intermedia, and spirochetes, particularly small spirochetes, are major subgingival components in this disease.[51]

Immunologic Findings. The majority of patients with rapidly progressing periodontitis have functional defects in either neutrophils or monocytes.[32] This manifests as either a suppression or an enhancement of chemotaxis. Neutrophils and, to a lesser extent, monocytes may play a role in the adverse response to the associated microflora.[51]

Although the exact significance of antibodies to oral bacteria is not known, elevated antibody titers occur to *P. gingivalis, A. actinomycetemcomitans, Capnocytophaga sputigena, C. rectus, Eubacterium brachyii, F. nucleatum,* and *Peptostreptococcus micros.*[32]

Prepubertal Periodontitis

Microbiologic Findings. The microflora seen in prepubertal periodontitis differs from that seen in juvenile periodontitis and rapidly progressing periodontitis.[32] Species of *Fusobacterium, Selenomonas, Campylobacter,* and *Capnocytophaga* and black-pigmented bacilli are frequently found in prepubertal periodontitis, whereas *A. actinomycetemcomitans, Haemophilus aphrophilus,* and *P. gingivalis* are infrequent subgingival inhabitants.

Immunologic Findings. In the generalized form, although peripheral white blood cell counts are elevated, patients have pronounced depression in neutrophil and monocyte chemotaxis and ability to adhere to surfaces. Although gingival biopsy specimens from adult periodontitis patients usually reveal inflammation, including extravascular leukocytes, leukocytes are rare in patients with generalized prepubertal periodontitis. It is thought that these functional defects play a role in the pathogenesis of this disease.

In the localized form, in comparison with the generalized form, defects in neutrophil and monocyte function are less frequent and less severe and do not occur simultaneously.

Refractory Periodontitis

Microbiologic Findings. Several microorganisms commonly are isolated from refractory periodontitis pockets.[42] In active sites, these include *Bacteroides forsythus, P. gingivalis, P. intermedia, C. rectus,* and *E. corrodens.* Inactive sites are characterized by increased numbers of facultative bacteria including *S. sanguis* and *Actinomyces.* The numbers of S. sanguis also increase in treated pockets.

Immunologic Findings. Patients with refractory periodontitis appear to have a reduced neutrophil function, similar to that observed in LJP.[30]

Acute Necrotizing Ulcerative Gingivitis

Microbiologic Findings. There is ample evidence to demonstrate that bacteria play an important role in the pathogenesis of ANUG. Although not routinely recommended for treatment, antibiotics such as metronidazole and penicillin lead to enhanced healing within a matter of days.

Early observations of smears from ANUG patients suggested that ANUG was caused by spirochetes and fusiform bacilli. The intermediate-size spirochete was called *Borrelia*

vincentii. Ultrastructural classification of spirochetes by Listgarten indicated that this spirochete was found only superficially, rather than within the lesion.

The principal bacteria associated with ANUG are *P. intermedia* and an unnamed intermediate-size spirochete.[17] *P. intermedia* constitutes a significant part of the microflora in ANUG, making up 8% to 15% of the total cell counts. Ultrastructurally, the disease is characterized by spirochetal invasion of the tissues.[16]

Although the role of the microorganisms in pathogenesis is not fully understood, both direct bacterial effects and indirect host responses may be important. Along with direct invasion of the gingival tissues, the bacterial counts and associated endotoxin concentrations may be important.

Immunologic Findings. In ANUG, both the cellular and humoral responses are affected. Sera collected from patients within a few days after onset of ANUG (acute phase) have elevated IgG and IgM antibody titers to intermediate-size oral spirochetes and elevated IgG titers to *P. gingivalis.*[5] These elevated titers suggest that these organisms proliferated weeks to months before the development of the lesions and indicate that they are pathogenically important agents. The significance of the elevated bacterial antibody titers in the pathogenesis of ANUG is unknown. The histopathologic changes, the large numbers of bacteria within the tissues, and the elevated levels of antibodies suggest the possibility of an immune complex disease. However, further studies are necessary.

At a cellular level, patients with ANUG have reduced PMN chemotaxis and phagocytosis.[6] Such dysfunction could play a role in the pathogenesis of ANUG, although this has not been proved. Whether leukocyte dysfunction results from the bacterial infection in ANUG or develops first, thus allowing the "explosion" in the bacterial flora to occur, is unknown.

AIDS-Related Periodontal Disease

Microbiologic Findings. Only initial microbiologic studies of periodontitis in AIDS patients have been reported; however, there appear to be similarities to and differences

---

Table 9–7. ASSAYS FOR STUDYING PERIODONTAL DISEASE

Plaque Assays

1. Phase and darkfield microscopy
2. Culture and isolation
3. Identification of bacterial enzymes and products in subgingival specimens
4. Immunofluorescence
5. Latex agglutination
6. Immunoperoxidase
7. ELISA
8. Immunoblotting
9. DNA probes

Indirect Assays on Sera

1. Immunofluorescence
2. ELISA

ELISA, Enzyme-linked immunosorbent assay.

from the flora seen in non-AIDS periodontitis patients.[56] Many of the same bacteria, including black-pigmented bacilli and *C. rectus,* may be found. In addition, there are relatively high numbers of a gram-positive bacillus and a gram-negative "wet-spreader" not usually seen in non-AIDS periodontitis (see Chapter 15).

ROLE OF BACTERIOLOGY AND IMMUNOLOGY IN THE DIAGNOSIS OF PERIODONTAL DISEASE

Numerous assays are being developed for studying periodontal disease (Table 9–7). These are described in Chapter 30.

REFERENCES

1. Altman LC, Page RC, Vandesteen GE, et al. Abnormalities of leukocyte chemotaxis in patients with various forms of periodontitis. J Periodont Res 20:553, 1985.
2. Asikainen S. Occurrence of *Actinobacillus actinomycetemcomitans* and spirochetes in relation to age in localized juvenile periodontitis. J Periodontol 57:537, 1986.
3. Bick PH, Carpenter AB, Holdeman LV, et al. Polyclonal B-cell activation induced by extracts of gram-negative bacteria isolated from periodontally diseased sites. Infect Immun 34:43, 1981.
4. Bolton RW, Kluever EA, Dyer JK. In vitro immunosuppression mediated by an extracellular polysaccharide from *Capnocytophaga ochracea.* J Periodont Res 20:251, 1985.
5. Chung CP, Nisengard RJ, Slots J, Genco RJ. Bacterial IgG and IgM antibody titers in acute necrotizing ulcerative gingivitis. J Periodontol 54:557, 1983.
6. Cogen RB, Stevens AW Jr, Cohen-Cole S, et al. Leukocyte function in the etiology of acute necrotizing ulcerative gingivitis. J Periodontol 54:402, 1983.
7. Christersson LA, Slots J, Zambon JJ, Genco RJ. Transmission and colonization of *Actinobacillus actinomycetemcomitans* in localized juvenile periodontitis patients. J Periodontol 56:127, 1985.
8. Dzink JL, Tanner ACR, Haffajee AD, Socransky SS. Gram negative species associated with active destructive periodontal lesions. J Clin Periodontol 12:648, 1985.
9. Ebersole JL, Taubman MA, Smith DJ, Haffajee AD. Effect of subgingival scaling on systemic antibody responses to oral microorganisms. Infect Immun 48:534, 1985.
10. Frank RM, Voegel JC. Bacterial bone resorption in advanced cases of human periodontitis. J Periodont Res 13:251, 1978.
11. Genco RJ, Slots J. Host responses in periodontal disease. J Dent Res 63:441, 1984.
12. Holt SC. Bacterial surface structures and their role in periodontal disease. In Genco RJ, Mergenhagen SE, eds. Host-Parasite Interactions in Periodontal Disease. Washington, DC, American Society for Microbiology, 1982, p 139.
13. Kilian M. Degradation of immunoglobulins A1, A2, and G by suspected principal periodontal pathogens. Infect Immun 34:757, 1981.
14. Kornman KS. Age, supragingival plaque, and steroid hormones as ecological determinants of the subgingival flora. In Genco RJ, Mergenhagen SE, eds. Host-Parasite Interactions in Periodontal Disease. Washington, DC, American Society for Microbiology, 1982, p 132.
15. Kornman KS, Loesche WJ. The subgingival microbial flora during pregnancy. J Periodont Res 15:111, 1980.
16. Listgarten MA. Electron microscopic observations on the bacterial flora of acute necrotizing ulcerative gingivitis. J Periodontol 36:328, 1965.
17. Loesche WJ, Syed SA, Laughon BE, Stoll J. The bacteriology of acute necrotizing ulcerative gingivitis. J Periodontol 53:223, 1982.
18. Loesche WJ, Syed SA, Schmidt E, Morrison EC. Bacterial profiles of subgingival plaques in periodontitis. J Periodontol 56:447, 1985.
19. Mashimo PA, Yamamoto Y, Slots J, et al. The periodontal microflora of juvenile diabetics: Culture, immunofluorescence, and serum antibody studies. J Periodontol 54:420, 1983.
20. Mergenhagen SE. Thymocyte activating factor(s) in human gingival fluids. J Dent Res 63:461, 1984.
21. Newman MG. Current concepts of pathogenesis of periodontal disease. J Periodontol 56:734, 1985.
22. Newman HN, Addison IE. Gingival crevice neutrophil function in periodontosis. J Periodontol 53:578, 1982.
23. Newman MG, Grinenco V, Weiner M, et al. Predominant microbiota associated with periodontal health in the aged. J Periodontol 49:553, 1978.
24. Newman MG, Sims TN. The predominant cultivable microbiota of the periodontal abscess. J Periodontol 50:350, 1979.
25. Newman MG, Socransky SS, Savitt ED, et al. Studies of the microbiology of periodontosis. J Periodontol 47:373, 1976.

26. Nisengard RJ. The role of immunology in periodontal disease. J Periodontol 48:505, 1977.
27. Nisengard RJ, Blann DB. Detection of immune complexes in gingiva from periodontitis patients. J Dent Res 64:361, 1985.
28. O'Neil PA, Woodson DL. Lymphokine production by human gingival lymphocytes. J Periodont Res 21:338, 1986.
29. Oshrain HI, Telsey B, Mandel ID. A longitudinal study of periodontal disease in patients with reduced immunocapacity. J Periodontol 54:151, 1983.
30. Oshrain HI, Telsey B, Mandel ID. Neutrophil chemotaxis in refractory cases of periodontitis. J Clin Periodontol 14:52, 1986.
31. Page RC. Pathogenic mechanisms. In Schluger S, Youdelis R, Page RC, eds. Periodontal Disease: Basic Phenomena, Clinical Management and Restorative Interrelationships. Philadelphia, Lea & Febiger, 1977.
32. Page RC, Altman LC, Ebersole JL, et al. Rapidly progressive periodontitis: A distinct clinical condition. J Periodontol 54:197, 1983.
33. Page RC, Bowen T, Altman L, et al. Prepubertal periodontitis. I. Definition of a clinical disease entity. J Periodontol 54:257, 1983.
34. Preus HR. Possible exogenous source of Aa in rapid destructive periodontitis in man. Abstract. J Dent Res 66:195, 1987.
35. Saglie R, Newman MG, Carranza FA Jr, Pattison GL. Bacterial invasion of gingiva in advanced periodontitis in humans. J Periodontol 53:217, 1982.
36. Savitt ED, Socransky SS. Distribution of certain subgingival microbial species in selected periodontal conditions. J Periodont Res 19:111, 1984.
37. Schenkein HA. The complement system in periodontal disease. In Genco RJ, Mergenhagen SE, eds. Host-Parasite Interactions in Periodontal Disease. Washington, DC, American Society for Microbiology, 1982, p 299.
38. Seymour GJ, Cole KL, Powell RN, et al. Interleukin-2 production and bone-resorption activity in vitro by unstimulated lymphocytes extracted from chronically-inflamed human periodontal tissues. Arch Oral Biol 30:481, 1985.
39. Seymour GJ. Possible mechanisms involved in the immunoregulation of chronic inflammatory periodontal disease. J Dent Res 66:2, 1987.
40. Shenker BJ, DiRienzo JM. Suppression of human peripheral blood lymphocytes by *Fusobacterium nucleatum.* J Immunol 132:2357, 1984.
41. Slots J. Importance of black-pigmented *Bacteroides* in human periodontal disease. In Genco RJ, Mergenhagen SE, eds. Host-Parasite Interactions in Periodontal Disease. Washington, DC, American Society for Microbiology, 1982, p 27.
42. Slots J, Bragd L, Wikstrom M, Dahlen G. The occurrence of *Actinobacillus actinomycetemcomitans, Bacteroides gingivalis* and *Bacteroides intermedius* in destructive periodontal disease in adults. J Clin Periodontol 13:570, 1986.
43. Slots J, Genco RJ. Black-pigmented *Bacteroides* species, *Capnocytophaga* species, and *Actinobacillus actinomycetemcomitans* in human periodontal disease: Virulence factors in colonization, survival, and tissue destruction. J Dent Res 63:412, 1984.
44. Slots J, Rosling BG. Suppression of the periodontopathic microflora in localized juvenile periodontitis by systemic tetracycline. J Clin Periodontol 10:465, 1983.
45. Socransky SS, Holt SE, Tanner AC, et al. Present status of studies on the microbial etiology of periodontal diseases. In Genco RJ, Mergenhagen SE, eds. Host-Parasite Interactions in Periodontal Diseases. Washington, DC, American Society for Microbiology, 1982, p 1.
46. Sundqvist G, Carlsson J, Herrmann B, Tarnvik A. Degradation of human immunoglobulins G and M and complement factors C3 and C5 by black-pigmented *Bacteroides.* J Med Microbiol 19:85, 1985.
47. Suzuki JB, Collison BC, Falker WA Jr, Nauman RK. Immunologic profile of juvenile periodontitis. II. Neutrophil chemotaxis, phagocytosis and spore germination. J Periodontol 55:461, 1984.
48. Taubman MA, Ebersole JL, Smith DJ. Association between systemic and local antibody and periodontal disease. In Genco RJ, Mergenhagen SE, eds. Host-Parasite Interactions in Periodontal Disease. Washington, DC, American Society for Microbiology, 1982, p 283.
49. Taubman MA, Yoshie H, Ebersole JL, et al. Host response in experimental periodontal disease. J Dent Res 63:455, 1984.
50. Tew JG, Marshall DR, Moore WEC, et al. Serum antibody reactive with predominant organisms in the subgingival flora of young adults with generalized severe periodontitis. Infect Immun 48:303, 1985.
51. Vandesteen GE, Williams BL, Ebersole JL, et al. Clinical, microbiological and immunological studies of a family with a high prevalence of early-onset periodontitis. J Periodontol 55:159, 1984.
52. Van Dyke TE, Horoszewicz HU, Cianciola LJ, Genco RJ. Neutrophil chemotaxis dysfunction in human periodontitis. Infect Immun 27:124, 1980.
53. Van Dyke TE, Schweinebraten M, Cianciola LJ, et al. Neutrophil chemotaxis in families with localized juvenile periodontitis. J Periodont Res 20:503, 1985.
54. Wahl SM. Mononuclear cell-mediated alterations in connective tissue. In Genco RJ, Mergenhagen SE, eds. Host-Parasite Interactions in Periodontal Disease. Washington, DC, American Society for Microbiology, 1982, p 132.
55. Wilson ME, Zambon JJ, Suzuki JB, Genco RJ. Generalized juvenile periodontitis, defective neutrophil chemotaxis and *Bacteroides gingivalis* in a 13-year-old female. J Periodontol 56:457, 1985.
56. Zambon JJ. Overview of periodontal lesions and studies of subgingival microflora in HIV infected individuals. In Robertson P, Greenspan J, eds. Perspectives in Oral Manifestations of AIDS: Diagnosis and Management of HIV-Associated Infections. Littleton, MA, Procter and Gamble Oral Health Group, PSG Publishing, 1988, p 96.
57. Zambon JJ, Christersson LA, Slots J. *Actinobacillus actinomycetemcomitans* in human periodontal disease—prevalence in patient groups and distribution of biotypes and serotypes within families. J Periodontol 54:707, 1983.

10

Altered Leukocyte Function and Periodontal Disease

KENNETH T. MIYASAKI

Periodontal diseases involve (1) a local infection and (2) a host response that may result in connective tissue alterations. The immune system plays a key role in limiting the infections to the gingival crevice or the tissues within the immediate vicinity of the gingival crevice. The immune system also orchestrates the alterations of the connective tissues in a complex remodeling process involving cycles of destruction and reconstruction.[26,66] Leukocytes are critical to periodontal defense, as most potential periodontal pathogens are known to be resistant to the antimicrobial mechanisms of serum. This chapter will examine how leukocytes function in the periodontium and consider how leukocyte abnormalities relate to periodontal diseases.

CONTROL OF LOCAL INFECTION

Acute Inflammation

Histologic observations reveal that the three primary leukocytes participating in the immune response to periodontal diseases are neutrophils, monocytes, and lymphocytes. The leukocytes infiltrate the gingiva in a temporal and spatial order, suggesting that the strategy of host defense against periodontal infections is similar to that used to combat most other local infections.[55]

Neutrophils are the initial leukocytes recruited into the gingiva. Neutrophils exit the circulation and migrate into the junctional epithelium and gingival crevice, where they provide the first cellular host mechanism to contact and control periodontal bacteria (Fig. 10–1). Neutrophils are well adapted to function in hypoxic environments, because virtually all of their energy is derived from fermentation of stored glycogen rather than oxidative phosphorylation. They possess a large number of antimicrobial compounds, most of which do not depend on oxygen. Evidence suggests that neutrophils, in addition to their well-known antimicrobial roles, modulate the inflammatory activities of the chronic immune system.[39]

Chronic Inflammation

Chronic inflammation begins with the infiltration of *monocytes* and *lymphocytes.* Unlike neutrophils, monocytes

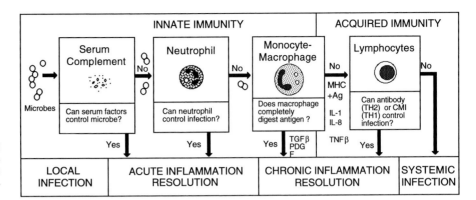

FIGURE 10-1. Host defense against local and systemic infections of periodontal origin. (Based on Miyasaki KT. The neutrophil: Mechanisms of controlling periodontal bacteria. J Periodontol *62*:761–774, 1991.)

and lymphocytes primarily infiltrate connective tissue and develop into tissue macrophages and activated lymphocytes. They seldom follow the neutrophil into the crevicular arena. Almost half of the energy of macrophages is derived from mitochondrial respiration and oxidative phosphorylation. The macrophages ingest particulate and soluble microbial antigens and may present partially digested antigen in association with major histocompatibility complex (MHC)–encoded class II molecules to lymphocytes. Lymphocytes, which predominate in the connective tissue infiltrate, may generate specific immunologic responses if presented with antigen-charged MHC class II molecules and a costimulatory signal such as membrane interleukin-1 (IL-1 or B7-1, B7-2, or B7-3). Chronic immune cells then elaborate cytokines, which induce the differentiation and activation of local immune cells and potentially signal the destruction or repair of the surrounding connective tissues. Chronic inflammation is aimed at preventing systemic infection, even if the price of such protection is local tissue injury.

NORMAL NEUTROPHIL FUNCTIONS

Neutrophils can crawl at a rate of about 400 μm/hr. This may seem fast, but it actually amounts to only about 40 cell lengths per hour. Hence, the neutrophil uses the circulatory system to travel rapidly about the body. Still, the primary role of the neutrophil is the destruction of pathogens that threaten tissues outside of the blood, including the periodontium. For this reason, leaving the blood, finding targets, and killing targets (Fig. 10–2) are important phagocyte functions in the defense of the periodontium.

Margination and Diapedesis

Neutrophils adhere to the luminal surface of the vascular endothelium (rolling, margination) and migrate across the endothelium (diapedesis, interendothelial transmigration).[36] There are two phases of leukocyte–endothelium adherence: the selectin-dependent phase (primarily involved in rolling) and the integrin-dependent phase (primarily involved in diapedesis).

Selectins

Selectins (Fig. 10–3*A*) are closely related to the regulators of complement activation (RCA) gene region products (such as CR1 and factor H). Like the regulators, they are encoded on chromosome 1 and possess complement regulatory (CR) motifs referred to as *short consensus repeats* that may be important in binding C3, C4, and C5 metabolites. In addition, the selectins possess lectin and epidermal growth factor (EGF)–like domains. Lectin activity (i.e., specific carbohydrate binding) is important in the adhesion of phagocytes to the endothelium. Some of the initial, reversible rolling contact between the leukocyte and uninflamed endothelium is mediated by L-selectin, which is constitutively expressed on the surface of the leukocyte. Inflammation causes endothelium to immediately express

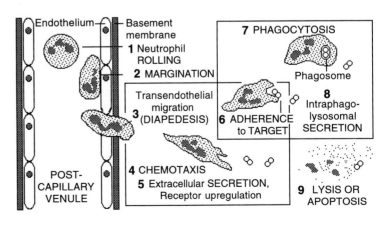

FIGURE 10-2. Normal neutrophil functions. Neutrophils continually make contact with the capillary wall to determine whether the endothelium expresses surface molecules that promote more firm contact and eventual egress of the neutrophils into the tissues. Neutrophils then seek targets by sensing chemical gradients. As neutrophils approach the target, they release molecules that can influence the behavior of other leukocytes. They finally neutralize the target by several mechanisms. (From Miyasaki K. Immunology for Dental Students. Unpublished.)

A. SELECTINS

B. LEUKOCYTE β2 INTEGRINS

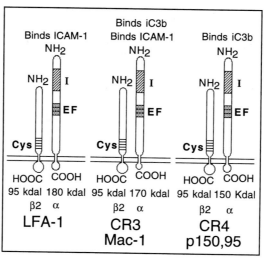

FIGURE 10–3. Leukocyte adhesion molecules. (From Miyasaki K. Immunology for Dental Students. Unpublished.)

P-selectin, which it stores in granules (Weibel-Palade bodies), and also induces the biosynthesis of E-selectin. Both P- and E-selectin strengthen the binding between the leukocyte and the endothelial cell and increase the number of leukocytes "rolling" in the inflamed postcapillary venule, the first manifestation of margination. P-selectin binds to the ligand gp150-Lewis x, and E-selectin binds to sialo-Lewis x, carbohydrate-bearing moieties found on leukocyte surfaces.

Inflammation also induces endothelium to produce the chemokine (intercrine), endothelial interleukin-8 (IL-8). Cytokines are dissipated rapidly by hemodynamic flow, and thus it is important that the leukocyte be temporarily immobilized by the selectins in order to be affected by the endothelial IL-8.

Leukocyte β_2-Integrins

IL-8 causes the leukocyte to shed L-selectin (and therefore was once referred to as *leukocyte adhesion inhibitor*) and to express the β_2-integrins, which are sequestered in the specific granules. The leukocyte β_2 integrins (Fig. 10–3B) include three related transmembranous glycoproteins consisting of a noncovalently associated heteroduplex structure. They share a common β_2 subunit and differ in the α subunit. The three leukocyte integrins are leukocyte function–associated antigen-1 (LFA-1; CD11a/CD18), Mac-1 (CD11b/CD18; complement receptor 3), and p150,95 (CD11c/CD18; complement receptor 4). The distribution of LFA-1 is greater than that of the other two leukocyte β_2-integrins, found on virtually all leukocytes (including lymphocytes) except some tissue macrophages. Both LFA-1 and Mac-1 are important in diapedesis. LFA-1 and Mac-1 interact with fairly widespread intercellular adhesion molecules (ICAMs), ICAM-1 and ICAM-2. The leukocyte β_2-integrins are particularly appealing as the molecular mediators of binding to endothelial cells, as their binding affinity can be increased or decreased as the leukocyte traverses the postcapillary venule.

At the beginning of transendothelial migration, neutrophils show distinct polarization, extending a pseudopod

between the endothelial cells while maintaining the nuclei and granules on the luminal side. The neutrophil eventually works its way to the serosal side of the endothelium, where it pauses briefly between the basement membrane and the endothelial cell before entering the connective tissues.

Chemotaxis

Chemotaxis is the directed movement of a cell along a chemical gradient. The neutrophil is attracted by chemical signals (chemotaxins) from multiple sources (Table 10–1). This multiplicity permits the neutrophil to respond to many different insults and also provides a redundant system that enables the neutrophil to respond to insult even if one receptor is defective. Both C5a and formyl peptides are likely to play a major role in attracting neutrophils into the gingival crevice. The gingival crevice contains 23% to 85% of the major complement components,[81] and activation has also been demonstrated in crevicular fluid.[82] Formyl peptides are the initial translation products of prokaryotic protein synthesis.

Chemotaxin Receptors

Chemotaxis requires that the phagocyte possess specific chemotaxin receptors for all of the molecules listed in Table 10–1. The most well-studied chemotaxin receptor is

Table 10–1. CHEMOATTRACTANTS FOR NEUTROPHILS

Source	Attractant
Macrophage/monocytes	Leukotriene B4
	IL-8
Many cells	Platelet activating factor
Serum/plasma	C5a, C5 *ades*Arg
Bacteria	f-Met peptides
Mast cells	Neutrophil chemotactic factor
Endothelium	Endothelial IL-8
B cells, macrophages	Interleukin 1

the receptor for formylmethionyl peptides, known as the *formylmethionyl peptide receptor* (FPR). The normal human neutrophil expresses about 50,000 FPRs per cell. The FPR is a transmembrane glycoprotein (about 32 kd, unglycosylated) and binds to formylated hydrophobic peptides derived from bacteria. The affinity of the FPR is modulated by a cytosolic, 40-kd guanosine triphosphate/guanosine diphosphate (GTP/GDP)–binding G protein. The G protein is sensitive to certain microbial toxins, and both cholera and pertussis toxins, which are adenosine diphosphate (ADP)-ribosylate G proteins, inhibit chemotaxis and high-affinity binding of formylmethionyleucyl-phenylalanine (FMLP) by the FPR.

The FPR belongs to a superfamily of G protein–coupled receptors (Fig. 10–4A) which includes light receptors, neuropeptide receptors, and more distantly, the receptors for neurotransmitters.[57] The chemotaxin receptors possess similar structures, as shown in Figure 10–4B. They are deeply imbedded within the cell membrane and feature three extracellular loops (designated EL-1, -2, and -3), three cytoplasmic loops (designated CL-1, -2, and -3), and seven transmembrane domains. The G proteins are coupled to CL-3.

Binding of Neutrophils to Targets: Opsonization

Opsonization refers to the process of coating a particle with recognizable molecules to enable phagocytic ingestion. Simplistically, there are two types of opsonins that should

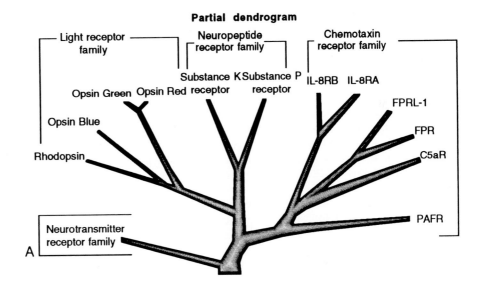

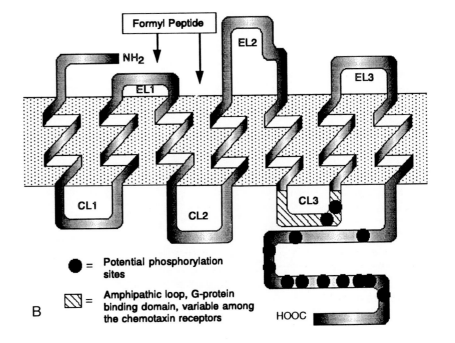

FIGURE 10–4. Chemotaxin receptors and their relatives in the G protein–coupled receptor superfamily. *A,* G protein receptor superfamily. (From Murphy PM, Özçelik T, Kenney RT, et al. A structural homologue of the N-formyl peptide receptor. J Biol Chem *267*:7637, 1992.) *B,* Formyl peptide receptor. (Redrawn from Snyderman R, Uhing RJ. Chemoattractant stimulus-responsive coupling. In Gallin JJ, Goldstein IM, Snyderman, R, eds. Inflammation: Basic Principles and Clinical Correlates. 2nd ed. New York, Raven Press, 1992.)

be considered: the complement metabolite, iC3b, and immunoglobulin G (IgG). Both the alternative and classic pathways of complement activation ultimately produce C3b bound covalently to the target surface. Once C3b is formed, its further metabolism is controlled by the regulators of complement activation, a group of related proteins encoded on chromosome 1. The phagocyte possesses a regulator, CR1, that serves as a cofactor (to a serum enzyme, factor I) that binds to C3b. In so doing, CR1 directs factor I to place a small "nick" in C3b to form iC3b. This abrogates the complement cascade and provides iC3b for endocytosis. (Amplification and opsonization are mutually exclusive.) Important in binding iC3b are the leukocyte β_2-integrins, Mac-1 (CR3) and p150,95 (CR4).

Phagocytic adhesion to targets may also be mediated by antibody using surface receptors collectively known as *Fc receptors.* The three main types of Fc receptors for the phagocytes are the IgG receptors FcγRI, FcγRII, and FcγRIII. FcγRI is a high-affinity receptor found mainly on macrophages. The other two are low-affinity receptors found on both macrophages and neutrophils. There are no known Fc receptors for immunoglobulin M (IgM).

The precise mechanism of phagocyte adhesion to targets may vary with disease states. Both gingivitis and adult periodontitis (AP) have been characterized primarily as involving alternative pathway activation,[82] which suggests that complement activation and opsonization in AP occur mainly via the alternative pathway. In localized juvenile periodontitis (LJP), probably in the later stages, C3, B, and C4 cleavage is observed. The complement cleavage patterns observed indicate greater classic pathway activation in LJP, which suggests a higher degree of opsonic antibody interacting with target antigen (i.e., *Actinobacillus actinomycetemcomitans*).

Antimicrobial Systems

Neutrophils have oxidative and nonoxidative mechanisms for exerting antimicrobial effects. Oxidative mechanisms are based on reduction of oxygen with resultant formation of toxic oxygen metabolites. Nonoxidative mechanisms in general appear to be based on membrane-disruptive antibi-

otic activities of peptides or peptide domains within larger proteins. Antimicrobial components localize to virtually every cellular compartment (Fig. 10–5).[55] Specific granules contain lactoferrin, lysozyme, and B_{12}-binding protein (cobalophilin) within their matrices and cytochrome *b* within their membrane. Azurophil granules contain myeloperoxidase; defensins; members of the neutral serine protease family, including cathepsin G, leukocyte elastase, proteinase 3, and azurocidin; lysozyme; and bactericidal/permeability-increasing protein. The cytosol contains a microbiostatic factor called *calprotectin,*[3] and the nucleus contains microbicidal histones.

The oxidative mechanisms include a nicotinamide-adenine dinucleotide phosphate (NADPH) oxidase and an enzyme, myeloperoxidase (MPO). Oxidative antibacterial effects are mediated by two main biochemical entities: the NADPH oxidase system and MPO. The NADPH oxidase system is required to transport electrons from the cytosolic NADPH to the external surface of the plasma membrane, where NADPH oxidase univalently or divalently reduces oxygen to superoxide anion or hydrogen peroxide, respectively. Hydrogen peroxide is mildly toxic to a number of oral pathogens. In the presence of hydrogen peroxide, MPO catalyzes the formation of a highly destructive bleach-like substance, hypochlorous acid, which is lethal to most microbes.

NEUTROPHIL ABNORMALITIES

Primary neutrophil defects are often associated with severe forms of periodontal disease and pyogenic infection of the host. Some of these diseases are listed in Table 10–2.

Neutropenia and Agranulocytosis

Neutropenia and agranulocytosis are signs of diseases or disease processes. An individual is said to be neutropenic if neutrophil counts are below 1500 mm[3] and to exhibit agranulocytosis if counts drop below 500 mm[3] (normal individuals have neutrophil counts between 5000 and 10,000/mm[3]). Some of the known causes of neutropenia in-

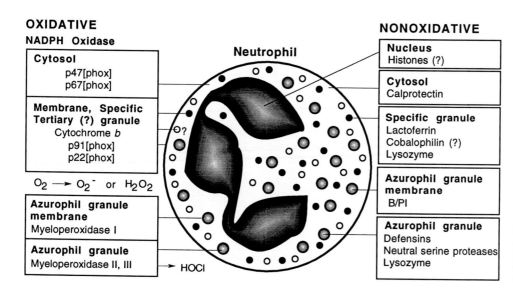

OXIDATIVE

NADPH Oxidase

Cytosol
p47[phox]
p67[phox]

Membrane, Specific Tertiary (?) granule
Cytochrome *b*
p91[phox]
p22[phox]

$O_2 \longrightarrow O_2^-$ or H_2O_2

Azurophil granule membrane
Myeloperoxidase I

Azurophil granule
Myeloperoxidase II, III

$\longrightarrow$ HOCl

Neutrophil

NONOXIDATIVE

Nucleus
Histones (?)

Cytosol
Calprotectin

Specific granule
Lactoferrin
Cobalophilin (?)
Lysozyme

Azurophil granule membrane
B/PI

Azurophil granule
Defensins
Neutral serine proteases
Lysozyme

FIGURE 10–5. Antimicrobial systems of neutrophils. (Based on Miyasaki KT. The neutrophil: Mechanisms of controlling periodontal bacteria. J Periodontol *62:*761–774, 1991.)

Table 10-2. PRIMARY DISORDERS OF PHAGOCYTES AND ASSOCIATED MANIFESTATIONS

Granulocyte Disorder	Periodontal Sign
Neutropenia	Severe periodontitis
Agranulocytosis	Severe periodontitis
Myelosuppression	Severe periodontitis
Hyperimmunoglobulinemia E (Job's syndrome)	Periodontitis, oral ulceration
Chédiak–Higashi syndrome	Severe periodontitis, oral ulceration
Papillon–Lefèvre syndrome	Severe periodontitis, both primary and secondary dentitions
Chronic granulomatous disease	Periodontitis? Oral ulceration
Specific granule deficiency	Severe periodontitis, oral ulceration
Leukocyte adhesion deficiency	Severe periodontitis, gingivitis, oral ulceration

clude drugs (idiosyncratic), infections, and autoimmune disorders in which the neutrophil is the target. Human immunodeficiency virus (HIV) infection has resulted in an increase in autoimmune neutropenia, as well as thrombocytopenia, a form of antibody-mediated cytotoxic autoimmunity (type II hypersensitivity reaction; see Chapter 8). As yet no association has been found between periodontal disease and HIV-induced autoimmune neutropenia, but this is a potential consideration. In any event, severe, intractable periodontal disease is fairly widely reported in circumstances in which the number of neutrophils has been diminished.[3,8,41,86]

Leukocyte Adhesion Deficiency

Type I

Leukocyte adhesion deficiency, type 1 (LAD-I) is an autosomal disorder (localized to chromosome 21q22.3) characterized by the inability of individuals to express the β_2 subunit (CD18) common to the leukocyte integrins LFA-1, Mac-1, and p150/95. The deficiency is profound, and individuals with LAD-I express leukocyte integrins at levels less than 6% of normal. Periodontal disease is related to whether one or two defective alleles are present.[99] Homozygotes exhibit generalized prepubertal periodontal (GPP), which affects both the deciduous and the permanent dentition. Heterozygotes appear to have normal prepubertal periodontal status. However, "post-LJP-like" lesions appear at some point postpubertally. The studies that associate GPP with LAD-I tend to suggest that LAD-I is the only contributor to GPP. This may not necessarily be true (except, perhaps, by definition), and several congenital neutrophil defects have been associated with severe periodontitis. Because of the rarity of these diseases, it cannot yet be stated that other congenital defects are associated with GPP.

Type II

There appears to be a selectin–ligand deficiency (i.e., the leukocytes do not express sialo-Lewis x or gp150-Lewis x), referred to as *leukocyte adhesion deficiency, type II* (LAD-II), in which neutrophil rolling does not increase in response to inflammation. Individuals with this deficiency suffer from recurrent bacterial infections, neutrophilia (20,000–70,000 neutrophils/mm^3), and severe, early-onset periodontitis.[65a]

Hyperimmunoglobulinemia E

Hyperimmunoglobulinemia (HIE; also known as *Job's syndrome*) is a rare, complex autosomal recessive disorder (possibly localized to chromosome 7q21) characterized by marked elevation of immunoglobulin E (IgE), variable defects in neutrophil chemotaxis, chronic dermatitis (eczematoid rash), "coarse facies," and serious, life-long bouts of recurrent infections with opportunistic organisms (*Staphylococcus aureus* and *Candida albicans*) that result in skin abscesses remarkable for their lack of erythema ("cold" abscesses). Abscesses can involve any organ. Invariably, infections are noted within the first 6 weeks of life. The term *Job's syndrome* is a Biblical reference to Job, who was afflicted with boils from head to foot. Coarse facial features include a broadened nasal bridge and irregularly proportioned cheeks and mandible. The cause of HIE is unclear, but it has been suggested that the balance between the T-cell elaboration of cytokines IL-4 and interferon-γ (INF-γ) (the two hormones involved in the regulation of IgE production) is defective. (IL-4 is protagonistic, and IFN-γ is antagonistic.) It has been proposed that the neutrophil chemotaxis defect may be related to defective IFN-γ production, as neutrophils from individuals with HIE apparently demonstrate improved chemotaxis when exposed to IFN-γ.[32]

Data suggest that cyclooxygenase pathway products can also produce osteoporotic changes in subjects with HIE.[43] Circulating immune complexes (ICs)—which appear to be IgG anti-IgE complexed against IgE Fc—are observed in the sera of afflicted individuals. ICs can impair leukocyte chemotaxis, suggesting a second mechanism of impaired leukocyte chemotaxis. Other investigators[10] provide evidence suggesting that mast cells, armed with IgE against inappropriate bacterial targets, release histamine when confronted by bacteria. Histamine also impairs neutrophil functions such as chemotaxis. Mononuclear cells from the blood of patients with HIE also release a 60-kd factor that impairs neutrophil function. Periodontal disease in individuals with HIE has been noted, and the preceding summary of HIE should suggest at least a few of the potential underlying mechanisms for this association.

Chédiak-Higashi Syndrome

Chédiak-Higashi syndrome (CHS) is a rare disease with an autosomal recessive mode of inheritance (possibly localized to chromosome 1q43). A structural defect, the fusion of azurophil and specific granules into giant granules called *megabodies,* is characteristic of neutrophils from individuals with this disease. Functional neutrophil defects include decreased chemotaxis, degranulation, and microbicidal activity. A biochemical defect, the relative lack of neutral serine proteases, has also been observed in CHS. Neutropenia and depressed inflammation are also observed. The depressed inflammation is thought to be due to decreased chemotaxis and secretion, not neutropenia. The formation of reduced oxygen metabolites is greatly exaggerated. Oral manifestations of this disease include severe periodontitis and oral ulceration.[10]

Specific Granule Deficiency

Specific granule deficiency (SGD) is a rare disease, probably autosomal recessive, which was originally described as a disease in which neutrophils lacked specific granules. Now it is clear that SGD represents a failure to package whole groups of proteins (both specific and azurophil granule proteins) into the granules. Specific granule proteins that are missing include lactoferrin, cobalophilin, cytochrome *b*, the FPR, C5a receptor, and CR3.

A deficiency of these components results in depressed respiratory burst activity, diminished ability to respond to chemotaxins, and poor phagocytosis. Packaging of defensins into azurophil granules is also defective in SGD. Therefore, intraphagolysosomal killing is predictably sluggish. Decreases in inflammation may also be predicted on the basis of the deficiency of chemotaxin receptors, both because these cells are less responsive chemotactically and because they do not secrete inflammatory mediators at normal levels. The disease is probably autosomal recessive, although there have been too few cases to analyze thoroughly. Oral manifestations of this disease include severe periodontitis and oral ulceration.[10]

Papillon-Lefèvre Syndrome

Papillon-Lefèvre syndrome (PLS) features rapid generalized destruction of alveolar bone (affecting both the primary and secondary dentition) and palmar-plantar hyperkeratosis. The exact immunologic abnormality (if any) that contributes to this condition is unknown; however, one report indicates that PLS may be associated with diminished neutrophil activity.[95] Neutrophils from an individual with PLS had decreased receptor affinity for chemotaxin ligands such as formyl peptides. Studies suggest that another systemic immunologic abnormality is an increase in circulating natural killer (NK) cells, although the periodontal lesions associated with PLS appear to be fairly typical plasma cell–dominated lesions.[26]

Chronic Granulomatous Disease

Chronic granulomatous disease (CGD) is clinically diagnosed by the presence of recurrent, indolent, pyogenic infections with certain bacteria. The cause of this problem is the inability of host phagocytes to mount a normal respiratory burst. The inability to rapidly dispatch bacteria, which then gain access to the connective tissues, leads to the formation of granulomas by the chronic immune cells. Several biochemical defects have been associated with CGD, including a deficiency in the membrane expression of cytochrome *b*, a transmembranous heterodimer that reduces oxygen to the antimicrobial oxidants superoxide anion and hydrogen peroxide. The X-linked form involves a mutation in the gene encoding the heavy subunit of cytochrome *b* (*p91phox*). An autosomal recessive form of CGD that mimics the X-linked form (i.e., the absence of cytochrome *b*)

involves the mutation of the small subunit of cytochrome *b* (*p22phox*) and is encoded on chromosome 16q24.[20] Two forms of CGD do not show diminished expression of cytochrome *b* but lack certain cytosolic proteins that shuttle electrons from NADPH to cytochrome *b*.[58,98]

These autosomal recessive forms have been associated with a defect in neutrophil cytosolic factors 1 and 2 (NCF-1 and NCF-2; also called *p47phox* and *p67phox*). The deficiency in NCF-1 has been localized to chromosome 7q11–23 and the deficiency in NCF-2 to chromosome 1q25.[91] Individuals with CGD exhibit greater than normal oral ulceration and gingivitis,[10] but CGD has not been strongly associated with severe periodontitis,[13] which suggests that oxidative antimicrobial mechanisms may not be very important in the gingival crevice and that the frequent regimen of antibiotics used in such cases has affected the periodontal ecology.

OTHER DISEASES ASSOCIATED WITH LEUKOCYTE DISORDERS

A number of disorders (e.g., Down syndrome, diabetes mellitus, and malnutrition) secondarily affect leukocyte function.[9,15,30,51,93] Many of these diseases also variably express severe periodontal disease. Because the correlation between these diseases and periodontal disease status is not perfect and because these individuals often have other biochemical problems, it is more difficult to assign relevance to the defective function of the phagocytes.

SEVERE PERIODONTAL DISEASES

Localized Juvenile Periodontitis

Chronic inflammatory adult periodontitis (AP) is a disease characterized by loss of attachment of between 0.072 and 0.36 mm/yr when averaged over many years and is usually associated with plaque and calculus. Several severe forms of periodontal diseases show much greater rates of attachment loss with less associated plaque and calculus. LJP is a severe form of periodontal disease that affects teenagers (usually near puberty). This disease is characterized by attachment loss (estimated rate of loss, 1.08 to 1.8 mm/yr), mainly about the secondary first molars and incisors (possibly reflecting eruption sequence), and very little macroscopic plaque (see Chapter 27).

The understanding of LJP represents an important step in the ability to comprehend the function of the immune system in periodontal diseases, because it provides a very important clue to the protective role of the neutrophil. Neutrophils from individuals with LJP possess an intrinsic defect in phagocytosis and chemotaxis (Table 10–3). Neutrophils from individuals with LJP also may exhibit increased levels of O_2 production, leading some to speculate that neutrophils may participate in the destruction of host tissues by generating toxic oxidants. It is probable that the disease can be caused by several different biochemical defects in the host neutrophil.

Neutrophils from individuals with LJP exhibit a selective decrease in ability to kill *A. actinomycetemcomitans*, de-

Table 10-3. LOCALIZED JUVENILE PERIODONTITIS AND RAPIDLY PROGRESSIVE PERIODONTITIS[31-37]

Periodontal Disorder	PMN Defect
Localized juvenile periodontitis (type 1)	Intrinsic chemotaxis (CTx) defect
	Decreased binding of chemotaxins
	40% decreased GP110
	Decreased phagocytosis
Localized juvenile periodontitis (type not specified)	Specific decreased ability to kill *A. actinomycetemcomitans*
Localized juvenile periodontitis (one case)	Decreased CTx to FMLP only
	Decreased FMLP receptor
Rapidly progressive periodontitis (adult)	Extrinsic CTx defect
	Phagocytosis defect without CTx defect
	Poor opsonization of *A. actinomycetemcomitans*
Generalized juvenile periodontitis	CTx defect, increased random migration

FMLP, Formylmethionyleucyl-phenylalanine; PMN, polymorphonuclear neutrophil.

spite normal phagocytosis, O_2 production, and secretion of specific granule components. It has been suggested that this defect lies in decreased ability of LJP neutrophils to undergo phagosome–lysosome fusion.

Neutrophils from individuals with the classic form of LJP (i.e., LJP-1) are characterized by a decrease in chemotactic responses to a variety of chemotactic factors, including C5a, FMLP (a formyl peptide), and leukotriene B_4.[60] The neutrophil dysfunction is associated with a functional decrease in chemotaxin receptors on the polymorphonuclear neutrophil (PMN) surface. The defect has been described as a *pan-receptor defect,* because all chemotaxin receptors appear to be decreased.

Van Dyke et al. have described about a 40% deficiency in a 110-kd membrane glycoprotein in LJP.[97] The exact function of GP110 is unknown, but antibodies against GP110 block neutrophil chemotaxis. Because GP110 is expressed late in cell differentiation at about the time that chemotaxin receptor expression occurs, it has been proposed that GP110 associates with all chemotaxin receptors, thus explaining the global aspect of the defect observed in LJP. The inheritance mode of LJP is still unclear; although some data suggest that it is inherited in an autosomal recessive manner, one report suggests an autosomal dominant mode of inheritance, localization to chromosome 4, and linkage to the gene involved in dentinogenesis imperfecta.[6]

A second form of LJP, dubbed *LJP-2,* has been described. This form manifests as clinical lesions identical to those seen in LJP-1; however, neither decreased chemotaxis, FMLP, or C5a receptors nor GP110 is observed in laboratory studies of patient neutrophils.

In one reported case, LJP may be associated with a defective FPR.[65] In this case the neutrophils were defective in their ability to migrate in response to FMLP but normal in their response to C5a. Furthermore, both secretory and respiratory burst activity was normal in response to FMLP. This unusual form of LJP is inconsistent with previous observations of a pan-receptor defect, diminished GP110, and genetic localization to chromosome 4 (the FPR is encoded on chromosome 19). This form of LJP may be a cleaner "natural experiment" and shows that the important lesion of LJP-1 is really the decreased expression of the FPR, and all the other neutrophil receptor defects associated with LJP are epiphenomenal (Fig. 10-6). The FPR of individuals

with LJP reported may differ from those of normal individuals.[17]

The reason that LJP is limited to certain sites is unknown. However, it has been proposed that the site limitation is a result of a time-dependent "window of opportunity." Antibody (with complement) is absolutely required for the opsonization of *A. actinomycetemcomitans.*[4] This indicates that antibody responses must be initiated before

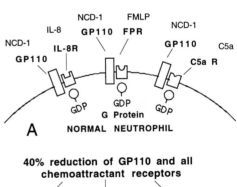

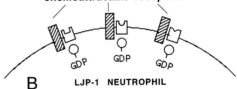

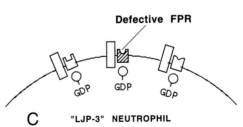

FIGURE 10-6. Normal *(A),* LJP-1 *(B),* and LJP-3 *(C)* neutrophils. *(B,* Data from Van Dyke TE, Wilson-Burrows C, Offenbacher S, Henson PM. Association of an abnormality of neutrophil chemotaxis in human periodontal disease with a cell surface protein. Infect Immun *55:*2262, 1987. *C,* Data from Perez HD, Kelly E, Elfman F, et al. Defective polymorphonuclear leukocyte formyl peptide receptor(s) in juvenile periodontitis. J Clin Invest *87:*971, 1991.) (From Miyasaki K. Immunology for Dental Students. Unpublished.)

neutrophils can kill this microbe. The time required to produce antibodies of the proper isotype, specificity, and affinity may be prolonged by immunosuppressive factors elaborated by the microbe[83] and represents a potential "window of opportunity" during which time the organism may be able to induce considerable local tissue changes.

Rapidly Progressive Periodontitis

Rapidly progressive periodontitis (RPP) is a severe form of periodontal disease afflicting young adults and/or postpubescent individuals.[70] Generalized juvenile periodontitis (GJP) has been associated with plaque and calculus, which suggests a somewhat different microbial etiology than LJP. Neutrophils from such individuals appear to exhibit chemotaxis disorders and no alteration in GP110. The chemotaxis disorders may result from some other phagocyte problem. Kishimoto has reported that serum from individuals with RPP, as well as serum from nondiseased individuals, did not support phagocytosis of *A. actinomycetemcomitans*.[36] RPP probably represents a mixture of several diseases, including rapidly progressive adult periodontitis (RAP).

Individuals with RAP have a mean age of about 40 years (range, 30 to 62). The chief diagnostic criterion appears to be subjective, and diagnosis is often based on the opinion of the referring periodontist (i.e., the attachment loss is inconsistent with age and plaque levels). One of the earliest studies found that in 3 of the 19 cases studied (16%), intrinsic defects in leukocyte chemotaxis could be observed (as in LJP-1). On the other hand, 6 of 19 (32%) exhibited factors in the serum that impaired leukocyte function. Some of these factors were immunoglobulins that functioned as cell-directed inhibitors (CDIs) of chemotaxis rather than as autoantibodies.[42] The difference between a CDI and an autoantibody is that the CDI functions via its Fc region rather than its Fab region by unexplained mechanisms. In one case an elevated factor in serum led to inactivation of the chemotaxin; this factor is known as a *chemotactic factor inactivator* (CFI). Extrinsic and intrinsic defects in cell function were not observed in 53% of the cases.

Intrinsic neutrophil defects have also been described in RAP. Abnormalities in leukocyte (neutrophil and monocyte) motility have been observed in some cases.[1] No defects in leukocyte motility could be observed in 13 RAP patients in Japan; instead, neutrophils from patients afflicted by RAP have impaired phagocytosis.[34]

Acquired Functional Neutrophil Defects

A number of pathogens secrete leukotoxins, Ig proteases, high-molecular-weight chemotaxis inhibitors (pertussis and cholera toxins, which catalyze the ribosylation of G proteins by ADP), inhibitors of phagosome–lysosome fusion, low-molecular-weight chemotaxis inhibitors, and lipo- and polysaccharides, all of which can affect immune function. Thus, the bacteria themselves can produce the dysfunction within the immune system. Of interest are the low-molecular-weight inhibitors. It has been reported that the periodontal organism *Capnocytophaga* can induce chemotactic defects in vivo.[84]

Although the factors responsible for this induced defect have never been identified, it has been suggested that *Cap-*

nocytophaga and other oral gram-negative bacteria produce low-molecular-weight factors that inhibit the binding of the chemotaxin FMLP to the formylmethionyl peptide receptor (FPR) and also inhibit neutrophil chemotaxis.[94]

Other acquired disturbances may be hormonal, drug or radiation induced, viral, immune, or autoimmune. For example, estradiol (but not progesterone) inhibits neutrophil chemotaxis.[54] Antihistamines and tranquilizers can impede neutrophil phagolysosomal fusion. Also, the phenothiazines (promethazine [an antihistamine] and trifluoperazine [a tranquilizer]) can block specific granule aggregation mediated by annexins and calcium.[52]

CHRONIC INFLAMMATORY CELLS

The term *chronic inflammatory cell system* is used to refer to a network of cells that includes monocytes, other antigen-presenting cells, and lymphocytes. The chronic inflammatory cell system performs three tasks with respect to the periodontium:

1. It protects the deep periodontal tissues from infection.
2. It orchestrates connective tissue destruction to prevent bone and systemic infection.
3. It orchestrates connective tissue repair and healing.

This section will first briefly describe the interactions among the chronic cells and then discuss how changes in the chronic inflammatory cell system may influence periodontopathogenesis.

Monocytes and Macrophages

Unlike neutrophils, which exit the bone marrow as terminally differentiated cells, monocytes exit the bone marrow in a functionally immature condition. As a result, monocytes arrive from blood to the tissues as multipotential cells capable of differentiating in a variety of different ways. Once in the tissues, they are referred to as *macrophages* and differentiate along many different pathways to kill pathogens, regulate clearance of tissue debris, regulate tissue remodeling, and process exogenously derived antigens.

Macrophages differentiate in response to environmental factors. For example, T cells release IFN-γ and may induce the differentiation of macrophages into antigen-processing and -presenting cells. These antigen-processing and antigen-presenting macrophages have somewhat limited proliferative abilities. Bacterial lipopolysaccharide (LPS) induces macrophages to further differentiate into activated macrophages. Fully activated macrophages are capable of adhering to and killing tumors by releasing a cytolytic protease (a 40-kd neutral serine protease secreted only by fully activated macrophages) and tumor necrosis factor-α (TNF-α). Fully activated macrophages are incapable of proliferation. Monocytic cells influence both tissue repair and lymphocyte activity by releasing IL-3, IL-6, IL-8, IFN-α, transforming growth factor-β (TGF-β), and TNF-α (see Chapter 8).

Antigen Processing and Presentation

Antigen processing is the partial degradation of proteins that results in antigen presentation. *Antigen presentation* refers to the expression of peptides (derived by processing) on the cell surface in association with molecules encoded within an important gene complex known as the major histocompatibility complex (MHC), located on the short arm of chromosome 6. MHC class I molecules are also referred to as *human leukocyte antigens A, B,* or *C* (HLA-A, HLA-B, or HLA-C). MHC class II molecules are known as HLA-DR, HLA-DQ, and HLA-DP.

There are two intracellular pathways for protein degradation. First, the protein may be degraded in the cytosol via a polymeric neutral serine protease structure referred to as a *proteasome* and transported into the endoplasmic reticulum by proteins that span the membrane of the endoplasmic reticulum (i.e., adenosine triphosphate (ATP)–binding cassette proteins). The genes for both the proteasome and ATP-binding cassette proteins are encoded and tightly linked within the MHC class II region. Second, the protein may be degraded within the endoplasmic reticulum, probably by the leader sequence-specific enzyme, called the *signal peptidase*. In part, protein chaperones of the heat shock protein 70 family may be involved, and these are also encoded within the MHC. In either pathway, the resultant peptides are bound by MHC class I molecules within the endoplasmic reticulum, and the peptide–MHC class I molecule complex is subsequently expressed on the cell surface.

Most frequently, cells degrade their own proteins and therefore usually express MHC class I molecules on their surfaces in association with self-peptides. Intracellular infection or neoplastic alteration may lead to the expression of different peptides associated with the MHC class I molecules on the cell surface.

MHC class II molecules may be produced by all cells but are usually limited in distribution to "professional" antigen-presenting cells, including mononuclear phagocytes, Langerhans cells, and B cells. A "professional" antigen-presenting cell is a cell that can process and present antigens derived from the extracellular milieu. Most bacterial infections are extracellular. The host uses an endolysosomal pathway to process and present antigens derived from extracellular sources. In this pathway the host ingests the antigen by phagocytosis or pinocytosis.

Macrophages ingest antigen by phagocytosis (binding the target particle using the iC3b receptor CR3 [Mac-1] or the IgG-binding Fcγ receptors) and digest it within a phagolysosome. MHC class II molecules are sequestered within the membrane of storage granules (lysosomes) and become available as a result of fusion between the lysosomal and phagosomal membranes. Peptides associate with MHC class II molecules in the phagolysosome, and this complex is expressed ("presented") on the phagocyte surface by exocytosis.

Extracellular antigens may also be ingested by antigen-specific B cells (pinocytosis initiated by patching and capping). B cells utilize a receptor complex known as the *B-cell antigen receptor* (BCR) to bind antigen specifically for endocytosis. The antigen-specific component of the BCR is a transmembranous immunoglobulin (antibody). Ingestion of univalent antigens (as most proteins would be) may be aided by complement receptor 2 (the Epstein-Barr virus receptor) and/or antibodies directed against a second epitope and the Fc receptor, FcγRII (CD32). The B cell processes

the antigen using lysosomal proteases (the neutral protease, cathepsin B, and the acid protease cathepsin D) within an endolysosome. Peptides derived from partially degraded protein associate with MHC class II molecules within multilaminar MHC class II molecule–containing compartments (MIIC) and are expressed by exocytosis on the B-cell surface in association with MHC class II molecules.

Processed peptides are bound in two "specificity pockets" within a wide groove of the MHC class I or class II molecules. The peptides are bound specifically at two anchor positions: P2-3 and P9 of a nonameric peptide). The intervening five to seven amino acids float on a "bed of water" and may be in almost any sequence; thus the MHC molecules are far less specific than antibodies, which recognize four to six contiguous residues).

Lymphocytes

NK cells possess receptors that recognize peptides associated with MHC class I molecules. The peptides are derived from self-proteins, which are highly conserved among many phyla (e.g., ribosomal, mitochondrial, and heat shock proteins). Recognition of antigen by the NK cell blocks the activation of the NK cell.

Cytocidal activity is initiated when an "altered" peptide derived from an analogous highly conserved protein from the intracellular parasite is presented to the NK cell. If the NK cell does not recognize (bind) the peptide antigen, it proceeds to kill the infected cell. Note that the level of conservation theoretically may allow a "foreign" peptide to exhibit anchor position residues identical to those of the peptides derived from the host, yet also possess one or two amino acid substitutions in nonanchor positions.

T cells possess specific antigen receptors referred to as *T-cell antigen receptors* (TCRs). TCRs recognize the peptides associated with MHC class I or class II molecules. In contrast to NK cells, T cells are activated when the TCR recognizes antigen associated with MHC class I or class II molecules. The CD4+ coreceptor binds MHC class II molecules, and the CD8+ coreceptor binds MHC class I molecules. Therefore, CD4+ T cells respond to peptide antigens associated with MHC class II molecules, and CD8+ T cells respond to antigens associated with MHC class I molecules. T cells require one additional signal—the costimulatory signal—to allow proliferation. Membrane IL-1 is expressed by the antigen-presenting cell only if the environment is appropriate, and this provides the costimulatory signal to T cells, enabling them to express receptors for growth hormones (e.g., IL-2). The costimulatory signal that enables the clonal expansion of CD8+ T cells is referred to as *B7-2* and interacts with CD28 on the CD+ T cell.

Why do humans have both NK cells and CD8+ T cells? Conceptually, almost any NK cell can respond to the loss of a self-molecule on the target cell surface. Therefore, NK cell responses can be rapid. In contrast, only a small proportion of CD8+ T cells can respond to a new antigen expressed on the target cell surface. In comparison with NK cells, such responses are slower to generate on first exposure; however, CD8+ T-cell responses are much more sensitive and rapid than NK responses on second exposure. Thus, it is advantageous to maintain a negative surveillance mechanism (the NK cells) because of the time and energy required to generate antigen-specific, positive surveillance responses.

CD4$^+$ T cells have been divided into functional subpopulations based on which cells they induce to proliferate. The two major subpopulations include the CD4$^+$ suppressor-inducer T cells and CD4$^+$ helper T cells. Helper T cells are the classic helpers that stimulate B-cell differentiation. Suppressor-inducer T cells usually appear later in the immune response and induce the proliferation of CD8$^+$ cytotoxic or suppressor T cells. CD4$^+$ T cells have also been divided into subpopulations based on stable cytokine production profiles (see Chapter 8). T_H1 cells produce IL-2, IFN-γ, IL-3, IL-12, granulocyte/macrophage colony-stimulating factor (GM-CSF), and TNF-β (lymphotoxin). T_H2 cells produce IL-3, IL-4, IL-5, IL-6, IL-10, and GM-CSF. Either CD4$^+$ or CD8$^+$ T cells can express these phenotypes. CD4$^+$ T_H1 cells mediate delayed-type hypersensitivity reactions. IL-2 is a general proliferative signal.

B cells elaborate substances (i.e., soluble immunoglobulins and cytokines) that serve to regulate antigen levels and inflammation. This effectory function of B cells requires T-cell signals. B cells process antigen by the endolysosomal pathway and present peptide antigen associated with MHC class II molecules to peptide-specific CD4$^+$ T cells. This results in the expression of a membrane glycoprotein, gp39, by the T cell, which serves as a costimulatory signal for B cells.

CHRONIC INFLAMMATORY CELLS IN THE PERIODONTIUM

Gingival T and B Cells

Part of the pathogenesis of periodontal diseases, including gingivitis and various forms of periodontitis, involves a net increase in the number of gingival lymphocytes and monocytes within the periodontal connective tissues. This infiltration is observed clearly in the early lesion (which is considered clinical gingivitis). In children, gingivitis is a stable lesion that does not progress to periodontitis. The dominant cell type within the subjacent connective tissue in childhood gingivitis happens to be T lymphocytes — that is, childhood gingivitis is a T-cell lesion.[79] In experimental gingivitis in adults, the dominant cells type for up to 3 weeks are B cells[63] or T cells.[80] Seymour and Greenspan[78] observed that the lymphocytic infiltrate in the subjacent connective tissues of adult periodontitis was primarily cells of the B lineage (both activated B blasts and plasma cells) and advanced the concept that periodontitis was a B-cell lesion. The proportion of cells of the B lineage in the connective tissues at sites of active periodontitis can be as high as 90%. The T-cell density in active periodontal lesions appears to be very similar to that seen in the healthy state. Thus, the T-cell–to–B-cell ratio decrease is due not to a decrease in T cells, but to an increase in B cells.[67]

Hypothetically, the goal of periodontal therapy is conversion of the B-cell lesion to a T-cell lesion. In clinical practice, of course, it is impossible to monitor a B-cell–to–T-cell conversion.

Changes in Intragingival T-Cell Subpopulations

The persistence of the T-cell populations in periodontitis and the increase in B-cell activity led to a postulation that T-cell regulation of B cells was altered (dysfunctional) in periodontal disease. Taubman et al.[89] observed that the number of lymphocytes recoverable from periodontally diseased tissues is almost three times greater than that from normal tissues (Fig. 10–7, *left panel*) and that the ratio of CD4$^+$ and CD8$^+$ T cells was 1:1 in both adult and juvenile periodontitis (Fig. 10–7, *middle panel*). The CD4-to-CD8 ratio is 2:1 in gingivitis in children[53] and in health. These observations suggested an immunoregulatory change and clearly revealed that juvenile periodontitis is similar to the adult form with respect to mononuclear cell (monocyte/lymphocyte) phenotype. The increased B-cell activation seems paradoxical in the presence of increased proportions of CD8$^+$ T cells (presumably suppressors).

The B-Cell Paradox

At least in part, the activation of B cells in the presence of "inverted" CD4-to-CD8 ratios may be explicable in terms of subpopulations of CD4$^+$ T cells. Although the CD4-to-CD8 ratio may be inverted, a decrease in suppressor-inducer activity (i.e., T_H1 cytokines) could lead to relatively "unchecked" B-cell activation, because T_H1 cells are required to shut down antibody production by suppressing B-cell differentiation and activating CD8$^+$ supressor T cells. Periodontal lesions have been examined using monoclonal antibodies designated 2H4 and 4B4.[89] 2H4 identifies CD45RA, a molecule associated with naive or virgin cells prior to activation by exposure to antigen. 4B4 reacts with CDw29, which is associated with previously activated (memory) cells. Naive cells have also been functionally associated with suppressor-inducer activity, and memory T cells seem to be important in helper activity. Both a decrease in proportion of 4B4 (helper) T cells and a predominance of CD4$^+$ double-labeled 2H4/4B4 cells were observed (Fig. 10–7, *right panel*). The function of the double-labeled cell type is unknown. However, the increased polyclonal activity of B cells in the presence of CD8$^+$ T cells cannot be attributed to increases in the 4B4 phenotype, suggesting that there may be a decrease in CD4$^+$ suppressor-inducer T-cell activity. The CD8$^+$ T supressors may simply proliferate without complete functional differentiation.

Polyclonal B-Cell Activation

T-cell "dysregulation" may result in the apparent activation of IgG-, IgA-, or IgE-bearing B cells in a polyclonal manner. Although it is clear that antibody within the periodontal tissues can be antigen specific and react with such pathogens as *A. actinomycetemcomitans,* the vast majority of the immunoglobulins found in the periodontal tissues do not appear to be reactive to specific antigens. Polyclonal B-cell activation can also explain this observation, as well as the B-cell aspect of the periodontal lesion. Importantly, the polyclonal nature of the antibody response in periodontitis has been suggested to preclude the formation of extensive

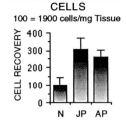

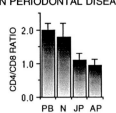

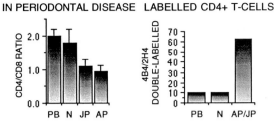

FIGURE 10−7. Characterization of gingival mononuclear cells. AP, Adult periodontitis; JP, juvenile periodontitis; PB, peripheral blood. (Data from Taubman MA, Stoufi ED, Seymour CJ, et al. Immunoregulatory aspects of periodontal disease. Adv Dent Res 2:328, 1988; and Armitt K. Identification of T-cell subsets in gingivitis in children. J Periodontol 57:3, 1986.)

insoluble immune complexes[12] and makes type III immunopathologic reactions (neutrophil-mediated attacks on immune complexes) unlikely. Perhaps a more important aspect of polyclonal B-cell activation is that it may lead to the production of soluble IL-1, which activates osteoclasts and impedes immunologic clearance of the pathogen.

Polyclonal activation of both naive, IgM-bearing B cells and IgG-, IgA-, and IgE-bearing B cells may also result from polyclonal B-cell activators (PBAs). PBAs are usually mitogenic (i.e., cause cell division ± T-cell help [cytokines]) and are usually T-independent antigens (i.e., can activate B cells specifically without T-cell help). The mechanism of interaction of PBAs probably differs with different activators. Some may be lectins that interact with B-cell surface glycoproteins; others may be charged carbohydrates. Usually, the B-cell mitogen is polyvalent. Dental plaque contains a number of components that can activate B cells in a polyclonal manner, including lipopolysaccharides, *Actinomyces viscosus, Fusobacterium nucleatum,* and *Porphyromonas gingivalis.*[64]

Localized Gingival Antibody Production

Gingival crevicular antibody does not originate as a serum exudate. Lally et al.[40] showed that gingival explants were capable of producing immunoglobulins in organ culture. Martin et al.[46] have demonstrated that organ culture antibody specificity is distinct from serum antibody specificity. Thus, both the subclass and specificity of the antibody response in periodontal tissues are distinct from those in serum. The periodontal lesion, as described previously, has a B-cell nature. Fifty-seven percent of the lymphocytic infiltrate in the connective tissues are plasma cells.

The gingiva in periodontitis is an organ of localized antibody production and is impregnated with very high levels of immunoglobulins (Table 10−4). Mackler et al[45] have demonstrated that there are differences in the immunoglobulin subclasses present in the inflamed gingivae and those present in serum. There is an enormous disparity between IgG2 and IgG4 subclasses in serum and the gingival tissues.

The amount of cytophilic antibody is about the same, but much of it appears to be IgG3 in the gingiva. Also, there is a relatively low proportion of IgG2, which suggests that polysaccharide antigens primarily induce IgM responses intragingivally. In total, these data clearly point to a significant separation of serum and gingival compartments.

Isotype switching involves B-cell activation and T-cell cytokines. B cells must be activated by "costimulatory signals" (e.g., gp39) or microbial components (e.g., dextran

plus IL-5) to be receptive to T-cell switch factors. For example, T$_H$2-cell−derived "B-cell switch factors"—IL-4, IL-5, and IL-6—can cause B cells to switch to IgG4 and IgA1 isotypes.[50]

Serologic Responses

Seroconversion (appearance of antibodies in the serum in response to antigenic challenge) is usually good immunologic evidence of an infection that was severe and protracted enough to elicit a regional lymph node response. Serologic studies have shown a good correlation between microbiologic culture of dental plaque in different periodontal diseases and serum antibody. Generally, individuals with AP possess antibodies to *P. gingivalis* and, to a lesser extent, *A. actinomycetemcomitans.*

Individuals with LJP possess antibodies to *A. actinomycetemcomitans* and, to a lesser extent, *P. gingivalis.*[22] Serum antibody appears to correlate with microorganisms cultured from sites approximately 80% of the time when the lesion is deemed active but only 20% of the time when the lesion is deemed inactive.

The strongest case can be made in LJP. There is a very strong correlation among antibodies to *A. actinomycetemcomitans,* LJP, and the culture of *A. actinomycetemcomitans.* LJP lesions appear to occur prior to seroconversion but nevertheless may progress locally (as a result of other complications) in the presence of high serum titers. The synthesis of antibody may be delayed until localized destruction is severe, as *A. actinomycetemcomitans* appears to elaborate an immunosuppressive factor that may extend the "window of opportunity" discussed previously.[83] Recent serologic data suggest that LJP also involves chronic exposure to *P. gingivalis.*[102]

Table 10−4. GINGIVAL ANTIBODY PRODUCTION

Subclass	Serum %	Gingival %	T$_{1/2}$ (days)	Functions
IgG1	70	40	20	Cytophilic; likely to interact with leukocytes; fix C
IgG2	18	2	24	Often produced against polysaccharides, LTA
IgG3	8	28	7	Cytophilic; likely to interact with leukocytes: fix C
IgG4	4	30		Variable homeostasis?

C, Complement; LTA, lipoteichoic acid.

It is unclear at what point in the infection and subsequent disease process initial seroconversion occurs, and it is also unknown how long serum titers remain elevated after the infection has subsided. In an attempt to address the latter issue, Ebersole et al.[21] examined the serum response in a longitudinal manner following subgingival scaling and aggressive treatment (multiple-site surgery and antibiotics; see later discussion). Interestingly, most patients manifest an increase in antibodies against certain pathogens after scaling. The increase in antibody titers peaks 100 to 200 days after scaling (Fig. 10–8). The reason for the antibody increase is unclear, but it may relate to the inoculation of microorganisms into the host tissues resulting from scaling. It may represent a more complex process involving a simplification of the microbial challenge. Therapy that includes surgery and antibiotics leads to a gradual decline in antibody. This decline in antibody titers takes about 1 year.

Natural Killer Cells

NK cells constitute between 3% and 7% of the total mononuclear cell infiltrate in periodontitis.[64] NK cells have been associated with the active B-cell lesion and are virtually absent in healthy gingivae.[101] The NK cell clearly has important immunoregulatory functions (e.g., production of IFN-γ). The role of the NK cell in periodontal disease is as yet unknown.

Cytokines

Cytokines are expressed by essentially all nucleated cells and platelets. However, certain cells are much more active at producing certain cytokines than are other cells. Bone, like all connective tissues, is continually broken down and remodeled. The chronic immune system cytokines may affect both osteoclastic bone resorption and osteoblastic bone formation and may stimulate net bone loss or net bone formation, increase both processes to increase the rate of remodeling, or decrease both processes to decrease the rate of remodeling.

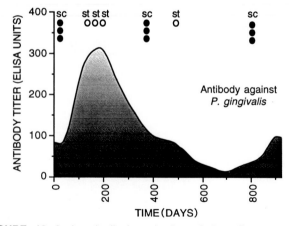

FIGURE 10–8. Longitudinal evaluation of the effectiveness of serum antibodies against periodontal bacteria. (Modified from Ebersole JL, Frey DE, Taubman MA, et al. Dynamics of systemic antibody responses in periodontal disease. J Periodont Res 22:184, 1987. © Munksgaard International Publishers Ltd, Copenhagen, Denmark.)

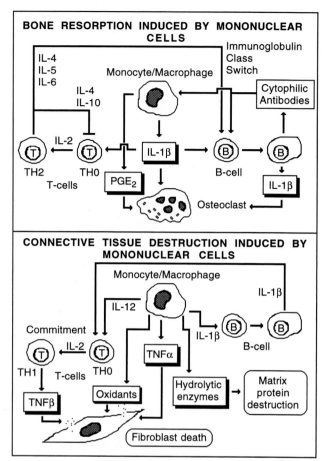

FIGURE 10–9. The central role of the monocyte/macrophage in alterations of bone and connective tissues. (From Miyasaki K. Immunology for Dental Students. Unpublished.)

Cytokines and Net Bone Loss

Dental scientists first revealed that IL-1b and the main osteoclast activating factor (OAF) were the same protein.[18] IL-1β, TNF-β, and TNF-α can induce osteoclastic bone resorption, and IL-1β and TNF-α interact synergistically in inducing bone resorption.

Interestingly, short-term exposure to IL-1β, TNF-β, and TNF-α can induce osteoblastic bone formation, whereas prolonged exposure to these cytokines inhibits osteoblastic bone formation. Importantly, IL-1β is known to be elevated in the crevicular fluid and gingival tissues at sites of periodontal lesions.[31,47] At periodontitis sites, bone resorptive and inhibitory cytokines (IL-1α, IL-1β, TNF-α) reach levels of 0.3, 11.7, and 0.4 ng/ml, respectively. Clinically healthy sites exhibit much lower levels of these cytokines (0.07, 3.1, and 0.03 ng/ml, respectively).[87] In terms of potency, IL-1β is 15 times more potent than IL-1α and 500 times more potent than TNF-α in stimulating bone resorption. Given its higher gingival levels and greater bone resorptive potency, it is clear that IL-1β is likely to be of the greatest importance in the pathogenesis of periodontal disease. IL-1β can also induce the production of collagenase and prostaglandin E$_2$ (PGE$_2$) from gingival fibroblasts.[71,72] Bone resorption is stimulated by the production of IL-1β (Fig. 10–9).

Bone Resorption

The Role of Interleukin-6

IL-6 has been shown to share bone resorptive effects with IL-1β.[70] IL-6 is produced by many cells, including bone marrow stromal cells and osteoblasts, and may play a central role in bone resorption. Inhibition of IL-6 production abrogates the bone resorptive effects of IL-1 and TNF-α.

The Role of Prostaglandin E_2

Activation of inflammatory cells causes a local release of arachidonic acid from the plasma membranes of cells. This activity is catalyzed by a phospholipase. Inflamed periodontal tissues exhibit a substantial elevation of free arachidonate.[23] The free arachidonate is metabolized oxidatively by mononuclear cells via the cyclooxygenase pathway, and a potent bone resorbing hormone, PGE_2, is produced. PGE_2 has been shown to be elevated in periodontitis lesions[27] and to correlate with periods of periodontal disease activity.[59]

HEALING

Gingival mononuclear cells (primarily monocytes and macrophages) are capable of stimulating healing. The healing that occurs within the periodontium can be either regenerative or reparative. For example, replacement of connective tissue by connective tissue is regenerative, but replacement of bone by connective tissue is reparative.

Negative Regulators of Inflammation

One of the first tasks of the immune system in healing is the shutdown of "proinflammatory" processes and the initiation of anti-inflammatory processes. Certain factors are thought to transmit the signal to initiate this conversion, including IL-1 receptor antagonist (IL-1ra), transforming growth factor β (TGF-β), and IFN-γ.[26]

Angiogenesis

Both IL-1β and TNF-α bridge the gap between inflammation and healing, participating in both processes as angiogenic factors. Although TNF-α is known for its cytotoxicity, the molecule can also induce endothelial proliferation. Angiogenic factors are made by cells of the monocyte/macrophage lineage.

Fibrogenic Cytokines

IL-1β and IL-1α are also involved in inducing fibroblast proliferation and collagen synthesis. This effect is not direct, and in vitro, the two appear to have very little capacity to stimulate fibroblasts. The addition of inflammatory cells seems to lead to in vitro fibrogenesis.[38] It has been proposed that this is due to the production of PGE_2 or secondary cytokines, especially platelet-derived growth factor (PDGF) and TGF-β (Fig. 10–10).

PDGF is a dimeric 30-kd cationic protein complex consisting of combinations of $\alpha\alpha$, $\alpha\beta$, and $\beta\beta$ chains and was originally isolated from the α granules of platelets.

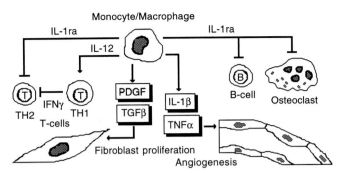

FIGURE 10–10. Mononuclear cell regulation of anti-inflammatory events and tissue regeneration. (From Miyasaki K. Immunology for Dental Students. Unpublished.)

Other important sources of PDGF are monocytes and macrophages. Other fibrogenic cytokines that may play a role include fibroblast growth factor (FGF), TGF-α, and TNF-α. The fibrogenic cytokines are produced mainly by cells of the monocyte/macrophage lineage.

Anti-inflammatory Activities and Bone

There are at least three ways in which the immune system (along with other tissues, such as bone tissue itself) can induce bone healing: blocking osteoclast activation by cytokines, blocking osteoclast formation, and activation of osteoblasts.

Blocking Cytokine-Induced Activation

NK and T_H1 cells can produce IFN-γ, which can inhibit osteoclast differentiation and proliferation.[56] The main effect of IFNγ appears to be inhibition of IL-1 and TNF-α–induced osteoclast activation. Another cytokine that inhibits osteoclastic bone resorption is IL-1ra. IL-1ra is produced by monocytes and monocyte-derived cells and is structurally related to IL-1α, IL-1β, and TNF-α. IL-1ra antagonizes the osteoclastic effects of all three.

Blocking Osteoclast Formation

Osteoclasts appear to remain active for about 10 days before disappearing, possibly by splitting into mononuclear cells.[56] TGF-β is a potent inhibitor of osteoclast formation. Therefore, by blocking osteoclast formation, it is possible to cause a marked decrease in osteoclastic activity within 10 days. Although monocytes can serve as a source of TGF-β, so can the bone matrix itself. The bone matrix contains TGF-β, which is released by osteoclastic resorption.

Activation of Osteoblasts

FGF, PDGF, and insulin-like growth factors I and II (IGF-I and IGF-II) are potent bone cell mitogens. The insulin-like factors induce osteoblast growth, differentiation, synthesis of type I collagen, and generation of alkaline phosphatase. Intriguingly, a single exposure to IGF-I plus PDGF has been used therapeutically in dogs to induce bone regeneration at the site of periodontal lesions.[44]

ABNORMALITIES AND ALTERATIONS IN CHRONIC CELL FUNCTION

Lymphosuppression

Hypofunction of the lymphocyte-monocyte-cytokine system does not appear to relate to severe forms of periodontitis as is observed in the case of hypofunction of neutrophils. Experimental lymphosuppression in animals with cyclosporin A or antithymocyte serum does not result in increased periodontal destruction. Similarly, there is no evidence that lymphosuppressed humans (e.g., as a result of azathioprine, corticosteroids, or prednisone) have a greater level of periodontal destruction. On the contrary, there have been reports that hyporesponsiveness may be related to less gingival inflammation (Table 10–5). These reports underscore the difference between the role of lymphocytes and that of neutrophils in periodontal disease.

Lymphocyte Hyperactivity

McAnulty et al.[48] suggested that individuals with severe periodontitis had an intrinsic problem—namely, hyperfunction—of their peripheral blood lymphocytes. Thus, in their view periodontal disease may partly be a result of predisposing factors residing within the lymphocyte-monocyte-cytokine system. This idea makes sense theoretically; however, the overwhelming opinion is that individuals with periodontal diseases such as adult periodontitis or LJP have a normal lymphocyte system.[66] Certain evidence does seem supportive. First, levamisole, a drug that enhances T-cell activity, aggravates gingival inflammation in humans.[29]

Second, dinitrochlorobenzene (DNB), a skin contact antigen, has been used to induce cell-mediated immune lesions in the gingiva of rats and dogs. The immunity to DNB could be passively transferred by spleen cells but not serum. The lesions were extensive and histologically resembled early gingivitis, except that they were dominated by mononuclear cells. No neutrophils participated in the lesion owing to the relative absence of microbial chemotactic factors.

Monocyte/Macrophage Hyperactivity

There are several studies that address whether increased monocyte activity results in accelerated periodontal destruc-

Table 10–5. LYMPHOCYTE DISORDERS AND PERIODONTAL DISEASES

Immune Disorder	Periodontal Status
Hypofunction	
IgA deficiency	Less gingival inflammation[78]
Hypogammaglobulinemia	Less gingival inflammation[79]
Lymphosuppression (e.g., with	Normal[80, 82, 83]
azathioprine, prednisone, or	Less periodontal disease[81]
corticosteroids)	
Hyperfunction	
Hyperproliferation of peripheral	Severe periodontitis[84]
blood lymphocytes to oral	
bacteria	

tion. Peripheral blood monocytes from individuals with periodontal disease appeared to spontaneously release two to three times as much soluble IL-1β (OAF) than monocytes from individuals without periodontal disease.[49] The increased IL-1β release in monocytes from periodontitis patients was also observed when the monocytes were stimulated by LPS, a part of bacterial outer membranes. Similarly, LPS-stimulated PGE_2 release was greater in monocytes from persons affected with periodontitis than in those from healthy individuals.[25] Interpretation of these findings requires caution, because it is not clear whether periodontal infection caused the increased monocyte activity or the increased monocyte activity resulted in severe periodontal destruction.[62] More studies are needed to determine whether these findings may be used to identify individuals at risk for periodontal disease.

HIV-Gingivitis and HIV-Periodontitis

Dentists and periodontists should remember that two of the most important clinical considerations regarding the handling of patients infected with HIV are blood platelet levels and clotting times. HIV-infected individuals may be thrombocytopenic (platelet counts below 50,000 mm^3) owing to autoimmune disease resulting from type II immunopathologic reactions. Petechiae and ecchymoses are indicative of a potential clotting (bleeding) disorder, to which the dentist should pay particular attention.

Periodontal diseases associated with HIV infection occur prior to drastic decreases in CD4 T-cell levels. Currently there are conflicting reports as to the association of severe forms of gingival inflammation and periodontal destruction with infection by HIV. HIV-gingivitis and HIV-periodontitis were first documented in the San Francisco Bay area.[100] The conflict is usually attributed to ill-defined regional differences, suggesting that either the primary etiologic agent of these diseases or the various cofactors of these diseases are unknown. Speculatively, cofactors of the disease may include smoking, use of recreational drugs, and other opportunistic infections.

HIV-gingivitis (HIV-G) is manifested clinically in HIV-seropositive individuals by intense erythema of the free gingiva (forming a characteristic 1- to 2-mm band of redness), attached gingiva, and alveolar mucosa. Erythema of the alveolar mucosa may have a punctate appearance.[89] Importantly, HIV-G is not responsive to conventional therapy (i.e., scaling and root planing). HIV-G is usually general in distribution rather than localized, although localized cases have been observed. The absolute circulating CD4 T-cell numbers, although modestly diminished, do not appear to be greatly reduced (that is, HIV-G occurs before acquired immunodeficiency syndrome [AIDS]). The CD4-to-CD8 ratio is considered to be within the range of low normals (0.9 to 1.7). Nevertheless, research has begun to characterize CD4$^+$ T-cell subpopulations, and there is emerging evidence of shifts in these subpopulations (by either the suppressor-inducer/helper T-cell criteria or the T_H1/T_H2 criteria).

HIV-periodontitis (HIV-P) is clinically defined as a form of periodontitis in which HIV-G can be observed in association with destructive periodontal changes, including all the usual indicators of periodontitis plus spontaneous bleeding welling up from the gingival crevice and the rapid destruction of periodontal tissues including necrosis of the gingival soft tissues and, frequently, the exposure of bone. Occasionally HIV-G precedes the onset of periodontitis by several months. Exposure of bone suggests that catabolic immune activities that normally prevent bone exposure (i.e., bone resorption) are dysfunctional. Bleeding gums (as evidenced, for example, by blood stains on pillowcases) are often the chief complaint.[100] Severe pain also distinguishes HIV-P from "regular" periodontitis.

The pain is not localized to the gums, as in necrotizing ulcerative gingivitis, but extends deep into the bones. The CD4-to-CD8 ratio is low (0.1 to 0.9). Serum antibodies to *Bacteroides gingivalis, Bacteroides intermedius, F. nucleatum, Eikenella corrodens,* and *A. actinomycetemcomitans* are observed, but the relationship of these antibodies to the disease process is not known. However, the presence of these antibodies suggests that these individuals were subjected to infections by these organisms at some point.

Nonsteroidal Anti-inflammatory Drugs

Currently it is unclear to what extent PGE_2 contributes to bone resorption in periodontitis. However, several studies suggest that the blockade of cyclooxygenase activity by aspirin and nonsteroidal anti-inflammatory drugs (NSAIDs) such as indomethacin can reduce alveolar bone loss by up to 28%.[69] Other NSAIDs, such as topical substituted oxazolopyridine derivative, topical ibuprofen, topical piroxicam, topical meclofenamic acid, oral flurbiprofen, and oral naproxen, appear to slow alveolar bone loss or reduce bleeding on probing. Not only are these observations clinically significant, but they also suggest that a percentage of alveolar bone loss in periodontal diseases is due to cyclooxygenase products of mononuclear cells.

From a clinical perspective, it is also interesting that certain aromatic oils (eugenol, guaiacol, thymol, creosol, and capsaicin) can block the formation of prostaglandins in vitro by up to 50%.[24] Eugenol (an oil from cloves) is particularly common in periodontal dressings and a variety of endodontic applications and has been popular primarily because of its antiseptic and anesthetic properties.

DRUG-INDUCED GINGIVAL FIBROGENESIS

A number of drugs, including phenytoin, the dihydropyridines, and cyclosporin A, frequently are associated with gingival hyperplasia. Of these, both phenytoin and cyclosporin A (CsA) are known to interact with the immune system. Although the relationship between their immunologic effects and gingival hyperplasia is unclear, it is plausible that inflammatory cells play a key role in the hyperplastic changes observed in the gingival connective tissues. It has been shown that phenytoin, a drug used to control seizures, increases the expression of PDGF in cultured monocytes, and this may explain the association of phenytoin with gingival connective tissue hyperplasia in almost 50% of users.[19] CsA is a fungal derivative with profound lymphosuppressive effects. It appears to interact with cy-

clophilins, cytosolic proteins that are broadly distributed in tissues.[76] It has been proposed that CsA functions as a "glue" that forms a complex between the cyclophilin and the intracellular protein phosphatase calcineurin. This interferes with the translocation of certain transactivating factors (proteins that induce the transcription of a number of other proteins) from the cytosol into the nucleus, resulting in an immunosuppressive effect. This immunosuppressive effect includes the blockade of macrophages and early T-cell activation,[7,28] resulting in the decreased elaboration of proinflammatory cytokines such as IL-1β. The significance of these immunosuppressive events in relationship to gingival hyperplasia is not understood; however, it has been proposed that inflammation is required for gingival hyperplasia.

MHC GENES AND PERIODONTAL DISEASE

The antigen-presenting, MHC-encoded molecules are extremely pleomorphic (i.e., exhibit many allotypes), and the MHC class I and class II molecules are particularly pleomorphic in the area of the specificity pockets. Different allotypes of the MHC molecules bind and present different peptides to T cells and thus dictate which specific T-cell clones respond to a given protein antigen. This is called *determinant selection* and is the main reason individuals of the same species exhibit diverse immunologic responses to the same antigens. Thus, the alleles of the MHC genes and their allotypic products are largely responsible for immune response pleomorphism.

MHC Class I Molecules

Many of the studies with regard to periodontal disease were performed in the 1970s, when only mixed lymphocyte assays were used to determine human leukocyte antigen (HLA) typing. These reactions primarily detect differences among the HLA-A and HLA-B allotypes. Reinholdt et al.[68] detected a positive association of localized juvenile periodontitis with HLA-A9, HLA-A28, and HLA-Bw15. Both Reinholdt et al.[68] and Terasaki et al.[90] detected a possible association between decreased frequency of HLA-A2 and LJP. The Reinholdt data are presented in Table 10–6. The Reinholdt data are interesting, because there is greater genetic homogeneity in Denmark than in the United States. These data also suggest either that cell-mediated processes are important in determining susceptibility to LJP or that these markers are in linkage disequilibrium with some other gene outside of these loci. Cell-mediated immunity may be used to combat periodontal pathogens, provided that at some point these pathogens exist as intracellular parasites.

Cullinan et al.[14] found differences in HLA-A28 and HLA-Bw15 (in contrast to Reinholdt et al.[68]) but detected no association of LJP with differing frequencies in HLA-A2 or HLA-A9. Furthermore, they suggested that differences observed in HLA-A28 and HLA-Bw15 were not statistically significant when corrected for sample size. Saxén and Koskimies[75] took a different approach. They decided to determine whether the HLA phenotype within a family dic-

Table 10–6. MHC CLASS I PHENOTYPE AND PERIODONTAL DISEASE

Group	n	HLA–A2 %	(P)	HLA–A9 %	(P)	HLA–A28 %	(P)	HLA–Bw15 %	(P)
LJP	39	43.6	(= .13)	38.5	(= .003)	23.1	(= .03)	38.5	(= .003)
AP	29	58.6	(>> .05)	6.9	(> .05)	10.3	(>> .05)	17.2	(>> .05)
Controls	1967	53.6		17.3		10.0		17.9	

LJP, Localized juvenile periodontitis; AP, adult periodontitis .
Data from Reinholdt J, Bay I, Svejgaard A. Association between HLA-antigens and periodontal disease. J Dent Res *56:*1261, 1977.

tated the presence or absence of LJP. They found that both healthy and diseased siblings expressed HLA-Bw15 and HLA-A9, which suggested that the "gene for LJP" was not linked to the HLA complex. These results are not surprising, as most investigations have associated LJP with a problem manifest in defective phagocyte motility. This defective behavior, although not necessarily the underlying cause of LJP, is not likely to be the result of an underlying problem that can be linked to the MHC.

MHC Class II Molecules

The MHC class II molecules are more closely associated with immune responses to infection by extracellular pathogens. Because periodontal disease is believed to result from extracellular pathogens, it seems reasonable that class II loci are more likely to influence the outcome of the bacteria–host interaction than are class I loci. Tantalizing data provided by a small study (10 subjects) suggest that there may be some association between RPP and the HLA-D phenotype.[35] An extremely strong association between HLA-DR4 and RPP was observed in Israel with both Ashkenazi and non-Ashkenazi groups. This HLA-DR4 phenotype is also found in high proportions in rheumatoid arthritis patients and HLA-DR3 or -DR4 are found in more than 90% of Scandinavian children with insulin-dependent diabetes mellitus (type I diabetes).[53] Type I diabetes has been associated with periodontal disease when normalized for age and plaque indices.[11]

MHC Class III Molecules

The MHC class III molecules include complement factors C2, C4, and B, which are encoded within the MHC. These molecules are also among the most pleomorphic molecules known. Because of the significance of these molecules in both alternative and classic pathway activation (see Chapter 6) and the importance of complement-mediated opsonization for phagocytic antigen presentation, it is possible that pleomorphism in these molecules may also affect immune responses. Currently there are no published reports regarding "complotypes" and periodontal diseases.

REFERENCES

1. Altman LC, Page RC, Vandesteen GE, et al. Abnormalities of leukocyte chemotaxis in patients with various forms of periodontitis. J Periodont Res *20:*553, 1985.
2. Armitt K. Identification of T-cell subsets in gingivitis in children. J Periodontol *57:*3, 1986.
3. Baehni PC, Payot P, Tsai C-C, Cimasoni G. Periodontal status associated with chronic neutropenia. J Clin Periodontol *10:*222, 1983.
4. Baker PJ, Wilson ME. Opsonic IgG antibody against *Actinobacillus actinomycetemcomitans* in localized juvenile periodontitis. Oral Microbiol Immunol *4:*98, 1990.
5. Boughman JA, Astemborski JA, Blitzer MG. Early onset periodontal disease: A genetic perspective. Crit Rev Oral Biol Med *1:*89, 1990.
6. Boughman JA, Halloran SL, Roulston D, et al. An autosomal-dominant form of juvenile periodontitis: Its localization to chromosome 4 and linkage to dentinogenesis imperfecta and Gc. J Craniofacial Genet Dev Biol *6:*341, 1986.
7. Camargo PM. Cyclosporin- and nifedipine-induced gingival enlargement: An overview. J West Soc Periodontol *37:*57, 1989.
8. Carrassi A, Abati S, Santarelli G, Vogel G. Periodontitis in a patient with chronic neutropenia. J Periodontol *60:*352, 1989.
9. Chandra RK. Iron-deficiency anaemia and immunologic response. Lancet *2:*1200, 1976.
10. Charon JA, Mergenhagen SE, Gallin JI. Gingivitis and oral ulceration in patients with neutrophil dysfunction. J Oral Pathol *14:*150, 1985.
11. Cianciola LJ, Park BH, Bruck E, et al. Prevalence of periodontal disease in insulin-dependent diabetes mellitus (juvenile diabetes). J Am Dent Assoc *104:*653, 1982.
12. Clagett JA, Page RC. Insoluble immune complexes and chronic periodontal disease in man and the dog. Arch Oral Biol *23:*153, 1978.
13. Cohen MS, Leong PA, Simpson DM. Phagocytic cells and periodontal defense. Periodontal status of patients with chronic granulomatous disease of childhood. J Periodontol *56:*611, 1985.
14. Cullinan MP, Sachs J, Wolf E, Seymour GJ. The distribution of HLA-A and -B antigens in patients and their families with periodontosis. J Periodont Res *15:*177, 1980.
15. Cutler CW, Eke P, Arnold RR, Van Dyke TE. Defective neutrophil function in an insulin-dependent diabetes mellitus patient. A case report. J Periodontol *62:*394, 1991.
16. Çelenligil H, Kansu E, Ruacan S, Eratalay K. Papillon-Lefèvre syndrome. Characterization of peripheral blood and gingival lymphocytes with monoclonal antibodies. J Clin Periodontol *19:*392, 1992.
17. DeNardin E, Deluca C, Levine MJ, Genco RJ. Antibodies directed to the chemotactic factor receptor detect differences between chemotactically normal and defective neutrophils from LJP patients. J Periodontol *61:*609, 1990.
18. Dewhirst FE, Stashenko PP, Mole JE, Tsurumachi T. Purification and partial sequence of human osteoclast-activating factor: Identity with interleukin 1b. J Immunol *135:*2562, 1985.
19. Dill RE, Miller EK, Weil T, et al. Phenytoin increases gene expression for platelet-derived growth factor B chain in macrophages and monocytes. J Periodontol *64:*169, 1993.
20. Dinauer MC, Pierce EA, Bruns GAP, et al. Human neutrophil cytochrome b light chain (p22-phox). Gene structure, chromosomal localization, and mutations in cytochrome-negative autosomal recessive chronic granulomatous disease. J Clin Invest *86:*1729, 1990.
21. Ebersole JL, Frey DE, Taubman MA, et al. Dynamics of systemic antibody responses in periodontal disease. J Periodont Res *22:*184, 1987.
22. Ebersole JL. Systemic humoral immune responses in periodontal disease. Crit Rev Oral Biol Med *1:*283, 1990.
23. El Attar TMA, Lin HS, Killoy WJ, et al. Hydroxy fatty acids and prostaglandin formation in diseased human periodontal pocket tissue. J Periodontal Res *21:*169, 1986.
24. El Attar TMA. Prostaglandins: Physiology, biochemistry, pharmacology and clinical applications. J Oral Pathol *7:*175, 1978.
25. Garrison SW, Nicholls FC. LPS-elicited secretory responses in monocytes: Altered release of PGE2 but not IL-1b in patients with adult periodontitis. J Periodont Res *24:*88, 1989.
26. Genco RJ. Host responses in periodontal tissues: Current concepts. J Periodontol *63:*338, 1992.
27. Goodson JM, Dewhirst FE, Brunetti A. Prostaglandin E2 level and human periodontal disease. Prostaglandins *6:*81, 1974.
28. Hassell TM, Hefti AF. Drug-induced gingival overgrowth: Old problem, new problem. Crit Rev Oral Biol Med *2:*103, 1991.
29. Ivanyi L, Lehner T. The effect of levamisole on gingival inflammation in man. Scand J Immunol *6:*219, 1977.

30. Izumi Y, Sugiyama S, Shinozuka O, et al. Defective neutrophil chemotaxis in Down's syndrome patients and its relationship to periodontal destruction. J Periodontol 60:238, 1989.

31. Jandinski JJ, Stashenko P, Feder LS, et al. Localization of interleukin-1β in human periodontal tissue. J Periodontol 62:36, 1991.

32. Jeppson JD, Jaffe HS, Hill HR. Use of recombinant human interferon gamma to enhance neutrophil chemotactic responses in Job syndrome of hyperimmunoglobulin E and recurrent infections. J Pediatr 118:383, 1991.

33. Kalmar JR, Arnold RR, Van Dyke TE. Direct interaction of *Actinobacillus actinomycetemcomitans* with normal and defective (LJP) neutrophils. J Periodont Res 22:179, 1987.

34. Katsuragi Y, Matsuda N, Nakamura M, Murayama Y. Neutrophil functions in patients with severe periodontal disease. Adv Dent Res 2:359, 1988.

35. Katz J, Goultshin J, Benoliel R, Brautbar C. Human leukocyte antigen (HLA) DR4. Positive association with rapidly progressive periodontitis. J Periodontol 58:607, 1987.

36. Kishimoto TK. A dynamic model for neutrophil localization to inflammatory sites. J NIH Res 3:75, 1991.

37. Kopp W. Density and localization of lymphocytes with natural-killer (NK) cell activity in periodontal biopsy. J Clin Periodontol 15:595, 1988.

38. Kovaks EJ. Fibrogenic cytokines: The role of immune mediators in the development of scar tissue. Immunol Today 12:17, 1991.

39. Lala R, Lindemann RA, Miyasaki KT. Effect of polymorphonuclear leukocyte secretions on lymphokine-activated killer cell activity. Oral Microbiol Immunol 7:89, 1992.

40. Lally ET, Baehni PC, McArthur WP. Local immunoglobulin synthesis in periodontal disease. J Periodont Res 15:159, 1980.

41. Lamster IB, Oshrain RL, Harper DS. Infantile agranulocytosis with survival into adolescence: periodontal manifestations and laboratory findings. A case report. J Periodontol 58:34, 1987.

42. Lavine WS, Maderazo EG, Stolman J, et al. Impaired neutrophil chemotaxis in patients with juvenile and rapidly progressive periodontitis. J Periodont Res 14:10, 1979.

43. Leung DYM, Geha RS. Clinical and immunologic aspects of the hyperimmunoglobulin E syndrome. Hematol/Oncol Clin North Am 2:81, 1988.

44. Lynch SE, Williams RC, Polson AM, et al. A combination of platelet-derived and insulin-like growth factors enhance periodontal regeneration. J Clin Periodontol 16:545, 1989.

45. Mackler BF, Faner RM, Schur P, et al. IgG subclasses in human periodontal disease. II. Cytophilic and membrane IgG subclass immunoglobulins. J Periodont Res 13:433, 1978.

46. Martin SA, Falkler WA, Vincent JW, et al. A comparison of the reactivity of *Eubacterium* species with localized and serum immunoglobulins from rapidly progressive and adult periodontitis. J Periodontol 59:32, 1988.

47. Masada MP, Persson R, Kenney JS, et al. Measurement of interleukin-1α and -1β in gingival crevicular fluid: implications for the pathogenesis of periodontal disease. J Periodont Res 25:156, 1990.

48. McAnulty R, Stone R, Hastings G, et al. Immunoregulation in severe generalized periodontitis. Clin Immunol Immunopathol 34:84, 1985.

49. McFarlane CG, Reynolds JJ, Meikle MC. The release of interleukin 1-β, tumor necrosis factor-α, and interferon-γ by cultured peripheral blood mononuclear cells from patients with periodontitis. J Periodont Res 25:207, 1990.

50. McGhee JR, Mestecky J, Elson CO, Kiyono H. Regulation of IgA synthesis and immune response by T cells and interleukins. J Clin Immunol 9:175, 1989.

51. McMullen JA, Van Dyke TE, Horoszewicz HU, Genco RJ. Neutrophil chemotaxis in individuals with advanced periodontal disease and a genetic predisposition to diabetes mellitus. J Periodontol 52:167, 1981.

52. Meers P, Ernst JD, Düzgünes N, et al. Synexin-like proteins from human polymorphonuclear leukocytes. Identification and characterization of granule-aggregating and membrane-fusing activities. J Biol Chem 262:7850, 1987.

53. Michelsen B, Wassmuth R, Ludvigsson J, et al. HLA heterozygosity in insulindependent diabetes is most frequent at the DQ locus. Scand J Immunol 31:405, 1990.

54. Miyagi M, Aoyama H, Morishita M, Iwamoto Y. Effects of sex hormones on chemotaxis of human peripheral polymorphonuclear leukocytes and monocytes. J Periodontol 63:28, 1992.

55. Miyasaki KT. The neutrophil: Mechanisms of controlling periodontal bacteria. J Periodontol 62:761, 1991.

56. Mundy GR. Inflammatory mediators and the destruction of bone. J Periodont Res 26:213, 1991.

57. Murphy PM, Özçelik T, Kenney RT, et al. A structural homologue of the N-formyl peptide receptor. J Biol Chem 267:7637, 1992.

58. Nunoi H, Rotrosen D, Gallin JI, Malech HL. Two forms of autosomal chronic granulomatous disease lack distinct neutrophil cytosolic factors. Science 242:1298, 1988.

59. Offenbacher S, Odle BM, Van Dyke TE. The use of crevicular fluid prostaglandin E2 levels as a predictor of periodontal attachment loss. J Periodont Res 21:101, 1986.

60. Offenbacher S, Scott SS, Odle BM, et al. Depressed leukotriene B4 chemotactic response of neutrophils from localized juvenile periodontitis patients. J Periodontol 58:602, 1987.

61. Oshrain HI, Telsey B, Mandel ID. Longitudinal study of patients with reduced immunocapacity. J Periodontol 54:151, 1983.

62. Page R. The role of inflammatory mediators in the pathogenesis of periodontal disease. J Periodontol 63:356, 1992.

63. Page RC, Schroeder HE. Pathogenesis of chronic inflammatory periodontal disease. A summary of current work. Lab Invest 33:235, 1976.

64. Page RC. Lymphoid responsiveness and human periodontitis. In: Genco RJ, Mergenhagen SE, eds. Host-Parasite Interactions in Periodontal Diseases. Washington, DC, American Society for Microbiology, 1982, p 217.

65. Perez HD, Kelly E, Elfman F, et al. Defective polymorphonuclear leukocyte formyl peptide receptor(s) in juvenile periodontitis. J Clin Invest 87:971, 1991.

65a. Price TH, Ochs HD, Gershoni-Baruch R, et al. In vivo neutrophil and lymphocyte function studies with leukocyte adhesion deficiency Type II. Blood 84:1635, 1994.

66. Ranney RR. Immunologic mechanisms of pathogenesis in periodontal diseases: An assessment. J Periodont Res 26:243, 1991.

67. Reinhardt RA, Bolton RW, McDonald TL, et al. In situ lymphocyte subpopulations from active versus stable periodontal sites. J Periodontol 59:656, 1988.

68. Reinholdt J, Bay I, Svejgaard A. Association between HLA-antigens and periodontal disease. J Dent Res 56:1261, 1977.

69. Research, Science, and Therapy Committee. Pharmacologic blocking of host responses as an adjunct in the management of periodontal diseases: A research update. Position paper, American Academy of Periodontology, 1992.

70. Research, Science, and Therapy Committee. Periodontal Diseases of Children and Adolescents. Position paper, American Academy of Periodontology, 1991.

71. Richards D, Rutherford RB. Interleukin-1 regulation of procollagenase mRNA and protein in periodontal fibroblasts in vitro. J Periodont Res 25:222, 1990.

72. Richards D, Rutherford RB. The effects of interleukin-1 on collagenolytic activity and prostaglandin-E secretion by human periodontal ligament and gingival fibroblast. Arch Oral Biol 33:237, 1988.

73. Robertson PB, Mackler BF, Wright TE, Levy BM. Periodontal status of patients with abnormalities of the immune system. II. Observations over a two-year period. J Periodontol 51:70, 1980.

74. Robertson PB, Wright TE, Mackler BF, et al. Periodontal status of patients with abnormalities of the immune system. J Periodont Res 13:37, 1978.

75. Saxén L, Koskimies S. Juvenile periodontitis—no linkage with HLA antigens. J Periodont Res 19:441, 1984.

76. Schreiber SL, Crabtree GR. The mechanism of action of cyclosporin A and FK506. Immunol Today 13:136, 1992.

77. Schuller PD, Freedman HL, Lewis DW. Periodontal status of renal transplant patients receiving immunosuppressive therapy. J Periodontol 44:167, 1973.

78. Seymour GJ, Greenspan JS. The phenotypic characterization of lymphocyte subpopulations in established human periodontal disease. J Periodont Res 14:39, 1979.

79. Seymour GJ, Crouch MS, Powell RN. The phenotypic characterization of lymphoid cell populations in gingivitis in children. J Periodont Res 16:582, 1981.

80. Seymour GJ, Powell RN, Cole KL, et al. Experimental gingivitis in humans. A histochemical and immunochemical characterization of lymphoid cell subpopulations. J Periodont Res 18:375, 1983.

81. Shenkein HA, Genco RJ. Gingival fluid and serum in periodontal disease. I. Quantitative study of immunoglobulins, complement, and other plasma proteins. J Periodontol 48:772, 1977.

82. Shenkein HA, Genco RJ. Gingival fluid and serum in periodontal disease. II. Evidence for cleavage of complement components C3, C3 proactivator (factor B), and C4 in gingival fluid. J Periodontol 48:778, 1977.

83. Shenker BJ, Vitale LA, Welham DA. Immune suppression induced by *Actinobacillus actinomycetemcomitans*. Effects on immunoglobulin production by human B cells. Infect Immun 58:3856, 1990.

84. Shurin SB, Socransky SS, Sweeney E, Stossel TP. A neutrophil disorder induced by Capnocytophaga, a dental micro-organism. N Engl J Med 301:849, 1979.

85. Sjöström K, Darveau R, Page R, et al. Opsonic antibody activity against *Actinobacillus actinomycetemcomitans* in patients with rapidly progressive periodontitis. Infect Immun 60:4819, 1992.

86. Stabholz A, Soskolne V, Machtei E, et al. Effect of benign familial neutropenia on the periodontium of Yemenite Jews. J Periodontol 61:51, 1990.

87. Stashenko P, Jandinski JJ, Fujiyoshi P, et al. Tissue levels of bone resorptive cytokines in periodontal disease. J Periodontol 62:504, 1991.

88. Sutton RBO, Smales FC. Cross-sectional study of the effects of immunosuppressive drugs on chronic periodontal disease in man. J Clin Periodontol 10:317, 1983.

89. Taubman MA, Stoufi ED, Seymour GJ, et al. Immunoregulatory aspects of periodontal disease. Adv Dent Res 2:328, 1988.

90. Terasaki PI, Kaslick RS, West TL, Chasens AI. Low HL-A2 frequency and periodontitis. Tissue Antigens 5:286, 1975.

91. The human genome. J NIH Res 4:153, 1992.

92. Tollefson T, Saltvedt E, Koppang HS. The effect of immunosuppressive agents on periodontal disease in man. J Periodont Res 13:240, 1978.

93. Van Dyke TE. Role of the neutrophil in oral disease; receptor deficiency in leukocytes from patients with juvenile periodontitis. Rev Infect Dis 7:419, 1985.

94. Van Dyke TE, Bartholomew E, Genco RJ, et al. Inhibition of neutrophil chemotaxis by soluble bacterial products. J Periodontol 53:502, 1982.

95. Van Dyke TE, Taubman MA, Ebersole JL, et al. The Papillon-Lefèvre syndrome: Neutrophil dysfunction with severe periodontal disease. Clin Immunol Immunopathol 31:419, 1984.

96. Van Dyke TE, Warbington M, Gardner M, Offenbacher S. Neutrophil surface protein markers as indicators of defective chemotaxis in LJP. J Periodontol 61:180, 1990.

97. Van Dyke TE, Wilson-Burrows C, Offenbacher S, Henson PM. Association of

an abnormality of neutrophil chemotaxis in human periodontal disease with a cell surface protein. Infect Immun *55:*2262, 1987.

98. Volpp BD, Nauseef WM, Clark RA. Two cytosolic neutrophil oxidase components absent in autosomal chronic granulomatous disease. Science *242:*1295, 1988.

99. Waldrop TC, Anderson DC, Hallmon WW, et al. Periodontal manifestations of the heritable Mac-1, LFA-1, deficiency syndrome. Clinical, histopathologic, and molecular characteristics. J Periodontol *58:*400, 1987.

100. Winkler JR, Grassi M, Murray PA. Clinical description and etiology of HIV-associated periodontal diseases. In Robertson PB, Greenspan JS, eds. Oral Manifestations of AIDS. Littleton, MA, PSG Publishing, 1988, p 49.

101. Wynne SE, Walsh LJ, Seymour GJ, Powell RN. In situ demonstration of natural killer (NK) cells in human gingival tissue. J Periodontol *57:*699, 1986.

102. Zafiropoulos G-GK, Flores-de-Jacoby L, Hungerer K-D, Nisengard RJ. Humoral antibody responses in periodontal disease. J Periodontol *63:*80, 1992.

11

Dental Calculus

FERMIN A. CARRANZA, Jr.

Calculus
Supragingival and Subgingival Calculus
Prevalence
Composition
Attachment to the Tooth Surface

Formation
Etiologic Significance
Materia Alba
Food Debris
Dental Stains

The cause of gingival inflammation is bacterial plaque (see Chapter 6). Several factors previously considered to be of direct etiologic significance in periodontal disease are now known to act only by favoring plaque accumulation. These include calculus, faulty restorations, partial removable prostheses, and food impaction. Calculus and other deposits are discussed in this chapter. Chapter 12 considers all other factors that favor plaque accumulation or that produce periodontal destruction by other mechanisms.

CALCULUS

Although acquired bacterial coatings have been demonstrated to be the major etiologic factor in periodontal disease, the presence of calculus is of great concern to the clinician. The primary effect of calculus is not, as was originally thought, due to mechanical irritation but is related to its always being covered by bacteria (Figs. 11–1 to 11–4). Experiments with germ-free animals have proved this point clearly (see Chapters 6 and 9). *However, these calcified deposits play a major role in maintaining and accentuating periodontal disease by keeping plaque in close contact with the gingival tissue and creating areas where plaque removal is impossible.* Therefore, the clinician must be extremely competent in the removal of calculus and the necrotic cementum to which it attaches.

Supragingival and Subgingival Calculus

Calculus is an adherent calcified or calcifying mass that forms on the surface of natural teeth and dental prostheses (Plate III). Ordinarily calculus consists of mineralized bac-

terial plaque. It is classified according to its relation to the gingival margin as supragingival or subgingival.

Supragingival calculus is located coronal to the gingival margin and therefore is visible in the oral cavity (Fig. 11–5 and Plate III). It is usually white or whitish yellow; has a hard, clay-like consistency; and is easily detached from the tooth surface. After removal it may recur rapidly, especially in the lingual area of the mandibular incisors. The color is affected by contact with such substances as tobacco and food pigments. It may localize on a single tooth or group of teeth, or it may be generalized throughout the mouth.

Supragingival calculus occurs most frequently and in greatest quantity on the buccal surfaces of the maxillary molars opposite Stensen's duct (Fig. 11–6) and on the lingual surfaces of the mandibular anterior teeth, particularly the centrals, opposite Wharton's duct (Fig. 11–7 and Plate III*B*). In extreme cases calculus may form a bridge-like structure over the interdental papilla of adjacent teeth (Fig. 11–8) or cover the occlusal surface of teeth without functional antagonists (Fig. 11–9).

Subgingival calculus is located below the crest of the marginal gingiva and therefore is not visible on routine clinical examination. Determination of the location and extent of subgingival calculus requires careful examination with an explorer (Fig. 11–10). It is usually dense, dark brown or greenish black, and hard or flint-like in consistency; it is firmly attached to the tooth surface (Figs. 11–11 and 11–12). Supragingival calculus and subgingival calculus generally occur together, but one may be present without the other. Microscopic studies demonstrate that the deposits usually extend near but do not reach the base of periodontal pockets in chronic periodontal lesions.

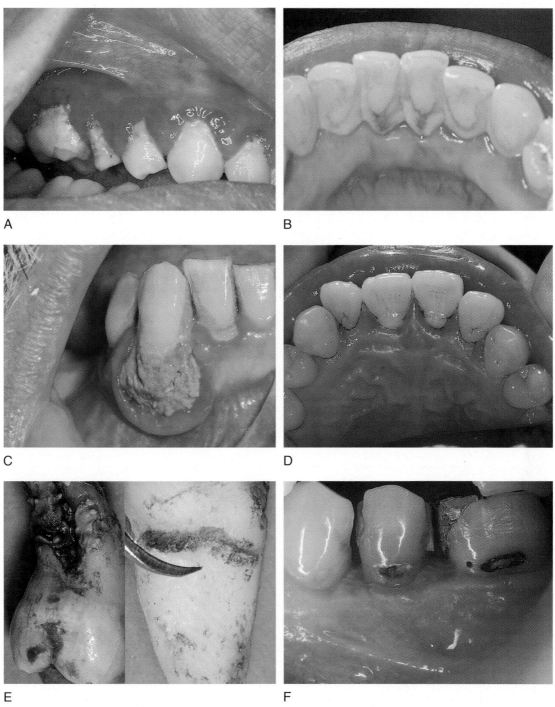

PLATE III. Local irritants. *A,* Heavy calculus deposits on facial surfaces of upper first molar and second premolar. Note the severe gingival inflammation in the entire quadrant. *B,* Calculus deposits on lingual surfaces of lower incisors forming a bridge over the interdental papillae. Gingival inflammation can also be seen. *C,* Heavy calculus deposit on facial surface of lower cuspid with associated gingival recession. *D,* Palatal view of upper anterior teeth with heavy calculus deposits, particularly in interdental spaces. *E,* Different shapes of calculus on extracted teeth. *F,* Overhanging margin of restoration and atrophied and inflamed gingival papilla.

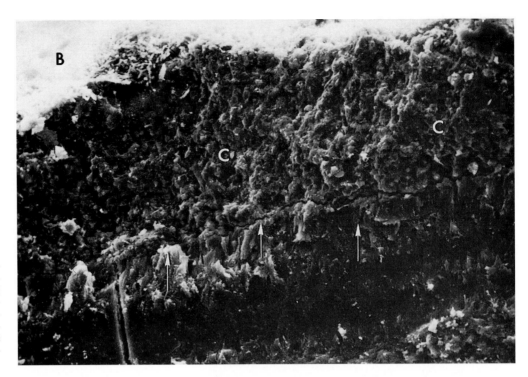

FIGURE 11-1. Scanning electron microscope view of an extracted human tooth, fractured experimentally. Subgingival calculus (C) is attached to the cementum surface *(arrows)*. Adherent plaque bacteria (B) is seen on calculus surface. (Courtesy of Dr. John Sottosanti.)

Supragingival calculus has also been referred to as *salivary calculus* and subgingival calculus as *serumal calculus,* based on the assumption that the former is derived from the saliva and the latter from the blood serum. This concept was overshadowed for a long time by the view that saliva was the sole source of all calculus. However, currently the consensus is that the saliva supplies the minerals for the formation of supragingival calculus, whereas the gingival fluid, which resembles serum, is the main mineral source for subgingival calculus.[33,81] The terms *salivary calculus* and *serumal calculus,* however, are no longer used.

When the gingival tissues recede, subgingival calculus becomes exposed and is classified as supragingival. Thus, supragingival calculus can be composed of both supragingival and subgingival types.

Prevalence

The following description is based on the longitudinal study of Anerud and coworkers in which Sri Lanka tea laborers and Norwegian academicians were followed for 15 years and all periodontal parameters recorded.[1] In the Sri

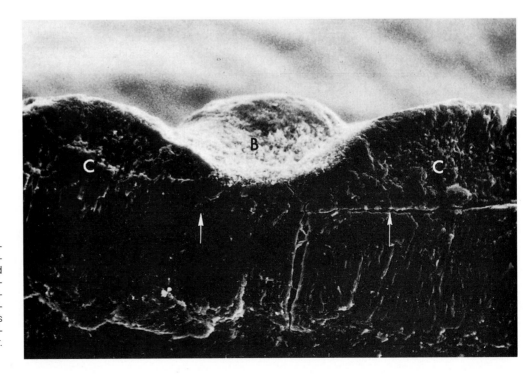

FIGURE 11-2. Scanning electron microscope view of an extracted human tooth, fractured experimentally. Subgingival calculus (C) is attached to the cementum surface *(arrows)*. Adherent plaque bacteria (B) is attached in depression on calculus surface. (Courtesy of Dr. John Sottosanti.)

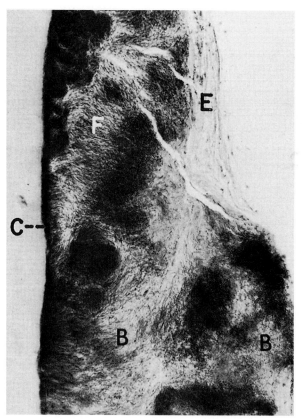

FIGURE 11–3. Detailed microscopic examination of calculus showing an inner structure (C), filamentous organisms (F), other bacteria (B), and desquamated epithelial cells (E).

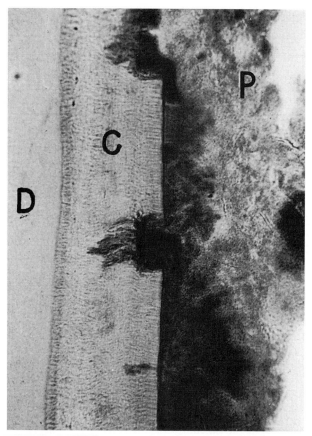

FIGURE 11–4. Calculus on tooth surface embedded within the cementum (C). Note the early stage of penetration shown in the lower portion of the illustration. D, Dentin; P, plaque attached to calculus.

Lanka individuals who had no oral hygiene or dental care, supragingival calculus formation started early in life, probably soon after tooth eruption. The first areas that showed calculus deposits were the facial aspects of maxillary molars and the lingual aspects of mandibular incisors. Supragingival calculus continued to accumulate with age, reaching a maximum at about 25 to 30 years. At this time most of the teeth were covered by calculus, although the facial surfaces had less calculus than the lingual or palatal surfaces. Calculus accumulation appeared to be symmetric, and by age 45 few teeth (usually the premolars) were without calculus.

Subgingival calculus appeared first either independently or on the interproximal aspects of areas where supragingival calculus already existed.[1] By age 30, all surfaces of all teeth had subgingival calculus without any pattern of predilection.[1]

The Norwegian academicians had good oral hygiene and frequent visits for dental care throughout their lives, resulting in markedly reduced accumulation of calculus. However, supragingival calculus still formed on facial surfaces of upper molars and lingual surfaces of lower incisors in 80% of teenagers; however, it did not extend to other teeth and did not increase with age.[1]

Supragingival calculus and subgingival calculus may be seen on radiographs (see Chapter 29). Supragingivally, well-calcified deposits are readily detectable, forming irregular contours on the radiographic crown. Interproximal cal-

culus, both supragingival and subgingival, is even more easily detectable, because these deposits form irregularly shaped projections into the interdental space. However, the sensitivity level of calculus detection by radiographs is low[14]; when it is detected, the location of calculus does not indicate the bottom of the periodontal pocket, because the most apical plaque is not sufficiently calcified to be radiographically visible.

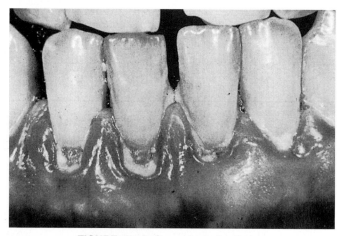

FIGURE 11–5. Supragingival calculus.

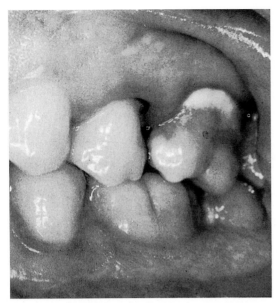

FIGURE 11–6. Calculus on molar opposite Stensen's duct.

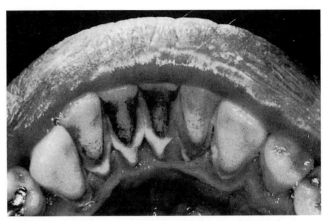

FIGURE 11–7. Calculus and stain on lingual surface in relation to orifice of submaxillary and sublingual glands.

Composition

Inorganic Content. Supragingival calculus consists of inorganic (70% to 90%[25]) and organic components. The inorganic portion consists of 75.9% calcium phosphate, $Ca_3(PO_4)_2$; 3.1% calcium carbonate, $CaCO_3$; and traces of magnesium phosphate, $Mg_3(PO_4)_2$, and other metals. The percentage of inorganic constituents in calculus is similar to that in other calcified tissues of the body. The principal inorganic components are calcium, 39%; phosphorus, 19%; carbon dioxide, 1.9%; magnesium, 0.8%; and trace amounts of sodium, zinc, strontium, bromine, copper, manganese, tungsten, gold, aluminum, silicon, iron, and fluorine.[57]

At least two thirds of the inorganic component is crystalline in structure.[40] The four main crystal forms and their percentages are

Hydroxyapatite, approximately 58%.
Magnesium whitlockite, approximately 21%.
Octacalcium phosphate, approximately 21%.
Brushite, approximately 9%.

Generally two or more crystal forms occur in a calculus sample, with hydroxyapatite and octacalcium phosphate being the most common (in 97% to 100% of all supragingival calculus) and occurring in the greatest amounts. Brushite is more common in the mandibular anterior region and magnesium whitlockite in the posterior areas. The incidence of the four crystal forms varies with the age of the deposit.[72]

Organic Content. The organic component of calculus consists of a mixture of protein-polysaccharide complexes, desquamated epithelial cells, leukocytes, and various types of microorganisms[50]; 1.9% to 9.1% of the organic component is carbohydrate, which consists of galactose, glucose, rhamnose, mannose, glucuronic acid, galactosamine, and sometimes arabinose, galacturonic acid, and glucosamine, all of which are present in salivary glycoprotein, except arabinose and rhamnose.[43,79]

Salivary proteins account for 5.9% to 8.2% of the organic component of calculus and include most of the amino acids.[43,48,79] Lipids account for 0.2% of the organic content in the form of neutral fats, free fatty acids, cholesterol, cholesterol esters, and phospholipids.[44]

The composition of subgingival calculus is similar to that of supragingival calculus, with some differences. It has the same hydroxyapatite content,[83] more magnesium whitlockite, and less brushite and octacalcium phosphate.[67] The ra-

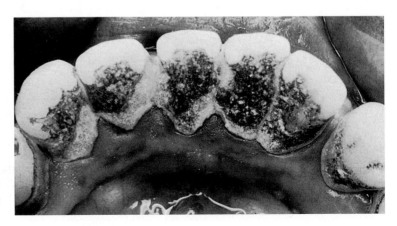

FIGURE 11–8. Calculus forming a bridge-like structure on the lingual surface of the mandibular anterior teeth.

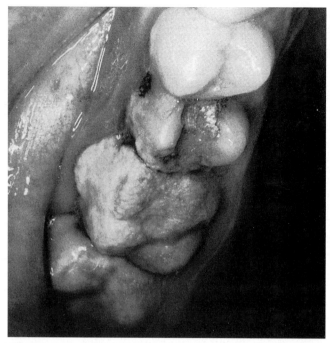

FIGURE 11-9. Calculus covering nonfunctioning maxillary molars and part of the second premolar. Compare with the first premolar, which has functional antagonists.

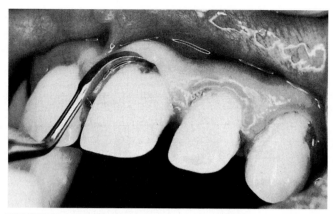

FIGURE 11-10. Subgingival calculus revealed by deflecting the pocket wall. Note the inflammation of the marginal gingiva on the adjacent lateral incisor and canine associated with supragingival calculus and subgingival calculus.

tio of calcium to phosphate is higher subgingivally, and the sodium content increases with the depth of periodontal pockets.[45] Salivary proteins present in supragingival calculus are not found subgingivally.[8] Dental calculus, salivary duct calculus, and calcified dental tissues are similar in inorganic composition.

Attachment to the Tooth Surface

Differences in the manner in which calculus is attached to the tooth surface affect the relative ease or difficulty encountered in its removal. Four modes of attachment have been described:[34,68,97] attachment by means of an organic pellicle (Fig. 11-13); penetration of calculus bacteria into cementum (this mode of attachment is not accepted by some investigators[34]); mechanical locking into surface irregularities, such as resorption lacunae and caries (Fig. 11-14); and close adaptation of calculus undersurface depressions to the gently sloping mounds of the unaltered cementum surface[80] (Fig. 11-15). Calculus embedded deeply in cementum may appear morphologically similar to cementum and has been termed *calculocementum*.[73,78]

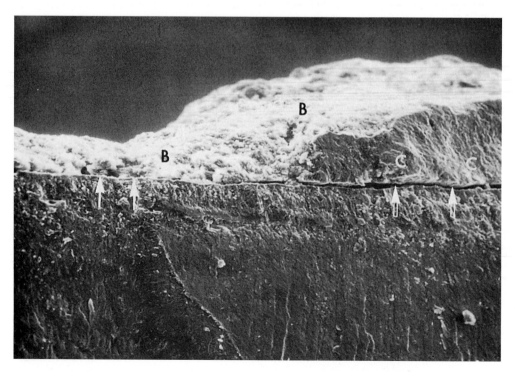

FIGURE 11-11. Scanning electron microscope view of an extracted human tooth, fractured experimentally, showing a cross section of subgingival calculus (C) that is not firmly attached to the cemental surface *(arrows).* Note bacteria (B) attached to calculus and cemental surface. (Courtesy of Dr. John Sottosanti.)

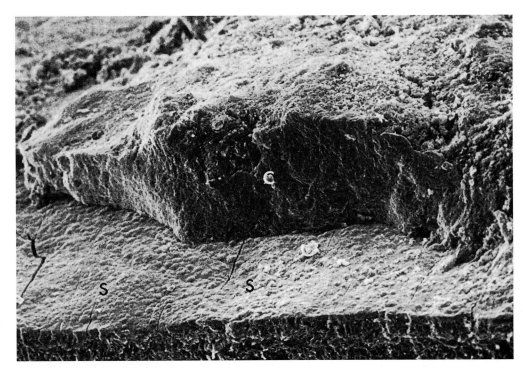

FIGURE 11-12. Scanning electron microscope view of an extracted human tooth, fractured experimentally, showing a cross section of subgingival calculus (C) attached to the cementum surface (S). (Courtesy of Dr. John Sottosanti.)

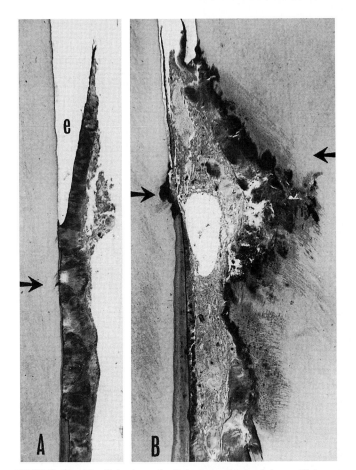

FIGURE 11-13. Calculus. *A,* Calculus attached to pellicle on enamel surface (e). The enamel was removed in the preparation of the specimen. Also note calculus attached to dentin and associated penetration of dental tubules *(arrows). B,* Interproximal area with early and advanced root caries of adjacent teeth and with calculus attached to carious surfaces *(arrows).*

Formation

Calculus is attached to dental plaque that has undergone mineralization. The soft plaque is hardened by precipitation of mineral salts, which usually starts between the first and the 14th day of plaque formation; however, calcification has been reported to occur in as little as 4 to 8 hours.[84] Calcifying plaques may become 50% mineralized in 2 days and 60% to 90% mineralized in 12 days.[54,69,75]

All plaque does not necessarily undergo calcification. Early plaque contains a small amount of inorganic material, which increases as the plaque develops into calculus. Plaque that does not develop into calculus reaches a plateau of maximal mineral content by 2 days.[54,70,75] Microorganisms are not always essential in calculus formation, as calculus occurs readily in germ-free rodents.[22,30]

Saliva is the mineral source for supragingival calculus, and the gingival fluid or exudate furnishes the minerals for subgingival calculus. Plaque has the ability to concentrate calcium at 2 to 20 times its level in saliva.[12] Early plaque of heavy calculus formers contains more calcium, three times more phosphorus, and less potassium than that of noncalculus formers, suggesting that phosphorus may be more critical than calcium in plaque mineralization.[50] Calcification entails the binding of calcium ions to the carbohydrate–protein complexes of the organic matrix[47] and the precipitation of crystalline calcium phosphate salts. Crystals form initially in the intercellular matrix and on the bacterial surfaces and, finally, within the bacteria.[26,98]

Calcification begins along the inner surface of the supragingival plaque (and in the attached component of subgingival plaque) adjacent to the tooth in separate foci that increase in size and coalesce to form solid masses of calculus (Fig. 11–16). It may be accompanied by alterations in the bacterial content and staining qualities of the plaque. With the occurrence of calcification, filamentous

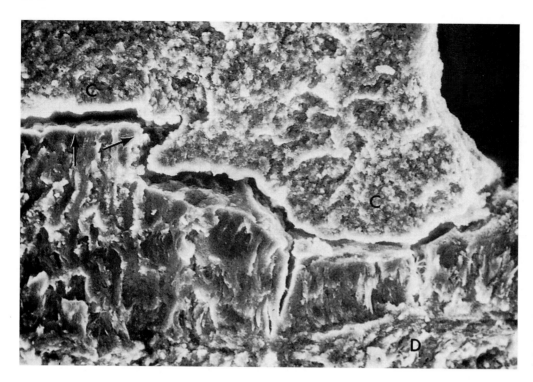

FIGURE 11–14. Subgingival calculus (C) embedded beneath the cementum surface *(arrows)* and penetrating to the dentin (D), making removal difficult. (Courtesy of Dr. John Sottosanti.)

bacteria increase in number. In the calcification foci there is a change from basophilia to eosinophilia; the staining intensity of groups exhibiting a positive periodic acid–Schiff reaction and of sulfhydryl and amino groups is reduced, and staining with toluidine blue, which is initially orthochromatic, becomes metachromatic and disappears.[92] Calculus is formed in layers, which are often separated by a thin cuticle that becomes embedded in the calculus as calcification progresses.[52]

Rate of Formation and Accumulation. The starting time and rates of calcification and accumulation of calculus

vary from person to person, in different teeth, and at different times in the same person.[56,85] On the basis of these differences, persons may be classified as heavy, moderate, or slight calculus formers or as non–calculus formers. The average daily increment in calculus formers is from 0.10% to 0.15% of dry weight.[75,85]

Calculus formation continues until it reaches a maximum, after which it may be reduced in amount. The time required to reach the maximal level has been reported as 10 weeks,[16] 18 weeks, and 6 months.[90] The decline from maximal accumulation (reversal phenomenon)[55,90] may be ex-

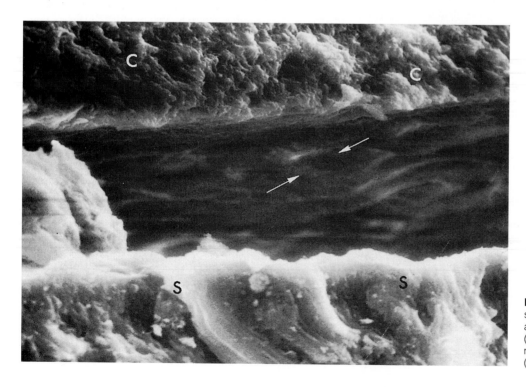

FIGURE 11–15. Undersurface of subgingival calculus (C) previously attached to the cementum surface (S). Note impression of cementum mounds in calculus *(arrows).* (Courtesy of Dr. John Sottosanti.)

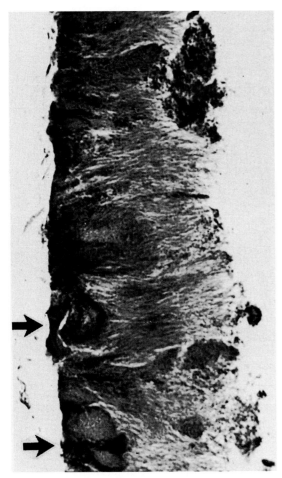

FIGURE 11-16. Five-day plaque, showing spherical calcification foci *(arrows)* and perpendicular alignment of filamentous organisms along the inner surface and colonies of cocci on the outer surface. (From Turesky S, Renstrup G, Glickman I. Histologic and histochemical observations regarding early calculus formation in children and adults. J Periodontol *32:*7, 1961.)

plained by the vulnerability of bulky calculus to mechanical wear from food and from the cheeks, lips, and tongue.

Anticalculus (antitartar) dentifrices claim to reduce the quantity and quality of calculus formed, making it easier to remove by the clinician. These products appear to be helpful for some patients.

Theories Regarding the Mineralization of Calculus. Theories regarding the mechanisms whereby plaque is mineralized to form calculus fit into two principal categories:[57]

1. *Mineral precipitation results from a local rise in the degree of saturation of calcium and phosphate ions,* which may be brought about in several ways:

   A rise in the pH of the saliva causes precipitation of calcium phosphate salts by lowering the precipitation constant. The pH may be elevated by the loss of carbon dioxide and by the formation of ammonia by dental plaque bacteria or by protein degradation during stagnation.[10,32,58]

   Colloidal proteins in saliva bind calcium and phosphate ions and maintain a supersaturated solution with respect to calcium phosphate salts. With stagnation of saliva, colloids settle out; the supersaturated state is no longer maintained, leading to precipitation of calcium phosphate salts.[63]

   Phosphatase liberated from dental plaque, desquamated epithelial cells, or bacteria precipitate calcium phosphate by hydrolyzing organic phosphates in saliva, thus increasing

the concentration of free phosphate ions.[15,94] Another enzyme, esterase, which is present in the cocci, filamentous organisms, leukocytes, macrophages, and desquamated epithelial cells of dental plaque, may initiate calcification by hydrolyzing fatty esters into free fatty acids.[4] The fatty acids form soaps with calcium and magnesium that are later converted into the less soluble calcium phosphate salts.

2. *Seeding agents induce small foci of calcification that enlarge and coalesce to form a calcified mass.*[59] This concept has been referred to as the *epitactic concept* or, more appropriately, *heterogeneous nucleation.* The seeding agents in calculus formation are not known, but it is suspected that the intercellular matrix of plaque plays an active role.[51,54,98] The carbohydrate–protein complexes may initiate calcification by removing calcium from the saliva (chelation) and binding with it to form nuclei that induce subsequent deposition of minerals.[47,91] Plaque bacteria have also been implicated as possible seeding agents (see following discussion).

Role of Microorganisms in the Mineralization of Calculus. Mineralization of plaque starts extracellularly around both gram-positive and gram-negative organisms[36]; it may also start intracellularly. Filamentous organisms, diphtheroids, and *Bacterionema* and *Veillonella* species have the ability to form intracellular apatite crystals. Calculus formation spreads until the matrix and bacteria are calcified.[26,66,98]

Some believe plaque bacteria actively participate in the mineralization of calculus by forming phosphatases, changing the plaque pH, or inducing mineralization,[19,47] but the prevalent opinion is that these bacteria are only passively involved[26,65,94] and are simply calcified along with other plaque components. The occurrence of calculus-like deposits in germ-free animals supports this opinion.[22,30] However, other experiments suggest that transmissible factors are involved in calculus formation and that penicillin in the diet of some of these animals reduces calculus formation.[5]

Etiologic Significance

It is difficult to separate the effects of calculus and plaque on the gingiva, because calculus is always covered with a nonmineralized layer of plaque.[70] There is a positive correlation between the presence of calculus and the prevalence of gingivitis,[64] but this correlation is not as great as that between plaque and gingivitis.[27] In young persons periodontal condition is more closely related to plaque accumulation than to calculus, but the situation is reversed with age.[27,41]

The incidence of calculus, gingivitis, and periodontal disease increases with age. It is extremely rare to find a periodontal pocket in adults without subgingival calculus, although in some cases subgingival calculus may be of microscopic proportion.

The nonmineralized plaque on the calculus surface is the principal irritant, but the underlying calcified portion may be a significant contributing factor. It does not irritate the gingiva directly, but it provides a fixed nidus for the continued accumulation of plaque and holds it against the gingiva.

Subgingival calculus may be the product rather than the cause of periodontal pockets. Plaque initiates gingival inflammation, which starts pocket formation, and the pocket in turn provides a sheltered area for plaque and bacterial accumulation. The increased flow of gingival fluid associated with gingival inflammation provides the minerals that convert the continually accumulating plaque into subgingival calculus.

Regardless of its primary or secondary relationship in pocket formation, and although the principal irritating feature of calculus is its surface plaque rather than its calcified interior, calculus is a significant pathogenic factor in periodontal disease.

MATERIA ALBA

Materia alba is a yellow or grayish white, soft, sticky deposit and is somewhat less adherent than dental plaque.[71] It is a concentration of microorganisms, desquamated epithelial cells, leukocytes, and a mixture of salivary proteins and lipids,[49,71,96] with few or no food particles,[62] and lacks the regular internal pattern observed in plaque. Materia alba is clearly visible without the use of disclosing agents and forms on tooth surfaces, restorations, calculus, and gingiva[49,54] (see Plate IIC). It tends to accumulate on the gingival third of the teeth and on malposed teeth. It can form on previously cleaned teeth within a few hours and during periods when no food is ingested.[62] Materia alba can be flushed away with a water spray, but mechanical cleansing is required to ensure complete removal.

The irritating effect of materia alba on the gingiva is caused by bacteria and their products. Materia alba has also been demonstrated to be toxic when injected into experimental animals after the bacterial component has been destroyed by heat.[9]

FOOD DEBRIS

Most food debris is rapidly liquefied by bacterial enzymes and cleared from the oral cavity within 5 minutes after eating, but some remains on the teeth and mucosa.[11,62] Salivary flow; mechanical action of the tongue, cheeks, and lips; and the form and alignment of the teeth and jaws affect the rate of food clearance, which is accelerated by increased chewing activity and the low viscosity of saliva.[35] Although it contains bacteria, food debris is different from the bacterial coatings (plaque and materia alba). Dental plaque is not a derivative of food debris, nor is food debris an important cause of gingivitis.[18] Food debris should be differentiated from fibrous strands trapped interproximally in areas of food impaction.

The rate of clearance from the oral cavity varies with the type of food and the individual. Liquids are cleared more readily than solids. For example, traces of sugar ingested in aqueous solution remain in the saliva for approximately 15 minutes, whereas sugar consumed in solid form is present for as long as 30 minutes after ingestion.[89] Sticky foods, such as figs, bread, toffee, and caramel, may adhere to tooth surfaces for more than 1 hour, whereas coarse foods such as raw carrots and apples are quickly cleared. Plain bread is cleared faster than bread with butter,[11,29] brown rye bread faster than white,[35] and cold foods slightly faster than hot. The chewing of apples and other fibrous foods can effectively remove most of the food debris from the oral cav-

ity, although it has no significant effect on the reduction of plaque.[12,42]

DENTAL STAINS

Pigmented deposits on the tooth surface are called *stains*. They are primarily an aesthetic problem. Stains result from the pigmentation of ordinarily colorless developmental and acquired dental coatings by chromogenic bacteria, foods, and chemicals. They vary in color and composition and in the firmness with which they adhere to the tooth surface.

Brown stain is a thin, translucent, acquired, usually bacteria-free, pigmented pellicle.[52,86-88] It occurs in individuals who do not brush sufficiently or who use a dentifrice with inadequate cleansing action. It is found most commonly on the buccal surface of the maxillary molars and on the lingual surface of the mandibular incisors. The brown color is usually due to the presence of tannin.

Tobacco stain is a tenacious dark brown or black surface deposit accompanied by brown discoloration of the tooth substance (see Figs. 11–7 and 11–8). Staining results from coal tar combustion products and from penetration of pits and fissures, enamel, and dentin by tobacco juices. The degree of staining is not necessarily proportional to the amount of tobacco consumed, but depends to a considerable degree on pre-existent acquired coatings that attach the tobacco products to the tooth surface.

Black stain occurs as a thin black line on facial and lingual surfaces of the teeth near the gingival margin and as a diffuse patch on the proximal surfaces. It is firmly attached, tends to recur after removal, is more common in women, and may occur in individuals with excellent hygiene. The black stain that occurs on human primary teeth is typically associated with a low incidence of caries in affected children.[76,82] Chromogenic bacteria have been implicated. The microflora of black stain is dominated by gram-positive rods, primarily *Actinomyces* species, and evidence implicates these bacteria as a probable cause. Isolated *Actinomyces* bacteria can produce black pigmentation, and in vitro investigations have demonstrated black pigment formation caused by *Actinomyces* in the dentin.[61,76] The chromogenic bacterial species *Prevotella melaninogenicus* accounts for less than 1% of isolated bacteria and is not considered an important cause of black stain.[76]

Green stain is a green or greenish yellow stain, sometimes of considerable thickness, that is common in children (see Plate IIF). It is considered to be the stained remnants of the enamel cuticle, but this has not been substantiated.[2] The discoloration has been attributed to fluorescent bacteria and fungi such as *Penicillium* and *Aspergillus*.[3] Green stain usually occurs on the facial surface of the maxillary anterior teeth, in the gingival half; it occurs more often in boys (65%) than in girls (43%).[37]

Orange stain is less common than green or brown stains. It may occur on both the facial and the lingual surfaces of anterior teeth. *Serratia marcescens* and *Flavobacterium lutescens* have been suggested as the responsible chromogenic organisms.[7]

Metallic stains are caused by metals and metallic salts, which may be introduced into the oral cavity in metal-containing dust inhaled by industrial workers or through orally administered drugs. The metals combine with acquired dental coatings (usually pellicle) to produce a surface stain or penetrate the tooth substance to cause permanent discoloration. Copper dust produces a green stain and iron dust a brown stain. Iron-containing medicines cause a black iron sulfite deposit. Other occasionally seen metallic stains are attributable to manganese (black), mercury (greenish black), nickel (green), and silver (black).

Chlorhexidine stain has been observed after prolonged use of this substance as a mouth rinse.[23,24,46,60] Chlorhexidine was introduced as a general disinfectant with a broad antibacterial action against gram-positive and gram-negative bacteria and fungi[23,46] (see Plate II*D* and Chapter 42). In vivo experiments using radioactive carbon-labeled chlorhexidine have shown retention of chlorhexidine in the human oral cavity.[12,22,23] This retention is attributed to chlorhexidine's affinity for sulfate and acidic groups such as those found in plaque constituents, carious lesions, pellicle, and bacterial cell walls.[13,23,31,60] Retention of chlorhexidine is concentration and time dependent and is not influenced by the temperature or pH of the rinsing solution.[13]

Chlorhexidine stain imparts a yellowish brown to brownish color to the tissues of the oral cavity.[20,23,24] The staining appears in the cervical and interproximal regions of the teeth, on restorations, in plaque, and on the surface of the tongue.[23,24,31,46,60] The presence of aldehydes and ketones, which are normally intermediates of both mammalian and microbial metabolism, appears to be essential for formation of discoloration by chlorhexidine.[60] No permanent staining of the enamel or dentin is observed clinically, because toothbrushing with a dentifrice or professional prophylaxis can remove any stain accumulating on the teeth.[60] A similar stain occurs with the use of alexidine.

REFERENCES

1. Anerud A, Loe H, Boysen H. The natural history and clinical course of calculus formation in man. J Clin Periodontol *18:*160, 1991.
2. Ayers P. Green stains. J Am Dent Assoc *26:*3, 1939.
3. Badanes BB. The role of fungi in deposits upon the teeth. Dent Cosmos *25:*795, 1939.
4. Baer PN, Burstone MS. Esterase activity associated with formation of deposits on teeth. Oral Surg *12:*1147, 1959.
5. Baer PN, Keyes PH, White CL. Studies on experimental calculus formation in the rat. XII. On the transmissibility of factors affecting dental calculus. J Periodontol *39:*86, 1968.
6. Barros L, Witkop CP. Oral and genetic study of Chileans, 1960. III. Periodontal disease and nutritional factors. Arch Oral Biol *8:*195, 1963.
7. Bartels HA. A note on chromogenic microorganisms from an organic colored deposit of the teeth. Int J Orthod *25:*795, 1939.
8. Baumhammers A, Stallard RE. A method for the labeling of certain constituents in the organic matrix of dental calculus. J Dent Res *45:*1568, 1966.
9. Beckwith TB, Williams A. Materia alba as toxic material. Am Dent Surg *29:*73, 1929.
10. Bibby BG. The formation of salivary calculus. Dent Cosmos *77:*668, 1935.
11. Bibby BG, Goldberg HJV, Chen E. Evaluation of caries producing potentialities of various foodstuffs. J Am Dent Assoc *42:*491, 1951.
12. Birkeland J, Jorkjend L. The effect of chewing apples on dental plaque and food debris. Commun Dent Oral Epidemiol *2:*161, 1974.
13. Bonesvell D, Lokken P, Rolla G. Influence of concentration, time, temperature and pH on the retention of chlorhexidine in the human oral cavity after mouth rinses. Arch Oral Biol *19:*1025, 1974.
14. Buchanan SA, Jenderseck RS, Granet MA, et al. Radiographic detection of dental calculus. J Periodontol *58:*747, 1987.
15. Citron S. The role of *Actinomyces israelii* in salivary calculus formation. J Dent Res *24:*87, 1945.
16. Conroy C, Sturzenberger O. The rate of calculus formation in adults. J Periodontol *39:*142, 1968.
17. Dawes C, Jenkins GN. Some inorganic constituents of dental plaque and their relationship to early calculus formation and caries. Arch Oral Biol *7:*161, 1962.
18. Egelberg J. Local effect of diet on plaque formation and development of gingivitis in dogs. III. Effect of frequency of meals and tube feeding. Odontol Revy *16:*50, 1965.
19. Ennever J. Microbiologic mineralization: A calcifiable cell-free extract from a calcifiable microorganism. J Dent Res *41:*1383, 1962.
20. Eriksen H, Gjermo P. Incidence of stained tooth surfaces in students using chlorhexidine-containing dentifrices. Scand J Dent Res *81:*533, 1973.
21. Everett FG, Tuchler H, Lu KH. Occurrence of calculus in grade school children in Portland, Oregon. J Periodontol *34:*54, 1963.
22. Gjermo P. Chlorhexidine in dental practice. J Clin Periodontol *1:*143, 1974.
23. Gjermo P, Basstad K, Rolla G. The plaque inhibiting capacity of eleven antibacterial compounds. J Periodont Res *5:*102, 1970.
24. Glas JE, Krasse B. Biophysical studies on dental calculus from germ free and conventional rats. Acta Odontol Scand *20:*127, 1962.
25. Glock GE, Murray MM. Chemical investigation of salivary calculus. J Dent Res *17:*257, 1938.
26. Gonzales F, Sognnaes RF. Electromicroscopy of dental calculus. Science *131:*156, 1960.
27. Greene JC. Oral hygiene and periodontal disease. Am J Public Health *53:*913, 1963.
28. Greene JC, Vermillion JR. The Oral Hygiene Index. J Am Dent Assoc *68:*7, 1964.
29. Grenby T. The influence of sticky foods of high sugar content on dental caries in the rat. Arch Oral Biol *14:*1259, 1969.
30. Gustafsson BE, Krasse B. Dental calculus in germ free rats. Acta Odontol Scand *20:*135, 1962.
31. Heyden G. Relation between locally high concentrations of chlorhexidine and staining as seen in the clinic. J Periodont Res *12*(suppl):76, 1973.
32. Hodge HC, Leung SW. Calculus formation. J Periodontol *21:*211, 1950.
33. Jenkins GN. The Physiology of the Mouth. Oxford, Blackwell Scientific Publications, 1966, p 495.
34. Kupczyk L, Conroy M. The attachment of calculus to root planed surfaces. Periodontics *6:*78, 1968.
35. Lanke LS. Influence on salivary sugar of certain properties of foodstuffs and individual oral conditions. Acta Odontol Scand *15*(suppl 23):3, 1957.
36. Leach SA, Saxton CA. An electron microscopic study of the acquired pellicle and plaque formed on the enamel of human incisors. Arch Oral Biol *11:*1081, 1966.
37. Leung SW. Naturally occurring stains on the teeth of children. J Am Dent Assoc *41:*191, 1950.
38. Leung SW. The uneven distribution of calculus in the mouth. J Periodontol *22:*7, 1951.
39. Leung SW. Role of calculus deposits in periodontal disease. In Muhler JC, Hine MK, eds. A Symposium on Preventive Dentistry. St Louis, CV Mosby, 1956, p 206.
40. Leung SW, Jensen AT. Factors controlling the deposition of calculus. Int Dent J *8:*613, 1958.
41. Lilienthal B, Amerena V, Gregory G. An epidemiological study of chronic periodontal disease. Arch Oral Biol *10:*553, 1965.
42. Lindhe J, Wicen P. The effects on the gingivae of chewing fibrous foods. J Periodont Res *4:*193, 1969.
43. Little MF, Bowman L, Casciani CA, Rowley J. The composition of dental calculus. III. Supragingival calculus. The amino acid and saccharide component. Arch Oral Biol *11:*385, 1966.
44. Little MF, Bowman LM, Dirksen TR. The lipids of supragingival calculus. J Dent Res *43:*836, 1964.
45. Little MF, Hazen SP. Dental calculus composition. 2. Subgingival calculus: Ash, calcium, phosphorus and sodium. J Dent Res *43:*645, 1964.
46. Löe H, Schiott C. The effect of mouth rinses and topical application of chlorhexidine on the development of dental plaque and gingivitis in man. J Periodont Res *5:*79, 1970.
47. Mandel ID. Calculus formation. The role of bacteria and mucoprotein. Dent Clin North Am *4:*731, 1960.
48. Mandel ID. Histochemical and biochemical aspects of calculus formation. Periodontics *1:*43, 1963.
49. Mandel ID. Dental plaque: Nature, formation, and effects. J Periodontol *37:*357, 1966.
50. Mandel ID. Biochemical aspects of calculus formation. J Periodont Res *4*(suppl):7, 1969.
51. Mandel ID, Levy BM, Wasserman BH. Histochemistry of calculus formation. J Periodontol *28:*132, 1957.
52. Manly RS. A structureless recurrent deposit on teeth. J Dent Res *22:*479, 1973.
53. Moskow BS. Calculus attachment in cemental separations. J Periodontol *40:*125, 1969.
54. Mühlemann HR, Schroeder H. Dynamics of supragingival calculus formation. Adv Oral Biol *1:*175, 1964.
55. Mühlemann HR, Villa PR. The Marginal Line Calculus Index. Helv Odontol Acta *11:*175, 1967.
56. Mühler JC, Ennever J. Occurrence of calculus through several successive periods in a selected group of subjects. J Periodontol *33:*22, 1962.
57. Mukherjee S. Formation and prevention of supragingival calculus. J Periodont Res *3*(suppl 2):1–33, 1968.
58. Naeslund C. A comparative study of the formation of concretions in the oral cavity and in the salivary glands and ducts. Dent Cosmos *68:*1137, 1926.
59. Neuman WF, Neuman MW. The Chemical Dynamics of Bone Mineral. Chicago, University of Chicago Press, 1958, p 209.

60. Nordno H. Discoloration of human teeth by a combination of chlorhexidine and aldehydes or ketones in vitro. Scand J Dent Res 79:356, 1971.
61. Onisi M, Nuckolls J. Description of *Actinomyces* and other pleomorphic organisms recovered from pigmented carious lesions of the dentine of human teeth. Oral Surg 11:910, 1958.
62. Parfitt GJ. Summary of the problem of the prevention of periodontal disease. Ala J Med Sci 5:305, 1968.
63. Prinz H. The origin of salivary calculus. Dent Cosmos 63:231, 369, 503, 619, 1921.
64. Ramfjord SP. The periodontal status of boys 11 to 17 years old in Bombay, India. J Periodontol 32:237, 1961.
65. Rizzo AA, Martin GR, Scott DB, Mergenhagen EE. Mineralization of bacteria. Science 135:439, 1962.
66. Rizzo AA, Scott DB, Bladen HA. Calcification of oral bacteria. Ann NY Acad Sci 109:14, 1963.
67. Rowles SL. The inorganic composition of dental calculus. In Blackwood HJJ, ed. Bone and Tooth. Oxford, Pergamon Press, 1964, p 175.
68. Schoff FR. Periodontia: An observation on the attachment of calculus. Oral Surg 8:154, 1955.
69. Schroeder HE. Inorganic content and histology of early dental calculus in man. Helv Odontol Acta 7:17, 1963.
70. Schroeder HE. Crystal morphology and gross structures of mineralizing plaque and of calculus. Helv Odontol Acta 9:73, 1965.
71. Schroeder HE. Formation and Inhibition of Dental Calculus. Berne, Hans Huber, 1969, p 12.
72. Schroeder HE, Bambauer HU. Stages of calcium phosphate crystallization during calculus formation. Arch Oral Biol 11:1, 1966.
73. Selvig J. Attachment of plaque and calculus to tooth surfaces. J Periodont Res 5:8, 1970.
74. Selvig KA. The formation of plaque and calculus on recently exposed tooth surfaces. J Periodont Res 4(suppl):10, 1969.
75. Sharawy A, Sabharwal K, Socransky SS, Lobene R. A quantitative study of plaque and calculus formation in normal and periodontally involved mouths. J Periodontol 37:495, 1966.
76. Slots J. The microflora of black stain on human primary teeth. Scand J Dent Res 82:484, 1974.
77. Sottosanti JS. A possible relationship between occlusion, root resorption, and the progression of periodontal disease. J West Soc Periodontol 25:69, 1977.
78. Sottosanti JS. Relationship of calculus to root surfaces. Personal communication, 1978.
79. Standford JW. Analysis of the organic portion of dental calculus. J Dent Res 45:128, 1966.
80. Stanton G. The relation of diet to salivary calculus formation. J Periodontol 40:167, 1969.
81. Stewart RT, Ratcliff PA. The source of components of subgingival plaque and calculus. Periodont Abstr 14:102, 1966.
82. Sutcliffe P. Extrinsic tooth stains in children. Dent Pract 17:175, 1967.
83. Theilade J, Schroeder HE. Recent results in dental calculus research. Int Dent J 16:205, 1966.
84. Tibbetts LS, Kashiwa HK. A histochemical study of early plaque mineralization. I.A.D.R. Abstracts, No. 616, 1970, p 202.
85. Turesky S, Renstrup G, Glickman I. Effects of changing the salivary environment on progress of calculus formation. J Periodontol 33:45, 1962.
86. Vallotton CF. An acquired pigmented pellicle of the enamel surface. I. Review of the literature. J Dent Res 24:161, 1945.
87. Vallotton CF. An acquired pigmented pellicle of the enamel surface. II. Clinical and histologic studies. J Dent Res 24:171, 1945.
88. Vallotton CF. An acquired pigmented pellicle of the enamel surface. III. Chemical studies. J Dent Res 24:183, 1945.
89. Volker JF, Pinkerton DM. Acid production in saliva carbohydrates. J Dent Res 26:229, 1947.
90. Volpe AR, Kupczak LJ, King WJ, et al. In vivo calculus assessment. Part IV. Parameters of human clinical studies. J Periodontol 40:76, 1969.
91. Von der Fehr F, Brudevold F. In vitro calculus formation. J Dent Res 39:1041, 1960.
92. Waerhaug J. The source of mineral salts in subgingival calculus. J Dent Res 34:563, 1955.
93. Waerhaug J. Effect of rough surfaces upon gingival tissue. J Dent Res 35:323, 1956.
94. Wasserman BH, Mandel JD, Levy BM. In vitro calcification of calculus. J Periodontol 29:145, 1958.
95. Wilkinson FC. A pathohistological study of the tissue to tooth attachment. Dent Record 55:105, 1935.
96. World Health Organization. Periodontal disease: Report of an expert committee on dental health. Int Dent J 11:544, 1961.
97. Zander HA. The attachment of calculus to root surfaces. J Periodontol 24:16, 1953.
98. Zander HA, Hazen SP, Scott DB. Mineralization of dental calculus. Proc Soc Exp Biol Med 103:257, 1960.

12

The Role of Iatrogenic and Other Local Factors

FERMIN A. CARRANZA, Jr.

IATROGENIC FACTORS

Faults in dental restorations and prostheses, referred to as *iatrogenic factors,* are common causes of gingival inflammation and periodontal destruction. Inadequate dental procedures may also injure the periodontal tissues. Six characteristics of restorations and partial dentures are important from a periodontal viewpoint: margins of restorations, contours, occlusion, materials, design of removable partial dentures, and restorative procedures themselves. They are described in this chapter because they play a role in the etiology of periodontal lesions; a more comprehensive review, with special emphasis on the recommended approach to restorative procedures, is presented in Chapter 67.

Margins of Restorations. Overhanging margins contribute to periodontal disease by (1) providing ideal locations for the accumulation of plaque and (2) changing the ecologic balance of the gingival sulcus area to one that favors the growth of disease-associated organisms (gram-negative anaerobic species) at the expense of the health-associated organisms (gram-positive facultative species)[60] (Figs. 12–1 and 12–2).

The frequency of overhanging margins of proximal restorations varies in different studies from 16.5% to 75%.[16,39,80] A highly significant statistical relationship was found between marginal defects and reduced bone height.[16,43,50] Removal of overhangs permits more effective control of plaque, resulting in the disappearance of gingival inflammation and increased alveolar bone support.[40,44]

The location of the gingival margin of a restoration is directly related to the periodontal health status.[97] Subgingivally located margins are associated with large amounts of plaque, more severe gingivitis, and deeper pockets. Margins placed at the level of the gingiva induce less severe conditions; and supragingival margins are associated with a degree of periodontal health similar to that seen with intact control surfaces.[32,97]

Numerous studies[39,47,52,88,100] have shown a positive correlation between subgingival margins and gingival inflammation. It has also been shown that even high-quality restorations, if placed subgingivally, will increase plaque accumulation, gingival inflammation,[61,74,89] and the rate of gingival fluid flow.[76]

Roughness in the subgingival area is considered to be the major cause of plaque buildup and the resultant inflammatory response.[97] The subgingival zone is made up of the crown and the margin of the restoration, the luting material, and the prepared tooth surface. Several sources of roughness have been described:[97] stripes and scratches in the surface of carefully polished acrylic resin, porcelain, or gold restorations (Fig. 12–3); separation of the cervical crown margin and the cervical margin of the finishing line by the luting material, exposing the rough surface of the prepared tooth (Fig. 12–4); dissolution and disintegration of the luting material, causing crater formation between the preparation and the restoration (Fig. 12–5); and inadequate marginal fit of the restoration.

The undersurface of pontics in fixed bridges should barely touch the mucosa. When this contact is excessive, it prevents cleaning. Plaque accumulates, causing inflammation and even pseudopocket formation (Fig. 12–6).

Contours. Overcontoured crowns and restorations tend to accumulate plaque and possibly prevent the self-cleaning mechanisms of the adjacent cheek, lips, and tongue[4,57,73,107] (Fig. 12–7). Previous claims that undercontouring of crowns may also have a deleterious effect as a result of lack of protection of the gingival margin during mastication have not been proved.[107]

Inadequate or improperly located proximal contacts and failure to reproduce the normal protective anatomy of the occlusal marginal ridges and developmental grooves lead to food impaction. Failure to re-establish adequate interproximal embrasures fosters the accumulation of irritants.

Occlusion. Restorations that do not conform to the occlusal patterns of the mouth cause occlusal disharmonies

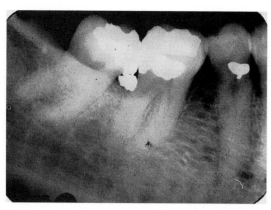

FIGURE 12–1. Amalgam excess, which is a source of irritation to the gingiva.

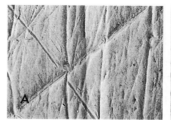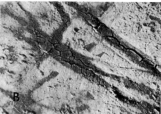

FIGURE 12–3. *A,* A polished gold alloy crown demonstrates surface scratches. *B,* A gold alloy crown that had been in the mouth for several years has scratches filled with deposits. (From Silness J. Fixed prosthodontics and periodontal health. Dent Clin North Am *24:*317, 1980.)

that may be injurious to the supporting periodontal tissues (see Chapter 24).

Materials. In general, restorative materials are not themselves injurious to the periodontal tissues.[4,53] One exception to this may be self-curing acrylics.[105]

Restorative materials differ in their capacity to retain plaque,[105] but all can be adequately cleaned if they are polished[75,91] and accessible to brushing. The composition of plaque formed on all types of restorative materials is similar, with the exception of that formed on silicate.[75] Plaque formed at the margins of restorations is similar to that formed on adjacent tooth surfaces.

Design of Removable Partial Dentures. Several investigations have shown that after the insertion of partial dentures, there is an increase in mobility of the abutment teeth, gingival inflammation, and periodontal pocket formation.[15,21,93] This is because partial dentures favor the accumulation of plaque, particularly if they cover the gingival tissue. Partial dentures that are worn night and day induce more plaque formation than those worn only during the day.[15] These observations emphasize the need for careful and personalized oral hygiene instruction to avoid harmful effects of partial dentures on the remaining teeth.[10]

The presence of removable partial dentures induces not only quantitative changes in dental plaque,[36] but also qualitative changes, promoting the development of spirilla and spirochetes.[37]

Restorative Dentistry Procedures. The use of rubber dam clamps, copper bands, matrix bands, and discs in such

a manner as to lacerate the gingiva results in varying degrees of inflammation. Although for the most part such transient injuries undergo repair, they are needless sources of discomfort to the patient. Injudicious tooth separation and excessively vigorous condensing of gold foil restorations are sources of injury to the supporting tissues of the periodontium that may be attended by acute symptoms such as pain and sensitivity to percussion.

PERIODONTAL PROBLEMS ASSOCIATED WITH ORTHODONTIC THERAPY

Orthodontic therapy may affect the periodontium by favoring plaque retention, by directly injuring the gingiva as a result of overextended bands, and by creating excessive and/or unfavorable forces on the supporting tooth structures.

Retention of Plaque. Orthodontic appliances not only tend to retain bacterial plaque and food debris, resulting in gingivitis (Fig. 12–8), but also are capable of modifying the gingival ecosystem. After tooth-banding, an increase in *Prevotella melaninogenica, P. intermedia,* and *Actinomyces odontolyticus* and a decrease in anaerobic/facultative flora in the gingival sulcus have been reported.[28]

Irritation From Orthodontic Bands. Orthodontic treatment is often started at a stage of tooth eruption when the

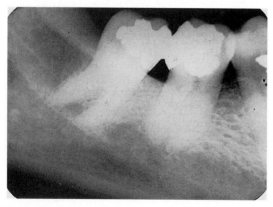

FIGURE 12–2. Amalgam excess removed (same case as in Fig. 12–1).

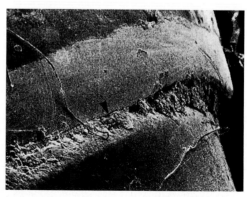

FIGURE 12–4. After cementation, luting material prevents approximation of the crown margin and the finishing line, leaving part of the prepared tooth uncovered *(area between arrowheads).* (From Silness J. Fixed prosthodontics and periodontal health. Dent Clin North Am *24:*317, 1980.)

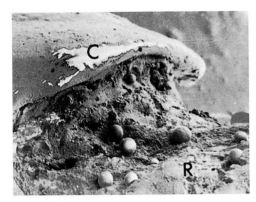

FIGURE 12–5. Craters have formed after dissolution and disintegration of the luting material. Spherical bodies are not identified. C, Crown; R, root. (From Silness J. Fixed prosthodontics and periodontal health. Dent Clin North Am *24*:317, 1980.)

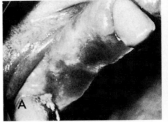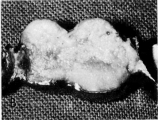

FIGURE 12–6. *A,* Red, inflamed soft tissues *(dark area on the ridge)* were found beneath the pontics after removal of a bridge that had been in the mouth for 12 years. *B,* The undersurfaces of the pontics were covered with a thick layer of plaque. (From Silness J. Fixed prosthodontics and periodontal health. Dent Clin North Am *24*:317, 1980.)

junctional epithelium is still on the enamel. The bands should not extend into the gingival tissues beyond the level of attachment. Forceful detachment of the gingiva from the tooth followed by apical proliferation of the junctional epithelium results in the increased gingival recession sometimes seen in orthodontically treated patients.[81] If gingival inflammation is present, the gingival margin is prevented from following the migrating epithelium, and pocket formation results.

Tissue Response to Orthodontic Forces. Orthodontic tooth movement is possible because the periodontal tissues are responsive to externally applied forces.[87,92] The bone is remodeled by an increase in osteoclasts and bone resorption in areas of pressure and by increased osteoblastic activity and bone formation in areas of tension. Orthodontic forces also produce vascular changes in the periodontal ligament that may influence bone resorptive and formative patterns.[23,38]

It is important to avoid excessive force and too rapid tooth movement in orthodontic treatment. Excessive force may produce necrosis of the periodontal ligament and adjacent alveolar bone, which ordinarily undergo repair. However, destruction of the periodontal ligament at the crest of the alveolar bone may lead to irreparable damage. If the periodontal fibers beneath the junctional epithelium are de-

stroyed by excessive force and the epithelium is stimulated to proliferate along the root by local irritants, the epithelium will cover the root and prevent re-embedment of the periodontal fibers in the course of repair. Excessive orthodontic forces also increase the risk of apical root resorption.

It has been reported that the marginal and attached gingivae are "pulled" when teeth are orthodontically rotated[29] and that relapse of the occlusion after orthodontic treatment can be reduced by surgical resection or removal of free gingival fibers, combined with a brief retention period.[17,72] Temporary separation of the reduced enamel epithelium on the tension side of orthodontically moved teeth and displacement and folding of the interdental papillae on the pressure side have also been noted.[8] A statistically significant, greater loss of attachment and of alveolar bone after orthodontic treatment has been reported[108,109] but has not been confirmed by other authors.[84,104]

FOOD IMPACTION

Food impaction is the forceful wedging of food into the periodontium by occlusal forces. It may occur interproximally or in relation to the facial or lingual tooth surfaces. Food impaction is a very common cause of gingival inflammation. Failure to recognize and eliminate food impaction

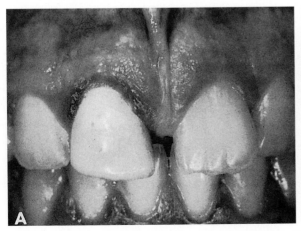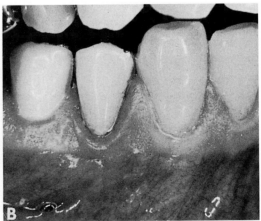

FIGURE 12–7. *A,* Gingival inflammation and recession associated with accumulated irritants on rough margin of crown. *B,* Inadequate mesial contour on first premolar restoration leads to accumulation of irritants and gingival inflammation.

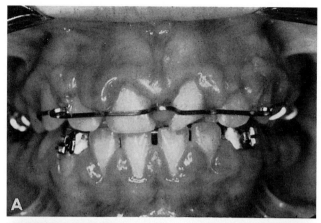

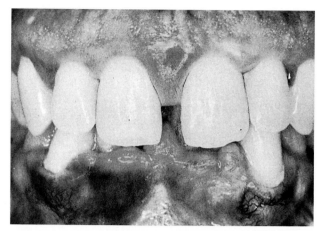

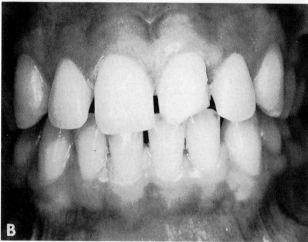

FIGURE 12-8. Gingival inflammation and enlargement associated with orthodontic appliance and poor oral hygiene. *A,* Gingival disease with orthodontic appliance in place. *B,* Appearance after removal of the appliance and periodontal treatment.

FIGURE 12-9. Inflammatory gingival enlargement in the mandibular anterior region associated with overbite and food impaction.

may be responsible for the unsuccessful outcome of an otherwise thoroughly treated case of periodontal disease.

Mechanism

Normally, the forceful wedging of food is prevented by the integrity and location of the proximal contacts, the contour of the marginal ridges and developmental grooves, and the contour of the facial and lingual surfaces. An intact, firm proximal contact relationship prevents the forceful wedging of food interproximally. The location of the contact is also important in protecting the tissues against food impaction. The optimal cervico-occlusal location of the contact is at the longest mesiodistal diameter of the tooth, close to the crest of the marginal ridge. The proximity of the contact point to the occlusal plane reduces the tendency toward food impaction in the smaller occlusal embrasure. The absence of contact or the presence of an unsatisfactory proximal relationship is conducive to food impaction.

The contour of the occlusal surface established by the marginal ridges and related developmental grooves normally serves to deflect food away from the interproximal spaces. As the teeth wear down and flattened surfaces replace the normal convexities, the wedging effect of the op-

posing cusp into the interproximal space is exaggerated, and food impaction results. Cusps that tend to forcibly wedge food interproximally are known as *plunger cusps.* The plunger cusp effect may occur with wear, as indicated, or be the result of a shift in tooth position after failure to replace missing teeth.

Excessive anterior overbite is a common cause of food impaction (Fig. 12-9). Forceful wedging of food into the gingiva on the facial surfaces of the mandibular anterior teeth and the lingual surfaces of the maxillary teeth produces varying degrees of periodontal involvement.

The classic analysis of the factors leading to food impaction was made by Hirschfeld,[45] who recognized the following factors: uneven occlusal wear, opening of the contact point as a result of loss of proximal support or from extrusion, congenital morphologic abnormalities, and improperly constructed restorations (Figs. 12-10 to 12-13).

However, the presence of the previously mentioned abnormalities does not necessarily lead to food impaction and periodontal disease. A study of interproximal contacts and

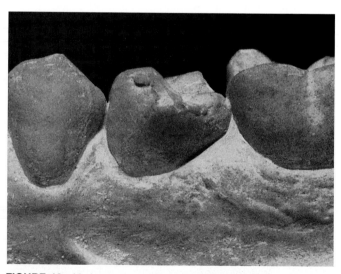

FIGURE 12-10. Improper proximal contact relationship associated with malposed premolar. Note the inclined "plateau" that directs food from the occlusal surface of the premolar into the distal interdental space.

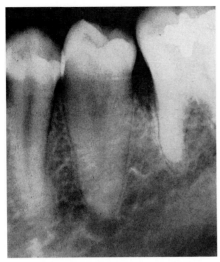

FIGURE 12–11. Bone loss in an area of food impaction associated with improper contact between the mandibular second premolar and molar.

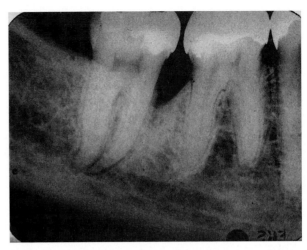

FIGURE 12–13. Food impaction and bone loss associated with restorations that fail to restore and maintain proximal contact.

marginal ridge relationships in three groups of periodontally healthy males revealed that from 61.7% to 76% of the proximal contacts were defective and that 33.5% of adjacent marginal ridges were uneven.[78]

Lateral Food Impaction. In addition to food impaction caused by occlusal forces, lateral pressure from the lips, cheeks, and tongue may force food interproximally. This is more likely to occur when the gingival embrasure is enlarged by tissue destruction in periodontal disease or by recession. Impaction results when food forced into such an embrasure during mastication is retained instead of passed through.

Sequelae

Food impaction serves to initiate gingival and periodontal disease and aggravates the severity of pre-existent

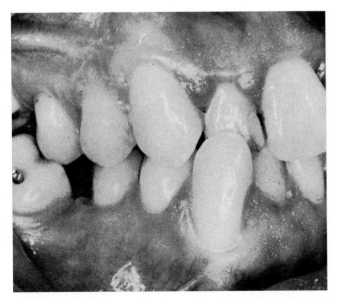

FIGURE 12–12. Malposed teeth with food impaction and gingival inflammation.

pathologic changes. The following signs and symptoms may occur in association with food impaction:

Feeling of pressure and the urge to dig the material from between the teeth

Vague pain that radiates deep in the jaws

Gingival inflammation, with bleeding and a foul taste in the involved area

Gingival recession

Periodontal abscess formation

Varying degrees of inflammatory involvement of the periodontal ligament, with an associated elevation of the tooth in its socket, prematurity in functional contact, and sensitivity to percussion

Destruction of the alveolar bone

Root caries

UNREPLACED MISSING TEETH

Failure to replace extracted teeth initiates a series of changes that produce various degrees of periodontal disease.[24,46] In isolated cases, spaces created by tooth extraction may not cause undesirable sequelae. *However, the frequency with which periodontal disease results from the failure to replace one or more missing teeth points to the advisability and prophylactic value of early prosthesis.*

The ramifications of failure to replace the first molar are sufficiently consistent to be recognized as a clinical entity. When the mandibular first molar is extracted, the initial change is a mesial drifting and tilting of the mandibular second and third molars and extrusion of the maxillary first molar. The distal cusps of the mandibular second molar are elevated and act as plungers, impacting food into the interproximal space between the extruded maxillary first molar and the maxillary second molar (Fig. 12–14). If there is no maxillary third molar, the distal cusps of the mandibular second molar act as a wedge that breaks the contact between the maxillary first and second molars and deflects the maxillary second molar distally. This results in food impaction, gingival inflammation, and bone loss in the interproximal area between the maxillary first and second molars. Tilting of the mandibular molars and extrusion of the maxillary molars alter the respective contact relationships

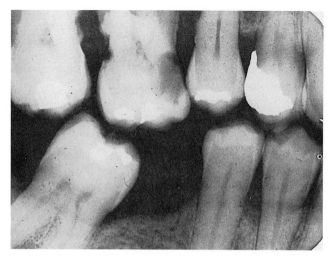

FIGURE 12–14. Tilted mandibular molar and extruded maxillary molar associated with unreplaced tooth. Note caries in the maxillary molar.

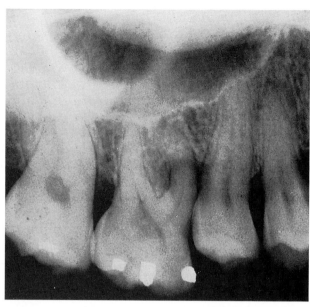

FIGURE 12–16. Extruded maxillary first molar with trifurcation involvement.

of these teeth, thereby favoring food impaction. Bone loss and pocket formation are commonly seen in relation to the extruded and tilted teeth (Figs. 12–15 to 12–17).

Tilting of the posterior teeth also results in a reduction in the vertical dimension and an accentuation of the anterior overbite. The mandibular anterior teeth slide gingivally along the palatal surfaces of the maxillary anterior teeth, resulting in a distal shift in the position of the mandible. In addition, there is food impaction and pocket formation in relation to the anterior teeth and a tendency toward labial migration and diastema formation in the maxilla. Distal drifting of the second premolar with food impaction and pocket formation in relation to the opened interproximal space between the premolars may be further complications. The aforementioned changes are accompanied by alterations in the functional relationships of the inclined cusps, with resultant occlusal disharmonies that are injurious to the periodontium. The changes associated with the unre-

placed mandibular first molar do not occur in all cases, nor are all the changes identified with failure to replace other teeth in the arch. In general, however, drifting and tilting of the teeth, with alterations in proximal contact, result from failure to replace teeth that have been extracted. These changes are common factors in the etiology of periodontal disease.

EXTRACTION OF IMPACTED THIRD MOLARS

Numerous clinical studies have reported that the extraction of impacted third molars often results in the creation of vertical defects distal to the second molars.[7] This iatrogenic effect is unrelated to flap design[25] and appears to occur more often when third molars are extracted in individu-

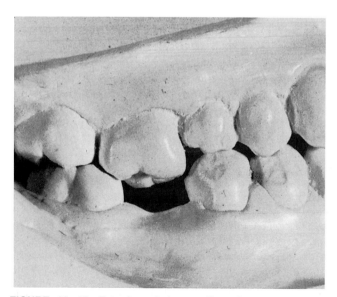

FIGURE 12–15. Extrusion of the maxillary first molar into the space created by unreplaced mandibular molar.

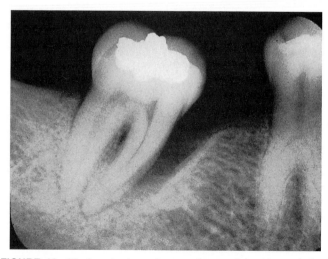

FIGURE 12–17. Angular bone loss on the mesial surface of tilted molar.

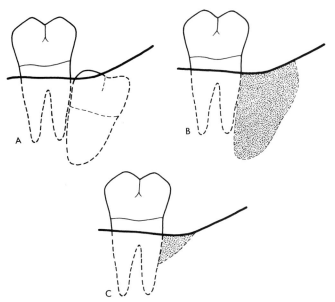

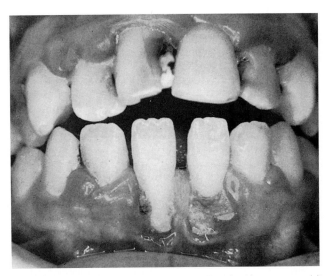

FIGURE 12–20. Chronic gingivitis associated with an open bite and accumulation of plaque and food debris.

FIGURE 12–18. *A,* Impacted third molar with little or no bone existing interdentally to the second molar. *B,* Third molar extraction results in a vertical osseous defect distal to the second molar *(C).*

als older than 25 years than in those younger than 25.[7,59,63] Other factors that appear to play a role in the development of distal lesions of second molars, particularly in those older than 25, are the presence of visible plaque, bleeding on probing, root resorption in the contact area between second and third molars, presence of a pathologically widened follicle, inclination of the third molar, and close proximity of the third molar to the second molar (Fig. 12–18).[59]

MALOCCLUSION

Depending on its nature, malocclusion exerts a varied effect on the etiology of gingivitis and periodontal dis-

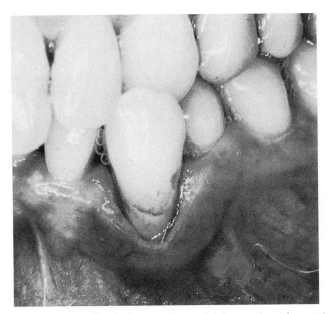

FIGURE 12–19. Gingival recession and inflammation of a malposed canine.

ease.[71,90] Irregular alignment of teeth will make plaque control difficult or even impossible. Several authors have found a positive correlation between crowding and periodontal disease,[18,80,103] although other investigators have found no correlation.[35] Uneven marginal ridges of contiguous posterior teeth have been found to have a low correlation with pocket depth, loss of attachment, plaque, calculus, and gingival inflammation.[55]

Gingival recession is associated with facially displaced teeth (Fig. 12–19). Occlusal disharmony associated with malocclusion results in injury to the periodontium.[77] The incisal edges of the anterior teeth often cause irritation to the gingiva in the opposing jaw in patients with a severe overbite. Open bite relationships lead to unfavorable periodontal changes caused by accumulation of plaque and an absence of or diminution in function (Fig. 12–20).[18,55] The prevalence and severity of periodontal disease are increased in children with bimaxillary protrusions.[48]

MOUTH BREATHING

Gingivitis is often associated with mouth breathing.[62] The gingival changes include erythema, edema, enlargement, and a diffuse surface shininess in the exposed areas (see Chapter 17). The maxillary anterior region is the common site of such involvement. In many cases, the altered gingiva is clearly demarcated from the adjacent unexposed normal mucosa (Fig. 12–21). The exact manner in which mouth breathing effects gingival changes has not been demonstrated. Its harmful effect is generally attributed to irritation from surface dehydration. However, comparable changes could not be produced by air drying the gingivae of experimental animals.[56]

Several studies have presented conflicting evidence with respect to the association of mouth breathing and gingivitis. The following findings have been reported:

1. Mouth breathing has no effect on the prevalence or extent of gingivitis except in patients with considerable calculus.[2]
2. Mouth breathers have more severe gingivitis than non–mouth breathers with similar plaque scores.[48]

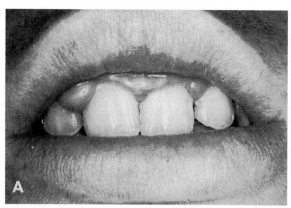
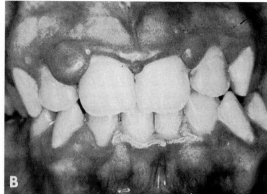

FIGURE 12–21. Gingivitis in mouth breather. *A,* High lip line in a mouth breather. *B,* Gingivitis and inflammatory gingival enlargement in an exposed area of gingiva.

3. There is no relationship between mouth breathing and prevalence of gingivitis, except a slight increase in severity.[103]
4. Crowding of teeth is associated with gingivitis only in mouth breathers.[49]

HABITS

Habit is an important factor in the initiation and progression of periodontal disease. Frequently the presence of an unsuspected habit is revealed in patients who have failed to respond to periodontal therapy. Habits of significance in the etiology of periodontal disease have been classified by Sorrin[101] as follows:

1. *Neuroses,* such as lip biting and cheek biting, which lead to extrafunctional positioning of the mandible; toothpick biting and wedging between the teeth; tongue thrusting; fingernail biting; pencil/pen biting; and occlusal neuroses.
2. *Occupational habits,* such as the holding of nails in the mouth, as practiced by cobblers, upholsterers, or carpenters; thread biting; and pressure of a reed during the playing of certain musical instruments.
3. *Miscellaneous habits,* such as pipe or cigarette smoking (Fig. 12–22), tobacco chewing, incorrect methods of toothbrushing, mouth breathing, and thumb sucking.

Habits such as bruxism, clenching, and tapping are discussed in Chapter 13.

Tongue Thrusting

Special mention should be made of tongue thrusting, because it is frequently undetected. Tongue thrusting entails persistent, forceful wedging of the tongue against the teeth, particularly in the anterior region. Instead of the dorsum of the tongue being placed against the palate with the tip behind the maxillary teeth during swallowing, the tongue is thrust forward against the anterior teeth, which tilt and also spread laterally (Fig. 12–23).

Tongue thrusting causes excessive lateral pressure, which may be traumatic to the periodontium.[22,96] It also causes spreading and tilting of the anterior teeth, with an open bite anteriorly, posteriorly, or in the premolar area (Fig. 12–23).

Numerous secondary sequelae may develop from tongue thrusting. The altered inclination of the maxillary anterior teeth results in a change in the direction of the functional forces so that lateral pressure against the crowns is in-

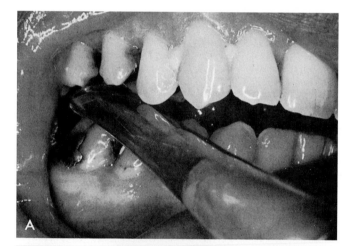
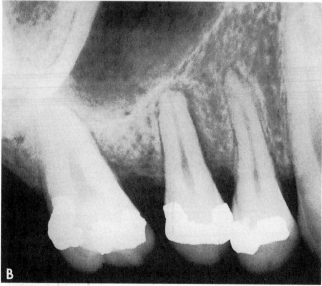

FIGURE 12–22. Trauma associated with holding a pipe in a fixed position. *A,* Pipe held by maxillary first and second premolars and molar. Note the intruded second premolar and tilted molar. *B,* Radiograph showing an intruded second premolar with apical resorption and widened periodontal ligament and angular bone destruction on the mesial surface. Note the widened periodontal ligament on the first premolar and the tilted molar.

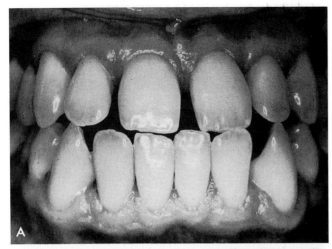
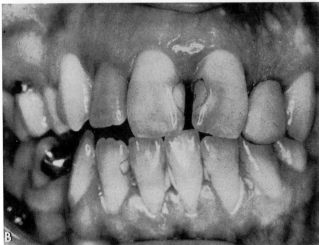

FIGURE 12–23. Tongue thrusting. *A,* Tilting and spreading of anterior teeth associated with tongue thrusting. *B,* Hypo-occlusion of the lateral incisor, canine, and premolar associated with tongue thrusting.

creased. This aggravates the labial drift and undesirable labiolingual rotational forces. The antagonism between forces that direct the tooth labially and inward pressure from the lip may lead to tooth mobility. The altered inclination of the teeth also interferes with food excursion and favors the accumulation of food debris at the gingival margin. The loss of proximal contact leads to food impaction. Tongue thrusting is an important contributing factor in pathologic tooth migration.[22,24]

Use of Tobacco

There is increasing scientific evidence that smoking has a detrimental effect on the progression of periodontal disease and healing after periodontal therapy. Heat and the accumulated products of combustion are particularly undesirable local irritants.

The following oral changes may occur in smokers:

1. Brownish, tar-like deposits and discoloration of tooth structure. Nicotine and its major metabolite, cotinine, are deposited on root surfaces.[26]
2. Diffuse grayish discoloration and leukoplakia of the gingiva may occur.
3. "Smoker's palate" (nicotinic stomatitis), characterized by

prominent mucous glands with inflammation of the orifices and a diffuse erythema or by a wrinkled, "cobblestone" surface, may occur.

4. The correlation between tobacco smoking and acute necrotizing ulcerative gingivitis (ANUG) has been clearly shown,[6] although a cause-and-effect relationship has not been proved. Both smoking and ANUG may be the result of underlying anxiety and tension.
5. Postsurgical healing is delayed.[51,70,85]
6. Smoking induces an immediate transient but marked increase in gingival fluid flow, probably as a result of blood flow changes induced by nicotine.[67]
7. More severe gingivitis and periodontitis have been reported in smokers,[5,34,41,42,102] probably because of increased plaque accumulation. Women between the ages of 20 and 39 and men between 30 and 59 who smoke cigarettes have about twice the chance of having periodontal disease or becoming edentulous as do nonsmokers.[98] More calculus has been reported in pipe smokers than in cigarette smokers.[34,82,83] A reduced bone height has been reported in smokers when compared with nonsmokers of similar age and oral hygiene status.[11]

Some reports, however, have produced controversial results. One study found that tobacco smoking has little or no effect on the rate of plaque formation,[9] and another reported that it results in less gingival inflammation.[27] Some early studies reported that when smokers and nonsmokers were matched with regard to age and oral hygiene levels, no difference was found in the degree of gingival inflammation and periodontal breakdown.[58,86,95]

A specific type of gingivitis, termed *gingivitis toxica*[83] and characterized by destruction of the gingiva and underlying bone, has been attributed to the chewing of tobacco.

The following laboratory findings may point to changes responsible for increased periodontal problems in smokers: Keratinized cells in the gingiva are increased in smokers,[20] but no changes other than altered oxygen consumption can be detected in the buccal mucosa. Nicotine metabolites have been found in saliva and crevicular fluid.[66] Oral polymorphonuclear leukocytes from smokers show a reduced ability to phagocytize particles.[54] Vascular reaction associated with plaque-induced gingivitis is suppressed in smokers.[12]

TOOTHBRUSH TRAUMA

Alterations in the gingiva as well as abrasions of the teeth may result from aggressive brushing in a horizontal or rotary fashion. The deleterious effect of abusive brushing is accentuated when excessively abrasive dentifrices are used.

The gingival changes attributable to toothbrush trauma may be acute or chronic. The acute changes are varied in appearance and duration and include scuffing of the epithelial surface with denudation of the underlying connective tissue to form a painful gingival bruise (Fig. 12–24). Punctate lesions are produced by penetration of the gingiva by perpendicularly aligned bristles. Painful vesicle formation in traumatized areas is also seen. Diffuse erythema and denudation of the attached gingiva throughout the mouth may be striking sequelae of overzealous brushing. The acute gingival changes noted commonly occur when the patient uses a new brush. A toothbrush bristle forcibly embedded

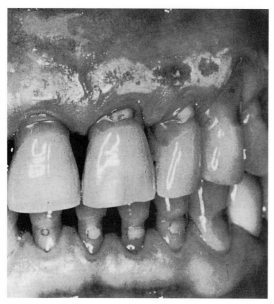

FIGURE 12–24. Toothbrush trauma. Surface erosion and hyperkeratosis caused by abusive toothbrushing.

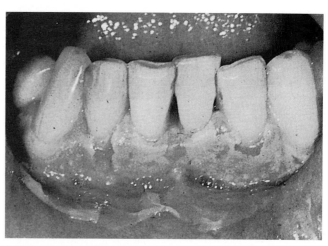

FIGURE 12–25. Chemical burn. Necrosis and sloughing produced by undiluted mouthwash.

and retained in the gingiva is a common cause of acute gingival abscess (see Chapter 22).

Chronic toothbrush trauma results in gingival recession with denudation of the root surface. Often the gingival margin is enlarged and appears to be "piled up," as if it were molded in conformity with the strokes of the toothbrush. Linear grooves that extend from the marginal to the attached gingivae may be present. The gingiva in such areas is usually pink and firm.

Improper use of dental floss, toothpicks, or wooden interdental stimulators may result in gingival inflammation. Creation of interproximal spaces by destruction of the gingiva

from overzealous use of toothpicks may lead to the accumulation of debris and to inflammatory changes.

CHEMICAL IRRITATION

Acute gingival inflammation may be caused by chemical irritation resulting from either sensitivity or nonspecific tissue injury. In allergic inflammatory states, the gingival changes range from simple erythema to painful vesicle formation and ulceration. Severe reactions to ordinarily innocuous mouthwashes, dentifrices, or denture materials are often explainable on this basis.

Acute inflammation with ulceration may be produced by the nonspecific injurious effect of chemicals on the gingival tissues. The indiscriminate use of strong mouthwashes (Figs. 12–25 and 12–26), application of aspirin tablets to

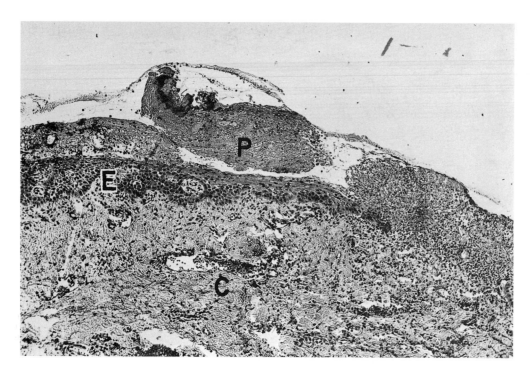

FIGURE 12–26. Biopsy specimen of a necrotic area produced by chemical burn. Note the inflamed connective tissue (C) and surface pseudomembrane (P). Of particular clinical importance is the newly formed sheet of epithelial cells (E), which undermines the necrotic pseudomembrane and separates it from the underlying connective tissue. This is an important feature of the healing process.

alleviate toothache (Fig. 12–27), injudicious use of escharotic drugs, and accidental contact with drugs such as phenol or silver nitrate are examples of the manner in which chemical irritation of the gingiva is commonly produced.

RADIATION

Patients with cancer of the oral cavity and adjacent regions who are treated with radiation initially develop erythema and desquamation of the oral mucosa, including the gingiva, which leads to ulcerations, infections, and suppuration. These lesions are nonspecific and heal slowly. Late changes include a thin mucous membrane with a thin, atrophic epithelium and dense fibrous connective tissue with a reduced number of blood vessels.[57] Irradiated bone demonstrates acellularity and avascularity with significant fibrosis and fatty degeneration, and atrophy of endosteum with loss of osteoclasts and osteoblasts.[14] These changes render the bone more susceptible to infections, and therefore, periodontal disease is considered a portal of entry for infection and the development of osteoradionecrosis after radiation therapy.

Radiation also induces atrophy of the salivary glands, leading to xerostomia and changes in the oral flora predisposing to dental caries.

Exposure of the entire body to radiation results in an acute radiation syndrome. This occurs after reactor accidents or atomic explosions. Changes include gastrointestinal, neurologic, and hematologic manifestations. In individuals studied after atomic bomb explosions in Japan,[13] oropharyngeal ulceration and ulcerative necrotizing gingivitis were frequent findings.

Studies in experimental animals exposed to single and multiple head or total body roentgen radiation in individual doses of 10 to 3000 rad to a total dosage of 11,000 rad[33,65,68,69] have reported changes that vary in severity from edema and bleeding of the gingiva and widening of the periodontal ligament with disrupted deposition of cementum to necrosis of the gingiva and periodontal ligament and resorption of alveolar bone, loosening and shedding of the teeth, and necrosis and sloughing of the oral mucosa.

The management of patients receiving radiation therapy for treatment of cancer is described in Chapter 34.

REFERENCES

1. Addy M, Dummer PMH, Hunter ML, et al. A study of the association of fraenal attachment, lip coverage and vestibular depth with plaque and gingivitis. J Periodontol 58:752, 1987.
2. Alexander AG. Habitual mouth breathing and its effect on gingival health. Parodontologie 24:49, 1970.
3. Anderson WS. The relationship of the tongue-thrust syndrome to maturation and other factors. Am J Orthod 49:264, 1963.
4. App GR. Effect of silicate, amalgam and cast gold on the gingiva. J Prosthet Dent 11:522, 1961.
5. Arno A, Schei O, Lovdal A, Waerhaug J. Alveolar bone loss as a function of tobacco consumption. Acta Odontol Scand 17:3, 1959.
6. Arno A, Waerhaug J, Lovdal A, Schei O. Incidence of gingivitis as related to sex, occupation, tobacco consumption, toothbrushing, and age. Oral Surg 11:587, 1958.
7. Ash MM Jr, Costich ER, Hayward JR. A study of periodontal hazards of third molars. J Periodontol 33:209, 1962.
8. Atherton JD, Kerr NW. Effect of orthodontic tooth movement upon the gingivae. Br Dent J 124:555, 1968.
9. Bastian RJ, Waite IM. Effects of tobacco smoking on plaque development and gingivitis. J Periodontol 49:480, 1978.
10. Bergman B, Hugoson A, Olsson C. Periodontal and prosthetic conditions in patients treated with removable partial dentures and artificial crowns. Acta Odontol Scand 29:621, 1971.
11. Bergstrom J, Eliasson S. Cigarette smoking and alveolar bone height in subjects with a high standard of oral hygiene. J Clin Periodontol 14:466, 1987.
12. Bergstrom J, Persson L, Preber H. Influence of cigarette smoking on vascular reaction during experimental gingivitis. Scand J Dent Res 96:34, 1988.
13. Bernier JL. The effect of atomic radiation on oral and pharyngeal mucosa. J Am Dent Assoc 39:647, 1949.
14. Beumer J III, Curtis TA, Firtell DN. Maxillofacial Rehabilitation; Prosthodontic and Surgical Considerations. St Louis, CV Mosby, 1979.
15. Bissada MF, Ibrahim SI, Barsoum WM. Gingival response to various types of removable partial dentures. J Periodontol 45:651, 1974.
16. Bjorn AL, Bjorn H, Grcovic B. Marginal fit of restorations and its relation to periodontal bone level. Odont Revy 20:311, 1969.
17. Brain WE. The effect of surgical transsection of free gingival fibers on the regression of orthodontically rotated teeth in the dog. Am J Orthod 55:50, 1969.
18. Buckley L. The relationship between malocclusion and periodontal disease. J Periodontol 43:415, 1972.
19. Burwasser P, Hill TJ. The effect of hard and soft diets on the gingival tissues of dogs. J Dent Res 18:389, 1939.
20. Calonius PEB. A cytological study on the variation of keratinization in the normal oral mucosa of young males. J West Soc Periodontol 10:69, 1962.
21. Carlsson GE, Hedegard B, Koivumaa K. Studies in partial dental prosthesis. IV. Final results of a four year longitudinal investigation of dentogingivally supported partial dentures. Acta Odontol Scand 23:443, 1965.
22. Carranza FA Sr, Carraro JJ. El empuje lingual como factor traumatizante en periodoncia. Rev Asoc Odontol Argent 47:105, 1959.
23. Castelli WA, Dempster WT. The periodontal vasculature and its responses to experimental pressures. J Am Dent Assoc 70:891, 1965.
24. Chaikin BS. Anterior periodontal destruction due to the loss of one or more unreplaced molars. Dent Items Int 61:17, 1939.
25. Chin Quee TA, Gosselin D, Millar EP, Stamm JW. Surgical removal of the fully impacted mandibular third molar. The influence of flap design and alveolar bone height. J Periodontol 56:625, 1985.
26. Cuff MJA, McQuade MJ, Scheidt MJ, et al. The presence of nicotine on root surfaces of periodontally diseased teeth in smokers. J Periodontol 60:564, 1989.
27. Danielsen B, Manji F, Nagelkerke N, et al. Effect of cigarette smoking on the transition dynamics in experimental gingivitis. J Clin Periodontol 17:159, 1990.
28. Diamanti-Kipioti A, Gusberti FA, Lang NP. Clinical and microbiological effects of fixed orthodontic appliances. J Clin Periodontol 14:326, 1987.

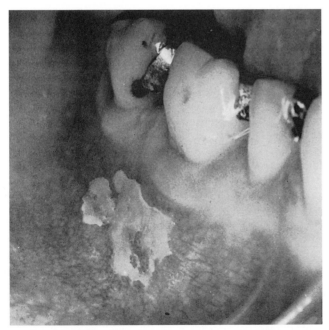

FIGURE 12–27. Aspirin burn. Necrosis of the mucosa produced by repeated application of aspirin tablets to relieve toothache.

29. Edwards JG. A study of the periodontium during orthodontic rotation of teeth. Am J Orthod *54:*441, 1968.

30. Ellinger F. Effects of ionizing radiation on the oral cavity. In Ellinger F, ed. Medical Radiation Biology. Springfield, IL, Charles C Thomas, 1957.

31. Flemmig TF, Sorensen JA, Newman MG, Nachnani S. Gingival enhancement in fixed prosthodontics. Part II. Microbiologic findings. J Prosthet Dent *65:*365, 1991.

32. Flores-de-Jacoby L, Zafiropoulos GG, Ciancio S. The effect of crown margin location on plaque and periodontal health. Int J Periodont Restor Dent *9:*197, 1989.

33. Frandsen AM. Periodontal tissue changes induced in young rats by roentgen irradiation of the molar regions of the head. Acta Odontol Scand *20:*393, 1962.

34. Frandsen AM, Pindborg JJ. Tobacco and gingivitis. III. Difference in the action of cigarette and pipe smoking. J Dent Res *28:*404, 1949.

35. Geiger A, Wasserman B, Turgeon L. Relationship of occlusion and periodontal disease. VIII. Relationship of crowding and spacing to periodontal destruction and gingival inflammation. J Periodontol *45:*43, 1974.

36. Ghamrawy E. Quantitative changes in dental plaque formation related to removable partial dentures. J Oral Rehabil *3:*115, 1976.

37. Ghamrawy E. Qualitative changes in dental plaque formation related to removable partial dentures. J Oral Rehabil *6:*183, 1979.

38. Gianelly AA. Force induced changes in the vascularity of the periodontal ligament. Am J Orthod *55:*5, 1969.

39. Gilmore N, Sheiham A. Overhanging dental restorations and periodontal disease. J Periodontol *42:*8, 1971.

40. Gorzo I, Newman HN, Strahan JD. Amalgam restoration, plaque removal and periodontal health. J Clin Periodontol *6:*98, 1979.

41. Goultschin J, Cohen HDS, Donchin M, et al. Association of smoking with periodontal treatment needs. J Periodontol *61:*364, 1990.

42. Haber J, Wattles J, Crowley M, et al. Evidence for cigarette smoking as a major risk factor for periodontitis. J Periodontol *64:*16, 1993.

43. Hakkarainen K, Ainamo J. Influence of overhanging posterior tooth restorations of alveolar bone height in adults. J Clin Periodontol *7:*114, 1980.

44. Highfield JE, Powell RN. Effects of removal of posterior overhanging metallic margins of restorations upon the periodontal tissues. J Clin Periodontol *5:*169, 1978.

45. Hirschfeld I. Food impaction. J Am Dent Assoc *17:*1504, 1930.

46. Hirschfeld I. Individual missing tooth. J Am Dent Assoc *24:*67, 1937.

47. Huttner G. Follow-up study of crowns and abutments with regard to the crown edge and the marginal periodontium. Dtsch Zahnarztl Z *26:*724, 1971.

48. Jacobson L. Mouth breathing and gingivitis. J Periodont Res *8:*269, 1973.

49. Jacobson L, Linder-Aronson S. Crowding and gingivitis: A comparison between mouth breathers and non–mouth breathers. Scand J Dent Res *80:*500, 1972.

50. Jeffcoat MK, Howell TH. Alveolar bone destruction due to overhanging amalgam in periodontal disease. J Periodontol *51:*599, 1980.

51. Jones J, Triplett R. The relationship of cigarette smoking to impaired intraoral wound healing: A review of evidence and implications for patient care. J Oral Maxillofac Surg *50:*237, 1992.

52. Karlsen K. Gingival reactions to dental restorations. Acta Odontol Scand *28:*895, 1970.

53. Kawakara H, Yamagani A, Nakamura M Jr. Biological testing of dental materials by means of tissue culture. Int Dent J *18:*443, 1968.

54. Kenney EB, Kraal JH, Saxe SR, Jones J. The effect of cigarette smoke on human oral polymorphonuclear leukocytes. J Periodont Res *12:*227, 1977.

55. Kepic TJ, O'Leary TJ. Role of marginal ridge relationships as an etiologic factor in periodontal disease. J Periodontol *49:*570, 1978.

56. Klingsberg J, Cancellaro BA, Butcher EO. Effects of air drying on rodent oral mucous membrane: A histologic study of simulated mouth breathing. J Periodontol *32:*38, 1961.

57. Koivumaa KK, Wennstrom A. A histological investigation of the changes in gingival margins adjacent to gold crowns. Odont T *68:*373, 1960.

58. Kreshover SJ. The effect of tobacco on the epithelial tissues of mice. J Am Dent Assoc *45:*528, 1952.

59. Kugelberg CF. Third molar surgery. Curr Opin Dent *2:*9, 1992.

60. Lang NP, Kiel RA, Anderhalden K. Clinical and microbiological effect of subgingival restorations with overhanging or clinically perfect margins. J Clin Periodontol *10:*563, 1983.

61. Leon AR. Amalgam restorations and periodontal disease. Br Dent J *140:*377, 1976.

62. Lite T, DiMaco DJ, Burman LR, et al. Gingival pathosis in mouth breathers. A clinical and histopathologic study and a method of treatment. Oral Surg *8:*382, 1955.

63. Marmary Y, Brayer L, Tzukert A, Feller L. Alveolar bone repair following extraction of impacted mandibular third molars. Oral Surg Oral Med Oral Pathol *61:*324, 1986.

64. Mayo J, Carranza FA Jr, Epper CE, Cabrini RL. The effect of total body irradiation on the oral tissues of the Syrian hamster. Oral Surg *15:*739, 1962.

65. McCarthy PL, Shklar G. Diseases of the Oral Mucosa. 2nd ed. Philadelphia, Lea & Febiger, 1980.

66. McGuire JR, McQuade MJ, Rossmann JA, et al. Cotinine in saliva and crevicular fluid of smokers with periodontal disease. J Periodontol *60:*176, 1989.

67. McLaughlin WS, Lovat FM, Macgregor IDM, Kelly PJ. The immediate effects of smoking on gingival fluid flow. J Clin Periodontol *20:*448, 1993.

68. Medak H, Burnett GW. The effect of x-ray irradiation on the oral tissues of the macaccus Rhesus monkey. Oral Surg *7:*778, 1954.

69. Meyer J, Shklar G, Turner J. A comparison of the effects of 200 kV radiation and dental structure of the white rat. Oral Surg *15:*1098, 1962.

70. Miller PD Jr. Root coverage with the free gingival graft. Factors associated with incomplete coverage. J Periodontol *58:*675, 1987.

71. Miller J, Hobson P. The relationship between malocclusion, oral cleanliness, gingival conditions and dental caries in school children. Br Dent J *111:*43, 1961.

72. Moffett BC. Remodeling changes of the facial sutures, periodontal and temporomandibular joints produced by orthodontic forces in Rhesus monkeys. Bull Pac Coast Soc Ortho *44:*46, 1969.

73. Morris ML. Artificial crown contours and gingival health. J Prosthet Dent *12:*1146, 1962.

74. Mueller HP. The effect of artificial crown margins on the periodontal conditions in a group of periodontally supervised patients treated with fixed bridges. J Clin Periodontol *13:*97, 1986.

75. Norman RD, Mehia RV, Swartz ML, Phillips RW. Effect of restorative materials on plaque composition. J Dent Res *51:*1596, 1972.

76. Normann W, Regolati B, Renggli HH. Gingival reaction to well-fitted subgingival proximal gold inlays. J Clin Periodontol *1:*120, 1974.

77. O'Leary TJ, Badell M, Bloomer R. Interproximal contact and marginal ridge relationships in periodontally healthy young males classified as to orthodontic status. J Periodontol *46:*6, 1975.

78. O'Leary TJ, Sosa CF. Signs of periodontal breakdown in patients with malocclusion. J Dent Educ *10:*172, 1955.

79. Pack ARC, Coxhead LJ, McDonald BW. The prevalence of overhanging margins in posterior amalgam restorations and periodontal consequences. J Clin Periodontol *17:*145, 1990.

80. Paunio K. The role of malocclusion and crowding in the development of periodontal disease. Int Dent J *23:*420, 1973.

81. Pearson LE. Gingival height of lower central incisors, orthodontically treated and untreated. Angle Orthod *38:*337, 1968.

82. Pindborg JJ. Tobacco and gingivitis. I. Statistical examination of the significance of tobacco in the development of ulceromembranous gingivitis and in the formation of calculus. J Dent Res *26:*261, 1947.

83. Pindborg JJ. Tobacco and gingivitis. II. Correlation between consumption of tobacco, ulceromembranous gingivitis and calculus. J Dent Res *28:*461, 1949.

84. Polson A, Reed BE. Long-term effect of orthodontic treatment on crestal alveolar bone levels. J Periodontol *55:*28, 1984.

85. Preber H, Bergstrom J. Effect of cigarette smoking on periodontal healing following surgical therapy. J Clin Periodontol *17:*324, 1990.

86. Preber H, Kant T, Bergstrom J. Cigarette smoking, oral hygiene and periodontal disease in Swedish army conscripts. J Clin Periodontol *7:*106, 1980.

87. Reitan K. Tissue changes following experimental tooth movement as related to the time factor. Dent Record *73:*559, 1953.

88. Renggli HH. The influence of subgingival proximal filling borders on the degree of inflammation of the adjacent gingiva. A clinical study. Schweiz Monatsschr Zahnheilkd *84:*181, 1974.

89. Renggli HH, Regolati B. Gingival inflammation and plaque accumulation by well-adapted supragingival and subgingival proximal restorations. Helv Odontol Acta *16:*99, 1972.

90. Rosenzweig KA, Langer A. Oral disease in Yeshiva students. J Dent Res *40:*993, 1961.

91. Sanchez-Sotres L, Van Huysen G, Gilmore HW. A histologic study of gingival tissue response to amalgam, silicate and resin restorations. J Periodontol *42:*8, 1969.

92. Schwartz AM. Tissue changes incidental to orthodontic tooth movement. Ortho Oral Surg Rad Int J *18:*331, 1932.

93. Scoman S. Study of the relationship between periodontal disease and the wearing of partial dentures. Aust Dent J *8:*206, 1963.

94. Severson HM. The effect of cigarette smoking on plaque formation. J Periodontol *50:*146, 1979.

95. Sheiham A. Periodontal disease and oral cleanliness in tobacco smokers. J Periodontol *42:*259, 1971.

96. Sheppard IM. Tongue dynamics. Dent Digest *59:*117, 1953.

97. Silness J. Fixed prosthodontics and periodontal health. Dent Clin North Am *24:*317, 1980.

98. Solomon H, Priore R, Bross I. Cigarette smoking and periodontal disease. J Am Dent Assoc *77:*1081, 1968.

99. Sorensen JA, Doherty FM, Newman MG, Flemmig TF. Gingival enhancement in fixed prosthodontics. Part I. Clinical findings. J Prosthet Dent *65:*100, 1991.

100. Sorensen J, Larsen IB, Jorgensen KD. Gingival and alveolar bone response to marginal fit of subgingival crown margins. Scand J Dent Res *94:*109, 1986.

101. Sorrin S. Habit: An etiologic factor of periodontal disease. Dent Digest *41:*290, 1935.

102. Summers CJ, Oberman A. Association of oral disease with twelve selected variables. I. Periodontal disease. J Dent Res *47:*457, 1968.

103. Sutcliffe P. Chronic anterior gingivitis: An epidemiological study in school children. Br Dent J *125:*47, 1968.

104. Tressello VK, Gianelly AA. Orthodontic treatment and periodontal status. J Periodontol *50:*665, 1979.

105. Waerhaug J, Zander HA. Reaction of gingival tissue to self-curing acrylic restorations. J Am Dent Assoc *54:*760, 1957.
106. Wise MD, Dykema RW. The plaque retaining capacity of four dental materials. J Prosthet Dent *33:*178, 1975.
107. Yuodelis RA, Weaver JD, Sapkos S. Facial and lingual contours of artificial complete crowns and their effect on the periodontium. J Prosthet Dent *29:*61, 1973.

108. Zachrisson BW, Alnaes L. Periodontal condition in orthodontically treated and untreated individuals. I. Loss of attachment, gingival pocket depth and clinical crown height. Angle Orthod *43:*402, 1973.
109. Zachrisson BW, Alnaes L. Periodontal condition in orthodontically treated and untreated individuals. II. Alveolar bone loss: Radiographic findings. Angle Orthod *44:*48, 1974.

13

Dental Occlusion

WILLIAM K. SOLBERG and DONALD A. SELIGMAN

Definition of Occlusion
Terminology
Mandibular Movement
Condyle Positions
Occlusion and Function
Mastication and Deglutition
Tooth Contacts and Forces in Chewing and Swallowing

Vertical Dimension of Occlusion
Dental Wear
Occlusal Parafunction: Bruxism

Recognition and correction of occlusal relationships that are injurious to the periodontium require an understanding of the principles of occlusion and masticatory function. Fundamentals of occlusal function are presented here; clinical application is described in Chapter 47.

DEFINITION OF OCCLUSION

The term *occlusion* refers to the contact relationships of the teeth resulting from neuromuscular control of the masticatory system (musculature, temporomandibular joints, mandible, and periodontium).[108] In the functional sense, normality or abnormality of an individual occlusion is determined by the manner in which an occlusion functions and by its effect on the periodontium, musculature, and temporomandibular joints, rather than by the alignment of the teeth in each arch and the static relationship of the arches to each other.

Three classes of functional occlusion have been identified:

Physiologic occlusion is an occlusion that exists in an individual who has no signs of occlusion-related pathosis. This implies a range of morphologic variability in the occlusion of the teeth and a sense of psychological and physical comfort. In fact, no occlusion that exists in a given mouth free of disease and dysfunction can be considered abnormal.[134]

Nonphysiologic occlusion is an occlusion judged to be associated with traumatic lesions or disturbances in the supporting structures of the teeth, muscles, and temporomandibular joints. The criterion that determines whether an occlusion is nonphysiologic is whether it contributes to injury, not how the teeth occlude.

Therapeutic occlusion is an occlusion used to counteract structural interrelationships related to traumatic occlusion. The term is also used to describe an occlusal scheme employed in restoring or replacing occlusal surfaces so that minimum physiologic and anatomic adaptation is required.

TERMINOLOGY

The terminology of occlusion was developed by workers in several biologic and dental specialties, which resulted in a heterogeneous terminology. To avoid confusion, the following terms used in this chapter are defined as follows:

Excursive movement: Movement occurring when the mandible moves away from the intercuspal position.

Intercuspal position (ICP): (1) The position of the mandible with maximum intercuspation of the teeth; (2) the most cranial point of all functional contact movement. *Synonyms:* centric occlusion (CO), habitual occlusion, acquired centric, habitual centric, maximum intercuspation.

Laterotrusion: Movement occurring when the mandible moves away from the midline. *Synonym:* working movement.

Laterotrusive side: The side of the dental arch that moves away from the midline in laterotrusion. *Synonyms:* working side, functional side.

Mediotrusion: Movement occurring when the mandible

moves toward the midline. *Synonyms:* non–working side movement, balancing movement.

Mediotrusive side: The side of the dental arch that moves toward the midline in mediotrusion. *Synonyms:* nonworking side, balancing side, nonfunctional side, idling side.

Muscular contact position (MCP): The position of the mandible when it has been lifted from its resting posture to the very first occlusal contact with a minimum of muscular effort. *Synonym:* physiologic rest contact position.

Protrusion: Movement occurring when the mandible moves anteriorly from the intercuspal position.

Retruded contact position (RCP): The end point of mandibular movement along the retruded path of closure. *Synonym:* centric relation contact (CRC).

Retruded position (RP): The most superior position along the retruded path of closure (transverse horizontal axis). *Synonyms:* centric relation (CR), terminal hinge position.

Retrusion: Movement occurring when the mandible moves posteriorly from the intercuspal position.

MANDIBULAR MOVEMENT

Jaw movement can be classified as border, contact, or intraborder. *Border movements* are the limits to which the mandible can move in any direction and are not common during mandibular function.[90] Posselt, in a classic study,[101] developed a rhomboid figure that represents boundaries of movement of the mandible (Fig. 13–1). This "envelope of motion" shows considerable variability within each individual and is not reproducible.[34]

Contact movement is the movement of the mandible with one or more of the opposing occlusal surfaces in contact (Fig. 13–2). ICP, RCP, and MCP are the most common contact reference positions. The difference between ICP and RCP is usually between 0 and 1.0 mm measured at the incisors, and between 0 and 0.5 mm measured at the mandibular condyles.[56,58,59,136,137] Moreover, ICP lies in a symmetric, forward position relative to RCP in 35% to

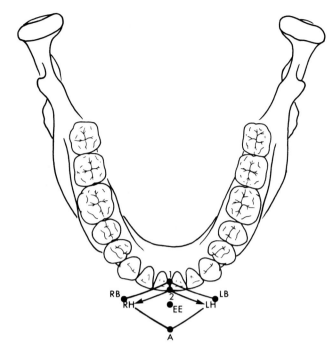

FIGURE 13–2. Movements of the mandible at the incisal point (infradentale). 1, Retruded contact position. 2, Intercuspal position. EE, Edge-to-edge position; A, Contact at maximal protrusion; RH and LH, Right and left habitual movement positions; RB and LB, Right and left border positions. Jaw undergoes maximum lateral movement at RB and LB.

85% of young adults (see Fig. 13–1).[2,137] In a small but significant percentage of individuals (10% to 30%), RCP and ICP are coincident or nearly coincident.

Although temporalis muscle effort is necessary to reach RCP,[78] most individuals with coincident RCP–ICP relationships show no discomfort when closing to full contact.[137] One of the characteristics of a physiologic occlusion is that the teeth normally contact directly in ICP when they are closed with a minimum muscular effort from the rest position. "Touch and slide" from MCP to ICP is a sign often found in patients with morphofunctional disharmony.[90]

Intraborder movement is any mandibular movement within the perimeter of border movement. Intraborder movement is chiefly associated with free movement, chewing, and phonation.[90]

Movements of the mandible with the teeth in contact, which are termed *excursions,* may be laterotrusive, protrusive, lateroprotrusive, or retrusive (Fig. 13–3). Laterotrusive (side-to-side) contacts of the mandibular posterior teeth along the buccal cusps of the maxillary teeth (lateral excursions) occur occasionally in chewing and swallowing[76] and often in bruxism.[38] Protrusive excursions are also part of the opening chewing cycle.[24,61]

In the lateral movements of the mandible, the laterotrusive side rotates about a vertical axis or combines lateral movement with rotation (Fig. 13–4). Lateral shift of the condyle (average, 0.2 mm)[14,43] is called the *Bennett movement* (see Fig. 13–4*B*). During Bennett movement the condyles rarely move purely horizontally, but instead translate and rotate in curvilinear paths in three planes of space simultaneously.[73] The condyle on the mediotrusive (nonworking) side moves downward, forward, and inward and

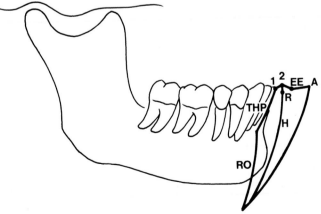

FIGURE 13–1. Rhomboid figure of mandibular movements in the sagittal plane (Posselt). 1, Retruded contact position. 2, Intercuspal position. THP, Terminal hinge path; EE, Edge-to-edge position; RO, Retruded path beyond terminal hinge opening. The condyles undergo both rotation and translation at this point. A, Border movement with maximum protrusion; H, Habitual (functional) pathway of the mandible; R, The rest (postural) position of the mandible.

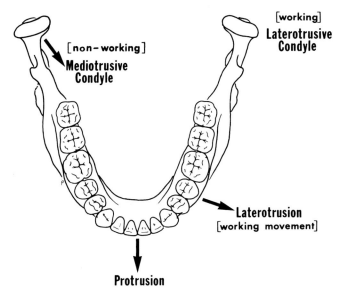

FIGURE 13–3. Mandibular movement is named after the direction of movement the mandible takes when it moves away from the intercuspal position. Functional parts of the mandible can also be identified by reference to the movement to which they are related.

describes the *Bennett angle* (with respect to a sagittal reference line) when viewed in the horizontal plane (see Fig. 13–4). To make the distinction between the two terms, it should be noted that the Bennett angle is always present but the Bennett movement may not be present.

The *Fisher angle* is formed by the inclinations of the straight protrusive and non–working side condylar paths as viewed in the sagittal plane.

CONDYLE POSITIONS

RCP is synonymous with the term CRC and refers to the end point of mandibular movement when it is moved along the retruded path of closure. The reproducibility of RCP is relative, as many studies have demonstrated that different RCPs can be established by different techniques.[131,152] It is generally agreed that the condyles in RCP are generally seated by way of the discs against the temporal bones, but this anatomic definition is less precise than the kinematically defined term RCP. Restraint on retrusive jaw movement is imposed by the lateral ligaments of the temporomandibular joints [4,10] and to some degree by the muscles of mastication.[82]

ICP is synonymous with the terms CO, habitual occlusion, and maximum intercuspation and refers to the position of the teeth at the most closed point. During contact movements from RCP to ICP, the condyles undergo slight anterior and inferior movement.[118] In some individuals, RCP and ICP are identical; hence, the position of the condyle does not change. When the mandible is in rest position, the condyles are usually anterior and inferior to their position in ICP.[58,116]

Jaw opening involves simultaneous rotation and downward and forward translation of the condyle. On maximal opening, the condyles glide along the posterior slope of the articular eminence to an average of 1 mm anterior to the inferior crest of the eminence.[116]

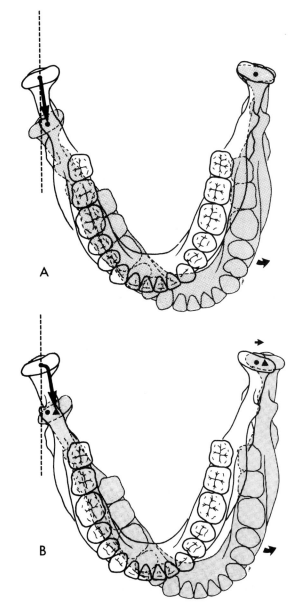

FIGURE 13–4. *A*, Pure left lateral rotation of the mandible (no Bennett movement). *B*, Lateral movement of the jaw incorporating Bennett movement.

The jaws ordinarily open and close directly into ICP rather than into RCP, unless the two positions are coincident. With the jaw opened wide, there may be a slight reduction (approximately 0.09 mm) in the width of the mandible in the molar area.[113] In making impressions of the teeth, it is therefore wise to keep the jaws at a minimal vertical opening while the mandibular impression material sets.

Condyle positions within the mandibular fossae at the ICP are highly variable.[114] Women are more often posterior of a centered condyle position, whereas men tend to be more anterior,[104,105,117] and this may reflect dimorphic angle class tendencies.[74] The condyle position does not appear to be related to overbite,[23,104] overjet,[23,104] dental midlines,[104] RCP–ICP discrepancies,[104,118] open bite,[97] or edentulousness.[51]

OCCLUSION AND FUNCTION

When the teeth are not in contact in mastication, swallowing, or speech, the lips are at rest and the jaws are apart. This is termed the *postural position of the mandible*, a term that is more appropriate[89] than *physiologic rest position*.[143] To maintain the mandible in this position, it is necessary to support it against the force of gravity. Thus, the masticatory muscles are in a mild state of contraction.[39,139] The postural position is not constant; it varies with the position of the head and body[46,99] and is affected by proprioceptive stimuli from the dentition, by prior jaw movements,[99] and by emotional factors.[102] Thus, there is no single, constant position of the mandible when the subject is at rest.[37]

The space between the mandibular and maxillary teeth when the mandible is in the postural position is called the *free way space* or the *vertical dimension of rest*. The postural position and free way space are fairly stable and reproducible but are not necessarily constant throughout life. They vary from individual to individual and even within the same individual with changes in the dentition.[110] A large free way space has been observed in subjects with a deep overbite, and a large sagittal difference between postural positions and ICP has been observed in subjects with marked overjet.[142] The average normal space is thought to be 1.7 mm,[42] but it has also been reported to be somewhat greater.[152] Generally, it ranges between 0 and 3 mm and may be related to facial type.[151] Aging, malocclusion, tooth mobility, periodontal disease, unreplaced posterior teeth, improperly constructed dental restorations, excessive occlusal wear, and unilateral chewing, which change the teeth and their functional relationships, may also change the muscle tonus, which in turn may alter the postural position and the free way space.[85,126]

The clinical rest position and the jaw position occurring at minimal electromyographic (EMG) activity (EMG rest position) have been compared.[19,35,39,42,99,139,146] The clinical rest position was always in a superior position relative to the point of minimal muscle activity[19,99,146] by an average distance of 8 to 12 mm.[139] The EMG rest position is also influenced by the history of jaw movement, previous jaw movements, head posture, and the choice of muscles being tested.[99] There is usually a rapid adaptation to an encroachment on the clinical rest position through an increase in the occlusal vertical dimension, with no increase or reduction in the EMG activity.[22] Of interest is the finding that the vertical dimension of the EMG rest position is significantly larger in men than in women.[122] Clinical norms for the free way space should not be applied using the values obtained at EMG rest.

MASTICATION AND DEGLUTITION

The pathway of the mandible in chewing is referred to as the *chewing* or *masticatory cycle*. The form of the chewing cycle has been observed using photography, graphic methods, radiography, and electrical and telemetric techniques.[13] The pathway of any point on the dental arch in chewing typically has a teardrop shape when viewed in

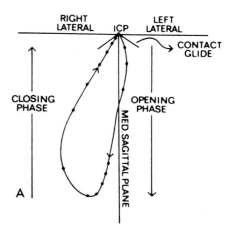

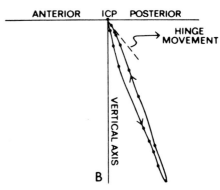

FIGURE 13–5. Incisal points during one chewing cycle. *A*, Frontal projection. *B*, Sagittal projection. ICP, intercuspal position. (From Ahlgren J. In Anderson DJ, Matthews B, eds. Mastication. Bristol, England, J. Wright & Sons, 1976.)

the frontal or sagittal plane (Fig. 13–5). The masticatory cycle consists of three phases: the *opening phase*, during which the mandible is depressed; the *closing phase*, during which the mandible is elevated; and the *intercuspal phase* (ICP).[63]

The chewing cycle can take many forms, and the classic teardrop shape is an oversimplification of reality.[88] There are wide variations even within a given individual that do not fit any one model.[153] To further complicate the pattern, differences in condyle movement between the chewing side and the nonchewing side during the chewing cycle are important and have not been taken into account in many chewing studies.[43,151] In the opening phase, the teeth and the condyles begin movement immediately downward and forward.[38] Early in the closing phase, the entire mandible moves laterally to the selected chewing side.[90] The chewing-side condyle moves to an upward and rearward position well in advance of the intercuspal phase (SRP, Fig. 13–6A–C). During the remainder of final closure to ICP, the chewing-side condyle usually demonstrates a slight forward (0.33 mm) and medial (Bennett) movement (0.2 mm).[129] The non–chewing-side condyle lags somewhat behind as it moves a considerable distance upward and backward to a condyle position dictated by ICP (Fig. 13–6D).[43]

There are about 15 chews in a series from the time of food entry until swallowing. Jaw opening is greatest when

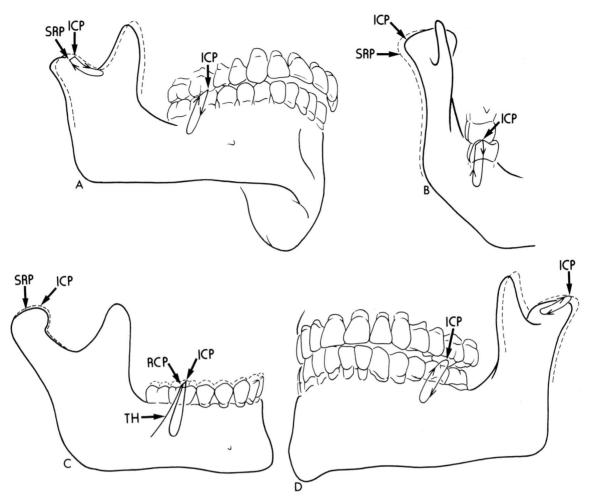

FIGURE 13-6. Masticatory cycle. *A,* Seen from the chewing side during one chewing cycle. The chewing-side condyle moves upward and rearward and reaches a superior, rearward position (SRP) before the teeth reach the intercuspal phase. The teeth then close along the lateroretrusive cusp inclines on the path to the intercuspal position (ICP). *B,* Frontal view of the chewing side, as in *A. C,* Sagittal component of the masticatory cycle (chewing side) seen in relation to the terminal hinge path (TH), the retruded contact position (RCP), and the intercuspal position (ICP). Note the retrusive component of the masticatory cycle on the chewing side. *D,* The masticatory cycle seen from the nonchewing side. The nonchewing-side condyle (mediotrusive condyle) moves a considerable distance upward and rearward to close directly to the intercuspal position (ICP). Note that closure is along the medioprotrusive maxillary cusp inclines on a path to the intercuspal position. The differences between the condyle paths and the paths of the cusps during the chewing cycle for the chewing side and those for the nonchewing side are significant and have not been taken into account in most chewing studies. (Courtesy of Dr. Harry Lundeen, and Dr. Charles Gibbs.)

food first enters the mouth and decreases in a somewhat linear fashion as chewing continues. The average jaw opening during chewing is between 16 and 20 mm, and the average lateral displacement on chewing is between 3 and 5 mm.[4] The duration of the masticatory cycle varies between 0.6 and 1.0 second. The duration is decreased and chewing forces are increased when the subject is stressed or in a hurry to eat.[119] Men chew faster and have a shorter occlusal phase than women.[65] The chewing pattern is also influenced by the consistency, shape, size, and taste of the bolus of food.[90,103,147] Tough foods typically precipitate an angulated, grinding movement, whereas soft foods favor a classic drop-shaped lenticular pattern.[103] The duration of the masticatory cycle is also affected by the bolus, with sticky and tough foods prolonging its duration.[4]

Chewing efficiency depends on many factors, and norms are difficult to establish because of large individual variation.[5] The number of posterior chewing units results in greater chewing efficiency and smaller bolus particle size,[148,156] and the number and extent of dental restorations[5] and the overall occlusal contact area also appear to be influential.[156]

Chewing-side preference is not predicted by any single variable[154]; in particular, it is not associated with the degree and distribution of ICP contacts[83,155] or by other occlusal factors.[100,103] Bilateral chewing is preferred and takes place on the right and left alternately, while the bolus is passed from side to side regularly and consistently according to the individual's particular pattern.[13,154]

The chewing-patterns of the adult and the child differ. In the adult, the opening stroke is medial to the wide lateral closing stroke, whereas in the child, the opening stroke is typically lateral to a less wide lateral closing stroke.[45] The change from the chewing pattern of the child to that of the adult appears to be related mostly to the eruption of the anterior teeth.[43] Children also chew with less velocity on closing than adults,[65] but there is a gradual return to reduced velocities with advancing age in adults.[63] The duration of the entire chewing cycle is particular for each individual and remains constant throughout life. This suggests a central control, referred to as a *central pattern generator.*[63]

Occlusion can be of significant importance for the development of masticatory movements,[4] and occlusal alterations or treatments can cause short-term changes in the chewing pattern.[13,43,66,158] The immediate response to an acute interference may be a pause in ICP and an increase in chewing intervals,[12] but a rapid adaptation without alteration in chewing patterns often results.[128] The occurrence of a deep overbite is associated with chopping chewing strokes, whereas in reduced lateral cuspal guidance, the chewing stroke assumes a more horizontal component.[4] Large discrepancies between RCP and ICP can also lengthen the expected chewing cycle and precipitate an earlier onset of temporalis muscle activity.[57]

Swallowing occurs approximately 600 times in a 24-hour period.[72] It occurs most frequently during eating and drinking, at a lesser rate during the usual indoor activities, and least frequently during sleep. The total time of tooth contact in chewing and swallowing in a 24-hour period has been estimated to be 17.5 minutes.

In swallowing, the palatal muscles seal off the oropharynx from the nasopharynx, the suprahyoid muscles raise and tilt the hyoid bone and larynx, and the tongue forcibly propels the food bolus or liquid posteriorly over the epiglottis into the esophagus. To provide firm anchorage for the action of the tongue and to oppose the depressing action of the suprahyoid muscles, the mandible is braced against the maxilla and cranium by the masseter, temporal, and medial pterygoid muscles.[47] A normal swallow, therefore, generally occurs with the teeth together,[96] and the muscle activity during swallowing can be influenced by occlusal factors.[85]

The act of swallowing may have a profound effect on the development of the orofacial structures, especially in the presence of an abnormal swallowing pattern, which may result from many factors, some of which are habitual, genetic, mechanical, or neurologic. Prolonged retention of an infantile swallow pattern with contiguous breathing and swallowing may contribute to the creation of a malocclusion[75] and incisor gingival recession in children.[79] Nevertheless, there is little evidence that abnormal swallowing habits (e.g., tongue thrusting) influence the periodontal condition in adults.[50]

Tooth Contacts and Forces in Chewing and Swallowing

It has been difficult to capture and record jaw movements and tooth contacts in the functioning dentition, despite the imaginative techniques used for this purpose (e.g., visual studies of attrition facets, photography, graphic methods, radiography, and electrical and telemetric techniques).[11,20] A review of these studies has been published by Bates and associates.[11-13]

There is some variation in the findings of photographic, graphic, and electronic techniques investigating tooth con-

tact in chewing and swallowing, but the preponderance of evidence indicates the following:

1. *Tooth contacts occur in chewing and swallowing in the majority of chewing cycles.* The RCP is rarely a terminal occlusal position in chewing or swallowing. Chewing cycles without tooth contact occur mainly at the beginning of the chewing sequence (i.e., the crushing strokes).[4]

2. *Almost all chewing contacts and most swallowing contacts involve contact in ICP, and this position is the usual terminal functional position during mastication.*[4,44] When full closure to ICP is attained, stoppage of movement for about 0.1 to 0.2 second occurs for the subject with stable occlusion, but the total contact time, which includes the gliding aspects of the feature, may be twice this time.[13] Subjects with pathologic occlusions, especially those with mobile teeth, are less likely to reach ICP and are less likely to demonstrate stoppage of jaw movement even when ICP is reached.[44] The chewing force is greatest during the short pause in ICP.[4,44] Chewing contacts in ICP are brief compared with the duration of swallowing contacts, and ICP forces during swallowing have been found to be greater than those during chewing.[43]

3. Gliding contact to and from ICP occurs frequently during mastication, with the average glide length being 1 mm at the incision point in both the opening and the closing strokes (see Fig. 13-6). These glides are less on the molar teeth because of cusp morphology and their proximity to the axes of jaw motion. The working-side molar closes from a rear and lateral direction with a small anterior component. The non-working-side molar closes from an anterior and medial direction with no anterior component. According to Gibbs and Lundeen,[43] steep anterior guidance does not appear to expose the teeth to extreme lateral forces. The tooth gliding contacts while entering and leaving the intercuspal position have been known to be of short duration and low magnitude when compared with the forces generated in ICP. In some individuals there is no tooth gliding contact at all, but merely a chopping stroke.

The occurrence of lateral tooth contact during the closing phase depends on the type of food and occlusion. The glide is significantly longer in aborigines chewing tough food. As dental wear proceeds, cuspal guidance is reduced, and the closing stroke assumes a more horizontal direction when moving into ICP.[4]

The angle of approach to and from ICP is steeper than the cuspal inclination; thus, the angle within the masticatory cycle always lies within the confines of that described by the cuspal inclines. The teeth are a major guiding factor in the closing phases of the masticatory cycle but exert little influence in the opening phases.[13]

Intercuspal Contacts

The teeth make contact in a variety of patterns, with fewer contacts[54,98] fewer ideal cusp-fossa or cusp-marginal ridge relationships,[54] and more asymmetry[68] than frequently believed. This suggests that ideal tooth contact relationships in natural dentitions are uncommon.[6,54,68,98,157]

Studies of Australian aborigines show that the anterior teeth should make very light contact or no contact.[18] However, in young American adults, firm contacts on the incisor teeth have been observed in many functionally asymptomatic individuals.[38,107] Therefore, a variety of interincisal contact schemes appear to be acceptable. In occlusal therapy, however, heavy anterior interincisal contact should be avoided because of the increased risk of creating bite discomfort, mandibular instability, and trauma from occlusion.[38] Heavy anterior contact can be felt as *fremitus,* which is a perceptible vibration on palpating the facial surface of the teeth when they come into contact.

In asymptomatic individuals, simultaneous posterior contacts on the existing posterior teeth are the norm during firm ICP closure. Absence of contact on the posterior teeth should arouse the attention of the clinician. There are significantly more contacts with hard pressure than with light pressure, and ICP patterns can vary slightly according to occlusal force.[132] Furthermore, occlusal contacts show diurnal variation, sometimes being more diffuse in the morning and more specific in the evening[15,86] but at other times showing random variation.[87] The patterns depend on the status of the masticatory muscles,[16] as well as the mental state.[15]

Although individual posterior supporting cusps occlude with variable stability on marginal ridges and in fossae, maximum total arch stability is rendered when the combined effect of multiple, simultaneous contacts has an overall horizontal vector of 0 at the ICP. Objective reporting of the frequency and distribution of ICP contact should include documentation of the results of ultrathin feeler gauge testing in the molar, premolar, canine, and incisal zones of each half of the dental arch.[107]

Supracontacts

Supracontact is a general term for any contact that hinders the remaining occlusal surfaces from achieving a many-pointed, stable contact. A supracontact is a morphologic relationship and does not necessarily imply a dysfunctional situation. Moreover, a supracontact in relation to one mandibular contact situation is not necessarily a supracontact in relation to others.[69]

Untoward supracontacts may be capable of injuring the supporting periodontal tissues or complicating mandibular movement. Altered forces generated by acute occlusal supracontacts are adapted primarily through responses in the alveolus and can result in changes in tooth position.[32] The mechanism is likely through increased pulpal blood flow initiated by a unilateral acute occlusal supracontact.[70] This can be manifested clinically as increased gingival bleeding.[40] Nevertheless, periodontal bone levels and pocket depth are not influenced by chronic occlusal supracontacts,[40,53] and tooth mobility does not seem to be affected.[40]

Iatrogenic new supracontacts that deflect closure in the retruded position are referred to as *retrusive supracontacts;* such supracontacts can alter muscle activity[77] and increase condylar loading.[67] Occlusal supracontacts that interfere with closure in ICP are called *intercuspal supracontacts.* Findings of persistent occlusal supracontacts in selected mandibular positions in almost 90% of otherwise normal individuals do not support the opinion that the mere presence of a supracontact is of great importance in the etiology of mandibular dysfunction.[2,21,91,92] In fact, chronic mediotrusive or laterotrusive supracontacts are common[2,91,92,144,157] and do not seem to alter chewing patterns[64,76] or muscle activity.[49] However, the abrupt introduction of an occlusal supracontact through operative treatment can lower pain thresholds,[55] reduce muscle activity,[60,123,127] and alter sleep patterns.[141]

VERTICAL DIMENSION OF OCCLUSION

The term *vertical dimension of occlusion* designates the distance between the maxilla and the mandible when the teeth are in ICP. The vertical dimension is maintained by a compensatory rate of both occlusal wear and continuous tooth eruption. Whereas the vertical dimension of occlusion should not be changed without a clear rationale, small changes in the course of dental therapy are usually rapidly accommodated by a re-establishment of the free way space.[22,52,80,160] Furthermore, increased vertical dimensions of up to 3 mm do not lead to signs of traumatic occlusion such as periodontal ligament width increases, tooth mobility, tooth impaction, or tooth abrasion.[55]

Evidence is lacking to suggest that the vertical dimension of occlusion should be changed in the presence of a large free way space, as there is considerable normal variation in this space. One serious problem in increasing the vertical dimension of occlusion could be the intrusion of teeth or a rapid resorption of alveolar bone under dentures. In this respect, it may be wise to err on the side of a reduced vertical dimension if no other means are available to assess the proper vertical dimension of occlusion.[109]

DENTAL WEAR

Attrition is the term used for dental wear caused by teeth against teeth. Such physical wearing patterns may occur on incisal, occlusal, and approximal tooth surfaces. A certain amount of tooth wear is physiologic, but accelerated wear may prevail with abnormal anatomic or unusual functional factors.

Occlusal or incisal surfaces worn by attrition are called *facets.* When active tooth gnashing occurs, the enamel rods are fractured and become highly reflective to light.[159] Thus, shiny, smooth, and curviplanar facets are usually the best indicator of ongoing frictional activity. If dentin is exposed, a yellowish brown discoloration is frequently present (Fig. 13–7). Facets vary in size and location depending on

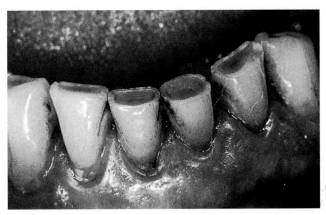

FIGURE 13–7. Occlusal wear. Flat, shiny, discolored surfaces produced by occlusal wear.

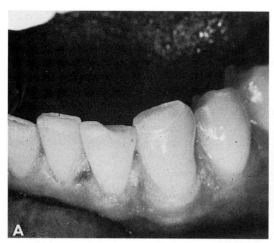
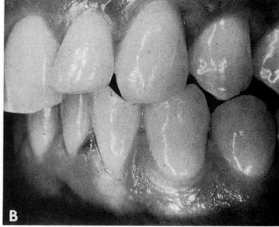

FIGURE 13–8. Wear facets. *A,* Flat facets worn on the incisal edges of the anterior teeth. Note the notch on the lateral incisor, also produced by wear. *B,* The maxillary canine fits into the notch on the lateral incisor produced by parafunctional mandibular movements.

whether they are produced by physiologic or abnormal wear[7,17,150] (Fig. 13–8). At least one significant wear facet has been reported in 92% of adults[130] and facet prevalence approaches universality.[140,157] Facets are usually not sensitive to thermal or tactile stimulation.

Facets generally represent functional and parafunctional wear as well as iatrogenic dental treatment through coronoplasty (occlusal adjustment). Coronoplasty, however, does not appear to contribute to higher ratings of wear.[130] Excessive wear may result in obliteration of the cusps and the formation of either a flat or a cuneiform (cupped-out) occlusal surface. Reversal of the occlusal plane of the premolars and first and second molars occurs in advanced stages of wear (Fig. 13–9). Contrary to earlier thought, attrition among young adults from modern societies is not age related.[31,37,115,130] This suggests that a significant amount of attrition, when present in young adults, is unlikely to occur from functional wear[71] and is probably the result of bruxing activity.[130] Attrition has been correlated with age when older adults are included.[3,138]

The angle of the facet on the tooth surface is of potential significance to the periodontium. Horizontal facets tend to direct forces in the vertical axis of the tooth, to which the periodontium can adapt most effectively. Angular facets direct occlusal forces laterally and increase the risk of periodontal consequences. However, gradual attrition may be compensated for by continuous tooth eruption without alveolar bone growth and is characterized by a lack of inflammatory changes on the alveolar bone surfaces.[148]

Erosion is wear to the nonoccluding tooth surfaces and includes sharply defined, wedge-shaped depressions in the facial cervical areas of the tooth. It is unique in being anatomically smooth and clean and is related to causative factors, such as digestive system regurgitation, bulimia, medicinal therapy, field of occupation (e.g., acid battery workers), and dietary habits (e.g., citrus fruits, carbonated drinks). *Idiopathic dental erosion* has long been the subject of much confusion. Some of these cases may be related to *frictional ablation,* a process caused by juxtaposition of natural and artificial dental surfaces and hyperfunctional oral soft tissues.[134,135] Frictional ablation is considered to be caused by the action of soft tissue and saliva against the dentition. It is generated through the vestibular pressures of

suction, swallowing, tongue motions, and the intervening forced flow of saliva.[135]

Abrasion implies wear caused by foreign substances, such as a hard-bristle toothbrush, coarse tooth powder, and toothpicks, or in ritual customs.[135] Cervical tooth abrasion

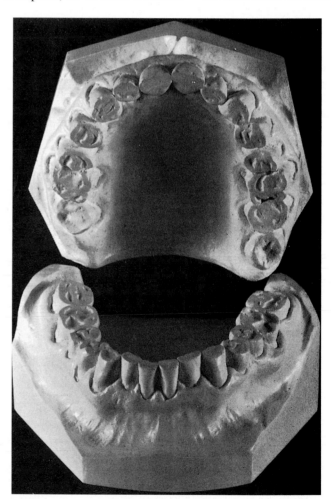

FIGURE 13–9. Reversed faciolingual occlusal plane (curve of pleasure). The normal occlusal plane is sometimes reversed by excessive wear, so that in the mandible the occlusal surfaces slope facially instead of lingually, and in the maxilla they are inclined lingually. The third molars are not usually affected.

was found to be more common in patients with periodontal disease.[41]

All of the preceding forms of dental wear exert influences that should be considered in the control and prevention of periodontal disease.

OCCLUSAL PARAFUNCTION: BRUXISM

Bruxism is the clenching or grinding of the teeth when the individual is not chewing or swallowing.[108] Bruxism can occur as brief, rhythmic strong contractions of the jaw muscles during eccentric lateral jaw movements or in maximum intercuspation, which is called *clenching*.[29] Bruxism may also take the form of tapping and tooth setting in a repetitive manner at isolated contact locations. Bruxism often occurs without any neurologic disorders or defects and can be viewed as a phenomenon present in healthy individuals. However, bruxism may lead to tooth wear, fractures of the teeth or dental restorations, or uncosmetic muscle hypertrophy.[81,95]

Tooth wear appears to be poorly associated with signs and symptoms of temporomandibular disorders (TMDs).[36,130] Therefore, the clinician should not assume that the presence of tooth wear in patients is necessarily causal.[106] Pullinger and Seligman[106] compared TMD patient diagnostic groups with asymptomatic controls and found that greater laterotrusive posterior wear was seen only in juvenile arthritis patients; such wear was interpreted to be the result of anterior open bite development from condylar autorepositioning resulting from rapid arthrosis.

Data from Rugh[125] indicate that 83% of a group of bruxers, when monitored, performed bilateral muscle contraction, whereas 17% performed unilateral contractions. Of clinical importance was the fact that bilateral contraction often occurred in an eccentric position. It has been proposed that bilateral eccentric bruxism may be harmful for the stomatognathic system and may be sufficient reason to generate full balance on nightguard appliances.[124]

Previously, nocturnal bruxism was not differentiated from daytime (diurnal) bruxism. It is now clear that these are two different phenomena with different causes requiring different treatment.[125] Most people are not aware of a bruxism habit until it is brought to their attention.[130] Only certain forms of bruxism are clearly audible. Wear from bruxism can be observed as facet patterns, but the observation of the degree of tooth wear does not necessarily indicate whether active bruxism is current. Because clenching is not related to attrition, the severity of bruxism is no doubt underestimated. Wear patterns on a well-adjusted bruxism splint are perhaps the most effective clinical tool for assessing current bruxism activity.

Sleep studies[112,126] have shown that bruxism can occur in any stage of sleep but is most common in stage II. Satoh and Harada[126] observed that bruxism tended to occur during the transition from a deeper stage of sleep to a lighter stage of sleep. Emerging evidence[125] suggests that bruxism occurring during rapid eye movement (REM) sleep may be the most damaging. Bruxism should not be considered a brain dysfunction, but rather a central nervous system instability that occurs idiopathically.[29]

Although bruxism occurs frequently among the population, its prevalence has been difficult to estimate. Currently there is no consensus as to what constitutes a bruxist event. Clark et al.[29] defined a bruxist event as a minimum level of 20% of maximum voluntary contraction of at least 2 seconds' duration; they found that some events even exceed the maximum voluntary contraction force and at a level to allow for crushing of enamel.

Most often bruxism goes unnoticed by the bruxer, and indirect measures observed on the teeth are not wholly reliable.[130] EMG sleep laboratory studies[130] suggest that bruxism is universal but with wide individual variations in severity. Rugh and Harlan[125] estimate that 5% of individuals brux to an unusually active extent at any one time. They further note that bruxism occurs equally as often in children as in adults, but it is not yet clear whether child bruxers continue to be bruxers when they become mature adults.

Bruxism and the periodontal condition appear to be independent phenomena, as no association has been shown between bruxism and periodontitis[52] or gingival inflammation.[27]

Certain types of individuals seem to be predisposed to bruxism. It has been reported that children of bruxist parents are more apt to be bruxers than children of nonbruxist parents.[1] Olkinuora[94] divided bruxers into two categories: those whose bruxism was associated with stressful events and those whose bruxism had no such association. He concluded that hereditary bruxism was much more common in the non–stress-related bruxism group.

Bruxism has been considered a multifactorial psychosomatic phenomenon, with individuals displaying aggressive, controlling, precise, energetic personality types on the one hand ("nonstress bruxists") and anxious, tense types on the other ("stress bruxists").[93] It is likely that these psychological characteristics fall within the normal limits of personality structure.[111] There is little evidence to suggest that bruxists have personality derangement or are mentally ill. However, it is interesting to note that brain-damaged children and mentally retarded individuals have a disproportionately higher rate of bruxism.[115]

The relationship between emotional states and muscle tension appears to be better understood. Reports have demonstrated that increased masseter muscle tension is directly related to stress situations during the day.[161] One study demonstrated that increased stress levels (as measured by urinary epinephrine content) are strongly correlated with increased levels of masseter muscle activity at night.[25] These studies have consistently shown a strong interrelationship between nonfunctional masseter muscle activity (bruxism) and stress. Nevertheless, the short-term muscle effects of sustained maximum clenching forces are probably innocuous, as rapid recovery without delayed onset muscle soreness is expected.[28]

Another aspect of bruxism concerns the perception of stress by bruxist patients. One study suggests that patients experiencing the greatest amount of bruxism have a diminished ability to recognize when they are under stress.[26] This may occur because chronic bruxism subjects are constantly overreacting to stress and therefore cannot determine when it increases. Alternatively, it may be that the bruxism subject simply has never learned to recognize or attend to the

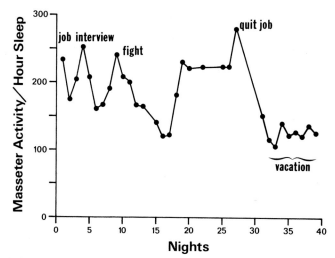

FIGURE 13–10. Electromyographic (EMG) data collected on bruxism patient. Nocturnal EMG recordings indicate that bruxist behavior may vary greatly from night to night and is correlated with the
previous day's stress level. (From Rugh JD, Solberg WK. Psychological implications in temporomandibular pain and dysfunction.
Oral Sci Rev *1:* 3, 1976. © 1976, Munksgaard International Publishers, Ltd., Copenhagen, Denmark.)

physiologic changes that occur in the body during stressful
situations.

Attempts to demonstrate the relationship between stress
and bruxism in the natural environment have involved the
use of portable EMG recording devices. The recordings indicate that bruxist behavior may vary greatly from night to
night and is correlated with the previous day's stress level
(Fig. 13–10).[121] Overall, it may be concluded that emotional stress acts together with other factors to produce
bruxism.

There is little support for the popular belief that occlusal
malrelationships or interferences may precipitate bruxism.
Artificial supracontacts intentionally placed did not elicit irreversible bruxism.[30,66,145] Two studies have shown that
bruxism cannot be stopped by means of occlusal adjustment.[9,62] These investigations indicate that occlusal therapy
for bruxism is likely to be unsuccessful.

Coronoplasty plays a role in occlusal treatments. However, invasive occlusal alterations in the form of extensive
occlusal adjustment, reconstruction, or orthodontic treatment are contraindicated as a means of controlling bruxism.
Splints are more significant in the management of the destructive effects of bruxism (see Chapter 47).

REFERENCES

1. Abe K, Shimakawa M. Genetic and developmental aspects of sleeptalking and
teeth grinding. Acta Paedopsychiatr *33:*336, 1966.
2. Agerberg G, Sandstrom R. Frequency of occlusal interferences: A clinical study
in teenagers and young adults. J Prosthet Dent *59:*212–217, 1988.
3. Agerberg G, Bergenholz A. Craniomandibular disorders in an adult population
of West Bothnia, Sweden. Acta Odontol Scand *47:*129–140, 1989.
4. Ahlgren J. Masticatory movements in man. In Anderson DJ, Mathews B, eds.
Mastication. Bristol, England, John Wright & Sons, 1976, p 119.
5. Akeel R, Nilner M, Nilner K. Masticatory efficiency in individuals with natural
dentitions. Swed Dent J *17:*191–198, 1993.
6. Anderson JR, Myers GE. Natural contacts in centric occlusion in 32 adults.
J Dent Res *50:*7, 1971.
7. Arstad T. The Capsular Ligaments of the Temporomandibular Joint and Retrusion Facets of the Dentition in Relationship to Mandibular Movements. Oslo,
Norway, Academisk Forlag, 1954.

8. Artun J, Hollender LG, Truelove EL. Relationship between orthodontic treatment, condylar position, and internal derangement in the temporomandibular
joint. Am J Orthod Dentofac Orthop *101:*48–53, 1992.
9. Bailey JO Jr, Rugh JD. Effect of occlusal adjustment on bruxism as monitored
by nocturnal EMG recordings. Abstract 199. J Dent Res *59:*317, 1980.
10. Bakke M, Moller E. Distortion of maximal elevator activity by unilateral premature contact. Scand J Dent Res *88:*67, 1980.
11. Bates JF, Stafford GD, Harrison A. Masticatory function: A review of the literature. I. The form of the masticatory cycle. J Oral Rehabil *2:*281, 1975.
12. Bates JF, Stafford GD, Harrison A. Masticatory function: A review of the literature. II. Speed of movement of the mandible, rate of chewing. J Oral Rehabil
*2:*349, 1975.
13. Bates JF, Stafford GD, Harrison A. Masticatory function: A review of the literature. III. Masticatory performance and efficiency. J Oral Rehabil *3:*57, 1976.
14. Bellanti ND, Martin KR. The significance of articular capability. Part II: The
prevalence of immediate sideshift. J Prosthet Dent *42:*255, 1979.
15. Berry DC, Singh BP. Daily variation in occlusal contacts. J Prosthet Dent
*50:*386–391, 1983.
16. Berry DC, Singh BP. Effect of EMG biofeedback therapy on occlusal contacts.
J Prosthet Dent *51:*397–403, 1984.
17. Beyron HL. Occlusal changes in the adult dentition. J Am Dent Assoc *48:*674,
1954.
18. Beyron HL. Occlusal relations and mastication in Australian aborigines. Acta
Odontol Scand *22:*597, 1964.
19. Burdette BH, Gale EN. Electromyographic activity of masticatory muscles of
MPD patients during opening. Abstract 1675. J Dent Res (special issue)
*68:*391.
20. Butler JH. Recent research on physiology of occlusion. Dent Clin North Am
*13:*555, 1969.
21. Butler JH, Folke LEA, Bandt CL. A descriptive survey of signs and symptoms
associated with the myofascial pain-dysfunction syndrome. J Am Dent Assoc
*90:*635–639, 1975.
22. Carlsson GE, Ingevall B, Kocak G. Effect of increasing vertical dimension on
the masticatory system in subjects with natural teeth. J Prosthet Dent *41:*284,
1979.
23. Castanada R, McNeill C, Guerrero A. Biomechanics in TMJ osteoarthritis: Part
II. Abstract 620. J Dent Res (special issue) *68:*259.
24. Christiansen LV, Hutchins MO. Methodological observations on positive and
negative work (teeth grinding) by human jaw muscles. J Oral Rehabil
*19:*399–411, 1992.
25. Clark GT. The relationship between stress, nocturnal masseter muscle activity
and symptoms of masticatory dysfunction. Master's thesis. University of
Rochester, Rochester NY, 1977.
26. Clark GT, Rugh JD, Beemsterboer P. Stress perception and nocturnal masseter
muscle activity. Abstract 436. J Dent Res (Special Issue B) *56:*161, 1977.
27. Clark GT, Love R. The effect of gingival inflammation on nocturnal masseter
muscle activity. J Am Dent Assoc *102:*319–322, 1981.
28. Clark GT, Jow RW, Lee JJ. Jaw pain and stiffness levels after repeated maximum voluntary clenching. J Dent Res *68:*69–71, 1989.
29. Clark GT, Koyano K, Browne PA. Oral motor disorders in humans. J Cal Dent
Assoc *21:*19–30, 1993.
30. Clark NG. Occlusion and myofascial pain dysfunction: Is there a relationship?
J Am Dent Assoc *104:*443–446, 1982.
31. Clark NG, Townsend GC, Carey SE. Bruxing patterns in man during sleep.
J Oral Rehabil *11:*123, 1984.
32. Curtis DA, Nielsen I, Kapila S, Miller AJ. Adaptability of the adult primate
craniofacial complex to asymmetrical lateral forces. Am J Orthod Dentofac Orthop *100:*266–273, 1991.
33. Curtis DA, Kapila S, Nielsen I, Miller AJ. Dentoalveolar adaptation to increased vertical dimension in adult rhesus monkeys. Abstract 204. J Dent Res
(special issue) *70:*291.
34. dos Santos J Jr, Ash MM Jr, Warshawsky P. Learning to reproduce a consistent
functional jaw movement. J Prosthet Dent *65:*294–302, 1991.
35. Drago CJ, Rugh JD. Measurement of vertical jaw relationship. In Lundeen HC,
Gibbs CH, eds. Advances in Occlusion. Postgraduate Dental Handbook Series,
Vol 14. Littleton MA, John Wright & Sons, 1982.
36. Droukas B, Lindee C, Carlsson GE. Occlusion and mandibular dysfunction: A
clinical study of patients referred for functional disturbances of the masticatory
system. J Prosthet Dent *53:*402, 1985.
37. Egermark-Eriksson I, Carlsson GE, Ingervall B. Prevalence of mandibular dysfunction and orofacial parafunction in 7-, 11-, and 15-year-old Swedish children. Eur J Orthop *3:*163, 1981.
38. Ehrlich J, Hochman N, Yaffe A. The masticatory pattern as an adjunct for diagnosis and treatment. J Oral Rehabil *19:*393–398, 1992.
39. Eriksson P-O, Stalberg E, Antoni L. Flexibility in motor-unit firing pattern in
the human temporal and masseter muscles related to type of activation and location. Arch Oral Biol *29:*707–712, 1984.
40. Ettala-Ylitalo UM, Markkanen H, Yli-Urpo A. Influence of occlusal interferences on the periodontium in patients treated with fixed prosthesis. J Prosthet
Dent *55:*252–255, 1986.
41. Furuya N, Cobb C, Pippin D. Cervical abrasion: correlation with periodontally
involved patients. Abstract 921. J Dent Res (special issue) *65:*271, 1986.
42. Garnick J, Ramfjord SP. Rest position. An electromyographic and clinical investigation. J Prosthet Dent *12:*895, 1962.
43. Gibbs CH, Lundeen HC. Jaw movements and forces during chewing and swal-

lowing and their clinical significance. In Lundeen HC, Gibbs CH, eds. Advances in Occlusion. Postgraduate Dental Handbook Series, Vol 14. Bristol, England, John Wright & Sons, 1982, pp 7, 22.

44. Gibbs CH, Messerman T, Reswick JB, Derda HJ. Functional movements of the mandible. J Prosthet Dent 26:604, 1971.
45. Gibbs CH, Wichwire NA, Jackobson AP, et al. Comparison of typical chewing patterns in normal children and adults. J Am Dent Assoc 105:33–42, 1982.
46. Goldstein DF, Kraus SW, Williams WB, Glasheen-Wray M. Influence of cervical posture on mandibular movement. J Prosthet Dent 52:421–426, 1984.
47. Guyton AC. Textbook of Medical Physiology. 2nd ed. Philadelphia, WB Saunders, 1961, pp 824–826.
48. Hanamura H, Houston F, Rylander H, et al. Periodontal status and bruxism: A comparative study of patients with periodontal disease and occlusal parafunction. J Periodontol 58:173–176, 1987.
49. Hannam AG, DeCou RE, Scott JD, Wood WW. The relationship between dental occlusion, muscle activity, and associated jaw movement in man. Arch Oral Biol 22:25–32, 1977.
50. Hanson ML, Andrianopoulos MV. Tongue thrust, occlusion, and dental health in middle-aged subjects: A pilot study. Int J Orofacial Myol 13:3–9, 1987.
51. Hatzigiogus CG, Gusins RJ, Fenster RK, Neff PA. A tomographic study of the temporomandibular joint of edentulous patients. J Prosthet Dent 57:354–358, 1987.
52. Hellsing G. Functional adaptation to changes in vertical dimension. J Prosthet Dent 52:867–870, 1984.
53. Hicks MJ, Brumfield FW, Devore CH, et al. Lack of relationship for occlusal prematurities with bone loss and probe depth. Abstract 1441. J Dent Res (special issue) 64:335, 1985.
54. Hochman N, Ehrlich J. Tooth contact location in intercuspal position. Quintess Int 18:193–196, 1987.
55. Ikeda T, Nakano M, Bando E. The effect of traumatic occlusal contact on tooth pain threshold. Abstract 519. J Dent Res (special issue) 70:330, 1991.
56. Ingervall B. Retruded contact position of the mandible. A comparison between children and adults. Odontol Revy 15:130, 1964.
57. Ingervall B, Egermark-Eriksson I. Function of temporal and masseter muscles in individuals with dual bite. Angle Orthodont 49:131–140, 1979.
58. Ingervall B. Studies of mandibular positions in children. Odontol Revy 19(suppl):15, 1968.
59. Johnston LE. Gnathologic assessment of centric slides in postretention orthodontic patients. J Prosthet Dent 60:712–715, 1988.
60. Joo HY, Kim KN. Influence of artificial occlusal interference on A. temporalis and masseter activity. Abstract 0-18. J Dent Res (special issue) 68:689, 1989.
61. Kang JH, Chung SC, Fricton JR. Normal movements of the mandible at the mandibular incisor. J Prosthet Dent 66:687–692, 1991.
62. Kardachi BJR, Bailey JO Jr, Ash MM Jr. A comparison of biofeedback and occlusal adjustment on bruxism. J Periodontol 49:367, 1978.
63. Karlsson S, Carlsson GE. Characteristics of mandibular masticatory movement in young and elderly dentate subjects. J Dent Res 69:473–476, 1990.
64. Karlsson S, Cho S-A, Carlsson GE. Changes in mandibular masticatory movements after insertion of non–working side interference. J Craniomandib Dis Fac Oral Pain 6:177–183, 1992.
65. Killiardes S, Karlsson S, Kjellberg H. Characteristics of masticatory mandibular movements and velocity in growing individuals and young adults. J Dent Res 70:1367–1370, 1991.
66. Kobayashi Y, Hansson TL. Auswirkung der Okklusion auf den menschlichen Koerper. Phillip J 5:255–263, 1988.
67. Korioth TWP, Hannam AG. Effect of bilateral asymmetric tooth clenching on load distribution at the mandibular condyle. J Prosthet Dent 64:62–73, 1990.
68. Korioth TWP. Number and location of occlusal contacts in intercuspal position. J Prosthet Dent 64:206–210, 1990.
69. Krogh-Poulsen WG, Olsson A. Management of the occlusion of the teeth. In Schwarz L, Chayes C, eds. Facial Pain and Mandibular Dysfunction. Philadelphia, WB Saunders, 1968.
70. Kvinnsland S, Kristiansen AB, Kvinnsland I, Heyeraas K. Effect of experimental traumatic occlusion on periodontal and pulpal blood flow. Acta Odontol Scand 50:211–219, 1992.
71. Lambrechts P, Braem M, Vuylsteke-Wanters M, Vanherle G. Quantitative in vivo wear of human enamel. J Dent Res 68:1752–1754, 1989.
72. Lear CSC, Flanagan JB Jr, Moorees CFA. The frequency of deglutition in man. Arch Oral Biol 10:83, 1965.
73. Lee RL. Anterior guidance. In Lundeen HC, Gibbs CH, eds. Advances in Occlusion. Postgraduate Dental Handbook Series, Vol 14. Bristol, England, John Wright & Sons, 1982, p 62.
74. Logsdon LC, Chaconas SJ. Laminographic evaluation of the temporomandibular joint. Abstract 556. J Dent Res (Special Issue A) 54:184, 1975.
75. Lous I, Sheik-Ol-Eslam A, Moller E. Postural activity in subjects with functional disorders of the chewing apparatus. Scand J Dent Res 78:404, 1970.
76. Lundeen H. Studies of condyle movements. Scientific Meeting of the American Academy of Craniomandibular Disorders, Chicago, February, 1983.
77. McCarroll RS, Naeije M, Kim YK, Hansson TL. Short term effect of a stabilization splint on the asymmetry of submaximal masticatory muscle activity. J Oral Rehabil 16:171–176, 1989.
78. MacDonald JWC, Hannam AG. Relationship between occlusal contacts and jaw closing muscles during tooth clenching: Part I. J Prosthet Dent 52:718–729, 1984.
79. Machtei E, Zubery Y, Brinstein E, Becker A. Open bite and oral habits in rela-

80. McNamara JA. An experimental study of increased vertical dimension in the growing face. Am J Orthod 4:382–395, 1977.
81. Magnusson T, Carlsson GE. Headache and mandibular dysfunction in two groups of dental patients. J Prosthet Dent 58:2296, 1979.
82. Mahan PA, Gibbs CJ, Mauderli A. Superior and inferior lateral pterygoid activity. Abstract. J Dent Res 61:272, 1982.
83. Martin G. Relationship between chewing side preference and distribution of occlusal contacts. Abstract 11. J Dent Res (special issue) 69:1077, 1990.
84. Matthews B. Mastication. In Lavelle CLB, ed. Applied Physiology of the Mouth. Bristol, England, John Wright & Sons, 1975, p 199.
85. Miralles R, Hevia R, Contreras L, et al. Patterns of electromyographic activity in subjects with different facial types. Angle Orthodont 61:277–283, 1991.
86. Molligoda MA, Berry DC, Gooding PG. Measuring diurnal variation in occlusal contact areas. J Prosthet Dent 56:487–492, 1986.
87. Molligoda M, Abuzar M, Berry D. Measuring diurnal variations in the dispersion of occlusal contacts. J Prosthet Dent 60:235–238, 1988.
88. Morel A, Albuisson E, Woda A. A study of human jaw movements deduced from scratches on occlusal wear facets. Arch Oral Biol 36:195–202, 1991.
89. Moyers RE. Some physiologic considerations of centric and other jaw relations. J Prosthet Dent 6:183, 1956.
90. Nielsen LL, Marcel T, Chun D, Miller AJ. Patterns of mandibular movements in subjects with craniomandibular disorders. J Prosthet Dent 30:202–217, 1990.
91. Nilner M, Lassing S-A. Prevalence of functional disturbances and diseases of the stomatognathic system in 7–14 year-olds. Swed Dent J 5:173–187, 1981.
92. Nilner M. Prevalence of functional disturbances and diseases of the stomatognathic system in 15–18 year-olds. Swed Dent J 5:189–197, 1981.
93. Olkinuora M. Psychosocial aspects in a series of bruxists compared with a group of non-bruxists. Proc Finn Dent Soc 68:200, 1972.
94. Olkinuora M. A psychosomatic study of bruxism with emphasis on mental strain and familial predisposition factors. Proc Finn Dent Soc 68:110, 1972.
95. Pameijer JHN, Brion M, Glickman I. Intraoral occlusal telemetry. Part IV. Tooth contact during swallowing. J Prosthet Dent 24:296–400, 1970.
96. Pavone BW. Bruxism and its effect on the natural teeth. J Prosthet Dent 53:692–696, 1985.
97. Pertes R, Vella M, Milone A. Vertical skeletal facial types and condylar position in TMJ patients. Abstract 109. J Dent Res (special issue) 68:195, 1989.
98. Plasmans PJJM, Knipers L, Vollenbrock HR, Vrijhoef MMA. The occlusal status of molars. J Prosthet Dent 60:500–503, 1988.
99. Plesh O, McCall W Jr, Gross A. The effect of prior jaw motion on the plot of electromyographic amplitude versus jaw position. J Prosthet Dent 60:369–373, 1988.
100. Pond LJ, Barghi N, Barnwell GM. Occlusion and chewing side preference. J Prosthet Dent 55:498–500, 1986.
101. Posselt V. Studies in the mobility of the human mandible. Acta Odontol Scand 10(suppl 10):1, 1952.
102. Preiskel HW. Some observations on the postural position of the mandible. J Prosthet Dent 15:625, 1965.
103. Proesdiel P, Hofmann M. Frontal chewing patterns of the incisor point and their dependence on resistance of food and type of occlusion. J Prosthet Dent 59:617–624, 1988.
104. Pullinger AG. Condyle position. Scientific Meeting of the American Academy of Craniomandibular Disorders, Chicago, February 1984.
105. Pullinger AG, Hollander L, Solberg WK, Petersson A. A tomographic study of mandibular condyle position in an asymptomatic population. J Prosthet Dent 53:706–713, 1985.
106. Pullinger AG, Seligman DA. The degree to which attrition characterizes diagnostic groups of temporomandibular disorders. J Orofac Pain 7:196–208, 1993.
107. Pullinger AG, Solberg WK, Xu YH. Epidemiological studies of occlusal contact in young adults. Unpublished data. UCLA School of Dentistry, Los Angeles, 1985.
108. Ramfjord SP, Kerr DA, Ash MM. World Workshop in Periodontics. Ann Arbor, MI, University of Michigan Press, 1966.
109. Ramfjord SP. Occlusion. Indent 1:19, 1973.
110. Ramfjord SP, Ash MM. Occlusion. 3rd ed. Philadelphia, WB Saunders, 1983.
111. Reding G, Zepelin H, Monroe L. Personality study of nocturnal tooth grinders. Precept Mot Skills 26:523, 1960.
112. Reding G, Zepelin H, Monroe LJ, et al. Sleep pattern of bruxism: Revision. Psychophysiology 4:396, 1967–1968.
113. Regli CP, Kelly EK. The phenomenon of decreased mandibular arch width in opening movements. J Prosthet Dent 17:49, 1967.
114. Rey R, Barghi N, Bailey JO Jr. Incidence of radiographic condylar concentricity in non-patients. Abstract 881. J Dent Res 60(suppl A): 530, 1981.
115. Richmond G, Rugh JD, Dolfi R, Wasilewsky JW. Survey of bruxism in an institutionalized mentally retarded population. Am J Ment Defic 88:418, 1984.
116. Ricketts RM. Variations of the temporomandibular joint as revealed by cephalometric laminography. Am J Orthod 36:877, 1950.
117. Rieder CE, Martinoff JT. Comparison of the multiphasic dysfunction profile with lateral transcranial radiographs. J Prosthet Dent 52:572–580, 1984.
118. Rokni A, Ismail YH. Radiographic comparative study of condyle position in centric relation and centric occlusion. Abstract 1070. J Dent Res (Special Issue A) 57:342, 1978.
119. Rugh JD. Variation in human masticatory behavior under temporal constraints. J Compar Physiol Psychol 80:169, 1972.

120. Rugh JD, Solberg WK. Electromyographic evaluation of bruxist behavior before and after treatment. Can Dent Assoc J 3:56, 1975.

121. Rugh JD, Solberg WK. Psychological implications in temporomandibular pain and dysfunction. Oral Sci Rev 1:3, 1976.

122. Rugh JD, Drago CJ. Vertical dimension: A study of clinical rest position and jaw muscle activity. J Prosthet Dent 45:670, 1981.

123. Rugh JD, Barghi N, Drago CJ. Experimental occlusal discrepancies and nocturnal bruxism. J Prosthet Dent 51:548–553, 1984.

124. Rugh JD. Lecture before the Danish Society of Craniomandibular Disorders, 1988, Grenaa, Denmark.

125. Rugh JD, Harlan J. Nocturnal bruxism and temporomandibular disorders. In Jankovic J, Tolosa T, eds. Advances in Neurology. Vol 49: Facial Dyskinesias. New York, Raven Press, 1988.

126. Satoh T, Harada Y. Tooth grinding during sleep as an arousal reaction. Experientia 27:785, 1971.

127. Schaerer P, Stallard RE, Zander HA. Occlusal interferences and mastication: An electromyographic study. J Prosthet Dent 17:438–449, 1967.

128. Schaerer P, Stallard E. The effect of an occlusal interference on the tooth contact occurrence during mastication. Helv Odont Acta 10:49–56, 1966.

129. Schulte JK, Wang SH, Erdman AG, Anderson GC. Three-dimensional analysis of cusp travel during non-working mandibular movement. J Prosthet Dent 53:839–843, 1985.

130. Seligman DA, Pullinger AG, Solberg WK. The prevalence of dental attrition and its association with factors of age, gender, and TMJ symptomology. J Dent Res 67:1323, 1988.

131. Serrano PT, Nicholis JI, Yuodelis RA. Centric relation change during therapy with corrective occlusion prosthesis. J Prosthet Dent 51:97–105, 1984.

132. Shinya A, Suganama T, Takahashi H, et al. Microdisplacement of the mandible during clench in an intercuspal position. Abstract 210. J Dent Res (special issue) 70:292, 1991.

133. Sochat P, Schwarz MS. Individualized occlusal adjustment. Part I. Rationale. J South Cal Dent Assoc 40:827, 1972.

134. Sognnaes R. Frictional ablation—a neglected factor in the mechanisms of hard tissue destruction? In Kuhlencordt F, Kruse HP, eds. Calcium Metabolism, Bone and Metabolic Bone Diseases. Berlin, Springer-Verlag, 1975.

135. Sognnaes R. Periodontal significance of intraoral frictional ablation. J West Soc Periodontol 25:112, 1977.

136. Solberg WK, Flint RT, Brantner JP. Temporomandibular joint pain and dysfunction. A clinical study of emotional and occlusal components. J Prosthet Dent 28:412, 1972.

137. Solberg WK, Woo M, Houston JB. Prevalence of mandibular dysfunction in young adults. J Am Dent Assoc 98:25, 1979.

138. Salonen L, Hellden L. Prevalence of signs and symptoms of dysfunction in the masticatory system: An epidemiologic study in an adult Swedish population. J Craniomandib Dis Fac Oral Pain 4:241–250, 1990.

139. Suvinen TI, Reade PC, Faulkner KDB. Masseter electromyography in normal and temporomandibular joint pain-dysfunction syndrome subjects. Abstract 109. J Dent Res 69:946, 1990.

140. Takenoshita Y, Ikebe T, Yamamoto M, Oka M. Occlusal contacts and temporomandibular symptoms. Oral Surg Oral Med Oral Pathol 72:388–394, 1991.

141. Takeda Y, Ishihara H, Kobayashi Y. Influence of occlusal interference on nocturnal sleep and masseter muscle activity. Abstract 561. J Dent Res (special issue) 68:936, 1989.

142. Talgren A. Muscle activity relative to changes in occlusal jaw relationship: Cephalometric and electromyographic correlation. In Rowe NH, ed. Occlusion: Research in Form and Function. Proceedings of Symposium, University of Michigan School of Dentistry. Ann Arbor, MI, University of Michigan Press, 1975, p 21.

143. Thompson JR. The rest position of the mandible and its significance to dental science. J Am Dent Assoc 33:151, 1946.

144. Tipton RT, Rinchuse DJ. The relationship between static occlusion and functional occlusion in a dental school population. Angle Orthodont 61:57–66, 1991.

145. Travell J. Myofascial trigger points: Clinical view. In Bonica J, DeAlbe-Fessards D, eds. Advanced Pain Research and Therapy. New York, Raven Press, 1976, pp 919–926.

146. Van Sickels JE, Rugh JD, Chu GW, Lemke RR. Electromyographic relaxed mandibular position in long-faced subjects. J Prosthet Dent 54:578–581, 1985.

147. Van der Bilt A, Van der Glas HW, Olthoff LW, Bosman F. The effect of particle size reduction on the jaw gape in human mastication. J Dent Res 70:931–937, 1991.

148. Van der Bilt A, Olthoff LW, Bosman F, Oosterhaven SP. The effect of missing postcanine teeth on chewing performance in man. Arch Oral Biol 38:423–429, 1993.

149. Varrela TM, Paunio K, Wouters FR, et al. Alveolar crest level in a population with advanced dental attrition. Abstract 698. J Dent Res (special issue) 68:954, 1989.

150. Weinberg LA. Diagnosis of facets in occlusal equilibration. J Am Dent Assoc 52:26, 1956.

151. Wessberg GA, Washburn MC, Epker BN, Dana KO. Evaluation of mandibular rest position in subjects with diverse dentofacial morphology. J Prosthet Dent 48:451–460, 1982.

152. Wessberg GA, Epker BN, Elliott AC. Comparison of mandibular rest positions induced by phonetics, transcutaneous electrical stimulation, and masticatory electromyography. J Prosthet Dent 49:100, 1983.

153. Wilding RJC, Lewin A. A computer analysis of normal human masticatory movements recorded with a sirognathograph. Arch Oral Biol 36:65–75, 1991.

154. Wilding RJC, Lewin A. A model for optimum functional human jaw movements based on values associated with preferred chewing patterns. Arch Oral Biol 36:519–523, 1991.

155. Wilding RJC, Adams LP, Lewin A. Absence of association between preferred chewing side and its area of functional occlusal contact in the human dentition. Arch Oral Biol 37:423–428, 1992.

156. Wilding RJC. The association between chewing efficiency and occlusal contact area in man. Arch Oral Biol 38:589–596, 1993.

157. Woda A, Gourdon AM, Faraj M. Occlusal contact and tooth wear. J Prosthet Dent 57:85–93, 1987.

158. Wood WW. A review of masticatory muscle function. J Prosthet Dent 57:222–232, 1987.

159. Xhonga FA. Bruxism and its effect on the teeth. J Oral Rehabil 4:65, 1977.

160. Yaffe A, Tal M, Ehrlich J. Effect of occlusal bite-raising splint on electromyogram motor unit histochemistry and myoneural dimensions in rats. J Oral Rehabil 18:343–351, 1991.

161. Yemm R. Neurophysiological studies of temporomandibular joint dysfunction. Oral Sci Rev 1:31, 1976.

14

Influence of Systemic Diseases on the Periodontium

FERMIN A. CARRANZA, JR.

This chapter will deal with the systemic diseases that have periodontal manifestations. In general, these diseases do not initiate chronic destructive periodontitis but may accelerate its progression and increase tissue destruction.

NUTRITIONAL DISEASES

The majority of opinions and research findings on the effects of nutrition on oral and periodontal tissues point to the following:

1. *There are nutritional deficiencies that produce changes in the oral cavity.* These changes include alterations of the lips, oral mucosa, and bone, as well as of the periodontal tissues. These changes are considered to be periodontal or oral manifestations of nutritional disease.
2. *There are no nutritional deficiencies that by themselves can cause gingivitis or periodontal pockets.* There are, however, nutritional deficiencies that can affect the condition of the periodontium and thereby aggravate the injurious effects of local irritants and excessive occlusal forces. Theoretically, it can be assumed that there may be a "border zone" in which local irritants of insufficient severity can cause gingival and periodontal disorders if their effect on the periodontium is aggravated by nutritional deficiencies. On the basis of this speculation, some clinicians enthusiastically adhere to the theory that assigns a key role in periodontal disease to nutritional deficiencies and imbalances.* Research conducted up to the present does not in general support this view, but numerous problems in experimental design and data interpretation may render these research findings inadequate.[2]

---

* Unfortunately, this area has been apt to be exploited by quacks and fraudulent claims that have somewhat discredited the role of nutrition in periodontal disease.[18a]

This section analyzes the existing knowledge in the field of nutrition as it relates to periodontal disease, with reference also made to other oral changes of nutritional origin.

Physical Character of the Diet

Numerous experiments in animals have shown that the physical character of the diet may play some role in the accumulation of plaque and the development of gingivitis.[57] Soft diets, although nutritionally adequate, may lead to plaque and calculus formation.[10,50,57] Hard and fibrous foods provide surface cleansing action and stimulation, which result in less plaque and gingivitis,[24,76] even if the diet is nutritionally inadequate.[45]

In humans, however, studies have been unable to demonstrate reduced plaque formation when hard foods are consumed.[46] The discrepancy may be related to differences in tooth anatomy and to the fact that hard foods are fed to experimental animals as the only diet, whereas humans also consume soft foods. Human diets also have a high sucrose content, which favors the production of a thick plaque.

Effect of Nutrition on Oral Microorganisms

Although dietary intake is generally thought of in terms of sustaining the individual, it is also the source of nutrients for bacteria.[7] By its effects on the oral bacteria, the diet may influence the relative distribution of types of organisms, their metabolic activity, and their pathogenic potential, which in turn affect the occurrence and severity of oral disease.

Sources of nutrients for the microorganisms can be endogenous and exogenous. Among the exogenous factors, the influence of the sugar content of the diet has been extensively studied, and it has been demonstrated that the amount and type of carbohydrates in the diet and the frequency of intake can influence bacterial growth.[13] Attachment and subsequent colonization of the tooth surface by certain microorganisms may also be made possible by components of the diet.

Fat-Soluble Vitamins

Vitamin A Deficiency. Deficiency of vitamin A results in ocular manifestations and keratinizing metaplasia of the epithelium.

The following periodontal changes have been reported in vitamin A–deficient rats: hyperplasia and hyperkeratinization of the gingival epithelium with proliferation of the junctional epithelium,[9] and retardation of gingival wound healing.[27] In the presence of local irritation, vitamin A–deficient rats develop periodontal pockets[8] that are deeper than those in non–vitamin A–deficient animals and exhibit associated epithelial hyperkeratosis.[32]

There is little information regarding the effects of vitamin A deficiency on the oral structures in humans. Several epidemiologic studies have failed to demonstrate any relation between this vitamin and periodontal disease.[73]

Vitamin D Deficiency. Vitamin D, or calciferol, is essential for the absorption of calcium from the gastrointestinal tract and for the maintenance of the calcium–phosphorus balance. Deficiency in vitamin D and/or imbalance in calcium–phosphorus intake results in rickets in the very young and osteomalacia in adults.

The effect of such deficiency or imbalance on the periodontal tissues of young dogs results in osteoporosis of alveolar bone[5]; osteoid that forms at a normal rate but remains uncalcified; failure of osteoid to resorb, which leads to its excessive accumulation; reduction in the width of the periodontal space; a normal rate of cementum formation, but defective calcification and some cementum resorption[74]; and distortion of the growth pattern of alveolar bone.

In osteomalacic animals, there is rapid, generalized, severe osteoclastic resorption of alveolar bone, proliferation of fibroblasts that replace bone and marrow, and new bone formation around the remnants of unresorbed bony trabeculae.[23]

Radiographically, there is generalized partial to complete disappearance of the lamina dura and reduced density of the supporting bone, loss of trabeculae, increased radiolucence of the trabecular interstices, and increased prominence of the remaining trabeculae. Microscopic and radiographic changes in the periodontium are almost identical with those seen in experimentally induced hyperparathyroidism.

Vitamin E Deficiency. No relationship has been demonstrated between deficiencies in vitamin E and oral disease,[54,56] but systemic vitamin E appears to accelerate gingival wound healing in the rat.[43]

Water-Soluble Vitamins

B Complex Deficiency. The vitamin B complex includes thiamine, riboflavin, niacin, pyridoxine (B_6), biotin, folic acid, and cobalamin (B_{12}). Oral disease is rarely due to a deficiency in just one component of the B complex group; the deficiency is generally multiple.

Oral changes common to B complex deficiencies are gingivitis, glossitis, glossodynia, angular cheilitis, and inflammation of the entire oral mucosa. The gingivitis in vitamin B deficiencies is nonspecific, as it is caused by bacterial plaque rather than by the deficiency, but it is subject to the modifying effect of the latter.[1]

The human manifestations of *thiamine deficiency,* called *beriberi,* are characterized by paralysis, cardiovascular symptoms (including edema), and loss of appetite. Frank beriberi is rare in the United States.

The following oral disturbances have been attributed to thiamine deficiency: hypersensitivity of the oral mucosa[51]; minute vesicles (simulating herpes) on the buccal mucosa, under the tongue, or on the palate; and erosion of the oral mucosa.[37]

The symptoms of *riboflavin deficiency (ariboflavinosis)* include glossitis, angular cheilitis, seborrheic dermatitis, and a superficial vascularizing keratitis. The glossitis is characterized by a magenta discoloration and atrophy of the papillae. In mild to moderate cases, the dorsum exhibits a patchy atrophy of the lingual papillae[1] and engorged fungiform papillae, which project as pebble-like elevations.[41] In severe deficiency, the entire dorsum is flat, with a dry and often fissured surface.

Angular cheilitis begins as an inflammation of the commissure of the lips, followed by erosion, ulceration, and fissuring. Riboflavin deficiency is not the only cause of angular cheilitis. Loss of vertical dimension, together with drooling of saliva into the angles of the lips, may produce a condition similar to angular cheilitis. Candidiasis may develop in the commissures of debilitated persons; this lesion has been termed *perlèche.*[36]

Changes observed in riboflavin-deficient animals include severe lesions of the gingivae, periodontal tissues, and oral mucosa (including noma).[15,67]

Niacin deficiency results in *pellagra,* which is characterized by dermatitis, gastrointestinal disturbances, neurologic and mental disturbances (dermatitis, diarrhea, and dementia), glossitis, gingivitis, and generalized stomatitis.

Glossitis and stomatitis may be the earliest clinical signs of niacin deficiency.[52] The gingiva may be involved in aniacinosis[44] with or without tongue changes. The most frequent finding is acute necrotizing ulcerative gingivitis, usually in areas of local irritation.

Oral manifestations of vitamin B complex and niacin deficiency in experimental animals include black tongue[1,21] and gingival inflammation with destruction of the gingiva, periodontal ligament, and alveolar bone.[6] Necrosis of the gingiva and other oral tissues and leukopenia are terminal features of niacin deficiency in experimental animals.

Folic acid deficiency results in macrocytic anemia with megaloblastic erythropoiesis, with oral changes and gastrointestinal lesions, diarrhea, and intestinal malabsorption.[22]

Folic acid–deficient animals demonstrate necrosis of the gingiva, periodontal ligament, and alveolar bone without inflammation.[61] The absence of inflammation is the result of deficiency-induced granulocytopenia. In humans with sprue and other folic acid deficiency states, there is generalized stomatitis, which may be accompanied by ulcerated glossitis and cheilitis. Ulcerative stomatitis is an early indication of the toxic effect of folic acid antagonists used in the treatment of leukemia.

In a series of human studies, a significant reduction of gingival inflammation has been reported after systemic or local use of folic acid, when compared with placebo.[70,71] This reduction occurred with no change in plaque accumulation. The same authors have postulated that the gingival changes associated with pregnancy and oral contraceptives may be partly related to suboptimal levels of folic acid in the gingiva.[69] In a clinical study of pregnant women,[55] a reduction in gingival inflammation occurred with the use of topical folate mouth rinses; no change was found with systemic folic acid. A relationship has also been assumed between phenytoin-induced gingival overgrowth and folic acid, based on the interference of folic acid absorption and utilization by phenytoin.[68]

Vitamin C (Ascorbic Acid) Deficiency. Severe vitamin C deficiency in humans results in *scurvy,* a disease characterized by hemorrhagic diathesis and retardation of wound healing. Vitamin C is required in the human diet but not in that of other animals except other primates, guinea pigs, and some rare flying mammals.[19] Vitamin C is abundant in fruits and vegetables. Scurvy is uncommon in countries that have adequate food supplies, but it may appear in infants in their first year of life if formulas are not fortified with vitamins and in the very elderly, especially those living alone and on restricted diets.[19] Alcoholism also may predispose an individual to scurvy.

Clinical manifestations of scurvy[19] include hemorrhagic lesions into the muscles of the extremities, the joints, and sometimes the nail beds; petechial hemorrhages, often around hair follicles; increased susceptibility to infections; and impaired wound healing. Bleeding, swollen gingivae, and loosened teeth are also common features of scurvy.

Vitamin C deficiency (scurvy) results in defective formation and maintenance of collagen, retardation or cessation of osteoid formation, and impaired osteoblastic function.[26,75] Vitamin C deficiency is also characterized by increased capillary permeability, susceptibility to traumatic hemorrhages, hyporeactivity of the contractile elements of the peripheral blood vessels, and sluggishness of blood flow.[48]

Possible Etiologic Relationships Between Ascorbic Acid and Periodontal Disease. It has been suggested that ascorbic acid may play a role in periodontal disease by one or more of the following mechanisms:[76]

1. *Low levels of ascorbic acid influence the metabolism of collagen within the periodontium, thereby affecting the ability of the tissue to regenerate and repair itself.* There is no experimental evidence to support this view of the role of ascorbic acid; furthermore, it has been shown that collagen fibers in the periodontal ligament of scorbutic monkeys are the last affected prior to death of the animals.[72]

2. *Ascorbic acid deficiency interferes with bone formation, leading to loss of periodontal bone.* Changes that do occur in alveolar bone and other bones as a result of failure of the osteoblasts to form osteoid take place very late in the deficiency state.[29] Osteoporosis of alveolar bone in scorbutic monkeys occurs as a result of increased osteoclastic resorption and is not associated with periodontal pocket formation.[72]

3. *Ascorbic acid deficiency increases the permeability of the oral mucosa to tritiated endotoxin and tritiated inulin*[3,4] *and of normal human crevicular epithelium to tritiated dextran.* Optimal levels of this vitamin, therefore, would maintain the epithelium's barrier function to bacterial products.

4. *Increasing levels of ascorbic acid enhance both the chemotactic and the migratory action of leukocytes without influencing their phagocytic activity.*[34] Megadoses of vitamin C seem to impair the bactericidal activity of leukocytes.[62] The significance of these findings for the pathogenesis and treatment of periodontal diseases is not understood.

5. *An optimal level of ascorbic acid is apparently required to maintain the integrity of the periodontal microvasculature, as well as the vascular response to bacterial irritation and wound healing.*[12]

6. *Depletion of vitamin C may interfere with the ecologic equilibrium of bacteria in plaque and thus increase its pathogenicity.* However, there is no evidence that demonstrates this effect.

Epidemiologic Studies. Several studies in large populations[73] have analyzed the relationship between gingival or periodontal status and ascorbic acid levels. These studies used different methods for the biochemical analysis of ascorbic acid and various indices for the assessment of periodontal changes and were made in persons of different socioeconomic status, different races, and various ages. All the epidemiologic surveys failed to establish a causal relationship between the levels of vitamin C and the prevalence or severity of periodontal disease.[11,25,60] Megadoses of ascorbic acid have also been found to be unrelated to better periodontal health.[40,77]

Gingivitis. The legendary association of severe gingival disease with scurvy led to the presumption that vitamin C deficiency is an etiologic factor in gingivitis, which is common at all ages.

Gingivitis with enlarged, hemorrhagic, bluish red gingiva is described as one of the classic signs of vitamin C deficiency, but *gingivitis is not caused by vitamin C deficiency per se.* Vitamin C–deficient patients do not necessarily have gingivitis. Acute vitamin C deficiency does not cause or increase the incidence of gingival inflammation,[29,30] but it does increase its severity.[16] Gingivitis in vitamin C–deficient patients is caused by bacterial plaque. Vitamin C deficiency may aggravate the gingival response to plaque and worsen the edema, enlargement, and bleeding, and the severity of the disorder may be reduced by correcting the deficiency, but gingivitis will remain as long as bacterial irritation is present.

Periodontitis. Changes in the supporting periodontal tissues and gingiva in vitamin C deficiency have been documented extensively in experimental animals.[29,39,72]

Acute vitamin C deficiency results in edema and hemorrhage in the periodontal ligament, osteoporosis of the alveolar bone, and tooth mobility; hemorrhage, edema, and degeneration of collagen fibers occur in the gingiva. Vitamin C deficiency also retards gingival healing. The periodontal fibers that are least affected by vitamin C deficiency are those just below the junctional epithelium and above the alveolar crest, which explains the infrequent apical downgrowth of the epithelium.[72]

Vitamin C deficiency does not cause periodontal pockets; local bacterial factors are required for pocket formation to occur. However, acute vitamin C deficiency accentuates the destructive effect of gingival inflammation on the underlying periodontal ligament and alveolar bone.[30]

The exaggerated destruction results partly from inability to marshal a defensive delimiting connective tissue barrier reaction to the inflammation and partly from destructive tendencies caused by the deficiency itself, including inhibition of fibroblast formation and differentiation to osteoblasts and impaired formation of collagen and mucopolysaccharide ground substance.

Experimental studies conducted in humans[20,38,59] failed to show the dramatic clinical changes that have traditionally been described in scurvy. A case report published by Charbeneau and Hurt[16] showed worsening of a pre-existing moderate periodontitis with the development of scurvy.

In summary, analysis of the literature indicates that the microscopic signs of vitamin C deficiency are quite different from those that occur in plaque-induced periodontal disease in humans. Patients with acute or chronic vitamin C–deficient states and no plaque accumulation show minimal, if any, changes in their gingival health status.

Protein Deficiency

Protein depletion results in hypoproteinemia with many pathologic changes, including muscular atrophy, weakness, weight loss, anemia, leukopenia, edema, impaired lactation, decreased resistance to infection, slow wound healing, lymphoid depletion, and reduced ability to form certain hormones and enzyme systems.[13]

Protein deprivation causes the following changes in the periodontium of experimental animals:[17,28] degeneration of the connective tissue of the gingiva and periodontal ligament, osteoporosis of alveolar bone,[14] retardation in the deposition of cementum, delayed wound healing,[64] and atrophy of the tongue epithelium.[65] Similar changes occur in the periosteum and bone in other areas. Osteoporosis results from reduced deposition of osteoid, reduction in the number of osteoblasts, and retardation in the morphodifferentiation of connective tissue cells to form osteoblasts, rather than from increased osteoclasis.

These observations are of interest in that they reveal a loss of alveolar bone that is the result of the inhibition of normal bone-forming activity rather than of the introduction of destructive factors. Protein deficiency also accentuates the destructive effects of local irritants[65] and occlusal trauma[53] on the periodontal tissues, but the initiation of gingival inflammation and its severity depend on the local irritants.

Starvation

In a study of controlled semistarvation in young adults,[42] there were no changes in the oral cavity or skeletal system, despite a 24% loss of body weight. Another study, however, showed a reduction in Plaque Index scores and a considerable increase in Gingival Index scores as the fasting period lengthened.[63]

In experimental animals, acute starvation results in osteoporosis of alveolar bone and other bones, reduction in the height of alveolar bone, and accentuated bone loss associated with gingival inflammation.[33]

Mineral Deficiencies and Toxicities

Fluoride. Fluoride in drinking water in levels used to prevent tooth decay presents no health hazards. Observations in populations using fluoridated water supplies do not agree regarding the effects, if any, on the condition of the periodontium (see Chapter 5). Findings in experimental animals vary, with some investigators reporting that fluoride increases periodontal disease[47,58] and others noting that it decreases[18] or protects against periodontal disease.[54] (See Chapter 44 for a discussion of the local use of fluorides in periodontal therapy.)

ENDOCRINE DISEASES

Hormonal disturbances may affect the periodontal tissues directly, as periodontal manifestations of endocrine diseases; modify the tissue response to plaque in gingival and periodontal disease; or produce anatomic changes in the oral cavity that may favor plaque accumulation or trauma from occlusion.

Thyroid Gland

Hypothyroidism leads to cretinism in children and myxedema in adults. Aside from impaired development in cretinism, no notable periodontal changes occur in hypothyroidism.

In animals with thiouracil-induced hypothyroidism, apposition of alveolar bone is retarded,[35] and the size of the haversian systems is reduced,[24] but there is no evidence of periodontal disease. Animals with experimentally induced myxedema develop hyperparakeratosis with some keratosis of the gingival epithelium, edema, and disorganization of the collagen bundles in the connective tissue; hydropic degeneration and fragmentation of the fibers of the periodontal ligament; and osteoporosis of the alveolar bone.[4,97]

In experimental animals fed thyroid extract over a period of 1 to 16 weeks, the following have been reported: osteoporosis of the alveolar bone; lacunar resorption; and an increase in the size of the marrow spaces, with fibrosis of the marrow and an increase in the width and vascularity of the periodontal ligament.[4]

Pituitary Gland

In adults, *hyperpituitarism* results in acromegaly, which is characterized by a disproportionate overgrowth of the facial bones and overdeveloped sinuses. The face is large, with coarse features. The lips are greatly enlarged, and localized areas of hyperpigmentation are often seen along the nasolabial folds. A marked overgrowth of the alveolar process causes an increase in the size of the dental arch and consequently affects the spacing of the teeth. This may affect the periodontium by causing food impaction. Hypercementosis is another feature of the increased rate of growth.

Hypopituitarism results in decreased skeletal growth and leads to crowding and malposition of teeth.

The periodontal tissues of experimental animals with artificially induced hypopituitarism show increased gingival inflammation, resorption of cementum in the molar furcation areas, reduced apposition of cementum, decreased osteogenesis in interdental areas, reduced vascularity of the periodontal ligament, and degeneration of the ligament with cystic degeneration and calcification of many of the epithelial rests.[104,106]

Parathyroid Glands

Parathyroid hypersecretion produces generalized demineralization of the skeleton, increased osteoclasis with proliferation of the connective tissue in the enlarged marrow spaces, and formation of bone cysts and giant cell tumors.[119] The disease is called *osteitis fibrosa cystica* or *von Recklinghausen's bone disease.*

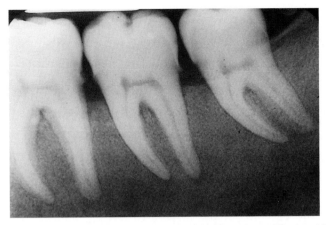

FIGURE 14–1. Secondary hyperparathyroidism in a 35-year-old woman with advanced kidney disease. This periapical radiograph shows ground-glass appearance of bone and loss of lamina dura. (Courtesy of Dr. L. Roy Eversole.)

Oral changes include malocclusion and tooth mobility, radiographic evidence of alveolar osteoporosis with closely meshed trabeculae, widening of the periodontal space, absence of the lamina dura, and radiolucent cyst-like spaces (Figs. 14–1 and 14–2). Bone cysts become filled with fibrous tissue with abundant hemosiderin-laden macrophages and giant cells. They have been called *brown tumors,* although they are not really tumors but reparative giant cell granulomas.

Loss of the lamina dura and giant cell tumors in the jaws are late signs of hyperparathyroid bone disease, which in itself is uncommon. Complete loss of the lamina dura does not occur often, and there is a danger of attaching too much diagnostic significance to it. Other diseases in which it may occur are Paget's disease, fibrous dysplasia, and osteomalacia.

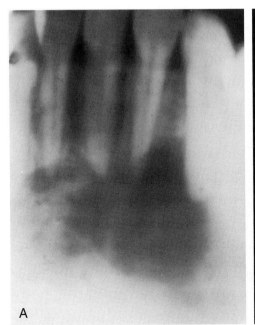
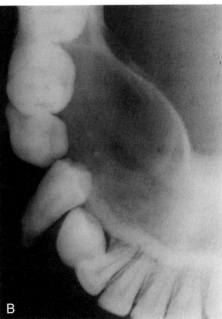

FIGURE 14–2. Periapical *(A)* and occlusal *(B)* radiographic views of brown tumors in a patient with hyperparathyroidism. (Courtesy of Dr. L. Roy Eversole.)

Different investigators report that 25%,[104] 45%,[96] and 50%[112] of patients with hyperparathyroidism have associated oral changes. A relationship has been suggested between periodontal disease in dogs and hyperparathyroidism secondary to calcium deficiency in the diet.[46] This has not been confirmed by other studies.[115]

Diabetes Mellitus

Diabetes is an extremely important disease from a periodontal standpoint. It is a complicated metabolic disease characterized by hypofunction or lack of function of the β cells of the islets of Langerhans in the pancreas, leading to high blood glucose levels and excretion of sugar in the urine. Two basic types of primary diabetes mellitus have been described: insulin-dependent and non–insulin-dependent.

Insulin-dependent diabetes mellitus (IDDM) (type I) is also known as *juvenile diabetes* or *juvenile-onset diabetes*, although it may sometimes appear at older ages. This type of diabetes results from an absolute lack of insulin, is very unstable and difficult to control, has a marked tendency toward ketosis and coma, is not preceded by obesity, and requires injected insulin to be controlled. Patients with the disease present with the symptoms traditionally associated with diabetes: polyphagia, polydipsia, polyuria, predisposition to infections, and anorexia.

Non–insulin-dependent diabetes mellitus (NIDDM) (type II) is the adult type (i.e., onset usually after age 45). It generally occurs in obese individuals and can often be controlled by diet or by oral hypoglycemic agents. The development of ketosis and coma is not common. Adult-onset diabetes has the same symptoms as juvenile diabetes but in a less severe form.

Other types of diabetes, classified as *secondary diabetes*, are those associated with other diseases that involve the pancreas and destroy the insulin-producing cells. Endocrine diseases such as acromegaly and Cushing's syndrome, tumors, pancreatectomy, and drugs and chemicals that cause hyperinsulinism are included in this group. Experimentally induced types of diabetes generally belong in this category rather than in one of the two classic categories of disease.

The prevalence of diabetes in the United States is between 2% and 4%, of which IDDM comprises between 7% and 10%.[84]

Oral Manifestations of Diabetes

Uncontrolled Diabetes. The following findings have been described in the oral mucosa: cheilosis and a tendency toward drying and cracking[41]; burning sensations[7]; decrease in salivary flow[70]; and alterations in the flora of the oral cavity, with greater predominance of *Candida albicans*, hemolytic streptococci, and staphylococci.[1] These changes, however, are not specific, and terms such as *diabetic stomatitis* should not be used.[74]

Perhaps the most striking changes in uncontrolled diabetes are the reduction in defense mechanisms and the increased susceptibility to infections leading to destructive periodontal disease. This topic is discussed in a subsequent section.

Controlled Diabetes. Control of diabetes may be attained by diet or by the administration of insulin and/or other drugs. In well-controlled diabetes, none of the previously mentioned changes is found. There is a normal tissue response,[116] no increase in the incidence of caries, a normally developed dentition, and a normal defense against infections. However, the possibility that the control of the disease may be inadequate makes it advisable to exercise special care in the periodontal treatment of individuals with controlled diabetes (Chapter 34).

Diabetes and the Periodontium

A variety of periodontal changes have been described in diabetic patients, such as a tendency toward abscess formation, diabetic periodontoclasia, enlarged gingiva, sessile or pedunculated gingival polyps, polypoid gingival proliferations, and loosened teeth[47] (Plate IV).

Studies in Humans

Clinical Aspects. The majority of well-controlled studies show a higher prevalence and severity of periodontal disease in diabetics than in nondiabetics with similar local irritation,[7,15,17,80,99,120] including greater loss of attachment, increased bleeding on probing, and increased tooth mobility (Fig. 14–3). However, other studies have not found a correlation between the diabetic state and the periodontal condition.[3,45,50,68,79,83] Probably the different degrees of diabetic involvement and control of the disease in patients examined and the diversity of indices and patient sampling are responsible for this lack of consistency.

A study of risk indicators for a group of 1426 patients 25 to 74 years of age revealed that individuals who are 45 years old or older and who are diabetic and smoke have a 20 times higher risk of periodontal disease than patients who do not have these indicators. If they are also infected subgingivally with *Bacteroides forsythus* or *Porphyromona gingivalis,* the risk increases to 30 to 50 times.[42]

Approximately 40% of adult Pima Indians in Arizona have NIDDM. A comparison of diabetics and nondiabetics in this Native American tribe[20] has shown a clear increase in prevalence of destructive periodontitis, as well as a 15% increase in edentulousness, in diabetic individuals. The risk of developing destructive periodontitis increases threefold in these individuals.[23]

Effect of Age. Periodontitis in IDDM appears to start after age 12.[16] The prevalence of periodontitis has been reported as being 9.8% in 13- to 18-year-olds, increasing to 39% in those 19 years and older. Insulin-dependent diabetic children tend to have more destruction around the first molars and incisors than elsewhere, but this destruction becomes more generalized at older ages.[16]

Other investigators have reported that the rate of periodontal destruction appears to be similar for diabetics and nondiabetics up to the age of 30[33,114]; after age 30 there is a greater degree of destruction in diabetics. Patients showing overt diabetes over a period of more than 10 years have greater loss of periodontal structures than those with a diabetic history of less than 10 years.[33,51]

Severity of Periodontal Changes. The extensive literature on this subject and the overall impression of clinicians point to the fact that *periodontal disease in diabetics follows no consistent pattern.* Very severe gingival inflamma-

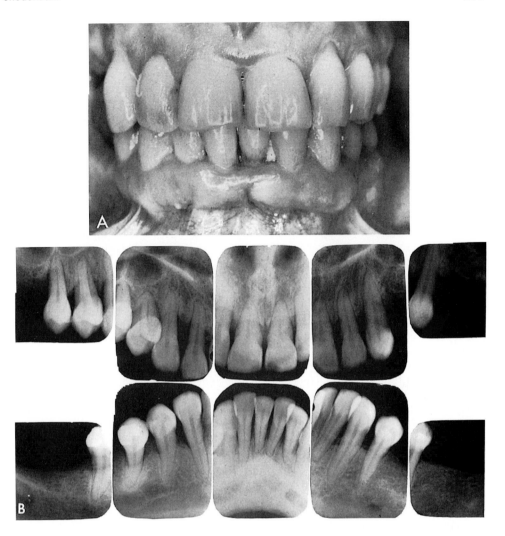

FIGURE 14–3. Diabetic patient. *A,* Gingival inflammation and periodontal pockets in a 34-year-old patient with diabetes of long duration. *B,* Extensive generalized bone loss in the patient shown in *A.* Failure to replace posterior teeth adds to the occlusal burden of the remaining dentition.

tion (Plate IV*C,D*), deep periodontal pockets, rapid bone loss,[2] and frequent periodontal abscesses often occur in diabetic patients with poor oral hygiene (Plate IV*E*). In juvenile diabetics there is often extensive periodontal destruction, which is noteworthy because of the age of these patients. However, in many other diabetic patients, both juvenile and adult, the gingival changes and bone loss are not unusual.

The distribution and severity of local irritants affect the severity of periodontal disease in diabetics. *Diabetes does not cause gingivitis or periodontal pockets, but there are indications that it alters the response of the periodontal tissues to local irritants (Plate IVA,B), hastening bone loss and retarding postsurgical healing of the periodontal tissues (Plate IVF). Frequent periodontal abscesses appear to be an important feature of periodontal disease in diabetics.*

Microscopic Aspects. Microscopic changes reported in the gingiva include thickening of the basement membrane and narrowing of the lumina of capillaries and precapillary arterioles,[13,49,55] with increased fuchsinophilia and periodic acid–Schiff–positive reaction of the vessel wall[75,111] but no osteosclerotic changes,[54] and reduced staining of acid mucopolysaccharides. Oxygen consumption in the gingiva and the oxidation of glucose are reduced.[14]

Among the microscopic changes described, thickening of the basement membrane of capillaries warrants special attention, because (1) this change in the vessel walls may hamper the transport of nutrients necessary for the maintenance of gingival tissues, and (2) it has been suggested that gingival biopsies may be an important aid in the detection of prediabetic and diabetic states.[49,54] Biopsies have also been used in other tissues.[29]

Statistically significant differences in the thickness of the basement membrane between diabetics and control subjects have been reported,[28,66] but the considerable overlap of the results between the two groups makes this very difficult to use as a diagnostic aid. The thickness of the basement membrane was found to be unrelated to inflammation, age, and duration of diabetes.[66]

Biochemical Studies. Comparison of the salivary and blood glucose levels with the periodontal condition of diabetics revealed that salivary glucose levels (measured 1 hour after breakfast) were higher in diabetics, but not to a degree that could be diagnostic.[77]

The glucose content of gingival fluid and blood is higher in diabetics than in nondiabetics with similar Plaque and Gingival Index scores.[26] The increased glucose in the gingival fluid and blood of diabetics could change the environment of the microflora, inducing qualitative changes in bacteria that could affect periodontal changes.

Gingival fluid from diabetics contains a reduced level of cyclic adenosine monophosphate (cAMP) when compared with that of nondiabetics.[43] Because cAMP reduces inflammation, this is another possible mechanism that could lead to increased severity of gingival inflammation in diabetics.

Microbiologic Studies. Insulin-dependent diabetic patients with periodontitis have been reported[44,72] to have a subgingival flora composed mainly of *Capnocytophaga,* anaerobic vibrios, and *Actinomyces* species; *P. gingivalis, Prevotella intermedia,* and *Actinobacillus actinomycetemcomitans,* which are common in periodontal lesions of nondiabetics, are present in low numbers in diabetics. Other studies, however, found scarce *Capnocytophaga*[70,100] and abundant *A. actinomycetemcomitans* and black-pigmented *Bacteroides,*[100] as well as *P. intermedia, Prevotella melaninogenica,* and *Campylobacter rectus.*[70]

Black-pigmented species, especially *P. gingivalis, P. intermedia,* and *C. rectus,* are prominent in severe periodontal lesions of Pima Indians with non–insulin-dependent diabetes.[31,122]

These results point to an altered flora in the periodontal pockets of diabetic patients. The exact role of these microorganisms has not been determined.

Immunologic Studies. The increased susceptibility of diabetics to infection has been hypothesized as being due to polymorphonuclear leukocyte deficiencies resulting in impaired chemotaxis,[76] defective phagocytosis,[87] or impaired adherence.[32] No alteration of immunoglobulins A, G, or M has been found in diabetics.[95]

Studies in Animals

There have been many studies of the periodontium in animals with diabetes induced by injection of toxic drugs[34] or partial pancreatectomy[11] and in hamsters[19,107] and mice[22] that developed the disease spontaneously. Animals in which diabetes is induced develop a secondary type of the disease, some features of which may differ from those of the spontaneous type.

Decreased collagen synthesis,[102] osteoporosis, and reduction in the height of alveolar bone occur in diabetic animals, with comparable osteoporosis in other bones.[34] The periodontal ligament and cementum are not affected, but glycogen is depleted in the gingiva. Other investigators report that gingival inflammation and bone destruction associated with local irritants are more severe in diabetic than in nondiabetic animals.[10] Generalized osteoporosis, resorption of the alveolar crest, and gingival inflammation and periodontal pocket formation associated with calculus have been described in Chinese hamsters with hereditary diabetes under insulin replacement therapy.[107]

Periodontal injury produced by excessive occlusal forces[38] and periodontal atrophy resulting from insufficient forces[55] are worsened in experimental diabetes, and postsurgical gingival healing is retarded.[40]

The Gonads

There are several types of gingival disease in which modification of the sex hormones is considered to be either the initiating or a complicating factor; these types of gingival alterations are associated with physiologic hormonal changes and are characterized by nonspecific inflammatory changes with a predominant vascular component leading clinically to a marked hemorrhagic tendency.

Experimental Studies. *Progesterone* administration to female dogs produces dilatation and increased permeability of the gingival microvasculature, which increases susceptibility to injury and exudation, but it does not affect the morphology of the gingival epithelium.[50]

Repeated injections of *estrogen* in female rats cause increased endosteal bone formation in the jaws[81,108] and decreased polymerization of mucopolysaccharide protein complexes in the bone ground substance.[8] Estrogen injections also counteract tendencies toward hyperkeratosis of the gingival epithelium and fibrosis of the vessel walls in castrated female animals and stimulate bone formation and fibroplasia, which compensate for destructive changes in the periodontium induced by the systemic administration of cortisone.[37] Locally applied progesterone, estrogen, and gonadotropin appear to reduce the acute inflammatory response to chemical irritation.[64]

Elevated levels of estrogen and progesterone increase gingival exudation in female dogs with and without gingivitis, most likely because of hormone-induced increased permeability of the gingival vessels.[65]

Ovariectomy results in osteoporosis of alveolar bone, reduced cementum formation, and reduced fiber density and cellularity of the periodontal ligament[36] in young adult mice, but not in older animals.[89] The gingival epithelium is atrophic in estrogen-deficient animals.[123]

Systemic administration of *testosterone* retards the downgrowth of sulcular epithelium over the cementum[98]; stimulates osteoblastic activity in alveolar bone; increases the cellularity of the periodontal ligament[109]; and restores osteoblastic activity, which is depressed by hypophysectomy.[110] The healing of oral wounds is accelerated by castration in males and is unaffected by ovariectomy.[12]

The Gingiva in Puberty

Puberty is frequently accompanied by an exaggerated response of the gingiva to local irritation.[113] Pronounced inflammation, bluish red discoloration, edema, and enlargement result from local irritants that would ordinarily elicit a comparatively mild gingival response (Fig. 14–4).

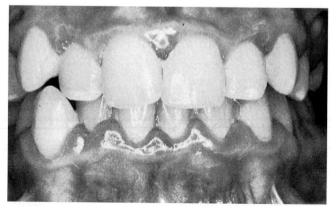

FIGURE 14–4. Gingivitis in puberty, with edema, discoloration, and enlargement.

As adulthood is approached, the severity of the gingival reaction diminishes, even when local irritants persist. However, complete return to normal requires removal of these irritants. Although the prevalence and severity of gingival disease are increased in puberty, gingivitis is not a universal occurrence during this period; with proper care of the mouth, it can be prevented (see also Chapter 18).

Gingival Changes Associated With the Menstrual Cycle

As a general rule, the menstrual cycle is not accompanied by notable gingival changes, but occasional problems do occur. Gingival changes associated with menstruation have been attributed to hormonal imbalances and in some instances may be accompanied by a history of ovarian dysfunction.

During the menstrual period, the prevalence of gingivitis increases. Some patients may complain of bleeding gums or a bloated, tense feeling in the gums in the days preceding menstrual flow. The exudate from inflamed gingiva is increased during menstruation, suggesting that existent gingivitis is aggravated by menstruation, but the crevicular fluid of normal gingiva is unaffected.[48] Tooth mobility does not change significantly during the menstrual cycle.[30] The salivary bacterial count is increased during menstruation and at ovulation 11 to 14 days earlier.[90]

Gingival Disease in Pregnancy

Gingival changes in pregnancy were described as early as 1898,[9] even before any knowledge about hormonal changes in pregnancy was available.

Pregnancy itself does not cause gingivitis. Gingivitis in pregnancy is caused by bacterial plaque, just as it is in nonpregnant individuals. Pregnancy accentuates the gingival response to plaque and modifies the resultant clinical picture (Figs. 14–5 to 14–7). No notable changes occur in the gingiva during pregnancy in the absence of local irritants.

The severity of gingivitis is increased during pregnancy beginning in the second or third month. Patients with slight chronic gingivitis that attracted no particular attention be-

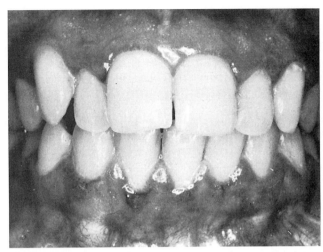

FIGURE 14–6. Gingiva in pregnancy, showing edema, discoloration, and bleeding.

fore the pregnancy become aware of the gingiva because previously inflamed areas become enlarged, edematous, and more noticeably discolored. Patients with a slight amount of gingival bleeding before pregnancy become concerned about an increased tendency to bleed (Plate V*A*).

Gingivitis becomes more severe by the eighth month and decreases during the ninth; plaque accumulation follows a similar pattern.[67] Some investigators report the greatest severity as being between the second and third trimesters.[18] The correlation between gingivitis and the quantity of plaque is greater after parturition than during pregnancy,[59] which suggests that pregnancy introduces other factors that aggravate the gingival response to local irritants.

The reported incidence of gingivitis in pregnancy in well-conducted studies varies from around 50%[67,69] to 100%.[69] Pregnancy affects the severity of previously inflamed areas; it does not alter healthy gingiva. Impressions of increased incidence may be created by the aggravation of previously inflamed but unnoticed areas.[94] Also increased in pregnancy are tooth mobility,[91] pocket depth, and gingival fluid.[50,61]

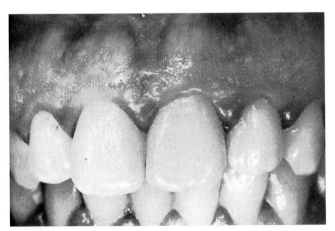

FIGURE 14–5. Early changes in the interdental papillae in pregnancy.

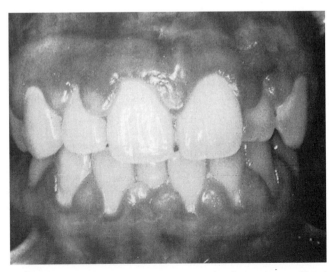

FIGURE 14–7. Gingiva in pregnancy, showing edema, discoloration, and enlargement.

There is partial reduction in the severity of gingivitis by 2 months post partum, and after 1 year the condition of the gingiva is comparable to that of patients who have not been pregnant.[18] However, the gingiva does not return to normal as long as local irritants are present. Also reduced after pregnancy are tooth mobility, gingival fluid, and pocket depth. In a longitudinal investigation of the periodontal changes during pregnancy and for 15 months post partum, no significant loss of attachment was observed.[18]

Clinical Features. Pronounced ease of bleeding is the most striking clinical feature. The gingiva is inflamed and varies in color from a bright red to a bluish red.[124,125] The marginal and interdental gingivae are edematous, pit on pressure, appear smooth and shiny, are soft and pliable, and sometimes present a raspberry-like appearance. The extreme redness results from marked vascularity, and there is an increased tendency to bleed (Plate V*A*). The gingival changes are usually painless unless complicated by acute infection. In some cases the inflamed gingiva forms discrete "tumor-like" masses, referred to as *pregnancy tumors* (described in Chapter 18) (Plate V*B–D*).

Histopathology. The microscopic picture[69,125] of gingival disease in pregnancy is one of nonspecific, vascularizing, proliferative inflammation. There is marked inflammatory cellular infiltration with edema and degeneration of the gingival epithelium and connective tissue. The epithelium is hyperplastic, with accentuated rete pegs, reduced surface keratinization,[118] and various degrees of intracellular and extracellular edema and infiltration by leukocytes. Newly formed engorged capillaries are present in abundance.

Microbiologic Studies. The possibility that bacterial–hormonal interactions may change the composition of plaque and lead to gingival inflammation has not been extensively explored. Kornman and Loesche[60] have reported that the subgingival flora changes to a more anaerobic flora as pregnancy progresses; the only microorganism that increases significantly during pregnancy is *P. intermedia*. This increase appears to be associated with elevations in systemic levels of estradiol and progesterone and to coincide with the peak in gingival bleeding.[60] It has also been suggested that during pregnancy a depression of the maternal T-lymphocyte response may be a factor in the altered tissue response to plaque.[85]

Correlation With Hormonal Levels. The aggravation of gingivitis in pregnancy has been attributed principally to the increased levels of progesterone, which produce dilatation and tortuosity of the gingival microvasculature, circulatory stasis, and increased susceptibility to mechanical irritation, all of which favor leakage of fluid into the perivascular tissues.[78,83] There is a marked increase in estrogen and progesterone during pregnancy and a reduction after parturition. The severity of gingivitis varies with the hormonal levels in pregnancy.[50]

The gingiva is a target organ for female sex hormones. Formicola and associates[27] have shown that radioactive estradiol injected into female rats appears not only in the genital tract but also in the gingiva.

It has also been suggested that the accentuation of gingivitis in pregnancy occurs in two peaks: during the first trimester, when there is overproduction of gonadotropins, and during the third trimester, when estrogen and progesterone levels are highest.[67] Destruction of gingival mast cells by the increased sex hormones and the resultant release of histamine and proteolytic enzymes may also contribute to the exaggerated inflammatory response to local irritants.[63]

Hormonal Contraceptives and the Gingiva

Hormonal contraceptives aggravate the gingival response to local irritants in a manner similar to that seen in pregnancy[21,62] and, when taken for a period of more than $1\frac{1}{2}$ years, increase periodontal destruction.[57]

Although some brands of oral contraceptives produce more dramatic changes than others,[88] no correlation has been found to exist on the basis of differences in progesterone or estrogen content in various brands.[69] Cumulative exposure to oral contraceptives apparently has no effect on gingival inflammation or oral Debris Index scores.[52]

Menopausal Gingivostomatitis (Senile Atrophic Gingivitis)

This condition occurs during menopause or in the postmenopausal period. Mild signs and symptoms sometimes appear, associated with the earliest menopausal changes. *Menopausal gingivostomatitis is not a common condition.* The term used for its designation has led to the erroneous impression that it invariably occurs associated with menopause, whereas the opposite is true. Oral disturbances are not a common feature of menopause.[121]

Clinical Features. The gingiva and remaining oral mucosa are dry and shiny, vary in color from abnormal paleness to redness, and bleed easily. There is fissuring in the mucobuccal fold in some cases,[93] and comparable changes may occur in the vaginal mucosa. The patient complains of a dry, burning sensation throughout the oral cavity, associated with extreme sensitivity to thermal changes; abnormal taste sensations described as "salty," "peppery," or "sour"[73]; and difficulty with removable partial prostheses.

Microscopically, the gingiva exhibits atrophy of the germinal and prickle cell layers of the epithelium and, in some instances, areas of ulceration.

The signs and symptoms of menopausal gingivostomatitis are in some degree comparable to those of chronic desquamative gingivitis (see Chapter 20). Signs and symptoms similar to those of menopausal gingivostomatitis occasionally occur after ovariectomy or sterilization by radiation in the treatment of malignant neoplasms.

Corticosteroid Hormones

In humans, systemic administration of cortisone and adrenocorticotropic hormone (ACTH) appears to have no effect on the incidence and severity of gingival and periodontal disease.[58] However, renal transplant patients who are receiving immunosuppressive therapy (prednisone or methylprednisone and azathioprine or cyclophosphamide)

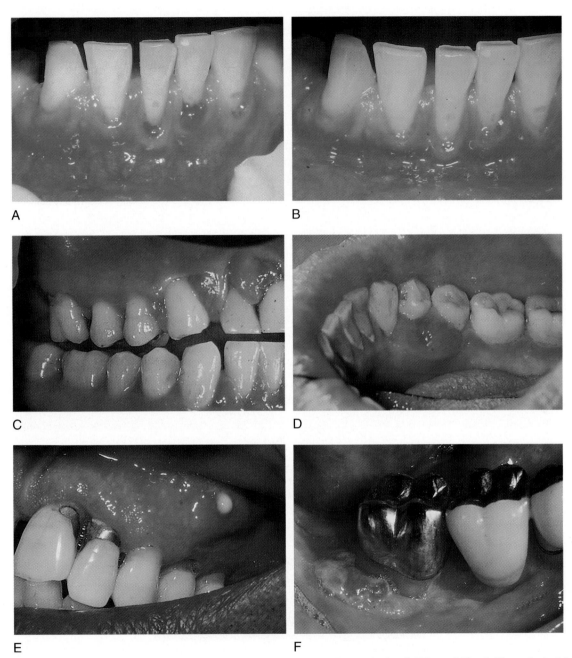

PLATE IV. Diabetes and periodontal disease. *A,* Adult diabetic patient: blood glucose level 400 mg/100 ml. Note gingival inflammation, spontaneous bleeding, and edema. *B,* Same patient as in *A* after 4 days of insulin therapy (glucose level less than 100 mg/100 ml). The clinical periodontal picture has improved in the absence of local therapy. *C,* Adult uncontrolled diabetic patient. Enlarged, smooth red gingiva with initial enlargement in anterior area. *D,* Lingual view of right mandibular area in same case as in C. Note the inflamed enlarged area around teeth #27–30. *E,* Suppurating abscess, facial of upper left area, in an uncontrolled diabetic. *F,* Adult uncontrolled diabetic patient showing delayed healing 7 weeks after surgery in tooth #31. (*A* and *B* courtesy of Dr. Joan Otomo-Corgel; *C–F* courtesy of Dr. T. N. Sims.)

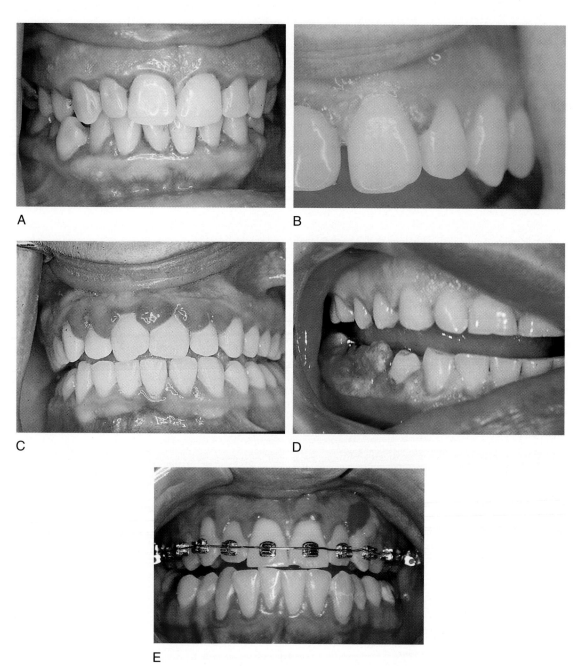

PLATE V. Pregnancy. *A,* Marginal redness and easily bleeding gingivae in 5-month-pregnant woman. *B,* Incipient gingival enlargement in papilla between teeth #9 and 10 in 4-month-pregnant woman. *C,* Generalized gingival enlargement in pregnancy, especially noticeable in upper anterior area. *D,* Localized discrete gingival enlargement in area facial of teeth #28–30 in a pregnant woman. *E,* Easily bleeding, marginal erythema with diffuse erythematous area between upper left lateral incisor and canine. Marginal edematous changes are seen, also easily bleeding around lower anterior teeth. Patient is 7 months pregnant. (*E* courtesy of Dr. Philip Melnick.)

have significantly less gingival inflammation than control subjects with similar amounts of plaque.[5,53,86,117]

The systemic administration of cortisone in experimental animals results in osteoporosis of alveolar bone; capillary dilatation and engorgement, with hemorrhage in the periodontal ligament and gingival connective tissue; degeneration and reduction in the number of collagen fibers of the periodontal ligament; and increased destruction of the periodontal tissues associated with inflammation caused by local irritation.[39]

HEMATOLOGIC DISEASES

Certain oral changes may suggest the existence of a blood disturbance; specific diagnosis, however, requires a complete physical examination and a thorough hematologic study. Comparable oral changes occur in more than one form of blood dyscrasia, and secondary inflammatory changes produce a wide range of variation in the oral signs.

Gingival and periodontal disturbances associated with blood dyscrasias must be thought of in terms of fundamental interrelationships between the oral tissues and the blood and blood-forming organs, rather than in terms of a simple association of dramatic oral changes with hematologic disease. Abnormal bleeding from the gingiva or other areas of the oral mucosa that is difficult to control is an important clinical sign suggesting a hematologic disorder. Hemorrhagic tendencies occur when the normal hemostatic mechanism is disturbed.

Leukemia

The leukemias are "malignant neoplasias of white blood cell precursors, characterized by (1) diffuse replacement of the bone marrow with proliferating leukemic cells; (2) abnormal numbers and forms of immature white cells in the circulating blood; and (3) widespread infiltrates in the liver, spleen, lymph nodes and other sites throughout the body."[51]

According to the type of white blood cell involved, leukemias can be *lymphocytic* or *myelocytic;* a subgroup of the myelocytic leukemias is *monocytic leukemia.* According to their evolution, leukemias can be *acute,* which is rapidly fatal; *subacute;* or *chronic.* The replacement of the bone marrow elements by leukemic cells reduces normal white blood cell and platelet production, leading to anemia and bleeding disorders. Some patients may have normal blood counts while leukemic cells are present in the bone marrow; this type of disease is called *aleukemic leukemia.*[23]

The Periodontium in Leukemic Patients

Oral and periodontal manifestations of leukemia consist of the following:

Leukemic Infiltration of the Periodontium. Leukemic cells can infiltrate the gingiva and, less frequently, the alveolar bone. Gingival infiltration often results in *leukemic gingival enlargement* (see Chapter 18).

A study of 1076 adult patients with leukemia[18] showed that 3.6% of the patients with teeth had leukemic gingival proliferative lesions, with the highest incidence in patients with acute monocytic leukemia (66.7%), followed by acute

myelocytic–monocytic leukemia (18.7%) and acute myelocytic leukemia (3.7%). It should be pointed out, however, that monocytic leukemia is an extremely rare form of the disease. Leukemic gingival enlargement is not found in edentulous patients or in patients with chronic leukemia. Leukemic gingival enlargement consists of a basic infiltration of the gingival corium by leukemic cells that creates gingival pockets where bacterial plaque accumulates, initiating a secondary inflammatory lesion that contributes also to the enlargement of the gingiva.

Clinically, the gingiva appears initially bluish red and cyanotic, with a rounding and tenseness of the gingival margin; then it increases in size, most often in the interdental papilla and partially covering the crowns of the teeth (Figs. 14–8 and 14–9).

Microscopically, the gingiva exhibits a dense, diffuse infiltration of predominantly immature leukocytes in the attached as well as the marginal gingiva. Occasional mitotic figures indicative of ectopic hematopoiesis may be seen. The normal connective tissue components of the gingiva are displaced by the leukemic cells (Fig. 14–10A). The nature of the cells depends on the type of leukemia. The cellular accumulation is denser in all the reticular connective tissue layer. In almost all cases, the papillary layer contains comparatively few leukocytes. The blood vessels are distended and contain predominantly leukemic cells, and the red blood cells are reduced in number. The epithelium presents a variety of changes. It may be thinned or hyperplastic. Degeneration associated with intercellular and intracellular edema and leukocytic infiltration with diminished surface keratinization are common findings.

The microscopic picture of the marginal gingiva differs from that of the remainder of the gingiva in that it usually exhibits a notable inflammatory component in addition to the leukemic cells. Scattered foci of plasma cells and lymphocytes with edema and degeneration are common findings. The inner aspect of the marginal gingiva is usually ulcerated, and marginal necrosis with pseudomembrane formation may also be seen.

The periodontal ligament and alveolar bone may also be involved in acute and subacute leukemia (Fig. 14–10B). The periodontal ligament may be infiltrated with mature and immature leukocytes. The marrow of the alveolar bone

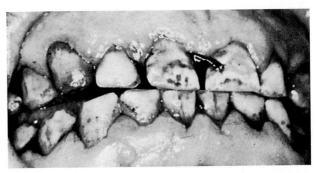

FIGURE 14–8. Acute lymphocytic leukemia. The gingiva is inflamed, edematous, and discolored and bleeds spontaneously.

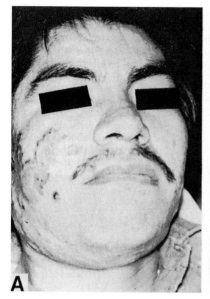

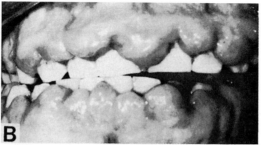

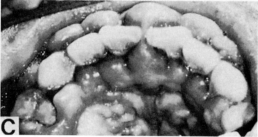

FIGURE 14–9. Acute myelocytic leukemia. *A,* View of patient's face. Note the elevated flat macules and papules (leukemia cutis) on the right cheek. *B,* Intraoral view showing the pronounced gingival enlargement *C,* Occlusal view of upper anterior teeth. Note the marked enlargement in both the facial and the palatal aspects. (Courtesy of Dr. Spencer Woolfe.)

exhibits a variety of changes, such as localized areas of necrosis, thrombosis of the blood vessels, infiltration with mature and immature leukocytes, occasional red blood cells, and replacement of the fatty marrow by fibrous tissue.

In leukemic mice, the presence of infiltrate in marrow spaces and the periodontal ligament results in osteoporosis of the alveolar bone with destruction of the supporting bone and disappearance of the periodontal fibers[11,14] (Fig. 14–11).

The abnormal accumulation of leukemic cells in the dermal and subcutaneous connective tissue is called *leukemia cutis* and forms elevated flat macules and papules[18,51] (see Fig. 14–9A).

Bleeding. Gingival hemorrhage is a common finding in leukemic patients (see Fig. 14–8), even in the absence of clinically detectable gingivitis. Bleeding gingiva can be an early sign of leukemia.[57] It is due to the thrombocytopenia that results from replacement of the bone marrow cells by leukemic cells and also from the inhibition of normal stem cell function by leukemic cells or their products.[51]

This bleeding tendency can also manifest itself in the skin and throughout the oral mucosa, where petechiae are frequently found, with or without leukemic infiltrates. Oral bleeding has been reported as a presenting sign in 17.7% of patients with acute leukemia and in 4.4% of patients with chronic leukemia.[36] This symptom can also result from the chemotherapeutic agents used.

Oral Ulcerations and Infections. The granulocytopenia

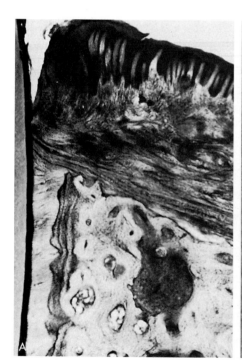

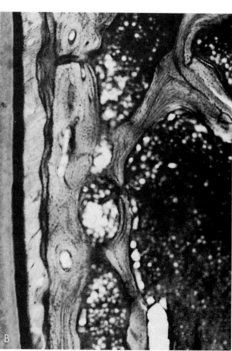

FIGURE 14–10. *A,* Leukemic infiltrate in gingiva and bone in a human autopsy specimen. *B,* Same case as in *A.* Note the dense infiltrate in marrow spaces and the lack of extension to the periodontal ligament.

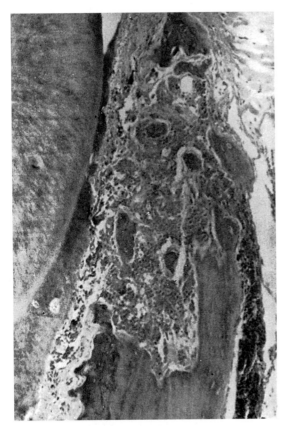

FIGURE 14–11. Leukemic infiltrate in alveolar bone in AKR mouse. Note the leukemic infiltrate producing destruction of bone and loss of periodontal ligament.

resulting from the replacement of bone marrow cells by leukemic cells reduces the tissue resistance to opportunistic microorganisms and leads to ulcerations and infections. Discrete, punched-out ulcers penetrating deeply into the submucosa and covered by a firmly attached white slough can be found in the oral mucosa.[4] These lesions occur in sites of trauma such as the buccal mucosa in relation to the line of occlusion or the palate. Patients with past history of herpes infection may develop herpetic oral ulcers, frequently in multiple sites and large atypical forms, after chemotherapy is instituted.[25]

Gingival bacterial infection in leukemic patients can be a primary bacterial infection or result from an increased severity of existing gingival or periodontal disease. Lesions of acute necrotizing ulcerative gingivitis may also be seen in terminal cases of leukemia.

In leukemia, the response to irritation is altered, so that the cellular component of the inflammatory exudate differs both quantitatively and qualitatively from that that occurs in nonleukemic individuals. There is pronounced infiltration of immature leukemic cells in addition to the usual inflammatory cells.

The inflamed gingiva differs clinically from inflamed gingiva in nonleukemic individuals. It is a peculiar bluish red, is markedly sponge-like and friable, and bleeds persistently on the slightest provocation or even spontaneously. This markedly altered and degenerated tissue is extremely susceptible to bacterial infection, which can be so severe as to cause acute gingival necrosis and pseudomembrane for-

mation. These are secondary oral changes superimposed on the oral tissues altered by the blood disturbance and produce associated disturbances that may be a source of considerable difficulty to the patient, such as systemic toxic effects, loss of appetite, nausea, blood loss from persistent gingival bleeding, and constant gnawing pain. By eliminating local irritants, it is possible to alleviate severe oral changes in leukemia.

Chronic Leukemia

In chronic leukemia, clinical oral changes suggesting a hematologic disturbance are very rare.

The microscopic changes in chronic leukemia may consist of replacement of the normal fatty marrow of the jaws by islands of mature lymphocytes or lymphocytic infiltration of the marginal gingiva without dramatic clinical manifestations.

Gingival Biopsy and Leukemia

The existence of leukemia is sometimes revealed by a gingival biopsy performed to clarify the nature of a troublesome gingival condition. In such cases, the gingival findings must be corroborated by medical examination and hematologic study. The absence of leukemic involvement in a gingival biopsy specimen does not rule out the possibility of leukemia. In chronic leukemia, the gingiva may simply present inflammatory changes, with no suggestion of a hematologic disturbance. In patients with recognized leukemia, the gingival biopsy indicates the extent to which leukemic infiltration is responsible for the altered clinical appearance of the gingiva. *Although such findings are of interest, their benefit to the patient is insufficient to warrant routine gingival biopsy studies in patients with leukemia.*

Anemias

Anemias are deficiencies in the quantity or quality of the blood as manifested by a reduction in the number of erythrocytes and in the amount of hemoglobin. Anemia may be the result of blood loss, defective blood formation, or increased blood destruction.

Anemias are classified according to cellular morphology and hemoglobin content as (1) macrocytic hyperchromic anemia (pernicious anemia), (2) microcytic hypochromic anemia (iron deficiency anemia), (3) sickle cell anemia, or (4) normocytic-normochromic anemia (hemolytic or aplastic anemia).

Pernicious anemia results in tongue changes in 75% of cases. The tongue appears red, smooth, and shiny owing to atrophy of the papillae. There is also marked pallor of the gingiva (Figs. 14–12 and 14–13).

Iron deficiency anemia induces similar tongue and gingival changes. A syndrome consisting of glossitis and ulceration of the oral mucosa and oropharynx, inducing dysphagia *(Plummer-Vinson syndrome),* has been described in patients with iron deficiency anemia.

Sickle cell anemia is a hereditary form of chronic hemolytic anemia that occurs almost exclusively in blacks. It is characterized by pallor, jaundice, weakness, rheumatoid manifestations, and leg ulcers. Oral changes include general-

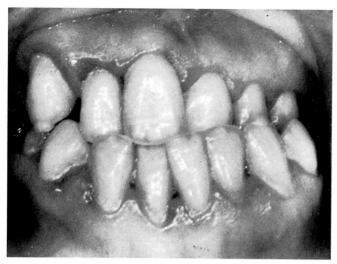

FIGURE 14–12. Diffuse pallor of the gingiva in a patient with anemia. The discolored, inflamed gingival margin stands out in sharp contrast to the adjacent pale, attached gingiva.

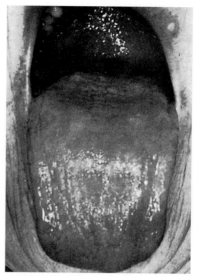

FIGURE 14–13. Smooth tongue in a patient with pernicious anemia.

ized osteoporosis of the jaws, with a peculiar stepladder alignment of the trabeculae of the interdental septa and pallor and yellowish discoloration of the oral mucosa. Periodontal infections may precipitate sickle cell crisis.[48] *Aplastic anemias* result from a failure of the bone marrow to produce erythrocytes. Their etiology is usually the effect of toxic drugs on the marrow. Oral changes include pale discoloration of the oral mucosa and increased susceptibility to infection owing to the concomitant neutropenia.

Thrombocytopenic Purpura

Thrombocytopenic purpura may be idiopathic (i.e., of unknown etiology, as in Werlhof's disease), or it may occur secondary to some known etiologic factor responsible for a reduction in the amount of functioning marrow and a resultant reduction in the number of circulating platelets. Such etiologic factors include aplasia of the marrow; crowding out of the megakaryocytes in the marrow, as, for example, in leukemia; replacement of the marrow by tumor; and destruction of the marrow by irradiation or radium or by drugs such as benzene, aminopyrine, and arsenical agents.

Thrombocytopenic purpura is characterized by a low platelet count, a prolonged clot retraction and bleeding time, and a normal or slightly prolonged clotting time. There is spontaneous bleeding into the skin or from mu-

cous membranes. Petechiae and hemorrhagic vesicles occur in the oral cavity, particularly in the palate and the buccal mucosa. *The gingivae are swollen, soft, and friable. Bleeding occurs spontaneously or on the slightest provocation and is difficult to control. Gingival changes represent an abnormal response to local irritation;* the severity of the gingival condition is dramatically alleviated by removal of the local irritants (Fig. 14–14).

IMMUNODEFICIENCY DISORDERS

Deficiencies in host defense mechanisms may lead to severely destructive periodontal lesions. These deficiencies may be primary, or inherited; or secondary, caused by immunosuppressive drug therapy or pathologic destruction of the lymphoid system. Leukemia, Hodgkin's disease, lymphomas, and multiple myeloma all may result in secondary immunodeficiency disorders.

Leukocyte Disorders

Disorders that affect production or function of leukocytes may result in severe periodontal destruction (see also Chapter 10).

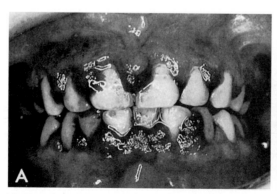
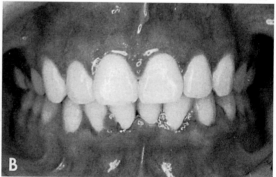

FIGURE 14–14. Thrombocytopenic purpura. *A,* Hemorrhagic gingivitis in patient with thrombocytopenic purpura. *B,* Marked reduction in severity of gingival disease after removal of surface debris and careful scaling.

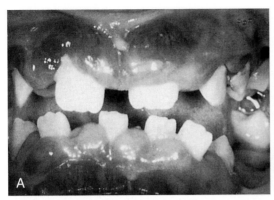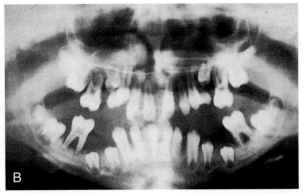

FIGURE 14–15. Prepubertal periodontitis, clinical picture *(A)* and panoramic radiograph *(B)*. The patient is a 10-year-old boy with cyclic neutropenia and agammaglobulinemia.

Agranulocytosis. *Agranulocytosis is characterized by a reduction in the number of circulating granulocytes and results in severe infections, including ulcerative necrotizing lesions of the oral mucosa, skin, and gastrointestinal and genitourinary tracts.* Less severe forms of the disease are called *neutropenia* or *granulocytopenia.*

Drug idiosyncrasy is the most common cause of agranulocytosis, but in some instances its etiology cannot be explained. Agranulocytosis has been reported after the administration of drugs such as aminopyrine,[34,50] barbiturates and their derivatives, benzene ring derivatives,[37] sulfonamides,[40] gold salts, or arsenical agents. It generally occurs as an acute disease, but it sometimes reappears in cyclic episodes *(cyclic neutropenia).* It may be periodic with recurring neutropenic cycles.[63]

The onset of the disease is accompanied by fever, malaise, general weakness, and sore throat. Ulceration in the oral cavity, oropharynx, and throat is characteristic. The mucosa exhibits isolated necrotic patches that are black and gray and are sharply demarcated from the adjacent uninvolved areas.[32,39] *The absence of a notable inflammatory reaction because of lack of granulocytes is a striking feature.* The gingival margin may or may not be involved. Gingival hemorrhage, necrosis, increased salivation, and fetid odor are accompanying clinical features. The occurrence of rapidly destructive periodontitis has been described in cyclic neutropenia (Fig. 14–15).[58]

The following microscopic changes have been described in the periodontium:[5] hemorrhage into the periodontal ligament with destruction of the principal fibers, osteoporosis of the cancellous bone with osteoclastic resorption, small fragments of necrotic bone in the hemorrhagic periodontal ligament, hemorrhage in the marrow adjacent to the teeth, areas in which the periodontal ligament is widened and consists of dense fibrous tissue with fibers parallel to the tooth surface, and the formation of new bony trabeculae. In cyclic neutropenia the gingival changes recur with recurrent exacerbation of the disease.[16]

Experimentally, neutropenia has been produced in dogs with heterologous antineutrophil serum. Neutrophilic granulocytes disappeared from the tissues, but ulcerative lesions and bacterial invasion were not observed, probably owing to the short duration of the experiment (4 days).[53]

Because infection is a common feature of agranulocyto-sis, differential diagnosis involves consideration of such conditions as acute necrotizing ulcerative gingivitis, diphtheria, noma, and acute necrotizing inflammation of the tonsils. Definitive diagnosis depends on the hematologic findings of pronounced leukopenia and almost complete absence of neutrophils.

Chédiak-Higashi Syndrome. Chédiak-Higashi syndrome is a rare disease that affects the production of organelles found in almost every cell. It affects mostly the melanocytes, platelets, and phagocytes and produces partial albinism, mild bleeding disorders, and recurrent bacterial infections,[2] including rapidly destructive periodontitis. It has been described as a genetically transmitted disease in ranch-raised mink[44] (see also Chapter 10).

Antibody Deficiency Disorders

Agammaglobulinemia. Agammaglobulinemia results from a deficiency in B cells; T-cell function remains normal. It can be congenital (X-linked or Bruton's agammaglobulinemia) or acquired. The disease is characterized by recurrent infections, including prepubertal destructive periodontitis (Fig. 14–15).

Acquired Immunodeficiency Syndrome. Acquired immunodeficiency syndrome (AIDS) is caused by the human immunodeficiency virus (HIV) and is characterized by destruction of lymphocytes, rendering the patient susceptible to opportunistic infections, including destructive periodontal lesions and malignancies. See Chapter 15.

CARDIOVASCULAR DISEASES

Arteriosclerosis

In aged individuals, arteriosclerotic changes characterized by intimal thickening, narrowing of the lumen, thickening of the media, and hyalinization of the media and adventitia, with or without calcification, are common in vessels throughout the jaws, as well as in areas of periodontal inflammation[24,47,65] (Fig. 14–16). Both periodontal disease and arteriosclerosis increase with age,[7,8] and it has been hypothesized that the circulatory impairment induced by vascular changes may increase the patient's susceptibility to periodontal disease.[4]

In experimental animals, partial ischemia of more than 10 hours' duration created by arteriolar occlusion produces

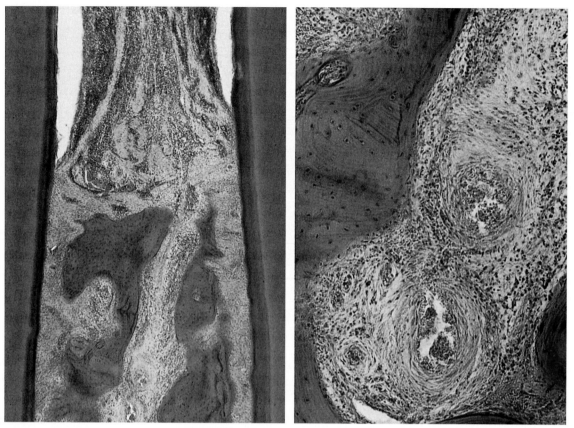

FIGURE 14–16. Vascular changes in an aged individual with periodontal disease. *A,* periodontitis, showing inflammation extending from the gingiva into the interdental septum. *B,* Detailed view, showing arterioles with thickened walls in the marrow space of the interdental septum.

changes in the oxidative enzymes and acid phosphatase activity and in the glycogen and lipid content of the gingival epithelium.[29] Focal necrosis, followed by ulceration, occurs in the epithelium, with the junctional epithelium least affected.[33] DNA duplication is depressed. Changes typical of periodontal disease do not occur. Ischemia is followed by hyperemia, which is accompanied by metabolic changes and increased DNA synthesis in the epithelium plus epithelial proliferation and thickening—all considered to be part of the gingival response to arteriolar occlusion.

Congenital Heart Disease

Gingival disease and other oral symptoms may occur in children with congenital heart disease.[10,31] In cases of *tetralogy of Fallot,* which is characterized by pulmonary stenosis, right ventricular enlargement, a defect in the interventricular septum, and malposition of the aorta to the right, the oral changes include a purplish red discoloration of the lips and gingiva and sometimes severe marginal gingivitis and periodontal destruction (Figs. 14–17 and 14–18). The discoloration of the lips and gingivae corre-

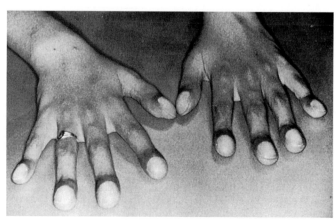

FIGURE 14–17. Extensive marginal inflammation with ulceronecrotic lesions and periodontal destruction in an adolescent with tetralogy of Fallot.

FIGURE 14–18. Characteristic clubbing of the fingers in the patient shown in Figure 14–17.

sponds to the general degree of cyanosis and returns to normal after corrective heart surgery. The tongue appears coated, fissured, and edematous, and there is extreme reddening of the fungiform and filiform papillae. The number of subepithelial capillaries is increased but will return to normal after heart surgery.[19]

In cases of *tetralogy of Eisenmenger,* there is pulmonary insufficiency and a diastolic murmur; the lips, cheeks, and buccal mucous membranes are cyanotic, but less markedly so than in tetralogy of Fallot. Severe generalized marginal gingivitis may be found. In cases in which there is *transposition of the aorta and superior vena cava,* cyanotic discoloration and marginal gingivitis of a lesser degree are noted. In *coarctation of the aorta,* there is narrowing of the vessel in the region where it is joined by the ductus arteriosus. Patients with this problem show marked inflammation of the gingiva in the anterior part of the mouth.

OTHER SYSTEMIC DISEASES

Metal Intoxications

The ingestion of metals such as mercury, lead, and bismuth in medicinal compounds and through industrial contact may result in oral manifestations owing to either intoxication or absorption without evidence of toxicity.

Bismuth Intoxication. Chronic bismuth intoxication is characterized by gastrointestinal disturbances, nausea, vomiting, and jaundice, as well as by an ulcerative gingivostomatitis, generally with pigmentation, accompanied by a metallic taste and a burning sensation of the oral mucosa. The tongue may be sore and inflamed. Urticaria, exanthematous eruptions of different types, bullous and purpuric lesions, and herpes zoster–like eruptions and pigmentation of the skin and mucous membranes are among the dermatologic lesions attributed to bismuth intoxication. Acute bismuth intoxication, which is less commonly seen, is accompanied by methemoglobin formation, cyanosis, and dyspnea.[28]

Bismuth pigmentation in the oral cavity usually appears as a narrow, bluish black discoloration of the gingival margin in areas of pre-existent gingival inflammation (see Chapter 17 and Fig. 17–11). Such pigmentation results from the precipitation of particles of bismuth sulfide associated with vascular changes in inflammation. It is not evidence of intoxication, but simply indicates the presence of bismuth in the blood stream. Bismuth pigmentation in the oral cavity also occurs in cases of intoxication. It assumes a linear form if the marginal gingiva is inflamed.

Lead Intoxication. Lead is slowly absorbed, and toxic symptoms are not particularly definitive when they do occur.[30] There is pallor of the face and lips and gastrointestinal symptoms consisting of nausea, vomiting, loss of appetite, and abdominal colic. Peripheral neuritis, psychological disorders, and encephalitis have been reported. Among the oral signs are salivation, coated tongue, a peculiar sweetish taste, gingival pigmentation, and ulceration. *The pigmentation of the gingiva is linear (burtonian line), steel gray, and associated with local irritation. Oral signs may occur without toxic symptoms.*

Mercury Intoxication. Mercury intoxication[1] is characterized by headache, insomnia, cardiovascular symptoms, pronounced salivation (ptyalism), and a metallic taste. *Gingival pigmentation in linear form results from the deposition of mercuric sulfide. The chemical also acts as an irritant, which accentuates the pre-existent inflammation and commonly leads to notable ulceration of the gingiva and adjacent mucosa and destruction of the underlying bone.* Mercurial pigmentation of the gingiva also occurs in areas of local irritation in patients without symptoms of intoxication.

Other Chemicals. Other chemicals, such as phosphorus,[56] arsenic, and chromium,[35] may cause necrosis of the alveolar bone with loosening and exfoliation of the teeth. Inflammation and ulceration of the gingiva are usually associated with destruction of the underlying tissues. Benzene intoxication is accompanied by gingival bleeding and ulceration with destruction of the underlying bone.[56]

Debilitating Diseases

Debilitating diseases such as syphilis, chronic nephritis, and tuberculosis may predispose the patient to periodontal disease by impairing tissue resistance to local irritants and creating a tendency toward gingivitis and alveolar bone loss.[13,48,54,60] However, the absence of periodontal disease in chronically ill patients has been presented as evidence that in individual cases systemic disease may exert no deleterious effect on the periodontium.[26,54,62] Patients with leprosy have nonspecific chronic destructive periodontitis, and *Mycobacterium leprae* has not been found in the gingiva.[63] However, pulmonary actinomycosis that originated in the periodontal flora has been described.[61]

PSYCHOSOMATIC DISORDERS

Harmful effects that result from psychic influences on the organic control of tissues are known as *psychosomatic disorders.*[27] There are two ways in which psychosomatic disorders may be induced in the oral cavity: through the development of habits that are injurious to the periodontium, and by the direct effect of the autonomic nervous system on the physiologic tissue balance.

Psychologically, the oral cavity is related directly or symbolically to the major human instincts and passions. In the infant, many oral drives find direct expression as oral receptive and oral aggressive trends and oral eroticism.[55] In the adult, most of the instinctive drives are normally suppressed by education and are satisfied in substitutive ways or are taken over by organs more appropriate than the mouth. *However, under conditions of mental and emotional duress, the mouth may subconsciously become an outlet for the gratification of basic drives in the adult.*

Gratification may be derived from neurotic habits, such as grinding or clenching the teeth,[12,21] nibbling on foreign objects (e.g., pencils or pipes), nail biting, or excessive use of tobacco, which are potentially injurious to the periodontium.[55] Self-inflicted gingival injuries have been described in children and adults and are often difficult diagnostic problems. Correlations have been reported between psychiatric and anxiety states and the occurrence of periodontal disease,[3,6,38,42] but these reports have been questioned by some investigators. Psychological factors in the etiology of acute necrotizing ulcerative gingivitis are discussed in Chapter 19.

HEREDITY IN THE ETIOLOGY OF PERIODONTAL DISEASE

In experimental animals, heredity appears to be a factor in calculus formation and periodontal disease.[43] Two studies made in human twins reported conflicting results: Ciancio and coworkers[15] found no evidence to support the concept that gingival recession; gingival crevice depth; and gingival, plaque, and calculus scores are inherited characteristics. However, Michalowicz and collaborators[41] identified significant genetic components for probing depth, attachment loss, gingivitis, and plaque.

Hypophosphatasia, an inherited disease characterized by rachitic-like skeletal changes, also presents as premature loss of the deciduous incisors and the surrounding alveolar bone by 10 months of age, sometimes without the skeletal changes.[46] Susceptibility to other forms of prepubertal and juvenile periodontitis is also suspected of being influenced by the host genotype. Specific heritable or genetic predisposing factors for slowly progressive adult periodontitis have not been identified.

REFERENCES

NUTRITIONAL DISEASES

1. Afonsky D. Oral lesions in niacin, riboflavin, pyridoxine, folic acid and pantothenic acid deficiencies in adult dogs. Oral Surg 8:207, 315, 867, 1955.
2. Alfano MC. Controversies, perspectives and clinical implications of nutrition in periodontal disease. Dent Clin North Am 20:519, 1976.
3. Alfano MC, Miller SA, Drummond JF. Effect of ascorbic acid deficiency on the permeability and collagen biosynthesis of oral mucosal epithelium. Ann NY Acad Sci 258:253, 1975.
4. Alvares O, Siegel I. Permeability of gingival sulcular epithelium in the development of scorbutic gingivitis. J Oral Pathol 10:40, 1981.
5. Becks H, Collins DA, Freytog RM. Changes in oral structures of the dog persisting after chronic overdoses of vitamin D. Am J Orthod 32:463, 1946.
6. Becks H, Wainwright WW, Morgan AF. Comparative study of oral changes in dogs due to deficiencies of pantothenic acid, nicotinic acid and unknowns of B vitamin complex. Am J Orthod 29:183, 1943.
7. Behbehani MJ, Jordan HV. Comparative colonization of human *Actinomyces* species in hamsters under different dietary conditions. J Periodont Res 15:395, 1980.
8. Boyle PE. Effect of vitamin A deficiency on the periodontal tissues. Am J Orthod 33:744, 1947.
9. Boyle PE, Bessey OA. The effect of acute vitamin A deficiency on the molar teeth and paradontal tissues, with a comment on deformed incisor-teeth in this deficiency. J Dent Res 20:236, 1941.
10. Burwasser P, Hill TJ. The effect of hard and soft diets on the gingival tissues of dogs. J Dent Res 18:389, 1939.
11. Buzina R, Brodarec A, Jušić M, et al. Epidemiology of angular stomatitis and bleeding gums. Int J Vitam Nutr Res 43:401, 1973.
12. Cabrini RL, Carranza FA Jr. Adenosine triphosphatase in normal and scorbutic wounds. Nature 200:1113, 1963.
13. Cannon PR. Some Pathologic Consequences of Protein and Amino Acid Deficiencies. Springfield, IL, Charles C Thomas, 1948.
14. Carranza FA Jr, Cabrini RL, Lopez Otero R, Stahl SS. Histometric analysis of interradicular bone in protein deficient animals. J Periodont Res 4:292, 1969.
15. Chapman OD, Harris AE. Oral lesions associated with dietary deficiencies in monkeys. J Infect Dis 69:7, 1941.
16. Charbeneau TD, Hurt WC. Gingival findings in spontaneous scurvy. A case report. J Periodontol 54:694, 1983.
17. Chawla TN, Glickman I. Protein deprivation and the periodontal structures of the albino rat. Oral Surg 4:578, 1951.
18. Costich ER, Hein JW, Hodge HC, Shourie KL. Reduction of hamster periodontal disease by sodium fluoride and sodium monofluorophosphate in drinking water. J Am Dent Assoc 55:617, 1957.
19. Cotran RS, Kumar V, Robbins SR. Robbins' Pathologic Basis of Disease. 4th ed. Philadelphia, WB Saunders, 1989.
20. Crandon JH, Lund CC, Dill DB. Experimental human scurvy. N Engl J Med 223:353, 1940.
21. Denton J. A study of tissue changes in experimental black tongue of dogs compared with similar changes in pellagra. Am J Pathol 4:341, 1928.
22. Dreizen S. Oral manifestations of human nutritional anemias. Arch Environ Health 5:66, 1962.
23. Dreizen S, Levy BM, Bernick S, et al. Studies of the biology of the periodontium of marmosets. III. Periodontal bone changes in marmosets with osteomalacia and hyperparathyroidism. Isr J Med Sci 3:731, 1967.
24. Egelberg J. Local effect of diet on plaque formation and development of gingivitis in dogs. I. Effect of hard and soft diets. Odont Revy 16:31, 1965.
25. Enwonwu CO, Edozien JC. Epidemiology of periodontal disease in western Nigerians in relation to socioeconomic status. Arch Oral Biol 15:1231, 1970.
26. Follis RH. The Pathology of Nutritional Disease. Springfield, IL, Charles C Thomas, 1948, p 134.
27. Frandsen AM. Periodontal tissue changes in vitamin A deficient young rats. Acta Odontol Scand 21:19, 1963.
28. Frandsen AM, et al. The effects of various levels of dietary protein on the periodontal tissues of young rats. J Periodontol 24:135, 1953.
29. Glickman I. Acute vitamin C deficiency and periodontal disease. I. The periodontal tissues of the guinea pig in acute vitamin C deficiency. J Dent Res 27:9, 1948.
30. Glickman I. Acute vitamin C deficiency and the periodontal tissues. II. The effect of acute vitamin C deficiency upon the response of the periodontal tissues of the guinea pig to artificially induced inflammation. J Dent Res 27:201, 1948.
31. Glickman I, Dines MM. Effect of increased ascorbic acid blood levels on the ascorbic acid level in treated and nontreated gingiva. J Dent Res 42:1152, 1963.
32. Glickman I, Stoller M. The periodontal tissues of the albino rat in vitamin A deficiency. J Dent Res 27:758, 1948.
33. Glickman I, Morse A, Robinson L. The systemic influence upon bone in periodontoclasia. J Am Dent Assoc 31:1435, 1944.
34. Goetzl EJ. Enhancement of random migration and chemotactic response of human leukocytes by ascorbic acid. J Clin Invest 53:813, 1974.
35. Frandsen AM, Becks H, Nelson MN, Evans HM. Protein deprivation in rats. J Dent Res 39:690, 1960.
36. Goodman MH. Perlèche: A consideration of its etiology and pathology. Bull Johns Hopkins Hosp 51:263, 1943.
37. Govier WM, Grieg ME. Prevention of oral lesions in B1 avitaminotic dogs. Science 98:216, 1943.
38. Hodges RE, Baker EM, Hood J, et al. Experimental scurvy in man. Am J Clin Nutr 22:535, 1969.
39. Hojer JA. Studies in scurvy. Acta Paediatr 3(suppl):119, 1924.
40. Ismail AI, Burt BA, Eklund SA. Relation between ascorbic acid intake and periodontal disease in the United States. J Am Dent Assoc 107:927, 1983.
41. Jeghers H. Riboflavin deficiency. IV. Oral changes. Advances in Internal Medicine I. New York, Interscience Publishers, 1942, p 257.
42. Keys A, Brožek J, Henschel A, et al. The Biology of Human Starvation. Vol 1. Minneapolis, University of Minnesota Press, 1950.
43. Kim JE, Shklar G. The effect of vitamin E on the healing of gingival wounds in rats. J Periodontol 54:305, 1983.
44. King JD. Vincent's disease treated with nicotinic acid. Lancet 2:32, 1940.
45. King JD, Glover NE. The relative effects of dietary constituents and other factors upon calculus formation and gingival disease in the ferret. J Pathol Bacteriol 57:353, 1945.
46. Krasse B, Brill N. Effect of consistency of diet on bacteria in gingival pockets in dogs. Odont Revy 11:152, 1960.
47. Kristoffersen T, Bang G, Meyer K. Lack of effect of high doses of fluoride in prevention of alveolar bone loss in rats. J Periodont Res 5:127, 1970.
48. Lee RE, Lee NZ. The peripheral vascular system and its reactions in scurvy: An experimental study. Am J Physiol 149:465, 1947.
49. Likins RC, Pakis G, McClure FJ. Effect of fluoride and tetracycline on alveolar bone resorption in the rat. J Dent Res 42:1532, 1963.
50. Lindhe J, Wicen PO. The effects on the gingivae of chewing fibrous foods. J Periodont Res 4:193, 1969.
51. Mann AW, Spies TD, Springer M. Oral manifestations of vitamin B complex deficiencies. J Dent Res 20:269, 1941.
52. Manson-Bahr P, Ransford ON. Stomatitis of vitamin B2 deficiency treated with nicotinic acid. Lancet 2:426, 1938.
53. Miller SC, Stahl SS, Goldsmith ED. The effects of vertical occlusal trauma on the periodontium of protein deprived young adult rats. J Periodontol 28:87, 1957.
54. Nelson MA, Chaudhry AP. Effects of tocopherol (vitamin E) deficient diet on some oral, para-oral and hematopoietic tissues of the rat. J Dent Res 45:1072, 1966.
55. Pack A, Thomson M. Effects of topical and systemic folic acid supplementation on gingivitis in pregnancy. J Clin Periodontol 7:402, 1980.
56. Parrish JH Jr, DeMarco TJ, Bissada NF. Vitamin E and periodontitis in the rat. Oral Surg 44:210, 1977.
57. Pelzer R. A study of the local oral effect of diet on the periodontal tissues and the gingival capillary structure. J Am Dent Assoc 27:13, 1940.
58. Ramseyer WF, Smith CAH, McCay CM. Effect of sodium fluoride administration on body changes in old rats. J Gerontol 12:14, 1957.
59. Restarski JS, Pijoan M. Gingivitis and vitamin C. J Am Dent Assoc 31:1323, 1944.
60. Russell AL. International nutrition surveys: A summary of preliminary dental findings. J Dent Res 42:233, 1963.

61. Shaw JH. The relation of nutrition to periodontal disease. J Dent Res *41*(suppl 1):264, 1962.

62. Shilotri PG, Bhat KS. Effect of megadoses of vitamin C on bacterial activity of leukocytes. Am J Clin Nutr *30:*1077, 1977.

63. Squire CF, Costley JM. Gingival status during prolonged fasting for weight loss. J Periodontol *28:*87, 1957.

64. Stahl SS. The effect of a protein-free diet on the healing of gingival wounds in rats. Arch Oral Biol *7:*551, 1962.

65. Stahl SS, Sandler HC, Cahn L. The effects of protein deprivation upon the oral tissues of the rat and particularly upon the periodontal structures under irritation. Oral Surg *8:*760, 1955.

66. Stralfors A, Thilander H, Bergenholtz A. Caries and periodontal disease in hamsters fed cereal foods varying in sugar content and hardness. Arch Oral Biol *12:*1681, 1967.

67. Topping NH, Fraser HF. Mouth lesions associated with dietary deficiencies in monkeys. Public Health Rep *54:*416, 1939.

68. Vogel R. Relationship of folic acid to phenytoin-induced gingival overgrowth. In Hassell TM, Johnson M, Dudley K, eds. Phenytoin-Induced Teratology and Gingival Pathology. New York, Raven Press, 1980.

69. Vogel R, Deasy M, Alfano M, Schneider L. The effect of folic acid on gingival health of women taking oral contraceptives. J Prev Dent *6:*221, 1980.

70. Vogel R, Fink R, Frank O, Baker H. The effect of topical application of folic acid on gingival health. J Oral Med *33:*20, 1978.

71. Vogel R, Fink R, Schneider L, et al. The effect of folic acid on gingival health. J Periodontol *47:*667, 1976.

72. Waerhaug J. Effect of C-avitaminosis on the supporting structures of the teeth. J Periodontol *29:*87, 1958.

73. Waerhaug J. Epidemiology of periodontal disease. Review of literature. In World Workshop in Periodontics. Ann Arbor, MI, American Academy of Periodontology and the University of Michigan Press, 1966, p 181.

74. Weinmann JP, Schour I. Experimental studies in calcification. Am J Pathol *21:*821, 1047, 1945.

75. Wolbach SB, Bessey OA. Tissue changes in vitamin deficiencies. Physiol Rev *22:*233, 1942.

76. Woolfe SN, Hume WR, Kenney EB. Ascorbic acid and periodontal disease: A review of the literature. J West Soc Periodontol *28:*44, 1980.

77. Woolfe SN, Kenney EB, Hume WR, Carranza FA Jr. Relationship of ascorbic acid levels of blood and gingival tissue with response to periodontal therapy. J Clin Periodontol *11:*159, 1984.

ENDOCRINE DISEASES

1. Adler P, Wegner H, Bohatka A. Influence of age and duration of diabetes on dental development in diabetic children. J Dent Res *52:*535, 1973.

2. Ainamo J, Lahtinen A, Vitto VJ. Rapid periodontal destruction in adult humans with poorly controlled diabetes. A report of two cases. J Clin Periodontol *17:*22, 1990.

3. Barnett ML, Baker RL, Yancey JM, et al. Absence of periodontitis in a population of insulin-dependent diabetes mellitus (IDDM) patients. J Periodontol *55:*402, 1984.

4. Baume LJ, Becks H. The effect of thyroid hormone in dental and paradental structures. Paradentologie *6:*89, 1952.

5. Been V, Engel D. The effects of immunosuppressive drugs on periodontal inflammation in human renal allograft patients. J Periodontol *53:*245, 1982.

6. Belting CM, Hinicker JJ, Dummett CO. Influence of diabetes mellitus on the severity of periodontal disease. J Periodontol *35:*476, 1964.

7. Bernick SM, Cohen DW, Baker L, Laster L. Dental disease in children with diabetes mellitus. J Periodontol *46:*241, 1975.

8. Bernick S, Ershoff BH. Histochemical study of bone in estrogen-treated rats. J Dent Res *42:*981, 1963.

9. Biro S. Studies regarding the influence of pregnancy upon caries. Vierteljahrschr Zahnheilk *14:*371, 1898.

10. Bissada NF, Schaffer EM, Laarow A. Effect of alloxan diabetes and local irritating factors on the periodontal structures of the rat. Periodontics *4:*233, 1966.

11. Borghelli RF, Devoto FCH, Foglia V, Erausquin J. Periodontal changes and dental caries in experimental prediabetes. Diabetes *16:*804, 1967.

12. Butcher EO, Klingsberg J. Age, gonadectomy and wound healing in the palatal mucosa. J Dent Res *40:*694, 1961.

13. Campbell MJA. An electron microscope study of the basement membrane of the small vessels from the gingival tissue of the diabetic and nondiabetic patient. J Dent Res *46:*1302, 1967.

14. Campbell MJA. The oxygen utilization and glucose oxidation rate of gingival tissue from nondiabetic and diabetic patients. Arch Oral Biol *15:*305, 1970.

15. Campbell MJA. Epidemiology of periodontal disease in the diabetic and the nondiabetic. Aust Dent J *17:*274, 1972.

16. Cianciola LJ, Park BH, Bruck E, et al. Prevalence of periodontal disease in insulin-dependent diabetes mellitus (juvenile diabetes). J Am Dent Assoc *104:*653, 1982.

17. Cohen DW, Friedman LA, Shapiro J, et al. Diabetes mellitus and periodontal disease: Two year longitudinal observations. Part I. J Periodontol *41:*709, 1970.

18. Cohen DW, Shapiro J, Friedman L, et al. A longitudinal investigation of the periodontal changes during pregnancy and fifteen months post-partum. J Periodontol *42:*653, 1971.

19. Cohen MM, Shklar G, Yerganian G. Periodontal pathology in a strain of Chinese hamster with hereditary diabetes mellitus. Am J Med *31:*864, 1961.

20. Diabetes and oral health. J Am Dent Assoc *115:*741, 1987.

21. El-Ashiry GM, El-Kafrawy AH, Nasr MF, Younis N. Comparative study of the influence of pregnancy and oral contraceptives on the gingivae. Oral Surg *30:*472, 1970.

22. El Geneldy AK, Stallard RE, Fillios LC, Goldman HM. Periodontal and vascular alterations: Their relationship to the changes in tissue glucose and glycogen in diabetic mouse. J Periodontol *45:*394, 1974.

23. Emrich LJ, Shlossman M, Genco RJ. Periodontal disease in non-insulin dependent diabetes mellitus. J Periodontol *62:*123, 1991.

24. English JA. Experimental effects of thiouracil and selenium on the teeth and jaws of dogs. J Dent Res *28:*172, 1949.

25. Ervasti T, Knuutila M, Pohjano L, Haukipuro K. Relation between control of diabetes and gingival bleeding. J Periodontol *56:*154, 1985.

26. Ficara AI, Levin MP, Grover MF, Kramer GD. A comparison of the glucose and protein content of gingival fluid from diabetics and nondiabetics. J Periodont Res *10:*171, 1975.

27. Formicola AJ, Weatherford T, Grupe H Jr. The uptake of H3-estradiol by the oral tissues in rats. J Periodont Res *5:*269, 1970.

28. Frantzis TG, Reeve CM, Brown JR. The ultrastructure of capillary basement membranes in the attached gingiva of diabetic and nondiabetic patients with periodontal disease. J Periodontol *42:*406, 1971.

29. Friederici HHR, Tucker WR, Schwartz TB. Observations on small blood vessels in normal and diabetic patients. Diabetes *15:*233, 1966.

30. Friedman LA. Horizontal tooth mobility and the menstrual cycle. J Periodont Res *7:*125, 1972.

31. Genco RJ, Shlossman M, Zambon JJ. Immunologic studies of periodontitis patients with type II diabetes (abstract). J Periodontol *66:*257, 1987.

32. Gillman CF, Berstein JM, Van Oss C. Increased phagocytosis associated with increased surface hydrophobicity of neutrophils of children with chronic infections (abstract). Fed Proc 35:227, 1976.

33. Glavind L, Lund B, Löe H. The relationship between periodontal state and diabetes duration, insulin dosage and retinal changes. J Periodontol *39:*341, 1968.

34. Glickman I. The periodontal structures in experimental diabetes. NY J Dent *16:*226, 1946.

35. Glickman I, Pruzansky S. Propylthiouracil hypothyroidism in the albino rat. J Dent Res *26:*471, 1947.

36. Glickman I, Quintarelli G. Further observations regarding the effect of ovariectomy upon the tissues of the periodontium. J Periodontol *31:*31, 1960.

37. Glickman I, Shklar G. The steroid hormones and the tissues of the periodontium. Oral Surg *8:*1179, 1955.

38. Glickman I, Smulow J, Moreau J. Effect of alloxan diabetes upon the periodontal response to excessive occlusal forces. J Periodontol *37:*146, 1966.

39. Glickman I, Stone IC, Chawla TN. The effect of cortisone acetate upon the periodontium of white mice. J Periodontol *24:*161, 1953.

40. Glickman I, Smulow J, Moreau J. Postsurgical periodontal healing in alloxan diabetes. J Periodontol *38:*93, 1967.

41. Gottsegen R. Dental and oral considerations in diabetes mellitus. NY J Med *62:*389, 1962.

42. Grossi SG, Zambon JJ, Norderyd OM, et al. Microbiological risk indicators for periodontal disease. Abstract 818. J Dent Res *72:*206, 1993.

43. Grower MF, Ficara AJ, Chandler DW, Kramer GD. Differences in cAMP levels in the gingival fluid of diabetics and nondiabetics. J Periodontol *46:*669, 1975.

44. Gusberti F, Grossman N, Löesche W. Puberty gingivitis in insulin-dependent diabetes. Abstract 199. J Dent Res (special issue) *61:*201, 1982.

45. Hayden P, Buckley LA. Diabetes mellitus and periodontal disease in an Irish population. J Periodont Res *24:*298, 1989.

46. Henrikson PA. Periodontal disease and calcium deficiency in the dog. Acta Odont Scand *26*(suppl 50), 1968.

47. Hirschfeld I. Periodontal symptoms associated with diabetes. J Periodontol *5:*37, 1934.

48. Holm-Pederson P, Löe H. Flow of gingival exudate as related to menstruation and pregnancy. J Periodont Res *2:*13, 1967.

49. Hove KA, Stallard RE. Diabetes and the periodontal patient. J Periodontol *41:*713, 1970.

50. Hugoson A. Gingival inflammation and female sex hormones. J Periodontol Res 5(suppl), 1970.

51. Hugoson A, Thorstensson H, Falk H, Kuylenstierna J. Periodontal conditions in insulin-dependent diabetics. J Clin Periodontol *16:*215, 1989.

52. Kalkwarf KL. Effect of oral contraceptive therapy on gingival inflammation in humans. J Periodontol *49:*560, 1978.

53. Kardachi BJR, Newcomb GM. A clinical study of gingival inflammation in renal transplant patients taking immunosuppressive drugs. J Periodontol *49:*307, 1978.

54. Keene JJ Jr. Observations of small blood vessels in human nondiabetic and diabetic gingiva. J Dent Res *48:*967, 1969.

55. Keene JJ Jr. An alteration in human diabetic arterioles. J Dent Res *41:*569, 1972.

56. Koronori A. Histological studies of the influence of occlusal function on the periodontal tissues of alloxan diabetic rats. Bull Tokyo Med Univ *11:*207, 1964.

57. Knight GM, Wade AB. The effects of hormonal contraceptives on the human periodontium. J Periodont Res *9:*18, 1974.

58. Krohn S. The effect of the administration of steroid hormones on the gingival tissues. J Periodontol *29:*300, 1958.

59. Kolodzinski E, Munoa N, Malatesta E. Clinical study of gingival tissue in pregnant women. Abstract. J Dent Res *53:*693, 1974.

60. Kornman KS, Loesche WJ. The subgingival microbial flora during pregnancy. J Periodont Res 15:111, 1980.
61. Lindhe J, Attstrom R. Gingival exudation during the menstrual cycle. J Periodont Res 2:194, 1967.
62. Lindhe J, Bjorn AL. Influence of hormonal contraceptives on the gingiva of women. J Periodont Res 2:1, 1967.
63. Lindhe J, Branemark PI. Changes in microcirculation after local application of sex hormones. J Periodont Res 2:185, 1967.
64. Lindhe J, Sonesson B. The effect of sex hormones on inflammation. II. Progestogen, oestrogen and chorionic gonadotropin. J Periodont Res 2:7, 1967.
65. Lindhe J, Attstrom R, Bjorn A. Influence of sex hormones on gingival exudation in gingivitis-free female dogs. J Periodont Res 3:272, 1968.
66. Listgarten MA, Ricker FH Jr, Laster L, et al. Vascular basement lamina thickness in the normal and inflamed gingiva of diabetics and nondiabetics. J Periodontol 45:676, 1974.
67. Löe H. Periodontal changes in pregnancy. J Periodontol 36:209, 1965.
68. MacKenzie RS, Millard HO. Interrelated effects of diabetes, arteriosclerosis and calculus on alveolar bone loss. J Am Dent Assoc 66:191, 1963.
69. Maier AW, Orban B. Gingivitis in pregnancy. Oral Surg 2:234, 1949.
70. Mascola B. The oral manifestations of diabetes mellitus: A review. NY Dent J 36:139, 1970.
71. Mandell RL, Dirienzo J, Kent R, et al. Microbiology of healthy and diseased periodontal sites in poorly controlled insulin-dependent diabetics. J Periodontol 63:274, 1992.
72. Mashimo P, Yamamoto Y, Slots J, et al. The periodontal microflora of juvenile diabetes—culture, immunofluorescence and serum antibody studies. J Periodontol 54:420, 1983.
73. Massler M, Henry J. Oral manifestations during the female climacteric. Alpha Omegan, September, p 105, 1950.
74. McCarthy P, Shklar G. Diseases of the Oral Mucosa. 2nd ed. Philadelphia, Lea & Febiger, 1980.
75. McMullen J, Gottsegen R, Camerini Davalos R. PAS fuchsinophilic thickening of small blood vessels in diabetic gingiva due to accumulation in the periendothelial area. J Periodontol 5:61, 1967.
76. McMullen JA, VanDyke TE, Horozewicz HU, Genco RJ. Neutrophil chemotaxis in individuals with advanced periodontal disease and a genetic predisposition to diabetes mellitus. J Periodontol 52:167, 1981.
77. Mehrotia KK, Chawla TN, Kumar A. Correlation of salivary sugar and blood sugar with periodontal health and oral hygiene status among diabetics and nondiabetics. J Indian Dent Assoc 40:287, 1968.
78. Mohammed AH, Waterhouse JP, Friederici HH. The microvasculature of the rat gingiva as affected by progesterone: An ultrastructural study. J Periodontol 45:50, 1974.
79. Nichols C, Laster AA, Bodak Gyovai LZ. Diabetes mellitus and periodontal disease. J Periodontol 49:85, 1978.
80. Novaes AB Jr, Pereira ALA, Moraes N, Novaes AB. Manifestations of insulin-dependent diabetes mellitus in the periodontium of young Brazilian patients. J Periodontol 62:116, 1991.
81. Nutlay AG, Bhaskar SN, Weinmann JP, Budy AM. The effect of estrogen on the gingiva and alveolar bone in rats and mice. J Dent Res 33:115, 1954.
82. Nyman S. Studies on the influence of estradiol and progesterone on granulation tissue. J Periodont Res 7(suppl), 1971.
83. O'Leary TM, Shannon I, Prigmore JR. Clinical and systemic findings in periodontal disease. J Periodontol 32:243, 1962.
84. Olefsky JM. Diabetes mellitus. In Wyngaarden JB, Smith LH Jr, Bennett JC, eds. Cecil Textbook of Medicine. 19th ed. Philadelphia, WB Saunders, 1992, pp 1291–1310.
85. O'Neil TCA. Maternal T-lymphocyte response and gingivitis in pregnancy. J Periodontol 50:178, 1979.
86. Oshrain HI, Mender S, Mandel ID. Periodontal status of patients with reduced immunocapacity. J Periodontol 50:185, 1979.
87. Phair J. Neutrophil dysfunction in diabetes mellitus. J Lab Clin Med 85:26, 1975.
88. Perry DA. Oral contraceptives and periodontal health. J West Soc Periodontol 29:72, 1981.
89. Piroshaw N, Glickman I. The effect of ovariectomy upon the tissues of the periodontium and skeletal bones. Oral Surg 10:133, 1957.
90. Prout RES, Hopps RM. A relationship between human oral bacteria and the menstrual cycle. J Periodontol 41:98, 1970.
91. Rateitschak KH. Tooth mobility changes in pregnancy. J Periodont Res 2:199, 1967.
92. Ray HG, Orban B. The gingival structures in diabetes mellitus. J Periodontol 21:85, 1950.
93. Richman JJ, Abarbanel AR. Effects of estradiol, testosterone, diethylstilbestrol and several of their derivatives upon the human mucous membrane. J Am Dent Assoc 30:913, 1943.
94. Ringsdorf WM, Powell BJ, Knight LA, Cheraskin E. Periodontal status and pregnancy. Am J Obstet Gynecol 83:258, 1962.
95. Robertson HD, Polk HC Jr. The mechanism of infection in patients with diabetes mellitus. A review of leukocyte malfunction. Surgery 75:123, 1974.
96. Rosenberg EH, Guralnick WC. Hyperparathyroidism. Oral Surg 15(suppl 2):84, 1962.
97. Rosenberg EH, Goldman HM, Garber E. The effects of experimental thyrotoxicosis and myxedema on the periodontium of rabbits. J Dent Res 40:708, 1961.

98. Rushton MA. Epithelial downgrowth: Effect of methyl testosterone. Br Dent J 93:27, 1952.
99. Safkan-Seppala B, Ainamo J. Periodontal conditions in insulin-dependent diabetes mellitus. J Clin Periodontol 19:24, 1992.
100. Sastrowijoto SH, Hillemans P, van Steenbergen TJM, et al. Periodontal condition and microbiology of healthy and diseased periodontal pockets in type I diabetes mellitus patients. J Clin Periodontol 16:316, 1989.
101. Sastrowijoto SH, van der Velde V, van Steenbergen TJ, et al. Improved metabolic control, clinical periodontal status and subgingival microbiology in insulin-dependent diabetes mellitus. A prospective study. J Clin Periodontol 17:233, 1990.
102. Schneir M, Imberman M, Ramamurthy N, Golub L. Streptozotocin-induced diabetes and the rat periodontium: Decreased relative collagen production. Coll Relat Res 8:221, 1988.
103. Schour I. The effects of hypophysectomy on the periodontal tissues. J Periodontol 5:15, 1934.
104. Silverman S, Gordon G, Grant T, et al. The dental structures in primary hyperparathyroidism. Oral Surg 15:426, 1962.
105. Shapiro S, Shklar G. The effect of hypophysectomy on the periodontium of the albino rat. J Periodontol 33:364, 1962.
106. Shklar G. The effect of adrenalectomy and cortisone replacement on the periodontium of the rat. Periodontics 3:239, 1965.
107. Shklar G, Cohen MM, Yerganian G. Periodontal disease in the Chinese hamster with hereditary diabetes. J Periodontol 33:14, 1962.
108. Shklar G, Glickman I. The effect of estrogenic hormone on the periodontium of white mice. J Periodontol 27:16, 1956.
109. Shklar G, Chauncey H, Peluso D. The effect of testosterone on the periodontium of the male albino rat. IADR Abstracts, 1962, p 68.
110. Shklar G, Chauncey H, Shapiro S. The effect of testosterone on the periodontium of normal and hypophysectomy rats. J Periodontol 38:203, 1967.
111. Stahl SS, Witkin GJ, Scopp IW. Degenerative vascular changes observed in selected gingival specimens. Oral Surg 15:1495, 1962.
112. Strock MS. The mouth in hyperparathyroidism. N Engl J Med 224:1019, 1945.
113. Sutcliffe P. A longitudinal study of gingivitis and puberty. J Periodont Res 7:52, 1972.
114. Sznajder N, Carraro JJ, Rugna S, Sereday M. Periodontal findings in diabetic and nondiabetic patients. J Periodontol 49:445, 1978.
115. Svanberg G, Lindhe J, Hugoson A, Grondahl HG. Effect of nutritional hyperparathyroidism on experimental periodontitis in the dog. Scand J Dent Res 81:155, 1973.
116. Tervonen T, Knuuttila M, Pohjamo L, Nukkala H. Immediate response to nonsurgical periodontal treatment in subjects with diabetes mellitus. J Clin Periodontol 18:65, 1991.
117. Tollefsen T, Saltvedt E, Koppang HS. The effect of immunosuppressive agents on periodontal disease in man. J Periodont Res 13:240, 1978.
118. Turesky S, Fisher B, Glickman I. A histochemical study of the attached gingiva in pregnancy. J Dent Res 37:1115, 1958.
119. Weinmann JP, Schour I. The effect of parathyroid hormone on the alveolar bone and teeth of the normal and rachitic rat. Am J Pathol 21:857, 1945.
120. Willershausen B, Barth S, Preac-Mursic V, Haslbeck M. Parodontalbefund und Mikroflora bei insulin–abhangigen (Typ I)–Diabetikern. Schweiz Monatsschr Zahnmed 101:1399, 1991.
121. Wingrove FA, Rubright WC, Kerber PE. Influence of ovarian hormone situation on atrophy, hypertrophy, and/or desquamation of human gingiva in premenopausal and postmenopausal women. J Periodontol 50:445, 1979.
122. Zambon JJ, Reynolds H, Fisher JB, et al. Microbiological and immunological studies of adult periodontitis in patients with non–insulin dependent diabetes mellitus. J Periodontol 59:23, 1988.
123. Ziskin DE, Blackberg SN. The effect of castration and hypophysectomy on the gingiva and oral mucous membranes of Rhesus monkeys. J Dent Res 19:381, 1940.
124. Ziskin DE, Blackberg SN. A study of the gingivae during pregnancy. J Dent Res 13:253, 1933.
125. Ziskin DE, Blackberg SN, Stout A. The gingivae during pregnancy: An experimental study and a histopathological interpretation. Surg Gynecol Obstet 57:719, 1933.
126. Ziskin RD, Stein G. The gingiva and oral mucous membrane of monkeys in experimental hypothyroidism. J Dent Res 21:296, 1942.

HEMATOLOGIC DISEASES

1. Akers LH. Ulcerative stomatitis following therapeutic use of mercury and bismuth. J Am Dent Assoc 23:781, 1936.
2. Babior BM. Disorders of neutrophil function. In Wyngaarden JB, Smith LH Jr, eds. Cecil Textbook of Medicine. 18th ed. Philadelphia, WB Saunders, 1988.
3. Baker EG, Crook GH, Schwabacher ED. Personality correlates of periodontal disease. J Dent Res 40:396, 1961.
4. Barrett P. Gingival lesions in leukemia. A classification. J Periodontol 55:585, 1984.
5. Bauer WH. Agranulocytosis and the supporting dental tissues. J Dent Res 25:501, 1946.
6. Belting CM, Gupta OP. The influence of psychiatric disturbances on the severity of periodontal disease. J Periodontol 32:219, 1961.
7. Bernick S. Age changes in the blood supply to human teeth. J Dent Res 46:544, 1967.

8. Bernick S, Levy BM, Patek PR. Studies on the biology of the periodontium of marmosets. VI. Arteriosclerotic changes in the blood vessels of the periodontium. J Periodontol *40:*355, 1969.

9. Biber O. Autonomic symptoms in psychoneurotics. Psychosom Med *3:*253, 1941.

10. Blitzer B, Sznajder N, Carranza FA Jr. Hallazgos clinicos periodontales en ninos con cardiopatias congenitas. Rev Assoc Odont Argent *63:*169, 1975.

11. Brown LR, Roth GD, Hoover D, et al. Alveolar bone loss in leukemic and non-leukemic mice. J Periodontol *40:*725, 1969.

12. Burstoen MS. The psychosomatic aspects of dental problems. J Am Dent Assoc *33:*862, 1946.

13. Cahn LR. Observations on the effect of tuberculosis on the teeth, gums and jaws. Dent Cosmos *67:*479, 1925.

14. Carranza FA Jr, Gravina O, Cabrini RL. Periodontal and pulpal pathosis in leukemic mice. Oral Surg *20:*374, 1965.

15. Ciancio S, Hazen S, Cunat J. Periodontal observations in twins. J Periodont Res *4:*42, 1969.

16. Cohen DW, Morris AL. Periodontal manifestations of cyclic neutropenia. J Periodontol *32:*159, 1961.

17. Dreizen S, McCredie KB, Keating MJ. Chemotherapy-associated oral hemorrhages in adult leukemics. Oral Surg *57:*494, 1984.

18. Dreizen S, McCredie KB, Keating MJ, Luna MA. Malignant gingival and skin infiltrates in adult leukemia. Oral Surg *55:*572, 1983.

18a. Editorial. J Am Dent Assoc *115:*679, 1987.

19. Forsslund G. Occurrence of subepithelial gingival blood vessels in patients with morbus caeruleus (tetralogy of Fallot). Acta Odontol Scand *20:*301, 1962.

20. Frantzell A, Törnquist R, Waldenström J. Examination of the tongue: A clinical and photographic study. Acta Med Scand *122:*207, 1945.

21. Frohman BS. Occlusal neuroses. Psychoanal Rev *19:*297, 1932.

22. Giddon DB. Psychophysiology of the oral cavity. J Dent Res *45:*1627, 1966.

23. Goldman HM. Acute aleukemic leukemia. Am J Orthod *26:*89, 1940.

24. Grant D, Bernick S. Arteriosclerosis in periodontal vessels of aging humans. J Periodontol *41:*170, 1970.

25. Greenberg MS, Cohen SB, Boosz B, Friedman H. Oral herpes infections in patients with leukemia. J Am Dent Assoc *114:*483, 1987.

26. Gruber IE. The condition of the teeth and the attachment apparatus in tuberculosis. J Dent Res *28:*483, 1949.

27. Gupta OP. Psychosomatic factors in periodontal disease. Dent Clin North Am *10:*11, 1966.

28. Higgins WH. Systemic poisoning with bismuth. JAMA *66:*648, 1916.

29. Itoiz ME, Litwack D, Kennedy JE, Zander HA. Experimental ischemia in monkeys: III. Histochemical analysis of gingival epithelium. J Dent Res *48:*895, 1969.

30. Jones RR. Symptoms in early stages of industrial plumbism. JAMA *104:*195, 1935.

31. Kaner A, Losch P, Green M. Oral manifestations of congenital heart disease. J Pediatr *29:*269, 1946.

32. Kastlin G. Agranulocytic angina. Am J Med Sci *173:*799, 1927.

33. Kennedy JE, Zander HA. Experimental ischemia in monkeys. I. Effect of ischemia on gingival epithelium. J Dent Res *48:*696, 1969.

34. Kracke RR. Granulopenia as associated with amidopyrine administration. Report made at the Annual Session of the AMA, June 1934.

35. Liberman H. Chrome ulcerations of the nose and throat. N Engl J Med *225:*132, 1941.

36. Lynch MA, Ship I. Initial oral manifestations of leukemia. J Am Dent Assoc *75:*932, 1967.

37. Madison FW, Squier TL. Primary granulocytopenia after administration of benzene chain derivatives. JAMA *102:*755, 1934.

38. Manhold JH. Report of a study on the relationship of personality variables to periodontal conditions. J Periodontol *24:*248, 1953.

39. Mark HA. Agranulocytic angina. Its oral manifestations. J Am Dent Assoc *21:*119, 1934.

40. Meyer A. Agranulocytosis. Report of a case caused by sulfadiazine. Calif West Med J *61:*54, 1944.

41. Michalowicz BS, Aeppli D, Virag JG, et al. Periodontal findings in adult twins. J Periodontol *62:*293, 1991.

42. Miller SC, Thaller JL, Soberman A. The use of the Minnesota Multiphasic Personality Inventory as a diagnostic aid in periodontal disease. A preliminary report. J Periodontol *27:*44, 1956.

43. Moskow BS, Rennert MC, Wasserman BH, Khurana H. Interrelationship of dietary factors and heredity in periodontal lesions in the gerbil. IADR Abstracts, 1970, p 134.

44. Page RC, Schroeder HE. Periodontitis in Man and Other Animals. A Comparative Review. Basel, S Karger, 1982.

45. Pattison GL. Self-inflicted gingival injuries: Literature review and case report. J Periodontol *54:*299, 1983.

46. Poland C III, Christian JC, Bixler D. Hypophosphatasia: An inherited oral disease. IADR Abstracts, 1970, p 228.

47. Quintarelli G. Histopathology of the human mandibular artery and arterioles in periodontal disease. Oral Surg *10:*1047, 1957.

48. Rada RE, Bronny AT, Hasiakos PS. Sickle cell crisis precipitated by periodontal infection. J Am Dent Assoc *11:*799, 1987.

49. Ramfjord S. Tuberculosis and periodontal disease, with special reference to the collagen fibers. J Dent Res *31:*5, 1952.

50. Randall CL. Granulocytopenia following barbiturates and amidopyrine. JAMA *102:*1137, 1934.

51. Robbins SL, Cotran RS, Kumar V. Pathologic Basis of Disease. 4th ed. Philadelphia, WB Saunders, 1989.

52. Ryan EJ. Psychobiologic Foundation in Dentistry. Springfield, IL, Charles C Thomas, 1946, p 27.

53. Rylander H, Attstrom R, Lindhe J. Influence of experimental neutropenia in dogs with chronic gingivitis. J Periodont Res *10:*315, 1975.

54. Sandler HC, Stahl SS. The influence of generalized diseases on clinical manifestations of periodontal disease. J Am Dent Assoc *49:*656, 1954.

55. Saul LJ. A note on the psychogenesis of organic symptoms. Psychoanal Q *4:*476, 1935.

56. Schour I, Sarnat BG. Oral manifestations of occupational origin. JAMA *120:*1197, 1942.

57. Scopp IW. Healthy periodontium in chronically ill patients. J Periodontol *28:*147, 1957.

58. Scully CE, MacFayden A, Campbell A. Oral manifestations in cyclic neutropenia. Br J Oral Surg *20:*96, 1982.

59. Shklar G, McCarthy PL. The Oral Manifestations of Systemic Disease. Boston, Butterworths, 1976.

60. Stahl SS, Wisan JM, Miller SC, et al. The influence of systemic diseases on alveolar bone. J Am Dent Assoc *45:*277, 1952.

61. Suzuki JB, Delisli AL. Pulmonary actinomycosis of periodontal origin. J Periodontol *55:*581, 1984.

62. Tanchester D, Sorrin S. Dental lesions in relation to pulmonary tuberculosis. J Dent Res *16:*69, 1937.

63. Telsey B, Beube FE, Zegarelli EV, Kutscher AH. Oral manifestations of cyclical neutropenia associated with hypergammaglobulinemia. Oral Surg *15:*540, 1962.

64. Tochichara Y. Pyorrhea alveolar as in leprosy. Nippar No Shikai *13:*165, 1933.

65. Wirthlin MR Jr, Ratcliff PA. Arteries, atherosclerosis and periodontics. J Periodontol *40:*341, 1969.

15

AIDS and the Periodontium

EDMUND CATALDO and TERRY D. REES

Epidemiology and Demographics
Classification and Staging
Oral and Periodontal Manifestations of
    HIV Infection
Oral Hairy Leukoplakia
Oral Candidiasis

Kaposi's Sarcoma
Bacillary (Epithelioid) Angiomatosis
Oral Hyperpigmentation
Atypical Ulcers and Delayed Healing
Adverse Drug Effects
Periodontal Disease

Acquired immunodeficiency syndrome (AIDS) is characterized by profound impairment of the immune system. The condition was first reported in 1981, and a viral pathogen, the human immunodeficiency virus (HIV), was identified in 1984.[75]

HIV has a strong affinity for cells of the immune system, most specifically those that carry the CD4 cell surface receptor molecule. Thus, helper T lymphocytes are most profoundly affected, but monocytes, macrophages, Langerhans cells, and some neuronal and glial brain cells may also be involved.[19] The overall effect of the virus is to gradually impair the immune system by interference with helper T lymphocytes and other immune cell functions.

B lymphocytes are not infected, but the altered function of infected T lymphocytes secondarily results in B-cell dysregulation. This may place the HIV-positive individual at increased risk for malignancy and disseminated infections with microorganisms such as viruses, mycobacterioses, and mycoses.[36,65,71,82] HIV-positive individuals are also at increased risk for adverse drug reactions owing to altered antigenic regulation.

HIV has been detected in most body fluids, although it is found in high quantities only in blood, semen, and cerebrospinal fluid. Transmission occurs almost exclusively by sexual contact or exposure to blood or blood products.

The high-risk population includes homosexual and bisexual men; users of illegal, injectable drugs; hemophiliacs or others with coagulation disorders; recipients of blood transfusions before April 1985; infants of HIV-infected mothers (in whom transmission occurs by fetal transmission, at delivery, or by breast feeding); promiscuous heterosexuals; and individuals who engage in unprotected sex with an HIV-positive individual. Heterosexual transmission is a common cause of AIDS in the world population and is increasing significantly in the United States. HIV transmission has also been reported to occur through organ transplantation and artificial insemination.[11]

EPIDEMIOLOGY AND DEMOGRAPHICS

As of June 1993, 310,680 AIDS cases had been reported in the United States. This number in part reflects a revision by the U.S. Centers for Disease Control (CDC) of its case definition criteria for AIDS. This modification markedly increased the number of reported AIDS cases.[9] The change was made to better identify HIV-positive individuals with failing immune systems. The World Health Organization (WHO) estimates that as many as 9 to 11 million individuals worldwide are infected with HIV. This number may increase to more than 40 million people by the beginning of the 21st century.[66]

AIDS affects individuals of all ages, but more than 90% of cases occur among adults ages 20 to 49 (mean age, 36.6 years). The majority of victims in the United States are men, 61% of whom are homosexuals or bisexuals and/or injectable drug users. More than 50% of infected women are injectable drug users, and more than one third reported sexual contact with men from high–AIDS-risk categories. Others were born in countries such as Haiti or one of several high-incidence African nations where heterosexual contact is the major mode of transmission. The percentage of individuals contracting AIDS from blood products or blood transfusion continues to decrease in the United States as a result of stringent controls established in blood banks. A disproportionately high number of black and Hispanic male homosexuals, women, children, and heterosexuals suffer from HIV infection. The major risk factor for this disparity appears to be a more frequent history of use of injectable drugs and needle sharing in these groups.[13,52,59]

CLASSIFICATION AND STAGING

In 1982 the CDC developed a surveillance case definition for AIDS based on the presence of opportunistic illnesses or malignancies secondary to defective cell-mediated immunity in HIV-positive individuals.[7] This definition was further expanded in 1985, 1987, and 1993.[8] The 1993 revision added invasive cervical cancer in women, bacillary tuberculosis, and recurrent pneumonia into the AIDS designation. Currently any of 25 specific clinical conditions found in HIV-positive individuals can establish the diagnosis of AIDS (Table 15–1). The most significant change in the new CDC case definition was the inclusion of severe immunodeficiency (CD4-T4 lymphocyte count of less than

Table 15-1. 1993 CDC AIDS SURVEILLANCE CASE DEFINITION CONDITIONS

- Candidiasis of bronchi, trachea, or lungs
- Candidiasis, esophageal
- Cervical cancer, invasive
- Coccidioidomycosis, disseminated or extrapulmonary
- Cryptococcosis, extrapulmonary
- Cryptosporidiosis, chronic intestinal (>1 month's duration)
- Cytomegalovirus disease (other than liver, spleen, or nodes)
- Cytomegalovirus retinitis (with loss of vision)
- Encephalopathy, HIV-related
- Herpes simplex: chronic ulcer(s) (>1 month's duration) or bronchitis, pneumonitis, or esophagitis
- Histoplasmosis, disseminated or extrapulmonary
- Isosporiasis, chronic intestinal (>1 month's duration)
- Kaposi's sarcoma
- Lymphoma, Burkitt's (or equivalent term)
- Lymphoma, immunoblastic (or equivalent term)
- Lymphoma, primary, of brain
- *Mycobacterium avium* complex or *Mycobacterium kansasii,* disseminated or extrapulmonary
- *Mycobacterium tuberculosis,* any site (pulmonary or extrapulmonary)
- *Mycobacterium,* other species or unidentified species, disseminated or extrapulmonary
- *Pneumocystis carinii* pneumonia
- Pneumonia, recurrent
- Progressive multifocal leukoencephalopathy
- *Salmonella* septicemia, recurrent
- Toxoplasmosis of brain
- Wasting syndrome owing to HIV

From Centers for Disease Control. 1993 Revised classification system for HIV infection and expanded surveillance case definition for AIDS among adolescents and adults. MMWR 41:RR-17, 1993.

$200/mm^3$ or a T4 lymphocyte percentage of less than 14% of total lymphocytes) as definitive for AIDS. This change was based on recognition that severe immunodeficiency results in increased risk for opportunistic life-threatening conditions.

A few weeks to a few months after exposure, some HIV-infected individuals may experience acute symptoms (e.g., sudden onset of an acute mononucleosis-like illness characterized by malaise, fatigue, fever, myalgia, erythematous cutaneous eruption, and thrombocytopenia).[23,47] This acute phase may last for up to 2 weeks, with seroconversion occurring 3 to 8 weeks later.[48] However, antigenic viremia may sometimes be present for an extended period of time before seroconversion occurs.[40] Some individuals experience asymptomatic HIV infection, whereas others may become asymptomatic after the initial acute infection. In any event, infected individuals eventually become seropositive for HIV antibody, but the mean time from infection until development of AIDS is estimated to be up to 11 or more years.

CDC Surveillance Case Classification (1993). AIDS patients have been grouped as follows:

Category A includes patients with acute symptoms or asymptomatic diseases, along with individuals with persistent generalized lymphadenopathy, with or without malaise, fatigue, or low-grade fever.

Category B patients have symptomatic conditions such as oropharyngeal or vulvovaginal candidiasis; herpes zoster; oral hairy leukoplakia; idiopathic thrombocytopenia; or constitutional symptoms of fever, diarrhea, and weight loss.

Category C patients are those with outright AIDS as manifested by life-threatening conditions identified by $CD4^+$. T4 lymphocyte levels of less than 200 per cubic millimeter.

These staging categories reflect progressive immunologic dysfunction, but patients do not necessarily progress serially through the three stages, and the predictive value of these categories is not known.

ORAL AND PERIODONTAL MANIFESTATIONS OF HIV INFECTION

Oral lesions are very common in HIV-infected patients.[5,16,21,25,38,62,63,69,79,81] More than 95% of AIDS patients have head and neck lesions,[76] and 55% of AIDS and AIDS-related complex patients have oral lesions.[49] Several reports have identified a strong correlation between HIV infection and oral candidiasis, oral hairy leukoplakia, atypical periodontal diseases, and oral Kaposi's sarcoma.[44,57,85,86]

The relationship between the presence of these oral conditions and HIV infection has been reaffirmed by an international consortium of authorities.[15] This group also added non-Hodgkin's lymphoma to the list of oral lesions strongly associated with HIV infection and recommended a significant modification to the terminology for HIV-related periodontal diseases, as will be discussed later. Oral lesions less strongly associated with HIV infection include melanotic hyperpigmentation, mycobacterial infections, necrotizing ulcerative stomatitis, miscellaneous oral ulcerations, and viral infections (herpes simplex virus, herpes zoster, condyloma acuminatum). Lesions seen in HIV-infected individuals but of undetermined frequency include less common viral infections (cytomegalovirus, molluscum contagiosum); recurrent aphthous stomatitis; and a newly described angiomatous disorder, bacillary angiomatosis (epithelioid angiomatosis).[15,23]

Oral Hairy Leukoplakia

Oral hairy leukoplakia (OHL) occurs in persons with HIV infection.[31] Found on the lateral borders of the tongue, it frequently has a bilateral distribution and may extend to the ventrum. This lesion is characterized by an asymptomatic, poorly demarcated keratotic area ranging in size from a few millimeters to several centimeters (Fig. 15-1). Often there are characteristic vertical striations, imparting a corrugated appearance, or the surface may be shaggy and, when dried, may appear "hairy" (Plate VI*A*). The lesion

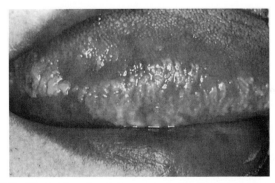

FIGURE 15-1. Hyperkeratotic areas in the lateral border of the tongue in a patient with AIDS.

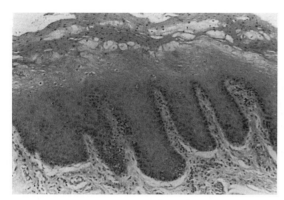

FIGURE 15–2. Microscopic view of hairy leukoplakia.

does not rub off and may resemble other keratotic oral lesions.

Microscopically, the lesion shows a hyperparakeratotic surface with projections that often resemble hairs. Beneath the parakeratotic surface there is some acanthosis and characteristic balloon cells resembling koilocytes (Fig. 15–2). It has been demonstrated that these cells contain virus particles of the human herpesvirus group; these particles have been interpreted as the Epstein-Barr virus (EBV).[31,33] Epithelial dysplasia is not a feature, and in most lesions there is little or no inflammatory infiltrate in the underlying connective tissue.

Hairy leukoplakia is found almost exclusively on the lateral borders of the tongue, although it has been reported on the dorsum of the tongue, the buccal mucosa, the floor of the mouth, the retromolar area, and the soft palate.[17,31,43] In addition, most of these lesions reveal surface colonization by *Candida* organisms, which are secondary invaders and not the cause of the lesion.

OHL was originally believed to be caused by the human papilloma virus, but subsequent evidence suggests that this condition is associated with EBV.[51] In the late 1980s a so-called pseudo-hairy leukoplakia was described in HIV- and EBV-negative individuals who manifested with lesions clinically identical to OHL. In addition, several case reports have described OHL in EBV-infected but HIV-negative individuals suffering from a variety of immunosuppressed conditions (e.g., acute myelogenous leukemia) or who are immunosuppressed as a result of organ transplantation or extensive systemic corticosteroid therapy.[34,42,93] Regardless, biopsy identification of a lesion suggestive of OHL should dictate that HIV testing be performed.

The differential diagnosis of hairy leukoplakia must consider white lesions of the mucosa, which include dysplasia, carcinoma, frictional and idiopathic keratosis, lichen planus, tobacco-related leukoplakia, psoriasiform lesions (e.g., geographic tongue), and hyperplastic candidiasis. However, the microscopic confirmation of hairy leukoplakia of the tongue in a high-risk patient is considered to be a specific early sign of HIV infection and a strong indicator that the patient will develop AIDS.[83] Survival analysis has shown that 83% of HIV-infected patients with hairy leukoplakia develop AIDS within 31 months,[32] and the number of patients with hairy leukoplakia who eventually develop AIDS approaches 100%.[35]

It should be emphasized that the severity of the lesion is not correlated with the likelihood of developing AIDS. Thus, small lesions are as diagnostically significant as extensive lesions.[83]

Oral Candidiasis

Candida, a fungus found in normal oral flora, under certain conditions proliferates in the surface of the oral mucosa. A major factor associated with overgrowth of *Candida* is diminished host resistance, as seen in debilitated patients or in patients receiving immunosuppressive therapy. The incidence of candidal infection has been demonstrated to progressively increase in relationship to diminishing immune competency.[20,41,53,54,81] Most oral candidal infections (85% to 95%) are associated with *Candida albicans,* but other species of *Candida* may be involved.[39]

Candidiasis is the most common oral lesion in HIV diseases and has been found in approximately 90% of AIDS patients.[67] It usually has one of four clinical presentations: pseudomembranous, erythematous, or hyperplastic candidiasis or angular cheilitis.

Pseudomembranous (thrush) candidiasis presents as painless or slightly sensitive white lesions that can be readily scraped and separated from the surface of the oral mucosa. This type is most common on the hard and soft palate.

Erythematous candidiasis may be present as a component of the pseudomembranous type, appearing as red patches on the buccal or palatal mucosa, or it may be associated with depapillation of the tongue (Fig. 15–3).

The *hyperplastic candidiasis* is the least common form and may be seen in the buccal mucosa and tongue. It is more resistant to removal than the other types (Fig. 15–4; Plate VI*D*).

In *angular cheilitis* the commissures appear erythematous with surface crusting and fissuring.

Diagnosis of candidiasis is made by microscopic examination of a tissue sample or smear of material scraped from

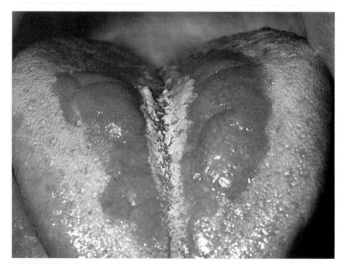

FIGURE 15–3. Depapillation of the tongue. A smear obtained from the tongue was positive for *Candida.*

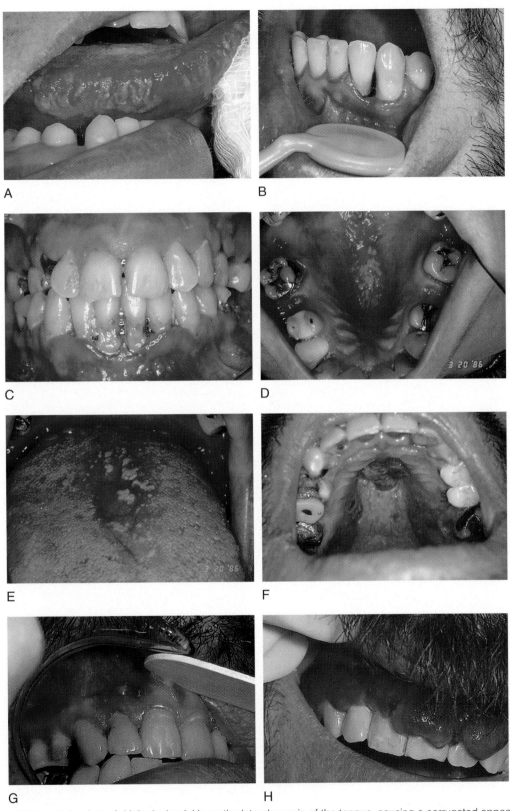

PLATE VI. AIDS and the periodontium. *A,* Hairy leukoplakia on the lateral margin of the tongue, causing a corrugated appearance. *B,* Painless ANUG-like lesion of several months' duration. The patient had a second ANUG-like lesion that was painful. *C–E,* ANUG-like lesion and candidiasis of the palate and tongue in a 29-year-old woman. *F,* Kaposi's sarcoma involving the anterior hard palate and right and left palatal mucosa. Candidiasis is also noted on the hard palate. *G,* Same patient as in *F,* with Kaposi's sarcoma of the labial gingiva presenting as a small purple nodule next to a parulis. *H,* Kaposi's sarcoma involving the anterior facial gingiva and producing a gingival enlargement. (Courtesy of Dr. Frank Lucatorto.)

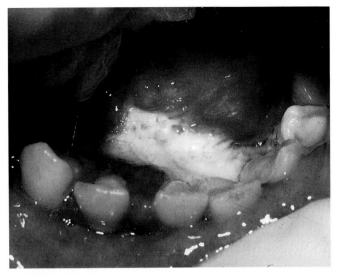

FIGURE 15–4. Large area of mucosal necrosis extending from the lingual gingival tissue onto the floor of the mouth in a 28-year-old patient with AIDS.

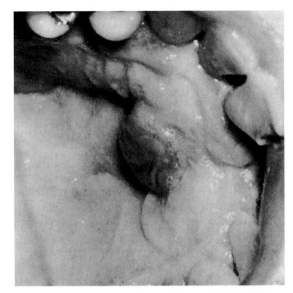

FIGURE 15–6. Kaposi's sarcoma of the palate extending to the gingiva. (Courtesy of Dr. Frank Lucatorto.)

the lesion, which shows hyphae and yeast forms of the organisms. When oral candidiasis appears in patients with no apparent predisposing causes, the clinician should be alerted to the possibility of HIV infection. Many patients at risk for HIV infection who present with oral candidiasis also have esophageal candidiasis, a diagnostic sign of AIDS.[94]

Although candidiasis in HIV-infected patients may respond to antifungal therapy, it is often refractory or recurrent.

Kaposi's Sarcoma

Kaposi's sarcoma (KS) is a rare, multifocal, vascular neoplasm; it was originally described in 1872 as occurring in the skin of the lower extremities of elderly men of Mediterranean origin. Although it is a malignant tumor, in its classic form it is a localized and slowly growing lesion. The KS that occurs in HIV-infected patients presents different clinical features (Figs. 15–5 to 15–7; Plate VIE). In these individuals it is a much more aggressive lesion and

frequently involves the oral mucosa, particularly the palate and the gingiva (see Plate VIH).

In the early stages the oral lesions are painless, reddish purple macules of the mucosa. As the lesions progress, they frequently become nodular and can easily be confused with other oral vascular entities such as hemangioma, hematoma, varicosity, or pyogenic granuloma (when occurring in the gingiva).[84]

Lesions manifest as nodules, papules, or nonelevated macules that are usually brown, blue, or purple in color. On occasion, however, lesions may display normal pigmentation. Diagnosis is based on histologic findings.[45,72,99]

Microscopically, KS consists of four components: endothelial cell proliferation, with the formation of atypical vascular channels; extravascular hemorrhage with hemosiderin deposition; spindle cell proliferation in association with atypical vessels; and a mononuclear inflammatory infiltrate consisting mainly of plasma cells[30] (Fig. 15–8).

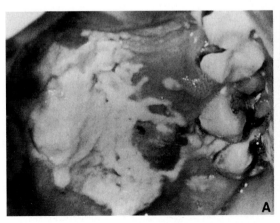
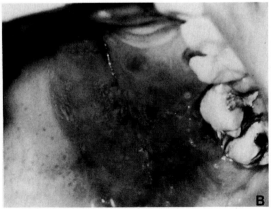

FIGURE 15–5. *A,* Kaposi's sarcoma of the palate and gingiva covered with *Candida. B,* After antifungal therapy, the candidiasis has disappeared, and the underlying sarcoma is more apparent. (Courtesy of Dr. Frank Lucatorto.)

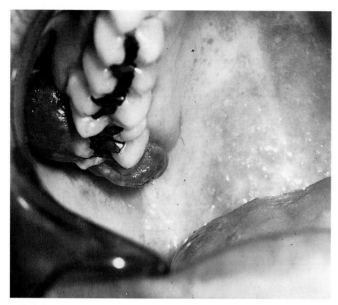

FIGURE 15–7. Kaposi's sarcoma of the gingiva in a 26-year-old man.

Regional and sex differences are becoming apparent as oral KS becomes more common in the United States than in Europe; it is found mainly in homosexual males in California and New York. The male-to-female ratio is 20:1.

The condition has also been reported in patients with lupus erythematosus who are receiving immunosuppressant therapy and in renal transplant patients and other individuals receiving corticosteroid or cyclosporin therapy. Case re-

ports describe gingival KS in HIV-negative patients experiencing cyclosporin-induced gingival enlargement.[70,89] In an HIV-positive individual, the presence of KS signifies transition to outright AIDS.

More than 50% of AIDS patients with KS display oral lesions, and the oral cavity may often be the first or only site of the lesion.[3] The incidence and severity of oral and generalized lesions may increase as CD4+ cells are depleted. Median survival time after onset of KS ranges from 7 to 31 months.[10]

The differential diagnosis of oral KS includes pyogenic granuloma, hemangioma, atypical hyperpigmentation, sarcoidosis, bacillary angiomatosis, angiosarcoma, pigmented nevi, and cat-scratch disease (skin).[72]

Bacillary (Epithelioid) Angiomatosis

Bacillary (epithelioid) angiomatosis (BA) is an infectious vascular proliferative disease with clinical and histologic features very similar to those of KS. BA is believed to be caused by a rickettsia-like organism, *Rochalimaea henselea*.[15,21,24,97] Skin lesions are similar to those seen in KS or cat-scratch disease. Gingival BA manifests as red, purple, or blue edematous soft tissue lesions that may cause destruction of periodontal ligament and bone (Fig. 15–9).

Differentiation of BA from KS is based on biopsy, which reveals an "epithelioid" proliferation of angiogenic cells accompanied by an acute inflammatory cell infiltrate. The causative organism in the biopsy specimen will sometimes react with Warthen-Starry silver stain.

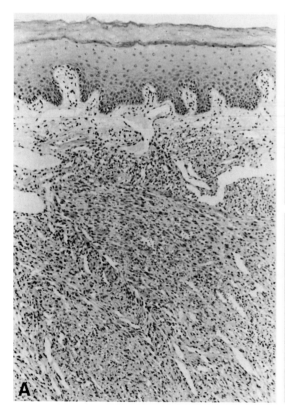

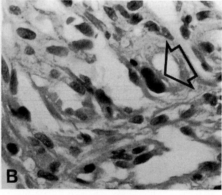

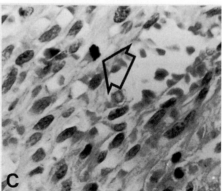

FIGURE 15–8. Kaposi's sarcoma of the palate in a patient with AIDS. *A*, Low-power view of hyperkeratotic epithelium overlying large vascular spaces and a dense tumoral mass. *B*, High-power view showing small blood vessels with occasional large hyperchromatic cells (*arrow*). *C*, High-power view showing dense endothelial cells with occasional mitotic figures (*arrow*). (Courtesy of Dr. Gerald Shklar.)

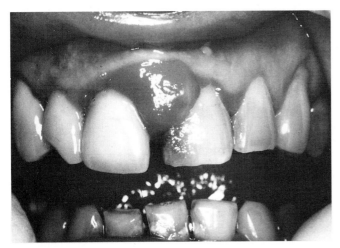

FIGURE 15–9. Bacillary angiomatosis in a 30-year-old HIV-positive male.

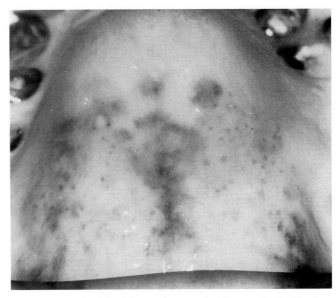

FIGURE 15–11. Palatal hyperpigmentation in a patient with drug-induced adrenocortical insufficiency.

Oral Hyperpigmentation

An increased incidence of oral hyperpigmentation has been described in HIV-infected individuals.[46] Oral pigmented areas often appear as spots or striations on the buccal mucosa, palate, gingiva, or tongue (Figs. 15–10 and 15–11). In some instances the pigmentation may relate to prolonged use of drugs such as ketoconazole and clofazimine.[100] Interestingly, prolonged use of zidovudine is associated with excessive pigmentation of the skin and nails. On occasion the pigmentation may be the result of adrenocorticoid insufficiency induced in an HIV-positive individual by prolonged use of ketoconazole or by *Pneumocystis carinii* infection or cytomegalovirus or other viral infections (see Fig. 15–11).

Atypical Ulcers and Delayed Healing

HIV-infected patients have a higher incidence of recurrent herpetic lesions and aphthous stomatitis (Figs. 15–12 and 15–13). Approximately 10% of HIV-infected patients have herpes infection,[67,91] and multiple episodes are common. Aphthae and aphthae-like lesions are seen in many patients when followed throughout the course of the disease.

In healthy patients these herpetic and aphthous lesions are self-limiting and relatively easy to diagnose by their characteristic clinical features (i.e., herpes on the keratinizing mucosa, aphthae on the non-keratinizing surfaces). In HIV-infected patients the clinical presentation and course of these lesions may be altered. Herpes may involve all mucosal surfaces and extend to the skin and may not heal in the expected 7 to 10 days but persist for months.[18] Currently the CDC includes mucocutaneous herpes present for more than 1 month as a sign of AIDS.[8]

The clinical features so characteristic of aphthae are quickly altered as the lesions persist and present as large, nonspecific, painful ulcers; other types of mucosal ulcers

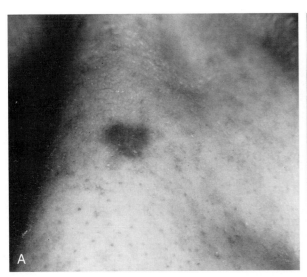

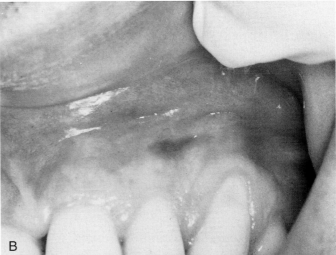

FIGURE 15–10. Oral hyperpigmentation in a 32-year-old AIDS patient with Kaposi's sarcoma of the skin. *A,* Kaposi's sarcoma of the bridge of the nose. *B,* Pigmented lesion of the alveolar mucosa. A biopsy specimen was negative for Kaposi's sarcoma.

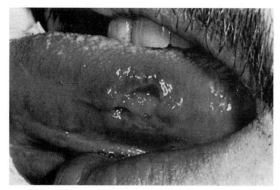

FIGURE 15–12. Ulcerous lesion in the tongue of a patient with AIDS.

may present similar clinical findings. As healing is delayed, these lesions develop secondary infections, often becoming indistinguishable from a persistent herpetic or aphthous lesion. These are probably best described as atypical ulcers.[73]

A wide variety of bacterial and viral infections may produce persistent and severe oral ulcerations in HIV infected individuals. Essentially, immunocompromised individuals are at risk from infectious agents endemic to the patient's geographic location. Atypical or nonhealing ulcers may require biopsy and/or microbial cultures to determine the etiology. Oral ulcerations have been described in association with enterobacterial organisms such as *Klebsiella pneumoniae, Enterobacter cloacae,* and *Escherichia coli.*[73] Such infections are rare and are usually associated with systemic involvement. Specific antibiotic therapy is indicated, and close coordination of oral therapy with the patient's physician is usually necessary.

Herpes simplex virus (HSV) and varicella-zoster virus (VZV) ulcerations may be severe and persistent in immunocompromised individuals. Cytomegalovirus (CMV) infection may produce large, nonhealing, painful oral ulcers, especially in patients with low CD4+ cell counts.[27] The presence of oral CMV-induced ulcers may be indicative of systemic CMV infection.

Recurrent aphthous stomatitis (RAS) has been described in HIV-infected individuals but the overall incidence may be no greater than that in the general population.[15] RAS may occur, however, as a component of the initial acute illness of HIV seroconversion.[55] The incidence of major aphthae may be increased, and the oropharynx, esophagus, or other areas of the gastrointestinal tract may be involved.[1,2]

Adverse Drug Effects

A number of adverse drug-induced effects have been reported in HIV-positive patients, and the dentist may be the first to recognize an oral drug reaction. Foscarnet, interferon, and 2'-3'-dideoxycytidine (DDC) occasionally induce oral ulcerations, and erythema multiforme has been reported with use of didanosine (DDI).[12] Zidovudine and ganciclovir may induce leukopenia and caries, resulting in oral ulcers.[56] Xerostomia and altered taste sensation have been described in conjunction with diethyldithiocarbamate (Dithiocarb). HIV-positive patients are believed to be generally more susceptible to drug-induced mucositis and lichenoid drug reactions than is the general population.[4,12,37,88] In some instances mouth ulcers and mucositis resolve if drug therapy is continued beyond 2 to 3 weeks, but when drug effects are severe or persistent, alternative therapy with different drugs should be used.

Periodontal Disease

Considerable interest has been directed toward the nature and incidence of periodontal diseases in HIV-infected individuals.

HIV Gingivitis. A persistent, linear, easily bleeding, erythematous gingivitis has been described in some HIV-positive patients. This may or may not serve as a precursor to a rapidly progressive necrotizing ulcerative periodontitis (NUP)[64,87,96] (Plate VI*B,C*; Fig. 15–14). Linear gingivitis lesions may be localized or generalized in nature. The erythematous gingivitis may (1) be limited to marginal tissue, (2) extend into attached gingiva in a punctate or a diffuse ery-

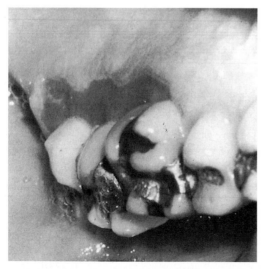

FIGURE 15–13. Nonhealing ulcer in the palatal gingiva of 6 weeks' duration. Biopsy revealed Kaposi's sarcoma. (Courtesy of Dr. Frank Lucatorto.)

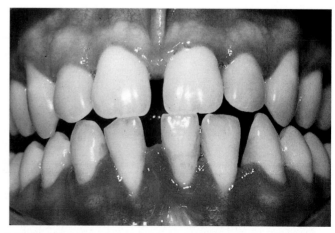

FIGURE 15–14. Marginal gingival erythema of the maxillary gingiva and diffuse erythema of the mandibular attached gingiva in a 28-year-old man. Early necrosis of some of the interdental papillae is seen.

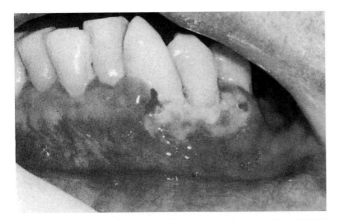

FIGURE 15–15. Acute necrotizing ulcerative gingivitis (ANUG)–like lesion and ulcer involving the facial gingiva. (Courtesy of Dr. Frank Lucatorto.)

thema, or (3) extend into the alveolar mucosa, representing a secondary candidal infection.

HIV-associated erythematous gingivitis is often unresponsive to corrective therapy, yet such lesions may undergo spontaneous remission. The condition was originally called *HIV-gingivitis* (HIV-G) shortly after its recognition, but the term *linear gingival erythema* is currently preferred.

Some reports have described an increased incidence of necrotizing ulcerative gingivitis (NUG) (Fig. 15–15) among HIV-infected individuals, although this has not been substantiated by other studies.[14,28,80,92]

A severely destructive, acutely painful necrotizing ulcerative stomatitis (NUS) has occasionally been reported in HIV-positive patients. NUS is characterized by necrosis of significant areas of oral soft tissue and underlying bone. It may occur separately or as an extension of NUP[15] and is commonly associated with severe depression of CD[+] immune cells.

HIV Periodontitis. A necrotizing, ulcerative, rapidly progressive form of periodontitis occurs more frequently among HIV-positive individuals than in the general population. Terms previously used to describe these lesions are

AIDS virus–associated periodontitis (AVAP) and *HIV-related periodontitis* (HIV-P), but the term *necrotizing ulcerative periodontitis* (NUP) is more appropriate, as such lesions were described long before the onset of the AIDS epidemic.

NUP is characterized by soft tissue necrosis and rapid periodontal destruction that often result in marked interproximal bone loss (Figs. 15–16 and 15–17). Lesions may occur anywhere in the dental arches and are usually localized to a few teeth, although generalized NUP is sometimes present after marked CD4[+] cell depletion. Bone is often exposed, resulting in necrosis and subsequent sequestration. NUP is severely painful at onset, and immediate treatment is necessary. On occasion, however, patients are encountered who have undergone spontaneous resolution of the necrotizing lesions, leaving painless deep interproximal craters that are difficult to clean and may lead to conventional periodontitis.

Some evidence suggests slight differences between the microbial flora found in NUP lesions and that found in chronic periodontitis,[58] but the bulk of data implicate a similar microbial component in both diseases.[28,60,61,78] The microbial flora described in association with linear gingival erythema in HIV-positive patients, however, is more typical of periodontal pockets than of conventional gingivitis.[60,61]

The periodontal health of HIV-infected individuals is subject to wide variations.[98] Riley and associates[77] examined 200 HIV-positive patients and found that 85 were periodontally healthy; none had NUG; 59 were suffering from gingivitis; 54 were experiencing mild, moderate, or advanced periodontitis; and only two had NUP. Using a different approach, Rowland and associates[80] studied 20 patients with NUG and found that seven were HIV positive, and two of those seven had CD4[+] lymphocyte depression (<400/mm³). They concluded that dentists should recognize NUG as a possible early marker for HIV infection. In contrast, Drinkard and associates[14] found no evidence of NUG in 106 HIV-positive individuals; 97 were asymptomatic, and nine exhibited Category B symptoms.

Swango and associates[92] reported early findings among 230 HIV-positive patients with relatively high CD4[+]

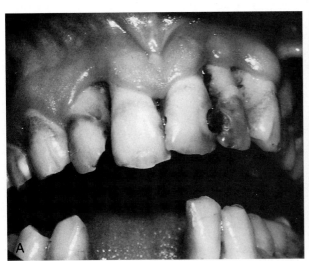
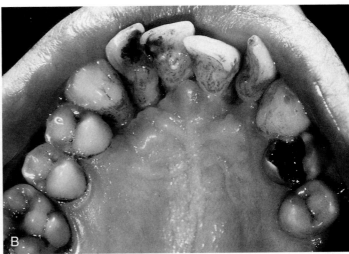

FIGURE 15–16. Necrotizing ulcerative periodontitis in an HIV-negative patient. *A,* Facial view. *B,* Lingual view.

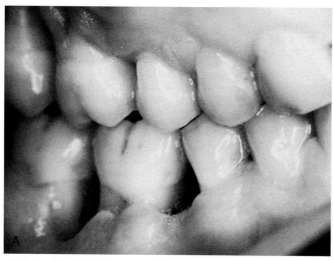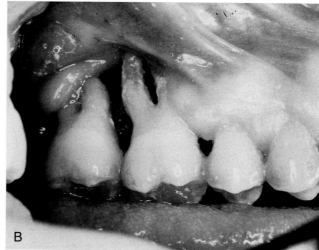

FIGURE 15–17. Necrotizing ulcerative periodontitis in a 30-year-old HIV-positive man. *A,* Mandibular/maxillary posterior facial view. *B,* Facial view of maxillary molars.

counts. They found no correlation between linear gingival erythema and $CD4^+$ T-cell levels in these patients, although 6% experienced NUG-like papillary destruction. Others have reported a relationship between NUP and decreased $CD4^+$ lymphocytes.[50,95] Glick and associates[28] reported on the incidence of periodontal diseases in 700 HIV-positive individuals. They found NUP in only 6.3% but concluded that NUP is a predictive marker for severe immune deficiency, because patients with NUP were 20.8 times as likely to have $CD4^+$ lymphocyte counts $<200/mm^3$.

It can be concluded from these studies that periodontal diseases can occur among HIV-infected patients in all categories, but susceptibility to periodontal infections increases as the immune system becomes more compromised. The majority of HIV-positive individuals experience periodontal disease in a manner similar to the general population. With proper home care and appropriate periodontal treatment and maintenance, HIV-positive individuals can anticipate reasonably good periodontal health throughout the course of their disease. The median period between initial HIV infection and outright AIDS is approximately 10 to 11 years, which means that HIV-infected patients are potential candidates for procedures such as periodontal surgery and implant placement.

Chapter 46 describes in detail the periodontal management of AIDS patients.

REFERENCES

1. Bach MC, Howell DA, Valenti AJ, et al. Aphthous ulceration of the gastrointestinal tract in patients with the acquired immunodeficiency syndrome (AIDS). Ann Intern Med *112:*465–467, 1990.
2. Bach MC, Valenti AJ, Howell DA, Smith TJ. Odynophagia from aphthous ulcers of the pharynx and oesophagus in the acquired immunodeficiency syndrome (AIDS). Ann Intern Med *108:*338–339, 1988.
3. Barrett AP, Bilous AM, Buckley DJ, et al. Clinicopathological presentations of oral Kaposi's sarcoma in AIDS. Aust Dent J *33*(5):395–399, 1988.
4. Bayard PJ, Berger TG, Jacobson MA. Drug hypersensitivity reactions and human immunodeficiency virus disease. J Acq Immune Defic Syn *5*(12):1237–1257, 1992.
5. Brahim JS, Katz RW, Roberts MW. Non-Hodgkin's lymphoma of the hard palate mucosa and buccal gingiva associated with AIDS. J Oral Maxillofac Surg *46:*328–330, 1988.
6. Brockmeyer NH, Kreugfelder E, Martins L, et al. Zidovudine therapy of asymptomatic HIV-1-infected patients and combined zidovudine-acyclovir therapy of HIV-1-infected patients with oral hairy leukoplakia. J Infect Dermatol *92:*647, 1989.
7. Centers for Disease Control. Update on AIDS—United States. MMWR *31:*507–514, 1982.
8. Centers for Disease Control. 1993 Revised classification system for HIV infection and expanded surveillance case definition for AIDS among adolescents and adults. MMWR *41:*RR-17, 1993.
9. Centers for Disease Control. Impact of the expanded AIDS surveillance case definition on AIDS case reporting—United States, first quarter, 1993. MMWR *42:*308–310, 1993.
10. Chachoua A, Krigel R, Lafleur F, et al. Prognostic factors and staging classification of Kaposi's sarcoma. J Clin Oncol *7:*774–780, 1989.
11. Chiasson MA, Stoneburner RL, Joseph SC. Human immunodeficiency virus transmission through artificial insemination. J Acq Immune Defic Syn *3:*69–72, 1990.
12. Coopman SA, Stern RS. Cutaneous drug reactions in human immunodeficiency virus infection. Arch Dermatol *127:*714–717, 1991.
13. DeRienzo B, Mongairdo N, Pellegrino F, et al. Heterosexual transmission of the human immunodeficiency virus: A seroepidemiological study. Arch Dermatol Res *281:*369–372, 1989.
14. Drinkard CR, Decher L, Little JW, et al. Periodontal status of individuals in early stages of human immunodeficiency virus infection. Commun Dent Oral Epidemiol *19:*281–285, 1991.
15. EC-Clearinghouse on Oral Problems Related to HIV Infection and WHO Collaborating Centre on Oral Manifestations of the Immunodeficiency Virus. Classification and diagnostic criteria for oral lesions in HIV infection. J Oral Pathol Med *22:*289–291, 1993.
16. Epstein JB, Silverman S. Head and neck malignancies associated with HIV infection. Oral Surg Oral Med Oral Pathol *73:*193–200, 1992.
17. Eversole LR, Jacobsen P, Stone CE, Freckleton V. Oral condyloma planus (hairy leukoplakia) among homosexual men. A clinico-pathologic study of thirty-six cases. Oral Surg *61:*249, 1986.
18. Eversole LR. Viral infections of the head and neck among HIV-seropositive patients. Oral Surg Oral Med Oral Pathol *73:*155, 1992.
19. Fauci AS, Schnittman SM, Poli G, et al. Immunopathogenic mechanisms in human immunodeficiency virus (HIV) infection. Ann Intern Med *114:*678–693, 1993.
20. Fetter A, Partisani M, Koenig H, et al. Asymptomatic oral *Candida albicans* carriage in HIV-infection: Frequency and predisposing factors. J Oral Pathol Med *22:*57–59, 1993.
21. Ficarra G. Oral lesions of iatrogenic and undefined etiology and neurologic disorders associated with HIV infection. Oral Surg Oral Med Oral Pathol *73:*201–211, 1992.
22. Ficarra G, Berson AM, Silverman S Jr, et al. Kaposi's sarcoma of the oral cavity: A study of 134 patients with a review of the pathogenesis, epidemiology, clinical aspects and treatment. Oral Surg Oral Med Oral Pathol *66:*543–550, 1988.
23. Gaines H, Von Sydow M, Pehrson PO, Lundbergh P. Clinical picture of primary HIV infection presenting as a glandular-fever-like illness. Br Med J *97:*1363–1368, 1988.
24. Glick M, Cleveland DB. Oral mucosal bacillary epithelioid angiomatosis in a patient with AIDS associated with rapid alveolar bone loss: A case report. J Oral Pathol Med *22:*235–239, 1993.
25. Glick M, Garfunkel AA. Common oral findings in two different diseases—

leukemia and AIDS: Part 1. Compend Contin Educ Dent *XIII*(6):432–447, 1992.

26. Glick M, Muzyka BC. Alternative therapies for major aphthous ulcers in AIDS patients. J Am Dent Assoc *123:*61–65, 1992.

27. Glick M, Muzyka BC, Lurie D, Salkin LM. Oral manifestations associated with HIV disease as markers for immune suppression and AIDS. Oral Surg Oral Med Oral Pathol *77:*344–349, 1994.

28. Glick M, Muzyka BC, Salkin LM, Lurie D. Necrotizing ulcerative periodontitis: A marker for immune deterioration and a predictor for the diagnosis of AIDS. J Periodontol. In press.

29. Gorin I, Vilette B, Gehanno P, Escande P. Thalidomide in hyperalgic pharyngeal ulceration of AIDS. Lancet *335:*1343, 1990.

30. Green TS, Beckstead JH, Lozada-Nur F, et al. Histopathologic spectrum of oral Kaposi's sarcoma. Oral Surg *58:*306, 1984.

31. Greenspan D, Conant M, Silverman S Jr, et al. Oral hairy leukoplakia in male homosexuals. Evidence of association with both papilloma virus and a herpesgroup virus. Lancet *2:*831, 1984.

32. Greenspan D, Greenspan JS, Hearst NG, et al. Relations of oral hairy leukoplakia with HIV and the risk of developing AIDS. J Infect Dis *155:*475, 1987.

33. Greenspan JS, Greenspan D, Lennette ET, et al. Replication of Epstein-Barr virus within the epithelial cells of oral hairy leukoplakia, and AIDS associated lesion. N Engl J Med *313:*1564, 1985.

34. Greenspan D, Greenspan JS, de Souza Y, et al. Oral hairy leukoplakia in an HIV-negative renal transplant recipient. J Oral Pathol Med *18:*32–34, 1989.

35. Greenspan D, Pindborg JJ, Greenspan JS, Schiodt M. AIDS and the Mouth. Copenhagen, Munksgaard, 1990.

36. Gupta G. Viral pathogenesis and opportunistic infections. CDA J *21*(9):29–36, 1993.

37. Harb GE, Alldredge BK, Coleman R, Jacobson MA. Pharmacoepidemiology of adverse drug reactions in hospitalized patients with human immunodeficiency virus disease. J Acq Immune Defic Syn *6:*919–926, 1993.

38. Haring JI. Oral manifestations of HIV infection, part I. Compend Contin Educ Dent *XI*(3):150–154, 1990.

39. Hauman CHJ, Thompson IOC, Theunissen F, Wolfaardt P. Oral carriage of *Candida* in healthy and HIV-seropositive persons. Oral Surg Oral Med Oral Pathol *76:*570–572, 1993.

40. Imagawa DT, Lee MH, Wolinsky SM, et al. Human immunodeficiency virus type 1 infection in homosexual men who remain seronegative for prolonged periods. N Engl J Med *320:*1458–1462, 1989.

41. Imam N, Carpenter CCJ, Mayer KH, et al. Hierarchical pattern of mucosal candida infections in HIV-seropositive women. Am J Med *89:*142–146, 1990.

42. Itin P, Rufli T, Huser B, Rudlinger R. Orale Haarleukoplakie bei Nierentransplantierten Patienten. Hautarzt *42:*487–491, 1991.

43. Kabani S, Greenspan D, DeSouza YD, et al. Oral hairy leukoplakia with extensive oral mucosal involvement: Report of two cases. Oral Surg Oral Med Oral Pathol *67:*411, 1989.

44. Klein RS, Harris CA, Small CB, et al. Oral candidiasis in high-risk patients as the initial manifestation of the acquired immunodeficiency syndrome. N Engl J Med *311:*354–358, 1984.

45. Kuntz AA, Gelderblum HR, Reichart PA. Ultrastructural findings on oral Kaposi's sarcoma (AIDS). J Oral Pathol *16:*372–379, 1987.

46. Langford A, Pohle HD, Gelderblum HR, et al. Oral hyperpigmentation in HIV-infected patients. Oral Surg Oral Med Oral Pathol *67:*301–307, 1989.

47. Leaf AN, Laubenstein LJ, Raphael B, et al. Thrombotic thrombocytopenic purpura associated with human immunodeficiency virus type I (HIV-1) infection. Ann Intern Med *109:*194–197, 1988.

48. Lindhardt BO, Ulrich K, Sindrup JH, et al. Seroconversion to human immunodeficiency virus (HIV) in persons attending an STD clinic in Copenhagen. Acta Derm Venereol (Stockh) *68:*250–253, 1988.

49. Lozada-Nur F, Silverman S Jr, Migliorati C, et al. The diagnosis of AIDS and AIDS related complex in the dental office, findings in 171 homosexual males. Calif Dent Assoc J *12:*21, 1984.

50. Lucht E, Helmdahl A, Nord CE. Periodontal disease in HIV-infected patients in relation to lymphocyte subsets and specific micro-organisms. J Clin Periodontol *18:*252–256, 1991.

51. Madinier I, Doglio A, Cagnon L, et al. Epstein-Barr virus DNA detection in gingival tissues of patients undergoing surgical extractions. Brit J Oral Maxillofac Surg *30:*237–243, 1992.

52. Marmor M, Krasinski K, Sanchez M, et al. Sex, drugs, and HIV infection in a New York city hospital outpatient population. J Acq Immune Defic Syn *3:*307–318, 1990.

53. McCarthy GM. Host factors associated with HIV-related oral candidiasis. Oral Surg Oral Med Oral Pathol *73:*181–186, 1992.

54. McCarthy GM, Mackie ID, Koval J, et al. Factors associated with increased frequency of HIV-related oral candidiasis. J Oral Pathol Med *20:*332–336, 1991.

55. McLeod AW. Dermatologic manifestations of AIDS. Med (North Am) *32:*4448–4454, 1986.

56. Medical Letter. Drugs for AIDS and associated infections. Med Lett *35:*79–86, 1993.

57. Melnick SL, Engel D, Truelove E, et al. Oral mucosal lesions: Association with the presence of antibodies to the human immunodeficiency virus. Oral Surg Oral Med Oral Pathol *68:*37–43, 1989.

58. Moore LVH, Moore WEC, Riley C, et al. Periodontal microflora of HIV-positive subjects with gingivitis or adult periodontitis. J Periodontol *64*(1):48–56, 1993.

59. Mulligan R. The changing profile of the HIV/AIDS epidemic. CDA J *21*(9):23–28, 1993.

60. Murray PA, Grassi M, Winkler JR. The microbiology of HIV-associated periodontal lesions. J Clin Periodontol *16:*636–642, 1989.

61. Murray PA, Winkler JR, Peros WJ, et al. DNA probe detection of periodontal pathogens in HIV-associated periodontal lesions. Oral Microbial Immunol *6:*34–40, 1991.

62. Navazesh M, Lucatorto F. Common oral lesions associated with HIV infection. CDA J *21*(9):37–42, 1993.

63. Oda D, McDougal L, Fritsche T, Worthington P. Oral histoplasmosis as a presenting disease in acquired immunodeficiency syndrome. Oral Surg Oral Med Oral Pathol *70:*631–636, 1990.

64. Overholser CD Jr. Significance of gingivitis in medically compromised patients. Am J Dent *2:*295–298, 1989.

65. Piliero PJ. HIV and hepatitis coinfection. AIDS Clin Care *5:*93–95, 102, 1993.

66. Pindborg JJ. Global aspects of the AIDS epidemic. Oral Surg Oral Med Oral Pathol *73:*138–141, 1992.

67. Phelan JA, Saltzman BR, Friedland GH, Klein RS. Oral findings in patients with acquired immuno-deficiency syndrome. Oral Surg *64:*50, 1987.

68. Plemons JM, Rees TD, Zachariah NY. Absorption of a topical steroid and evaluation of adrenal suppression in patients with erosive lichen planus. Oral Surg Oral Med Oral Pathol *69:*688–693, 1990.

69. Porter SR, Luker J, Scully C, et al. Orofacial manifestions of a group of British patients infected with HIV-1. J Oral Pathol Med *18:*47–48, 1989.

70. Qunibi WY, Akhtar M, Ginn E, Smith P. Kaposi's sarcoma in cyclosporine-induced gingival hyperplasia. Am J Kidney Dis *11:*349–352, 1988.

71. Rahman MA, Kingsley LA, Breinig MK, et al. Enhanced antibody responses to Epstein-Barr virus in HIV-infected homosexual men. J Infect Dis *159:*472–479, 1989.

72. Regezi JA, MacPhail LA, Daniels TE, et al. Oral Kaposi's sarcoma: A 10-year retrospective histopathologic study. J Oral Pathol Med *22:*292–297, 1993.

73. Reichart PA. Oral ulceration and iatrogenic disease in HIV infection. Oral Surg Oral Med Oral Pathol *73:*212–214, 1992.

74. Reichart PA, Langford A, Gelderblom HR, et al. Oral hairy leukoplakia: Observations in 95 cases and review of the literature. J Oral Pathol Med *18:*410–415, 1989.

75. Relman AS. Pathogenic human retroviruses. N Engl J Med *318:*243–246, 1988.

76. Richards JM. Notes on AIDS. Br Dent J *158:*199, 1985.

77. Riley C, London JP, Burmeister JA. Periodontal health in 200 HIV-positive patients. J Oral Pathol Med *21:*124–127, 1992.

78. Robinson P. Periodontal diseases and HIV infection. J Clin Periodontol *19:*609–614, 1992.

79. Rosenstein DL, Chiodo GT, Bartley MH. Unusual presentation of non-Hodgkin's lymphoma in a patient with HIV. Gen Dent *41:*40–42, 1992.

80. Rowland RW, Escobar MR, Friedman RB, Kaplowitz LG. Painful gingivitis may be an early sign of infection with the human immunodeficiency virus. Clin Infect Dis *16*(2):233–236, 1993.

81. Royce RA, Luckmann RS, Fusaro RE, Winkelstein W Jr. The natural history of HIV-1 infection: Staging classifications of disease. AIDS *5:*355–364, 1991.

82. Safai B, Diaz B, Schwartz J. Malignant neoplasms associated with human immunodeficiency virus infection. AIDS Patient Care *October:*262–274, 1993.

83. Schiodt M, Greenspan D, Daniels TE, Greenspan JS. Clinical and histologic spectrum of oral hairy leukoplakia. Oral Surg Oral Med Oral Pathol *64:*716–720, 1987.

84. Sciubba JJ. Recognizing the oral manifestations of AIDS. Oncology *6:*64, 1992.

85. Schulten EAJM, ten Kate RW, van der Waal I. Oral manifestations of HIV infection in 75 Dutch patients. J Oral Pathol Med *18:*42–46, 1989.

86. Schulten EAJM, ten Kate RW, van der Waal I. Oral findings in HIV-infected patients attending a department of internal medicine: The contribution of intraoral examination towards the clinical management of HIV disease. Q J Med New Series *76*(279):741–745, 1990.

87. Scully C, Epstein JB, Porter S, Luker J. Recognition of oral lesions of HIV infection. Part 3. Gingival and periodontal disease and less common lesions. Br Dent J *169:*370–372, 1990.

88. Scully C, McCarthy G. Management of oral health in persons with HIV infection. Oral Surg Oral Med Oral Pathol *73:*215–225, 1992.

89. Siegal B, Levinton-Kriss S, Schiffer A, et al. Kaposi's sarcoma in immunosuppression. Possibly the result of a dual viral infection. Cancer *65:*492–498, 1990.

90. Silverman S. Color Atlas of Oral Manifestations of AIDS. Toronto, Decker, 1989.

91. Silverman S Jr, Migliorati CA, Lozada-Nur F, et al. Oral findings in people with or at risk for AIDS: A study of 375 homosexual males. J Am Dent Assoc *112:*187, 1986.

92. Swango PA, Kleinman DV, Konzelman JL. HIV and periodontal health. A study of military personnel with HIV. J Am Dent Assoc *122:*49–54, 1991.

93. Syrjanen S, Laine P, Niemela M, Happonen R-P. Oral hairy leukoplakia is not a specific sign of HIV-infection but related to immunosuppression in general. J Oral Pathol Med *18:*28–31, 1989.

94. Tavitian A, Raufman J-P, Rosenthal LE. Oral candidiasis as a marker for esophageal candidiasis in the acquired immuno-deficiency syndrome. Ann Intern Med *104:*54, 1986.

95. Tenenbaum HC, Mock D, Simor AE. Periodontitis as an early presentation of HIV infection. Can Med Assoc J *144*(10):1265–1269, 1991.

96. Tukutuku K, Muyembe-Tamfum L, Kayembe K, et al. Prevalence of dental caries, gingivitis, and oral hygiene in hospitalized AIDS cases in Kinshasa, Zaire. J Oral Pathol Med *19:*271–272, 1990.

97. Welch DF, Pickett DA, Slater LN, et al. *Rochalimaea henselae* sp. nov., a cause of septicemia, bacillary angiomatosis and parenchymal bacillary peliosis. J Clin Microbiol *30:*275–280, 1992.

98. Yeung SCH, Stewart GJ, Cooper DA, Sindhusake D. Progression of periodontal disease in HIV seropositive patients. J Periodontol *64*(7):651–657, 1993.

99. Zhang X, Langford A, Gelderblom H, Reichart P. Ultrastructural findings in clinically uninvolved oral mucosa of patients with HIV infection. J Oral Pathol Med *18:*35–41, 1989.

100. Zhang X, Langford A, Gelderblom H, Reichart P. Ultrastructural findings in oral hyperpigmentation of HIV-infected patients. J Oral Pathol Med *18:* 471–474, 1989.

Section Four

Periodontal Pathology

MMP = Metal Matrix Proteases?

16

Gingival Inflammation

FERMIN A. CARRANZA, Jr. and JOHN W. RAPLEY

Inflammation itself produces collagenase — the one thing its trying to overcome.

Stage I Gingivitis: The Initial Lesion
Stage II Gingivitis: The Early Lesion
Stage III Gingivitis: The Established Lesion
Stage IV Gingivitis: The Advanced Lesion

Pathologic changes in gingivitis are associated with the presence of microorganisms in the gingival sulcus (see Chapters 6 and 7). These organisms are capable of synthesizing products (e.g., collagenase, hyaluronidase, protease, chondroitin sulfatase, or endotoxin[9,48]) that cause damage to epithelial and connective tissue cells and to intercellular constituents, such as collagen, ground substance, and glycocalyx (cell coat). The resultant widening of the spaces between the junctional epithelial cells during early gingivitis may permit injurious agents derived from bacteria or bacteria themselves[43] to gain access to the connective tissue.

Microbial products activate monocytes and macrophages to produce vasoactive substances such as prostaglandin E_2, interferon, tumor necrosis factor, or interleukin-1.[25,35]

The sequence of events in the development of gingivitis is analyzed in three different stages (Table 16–1).[38] Obviously, one stage evolves into the next, with no clear-cut dividing lines.

STAGE I GINGIVITIS: THE INITIAL LESION

no clinical signs, just histological

The first manifestations of gingival inflammation are vascular changes consisting essentially of dilation of capillaries and increased blood flow. Clinically, this initial response of the gingiva to bacterial plaque (*subclinical gingivitis*[27]) is not apparent.

dilation; permeability, hyperemia

Microscopically, some classic features of acute inflammation can be seen in the connective tissue beneath the junctional epithelium. Changes in blood vessel morphologic features[10,11,50] (e.g., widening of capillaries and venules) and adherence of neutrophils to vessel walls (margination) occur within 1 week and sometimes as early as 2 days after plaque has been allowed to accumulate[19,39] (Fig. 16–1). Leukocytes, mainly polymorphonuclear neutrophils (PMNs),

leave the capillaries by migrating through the walls (diapedesis, emigration)[29,42,52] (Fig. 16–2). They can be seen in increased quantities in the connective tissue, the junctional epithelium, and the gingival sulcus (Figs. 16–3 and 16–4).[2,3,26,34,39,45,46] Exudation of fluid from the gingival sulcus[17] and extravascular serum proteins are present.[22,23]

Subtle changes can also be detected in the junctional epithelium and the perivascular connective tissue at this early stage. Lymphocytes soon begin to accumulate (see Fig. 16–3D). The increase in the migration of leukocytes and their accumulation within the gingival sulcus may be correlated with an increase in the flow of gingival fluid into the sulcus.[4]

The character and intensity of the host response determines whether the initial lesion resolves rapidly, with restoration of the tissue to a normal state, or evolves into a chronic inflammatory lesion. If the latter occurs, an infiltrate of macrophages and lymphoid cells appears within a few days.

STAGE II GINGIVITIS: THE EARLY LESION

clinical signs

As time goes on, clinical signs of erythema may appear, mainly owing to the proliferation of capillaries and increased formation of capillary loops between rete pegs or ridges. Bleeding on probing may also be evident.[1]

Microscopic examination of the gingiva reveals a leukocyte infiltration in the connective tissue beneath the junctional epithelium consisting primarily of lymphocytes (75%, with the majority of them T cells),[39,46] but also composed of some migrating neutrophils, as well as macrophages, plasma cells, and mast cells. All the changes seen in the initial lesion continue to intensify.[16,28,31,39,47] The junc-

Periostat = enzyme suppressor (stops collagenase)

Table 16-1. STAGES OF GINGIVITIS

Stage	Time (Days)	Blood Vessels	Junctional and Sulcular Epithelium	Predominant Immune Cells	Collagen	Clinical Findings
I. Initial Lesion	2–4	Vascular dilation Vasculitis	Infiltrated by PMNs	PMNs	Perivascular loss	Gingival fluid flow
II. Early Lesion	4–7	Vascular proliferation	Same as Stage I Rete peg formation Atrophic areas	Lymphocytes	Increased loss around infiltrate	Erythema Bleeding on probing
III. Established Lesion	14–21	Same as Stage II, plus blood stasis	Same as Stage II but more advanced	Plasma cells	Continued loss	Changes in color, size, texture, etc.

PMNs, Polymorphonuclear leukocytes.

tional epithelium becomes densely infiltrated with neutrophils, as does the gingival sulcus, and the junctional epithelium starts to show development of rete pegs or ridges.

There is an increase in the amount of collagen destruction[12,28,47]; 70% of the collagen is destroyed around the cellular infiltrate. The main fiber groups affected appear to be the circular and dentogingival fiber assemblies. Alterations in blood vessel morphologic features and vascular bed patterns have also been described.[19,21]

Cementum & bone = 90% protein

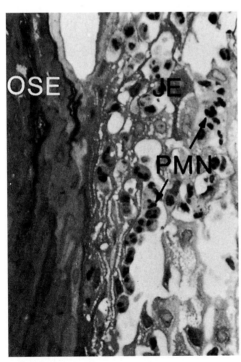

FIGURE 16-1. Human biopsy, experimental gingivitis. After 4 days of plaque accumulation, the blood vessels immediately adjacent to the junctional epithelium (JE) are distended and contain polymorphonuclear leukocytes (PMNs). Neutrophils have also migrated between the cells of the junctional epithelium. OSE, oral sulcular epithelium. ×500. (From Payne WA, Page RC, Ogilvie AL, et al. Histopathologic features of the initial and early stages of experimental gingivitis in man. J Periodont Res *10*:51, 1975. ©1975 Munksgaard International Publisher LTD., Copenhagen, Denmark.)

*acute = 24 hrs.
longer is chronic*

PMNs that have left the blood vessels in response to chemotactic stimuli from plaque components travel to the epithelium, cross the basement lamina, and are found in the epithelium and emerging in the pocket area (see Fig. 16-2). PMNs are attracted to bacteria and engulf them in a process of phagocytosis (Fig. 16-5). PMNs release their lysosomes in association with the ingestion of bacteria.[24] Fibroblasts show cytotoxic alterations[38] with a decreased capacity for collagen production.

STAGE III GINGIVITIS: THE ESTABLISHED LESION

vessels become engorged & congested.

In chronic gingivitis (stage III), the blood vessels become engorged and congested, venous return is impaired, and the blood flow becomes sluggish. The result is localized gingival anoxemia, which superimposes a somewhat bluish hue on the reddened gingiva.[18] Extravasation of red blood cells into the connective tissue and breakdown of hemoglobin into its component pigments can also deepen the color of the chronically inflamed gingiva.

The established lesion can be described clinically as moderately to severely inflamed gingiva.

In histologic sections an intense, chronic inflammatory reaction is observed. Several detailed cytologic studies have been carried out on chronically inflamed gingiva.[13,15,16,37,44,49,51] A key feature that differentiates the established lesion from the early lesion is the increase in the number of plasma cells, which become the preponderant inflammatory cell type. Plasma cells invade the connective tissue not only immediately below the junctional epithelium, but also deep into the connective tissue, around blood vessels, and between bundles of collagen fibers; extravascular immunoglobulins are present in the connective tissue and junctional epithelium.[7] The junctional epithelium reveals widened intercellular spaces filled with granular cellular debris, including lysosomes derived from disrupted neutrophils, lymphocytes, and monocytes (Fig. 16-6). The lysosomes contain acid hydrolases that can destroy tissue components. The junctional epithelium develops rete pegs or ridges that protrude into the connective tissue, and the basal lamina is destroyed in some areas. In the connective tissue, collagen

localized passive hyperemia

SPPD - Slow progressive periodontal disease

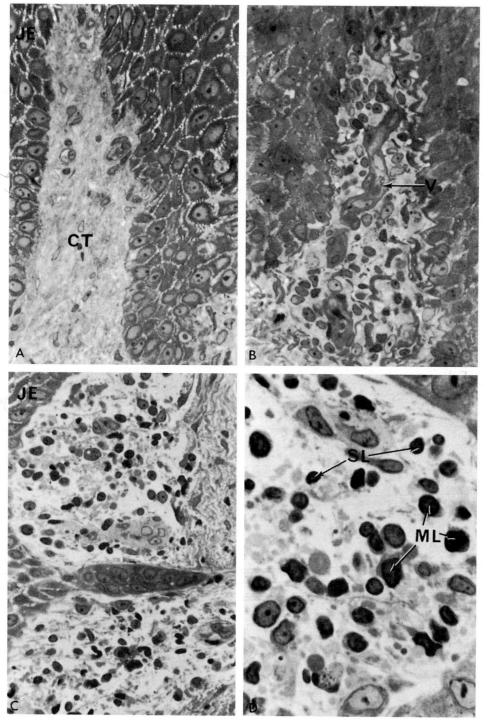

FIGURE 16–2. Human biopsy, experimental gingivitis. *A,* Control biopsy specimen from a patient with good oral hygiene and no detectable plaque accumulation. The junctional epithelium (JE) is at the left. The connective tissue (CT) shows few cells other than fibroblasts, blood vessels, and a dense background of collagen fibers. ×500. *B,* Biopsy specimen taken after 8 days of plaque accumulation. The connective tissue is infiltrated with inflammatory cells, which displace the collagen fibers. A distended blood vessel (V) is seen in the center. ×500. *C,* After 8 days of plaque accumulation, the connective tissue next to the junctional epithelium (JE) at the base of the sulcus shows a mononuclear cell infiltrate and evidence of collagen degeneration (clear spaces around cellular infiltrate). ×500. *D,* The inflammatory cell infiltrate at higher magnification. After 8 days of plaque accumulation, numerous small lymphocytes (SL) and medium size lymphocytes (ML) are seen within the connective tissue. Most of the collagen fibers around these cells have disappeared, presumably as a result of enzymatic digestion. ×1250. (From Payne WA, Page RC, Ogilvie AL, et al. Histopathologic features of the initial and early stages of experimental gingivitis in man. J Periodont Res *10:*51, 1975. ©1975 Munksgaard International Publisher LTD., Copenhagen, Denmark.)

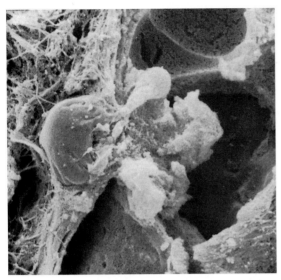

FIGURE 16-3. Scanning electron micrograph showing a leukocyte traversing the vessel wall to enter into the gingival connective tissue.

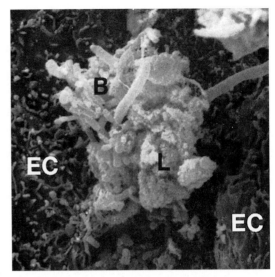

FIGURE 16-5. Scanning electron micrograph of a leukocyte (L) emerging into a pocket wall and covered with bacteria (B) and extracellular lysosomes. EC, Epithelial cells.

remember

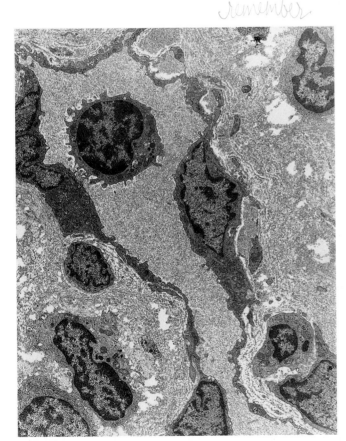

FIGURE 16-4. Early human gingivitis lesion. Area of lamina propria subjacent to the crevicular epithelium showing a capillary with several extravascular lymphocytes and one lymphocyte within the lumen. The specimen also exhibits considerable loss of perivascular collagen density. ×2500. (Courtesy of Dr. Charles Cobb.)

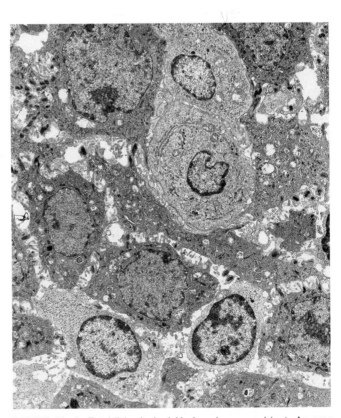

FIGURE 16-6. Established gingivitis in a human subject. An area of crevicular epithelium exhibiting enlarged intercellular spaces with numerous microvilli and desmosomal junctions. Several lymphocytes, both small and large, are seen migrating through the epithelial layer. ×3000. (Courtesy of Dr. Charles Cobb.)

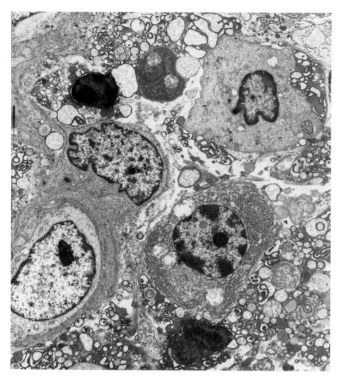

FIGURE 16–7. Advanced gingivitis in a human subject. Specimen from the lamina propria exhibiting plasma cell degeneration with abundant cellular debris visible. ×3000. (Courtesy of Dr. Charles Cobb.)

fibers are destroyed around the infiltrate of intact and disrupted plasma cells, neutrophils, lymphocytes, monocytes, and mast cells (Fig. 16–7).

There appears to be an inverse relationship between the number of intact collagen bundles and the number of inflammatory cells.[49] Collagenolytic activity is increased in inflamed gingival tissue[14] by the enzyme collagenase. Collagenase is normally present in gingival tissues[6] and is produced by some oral bacteria and by PMNs.

Enzyme histochemistry studies have shown that chronically inflamed gingiva has elevated levels of acid and alkaline phosphatase,[53] β-glucuronidase, β-glucosidase, β-galactosidase, esterases,[30] aminopeptidase,[33,40] cytochrome oxidase,[8] elastase,[20] lactic dehydrogenase, and aryl sulfatase,[22] all of which result from bacterial and tissue destruction. Neutral mucopolysaccharide levels are decreased,[51] presumably as a result of degradation of the ground substance.

STAGE IV GINGIVITIS: THE ADVANCED LESION

Extension of the lesion into alveolar bone characterizes a fourth stage that has been named the *advanced lesion*[37] or *phase of periodontal breakdown.*[28] This is described in detail in Chapters 22 and 23.

REFERENCES

1. Amato R, Caton J, Polson A, Espeland M. Interproximal gingival inflammation related to the conversion of a bleeding to a nonbleeding state. J Periodontol 57:63, 1986.
2. Attstrom R. Studies on neutrophil polymorphonuclear leukocytes at the dentogingival junction in gingival health and disease. J Periodont Res 8(suppl):6, 1971.
3. Attstrom R. The roles of gingival epithelium and phagocytosing leukocytes in gingival defense. J Clin Periodontol 2:25, 1975.
4. Attstrom R, Egelberg J. Emigration of blood neutrophils and monocytes into the gingival crevices. J Periodont Res 5:48, 1970.
5. Baehni P, Tsai CC, Taichman NS, McArthur W. Interaction of inflammatory cells and oral microorganisms. TEM and biochemical study on the mechanisms of release of lysosomal constituents of human PMN leukocytes exposed to dental plaque. J Periodont Res 13:333, 1978.
6. Beutner EH, Triftshauser C, Hazen SP. Collagenase activity of gingival tissue from patients with periodontal disease. Proc Soc Exp Biol Med 121:1082, 1966.
7. Brecx M. Histophysiology and histopathology of the gingiva. J West Soc Periodontol 39:33, 1991.
8. Burstone MS. Histochemical study of cytochrome oxidase in normal and inflamed gingiva. Oral Surg 13:1501, 1960.
9. Caffesse RG, Nasjleti C. Enzymatic penetration through intact sulcular epithelium. J Periodontol 47:391, 1976.
10. Egelberg J. Permeability of the dentogingival blood vessels. III. Chronically inflamed gingivae. J Periodont Res 1:287, 1966.
11. Egelberg J. The topography and permeability of vessels at the dentogingival junction in dogs. J Periodont Res 1(suppl):2, 1967.
12. Flieder DE, Sun CN. Chemistry of normal and inflamed human gingival tissues. Periodontics 4:302, 1966.
13. Freedman HL, Listgarten MA, Taichman NS. Electron microscopic features of chronically inflamed human gingiva. J Periodont Res 3:313, 1968.
14. Fullmer H, Gibson W. Collagenolytic activity in gingivae of man. Nature 209:728, 1966.
15. Garant PR, Mulvihill JE. The fine structure of gingivitis in the beagle. III. Plasma cell infiltration of the subepithelial connective tissue. J Periodont Res 7:161, 1971.
16. Gavin JR. Ultrastructural features of chronic marginal gingivitis. J Periodont Res 5:19, 1970.
17. Hancock E, Cray R, O'Leary T. The relationship between gingival crevicular fluid and gingival inflammation. A clinical and histologic study. J Periodontol 50:13, 1979.
18. Hanioka T, Shizukuishi S, Tsunemitsu A. Changes in hemoglobin concentration and oxygen saturation in human gingiva with decreasing inflammation. J Periodontol 62:366, 1991.
19. Hock J, Nuki K. A vital microscopy study of the morphology of normal and inflamed gingiva. J Periodont Res 6:81, 1971.
20. Huynh C, Roch-Arveiller M, Meyer J, Giroud J. Gingival crevicular fluid of patients with gingivitis or periodontal disease: Evaluation of elastase-a1 proteinase inhibitor complex. J Clin Periodontol 19:187, 1992.
21. Kindlova M. Changes in the vascular bed of the marginal periodontium in periodontitis. J Dent Res 44:456, 1965.
22. Lamster I, Hartley L, Vogel R. Development of a biochemical profile for gingival crevicular fluid. Methodological considerations and evaluation of collagen-degrading and ground substance–degrading enzyme activity during experimental gingivitis. J Periodontol Special Issue:13, 1985.
23. Lamster I, Vogel R, Hartley L, et al. Lactate dehydrogenase, b-glucuronidase and arylsulfatase activity in gingival fluid associated with experimental gingivitis in man. J Periodontol 56:139, 1985.
24. Lange D, Schroeder HE. Cytochemistry and ultrastructure of gingival sulcus cells. Helv Odontol Acta 15(suppl 6):65, 1971.
25. Lindemann R, Economou J. *Actinobacillus actinomycetemcomitans* and *Bacteroides gingiovalis* activate human peripheral monocytes to produce interleukin-1 and tumor necrosis factor. J Periodontol 59:728, 1988.
26. Levy BM, Taylor AC, Bernick S. Relationship between epithelium and connective tissue in gingival inflammation. J Dent Res 48:625, 1969.
27. Lindhe J, Hamp SE, Löe H. Experimental periodontitis in the beagle dog. J Periodont Res 8:1, 1973.
28. Lindhe J, Schroeder HE, Page RC, et al. Clinical and stereologic analysis of the course of early gingivitis in dogs. J Periodont Res 9:314, 1974.
29. Lindhe J, Socransky SS. Chemotaxis and vascular permeability produced by human periodontopathic bacteria. J Periodont Res 14:138, 1979.
30. Lisanti VF. Hydrolytic enzymes in periodontal tissues. Ann NY Acad Sci 85:461, 1960.
31. Listgarten MA, Ellegaard B. Experimental gingivitis in rhesus monkeys. J Periodont Res 8:199, 1973.
32. Löe H, Theilade E, Jensen S. Experimental gingivitis in man. J Periodontol 36:177, 1965.
33. Mori M, Kishiro A. Histochemical observation of aminopeptidase activity in the normal and inflamed oral epithelium. J Osaka Univ Dent Sch 1:39, 1961.
34. Oliver RC, Holm-Pedersen P, Löe H. The correlation between clinical scoring, exudate measurements, and microscopic evaluation of inflammation of the gingiva. J Periodontol 40:201, 1969.

35. Page RC. The role of inflammatory mediators in the pathogenesis of periodontal disease. J Periodont Res 26:230, 1991.
36. Page RC. Host response testing for diagnosing periodontal disease. J Periodontol 63:356, 1992.
37. Page RC, Ammons WF, Simpson DM. Host tissue response in chronic inflammatory periodontal disease. IV. The periodontal and dental status of a group of aged great apes. J Periodontol 46:144, 1975.
38. Page RC, Schroeder HE. Pathogenic mechanisms. In Schluger S, Youdelis R, Page RC, eds. Periodontal Disease: Basic Phenomena, Clinical Management and Restorative Interrelationships. Philadelphia, Lea & Febiger, 1977.
39. Payne WA, Page RC, Ogilvie AL, Hall WB. Histopathologic features of the initial and early stages of experimental gingivitis in man. J Periodont Res 10:51, 1975.
40. Quintarelli G. Histochemistry of gingiva. III. The distribution of aminopeptidase in normal and inflammatory conditions. Arch Oral Biol 2:271, 1960.
41. Rizzo AA, Mergenhagen SE. Host responses in periodontal disease. In Proceedings of the International Conference on Research on the Biology of Periodontal Disease, Chicago, June 12–15, 1977.
42. Saglie R, Newman MG, Carranza FA Jr. Scanning electron microscopy study of the interaction of leukocytes and bacteria in human periodontitis. J Periodontol 53:752, 1982.
43. Saglie R, Newman MG, Carranza FA Jr, Pattison GL. Bacterial invasion of gingiva in advanced periodontitis in humans. J Periodontol 53:217, 1982.
44. Schectman LR, Ammons WF, Simpson DM, Page RC. Host tissue response in chronic periodontal disease. II. Histologic features of the normal periodontium, and histopathologic and ultrastructural manifestations of disease in the marmoset. J Periodont Res 7:195, 1972.
45. Schroeder HE. Transmigration and infiltration of leucocytes in human junctional epithelium. Helv Odontol Acta 17:6, 1973.
46. Schroeder HE, Graf de Beer M, Attstrom R. Initial gingivitis in dogs. J Periodont Res 10:128, 1975.
47. Schroeder HE, Munzell-Pedrazzoli S, Page RC. Correlated morphological and biochemical analysis of gingival tissue in early chronic gingivitis in man. Arch Oral Biol 18:899, 1973.
48. Schwartz J, Stinson F, Parker R. The passage of bacterial endotoxin across intact gingival crevicular epithelium. J Periodontol 43:270, 1972.
49. Simpson DM, Avery BE. Histopathologic and ultrastructural features of inflamed gingiva in the baboon. J Periodontol 45:500, 1974.
50. Soderholm G, Egelberg J. Morphological changes in gingival blood vessels during developing gingivitis in dogs. J Periodont Res 8:16, 1973.
51. Thilander H. Epithelial changes in gingivitis. An electron microscopic study. J Periodont Res 3:303, 1968.
52. Wennstrom J, Heijl L, Lindhe J, Socransky SS. Migration of gingival leukocytes mediated by plaque bacteria. J Periodont Res 15:363, 1980.
53. Winer RA, O'Donnell LS, Chauncey HH, et al. Enzyme activity in periodontal disease. J Periodontol 41:449, 1970.

17

Clinical Features of Gingivitis

FERMIN A. CARRANZA, JR.

Course and Duration
Distribution
Clinical Findings
Gingival Bleeding
Color Changes in the Gingiva

Changes in the Consistency of the Gingiva
Changes in the Surface Texture of the Gingiva
Changes in the Position of the Gingiva
Changes in Gingival Contour

COURSE AND DURATION

Acute gingivitis is a painful condition that comes on suddenly and is of short duration.

Subacute gingivitis is a less severe phase of the acute condition.

Recurrent gingivitis reappears after having been eliminated by treatment or disappears spontaneously and then reappears.

Chronic gingivitis comes on slowly, is of long duration, and is painless unless complicated by acute or subacute exacerbations. Chronic gingivitis is the type most commonly encountered (Fig. 17–1). Patients seldom recollect having had any acute symptoms. Chronic gingivitis is a fluctuating disease in which inflammation persists or resolves and normal areas become inflamed.[14,15]

DISTRIBUTION

Localized gingivitis is confined to the gingiva in relation to a single tooth or group of teeth.

Generalized gingivitis involves the entire mouth.

Marginal gingivitis involves the gingival margin but may include a portion of the contiguous attached gingiva.

Papillary gingivitis involves the interdental papillae and often extends into the adjacent portion of the gingival margin. Papillae are involved more frequently than is the gingival margin, and the earliest signs of gingivitis most often occur in the papillae.

Diffuse gingivitis affects the gingival margin, the attached gingiva, and the interdental papillae.

The distribution of gingival disease in individual cases is described by combining the preceding terms, as follows:

Localized marginal gingivitis is confined to one or more areas of the marginal gingiva (Fig. 17–2).

Localized diffuse gingivitis extends from the margin to the mucobuccal fold but is limited in area (Fig. 17–3; Plate VIIA).

Localized papillary gingivitis is confined to one or more interdental spaces in a limited area (Fig. 17–4; Plate VIIB).

Generalized marginal gingivitis involves the gingival margins in relation to all the teeth. The interdental papillae are usually also affected in generalized marginal gingivitis (Fig. 17–5; Plate VIIC).

Generalized diffuse gingivitis involves the entire gingiva.

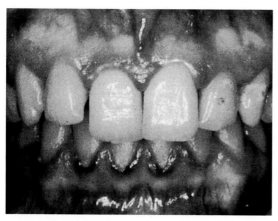

FIGURE 17–1. Chronic gingivitis. The marginal and interdental gingivae are smooth, edematous, and discolored.

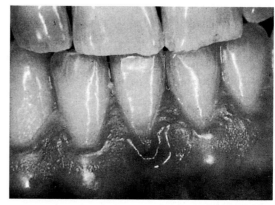

FIGURE 17–3. Localized diffuse gingivitis involving both the marginal and the attached gingiva.

The alveolar mucosa is usually also affected, so the demarcation between it and the attached gingiva is obliterated (Fig. 17–6; Plate VII*D*). Systemic conditions are involved in the etiology of generalized diffuse gingivitis, except in cases caused by acute infection or generalized chemical irritation.

CLINICAL FINDINGS

In evaluating the clinical features of gingivitis, it is necessary to be *systematic.* Attention should be focused on subtle tissue alterations, because these may be of great diagnostic significance. A systematic clinical approach requires an orderly examination of the gingiva for color, size and shape, consistency, surface texture, position, ease and severity of bleeding, and pain. These clinical characteristics and the microscopic changes responsible for each are discussed in this chapter.

Gingival Bleeding

The two earliest symptoms of gingival inflammation, which precede established gingivitis, are (1) increased gingival fluid production rate and (2) bleeding from the gingival sulcus on gentle probing (Fig. 17–7; Plate VII*G,H*). Gingival fluid is discussed in detail in Chapter 7.

Gingival bleeding varies in severity, duration, and the ease with which it is provoked. *Bleeding on probing is easily detectable clinically and therefore is of great value for the early diagnosis and prevention of more advanced gingivitis.* It has been shown that bleeding on probing appears earlier than change in color or other visual signs of inflammation[15,16,19]; moreover, the use of bleeding rather than color changes to diagnose early gingival inflammation has an advantage in that bleeding is a more objective sign that requires less subjective estimation by the examiner. Several gingival indices based on bleeding have been developed[1,6,25] and are described in Chapter 5. (For further considerations on probing, see Chapter 28.)

Gingival Bleeding Caused by Local Factors

Chronic and Recurrent Bleeding

The most common cause of abnormal gingival bleeding is chronic inflammation.[22] The bleeding is chronic or recur-

Boards

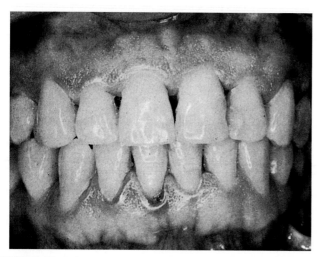

FIGURE 17–2. Localized marginal gingivitis in the mandibular anterior region.

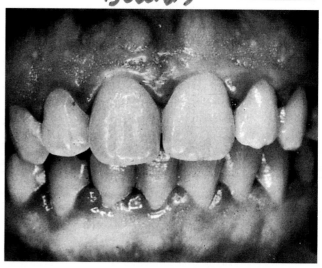

FIGURE 17–4. Papillary gingivitis.

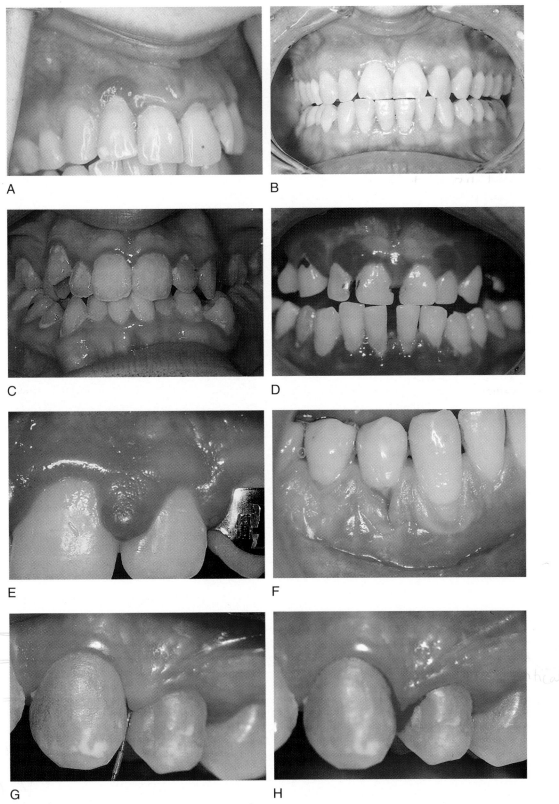

PLATE VII. Gingivitis: clinical features. *A,* Localized, diffuse, intensely red area facial of tooth #7 and dark pink marginal changes in the remaining anterior teeth. *B,* Generalized papillary gingivitis. *C,* Generalized marginal inflammatory lesion. *D,* Generalized diffuse inflammatory lesion. *E,* Papillary gingival enlargement. *F,* Different degrees of recession. Recession is slight in teeth #26 and 29 and marked in #27 and 28. Note the irregular contours of the gingiva in #28 and the lack of attached gingiva in #27. *G,* Insertion of a probe into the gingival sulcus. Note the lack of stippling, the slightly rolled margins, and the dark red color. *H,* Bleeding appears about 30 seconds after probing.

Stage I = neutrophil
II = lymphocytes
III = plasma cells

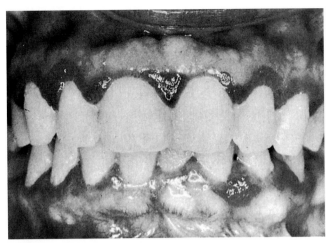

FIGURE 17-5. Generalized marginal gingivitis. The interdental papillae are also involved.

rent and is provoked by mechanical trauma (e.g., from toothbrushing, toothpicks, or food impaction) or by biting into solid foods such as apples.

In gingival inflammation, the following histopathologic alterations result in abnormal gingival bleeding: dilation and engorgement of the capillaries and thinning or ulceration of the sulcular epithelium (Fig. 17-8). Because the capillaries are engorged and closer to the surface and the thinned, degenerated epithelium is less protective, stimuli that are ordinarily innocuous cause rupture of the capillaries and gingival bleeding.

Sites that bleed on probing have a greater area of inflamed connective tissue (i.e., cell-rich, collagen-poor tissue) than do sites that do not bleed. In most cases the cellular infiltrate of sites that bleed on probing is predominantly lymphocytic (a characteristic of stage II, or early, gingivitis).[2,7,11]

The severity of the bleeding and the ease with which it is

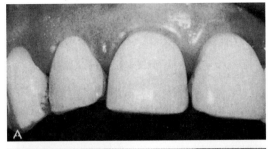

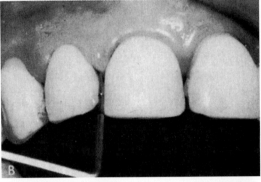

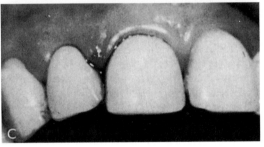

FIGURE 17-7. Bleeding on probing. *A*, Mild gingivitis with slight edema. *B*, Introduction of the periodontal probe to the bottom of the gingival sulcus. *C*, Bleeding appears after a few seconds. (Courtesy of Dr. Joseph Hsiou.)

provoked depend on the intensity of the inflammation. After the vessels rupture, a complex of mechanisms induces hemostasis.[33] The vessel walls contract, and blood flow is diminished; blood platelets adhere to the edges of the tissue; and a fibrous clot is formed, which contracts and results in approximation of the edges of the injured area. Bleeding recurs, however, when the area is irritated.

In cases of moderate or advanced periodontitis the presence of bleeding on probing is considered a sign of active tissue destruction (see Chapter 22).

Acute Bleeding — many factors

Acute episodes of gingival bleeding are caused by injury or occur spontaneously in acute gingival disease. Laceration of the gingiva by toothbrush bristles during aggressive toothbrushing or by sharp pieces of hard food causes gingival bleeding even in the absence of gingival disease. Gingival burns from hot foods or chemicals increase the ease of gingival bleeding.

Spontaneous bleeding or bleeding on slight provocation occurs in acute necrotizing ulcerative gingivitis. In this condition, engorged blood vessels in the inflamed connective tissue are exposed by ulceration of the necrotic surface epithelium.

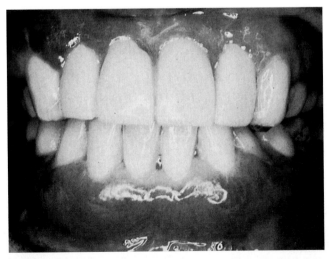

FIGURE 17-6. Generalized diffuse gingivitis. The marginal, interdental, and attached gingivae are involved in chronic desquamative gingivitis.

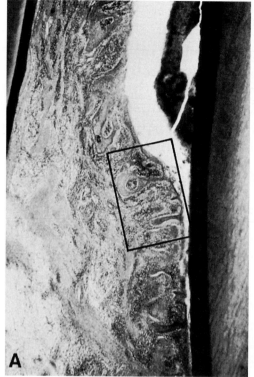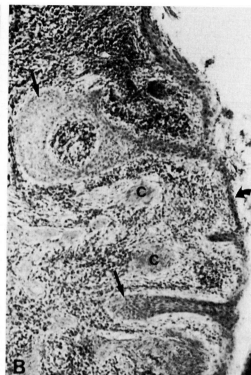

FIGURE 17–8. *A,* Microscopic view of interdental space in a human autopsy specimen. *B,* Higher magnification of the area within the rectangle in *A.* Note the dense inflammatory infiltrate, the thinned epithelium (*curved arrow*), the extension of rete pegs (*straight arrows*), and the remnants of collagen fibers (c).

Gingival Bleeding Associated with Systemic Disturbances

In some systemic disorders gingival hemorrhage occurs spontaneously, unprovoked by mechanical irritation, or occurs after irritation and is excessive and difficult to control. These hemorrhagic diseases represent a wide variety of conditions that vary in etiology and clinical manifestations. Such conditions have one feature in common: namely, abnormal bleeding in the skin, internal organs, and other tissues, as well as in the oral mucous membrane.

The hemorrhagic tendency may be due to failure of one or more of the hemostatic mechanisms.[31] Hemorrhagic disorders in which abnormal gingival bleeding is encountered include vascular abnormalities (vitamin C deficiency or allergy such as Schönlein-Henoch purpura), platelet disorders (idiopathic thrombocytopenic purpura or thrombocytopenic purpura caused by diffuse injury to the bone marrow), hypoprothrombinemia (vitamin K deficiency resulting from liver disease or sprue), other coagulation defects (hemophilia, leukemia, Christmas disease), deficient platelet thromboplastic factor (PF3) resulting from uremia,[20] multiple myeloma and postrubella purpura.[12] Bleeding may follow the administration of excessive amounts of drugs such as salicylates and the administration of anticoagulants such as dicumarol and heparin. (Periodontal involvement in hematologic disorders is considered in Chapter 14.)

Color Changes in the Gingiva

Color Changes in Chronic Gingivitis

Change in color is an important clinical sign of gingival disease. The normal gingival color is "coral pink" and is produced by the tissue's vascularity and modified by the overlying epithelial layers. For this reason, the gingiva becomes redder when there is an increase in vascularization or the degree of epithelial keratinization becomes reduced or disappears. The color becomes paler when vascularization is reduced (in association with fibrosis of the corium) or epithelial keratinization increases.

Thus, chronic inflammation intensifies the red or bluish red color; this is caused by vascular proliferation and reduction of keratinization owing to epithelial compression by the inflamed tissue. Venous stasis will add a bluish hue. Originally a light red, the color changes through varying shades of red, reddish blue, and deep blue with increasing chronicity of the inflammatory process. The changes start in the interdental papillae and gingival margin and spread to the attached gingiva (see Fig. 17–1). Proper diagnosis and treatment require an understanding of the tissue changes that alter the color of the gingiva at the clinical level.

Small, crescent-shaped, bluish red areas may appear in the marginal gingiva. These were at one time attributed to trauma from occlusion (Fig. 17–9), but they are now known to be chronic inflammatory lesions caused by local irritants. The suspected contributory role of excessive occlusal forces has never been demonstrated.

Color Changes in Acute Gingivitis

Color changes in acute gingival inflammation differ in both nature and distribution from those in chronic gingivitis. The color changes may be marginal, diffuse, or patch-like, depending on the underlying acute condition. In acute necrotizing ulcerative gingivitis, the involvement is marginal; in herpetic gingivostomatitis, it is diffuse; and in

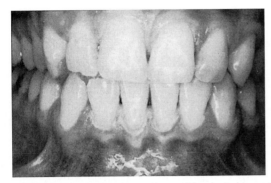

FIGURE 17–9. Crescent-shaped changes. Marginal areas of gingival erythema in the anterior mandibular region.

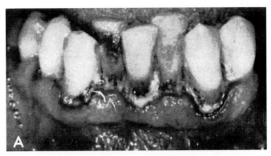

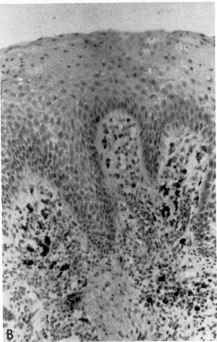

FIGURE 17–11. Bismuth line. *A,* Linear discoloration of the gingiva in relation to local irritation in a patient receiving bismuth therapy. *B,* Biopsy specimen showing bismuth particles engulfed by macrophages.

acute reactions to chemical irritation, it is patch-like or diffuse.

Color changes vary with the intensity of the inflammation. In all instances there is an initial bright red erythema. If the condition does not worsen, this is the only color change until the gingiva reverts to normal. In severe acute inflammation, the red color changes to a shiny slate gray, which gradually becomes a dull whitish gray. The gray discoloration produced by tissue necrosis is demarcated from the adjacent gingiva by a thin, sharply defined erythematous zone. Detailed descriptions of the clinical and pathologic features of the various forms of acute gingivitis are found in Chapter 19.

Metallic Pigmentation

Heavy metals absorbed systemically from therapeutic use or occupational environments may discolor the gingiva and other areas of the oral mucosa.[18] This is different from tattooing produced by the accidental embedding of amalgam or other metal fragments[5] (Fig. 17–10).

Bismuth, arsenic, and mercury produce a black line in the gingiva that follows the contour of the margin (Fig. 17–11). The pigmentation may also appear as isolated black blotches involving the marginal, interdental, and attached gingivae. Lead results in a bluish red or deep blue linear pigmentation of the gingival margin (burtonian line).[8]

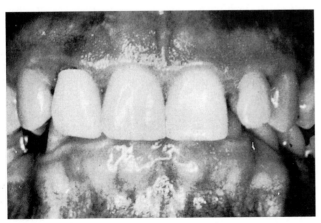

FIGURE 17–10. Discoloration of gingiva over the lateral incisor caused by embedded metal particles.

Exposure to silver (argyria) causes a violet marginal line, often accompanied by a diffuse bluish gray discoloration throughout the oral mucosa.[29]

Gingival pigmentation from systemically absorbed metals results from perivascular precipitation of metallic sulfides in the subepithelial connective tissue. Gingival pigmentation is not a result of systemic toxicity. It occurs only in areas of inflammation, where the increased permeability of irritated blood vessels permits seepage of the metal into the surrounding tissue. In addition to inflamed gingiva, mucosal areas irritated by biting or abnormal chewing habits (e.g., the inner surface of the lips, the cheek at the level of the occlusal line, and the lateral border of the tongue) are common pigmentation sites.

Gingival or mucosal pigmentation is eliminated by removing the local irritating factors and restoring tissue health; any metal-containing drugs required for therapeutic purposes do not necessarily have to be discontinued. Temporary correction is obtained by topical application of concentrated peroxide or by insufflation of the gingiva with oxygen to oxidize the dark metallic sulfides. The discoloration reappears unless the procedures are repeated.

Color Changes Associated With Systemic Factors

Many systemic diseases may cause color changes in the oral mucosa, including the gingiva.[9] In general, these abnormal pigmentations are nonspecific in nature and should stimulate further diagnostic efforts or referral to the appropriate specialist.[30]

Endogenous oral pigmentations can be due to melanin, bilirubin, or iron.[29] Melanin oral pigmentations can be normal physiologic pigmentations; they are commonly found in darker races (see Chapter 1), as well as in dark-haired whites. Diseases that increase melanin pigmentation include Addison's disease, which is caused by adrenal dysfunction and produces isolated patches of discoloration varying from bluish black to brown; Peutz-Jeghers syndrome, which produces intestinal polyposis and melanin pigmentation in the oral mucosa and lips; and Albright's syndrome (polyostotic fibrous dysplasia) and von Recklinghausen's disease (neurofibromatosis), both of which produce areas of oral melanin pigmentation.

Skin and mucous membranes can also be stained by bile pigments. Jaundice is best detected by examination of the sclera, but the oral mucosa may also acquire a yellowish color. The deposition of iron in hemochromatosis may produce a blue-gray pigmentation of the oral mucosa. Several endocrine and metabolic disturbances, including diabetes and pregnancy, may result in color changes. Blood dyscrasias such as anemia, polycythemia, and leukemia may also induce color changes.

Exogenous factors capable of producing color changes in the gingiva include atmospheric irritants such as coal and metal dust and coloring agents in food or lozenges. Tobacco causes a gray hyperkeratosis of the gingiva. Localized bluish black areas of pigment are commonly due to amalgam implanted in the mucosa (Fig. 17–12).

Changes in the Consistency of the Gingiva

Both chronic and acute inflammations produce changes in the normal firm, resilient consistency of the gingiva. As noted in the preceding discussion, in chronic gingivitis both

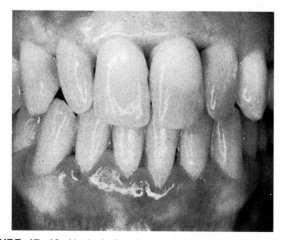

FIGURE 17–12. Vertical discoloration of marginal and attached gingivae associated with periodontal pockets.

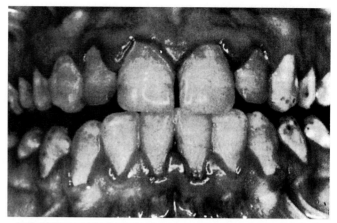

FIGURE 17–13. Chronic gingivitis, showing swelling and discoloration produced when inflammatory exudate and tissue degeneration are the predominant microscopic changes. The gingiva is soft and friable and bleeds easily. Note the mottled teeth.

destructive (edematous) and reparative (fibrotic) changes coexist, and the consistency of the gingiva is determined by their relative predominance (Figs. 17–13 and 17–14). Table 17–1 summarizes the clinical alterations in the consistency of the gingiva and the microscopic changes that produce them.

Calcified Masses in the Gingiva. Calcified microscopic masses may be found in the gingiva.[4] They can occur singly or in groups and vary in size, location, shape, and structure. Such masses may be calcified material removed from the tooth and traumatically displaced into the gingiva during scaling,[24] root remnants, cementum fragments, or cementicles (Fig. 17–15). Chronic inflammation and fibrosis and occasionally foreign body giant cell activity occur in relation to these masses. They are sometimes enclosed in an osteoid-like matrix. Crystalline foreign bodies have also been described in the gingiva, but their origin has not been determined.[28]

Changes in the Surface Texture of the Gingiva

Loss of surface stippling is an early sign of gingivitis. In chronic inflammation the surface is either smooth and shiny or firm and nodular, depending on whether the dominant changes are exudative or fibrotic. Smooth surface texture is also produced by epithelial atrophy in senile atrophic gingivitis, and peeling of the surface occurs in chronic desquamative gingivitis. Hyperkeratosis results in a leathery texture, and noninflammatory gingival hyperplasia produces a minutely nodular surface.

Changes in the Position of the Gingiva

Actual and Apparent Positions of the Gingiva

Recession is exposure of the root surface by an apical shift in the position of the gingiva. To understand what is

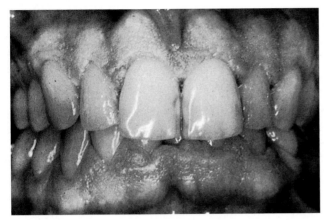

FIGURE 17–14. Chronic gingivitis, showing a firm gingiva with a minutely nodular surface produced when fibrosis predominates in the inflammatory process.

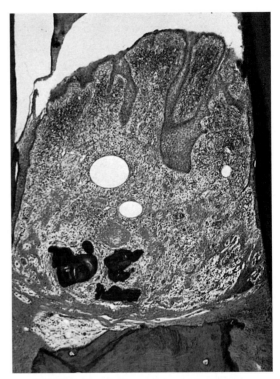

FIGURE 17–15. Cementicles in the gingiva.

meant by recession, one must distinguish between the actual and apparent positions of the gingiva. The *actual position* is the level of the epithelial attachment on the tooth (Fig. 17–16), whereas the *apparent position is* the level of the crest of the gingival margin. *The severity of recession is determined by the actual position of the gingiva, not its apparent position.*

There are two types of recession: visible, which is clinically observable, and hidden, which is covered by gingiva and can be measured only by inserting a probe to the level of epithelial attachment (see Fig. 17–16). For example, in periodontal disease part of the denuded root is covered by

the inflamed pocket wall; thus, some of the recession is hidden, and some may be visible (see Fig. 17–16). The total amount of recession is the sum of the two.

Recession refers to the location of the gingiva, not

Table 17–1. CLINICAL AND HISTOPATHOLOGIC CHANGES IN GINGIVAL CONSISTENCY

Chronic Gingivitis

Clinical Changes	Underlying Microscopic Features
1. Soggy puffiness that pits on pressure	1. Infiltration by fluid and cells of inflammatory exudate
2. Marked softness and friability, with ready fragmentation on exploration with probe and pinpoint surface areas of redness and desquamation	2. Degeneration of connective tissue and epithelium associated with injurious substances that provoke the inflammation and inflammatory exudate; change in connective tissue–epithelium relationship, with the inflamed, engorged connective tissue expanding to within a few epithelial cells of surface; thinning of epithelium and degeneration associated with edema and leukocytic invasion, separated by areas in which rete pegs are elongated to connective tissue.
3. Firm, leathery, consistency	3. Fibrosis and epithelial proliferation associated with longstanding chronic inflammation

Acute Gingivitis

Clinical Changes	Underlying Microscopic Features
1. Diffuse puffiness and softening	1. Diffuse edema of acute inflammatory origin; fatty infiltration in xanthomatosis
2. Sloughing with grayish flake-like particles of debris adhering to eroded surface	2. Necrosis with formation of a pseudomembrane composed of bacteria, PMNs, and degenerated epithelial cells in a fibrinous meshwork
3. Vesicle formation	3. Inter- and intracellular edema with degeneration of nucleus and cytoplasm and rupture of cell wall

PMN, Polymorphonuclear neutrophils.

Recession   **Position of Gingiva**

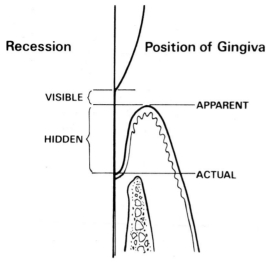

VISIBLE

HIDDEN

APPARENT

ACTUAL

FIGURE 17–16. Diagram illustrating the apparent and actual positions of the gingiva and visible and hidden recession.

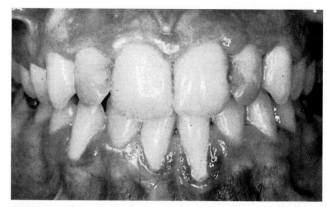

FIGURE 17–18. Recession around malposed anterior teeth. The gingiva is markedly inflamed.

its condition. Receded gingiva is often inflamed (Figs. 17–17 and 17–18) but may be normal except for its position (Fig. 17–19). Recession may be localized to one tooth (Fig. 17–20) or a group of teeth or may be generalized throughout the mouth (Fig. 17–21; see also Plate VII*F*).

Etiology of Recession. Gingival recession increases with age; the incidence varies from 8% in children to 100% after the age of 50 years.[38] This has led some investigators to assume that recession may be a physiologic process related to aging. However, convincing evidence for a physiologic shift of the gingival attachment has never been presented.[17] The gradual apical shift is most probably the result of the cumulative effect of minor pathologic involvement and/or repeated minor direct trauma to the gingiva.

The following factors have been implicated in the etiology of gingival recession: faulty toothbrushing technique (gingival abrasion), tooth malposition, friction from soft tissues (gingival ablation),[32] gingival inflammation, and high frenum attachment. Trauma from occlusion has also been suggested, but its mechanism of action has never been demonstrated. Orthodontic movement in a labial direction has been shown in monkeys to result in loss of marginal bone and connective tissue attachment, as well as in gingival recession.[34]

Although toothbrushing is important for gingival health, faulty toothbrushing may cause gingival recession. Recession tends to be more frequent and severe in patients with comparatively healthy gingiva, little bacterial plaque, and good oral hygiene.[10,26,27]

Susceptibility to recession is influenced by the position of teeth in the arch,[37] the root–bone angle, and the mesiodistal curvature of the tooth surface.[23] On rotated, tilted, or facially displaced teeth, the bony plate is thinned or reduced in height. Pressure from mastication or moderate toothbrushing wears away the unsupported gingiva and produces recession. The effect of the angle of the root in the bone on recession is often observed in the maxillary molar area (Fig. 17–22). If the lingual inclination of the palatal root is prominent or the buccal roots flare outward, then the bone in the cervical area is thinned or shortened,

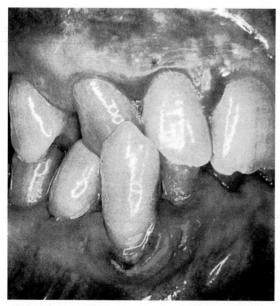

FIGURE 17–17. Recession on prominent canine. Note the severe inflammatory reaction to local irritation.

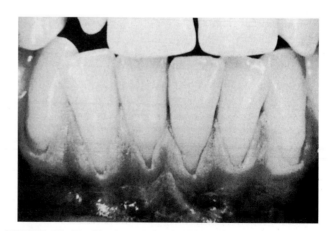

FIGURE 17–19. Gingival recession. Note the excellent condition of the gingiva.

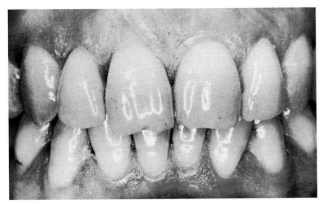

FIGURE 17-20. Localized recession on the maxillary central incisor associated with aggressive toothbrushing.

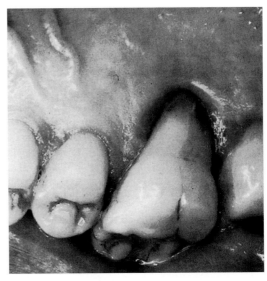

FIGURE 17-22. Accentuated recession on a maxillary first molar aggravated by the angulation of the prominent palatal root in the bone.

and recession results from wear of the unsupported marginal gingiva.

Clinical Significance. Several aspects of gingival recession make it clinically significant. Exposed root surfaces are susceptible to caries. Wearing away of the cementum exposed by recession leaves an underlying dentinal surface that is extremely sensitive, particularly to the touch. Hyperemia of the pulp and associated symptoms may also result from exposure of the root surface.[21] Interproximal recession creates spaces in which plaque, food, and bacteria can accumulate.

Changes in Gingival Contour

Changes in gingival contour are for the most part associated with gingival enlargement (see Chapter 18), but such changes may also occur in other conditions.

Stillman's Clefts *Know def.*

Stillman's clefts are apostrophe-shaped indentations extending from and into the gingival margin for varying distances. The clefts generally occur on the facial surface (Fig. 17-23). One or two may be present in relation to a single tooth. The margins of the clefts are rolled underneath the linear gap in the gingiva, and the remainder of the gingival

margin is blunt instead of knife edged. Originally described by Stillman[35] and considered to be the result of occlusal trauma, these clefts were subsequently described by Box[4] as pathologic pockets in which the ulcerative process had extended to the facial surface of the gingiva. The clefts may repair spontaneously or persist as surface lesions of deep periodontal pockets that penetrate into the supporting tissues. Their association with trauma from occlusion has not been substantiated.

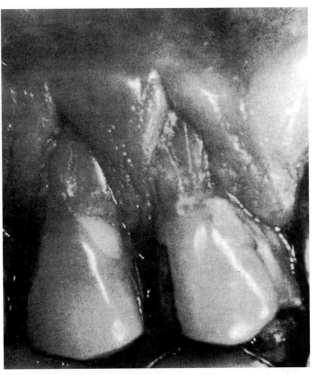

FIGURE 17-23. Stillman's clefts in the gingiva.

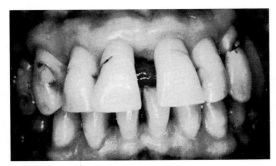

FIGURE 17-21. Generalized recession resulting from chronic periodontal disease.

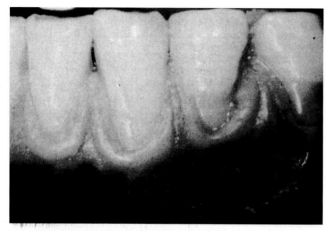

FIGURE 17–24. McCall's festoons showing characteristic rim-like enlargement of the gingival margin.

The clefts are divided into simple clefts, in which cleavage occurs in a single direction (the most common type), and compound clefts, in which cleavage occurs in more than one direction.[36] The clefts vary in length from a slight break in the gingival margin to a depth of 5 to 6 mm or more.

McCall's Festoons

McCall's festoons are life preserver–shaped enlargements of the marginal gingiva that occur most frequently in the canine and premolar areas on the facial surface. In the early stages, the color and consistency of the gingiva are normal. However, accumulation of food debris leads to secondary inflammatory changes (Fig. 17–24).

REFERENCES

1. Ainamo J, Bay I. Problems and proposals for recording gingivitis and plaque. Int Dent J 25:229, 1975.
2. Amato R, Caton JG, Polson AM, Espeland M. Interproximal gingival inflammation related to the conversion of a bleeding to a nonbleeding state. J Periodontol 57:63, 1986.
3. Bennett SH, Shankar S. Gingival bleeding as the presenting feature of multiple myeloma. Br Dent J 157:101, 1984.
4. Box HK. Gingival clefts and associated tracts. NY State Dent J 16:3, 1950.
5. Buchner A, Hansen LA. Amalgam pigmentation (amalgam tattoo) of the oral mucosa. A clinicopathologic study of 268 cases. Oral Surg 49:139, 1980.
6. Carter HG, Barnes GP. The gingival bleeding index. J Periodontol 45:801, 1974.
7. Cooper PG, Caton JG, Polson AM. Cell populations associated with gingival bleeding. J Periodontol 54:497, 1983.
8. Dummett CO. Abnormal color changes in gingivae. Oral Surg 2:649, 1949.
9. Dummett CO. Oral tissue color changes. Ala J Med Sci 16:274, 1979.
10. Gorman NJ. Prevalence and etiology of gingival recession. J Periodontol 38:316, 1967.
11. Greenstein PG, Caton JG, Polson AM. Histologic characteristics associated with bleeding after probing and ritual signs of inflammation. J Periodontol 52:420, 1981.
12. Haeb HP. Postrubella thrombocytopenic purpura. A report of cases with discussion of hemorrhagic manifestations of rubella. Clin Pediatr (Phila) 7:350, 1968.
13. Hirschfeld I. A study of skulls in the American Museum of Natural History in relation to periodontal disease. J Dent Res 5:241, 1923.
14. Hoover DR, Lefkowitz W. Fluctuation in marginal gingivitis. J Periodontol 36:310, 1965.
15. Larato D, Stahl SS, Brown R Jr, et al. The effect of a prescribed method of toothbrushing on the fluctuation of marginal gingivitis. J Periodontol 40:142, 1969.
16. Lenox JA, Kopczyk RA. A clinical system for scoring a patient's oral hygiene performance. J Am Dent Assoc 86:849, 1973.
17. Löe H. The structure and physiology of the dentogingival junction. In Miles AE, ed. Structural and Chemical Organization of Teeth. Vol 2. New York, Academic Press, 1967.
18. McCarthy FP, Dexter SO Jr. Oral manifestations of bismuth. N Engl J Med 213:345, 1935.
19. Meitner SW, Zander H, Iker HP, et al. Identification of inflamed gingival surfaces. J Clin Periodontol 6:93, 1979.
20. Merril A, Peterson LJ. Gingival hemorrhage secondary to uremia. Review and report of a case. Oral Surg 29:530, 1970.
21. Merritt AA. Hyperemia of the dental pulp caused by gingival recession. J Periodontol 4:30, 1933.
22. Milne AM. Gingival bleeding in 848 army recruits. An assessment. Br Dent J 122:111, 1967.
23. Morris ML. The position of the margin of the gingiva. Oral Surg 11:969, 1958.
24. Moskow BS. Calcified material in human gingival tissues. J Dent Res 40:644, 1961.
25. Muhlemann HR, Son S. Gingival sulcus bleeding, a leading symptom in initial gingivitis. Helv Odontol Acta 15:107, 1971.
26. O'Leary TJ, Drake RV, Crump P, Allen NF. The incidence of recession in young males—a further study. J Periodontol 42:264, 1971.
27. O'Leary TJ, Drake RV, Jividen GJ, Allen NF. The incidence of recession in young males: relationship to gingival and plaque scores. USAF School of Aerospace Medicine. SAM-TR-67–97:1, November 1967.
28. Orban B. Gingival inclusions. J Periodontol 16:16, 1945.
29. Prinz H. Pigmentations of oral mucous membrane. Dent Cosmos 74:554, 1932.
30. Shklar G, McCarthy PL. The Oral Manifestations of Systemic Disease. Boston, Butterworths, 1976.
31. Sodeman WA Jr, Sodeman WA. Pathologic Physiology: Mechanisms of Disease. 7th ed. Philadelphia, WB Saunders, 1985.
32. Sognnaes RF. Periodontal significance of intraoral frictional ablation. J West Soc Periodontol 25:112, 1977.
33. Stefanini M, Dameshek W. The Hemorrhagic Disorders. 2nd ed. New York, Grune & Stratton, 1962, p 78.
34. Steiner GG, Person JK, Ainamo J. Changes of the marginal periodontium as a result of labial tooth movement in monkeys. J Periodontol 52:314, 1981.
35. Stillman PR. Early clinical evidence of disease in the gingiva and the pericementum. J Dent Res 3:25, 1921.
36. Tishler B. Gingival clefts and their significance. Dent Cosmos 49:1003, 1927.
37. Trott JR, Love B. An analysis of localized gingival recession in 766 Winnipeg high school students. Dent Pract (Bristol) 16:209, 1966.
38. Woofter C. The prevalence and etiology of gingival recession. Periodont Abstr 17:45, 1969.

18

Gingival Enlargement

FERMIN A. CARRANZA, JR.

Gingival enlargement (increase in size) is a common feature of gingival disease. There are many types of gingival enlargement, and these types vary according to the etiologic factors and pathologic processes that produce them (Plate VIII).

CLASSIFICATION

Gingival enlargement is classified according to etiologic factors and pathologic changes as follows:

I. Inflammatory enlargement
   A. Chronic
   B. Acute
II. Fibrotic enlargement (gingival hyperplasia)
   A. Drug-induced
   B. Idiopathic
III. Combined enlargement (inflammatory + fibrotic)
IV. Enlargements associated with systemic diseases/conditions
   A. Conditioned enlargement
      1. Pregnancy
      2. Puberty
      3. Vitamin C deficiency
      4. Plasma cell gingivitis
      5. Nonspecific conditioned enlargement (granuloma pyogenicum)
   B. Systemic diseases causing gingival enlargement
      1. Leukemia
      2. Granulomatous diseases (Wegener's granulomatosis, sarcoidosis, etc.)
V. Neoplastic enlargement (gingival tumors)
   A. Benign tumors
   B. Malignant tumors
VI. False enlargement

LOCATION AND DISTRIBUTION

Using the criteria of location and distribution, gingival enlargement is designated as follows:

Localized: Limited to the gingiva adjacent to a single tooth or group of teeth
Generalized: Involving the gingiva throughout the mouth
Marginal: Confined to the marginal gingiva
Papillary: Confined to the interdental papilla
Diffuse: Involving the marginal and attached gingivae and papillae
Discrete: An isolated sessile or pedunculated tumor-like enlargement

INFLAMMATORY ENLARGEMENT

Gingival enlargement may result from chronic or acute inflammatory changes. The former is by far the more common cause.

Chronic Inflammatory Enlargement

Clinical Features. Chronic inflammatory gingival enlargement originates as a slight ballooning of the interdental papilla and/or the marginal gingiva. In the early stages it produces a life preserver–like bulge around the involved teeth. This bulge increases in size until it covers part of the crowns. The enlargement is generally papillary or marginal and may be localized (Fig. 18–1) or generalized (Fig. 18–2). It progresses slowly and painlessly unless it is complicated by acute infection or trauma.

Occasionally, chronic inflammatory gingival enlargement occurs as a discrete sessile or pedunculated mass resembling a tumor. It may be interproximal or on the marginal or attached gingiva (see Plate VIII*A*). The lesions are slow growing and usually painless. They may undergo spontaneous reduction in size, followed by exacerbation and continued enlargement. Painful ulceration sometimes occurs in the fold between the mass and the adjacent gingiva.

Histopathology (Fig. 18–3). Chronic inflammatory gingival enlargements show exudative and proliferative features of chronic inflammation. Lesions that are clinically deep red

233

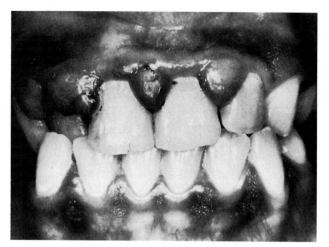

FIGURE 18–1. Chronic inflammatory gingival enlargement localized to the anterior region, associated with irregularity of teeth.

FIGURE 18–3. Survey section of chronic inflammatory gingival enlargement showing the central connective tissue core (C) and thickened epithelium at the periphery (E). Note the ulceration of the epithelial surface at the lower border of the mass that was adjacent to the tooth surface.

or bluish red, are soft and friable with a smooth shiny surface, and bleed easily have a preponderance of inflammatory cells and fluid with vascular engorgement, new capillary formation, and associated degenerative changes. Lesions that are relatively firm, resilient, and pink have a greater fibrotic component, with an abundance of fibroblasts and collagen fibers.

Etiology. Chronic inflammatory gingival enlargement is caused by prolonged exposure to dental plaque. Factors that favor plaque accumulation and retention[49] include poor oral hygiene (Fig. 18–4), abnormal relationships of adjacent teeth and opposing teeth, lack of tooth function, cervical cavities, overhanging margins of dental restorations, improperly contoured dental restorations or pontics, food impaction, irritation from clasps or saddle areas of removable prostheses, nasal obstruction, orthodontic therapy involving repositioning of the teeth, and habits such as mouth breathing and pressing the tongue against the gingiva.

Gingival Changes Associated With Mouth Breathing. Gingivitis and gingival enlargement are often seen in mouth breathers.[70] The gingiva appears red and edematous, with a diffuse surface shininess of the exposed area. The maxillary anterior region is the common site of such involvement. In many cases the altered gingiva is clearly demarcated from the adjacent unexposed normal gingiva (Fig. 18–5; Plate VIIIB). The exact manner in which mouth

breathing affects gingival changes has not been demonstrated. Its harmful effect is generally attributed to irritation from surface dehydration. However, comparable changes could not be produced by air drying the gingiva of experimental animals.[63]

Acute Inflammatory Enlargement

Gingival Abscess. A gingival abscess is a localized, painful, rapidly expanding lesion that is usually of sudden onset. It is generally limited to the marginal gingiva or interdental papilla. In its early stages it appears as a red swelling with a smooth, shiny surface. Within 24 to 48 hours, the lesion usually becomes fluctuant and pointed, with a surface orifice from which a purulent exudate may be expressed. The adjacent teeth are often sensitive to percussion. If permitted to progress, the lesion generally ruptures spontaneously.

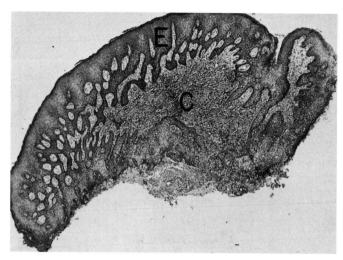

FIGURE 18–4. Chronic inflammatory gingival enlargement associated with plaque accumulation around an orthodontic appliance.

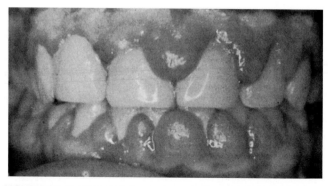

FIGURE 18–2. Chronic inflammatory gingival enlargement.

Pus is a SIGN, but not an indicator of the severity of disease.

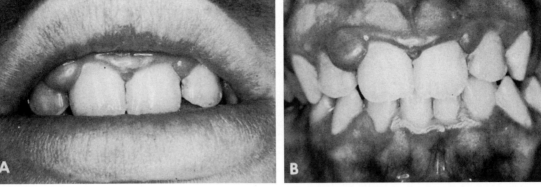

FIGURE 18-5. Gingivitis in a mouth breather. *A,* High lip line in a mouth breather. *B,* Gingivitis and inflammatory gingival enlargement in the exposed area of the gingiva.

Histopathology. The gingival abscess consists of a purulent focus in the connective tissue surrounded by a diffuse infiltration of polymorphonuclear leukocytes, edematous tissue, and vascular engorgement. The surface epithelium has varying degrees of intra- and extracellular edema, invasion by leukocytes, and ulceration.

Etiology. Acute inflammatory gingival enlargement results from bacteria carried deep into the tissues when a foreign substance such as a toothbrush bristle, a piece of apple core, or a lobster shell fragment is forcefully embedded into the gingiva. The lesion is confined to the gingiva and should not be confused with periodontal or lateral abscesses.

Periodontal (Lateral) Abscess. Periodontal abscesses generally produce enlargement of the gingiva, but they also involve the supporting periodontal tissues. For a detailed description of periodontal abscesses, see Chapter 22.

FIBROTIC ENLARGEMENT (GINGIVAL HYPERPLASIA)

The term *hyperplasia* refers to an increase in the size of a tissue or an organ produced by an increase in the number

of its component cells. Noninflammatory gingival hyperplasia is produced by factors other than local irritation. It is not common, and most cases occur after therapy with drugs such as phenytoin, cyclosporine, and nifedipine.

Drug-Induced Gingival Hyperplasia

Phenytoin

Enlargement of the gingiva caused by phenytoin (Dilantin), an anticonvulsant used in the treatment of epilepsy, occurs in some patients receiving the drug. Its reported incidence varies from 3% to 84.5%,[2,38,87] and it occurs more frequently in younger patients.[3] Its occurrence and severity are not necessarily related to the dosage, the concentration of phenytoin in serum or saliva, or the duration of drug therapy, although some reports indicate a definite relation between the dosage of the drug and the degree of gingival hyperplasia.[57,62]

Clinical Features. The primary or basic lesion starts as a painless, bead-like enlargement of the facial and lingual gingival margins and interdental papillae (Fig. 18-6). As the condition progresses, the marginal and papillary enlargements unite; they may develop into a massive tissue fold covering a considerable portion of the crowns, and they may interfere with occlusion (Fig. 18-7; Plate VIII*C,D*). When uncomplicated by inflammation, the lesion is mulberry shaped, firm, pale pink, and resilient, with a minutely lobulated surface and no tendency to bleed. The enlargement characteristically appears to project from beneath the gingival margin, from which it is separated by a linear groove.

Phenytoin-induced hyperplasia may occur in mouths devoid of local irritants and may be absent in mouths in which local irritants are profuse. The hyperplasia is usually generalized throughout the mouth but is more severe in the maxillary and mandibular anterior regions. It occurs in areas in which teeth are present, not in edentulous spaces, and the enlargement disappears in areas from which teeth are extracted. Hyperplasia of the mucosa in edentulous mouths has been reported but is rare.[30,31]

The enlargement is chronic and slowly increases in size. When surgically removed, it recurs. Spontaneous disappearance occurs within a few months after discontinuation of the drug (see Chapter 60).

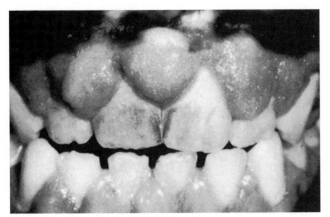

FIGURE 18-6. Gingival enlargement associated with phenytoin therapy. Note the prominent papillary lesions and the firm, nodular surface. Black patches in attached gingiva are melanin-pigmented areas.

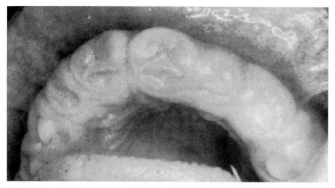

FIGURE 18–7. Massive phenytoin-associated gingival enlargement in a 5-year-old patient. The teeth are almost completely covered by firm, dense tissue.

The presence of the enlargement makes plaque control difficult, resulting in a secondary inflammatory process that complicates the gingival hyperplasia caused by the drug. *It is important to distinguish between the increase in size caused by the phenytoin-induced hyperplasia and the complicating inflammation caused by bacteria.* Secondary inflammatory changes add to the size of the lesion caused by phenytoin, produce red or bluish red discoloration, obliterate the lobulated surface demarcations, and result in an increased tendency toward bleeding.

Histopathology. The enlargement entails pronounced hyperplasia of the connective tissue and epithelium (Fig. 18–8). There is acanthosis of the epithelium, and elongated rete pegs extend deep into the connective tissue, which exhibits densely arranged collagen bundles with an increase in the number of fibroblasts and new blood vessels. The "mature" phenytoin enlargement has a fibroblast-to-collagen ratio equal to that of normal gingiva from normal individuals,[47] suggesting that at some point in the development of the lesion there must have been an abnormally high fibroblastic proliferation.[47] Oxytalan fibers are numerous beneath the epithelium and in areas of inflammation.[6] Inflammation is common along the sulcular surfaces of the gingiva.

Recurrent enlargements appear as granulation tissue composed of numerous young capillaries and fibroblasts and irregularly arranged collagen fibrils with occasional lymphocytes (Figs. 18–9 and 18–10).

Nature of the Lesion. *The enlargement is basically a hyperplastic reaction initiated by the drug, with inflammation being a secondary complicating factor.* Some investigators believe that inflammation is a prerequisite for development of the hyperplasia, and therefore, hyperplasia can be prevented by the removal of local irritants and fastidious oral hygiene.[41,67,86] However, oral hygiene by means of toothbrushing[32] or the use of a chlorhexidine toothpaste[95] reduces the inflammation but does not lessen or prevent the hyperplasia.

Tissue culture experiments indicate that phenytoin stimulates proliferation of fibroblast-like cells[101] and epithelium.[81] Two analogues of phenytoin (1-allyl-5-phenylhydantoinate and 5-methyl-5-phenylhydantoinate) have a similar effect on fibroblast-like cells.[101] Fibroblasts from a phenytoin-induced gingival hyperplasia show increased synthesis of sulfated glycosaminoglycans in vitro.[56] Phenytoin may induce a decrease in collagen degradation as a result of the production of an inactive fibroblastic collagenase.[45]

Experimental attempts to induce gingival enlargement with phenytoin administration in laboratory animals have been successful only in the cat,[52] the ferret, and the *Macaca speciosa* monkey.[106] In experimental animals, phenytoin causes gingival enlargement that is independent of local inflammation.

Phenytoin-induced enlargement begins as hyperplasia of the connective tissue core of the marginal gingiva, followed

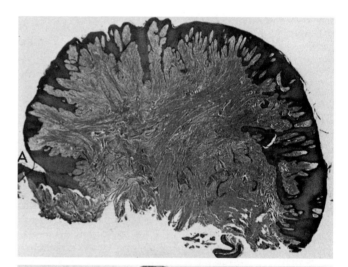

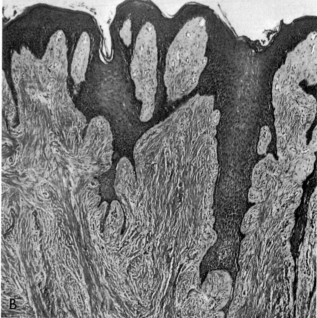

FIGURE 18–8. Gingival enlargement associated with phenytoin therapy. *A,* Survey section showing bulbous gingival enlargement. *B,* Detailed view showing hyperplasia and acanthosis of the epithelium with extension of deep rete pegs into the connective tissue. The connective tissue is densely collagenous. There is little evidence of inflammation.

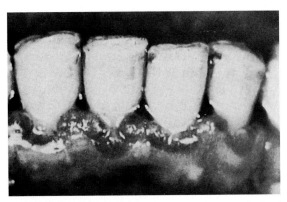

FIGURE 18–9. Early recurrence after surgical removal of enlarged gingiva in a patient receiving phenytoin therapy.

by proliferation of the epithelium.[52] The enlargement increases by proliferation and expansion of the central core beyond the crest of the gingival margin.

In cats, one of the metabolic products of phenytoin is 5-(parahydroxyphenyl)-5-phenylhydantoin; administration of this metabolite to cats also induces gingival enlargement in some cases.[46] This led Hassell and Page[46] to hypothesize that gingival hyperplasia may result from the genetically determined ability or inability of the host to deal effectively with prolonged administration of phenytoin.

Phenytoin occurs in the saliva. There is no consensus, however, on whether the severity of the hyperplasia is related to the levels of phenytoin in plasma or saliva.[2,4,118]

Systemic administration of phenytoin accelerates the healing of gingival wounds in nonepileptic humans[104] and increases the tensile strength of healing abdominal wounds in rats.[103] The administration of phenytoin may precipitate a megaloblastic anemia[73] and a folic acid deficiency.[107] For further information on this topic, the reader is referred to the monograph by Hassell.[44]

Cyclosporine

Cyclosporine is a fairly potent immunosuppressive agent used to prevent organ transplant rejection and to treat several diseases of autoimmune origin.[23] Its exact mechanism of action is not well known, but it appears to selectively and reversibly inhibit T helper cells, which play a role in cellular and humoral immune responses. Cyclosporine is administered intravenously or by mouth, and dosages >500 mg/day have been reported to induce gingival overgrowth.[28]

Clinically, the gingival hyperplasia induced by cyclosporine is similar to that induced by phenytoin.[22] The growth starts in the interproximal papillae (Fig. 18–11; Plate VIII*E*), more frequently in anterior facial areas, partially covering the crowns.[90] The tissue is usually pink, dense, and resilient, with a stippled or granular surface and little bleeding tendency. In some cases it may be of a more inflammatory character.

Clinically obvious cyclosporine-induced gingival enlargement occurs in approximately 30% of patients receiving the drug, and its magnitude appears to be related more to the plasma concentration than to the patient's periodontal status.[100]

Histopathology. The histologic features are similar to those observed in phenytoin-induced hyperplasia (collagenous overgrowth covered by a parakeratinized, multilayered epithelium with elongated rete pegs), although the connective tissue appears highly vascularized and with foci of chronic inflammatory cells,[91,116] particularly plasma cells.[66] The latter finding plus the presence of an abundant amorphous extracellular substance has suggested that the enlargement is a hypersensitivity response to cyclosporine.[76]

Nifedipine

Nifedipine is a calcium channel blocker that induces direct dilation of the coronary arteries and arterioles, improving oxygen supply to the heart muscle; it also reduces hypertension by dilating the peripheral vasculature. It is used primarily in the treatment of acute and chronic coronary insufficiency, including angina pectoris and refractory hypertension.[42] It is also used with cyclosporine in kidney transplant recipients.

Gingival overgrowth occurs in about 20% of cases.[7] The clinical and histologic features of nifedipine-induced hyperplasia are similar to those observed in phenytoin-induced overgrowth.[68,72,84] Nitrendipine, an analogue of nifedipine, has also been reported to induce gingival enlargement.[16,29]

Idiopathic Gingival Fibromatosis

Idiopathic gingival fibromatosis is a rare condition of undetermined etiology. It has been designated by such terms as gingivomatosis, elephantiasis,[5] diffuse fibroma,[20] familial elephantiasis, idiopathic fibromatosis,[122] hereditary gingival hyperplasia,[94,115] hereditary gingival fibromatosis,[120] and congenital familial fibromatosis.

Clinical Features. The enlargement affects the attached

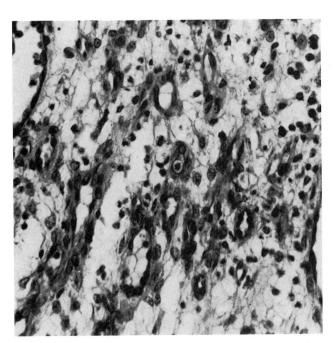

FIGURE 18–10. Biopsy specimen of the recurrent gingival enlargement shown in Figure 18–9. Note the abundance of new blood vessels.

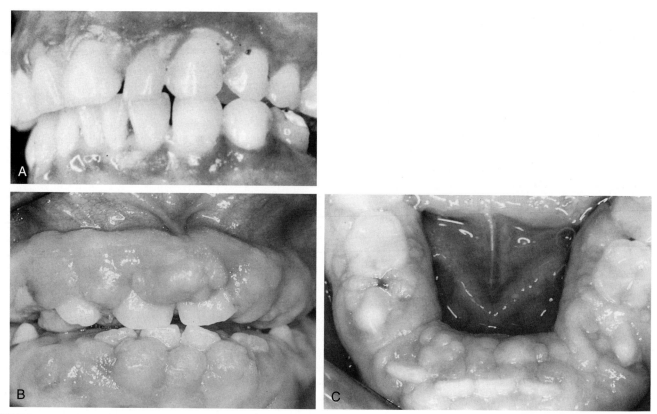

FIGURE 18–11. Cyclosporine-associated gingival enlargement. *A,* Mild involvement located particularly on papillae between teeth # 9 and 10 and 10 and 11. *B,* Advanced enlargement covering most of the crowns of the teeth. *C,* Occlusal view of the same case shown in *B.*

gingiva as well as the gingival margin and interdental papillae, in contrast to phenytoin-induced hyperplasia, which is often limited to the gingival margin and interdental papillae. The facial and lingual surfaces of the mandible and maxilla are generally affected, but the involvement may be limited to either jaw. The enlarged gingiva is pink, firm, and almost leathery in consistency and has a characteristic minutely pebbled surface (Fig. 18–12). In severe cases the teeth are almost completely covered, and the en-

largement projects into the oral vestibule (Plate VIII*F*). The jaws appear distorted because of the bulbous enlargement of the gingiva. Secondary inflammatory changes are common at the gingival margin.

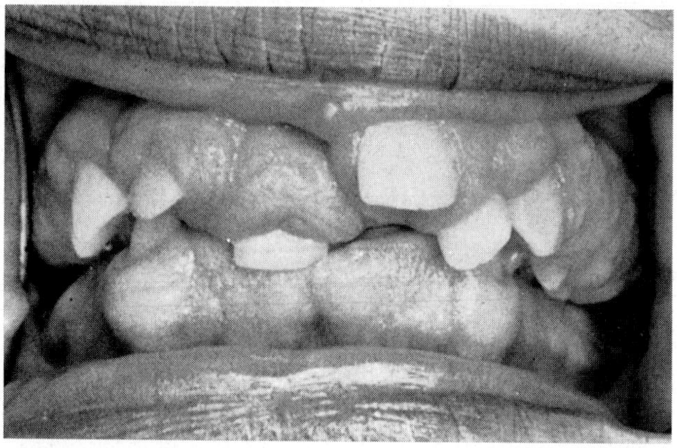

Histopathology. There is a bulbous increase in the amount of connective tissue that is relatively avascular and consists of densely arranged collagen bundles and numerous fibroblasts. The surface epithelium is thickened and acanthotic, with elongated rete pegs.

Etiology. The etiology is unknown, and thus the hyperplasia is designated as idiopathic. Some cases have a hereditary basis,[33,120,122] but the genetic mechanisms involved are not well understood. A study of several families found the mode of inheritance to be autosomal recessive in some cases and autosomal dominant in others.[55,90] In some families the gingival hyperplasia may be linked to retardation of physical development.[61] The enlargement usually begins with the eruption of the primary or secondary dentition and may regress after extraction, suggesting the possibility that the teeth (or the plaque attached to them) may be initiating factors. Nutritional and hormonal causes have been explored but have not been substantiated.[82] Local irritation is a complicating factor. Gingival hyperplasia has been described in tuberous sclerosis, which is an inherited condition characterized by a triad of epilepsy, mental deficiency, and cutaneous angiofibromas.[109,114]

FIGURE 18–12. Idiopathic hyperplastic gingival enlargement. The gingiva is firm, with a nodular, pebbled surface. The hyperplastic gingiva deflects the erupting teeth from proper alignment. (Courtesy of Dr. E. I. Ball.)

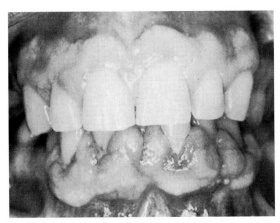

FIGURE 18–13. Combined gingival enlargement in a patient receiving phenytoin therapy. The basic hyperplasia is complicated by secondary inflammatory involvement. Note the edema and discoloration produced by the inflammation.

COMBINED ENLARGEMENT

Combined enlargement results when gingival hyperplasia is complicated by secondary inflammatory changes. Gingival hyperplasia produces conditions favorable for the accumulation of plaque and materia alba by accentuating the depth of the gingival sulcus, by interfering with effective hygienic measures, and by deflecting the normal excursive pathways of food. The secondary inflammatory changes increase the size of the pre-existing gingival hyperplasia and produce combined gingival enlargement. In many instances secondary inflammation obscures the features of the pre-existent noninflammatory hyperplasia to the extent that the entire lesion appears to be inflammatory (Fig. 18–13).

It is essential that the nature of combined gingival enlargement be understood. It consists of two components: *a primary or basic hyperplasia of connective tissue and epithelium* (the origin of which is unrelated to inflammation) *and a secondary complicating inflammatory component.* The removal of local irritation eliminates the secondary inflammatory component and reduces the size of the lesion proportionately, but the noninflammatory hyperplasia remains. Elimination of the noninflammatory hyperplasia requires correction of the causative factors.

ENLARGEMENTS ASSOCIATED WITH SYSTEMIC DISEASES/CONDITIONS

Numerous systemic diseases can develop oral manifestations that may include gingival enlargement. These diseases and/or conditions can affect the periodontium by two different mechanisms:

1. Magnification of an existing inflammation initiated by dental plaque. This group of diseases includes some hormonal conditions (e.g., pregnancy and puberty), nutritional diseases such as vitamin C deficiency (both of which are examples of conditioned enlargement), and some cases in which systemic influence is not identified (nonspecific conditioned enlargement).
2. Manifestation of the systemic disease independently of the inflammatory status of the gingiva. This group will be de-

scribed under "Systemic Diseases Causing Gingival Enlargement" and under "Neoplastic Enlargement (Gingival Tumors)."

Conditioned Enlargement

Conditioned enlargement occurs when the systemic condition of the patient exaggerates or distorts the usual gingival response to dental plaque, and a corresponding modification of the usual clinical features of chronic gingivitis occurs. The specific manner in which the clinical picture of conditioned gingival enlargement differs from that of chronic gingivitis depends on the nature of the modifying systemic influence. *Local irritation is necessary for the initiation of this type of enlargement.* However, plaque does not solely determine the nature of the clinical features. There are three types of conditioned gingival enlargement: hormonal (pregnancy, puberty), nutritional (associated with vitamin C deficiency), or allergic. Nonspecific conditioned enlargement is also seen.

Enlargement in Pregnancy

In pregnancy, gingival enlargement may be marginal and generalized or may occur as single or multiple tumor-like masses (see also Chapter 14).

Marginal Enlargement. Marginal gingival enlargement during pregnancy results from the aggravation of previous inflammation, and its incidence has been reported as 10%[21] and 70%.[121] However, the gingival enlargement does not occur without clinical evidence of local irritation. Pregnancy does not cause the condition; the altered tissue metabolism in pregnancy accentuates the response to local irritants.[50]

Clinical Features. The clinical picture varies considerably. The enlargement is usually generalized and tends to be more prominent interproximally than on the facial and lingual surfaces. The enlarged gingiva is bright red or magenta, soft, and friable and has a smooth, shiny surface. Bleeding occurs spontaneously or on slight provocation.[98]

Tumor-like Gingival Enlargement. The so-called pregnancy tumor is not a neoplasm; it is an inflammatory response to local irritation and is modified by the patient's condition. It usually appears after the third month of pregnancy but may occur earlier.[69] The reported incidence is 1.8% to 5%.[74]

Clinical Features. The lesion appears as a discrete, mushroom-like, flattened spherical mass that protrudes from the gingival margin or, more frequently, from the interproximal space and is attached by a sessile or pedunculated base (Fig. 18–14). It tends to expand laterally, and pressure from the tongue and the cheek perpetuates its flattened appearance. Generally dusky red or magenta, it has a smooth, glistening surface that frequently exhibits numerous deep red, pinpoint markings. It is a superficial lesion and ordinarily does not invade the underlying bone. The consistency varies; the mass is usually semifirm, but it may have various degrees of softness and friability. It is usually painless unless its size and shape foster accumulation of debris under its margin or interfere with occlusion, in which case painful ulceration may occur.

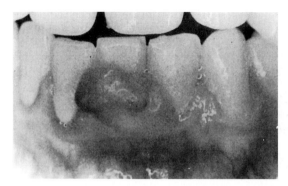

FIGURE 18–14. Conditioned gingival enlargement in pregnancy.

Histopathology. Both marginal and tumor-like enlargements consist of a central mass of connective tissue, the periphery of which is outlined with stratified squamous epithelium. The connective tissue consists of numerous diffusely arranged, newly formed, and engorged capillaries lined by cuboid endothelial cells (Fig. 18–15). Between the capillaries is a moderately fibrous stroma with varying degrees of edema and leukocytic infiltration. The stratified squamous epithelium is thickened, with prominent rete pegs. The basal epithelium exhibits some degree of intracellular and extracellular edema; there are prominent intercellular bridges and leukocytic infiltration. The surface of the epithelium is generally keratinized. There is generalized chronic inflammatory involvement, usually with a surface zone of acute inflammation.

Gingival enlargement in pregnancy is termed *angiogranuloma*, which avoids the implication of neoplasm implicit in terms such as *fibrohemangioma* or *pregnancy tumor*. Prominent endothelial proliferation with capillary formation and associated inflammation are its characteristic features. The capillary formation exceeds the usual gingival response to chronic irritation and accounts for the enlargement. Although the microscopic findings are characteristic of gingival enlargement in pregnancy, they are not pathognomonic because they cannot be used to differentiate pregnant and nonpregnant patients.[74]

Most gingival disease during pregnancy can be prevented by the removal of local irritants and the institution of fastidious oral hygiene at the outset. In pregnancy, treatment of the gingiva that is limited to the removal of tissue, without complete elimination of local irritants, is followed by recurrence of gingival enlargement. Although spontaneous reduction in the size of gingival enlargement commonly follows the termination of pregnancy, complete elimination of the residual inflammatory lesion requires the removal of all forms of local irritation.

Enlargement in Puberty

Enlargement of the gingiva is sometimes seen during puberty (see also Chapter 14). It occurs in both male and female adolescents and appears in areas of local irritation.

Clinical Features. The size of the gingival enlargement far exceeds that usually seen in association with comparable local factors. It is marginal and interdental and is characterized by prominent bulbous interproximal papillae (Fig. 18–16). Frequently, only the facial gingivae are enlarged, and the lingual surfaces are relatively unaltered. This is because the mechanical action of the tongue and the excursion of food prevent a heavy accumulation of local irritants on the lingual surface.

Gingival enlargement during puberty has all of the clinical features generally associated with chronic inflammatory gingival disease. It is the degree of enlargement and the tendency to develop massive recurrence in the presence of relatively little local irritation that distinguish pubertal gingival enlargement from uncomplicated chronic inflammatory gingival enlargement. After puberty, the enlargement undergoes spontaneous reduction but does not disappear until local irritants are removed.

A longitudinal study of 127 children 11 to 17 years of age showed a high initial prevalence of gingival enlargement that tended to decline with age.[110] When the mean

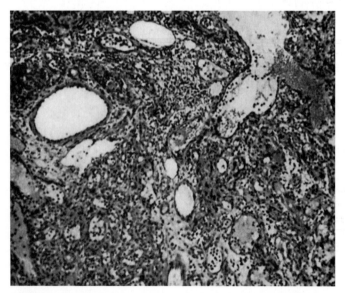

FIGURE 18–15. Microscopic view of gingival enlargement in pregnancy showing an abundance of blood vessels and interspersed inflammatory cells.

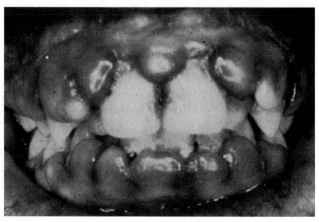

FIGURE 18–16. Conditioned gingival enlargement in puberty in a 13-year-old boy.

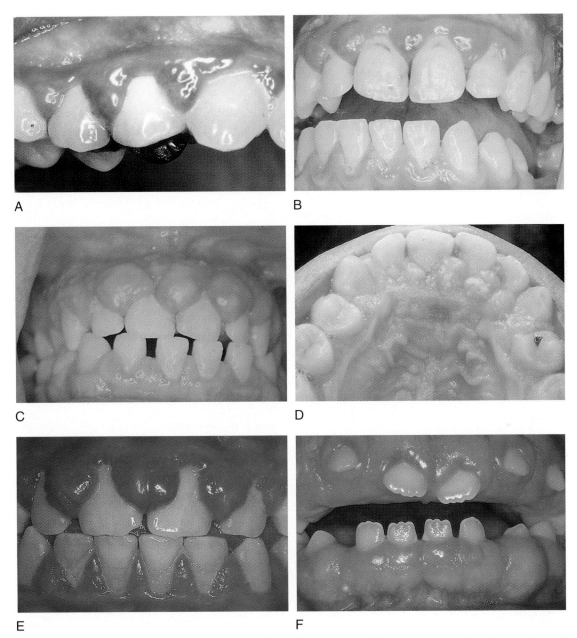

PLATE VIII. Gingival enlargements. *A,* Chronic inflammatory gingival enlargement in a 27-year-old woman. Note the papillary enlargement and the red, smooth surface. *B,* Gingival enlargement associated with mouth breathing, typically localized to the marginal and papillary areas of teeth #6–11, in an 18-year-old man. *C,* Phenytoin-associated gingival enlargement in a 21-year-old man. In the maxilla, note the bulbous papillary enlargement, leaving a trough between enlarged papillae, and the pink, stippled surface. *D,* Occlusal view of same case shown in *C. E,* Cyclosporine-associated gingival enlargement in a 14-year-old boy. Note the enlarged papillae and margin, the deep red color, and the smooth surface. *F,* Gingival fibromatosis in a 16-year-old boy. Dense fibrotic enlargement partially covers the crowns of the teeth, and the pink, stippled surface shows minor marginal inflammatory changes.

number of inflamed gingival sites per child was determined and was correlated with the time at which the maximal number of inflamed sites was observed and the oral hygiene index at that time, it could be clearly seen that a pubertal peak in gingival inflammation that was unrelated to oral hygiene factors occurred. A longitudinal study of subgingival microbiota of children between the ages of 11 and 14 and their association with clinical parameters has implicated *Capnocytophaga* sp. in the initiation of pubertal gingivitis.[79]

Histopathology. Because the enlargement is predominantly inflammatory in nature, it is difficult to discern the conditioning systemic influence in terms of specific histologic changes. The microscopic picture is that of chronic inflammation with prominent edema and associated degenerative changes.

Vitamin C Deficiency

Enlargement of the gingiva is generally included in classic descriptions of scurvy. It is important to recognize that such enlargement is essentially a conditioned response to bacterial plaque. Acute vitamin C deficiency does not of itself cause gingival inflammation, but it does cause hemorrhage, collagen degeneration, and edema of the gingival connective tissue. These changes modify the response of the gingiva to plaque to the extent that the normal defensive delimiting reaction is inhibited, and the extent of the inflammation is exaggerated.[36] The combined effect of acute vitamin C deficiency and inflammation produces the massive gingival enlargement in scurvy (Fig. 18–17) (see also Chapter 14).

Clinical Features. Gingival enlargement in vitamin C deficiency is marginal; the gingiva is bluish red, soft, and friable and has a smooth, shiny surface. Hemorrhage, occurring either spontaneously or on slight provocation, and surface necrosis with pseudomembrane formation are common features.

Histopathology. The gingiva has a chronic inflammatory cellular infiltration with a superficial acute response. There

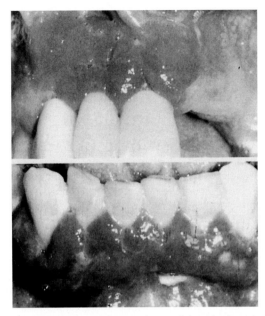

FIGURE 18–18. Plasma cell granuloma of the gingiva. *A,* Diffuse lesions on the facial surface of the anterior maxilla. *B,* Mandibular lesions. (Courtesy of Dr. Kim D. Zussman.)

are scattered areas of hemorrhage, with engorged capillaries. Marked diffuse edema, collagen degeneration, and scarcity of collagen fibrils or fibroblasts are striking findings.

Plasma Cell Gingivitis

Plasma cell gingivitis is also referred to as *atypical gingivitis* and *plasma cell gingivostomatitis* and frequently consists of a mild marginal gingival enlargement that extends to the attached gingiva. A localized lesion, referred to as *plasma cell granuloma,* has also been described.[15]

Clinically, the gingiva appears red, friable, and sometimes granular and bleeds easily; usually it does not induce a loss of attachment (Fig. 18–18). This lesion is located in the oral aspect of the attached gingiva and therefore differs from plaque-induced gingivitis.

Microscopically, the oral epithelium is parakeratinized and ultrastructurally shows signs of damage in the lower spinous layers and the basal layers. The underlying connective tissue contains a dense infiltrate of plasma cells that also extends to the oral epithelium, inducing a dissecting type of injury.[83]

An associated cheilitis and glossitis have been reported.[60,105] Plasma cell gingivitis is thought to be allergic in origin, possibly related to components of chewing gum, dentifrices, or various diet components. Cessation of exposure to the allergen brings resolution of the lesion.

In rare instances, marked inflammatory gingival enlargements with a predominance of plasma cells can appear associated with rapidly progressive periodontitis.[85]

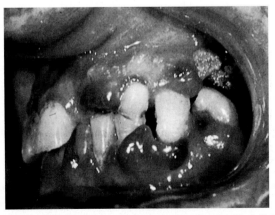

FIGURE 18–17. Gingival enlargement in vitamin C deficiency. Note the prominent hemorrhagic areas.

Nonspecific Conditioned Enlargement (Granuloma Pyogenicum)

Granuloma pyogenicum is a tumor-like gingival enlargement that is considered an exaggerated conditioned response to minor trauma (Fig. 18–19). The exact nature of the systemic conditioning factor has not been identified.[59]

Clinical Features. The lesion varies from a discrete spherical, tumor-like mass with a pedunculated attachment to a flattened, keloid-like enlargement with a broad base. It is bright red or purple and either friable or firm, depending on its duration; in the majority of cases it presents with surface ulceration and purulent exudation. The lesion tends to involute spontaneously to become a fibroepithelial papilloma or persists relatively unchanged for years.

Histopathology. Granuloma pyogenicum appears as a mass of granulation tissue with chronic inflammatory cellular infiltration. Endothelial proliferation and the formation of numerous vascular spaces are the prominent features. The surface epithelium is atrophic in some areas and hyperplastic in others. Surface ulceration and exudation are common features.

Treatment consists of removal of the lesions plus the elimination of irritating local factors. The recurrence rate is about 15%.[14] Granuloma pyogenicum is similar in clinical and microscopic appearance to the conditioned gingival enlargement seen in pregnancy.[69] Differential diagnosis depends on the patient's history.

Systemic Diseases Causing Gingival Enlargement

Several systemic diseases may, by different mechanisms, result in gingival enlargement. These are uncommon cases and will be only briefly discussed.

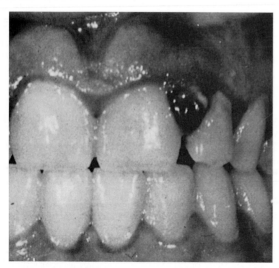

FIGURE 18–19. Pyogenic granuloma in a young woman.

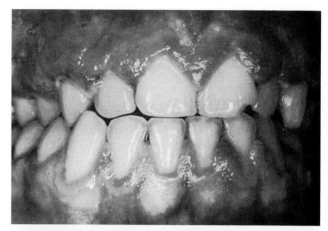

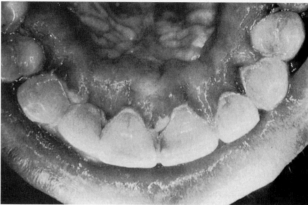

FIGURE 18–20. Leukemic gingival enlargement. *Top,* Leukemic gingival enlargement in a patient with acute myelocytic leukemia. Note that the enlargement is more prominent in the maxilla and is associated with greater local irritation. *Bottom,* Lingual view of gingival enlargement in a patient with subacute monocytic leukemia, showing a bulbous increase in size with discoloration and a smooth, shiny surface. Note the difference between the enlarged gingiva and the adjacent palatal mucosa.

Leukemia

Leukemic enlargement may be diffuse or marginal, localized or generalized (see also Chapter 14). It may appear as a diffuse enlargement of the gingival mucosa (Fig. 18–20), an oversized extension of the marginal gingiva, or a discrete tumor-like interproximal mass. In leukemic enlargement the gingiva is generally bluish red and has a shiny surface. The consistency is moderately firm, but there is a tendency toward friability and hemorrhage, occurring either spontaneously or on slight irritation. Acute painful necrotizing ulcerative inflammatory involvement sometimes occurs in the crevice formed at the junction of the enlarged gingiva and the contiguous tooth surfaces.

Leukemic patients may also have a simple chronic inflammation without the involvement of leukemic cells and presenting with the same clinical and microscopic features seen in nonleukemic patients. Most cases reveal features of both simple chronic inflammation and a leukemic infiltrate.

True leukemic enlargement occurs commonly in acute leukemia but may also be seen in subacute leukemia. It seldom occurs in chronic leukemia.

Histopathology. Gingival enlargements in leukemic patients show various degrees of chronic inflammation with mature leukocytes and areas of connective tissue infiltrated with a dense mass of immature and proliferating leukocytes, the specific nature of which varies with the type of leukemia. Engorged capillaries, edematous and degenerated connective tissue, and epithelium with various degrees of leukocytic infiltration and edema are found. Isolated surface areas of acute necrotizing inflammation with a pseudomembranous meshwork of fibrin, necrotic epithelial cells, polymorphonuclear neutrophils (PMNs), and bacteria are frequently seen.

Granulomatous Diseases

Wegener's Granulomatosis

Wegener's granulomatosis is a rare disease characterized by acute granulomatous necrotizing lesions of the respiratory tract, including nasal and oral defects. Renal lesions develop, and acute necrotizing vasculitis affects the blood vessels. The initial manifestations of Wegener's granulomatosis may involve the orofacial region and include oral mucosal ulceration, gingival enlargement, abnormal tooth mobility, exfoliation of teeth, and delayed healing response.[19]

Clinically, the granulomatous papillary enlargement is reddish purple and bleeds easily on stimulation.

Histopathology. Chronic inflammation occurs, with scattered giant cells and foci of acute inflammation and microabscesses covered by a thin acanthotic epithelium. Vascular changes have not been described, probably owing to the small size of the gingival blood vessels.[53]

The etiology of Wegener's granulomatosis is unknown, but the condition is considered an immunologically mediated tissue injury.[26] At one time the usual outcome was death from kidney failure within a few months, but more recently the use of immunosuppressive drugs has produced prolonged remissions in more than 90% of cases.[64]

Sarcoidosis

Sarcoidosis is a granulomatous disease of unknown etiology. It starts in individuals in their twenties or thirties and can involve almost any organ, including the gingiva, where a red, smooth enlargement may appear (Fig. 18–21).

Sarcoid granulomas consist of whorls of epithelioid cells and multinucleated Langhans giant cells with peripheral mononuclear cells.

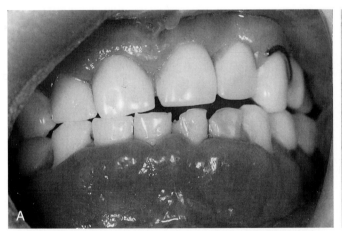

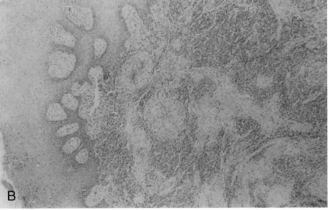

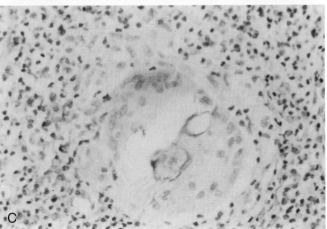

FIGURE 18–21. *A,* Gingival enlargement in a case of sarcoidosis. Low power *(B)* and high-power *(C)* microscopic view of sarcoid granuloma. (Courtesy Dr. Silvia Oreamuno.)

NEOPLASTIC ENLARGEMENT (GINGIVAL TUMORS)

Benign Tumors of the Gingiva

Epulis is a generic term used clinically to designate all discrete tumors and tumor-like masses of the gingiva. It serves to locate the tumor but not to describe it. Most lesions referred to as *epulis* are inflammatory rather than neoplastic.

Neoplasms account for a comparatively small proportion of gingival enlargements and make up a small percentage of the total number of oral neoplasms. In a survey of 257 oral tumors,[77] approximately 8% occurred on the gingiva. In another study[10] of 868 growths of the gingiva and palate, of which 57% were neoplastic and the remainder inflammatory, the following incidence of tumors was noted: carcinoma, 11.0%; fibroma, 9.3%; giant cell tumor, 8.4%; papilloma, 7.3%; leukoplakia, 4.9%; mixed tumor (salivary gland type), 2.5%; angioma, 1.5%; osteofibroma, 1.3%; sarcoma, 0.5%; melanoma, 0.5%; myxoma, 0.45%; fibropapilloma, 0.4%; adenoma, 0.4%; and lipoma, 0.3%.

Fibroma. Fibromas of the gingiva arise from the gingival connective tissue or from the periodontal ligament. They are slow-growing, spherical tumors that tend to be firm and nodular but may be soft and vascular. Fibromas are usually pedunculated. Hard fibromas of the gingiva are rare; most of the lesions diagnosed clinically as fibromas are inflammatory hyperplasias.[96]

Histopathology. The hard fibroma is composed of densely arranged bundles of well-formed collagen fibers with a scattering of flattened elliptical fibrocytes. It is a relatively avascular tumor. In the soft fibroma, fibroblasts are comparatively more numerous and stellate. Collagen is present but is less densely arranged. Various degrees of vascularity are also seen. Bone formation within fibromas is a frequent finding. The bone appears as irregularly arranged trabeculae with osteoblasts and osteoid along the margins. Lipofibroma,[75] myxofibroma,[11] and peripheral odontogenic fibroma[78] of the gingiva and alveolar mucosa have also been described.

Papilloma. Papilloma of the gingiva appears as a hard, wart-like protuberance from the gingival surface (Fig. 18–22). The lesion may be small and discrete or may appear as a broad, hard elevation of the gingiva with minutely irregular surfaces.

Histopathology. The lesion has a central core of connective tissue with marked proliferation and hyperkeratosis of the epithelium.

Peripheral Giant Cell Granuloma. Giant cell lesions of the gingiva arise interdentally or from the gingival margin, occur most frequently on the labial surface, and may be sessile or pedunculated. They vary in appearance from smooth, regularly outlined masses to irregularly shaped, multilobulated protuberances with surface indentations (Fig. 18–23). Ulceration of the margin is occasionally seen. The

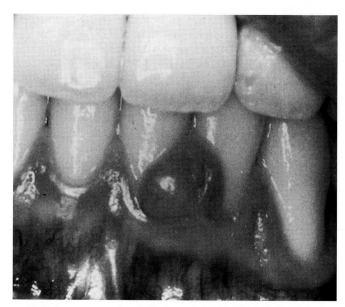

FIGURE 18–22. Papilloma of the gingiva in a 26-year-old man.

lesions are painless, vary in size, and may cover several teeth. They may be firm or spongy, and the color varies from pink to deep red or purplish blue. There are no pathognomonic clinical features whereby these lesions can be differentiated from other forms of gingival enlargement. Microscopic examination is required for definitive diagnosis (Figs. 18–24 and 18–25).

In the past, giant cell lesions of the gingiva have been referred to as *giant cell epulides* or *peripheral giant cell tumors*. Most often, however, these gingival lesions are essentially responses to local injury and not neoplasms. When they occur on the gingiva, they should be referred to as *peripheral giant cell granulomas*[89,94] to differentiate them from comparable lesions that originate within the jaw bone (i.e., *central giant cell granulomas*).[54]

In some instances, the giant cell granuloma of the gingiva is locally invasive and causes destruction of the under-

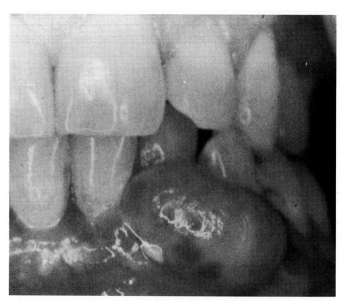

FIGURE 18–23. Gingival giant cell granuloma.

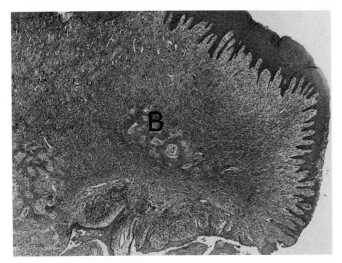

FIGURE 18–24. Microscopic survey of peripheral giant cell reparative granuloma. Trabeculae of newly formed bone (B) are contained within the mass.

lying bone (Fig. 18–26). Complete removal leads to uneventful recovery.

Histopathology. The giant cell granuloma has numerous foci of multinuclear giant cells and hemosiderin particles in a connective tissue stroma. Areas of chronic inflammation are scattered throughout the lesion, with acute involvement occurring at the surface. The overlying epithelium is usually hyperplastic, with ulceration at the base. Bone formation occasionally occurs within the lesion (see Figs. 18-24 and 18-25).

Central Giant Cell Granuloma. These lesions arise within the jaws and produce central cavitation. They occasionally create deformity of the jaw such that the gingiva appears enlarged.

Mixed tumors, salivary gland type tumors, eosinophilic granulomas, and plasmacytomas of the gingiva have also been described but are not often seen.

Leukoplakia. Leukoplakia of the gingiva varies in appearance from a grayish white, flattened, scaly lesion to a thick, irregularly shaped, keratinous plaque (Fig. 18–27).

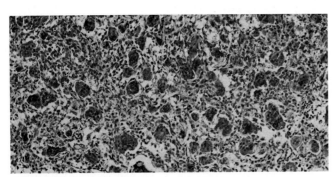

FIGURE 18–25. High-power study of the lesion shown in Figure 18–24 demonstrating the giant cells and intervening stroma that make up the major portion of the mass.

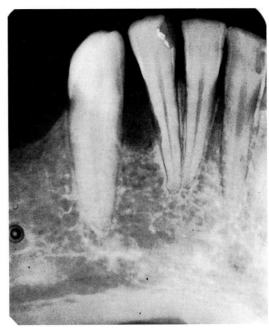

FIGURE 18–26. Bone destruction in the interproximal space between the canine and lateral incisor caused by the extension of a peripheral giant cell reparative granuloma of the gingiva. (Courtesy of Dr. Sam Toll.)

Histopathology. Leukoplakia exhibits thickening of the epithelium with hyperkeratosis, acanthosis, and some degree of dyskeratosis. Inflammatory involvement of the underlying connective tissue is a commonly associated finding. Leukoplakia is caused by chronic irritation. Its capacity for malignant transformation must be borne in mind.

Gingival Cyst. Gingival cysts of microscopic proportions are common, but they seldom reach a clinically significant size.[80] When they do, they appear as localized enlargements that may involve the marginal and attached gingivae.[92] They occur in the mandibular canine and premolar areas, most often on the lingual surface. They are painless, but with expansion they may cause erosion of the surface of the alveolar bone. The cysts develop from odontogenic epithelium or from surface or sulcular epithelium traumatically implanted in the area. Removal is followed by uneventful recovery.

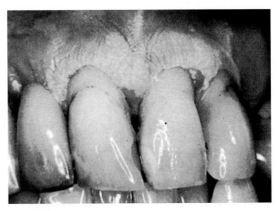

FIGURE 18–27. Leukoplakia of the gingiva.

Microscopically, there is a cyst cavity lined by a thin, flattened epithelium with or without localized areas of thickening. Less frequently, the following types of epithelium can be found: unkeratinized stratified squamous epithelium, keratinized stratified squamous epithelium, and parakeratinized epithelium with palisading basal cells.[18]

Other benign tumors have also been described as rare or infrequent findings in the gingiva. They include nevus,[12] myoblastoma,[40,58] hemangioma[9,111] (Fig. 18–28), mucus-secreting cysts (mucoceles),[116] and ameloblastoma.[108]

Malignant Tumors of the Gingiva

Carcinoma. The gingiva is not a frequent site of oral malignancy. *Squamous cell carcinoma is the most common malignant tumor of the gingiva.* Oral cancer accounts for 5% of all malignant tumors in the body; of these, 6% occur in the gingiva.[65]

Carcinomas may be exophytic or verrucous, both of which are outgrowths from the gingival surface, or ulcerative, which appear as flat, erosive lesions. They are locally invasive, involving the underlying bone and adjacent mucosa (Fig. 18–29). Often symptom free, they frequently go unnoticed until complicated by painful inflammation. The inflammatory changes may mask the neoplasm. Metastasis is usually confined to the region above the clavicle; however, more extensive involvement may include the lung, liver, or bone.

Malignant Melanoma. Malignant melanoma is a rare oral tumor that tends to occur in the gingiva of the anterior maxilla.[8] It is usually darkly pigmented and is often preceded by the occurrence of localized pigmentation.[24] It may be flat or nodular and is characterized by rapid growth and early metastasis. It arises from melanoblasts in the gingiva, cheek, or palate. An unpigmented malignant melanoma of the gingiva has been reported.[71] Infiltration into the underlying bone and metastasis to cervical and axillary lymph nodes are common.

Sarcoma. Fibrosarcoma, lymphosarcoma, and reticulum cell sarcoma of the gingiva are rare; only isolated cases have been described in the literature.[39,113] Kaposi's sarcoma occurs frequently in the oral cavity of acquired immunodeficiency syndrome (AIDS) patients, particularly in the palate and the gingiva (see Chapter 15).

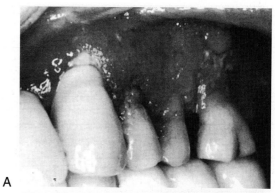

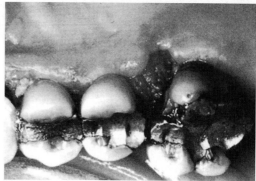

FIGURE 18–29. Squamous cell carcinoma of the gingiva. *A,* Facial view. Note the extensive verrucous involvement. *B,* Palatal view. Note the mulberry-like tissue emerging between the second premolar and the first molar.

Metastasis. Tumor metastasis to the gingiva is not common. Such metastasis has been reported with various tumors, including adenocarcinoma of the colon,[51] lung carcinoma, primary hepatocellular carcinoma,[117] renal cell carcinoma,[5] hypernephroma,[88] chondrosarcoma,[112] and testicular tumor.[34]

One must not be misled by the low incidence of malignancy of the gingiva. *Ulcerations that do not respond to therapy in the usual manner and all gingival tumors and tumor-like lesions must undergo biopsy and be submitted for microscopic diagnosis* (see Chapter 29).

The reader is referred to textbooks in oral pathology for more complete information on benign and malignant tumors of the gingiva.

FALSE ENLARGEMENT

False enlargements are not true enlargements of the gingival tissues but may appear as such as a result of increases in size of the underlying osseous or dental tissues. The gingiva usually presents with no abnormal clinical features except the massive increase in size of the area.

Underlying Osseous Lesions. Enlargement of the bone subjacent to the gingival area occurs most commonly in tori and exostoses, but it can also occur in Paget's disease, fibrous dysplasia, cherubism, central giant cell granuloma, ameloblastoma, osteoma, and osteosarcoma. One example of this type of enlargement is shown in Figure 18–30. In this case a fibrous dysplasia (florid type) in a 38-year-old black female induced an osseous enlargement in the

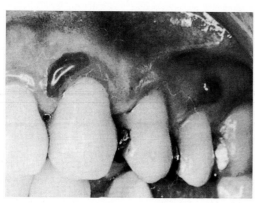

FIGURE 18–28. Hematomas produced by trauma.

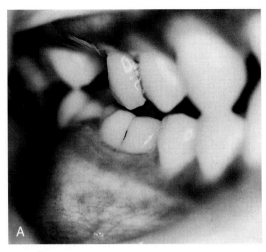 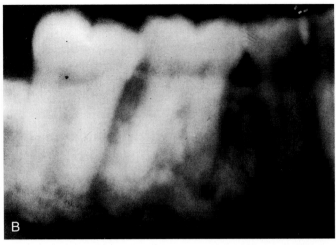

FIGURE 18–30. *A,* Apparent gingival enlargement associated with bone augmentation in a case of fibrous dysplasia. *B,* Radiograph of the case shown in *A,* depicting a ground-glass, mottled radiographic pattern.

mandibular molar area that appeared as a gingival enlargement. The gingival tissue can appear normal or may have unrelated inflammatory changes.

Underlying Dental Tissues. During the various stages of eruption, particularly of the primary dentition, the labial gingiva may show a bulbous marginal distortion caused by superimposition of the bulk of the gingiva on the normal prominence of the enamel in the gingival half of the crown. This enlargement has been termed *developmental enlargement* and often persists until the junctional epithelium has migrated from the enamel to the cementoenamel junction.

In a strict sense, developmental gingival enlargements are physiologic and ordinarily present no problems. However, when such enlargement is complicated by marginal inflammation, the composite picture gives the impression of extensive gingival enlargement (Fig. 18–31). Treatment to alleviate the marginal inflammation, rather than resection of the enlargement, is sufficient in these cases.

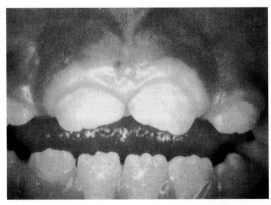

FIGURE 18–31. Developmental gingival enlargement. The normal bulbous contour of the gingiva around the incompletely erupted anterior teeth is accentuated by chronic inflammation.

REFERENCES

1. Aas E. Hyperplasia Gingivae Diphenylhydantoinea. Oslo, Norway, Universitetsforlaget, 1963.
2. Angelopoulos AP, Goaz PW. Incidence of diphenylhydantoin gingival hyperplasia. Oral Surg *34:*898, 1972.
3. Babcock JR. Incidence of gingival hyperplasia associated with dilantin therapy in a hospital population. J Am Dent Assoc *71:*1447, 1965.
4. Babcock JR, Nelson GH. Gingival hyperplasia and Dilantin content of saliva. J Am Dent Assoc *68:*195, 1964.
5. Ball EI. Case of gingivomatosis or elephantiasis of the gingiva. J Periodontol *12:*96, 1941.
6. Baratieri A. The oxytalan connective tissue fibers in gingival hyperplasia in patients treated with sodium diphenylhydantoin. J Periodont Res *2:*106, 1967.
7. Barclay S, Thomason JM, Idle JR, Seymour RA. The incidence and severity of nifedipine-induced gingival overgrowth. J Clin Periodontol *19:*311, 1992.
8. Baxter HA, Brown JB, Byars LT. Malignant melanomas. Am J Orthod *27:*90, 1941.
9. Bellinger DH. Blood and lymph vessel tumors involving the mouth. J Oral Surg *2:*141, 1944.
10. Bernick S. Growth of the gingiva and palate. II. Connective tissue tumors. Oral Surg *1:*1098, 1948.
11. Bernier JL, Ash JE. Atlas of Dental and Oral Pathology. Washington, DC, Registry Press, 1948.
12. Bernier JL, Tiecke RW. Nevus of the gingiva. J Oral Surg *8:*165, 1950.
13. Bhaskar SN, Bernier JL, Godby F. Aneurysmal bone cyst and other giant cell lesions of the jaws. Report of 104 cases. J Oral Surg *17:*30, 1959.
14. Bhaskar SN, Jacoway JR. Pyogenic granuloma: Clinical features, incidence, histology and result of treatment. J Oral Surg *24:*391, 1966.
15. Bhaskar SN, Levin MP, Frisch J. Plasma cell granuloma of periodontal tissues. Report of 45 cases. Periodontics *6:*272, 1968.
16. Brown RS, Sein P, Corio R, Bottomley WK. Nitrendipine-induced gingival hyperplasia. Oral Surg *70:*593, 1990.
17. Buchner A, Begleiter A. Metastatic renal cell carcinoma in the gingiva mimicking a hyperplastic lesion. J Periodontol *51:*413, 1980.
18. Buchner A, Hansen AS. The histomorphologic spectrum of the gingival cyst in the adult. Oral Surg *48:*532, 1979.
19. Buckley DJ, Barrett AP, Bilous AM, Despas PJ. Wegener's granulomatosis— are gingival lesions pathognomonic? J Oral Med *42:*169, 1987.
20. Buckner HJ. Diffuse fibroma of the gums. J Am Dent Assoc *24:*2003, 1937.
21. Burket LW. Oral Medicine. Philadelphia, JB Lippincott, 1946, p 295.
22. Butler RT, Kalkwarf KL, Kaldhal WB. Drug-induced gingival hyperplasia: Phenytoin, cyclosporine and nifedipine. J Am Dent Assoc *114:*56, 1987.
23. Calne R, Rolles K, White DJ, et al. Cyclosporin-A initially as the only immunosuppressant in 34 recipients of cadaveric organs: 32 kidneys, 2 pancreas and 2 livers. Lancet *2:*1033, 1979.
24. Chaudry AP, Hampel A, Gorlin RJ. Primary malignant melanoma of the oral cavity: A review of 105 cases. Cancer *11:*923, 1958.
25. Ciancio SG, Yaffe SJ, Catz CC. Gingival hyperplasia and diphenylhydantoin. J Periodontol *7:*411, 1972.
26. Cotran RS, Kumar V, Robbins SL. Robbins' Pathologic Basis of Disease. 4th ed. Philadelphia, WB Saunders, 1989.
27. Daley TD, Nartey NO, Wysocki GP. Pregnancy tumor: An analysis. Oral Surg *72:*196, 1991.

28. Daley TD, Wysocki GP, Day C. Clinical and pharmacologic correlations in cyclosporine-induced gingival hyperplasia. Oral Surg 62:417, 1986.

29. Heijl L, Sundin Y. Nitrendipine-induced gingival overgrowth in dogs. J Periodontol 60:104, 1989.

30. Dallas BM. Hyperplasia of the oral mucosa in an edentulous epileptic. NZ Dent J 59:54, 1963.

31. Dreyer WP, Thomas CJ. DPH-induced hyperplasia of the masticatory mucosa in an edentulous epileptic patient. Oral Surg 45:701, 1978.

32. Elzay RP, Swenson HM. Effect of an electric toothbrush on Dilantin sodium induced gingival hyperplasia. NY J Dent 34:13, 1964.

33. Emerson TG. Hereditary gingival hyperplasia. A family pedigree of four generations. Oral Surg 19:1, 1965.

34. Fantasia JE, Chen A. A testicular tumor with gingival metastasis. Oral Surg 48:64, 1979.

35. Glickman I. The periodontal tissues of the guinea pig in vitamin C deficiency. J Dent Res 27:9, 1948.

36. Glickman I. The effect of acute vitamin C deficiency upon the response of the periodontal tissues of the guinea pig to artificially induced inflammation. J Dent Res 27:201, 1948.

37. Glickman I. A basic classification of gingival enlargement. J Periodontol 21:131, 1950.

38. Glickman I, Lewitus M. Hyperplasia of the gingiva associated with Dilantin (sodium diphenyl hydantoinate) therapy. J Am Dent Assoc 28:199, 1941.

39. Goldman HM. Sarcoma. Am J Orthod 30:311, 1944.

40. Hagen JD, Soule EH, Gores RJ. Granular cell myoblastoma of the oral cavity. Oral Surg 14:454, 1961.

41. Hall WB. Dilantin hyperplasia: A preventable lesion. J Periodont Res 4(suppl):36, 1969.

42. Hancock RH, Swan RH. Nifedipine-induced gingival overgrowth. J Clin Periodontol 19:12, 1992.

43. Hardman FG. Secondary sarcoma presenting clinical appearance of fibrous epulis. Br Dent J 86:109, 1949.

44. Hassell TM. Epilepsy and the Oral Manifestations of Phenytoin Therapy. Monographs in Oral Science. Vol 9. New York, S Karger, 1981.

45. Hassell TM. Evidence for production of an inactive collagenase by fibroblasts from phenytoin-enlarged human gingiva. J Oral Pathol 11:310, 1982.

46. Hassell TM, Page RC. The major metabolite of phenytoin (Dilantin) induces gingival overgrowth in cats. J Periodont Res 13:280, 1978.

47. Hassell TM, Page RC, Lindhe J. Histologic evidence of impaired growth control in diphenylhydantoin gingival overgrowth in man. Arch Oral Biol 23:381, 1978.

48. Henefer EP, Kay LA. Congenital idiopathic gingival fibromatosis in the deciduous dentition. Oral Surg 24:65, 1967.

49. Hirschfeld I. Hypertrophic gingivitis; its clinical aspect. J Am Dent Assoc 19:799, 1932.

50. Hugoson A. Gingival inflammation and female sex hormones. J Periodont Res, Suppl. 5, 1970.

51. Humphrey AA, Amos NH. Metastatic gingival adenocarcinoma from primary lesion of colon. Am J Cancer 28:128, 1936.

52. Ishikawa J, Glickman I. Gingival response to the systemic administration of sodium diphenyl hydantoinate (Dilantin) in cats. J Periodontol 32:149, 1961.

53. Israelson H, Binnie WH, Hurt WC. The hyperplastic gingivitis of Wegener's granulomatosis. J Periodontol 52:81, 1981.

54. Jaffe HL. Giant cell reparative granuloma, traumatic bone cyst, and fibrous (fibroousseous) dysplasia of the jaw bones. Oral Surg 6:159, 1953.

55. Jorgenson RJ, Cocker ME. Variation in the inheritance and expression of gingival fibromatosis. J Periodontol 45:472, 1974.

56. Kantor ML, Hassell TM. Increased accumulation of sulfated glycosaminoglycans in cultures of human fibroblasts from phenytoin-induced gingival overgrowth. J Dent Res 62:383, 1983.

57. Kapur RN, Grigis S, Little TM, Masotti RE. Diphenylhydantoin induced gingival hyperplasia: Its relation to dose and serum level. Dev Med Child Neurol 15:483, 1973.

58. Kerr DA. Myoblastic myoma. Oral Surg 2:41, 1949.

59. Kerr DA. Granuloma pyogenicum. Oral Surg 4:155, 1951.

60. Kerr DA, McClatchey KD, Regezi JA. Allergic gingivostomatitis (due to gum chewing). J Periodontol 42:709, 1971.

61. Kilpinen E, Raeste AM, Collan Y. Hereditary gingival hyperplasia and physical maturation. Scand J Dent Res 86:118, 1978.

62. Klar LA. Gingival hyperplasia during Dilantin therapy: A survey of 312 patients. J Public Health Dent 33:180, 1973.

63. Klingsberg J, Cancellaro LA, Butcher EO. Effects of air drying in rodent oral mucous membrane. A histologic study of simulated mouth breathing. J Periodontol 32:38, 1961.

64. Kornblut AD, Wolff SM, de Fries HE, Fauci AS. Wegener's granulomatosis. Laryngoscope 90:1453, 1980.

65. Krolls SO, Hoffman S. Squamous cell carcinomas of the oral soft tissues: A statistical analysis of 14,253 cases by age, sex and race of patients. J Am Dent Assoc 92:571, 1976.

66. Lamborghini Deliliers G, Santoro F, Polli N, et al. Light and electron microscopic study of cyclosporin-A induced gingival hyperplasia. J Periodontol 57:771, 1986.

67. Larmas LA, Mackinen KK, Paunio KU. A histochemical study of amylaminopeptidase in hydantoin induced hyperplastic, healthy and inflamed human gingiva. J Periodont Res 8:21, 1973.

68. Lederman D, Lummerman H, Reuben S, Freedman PD. Gingival hyperplasia associated with nifedipine therapy. Oral Surg 57:620, 1984.

69. Lee KW. The fibrous epulis and related lesions. Granuloma pyogenicum, "pregnancy tumor," fibroepithelial polyp and calcifying fibroblastic granuloma. A clinicopathological study. Periodontics 6:277, 1968.

70. Lite T, Dimaio DJ, Burman LR. Gingival patterns in mouth breathers. A clinical and histopathologic study and a method of treatment. Oral Surg 8:382, 1955.

71. Loscalzo LJ. Unpigmented melanocarcinoma of the gingivae. Report of a case. Oral Surg 11:646, 1958.

72. Lucas RM, Howell LP, Wall RA. Nifedipine-induced gingival hyperplasia. A histochemical and ultrastructural study. J Periodontol 56:211, 1985.

73. Lustberg A, Goldman D, Dreskin OH. Megaloblastic anemia due to Dilantin therapy. Ann Intern Med 54:153, 1961.

74. Maier AW, Orban B. Gingivitis in pregnancy. Oral Surg 2:334, 1949.

75. Marfino NR. Developing fibrolipoma of the free gingiva. Oral Surg 12:489, 1959.

76. Mariani G, Calastrini C, Carinci F, et al. Ultrastructural features of cyclosporine A-induced gingival hyperplasia. J Periodontol 64:1092, 1993.

77. McCarthy FP. A clinical and pathological study of oral disease. JAMA 116:16, 1941.

78. Michaelides PL. Recurrent peripheral odontogenic fibroma of the attached gingiva: A case report. J Periodontol 63:645, 1992.

79. Mombelli A, Lang NP, Burgin WB, Gusberti FA. Microbial changes associated with the development of puberty gingivitis. J Periodont Res 25:331, 1990.

80. Moskow BS. The pathogenesis of the gingival cyst. Periodontics 4:23, 1966.

81. Nease WJ. Effect of sodium diphenylhydantoinate on tissue cultures of human gingiva. J Periodontol 36:22, 1965.

82. Newby CD. A report on a case of hypertrophied gum tissue. J Can Dent Assoc 6:183, 1940.

83. Newcomb GM, Seymour GJ, Adkins KF. An unusual form of chronic gingivitis: An ultrastructural, histochemical and immunologic investigation. Oral Surg 53:488, 1982.

84. Nishikawa S, Tada H, Hamasaki A, et al. Nifedipine-induced gingival hyperplasia: A clinical and in vitro study. J Periodontol 62:30, 1991.

85. Nitta H, Kameyama Y, Ishikawa I. Unusual gingival enlargement with rapidly progressive periodontitis. Report of a case. J Periodontol 64:1008, 1993.

86. Nuki K, Cooper SH. The role of inflammation in the pathogenesis of gingival enlargement during the administration of diphenylhydantoin sodium in cats. J Periodont Res 7:91, 1972.

87. Panuska HJ, Gorlin RJ, Bearman JE, Mitchell DF. The effect of anticonvulsant drugs upon the gingiva. A series of 1048 patients. II. J Periodontol 32:15, 1961.

88. Persson PA, Wallenino K. Metastatic renal carcinoma (hypernephroma) in the gingiva of the lower jaw. Acta Odontol Scand 19:289, 1961.

89. Phillips RL, Shafer WG. An evaluation of the peripheral giant cell tumor. J Periodontol 26:216, 1955.

90. Raeste AM, Collan Y, Kilpinen E. Hereditary fibrous hyperplasia of the gingiva with varying penetrance and expressivity. Scand J Dent Res 86:357, 1978.

91. Rateitschak-Pluss EM, Hefti A, Lortscher R, Thiel G. Initial observation that cyclosporin A induces gingival enlargement in man. J Clin Periodontol 10:237, 1983.

92. Rickles NH, Everett FG. Gingival and lateral periodontal cysts. Parodontologie 14:41, 1960.

93. Rostock MH, Fry HR, Turner JE. Severe gingival overgrowth associated with cyclosporine therapy. J Periodontol 57:294, 1986.

94. Rushton MA. Hereditary or idiopathic hyperplasia of the gums. Dent Pract 7:136, 1957.

95. Russell BJ, Bay LM. Oral use of chlorhexidine gluconate toothpaste in epileptic children. Scand J Dent Res 86:52, 1978.

96. Schneider LC, Weisinger E. The true gingival fibroma; an analysis of 129 fibrous gingival lesions. J Periodontol 49:423, 1978.

97. Serio FG, Siegel MA, Slade BE. Plasma cell gingivitis of unusual origin. A case report. J Periodontol 62:390, 1991.

98. Setia AP. Severe bleeding from a pregnancy tumor. Oral Surg 36:192, 1973.

99. Seymour RA, Jacobs DJ. Cyclosporine and the gingival tissues. J Clin Periodontol 19:1, 1992.

100. Seymour RA, Smith DG, Rogers SR. The comparative effects of azathioprine and cyclosporine on some gingival health parameters of renal transplant patients. J Clin Periodontol 14:610, 1987.

101. Shafer WG. Effect of Dilantin sodium analogues on cell proliferation in tissue culture. Proc Soc Exp Biol Med 106:205, 1960.

102. Shafer WG. Effect of Dilantin sodium on various cell lines in tissue culture. Proc Soc Exp Biol Med 108:694, 1961.

103. Shafer WG, Beatty RE, Davis WB. Effect of Dilantin sodium on tensile strength of healing wounds. Proc Soc Exp Biol Med 98:348, 1958.

104. Shapiro M. Acceleration of gingival wound healing in nonepileptic patients receiving diphenylhydantoin sodium. Exp Med Surg 16:41, 1958.

105. Silverman S Jr, Lozada F. An epilogue to plasma cell gingivostomatitis (allergic gingivostomatitis). Oral Surg 43:211, 1977.

106. Staple PH, Reed MJ, Mashimo PA. Diphenylhydantoin gingival hyperplasia in *Macaca arctoides:* A new human model. J Periodontol 48:325, 1977.

107. Stein GM, Lewis H. Oral changes in a folic acid deficient patient precipitated by anticonvulsant drug therapy. J Periodontol 44:645, 1973.

108. Stevenson ARL, Austin BW. A case of ameloblastoma presenting as an exophytic gingival lesion. J Periodontol 61:378, 1990.

109. Stirrups D, Inglis J. Tuberous sclerosis with nonhydantoin gingival hyperplasia. Report of a case. Oral Surg *49:*211, 1980.
110. Sutcliffe P. A longitudinal study of gingivitis and puberty. J Periodont Res *7:*52, 1972.
111. Sznajder N, Dominguez FV, Carraro JJ, Lis G. Hemorrhagic hemangioma of the gingiva: Report of a case. J Periodontol *44:*579, 1973.
112. Taicher S, Mazar A, Hirschberg A, Dayan D. Metastatic chondrosarcoma of the gingiva mimicking a reactive exophytic lesion: A case report. J Periodontol *623:*223, 1991.
113. Thoma KH, Holland DJ, Woodbury HW, et al. Malignant lymphoma of the gingiva. Oral Surg *1:*57, 1948.
114. Thomas D, Rapley J, Strathman R, Parker R. Tuberous sclerosis with gingival overgrowth. J Periodontol *63:*713, 1992.
115. Thukral PP. Idiopathic gingival hyperplasia. J Indian Dent Assoc *44:*109, 1972.
116. Traeger KA. Cyst of the gingiva (mucocele): Report of a case. Oral Surg *14:*243, 1961.
117. Wedgwood D, Rusen D, Balk S. Gingival metastases from primary hepatocellular carcinoma. Oral Surg *47:*263, 1979.
118. Westphal P. Salivary secretion and gingival hyperplasia in diphenylhydantoin-treated guinea pigs. Sven Tandlak Tidskr *62:*505, 1969.
119. Wysocki G, Gretsinger HA, Laupacis A, et al. Fibrous hyperplasia of the gingiva: A side effect of cyclosporin A therapy. Oral Surg *55:*274, 1983.
120. Zackin SJ, Weisberger D. Hereditary gingival fibromatosis. Oral Surg *14:*828, 1961.
121. Ziskin DE, Blackberg SM, Stout AP. The gingivae during pregnancy. Surg Gynecol Obstet *57:*719, 1933.
122. Ziskin DE, Zegarelli E. Idiopathic fibromatosis of the gingivae. Ann Dent *2:*50, 1943.

19

Acute Gingival Infections

FERMIN A. CARRANZA, JR.

Acute Necrotizing Ulcerative Gingivitis	Communicability
Clinical Features	**Acute Herpetic Gingivostomatitis**
Acute Necrotizing Ulcerative Gingivitis and Chronic Destructive Periodontitis	Etiology
Relation of Bacteria to the Characteristic Lesion	Clinical Features
Bacterial Flora	Diagnosis
Diagnosis	Differential Diagnosis
Differential Diagnosis	Communicability
Etiology	**Pericoronitis**
Epidemiology and Prevalence	Clinical Features
	Complications

ACUTE NECROTIZING ULCERATIVE GINGIVITIS

Acute necrotizing ulcerative gingivitis (ANUG)* is an inflammatory destructive disease of the gingiva that presents characteristic signs and symptoms. It was recognized as far back as the fourth century BC by Xenophon, who mentioned that Greek soldiers were affected with "sore mouth" and foul-smelling breath. In 1778 John Hunter described the clinical findings and differentiated ANUG from scurvy and chronic destructive periodontal disease. ANUG occurred in epidemic form in the French army in the 19th century, and in 1886 Hersch, a German pathologist, discussed some of the features associated with the disease, such as enlarged lymph nodes, fever, malaise, and increased salivation. In the 1890s Plaut[56] and Vincent[79] described the disease and attributed its origin to fusiform bacilli and spirochetes. It was commonly known as *Vincent's infection* during the first half of the 20th century, but its current designation is acute necrotizing ulcerative gingivitis.

Clinical Features

Classification. Necrotizing ulcerative gingivitis most often occurs as an acute disease. Its relatively mild and more persistent form is referred to as *subacute* disease. *Recurrent* disease is marked by periods of remission and exacerbation. Reference is also sometimes made to *chronic* necrotizing ulcerative gingivitis. However, it is difficult to justify this designation as a separate entity, because most periodontal pockets with ulceration and destruction of gingival tissue have comparable microscopic and clinical features.

History. ANUG is characterized by sudden onset, sometimes following an episode of debilitating disease or acute respiratory tract infection. A change in living habits, protracted work without adequate rest, and psychological stress are frequent features of the patient's history.

Oral Signs. Characteristic lesions are punched out, crater-like depressions at the crest of the interdental papillae, subsequently extending to the marginal gingiva. The surface of the gingival craters is covered by a gray, pseudomembranous slough demarcated from the remainder

---

* Other terms for this condition include Vincent's infection, acute ulceromembranous gingivitis, trench mouth, ulcerative gingivitis, Vincent's stomatitis, Plaut-Vincent stomatitis, stomatitis ulcerosa, fusospirillary gingivitis, fetid stomatitis, putrid stomatitis, acute septic gingivitis, pseudomembranous angina, and spirochetal stomatitis.

of the gingival mucosa by a pronounced linear erythema (Plate IX*A*). In some instances, the lesions are denuded of the surface pseudomembrane, exposing the gingival margin, which is red, shiny, and hemorrhagic. *The characteristic lesions progressively destroy the gingiva and underlying periodontal tissues* (Plate IX*B*).

Spontaneous gingival hemorrhage or pronounced bleeding on the slightest stimulation are additional characteristic clinical signs (Plate IX*C*). Other signs frequently found are fetid odor and increased salivation.[1,71]

ANUG can occur in otherwise disease-free mouths or can be superimposed on chronic gingivitis (Plate IX*D*) *or periodontal pockets.* Involvement may be limited to a single tooth or group of teeth (Fig. 19–1) or may be widespread throughout the mouth. It is rare in edentulous mouths, but isolated spherical lesions occasionally occur on the soft palate.

Oral Symptoms. The lesions are extremely sensitive to touch, and the patient complains of a constant radiating, gnawing pain that is intensified by spicy or hot foods and chewing. There is a metallic foul taste, and the patient is conscious of an excessive amount of "pasty" saliva.

Extraoral and Systemic Signs and Symptoms. Patients are usually ambulatory and have a minimum of systemic complications. Local lymphadenopathy and a slight elevation in temperature are common features of the mild and moderate stages of the disease. In severe cases there are marked systemic complications such as high fever, increased pulse rate, leukocytosis, loss of appetite, and general lassitude. Systemic reactions are more severe in children. Insomnia, constipation, gastrointestinal disorders, headache, and mental depression sometimes accompany the condition.

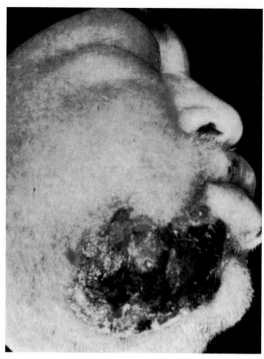

FIGURE 19–2. Noma following acute necrotizing ulcerative gingivitis in a 50-year-old man with severe anemia.

In very rare cases, severe sequelae such as noma or gangrenous stomatitis[2,3,21] (Fig. 19–2), fusospirochetal meningitis and peritonitis, pulmonary infections,[48] toxemia, and fatal brain abscess may occur.[74]

Clinical Course. The clinical course is indefinite. If untreated, ANUG may result in progressive destruction of the periodontium and denudation of the roots, accompanied by an increase in the severity of toxic systemic complications. It often undergoes a diminution in severity, leading to a subacute stage with varying degrees of clinical symptoms. *The disease may subside spontaneously without treatment.* Such patients generally have a history of repeated remissions and exacerbations. Recurrence of the condition in previously treated patients is also frequent.

Histopathology. Microscopically, the lesion appears as a nonspecific acute necrotizing inflammation at the gingival margin involving both the stratified squamous epithelium and the underlying connective tissue. The surface epithelium is destroyed and is replaced by a pseudomembranous meshwork of fibrin, necrotic epithelial cells, polymorphonuclear neutrophils (PMNs), and various types of microorganisms (Fig. 19–3). This is the zone that appears clinically as the surface pseudomembrane. The underlying connective tissue is markedly hyperemic, with numerous engorged capillaries and a dense infiltration of PMNs. This acutely inflamed hyperemic zone appears clinically as the linear erythema beneath the surface pseudomembrane. Numerous plasma cells may appear in the periphery of the infiltrate; this is interpreted as an area of established chronic marginal gingivitis on which the acute lesion became superimposed.[35]

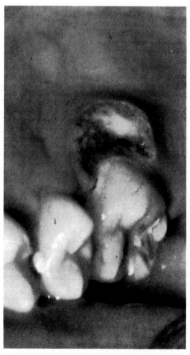

FIGURE 19–1. Localized zone of acute necrotizing ulcerative gingivitis.

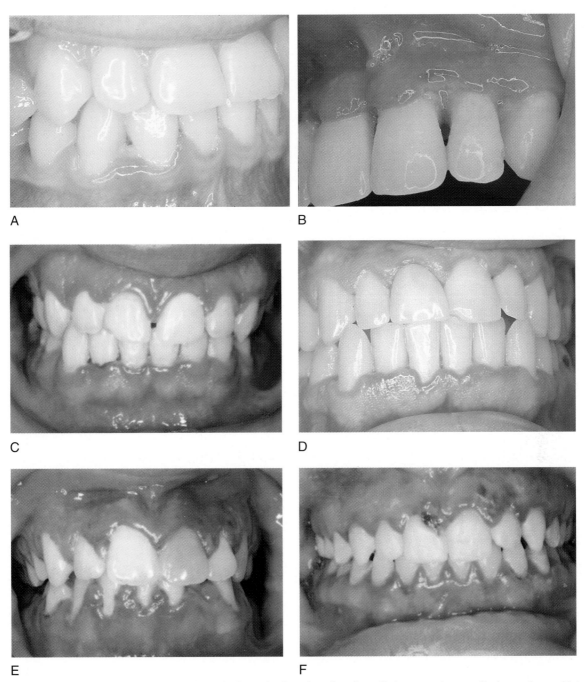

PLATE IX. *A,* Acute necrotizing ulcerative gingivitis: typical punched-out interdental papilla between the mandibular canine and lateral incisor. *B,* Acute necrotizing ulcerative gingivitis: typical lesions with progressive tissue destruction. *C,* Acute necrotizing ulcerative gingivitis: typical lesions with spontaneous hemorrhage. *D,* Acute necrotizing ulcerative gingivitis: typical lesions have produced irregular gingival contour. *E,* Acute herpetic gingivostomatitis: typical diffuse erythema. *F,* Acute herpetic gingivostomatitis: vesicles on the gingiva.

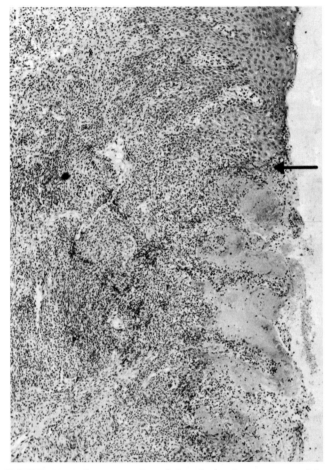

FIGURE 19–3. Survey section of the gingiva in acute necrotizing ulcerative gingivitis. The portion of the section below the arrow shows ulceration and accumulation of leukocytes, fibrin, and necrotic tissue that form the gray marginal pseudomembrane.

The epithelium and connective tissue have decreasing alterations in appearance as the distance from the necrotic gingival margin increases. There is a gradual blending of the epithelium from the uninvolved gingiva to the necrotic lesion. At the immediate border of the necrotic pseudomembrane, the epithelium is edematous, and the individual cells exhibit varying degrees of hydropic degeneration. In addition, there is an infiltration of PMNs in the intercellular spaces. The inflammatory involvement in the connective tissue diminishes as the distance from the necrotic lesion increases, until the involved tissue blends in appearance with the uninvolved connective tissue stroma of the normal gingival mucosa.

It is noteworthy that the microscopic appearance of ANUG is nonspecific. Comparable changes result from trauma, chemical irritation, or the application of escharotic drugs.

Acute Necrotizing Ulcerative Gingivitis and Chronic Destructive Periodontitis

It is important to understand the relationship between ANUG and chronic destructive periodontal disease. As pointed out earlier, ANUG may occur in a mouth devoid of pre-existing gingival disease, or it may be superimposed on underlying chronic gingivitis and periodontal pockets. However, it does not usually lead to conventional periodontal pocket formation because the necrotic changes involve the junctional epithelium; a viable junctional epithelium is needed for pocket deepening (see Chapter 22).

ANUG can, however, progress to cause destruction of the supporting structures. When bone loss occurs the condition is called *necrotizing ulcerative periodontitis* (see Chapter 26).

Relation of Bacteria to the Characteristic Lesion

The light microscope and the electron microscope have been used to study the relationship of bacteria to the characteristic lesion of ANUG. The exudate on the surface of the necrotic lesion appears to contain microorganisms that morphologically resemble cocci, fusiform bacilli, and spirochetes.[76] The layer between the necrotic and the living tissue contains enormous numbers of fusiform bacilli and spirochetes, in addition to leukocytes and fibrin. Spirochetes and other bacteria[6,13,19,40] invade the underlying living tissue; however, not all organisms seen on the surface penetrate the tissue.

Listgarten[40] described the following four zones, which blend with each other and may not all be present in every case:

> *Zone 1: Bacterial zone.* The most superficial; consists of varied bacteria, including a few spirochetes of the small, medium, and large types.
> *Zone 2: Neutrophil-rich zone.* Contains numerous leukocytes, preponderantly neutrophils, with bacteria, including many spirochetes of various types, between the leukocytes.
> *Zone 3: Necrotic zone.* Consists of disintegrated tissue cells, fibrillar material, remnants of collagen fibers, and numerous intermediate and large type spirochetes, with few other organisms.
> *Zone 4: Zone of spirochetal infiltration.* Consists of well-preserved tissue infiltrated with intermediate and large spirochetes, without other organisms.

Spirochetes have been found as deep as 300 μm from the surface. The majority of spirochetes in the deeper zones are morphologically different from cultivated strains of *Treponema macrodentium*. They occur in non-necrotic tissue before other types of bacteria and may be present in high concentrations intercellularly in the epithelium adjacent to the ulcerated lesion and in the connective tissue.[40]

Bacterial Flora

Smears from the lesions (Fig. 19–4) demonstrate scattered bacteria, predominantly spirochetes and fusiform bacilli, desquamated epithelial cells, and occasional PMNs. A smear containing only spirochetes and fusiform bacilli is rarely seen. Usually these two organisms are seen with other oral spirochetes, vibrios, streptococci, and filamentous organisms. The spirochetal organisms form a light-staining,

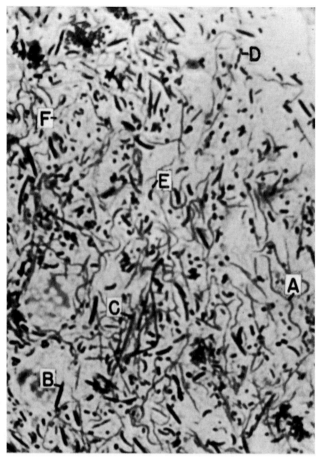

FIGURE 19-4. Bacterial smear from a lesion in acute necrotizing ulcerative gingivitis. A, Spirochete; B, *Bacillus fusiformis;* C, filamentous organism (*Actinomyces* or *Leptotrichia*); D, *Streptococcus;* E, *Vibrio;* F, *Treponema macrodentium.*

conspicuous, interlacing network throughout the microscopic field.

Electron microscopic studies indicate that the spirochetes may be classified into three morphologic groups: small (7% to 39% of the total spirochetes present), intermediate (43.9% to 90%), and large (0% to 20%).[41] It was also suggested that intermediate spirochetes are present in greater

numbers in pooled scrapings from lesions of ANUG and are found in greater percentages in deeper portions of the lesions.

The mean fusiform bacillus count in the saliva of patients with ANUG is higher than that in the saliva of "normal" persons. *Fusobacterium* species account for the majority of the total fusiform bacilli in both groups.

Diagnosis

Diagnosis is based on clinical findings. A bacterial smear may be used to corroborate the clinical diagnosis, but it is not necessary or definitive because the bacterial picture is not appreciably different from that in marginal gingivitis, periodontal pockets, pericoronitis, or herpetic gingivostomatitis.[60] Bacterial studies are useful, however, in the differential diagnosis of ANUG and specific infections of the oral cavity such as diphtheria, thrush, actinomycosis, and streptococcal stomatitis.

Microscopic examination of the biopsy specimen is not sufficiently specific to be diagnostic. It can be used to differentiate ANUG from specific infections such as tuberculosis or from neoplastic disease, but it does not differentiate ANUG from other acute necrotizing conditions of nonspecific origin, such as those produced by trauma or escharotic drugs.

Differential Diagnosis

Necrotizing ulcerative gingivitis should be differentiated from other conditions that resemble it in some respects, such as acute herpetic gingivostomatitis (Table 19-1), chronic periodontal pockets, desquamative gingivitis (Table 19-2), streptococcal gingivostomatitis, aphthous stomatitis, gonococcal gingivostomatitis, diphtheritic and syphilitic lesions (Table 19-3), tuberculous gingival lesions, candidiasis, agranulocytosis, dermatoses (pemphigus, erythema multiforme, and lichen planus), and stomatitis venenata. See Chapter 20 for a description of most of these conditions.

Streptococcal gingivostomatitis[45] is a rare condition characterized by a diffuse erythema of the posterior areas of the oral mucosa, sometimes including the gingiva. Necrosis of

Table 19-1. DIFFERENTIATION OF ACUTE NECROTIZING ULCERATIVE GINGIVITIS FROM ACUTE HERPETIC GINGIVOSTOMATITIS

Acute Necrotizing Ulcerative Gingivitis	Acute Herpetic Gingivostomatitis
Etiology: interaction between host and bacteria, most probably fusospirochetes	Specific viral etiology
Necrotizing condition	Diffuse erythema and vesicular eruption
Punched out gingival margin; pseudomembrane that peels off, leaving raw areas; marginal gingiva affected, other oral tissues rarely involved	Vesicles rupture and leave slightly depressed oval or spherical ulcer
	Diffuse involvement of gingiva; may include buccal mucosa and lips
Rare in children	Occurs more frequently in children
No definite duration	Duration of 7 to 10 days
No demonstrated immunity	An acute episode results in some degree of immunity
Contagion not demonstrated	Contagious

Table 19–2. DIFFERENTIATION AMONG ACUTE NECROTIZING ULCERATIVE GINGIVITIS, CHRONIC DESQUAMATIVE GINGIVITIS, AND CHRONIC PERIODONTAL DISEASE

Acute Necrotizing Ulcerative Gingivitis	Desquamative Gingivitis	Chronic Destructive Periodontal Disease
Bacterial smears show fusospirochetal complex	Bacterial smears reveal numerous epithelial cells, few bacterial forms	Bacterial smears are variable
Marginal gingiva affected	Diffuse involvement of marginal and attached gingivae and other areas of oral mucosa	Marginal gingiva affected
Acute history	Chronic history	Chronic history
Painful	May or may not be painful	Painless if uncomplicated
Pseudomembrane	Patchy desquamation or gingival epithelium	No desquamation generally, but purulent material may appear from pockets
Papillary and marginal necrotic lesions	Papillae do not undergo necrosis	Papillae do not undergo notable necrosis
Affects adults of both sexes, occasionally children	Affects adults, most often women	Generally in adults, occasionally in children
Characteristic fetid odor	None	Some odor present but not strikingly fetid

the gingival margin is not a feature of this disease, and there is no notably fetid odor. Bacterial smears show a preponderance of streptococcal forms, which on culture appear as *Streptococcus viridans*.

Gonococcal stomatitis is rare and is caused by *Neisseria gonorrhoeae*. The oral mucosa is covered with a grayish membrane that sloughs off in areas to expose an underlying raw, bleeding surface.[45] It is most common in newborns and is caused by transmission of infection from the maternal passages, but cases in adults resulting from direct contact have been described.

Agranulocytosis is characterized by ulceration and necrosis of the gingiva that resembles ANUG. The oral condition in agranulocytosis is primarily necrotizing. Because of the diminished defense mechanisms in agranulocytosis, the clinical picture is not marked by the severe inflammatory reaction seen in ANUG. Blood studies are used to differentiate necrotizing ulcerative gingivitis from the gingival necrosis in agranulocytosis.

Vincent's angina is a fusospirochetal infection of the oropharynx and throat, as distinguished from ANUG, which affects the marginal gingiva. In Vincent's angina there is a painful membranous ulceration of the throat, with edema and hyperemic patches breaking down to form ulcers covered with pseudomembranous material. The process may extend to the larynx and middle ear.

ANUG in leukemia is not produced by leukemia per se. However, ANUG may be superimposed on gingival tissue alterations caused by leukemia. The differential diagnosis consists not in distinguishing between ANUG and leukemic gingival changes, but rather in determining whether leukemia is a predisposing factor in a mouth in which ANUG is present. For example, if a patient with acute necrotizing involvement of the gingival margin also has generalized diffuse discoloration and edema of the attached gingiva, the possibility of an underlying, systemically induced gingival change should be considered. Leukemia is one of the conditions that would have to be ruled out (see Chapter 14).

ANUG in acquired immunodeficiency syndrome (AIDS) has the same clinical features, although it reportedly follows a very destructive course leading to the loss of soft tissue and bone and to the formation of sequestra[30] (see Chapter 15).

Table 19–3. DIFFERENTIATION AMONG ACUTE NECROTIZING ULCERATIVE GINGIVITIS, DIPHTHERIA, AND SECONDARY STAGE OF SYPHILIS

Acute Necrotizing Ulcerative Gingivitis	Diphtheria	Secondary Stage of Syphilis (Mucous Patch)
Etiology: interaction between host and bacteria, possibly fusospirochetes	Specific bacterial etiology: *Corynebacterium diphtheriae*	Specific bacterial etiology: *Treponema pallidum*
Affects marginal gingiva	Rarely affects marginal gingiva	Rarely affects marginal gingiva
Membrane removal easy	Membrane removal difficult	Membrane not detachable
Painful condition	Less painful	Minimal pain
Marginal gingiva affected	Throat, fauces, tonsils affected	Any part of mouth affected
Serologic findings normal	Serologic findings normal	Serologic findings abnormal (Wasserman, Kahn, VDRL)
Immunity not conferred	Immunity conferred by an attack	Immunity not conferred
Doubtful contagiosity	Contagious	Only direct contact will communicate disease
Antibiotic therapy relieves symptoms	Antibiotic treatment has little effect	Antibiotic therapy has excellent results

VDRL, Venereal Disease Research Laboratory (test).

Etiology

Role of Bacteria. Plaut[56] and Vincent,[79] in 1894 and 1896, respectively, introduced the concept that ANUG is caused by specific bacteria—namely, a fusiform bacillus and a spirochetal organism.

Opinions still differ regarding whether bacteria are the primary causative factors in ANUG. Several observations support this concept: spirochetal organisms and fusiform bacilli are always found in the disease; other organisms are also involved. Rosebury and coworkers[60] described a fusospirochetal complex consisting of *T. macrodentium,* intermediate spirochetes, vibrios, fusiform bacilli, and filamentous organisms in addition to several *Borrelia* species.

More recently Loesche and colleagues[42] described a constant flora and a variable flora associated with ANUG. The constant flora is composed of fusospirochetal organisms and also *Bacteroides melaninogenicus* subsp. *intermedius* and possibly *Actinomyces odontolyticus* and various spirilla-like *Selenomonas* species. The variable flora consists of a heterogeneous array of bacterial types.

Treatment with metronidazole results in a significant reduction of *Treponema* species, *B. melaninogenicus* subsp. *intermedius,* and *Fusobacterium,* with resolution of the clinical symptoms.[18,42] Given the antibacterial spectrum of this drug, the anaerobic members of the flora mentioned are thought to be responsible for the symptoms.

These bacteriologic findings have been supported by immunologic data presented by Chung et al.,[10] who reported increased immunoglobulin G and M (IgG; IgM) antibody titers to intermediate spirochetes and *B. melaninogenicus* subsp. *intermedius* in ANUG patients compared with titers in those with chronic gingivitis and healthy controls. Cogen and coworkers[11] described a depression in host defense mechanisms, particularly in PMN chemotaxis and phagocytosis, in ANUG patients. For further details on host–bacteria interactions in ANUG, see Chapters 6, 9, and 10.

ANUG has not been produced experimentally in humans or animals by inoculation of bacterial exudates from the lesions. Exudates from ANUG produce fusospirochetal abscesses when inoculated subcutaneously in experimental animals, and the infection is freely transmissible in series.[59] Local intracutaneous injection of a hyaluronidase- and chondroitinase-containing cell-free filtrate of oral microaerophilic diphtheroid bacilli aggravated spirochetal lesions produced by oral treponemes.[33] In only one animal experiment has the transmission of lesions comparable to those seen in humans been reported.[2]

The specific cause of ANUG has not been established. The prevalent opinion is that it is produced by a complex of bacterial organisms but requires underlying tissue changes to facilitate the pathogenic activity of the bacteria.

Local Predisposing Factors. Pre-existing gingivitis, injury to the gingiva, and smoking are important predisposing factors. Although ANUG may appear in an otherwise disease-free mouth, it most often occurs superimposed on pre-existing chronic gingival disease and periodontal pockets. Deep periodontal pockets and pericoronal flaps are particularly vulnerable areas for the occurrence of the disease, because they offer a favorable environment for the proliferation of anaerobic fusiform bacilli and spirochetes. Areas of the gingiva traumatized by opposing teeth in malocclusion,

such as the palatal surface behind the maxillary incisors and the labial gingival surface of the mandibular incisors, are frequent sites of ANUG.

The relationship between ANUG and smoking has been frequently mentioned in the literature. Pindborg[54] reported that 98% of his ANUG patients were smokers and that the frequency of ANUG increased with an increasing exposure to tobacco smoke. It has not been established whether this correlation occurs because (1) tobacco smoke has a direct toxic effect on the gingiva, (2) vascular or other changes are induced by nicotine or other substances, or (3) smoking and ANUG are both reflections of stress.

Systemic Predisposing Factors. ANUG is often superimposed on gingival alterations caused by severe systemic disease.

Nutritional Deficiency. Necrotizing gingivitis has been produced in animals fed nutritionally deficient diets.[8,38,48,75,78] Several researchers found an increase in the fusospirochetal flora in the mouths of the experimental animals, but the bacteria were regarded as opportunistic, proliferating only when the tissues were altered by the deficiency.

Conditioning Effect of Nutritional Deficiency on Bacterial Pathogenicity. Nutritional deficiencies (e.g., vitamin C, vitamin B_2) accentuate the severity of the pathologic changes induced when the fusospirochetal bacterial complex is injected into animals.[69]

Debilitating Disease. Debilitating systemic disease may predispose patients to the development of ANUG. Included among these systemic disturbances are chronic diseases such as syphilis and cancer, severe gastrointestinal disorders such as ulcerative colitis, blood dyscrasias such as the leukemias and anemia, and AIDS. Nutritional deficiency resulting from debilitating disease may be an additional predisposing factor. Experimentally induced leukopenia in animals may produce ulcerative gangrenous stomatitis.[48,72,73,77] Necrotizing gingivitis and stomatitis occurred in 74% of animals with experimentally induced renal insufficiency.[28] Ulceronecrotic lesions appear in the gingival margins of hamsters exposed to total body irradiation[44]; these lesions can be prevented by systemic antibiotics.[43]

Psychosomatic Factors. Psychological factors appear to be important in the etiology of ANUG. The disease often occurs in association with stress situations (e.g., induction into the armed forces or school examinations).[20,27] Psychological disturbances,[28] as well as increased adrenocortical secretion,[65] are common in patients with the disease.

Significant correlation between disease incidence and two personality traits—dominance and abasement—suggests the presence of an ANUG-prone personality.[24] The mechanisms whereby psychological factors create or predispose to gingival damage have not been established, but alterations in digital and gingival capillary responses suggestive of increased autonomic nervous activity have been demonstrated in patients with ANUG.[26]

Cohen-Cole and coworkers[12] suggested that a psychiatric disturbance (e.g., trait anxiety, depression, and psychopathic deviance) and the impact of negative life events (stress) may lead to activation of the hypothalamic-pituitary-adrenal axis. This results in elevation of serum and urine cortisol levels, which is associated with a depression of lymphocyte and PMN function that may predispose to ANUG.

Epidemiology and Prevalence

ANUG often occurs in groups in an epidemic pattern. At one time it was considered contagious, but this has not been substantiated.[62]

The prevalence of ANUG appears to have been rather low in the United States and Europe prior to 1914. During World Wars I and II there were numerous epidemics among the Allied troops, but German soldiers did not seem to be similarly affected. There have also been epidemic-like outbreaks among civilian populations. In a study conducted at a dental clinic in Prague, Czech Republic, the incidence of ANUG was reported as 0.08% in patients 15 to 19 years old, 0.05% in those 20 to 24 years old, and 0.02% in persons 25 to 29 years old.[68]

ANUG occurs at all ages,[15] with the highest incidence reported between the ages of 20 and 30[16,70] and 15 and 20 years.[41] It is not common in children in the United States, Canada, and Europe, but it has been reported in children from low socioeconomic groups in underdeveloped countries.[37] In India, 54%[54] and 58%[55] of the patients in two studies were younger than 10 years old. In a random school population in Nigeria, ANUG occurred in 11.3% of children between the ages of 2 and 6 years,[66] and in a Nigerian hospital population, it was present in 23% of children less than 10 years old.[20] It has been reported in several members of the same family in low socioeconomic groups. ANUG is more common in children with Down syndrome than in other retarded children.[4]

Opinions differ as to whether ANUG is more common during the winter,[52] summer, or fall,[68] or whether there is a peak seasonal incidence.[16,80]

Communicability

A distinction must be made between communicability and transmissibility when referring to the characteristics of disease. The term *transmissible* denotes a capacity for the maintenance of an infectious agent in successive passages through a susceptible animal host.[58] The term *communicable* signifies a capacity for the maintenance of infection by natural modes of spread (e.g., direct contact through drinking water, food, and eating utensils; the airborne route; or arthropod vectors). A disease that is communicable is described as contagious. Disease associated with the fusospirochetal bacterial complex is transmissible but *has not been shown to be communicable or contagious.*

Attempts have been made to spread ANUG from human to human, without success.[36] King[38] traumatized an area in his gingiva and introduced debris from a patient with a severe case of ANUG. There was no response until he happened to fall ill shortly thereafter; subsequent to his illness, he observed the characteristic lesion in the experimental area. It may be inferred from this experiment, with reservation, that systemic debility is a prerequisite for the development of ANUG.

It is a common impression that because ANUG often occurs in groups of people who use the same kitchen facilities, the disease is spread by bacteria on eating utensils. Growth of fusospirochetal organisms requires carefully controlled conditions and an anaerobic environment; they do not ordinarily survive on eating utensils.[14]

The occurrence of the disease in epidemic-like outbreaks does not necessarily mean that it is contagious. The affected groups may be afflicted by the disease because of common predisposing factors rather than because of its spread from person to person. In all likelihood both a predisposed host and the presence of appropriate bacteria are necessary for the production of this disease.

ACUTE HERPETIC GINGIVOSTOMATITIS

Etiology

Acute herpetic gingivostomatitis is the primary infection of the oral cavity caused by the herpes simplex virus (HSV) type 1.[17,46,64] It occurs most frequently in infants and children younger than 6 years of age,[64] but it is also seen in adolescents and adults. It occurs with equal frequency in males and females. In most people (88% to 99%), however, this primary infection is asymptomatic.

After the primary infection, the virus ascends through sensory or autonomic nerves and persists in neuronal ganglia that innervate the site as a latent HSV. In approximately one third of the world's population, secondary manifestations occur as a result of various stimuli such as sunlight, trauma, fever, or stress. These secondary manifestations include recurrent herpes labialis (Fig. 19–5), herpes genitalis, ocular herpes, and herpes encephalitis.[51]

Clinical Features

Oral Signs. Acute herpetic gingivostomatitis appears as a diffuse, erythematous, shiny involvement of the gingiva and the adjacent oral mucosa, with varying degrees of edema and gingival bleeding (see Plate IX*E*). In its initial stage it is characterized by the presence of discrete, spherical gray vesicles (see Plate IX*F*), which may occur on the gingiva, the labial and buccal mucosae, the soft palate, the pharynx, the sublingual mucosa, and the tongue (Fig. 19–6). After approximately 24 hours the vesicles rupture and form painful small ulcers with a red, elevated, halo-like margin and a depressed yellowish or grayish white central portion. These occur either in widely separated areas or in clusters where confluence occurs (Fig. 19–7).

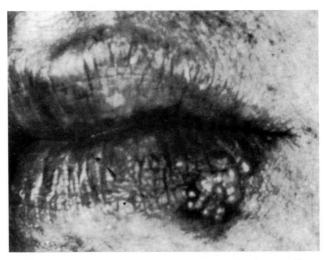

FIGURE 19–5. Cluster of herpetic vesicles ("cold sores").

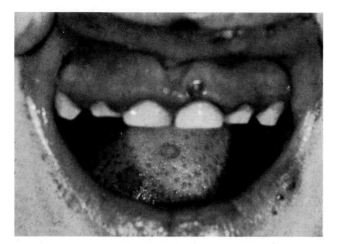

FIGURE 19-6. Vesicles on the tongue in acute herpetic gingivostomatitis.

Occasionally, acute herpetic gingivitis may occur without overt vesiculation. Diffuse, erythematous, shiny discoloration and edematous enlargement of the gingivae with a tendency toward bleeding make up the clinical picture.

The course of the disease is limited to 7 to 10 days. The diffuse gingival erythema and edema that appear early in the disease persist for several days after the ulcerative lesions have healed. Scarring does not occur in the areas of healed ulcerations.

Oral Symptoms. The disease is accompanied by generalized "soreness" of the oral cavity that interferes with eating and drinking. The ruptured vesicles are the focal sites of pain and are particularly sensitive to touch, thermal changes, foods such as condiments and fruit juices, and the action of coarse foods. In infants the disease is marked by irritability and refusal to take food.

Extraoral and Systemic Signs and Symptoms. Cervical adenitis, fever as high as 101°F to 105°F (38.3°C to 40.6°C), and generalized malaise are common.

History. Recent acute infection is a common feature of the history of patients with acute herpetic gingivostomatitis.[17] The condition frequently occurs during and immediately after an episode of such febrile diseases as pneumonia, meningitis, influenza, and typhoid. It also tends to occur during periods of anxiety, strain, or exhaustion and during menstruation. A history of exposure to patients with herpetic infection of the oral cavity or lips may also be elicited. Acute herpetic gingivostomatitis often occurs in the early stage of infectious mononucleosis.[49]

Histopathology. The discrete ulcerations of herpetic gingivostomatitis that result from rupture of the vesicles have a central portion of acute inflammation, with ulceration and various degrees of purulent exudate, surrounded by a zone rich in engorged blood vessels. The microscopic picture of the vesicles is characterized by extra- and intracellular edema and degeneration of the epithelial cells. The cell cytoplasm appears liquefied and clear; the cell membrane and nucleus stand out in relief. The nucleus later degenerates, loses its affinity for stain, and finally disintegrates. The vesicle formation results from fragmentation of the degenerated epithelial cells.

The fully developed vesicle is a cavity in the epithelial cells with occasional PMNs. The base of the vesicle is formed by edematous epithelial cells of the basal and prickle cell layers. The superficial surface of the vesicle is formed by compressed upper layers of prickle cells of the stratum granulosum and the stratum corneum. Occasionally, rounded eosinophilic inclusion bodies[39] are found in the nuclei of epithelial cells bordering vesicles (Fig. 19-8). Inclusion bodies may be a colony of virus particles, degenerated protoplasm remnants of the affected cell, or a combination of both.[50]

Diagnosis

The diagnosis is usually established from the patient's history and the clinical findings. Material may be obtained from the lesions and submitted to the laboratory for confirmatory tests, including virus culture and immunologic tests

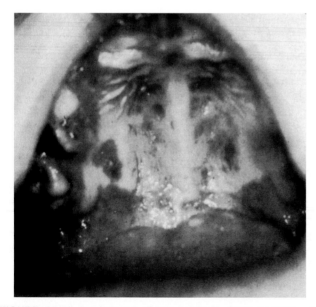

FIGURE 19-7. Involvement of the palate in acute herpetic gingivostomatitis.

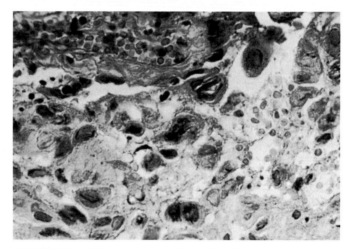

FIGURE 19-8. Biopsy showing giant cells with inclusion bodies at the base of a herpetic lesion.

using monoclonal antibodies or DNA hybridization techniques.[7,25,57]

Differential Diagnosis

Acute herpetic gingivostomatitis must be differentiated from several conditions.

ANUG can be differentiated in several ways (see Table 19–1).

Erythema multiforme can be differentiated because the vesicles in erythema multiforme are generally more extensive than those in acute herpetic gingivostomatitis and on rupture demonstrate a tendency toward pseudomembrane formation. In addition, the tongue in the former condition usually is markedly involved, with infection of the ruptured vesicles resulting in varying degrees of ulceration. Oral involvement in erythema multiforme may be accompanied by skin lesions. The duration of erythema multiforme may be comparable to that of acute herpetic gingivostomatitis, but prolonged involvement for a period of weeks is not uncommon.

Stevens-Johnson syndrome is a comparatively rare form of erythema multiforme characterized by vesicular hemorrhagic lesions in the oral cavity, hemorrhagic ocular lesions, and bullous skin lesions.

Bullous lichen planus is a painful condition characterized by large blisters on the tongue and cheek that rupture and undergo ulceration; it runs a prolonged, indefinite course. Patches of linear, gray, lace-like lesions of lichen planus are often interspersed among the bullous eruptions. Coexistent involvement of the skin in lichen planus affords a basis for differentiation between bullous lichen planus and acute herpetic gingivostomatitis.

Desquamative gingivitis is characterized by diffuse involvement of the gingiva, with varying degrees of "peeling" of the epithelial surface and exposure of the underlying tissue. It is a chronic condition.

Lesions of *recurrent aphthous stomatitis* (RAS)[22] (Fig. 19–9) range from occasional small (0.5 to 1 cm in diameter), well-defined round or ovoid shallow ulcers with a gray-yellowish central area surrounded by an erythematous halo, which heal in 7 to 10 days without scarring, to larger (1 to 3 cm in diameter) oval or irregular ulcers, which persist for weeks and heal with scarring. The etiol-

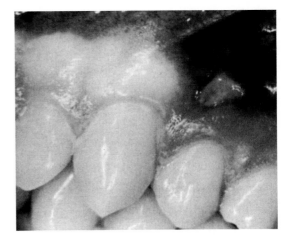

FIGURE 19–9. Aphthous lesion in the mucobuccal fold. The depressed gray center is surrounded by an elevated red border.

ogy is unknown, although immunopathologic mechanisms appear to play a role. RAS is a different clinical entity from acute herpetic gingivostoma-titis. The ulcerations may look the same in the two conditions, but diffuse erythematous involvement of the gingiva and acute toxic systemic symptoms do not occur in RAS.

Communicability

Acute herpetic gingivostomatitis is contagious.[9,39] Most adults have developed immunity to HSV as a result of infection during childhood,[5] which in most instances is subclinical. For this reason acute herpetic gingivostomatitis usually occurs in infants and children. Although recurrent herpetic gingivostomatitis has been reported,[31] it does not ordinarily recur unless immunity is destroyed by debilitating systemic disease. Herpetic infection of the skin, such as herpes labialis, does recur.[67]

PERICORONITIS

The term *pericoronitis* refers to inflammation of the gingiva in relation to the crown of an incompletely erupted tooth (Fig. 19–10). It occurs most frequently in the

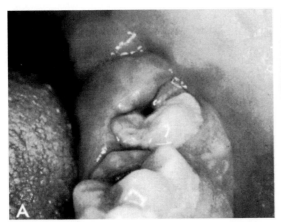
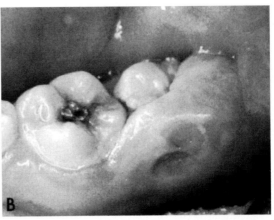

FIGURE 19–10. Pericoronitis. *A,* Third molar partially covered by an infected flap. *B,* Lingual view showing sinus draining from an infected flap.

mandibular third molar area. Pericoronitis may be acute, subacute, or chronic.

Clinical Features

The partially erupted or impacted mandibular third molar is the most common site of pericoronitis. The space between the crown of the tooth and the overlying gingival flap is an ideal area for the accumulation of food debris and bacterial growth. Even in patients with no clinical signs or symptoms, the gingival flap is often chronically inflamed and infected, with various degrees of ulceration along its inner surface. Acute inflammatory involvement is a constant possibility.

Acute pericoronitis is identified by various degrees of involvement of the pericoronal flap and adjacent structures, as well as systemic complications. An influx of inflammatory fluid and cellular exudate results in an increase in the bulk of the flap, which interferes with complete closure of the jaws. The flap is traumatized by contact with the opposing jaw, and the inflammatory involvement is aggravated.

The resultant clinical picture is that of a markedly red, swollen, suppurating lesion that is exquisitely tender, with radiating pains to the ear, throat, and floor of the mouth. The patient is extremely uncomfortable because of the pain, a foul taste, and an inability to close the jaws. Swelling of the cheek in the region of the angle of the jaw and lymphadenitis are common findings. The patient may also have toxic systemic complications such as fever, leukocytosis, and malaise.

Complications

The involvement may become localized in the form of a pericoronal abscess. It may spread posteriorly into the oropharyngeal area and medially to the base of the tongue, making it difficult for the patient to swallow. Depending on the severity and extent of the infection, there is involvement of the submaxillary, posterior cervical, deep cervical, and retropharyngeal lymph nodes.[36,53] Peritonsillar abscess formation, cellulitis, and Ludwig's angina are infrequent but nevertheless potential sequelae of acute pericoronitis.

REFERENCES

1. Barnes GP, Bowles WF III, Carter HG. Acute necrotizing ulcerative gingivitis: A survey of 218 cases. J Periodontol *44:*35, 1973.
2. Berke JD. Experimental study of acute ulcerative stomatitis. J Am Dent Assoc *63:*86, 1961.
3. Box HK. Necrotic Gingivitis. Toronto, University of Toronto Press, 1930.
4. Brown RH. Necrotizing ulcerative gingivitis in mongoloid and nonmongoloid retarded individuals. J Periodont Res *8:*290, 1973.
5. Burnet FM, Williams SW. Herpes simplex: New point of view. Med J Aust *1:*637, 1939.
6. Cahn LR. The penetration of the tissue by Vincent's organisms. A report of a case. J Dent Res *9:*695, 1929.
7. Cawson RA. Infections of the oral mucous membrane. In Cohen B, Kramer IRH, eds. Scientific Foundations of Dentistry. Chicago, Year Book Medical Publishers, 1976.
8. Chapman OD, Harris AE. Oral lesions associated with dietary deficiencies in monkeys. J Infect Dis *69:*7, 1941.
9. Chilton NW. Herpetic stomatitis. Am J Orthod Oral Surg *30:*335, 1944.
10. Chung CP, Nisengard RJ, Slots J, Genco RG. Bacterial IgG and IgM antibody titers in acute necrotizing ulcerative gingivitis. J Periodontol *54:*557, 1983.
11. Cogen RB, Stevens AW Jr, Cohen-Cole SA, et al. Leukocyte function in the etiology of acute necrotizing ulcerative gingivitis. J Periodontol *54:*402, 1983.
12. Cohen-Cole SA, Cogen RB, Stevens AW Jr, et al. Psychiatric, psychosocial and endocrine correlates of acute necrotizing ulcerative gingivitis (trench mouth): A preliminary report. Psychiatr Med *1:*215, 1983.
13. Curtois GJ III, Cobb CM, Killoy WJ. Acute necrotizing ulcerative gingivitis. A transmission electron microscope study. J Periodontol *54:*671, 1983.
14. Coutley RL. Vincent's infection. Br Dent J *74:*34, 1943.
15. Daley FH. Studies of Vincent's infection at the clinic of Tufts College Dental School from October, 1926 to February, 1928. J Dent Res *8:*408, 1928.
16. Dean HT, Singleton JE Jr. Vincent's infection—a wartime disease. Am J Public Health *35:*433, 1945.
17. Dodd K, Johnston LM, Buddingh GJ. Herpetic stomatitis. J Pediatr *12:*95, 1938.
18. Duckworth R, Waterhouse JP, Britton DG, et al. Acute ulcerative gingivitis. A double blind controlled clinical trial with metronidazole. Br Dent J *120:*599, 1966.
19. Ellerman V. Vincent's organisms in tissue. Z Hyg Infekt Pr *56:*453, 1907.
20. Emslie RD. Cancrum oris. Dent Pract *13:*481, 1963.
21. Enwonwu CO. Epidemiological and biochemical studies of necrotizing ulcerative gingivitis and noma (cancrum oris) in Nigerian children. Arch Oral Biol *17:*1357, 1972.
22. Eversole LR. Diseases of the oral mucous membranes. Review of the literature. In Millard HD, Mason DK, eds. World Workshop on Oral Medicine. Chicago, Year Book Medical Publishers, 1989.
23. Falkler WA Jr, Martin SA, Vincent JW, et al. A clinical, demographic and microbiologic study of ANUG patients in an urban dental school. J Clin Periodontol *14:*307, 1987.
24. Formicola AJ, Witte ET, Curran PM. A study of personality traits and acute necrotizing ulcerative gingivitis. J Periodontol *41:*36, 1970.
25. Gardner PS, McQuillin J, Black MM, Richardson J. Rapid diagnosis of herpesvirus hominis infections in superficial lesions by immunofluorescent antibody techniques. Br Med J *4:*89, 1968.
26. Giddon DB. Psychophysiology of the oral cavity. J Dent Res *45*(suppl 6):1627, 1966.
27. Giddon DB, Zackin SJ, Goldhaber P. Acute necrotizing gingivitis in college students. J Am Dent Assoc *68:*381, 1964.
28. Goldhaber P, Giddon DB. Present concepts concerning the etiology and treatment of acute necrotizing ulcerative gingivitis. Int Dent J *14:*468, 1964.
29. Greenberg MS, Brightman VJ, Ship II. Clinical and laboratory differentiation of recurrent intraoral herpes simplex virus infections following fever. J Dent Res *48:*385, 1969.
30. Greenspan D, Pindborg JJ, Greenspan JS, Schiodt M. AIDS and the Dental Team. Copenhagen, Munksgaard, 1986.
31. Griffin JW. Recurrent intraoral herpes simplex virus infection. Oral Surg Oral Med Oral Pathol *19:*209, 1965.
32. Grinspan D. Enfermedades de la Boca. Vol 2: Patologia Clinica y Terapeutica de la Mucosa Bucal. Buenos Aires, Ed Mundi, 1972.
33. Hampp EG, Mergenhagen SE. Experimental infection with oral spirochetes. J Infect Dis *109:*43, 1961.
34. Harding J, Berry WC, Marsh C, Jolliff CR. Salivary antibodies in acute gingivitis. J Periodontol *51:*63, 1980.
35. Hooper PA, Seymour GJ. The histopathogenesis of acute ulcerative gingivitis. J Periodontol *50:*419, 1979.
36. Jacobs MH. Pericoronal and Vincent's infections: Bacteriology and treatment. J Am Dent Assoc *30:*392, 1943.
37. Jimenez M, Baer PN. Necrotizing ulcerative gingivitis in children: A 9 year clinical study. J Periodontol *46:*715, 1975.
38. King JD. Nutritional and other factors in trench mouth with special reference to the nicotinic acid component of vitamin B complex. Br Dent J *74:*113, 1943.
39. Levine HD, et al. Vesicular pharyngitis and stomatitis. JAMA *112:*2020, 1939.
40. Listgarten MA. Electron microscopic observations on the bacterial flora of acute necrotizing ulcerative gingivitis. J Periodontol *36:*328, 1965.
41. Listgarten MA, Lewis DW. The distribution of spirochetes in the lesion of acute necrotizing ulcerative gingivitis: An electron microscopic and statistical survey. J Periodontol *38:*379, 1967.
42. Loesche WJ, Syed SA, Langhorn BE, Stoll J. The bacteriology of acute necrotizing ulcerative gingivitis. J Periodontol *53:*223, 1982.
43. Mayo J, Carranza FA Jr, Cabrini RL. Comparative study of the effect of antibiotics, bone marrow and cysteamine on oral lesions produced in hamsters by total body irradiation. Experientia *20:*403, 1964.
44. Mayo J, Carranza FA Jr, Epper CE, Cabrini RL. The effect of total-body irradiation on the oral tissues of the Syrian hamster. Oral Surg Oral Med Oral Pathol *15:*739, 1962.
45. McCarthy PL, Shklar G. Diseases of the Oral Mucosa. 2nd ed. Philadelphia, Lea & Febiger, 1980.
46. McNair ST. Herpetic stomatitis. J Dent Res *29:*647, 1950.
47. Miglani DC, Sharma OP. Incidence of acute necrotizing gingivitis and periodontosis among cases seen at the government hospital, Madras. J All India Dent Assoc *37:*183, 1965.
48. Miller DK, Rhoads CP. The experimental production in dogs of acute stomatitis associated with leukopenia and a maturation defect of the myeloid elements of the bone marrow. J Exp Med *61:*173, 1935.
49. Nathanson I, Morin GE. Herpetic stomatitis. An aid in the early diagnosis of infectious mononucleosis. Oral Surg Oral Med Oral Pathol *6:*1284, 1953.
50. Nicolau S, Kopciowska L. Inclusion bodies in experimental herpes. Ann Inst Pasteur *60:*401, 1938.

51. Park N-H. Virology. In Newman MG, Nisengard R, eds. Oral Microbiology and Immunology. Philadelphia, WB Saunders, 1988.
52. Pedler JA, Radden BG. Seasonal influence of acute ulcerative gingivitis. Dent Pract 8:23, 1957.
53. Perkins AE. Acute infections around erupting mandibular third molar. Br Dent J 76:199, 1944.
54. Pindborg JJ. Gingivitis in military personnel with special reference to ulceromembranous gingivitis. Odontol Tidskr 59:407, 1951.
55. Pindborg JJ, Bhat M, Devanath KR, et al. Occurrence of acute necrotizing gingivitis in South Indian children. J Periodontol 37:14, 1966.
56. Plaut HC. Studien zur bakteriellen Diagnostik der Diphtherie und der Anginen. Dtsch Med Wochenschr 20:920, 1894.
57. Regezi JA, Sciubba JJ. Oral Pathology. Clinical-Pathologic Correlations. Philadelphia, WB Saunders, 1989.
58. Rosebury T. Is Vincent's infection a communicable disease? J Am Dent Assoc 29:823, 1942.
59. Rosebury T, Foley G. Experimental Vincent's infection. J Am Dent Assoc 26:1978, 1939.
60. Rosebury T, MacDonald JB, Clark A. A bacteriologic survey of gingival scrapings from periodontal infections by direct examination, guinea pig inoculation and anaerobic cultivation. J Dent Res 29:718, 1950.
61. Roy S, Wolman L. Electron microscopic observations on the virus particles in herpes simplex encephalitis. J Clin Pathol 22:51, 1969.
62. Schluger S. Necrotizing ulcerative gingivitis in the army. Incidence, communicability, and treatment. J Am Dent Assoc 38:174, 1949.
63. Schwartzman J, Grossman L. Vincent's ulceromembranous gingivostomatitis. Arch Pediatr 58:515, 1941.
64. Scott TFM, Steigman AS, Convey JH. Acute infectious gingivostomatitis: Etiology, epidemiology, and clinical picture of common disorders caused by virus of herpes simplex. JAMA 117:999, 1941.
65. Shannon IL, Kilgore WG, Leary TJ. Stress as a predisposing factor in necrotizing ulcerative gingivitis. J Periodontol 40:240, 1969.

66. Sheiham A. An epidemiological study of oral disease in Nigerians. J Dent Res 44:1184, 1965.
67. Ship II, Brightman VJ, Laster LL. The patient with recurrent aphthous ulcers and the patient with recurrent herpes labialis: A study of two population samples. J Am Dent Assoc 75:645, 1967.
68. Skach M, Zabrodsky S, Mrklas L. A study of the effect of age and season on the incidence of ulcerative gingivitis. J Periodont Res 5:187, 1970.
69. Smith DT. Spirochetes and Related Organisms in Fusospirochetal Disease. Baltimore, Williams & Wilkins, 1932.
70. Stammers AF. Vincent's infection. Br Dent J 76:171, 1944.
71. Stevens AWJ, Cogen RB, Cohen-Cole SA, Freeman A. Demographic and clinical data associated with acute necrotizing ulcerative gingivitis in a dental school population. J Clin Periodontol 11:487, 1984.
72. Swenson HM. Induced Vincent's infection in dogs. J Dent Res 23:190, 1944.
73. Swenson HM, Muhler JC. Induced fusospirochetal infection in dogs. J Dent Res 26:161, 1947.
74. Thompson LE. A fatal case of brain abscess from Vincent's angina. Dent Digest 35:821, 1929.
75. Topping NH, Fraser HF. Mouth lesions associated with dietary deficiencies in monkeys. US Public Health Rep 54:431, 1939.
76. Tunnicliff R, Fink EB, Hammond C. Significance of fusiform bacilli and spirilla in gingival tissue. J Am Dent Assoc 23:1959, 1936.
77. Tunnicliff R, Hammond C. Abscess production by fusiform bacilli in rabbits and mice by the use of scillaren-B or mucin. J Dent Res 16:479, 1937.
78. Underhill FP, Mendel LB. Further experiments on the pellagra-like syndrome in dogs. Am J Physiol 83:589, 1928.
79. Vincent H. Sur l'etiologie et sur les lesions anatomopathologiques, de la pourriture d'hopital. Ann de l'Inst Pasteur 10:448, 1896.
80. Wilkie R. An etiology of Vincent's gingivitis. Br Dent J 78:65, 1945.
81. Wilton JMA, Ivanyi A, Lehner T. Cell-mediated immunity and humoral antibodies in acute ulcerative gingivitis. J Periodont Res 6:9, 1971.

20

Desquamative Gingivitis and Oral Mucous Membrane Diseases

GERALD SHKLAR

Chronic Desquamative Gingivitis
Dermatoses
Lichen Planus
Pemphigus
Bullous Pemphigoid
Mucous Membrane Pemphigoid
Erythema Multiforme
Lupus Erythematosus

Scleroderma
Chronic Bacterial Infections
Drug Eruptions
Mycotic Diseases
Acute Candidiasis (Moniliasis, Thrush)
Chronic Candidiasis
Other Chronic Mycotic Diseases

For many years erosive and desquamating lesions of the gingiva were termed *desquamative gingivitis,* and a specific disease entity was postulated. It is now understood that desquamative gingivitis encompasses a variety of different oral mucous membrane diseases. The extensive literature in which the term *desquamative gingivitis* is used has resulted in considerable confusion over the years, but the term is so common that it continues to be used and thus will be used in this chapter as well.

The large majority of cases of so-called chronic desquamative gingivitis represent oral manifestations of one of the following dermatoses: lichen planus, mucous membrane pemphigoid, bullous pemphigoid, or pemphigus. Other conditions that must be considered when gingival desquamative lesions are present include endocrine imbalances, chronic infections, and drug reactions.

CHRONIC DESQUAMATIVE GINGIVITIS

Chronic desquamative gingivitis is characterized by intense redness and desquamation of the surface epithelium of the attached gingiva. Initially the cause of the condition was unknown, and a variety of etiologic influences were suggested. Some form of endocrine imbalance was particularly suspected, because most cases were described in postmenopausal females.[22,29,50,57,77,88,89] However, in 1960 McCarthy and colleagues,[48] in a study of 40 cases, clarified that *desquamative gingivitis is not a specific disease entity, but a nonspecific gingival manifestation of a variety of systemic disturbances.* The concept of desquamative gingivitis as a nonspecific but unusual manifestation of a variety of diseases, rather than a specific disease entity, has been confirmed in other studies dealing with oral mucous membrane diseases and their diagnosis by immunopathologic techniques.[40,54,59,75]

The microscopic changes described in so-called desquamative gingivitis are consistent with those of either lichen planus or mucous membrane pemphigoid. All cases of mucous membrane pemphigoid[71] and of bullous pemphigoid with oral involvement[73] present a desquamative or erosive gingivitis. *However, because mucous membrane pemphigoid is a relatively rare disease, it is probable that the majority of cases of so-called desquamative gingivitis are in fact lichen planus.* A desquamative gingivitis is an uncommon manifestation of lichen planus (10% to 20% of cases),[74] but lichen planus is a relatively common disease of the mouth, and therefore, the incidence of gingival lichen planus should be higher than that of mucous membrane pemphigoid.

Careful examination of the mouth in cases of lichen planus should reveal other manifestations of lichen planus, such as reticulate lesions of the buccal mucosa. However, some cases start with gingival involvement, and other lesions may appear as the disease progresses. Diagnosis may be possible by histologic studies.

In mucous membrane pemphigoid, there may be conjunctival lesions as well as involvement of other mucous membrane sites, such as the nasal mucosa, vagina, rectum, and urethra. However, the involvement may be confined to the gingiva in the early stages of the disease, and other oral lesions may follow. Biopsy studies may reveal the characteristic clean separation of the epithelium from the underlying connective tissue.

Clinical Features. The clinical features of so-called desquamative gingivitis vary in severity, and mild, moderate, and severe forms have been described.[27]

Mild Form. In its mildest form, there is diffuse erythema of the marginal, interdental, and attached gingivae; the condition is usually painless and comes to the attention of the patient or dentist because of the overall discoloration. The mild form occurs most frequently in females between 17 and 23 years of age.

Moderate Form. This is a more advanced form that presents as a patchy distribution of bright red and gray areas involving the marginal and attached gingivae (Fig. 20–1A). The surface is smooth and shiny, and the normally resilient gingiva becomes soft. There is slight pitting with pressure, and the epithelium is not firmly adherent to the underlying tissues. Massaging the gingiva with the finger results in peeling of the epithelium and exposure of the underlying bleeding connective tissue surface.

The oral mucosa in the remainder of the mouth is ex-

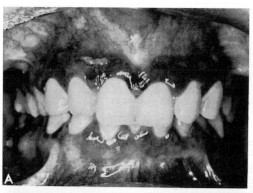
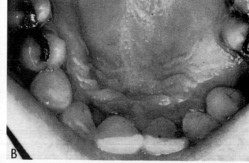
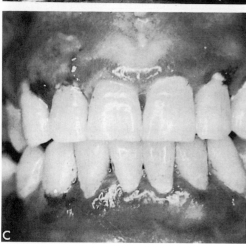
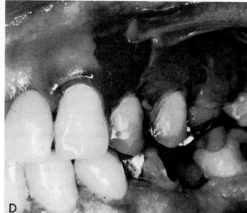

FIGURE 20–1. Chronic desquamative gingivitis of varied severity. *A,* Moderate, with generalized edema and erythema associated with inflammation and exposure of underlying connective tissue. *B,* Lingual view of patient shown in *A.* Aside from slight marginal erythema, there is little evidence of change in the gingiva and adjacent mucosa. *C,* Severe, with scattered, irregularly shaped, denuded areas producing a mosaic appearance. Note the ulceration between the right maxillary lateral and canine teeth. *D,* Severe, with complete denudation of the epithelium and exposure of underlying erythematous inflamed connective tissue.

tremely smooth and shiny. This condition is seen most frequently in persons between 30 and 40 years of age. Patients complain of a burning sensation and sensitivity to thermal changes, and inhalation of air is painful. The patient cannot tolerate condiments, and toothbrushing causes painful denudation of the gingival surface.

In this and other forms of desquamative gingivitis, the lingual surface is usually less severely involved than the labial surface (Fig. 20–1*B*), because the tongue and friction from food excursion reduce the accumulation of local irritants and limit the inflammation.

Severe Form. This form is characterized by scattered, irregularly shaped areas in which the gingiva is denuded and strikingly red in appearance (Fig. 20–1*C*). Because the gingiva separating these areas is grayish blue, in overall appearance the gingiva seems to be speckled. The surface epithelium seems shredded and friable and can be peeled off in small patches (Fig. 20–1*D*).

Occasionally there are surface vessels that rupture, releasing a thin, aqueous fluid and exposing an underlying surface that is red and raw. A blast of air directed at the gingiva causes elevation of the epithelium and the consequent formation of a bubble. The areas of involvement seem to shift to different locations on the gingiva. The mucous membrane other than the gingiva is smooth and shiny and may present a fissuring in the cheek adjacent to the line of occlusion.

The condition is extremely painful. The patient cannot tolerate coarse foods, condiments, or temperature changes. There is a constant dry, burning sensation throughout the oral cavity that is accentuated in the denuded gingival zones.

Histopathology. Microscopically, so-called desquamative gingivitis often appears as one of two types:[28] bullous lesions, resembling the histopathologic features of mucous membrane pemphigoid (Fig. 20–2), or lichenoid lesions, with features similar to those of lichen planus (Fig. 20–3). Occasionally there will be a thin, atrophic epithelium with little or no keratin at the surface and a dense, diffuse infiltration of chronic inflammatory cells in the underlying connective tissue. This tends to be the histopathologic picture in those rare cases of desquamative gingivitis that are a result of menopausal alterations or the atrophic changes of aging.

Histochemical[21,76] and ultrastructural studies have not contributed significant information. The electron microscopic changes described are extremely variable and resemble many of the changes seen in lichen planus[32,58] or mucous membrane pemphigoid[53,85] Separation of the epithelium and connective tissue was seen to start with a separation of collagen fibrils and a decrease in the number of anchoring fibrils.

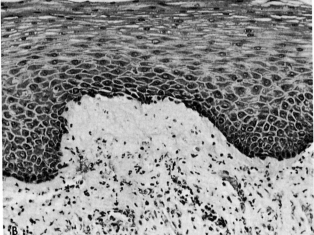

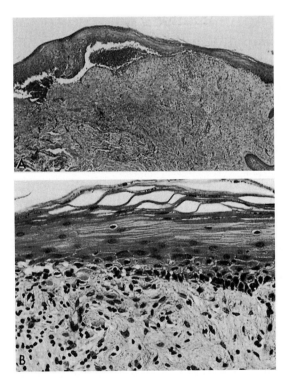

FIGURE 20–2. Chronic desquamative gingivitis: bullous type. *A,* There is massive replacement of the papillary and reticular connective tissue by inflammatory exudate, disruption of the epithelial–connective tissue junction, and formation of large subepithelial bullae. *B,* Detailed view showing blunting of epithelial rete pegs and inflammatory exudate of edema, fibrin, and leukocytes that have replaced the connective tissue.

FIGURE 20–3. Chronic desquamative gingivitis: lichenoid type. *A,* The epithelium is atrophic, the connective tissue is inflamed, and the epithelium is separated from the connective tissue by a subepithelial vesicle. *B,* Detailed view showing atrophic parakeratotic epithelium with vacuolization of the basal cells and microvesicle formation at the epithelial–connective tissue junction.

Therapy. The therapy for so-called desquamative gingivitis must be based, if possible, on an understanding of the basic disease process causing the gingival reaction.

A careful oral examination must be carried out so that other lesions may be discovered. In lichen planus, the gingiva is rarely affected without other oral mucosal lesions being present.

A complete history should be taken to uncover possible coexistent extraoral disease. Conjunctivitis and symptoms of burning on urination or vaginal irritation may suggest multiple sites of mucosal disease, indicating mucous membrane pemphigoid. The presence of papular skin lesions, particularly on sites such as wrists or ankles, suggests lichen planus. Menopausal history or a history of hysterectomy suggests a possible hormonal etiology.

Biopsy studies often point to the diagnosis of lichen planus or mucous membrane pemphigoid. They will also reveal those unusual cases in which a desquamative gingivitis represents a chronic bacterial infection such as tuberculosis or a mycotic infection such as candidiasis.

Local Treatment. Local treatment is essential for all forms of desquamative gingivitis. The patient must be carefully instructed in plaque control using a soft toothbrush, because the gingival surface is easily abraded with a hard brush. Oxidizing mouthwashes (hydrogen peroxide 3% diluted to one part peroxide and two parts warm water) should be used twice daily. A reduction in marginal gingivitis results in reduced inflammation and desquamation of the attached gingiva. Topical corticosteroid ointments[30] and creams may be used, but their success has been limited. The gingival tissue is gently dried with a sterile sponge, and an ointment or cream such as triamcinolone (Kenalog, Aristocort) 0.1%, fluocinonide (Lidex) 0.05%, or desonide (Tridesilon) 0.05% is applied and gently rubbed into the gingiva several times daily.

Systemic Therapy. Systemic therapy may be used in cases of severe gingival involvement. Systemic corticosteroid therapy should not be considered lightly, because a variety of side effects are possible. The patient's general health should be discussed with his or her physician prior to the use of systemic corticosteroids. If a diagnosis of mucous membrane pemphigoid is considered, moderate doses of corticosteroids are often helpful in alleviating discomfort and improving the tissue response. Prednisone can be used in a daily or every-other-day dose of 30 to 40 mg and gradually reduced to a daily maintenance dose of 5 to 10 mg or every-other-day maintenance dose of 10 to 20 mg. Other steroids can be used in comparable doses. Systemic steroid therapy in lichen planus is helpful only in rare cases.

Conclusion. In many cases of desquamative gingivitis it may not be possible to determine the basic etiology. However, local therapy together with diligence and patience will eventually improve the condition, and the etiologic background may be discovered on the eventual appearance of other lesions or symptoms. Particular care and patience are required in the atrophic gingivitis of aging, because no systemic therapy has been found to be useful other than nutritional supplementation if the patient's nutritional status is deficient. Such supplements may be of value if the patient suffers from a true nutritional deficiency, such as vitamin B deficiency.

DERMATOSES

Many dermatologic diseases may be accompanied by involvement of the oral mucous membrane, as well as of other mucosal sites. Although oral and skin lesions often occur together in dermatologic disease, changes in the oral cavity may mark the onset of the disease and precede the skin lesions by months or years. In many conditions (e.g., lichen planus, erythema multiforme, and pyostomatitis vegetans), oral lesions may constitute the only manifestation. Oral manifestations in the absence of skin involvement often result from drugs capable of causing dermatoses. Gingival involvement in dermatologic disorders and in drug reactions presents a challenging diagnostic and therapeutic problem.

Plate X illustrates some common desquamative lesions of the oral mucosa.

Lichen Planus

Lichen planus is an inflammatory disease of skin and mucous membranes characterized by the eruption of papules. The papules are violaceous and pointed on the skin, but tend to be white and flattened on the mucosa. When the disease is confined to the skin, it may be acute, subacute, or chronic; oral involvement is usually chronic.

There is a strong indication that lichen planus is an autoimmune disease. The association of host T lymphocytes with self-antigen has been demonstrated in several publications.[10,34,47]

Oral Lesions. Lichen planus may be confined to the skin or oral mucosa or may develop in both locations.[49] However, a large percentage of cases remain confined to the oral cavity, and the lesions often present a diagnostic problem because of their variability in clinical appearance.[49]

Frictional factors play a role in determining the location of lesions of lichen planus; the most common oral sites are the buccal mucosa in relation to the occlusal plane of the teeth, the lateral borders of the tongue, the labial and buccal surfaces of the attached gingiva, the hard palate, and the lower lip.

The lesions are often symmetric and tend to be dendritic and papular. *Dendritic* or *reticulate lesions* consist of grayish white, linear, lace-like elevations composed of large numbers of small, individual papules. Isolated *papules* of pinhead size may also be observed (Figs. 20–4 to 20–6). In addition to raised dendritic lesions, there may also be raised plaque-like lesions and reddened areas of erosion and ulceration.

Vesicles and *bullae* may also appear in lichen planus and will confuse the clinical picture by suggesting the possibility of a vesiculobullous dermatosis such as pemphigus or pemphigoid. The bullae eventually rupture, leaving areas of ulceration and erosion or desquamation. The great variability in the clinical appearance of the oral lesions of lichen planus depends on the unique microscopic alterations and the severity of the degenerative changes in the basal layer of the epithelium.

The skin involvement of lichen planus usually results in pruritus, but the oral lesions tend to be asymptomatic unless erosion or ulceration is present. These areas may be sensitive to hot, acidic, or spicy foods, and extensive areas

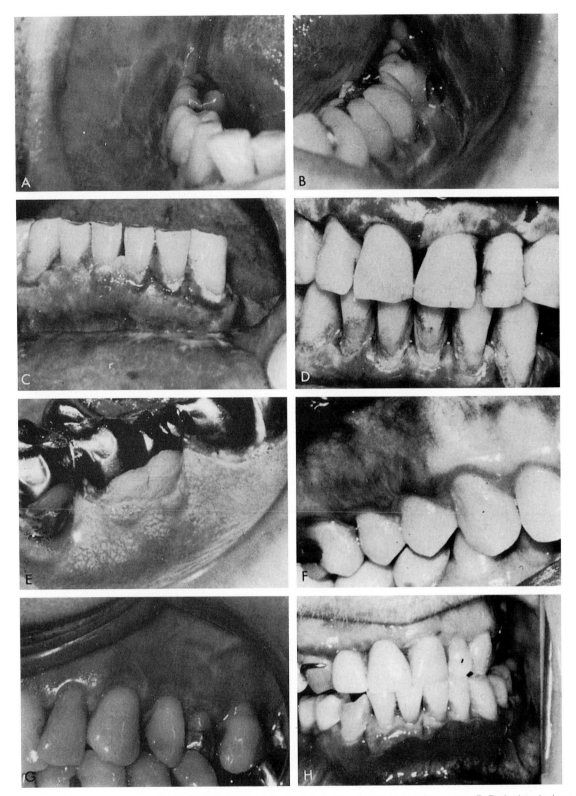

FIGURE 20–4. Different clinical patterns of oral lichen planus. *A,* Reticulate lesions on the buccal mucosa. *B,* Reticulate lesions on the gingiva. *C,* Reticulate and plaque-like lesions on the gingiva and labial mucosa. *D,* Plaque-like and erosive lesions on the gingiva. *E,* Papular lesions on the gingiva. *F,* Erosive and striated lesions on the gingiva. *G,* Erosive and desquamative lesions on the gingiva. *H,* Bullous involvement of the mandibular gingiva. A large bulla has ruptured, leaving extensive ulceration.

of ulceration may be painful. The disease tends to run a chronic or subacute course, with the duration varying from several months to many years. Periods of exacerbation of lesions tend to correspond to episodes of emotional stress.

Gingival Lesions. The gingival tissue is often involved in oral lichen planus, and the pattern is extremely variable.[35,74] Lesions may occur as one or more types of four distinctive patterns:

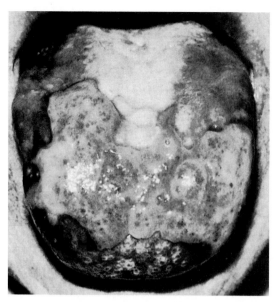

FIGURE 20–5. Bullous lichen planus of the tongue. A ruptured bulla appears anteriorly, and plaque-like lesions are seen posteriorly.

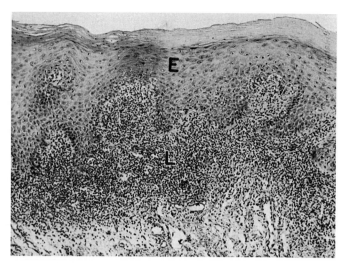

FIGURE 20–7. Microscopic appearance of lichen planus. Biopsy specimen from lesion on the gingiva showing hyperkeratosis and acanthosis of the epithelium (E), as well as extension of rete pegs. There is dense lymphocytic infiltration of the lamina propria (L) confined to a broad zone immediately beneath the epithelium.

1. *Keratotic lesions.* These raised white lesions may present as groups of individual papules, as linear or reticulate lesions, or as plaque-like configurations (Fig. 20–4B–E).
2. *Erosive or ulcerative lesions.* These red areas may present as a patchy distribution among keratotic lesions or as extensive involvement. They may be hemorrhagic with slight trauma (e.g., toothbrushing) (Fig. 20–4F,G).
3. *Vesicular or bullous involvement.* Raised, fluid-filled lesions will rupture, leaving ulceration (Fig. 20–4H).
4. *Atrophic involvement.* Atrophic forms of lichen planus usually occur on the tongue or gingiva. Atrophic involvement of the dorsum of the tongue is characterized by the loss of filiform and fungiform papillae. Atrophic involvement of the gingiva causes thinning of the epithelium and a resulting erosive or desquamative gingivitis. Because lichen planus is a common disease of the oral mucosa, most cases of so-called desquamative gingivitis are actually cases of erosive gingival lichen planus. If the mouth is carefully examined, lesions in sites other than the gingiva are usually found. In a small number of cases of oral lichen planus (less than 10%), the involvement is confined to the gingiva, and the clinical pattern is one of erosion and desquamation.

Histopathology. Microscopically, oral lichen planus is characterized by three main features: hyperkeratosis or parakeratosis, hydropic degeneration of the basal layer of the stratum germinativum, and a dense infiltration of lymphocytes as a broad band in the upper corium adjacent to the epithelium (Figs. 20–7 and 20–8). Occasionally there may be extension of rete pegs in a sawtooth pattern, but this feature is more typical of lesions on the skin. Hydropic degeneration of the basal layer of the epithelium may be sufficiently extensive that the epithelium becomes thin and atrophic or lifts off the underlying corium and produces either a subepithelial vesicle or an ulcer.

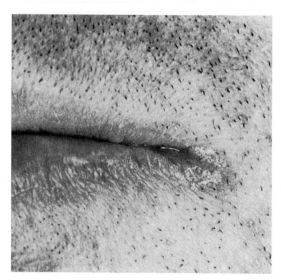

FIGURE 20–6. Lichen planus at the labial commissure showing typical papules.

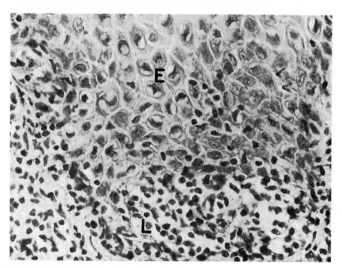

FIGURE 20–8. High-power view of Figure 20–7 showing hydropic degeneration in the basal layer of the epithelium (E) with lymphocytic infiltration of the lamina propria (L).

The nature of the clinical lesion depends on the microscopic pattern. The white papular or reticulate lesions demonstrate hyperkeratosis or parakeratosis and lymphocytic infiltration. Erosive or ulcerative lesions demonstrate extensive degeneration of the basal layer and patchy loss of epithelium. Vesicular lesions show degenerative and epithelial separation from underlying connective tissue. Atrophic lesions show a thin, degenerating epithelium.

A microscopic diagnosis can usually be made of oral lesions of lichen planus, but the characteristic pattern is found in the keratotic lesions, and biopsy specimens should be obtained from these areas if possible. Oral lesions of lichen planus change in pattern, and in certain unusual cases a second or even third biopsy may be necessary before a definitive diagnosis can be made.

Electron microscopic studies indicate that lichen planus can be divided into three stages. The earliest stage is degeneration of the cytoplasm of the epithelial cells, with aggregation of particulate material. The intercellular spaces are enlarged, accompanied by lymphocytic infiltration. In the second stage there is loss of collagen fibers in the superficial lamina propria. The final stage shows degeneration and necrosis of the basal and lower spinous layers of the epithelium, except for the desmosomes, which for the most part are structurally unaltered. The superficial lamina propria is also degenerated and necrotic, and the basement lamina is no longer visible. Secondary bacterial involvement of the necrotic tissue is often observed.[84] Separation of the basal lamina from the basal cell layer is an early manifestation of lichen planus.[66]

Differential Diagnosis. Among the conditions to be considered in the differential diagnosis of oral lichen planus are leukoplakia, white sponge nevus, chronic discoid lupus erythematosus, pemphigus, and mucous membrane pemphigoid.

Leukoplakia. Leukoplakia usually appears on the oral mucosa as raised plaques of variable size (Fig. 20–9). Linear lesions of oral leukoplakia can resemble the reticulate lesions of lichen planus, and the more common discrete lesions of leukoplakia can resemble plaque-like configurations of lichen planus. However, in lichen planus lesions, the papular structure can usually be discerned grossly. Microscopic study will differentiate the two diseases. Leukoplakia presents hyperkeratosis, with dysplasia in some cases. Leukoplakia usually occurs in heavy smokers.[49]

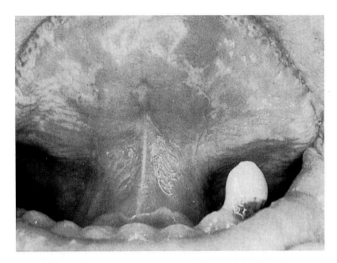

FIGURE 20–10. White sponge nevus (white folded gingivostomatitis) showing thickened epithelium with minute surface folds on the tongue and lips.

White Sponge Nevus (White Folded Gingivostomatitis). This is a benign genetic disease manifested at birth or during childhood by the development of white, plaque-like areas on the oral mucosa (Fig. 20–10). Microscopic examination shows a thickened epithelium characterized by extensive spongiosis.

Chronic Discoid Lupus Erythematosus. Coexistent skin lesions on the face are present in almost all cases, so the oral lesions, when present, do not present a significant diagnostic problem. They appear as slightly raised white plaques or white linear configurations and present a characteristic histopathologic pattern. Biopsy studies reveal parakeratosis or hyperkeratosis, hydropic degeneration of the basal layer, collagen degeneration, and a perivascular lymphocytic infiltrate.

Pemphigus. Pemphigus may resemble bullous or ulcerative lesions of oral lichen planus. However, the characteristic clinical white striations of lichen planus are usually evident even in cases of bullous lichen planus. Diagnosis of pemphigus can be made by the microscopic finding of acantholysis and is usually confirmed by immunofluorescent antibody studies.

Mucous Membrane Pemphigoid. Mucous membrane pemphigoid may resemble oral lichen planus of the bullous type. In addition, pemphigoid invariably presents as an ero-

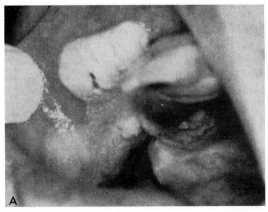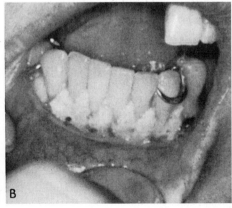

FIGURE 20–9. Leukoplakia of buccal mucosa *(A)* and leukoplakia of gingiva *(B)* in a 53-year-old woman. Microscopic examination revealed evidence of dysplasia.

sive or desquamative gingivitis, and this type of gingival reaction may also appear in lichen planus. Microscopic evaluation of the oral lesions of pemphigoid reveals a subepithelial vesiculation without hydropic degeneration of the basal layer. In oral lichen planus of the bullous or ulcerative variety, the keratotic white striations can usually be found at the periphery of the ulcerated areas.

Therapy. The most important aspect of the management of oral lichen planus is definitive diagnosis so that a specific cause can be determined and the patient can be reassured that the condition is not infectious, contagious, or precancerous.

If the oral lesions are of the keratotic variety, no therapy is required. Skin lesions of lichen planus are often characterized by pruritus, but oral keratotic lesions usually present no discomfort.

If the oral lesions are erosive, bullous, or ulcerative, they may be painful and uncomfortable. Peroxide mouthwashes two or three times daily are recommended. If the ulcerative areas are well defined and reasonably localized, they can be dried with a sterile sponge and a corticosteroid ointment or cream rubbed gently into the lesions several times daily. Intralesional injections of corticosteroids are occasionally beneficial. For severe discomfort, topical anesthetics or a rinse comprising a 50:50 mixture of diphenhydramine (Benadryl elixir) and magnesium hydroxide–aluminum hydroxide (Maalox) can be used. In severe, widespread lesions, systemic corticosteroids may be helpful (30 to 40 mg of prednisone every other day, reduced to a 10- to 20-mg, every-other-day maintenance dose after 2 weeks). This low maintenance dose can be used for many months without evidence of steroid side effects.

Pemphigus

Pemphigus is a chronic vesiculobullous lesion involving the skin and mucous membranes. The oral mucosa is invariably affected, and oral lesions usually precede the extensive skin involvement. Early diagnosis of pemphigus is of considerable value, as therapy is simplified if the disease is confined to the mouth. Systemic corticosteroid therapy at this point in the natural history of the disease may prevent the development of skin lesions, and a lower maintenance dose of steroids may be used successfully. Pemphigus has a distinctive microscopic appearance, and a definitive diagnosis can usually be made from an oral biopsy specimen.

The etiology of pemphigus is currently considered to be autoimmune, and antibodies can be demonstrated with immunofluorescent techniques. The antibodies appear to relate directly to the major pathologic changes in pemphigus,[3] and the changes can be induced in experimental animals by passive transfer of immunoglobulin G (IgG) from patients with the disease.[8] The immune changes in pemphigus also have a genetic origin.[1]

Ahmed and associates[2,4,5] have demonstrated that pemphigus has a genetic predisposition and that in Jewish patients the gene is linked to human leukocyte antigen (HLA) genes DR4 and B38DR4. This is consistent with a dominant expression of a class 11 (D region or D region–linked susceptibility gene). Evidence that the major histocompatibility complex (MHC) susceptibility gene for pemphigus vulgaris in Jews is inherited as a dominant trait is entirely

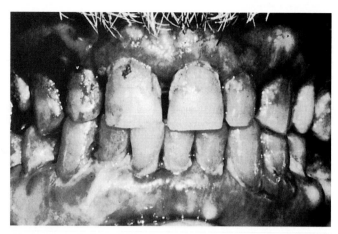

FIGURE 20–11. Pemphigus of the gingiva. Note the ruptured bulla.

consistent with its being an immune response gene for the intraepidermal intercellular cement substance antigen.

Oral Lesions. Oral lesions of pemphigus range from small vesicles to large bullae (Fig. 20–11). The bullae rupture, leaving extensive areas of ulceration. Any region of the mouth can be involved, but lesions often develop at sites of irritation or trauma, such as the occlusal line of the buccal mucosa or edentulous alveolar ridges. An erosive or desquamative type of gingivitis is occasionally seen as a manifestation of oral pemphigus.

Histopathology. Lesions of pemphigus demonstrate acantholysis, a separation of the epithelial cells of the lower stratum spinosum.[18,45,87] The upper layers of the epithelium separate from the basal layer, which remains attached to the underlying corium. The intraepithelial vesiculation begins as a microscopic alteration (Fig. 20–12) and gradually results in a grossly visible lesion as a fluid-filled bulla is formed. The separating cells of the stratum spinosum present degenerative changes: The cell outlines are round rather than polyhedral, the intercellular bridges are lost, and the nuclei are large and hyperchromatic. Many of these acantholytic cells are found within the clear fluid of the vesicle. The underlying connective tissue is densely infiltrated with chronic inflammatory cells, which may also enter the vesicular fluid. As the vesicle or bulla ruptures, the ulcerated lesion becomes infiltrated with polymorphonuclear leukocytes, and the surface may show suppuration.

Cytology. Cytologic smears of oral pemphigus lesions may be used as corroborating evidence for a definitive diagnosis. A positive smear will show large numbers of rounded acantholytic cells with serrated borders and large, hyperchromatic nuclei.[13,63]

Electron Microscopy. Electron microscopic studies indicate that breakdown of the epithelial intercellular cement substance is the first stage in the development of acantholysis. Other investigators believe that the destruction starts in the tonofilaments[32] or in the desmosomes[67] (Fig. 20–13).

Immunofluorescence. The presence of antibodies can be demonstrated in the oral mucosa of patients with oral pem-

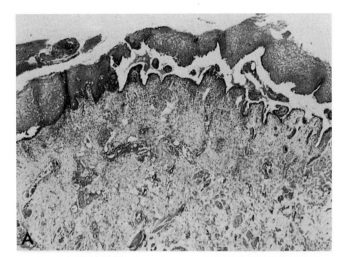

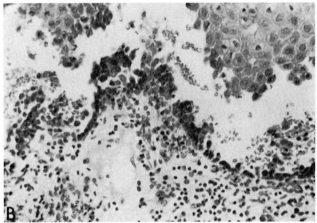

FIGURE 20–12. Pemphigus vulgaris. *A,* Oral mucosa showing acantholysis and an intraepithelial vesicle. *B,* Detailed view of an intraepithelial vesicle in pemphigus vulgaris.

phigus by the use of immunofluorescent techniques.[12] In the direct fluorescent technique, an oral biopsy specimen is incubated with fluorescein-labeled IgG from the patient's serum. In the indirect technique, a piece of oral or esophageal mucosa from a laboratory animal such as a rhesus monkey is first incubated with the patient's serum to attach the serum antibodies to the mucosal tissue. The tissue is then incubated with fluorescein-labeled antihuman IgG serum. The test is positive if the immunofluorescence is observed in the intercellular spaces of the stratified squamous epithelium of the mucosa. The indirect technique is less sensitive than the direct technique.

Varieties of Pemphigus. The common form of pemphigus is referred to as *pemphigus vulgaris.* A variant, *pemphigus vegetans,* may be considered a subacute form of pemphigus vulgaris with comparable but somewhat less severe clinical features. This form of the disease may be confined to the oral cavity for several weeks or months before the skin is involved. In the vegetative type of pemphigus, oral lesions dominate the picture, with crusted lesions of the skin being seen in intertriginous areas. However, the vegetating or hyperplastic lesions do not occur in the mouth; instead, the oral lesions are of the common vesiculobullous and ulcerative form (Plate X*E,F*).

Differential Diagnosis. The oral lesions of erythema

multiforme are frequently similar to those seen in pemphigus. In the former condition, however, there are recurrent active episodes of comparatively short duration, followed by long intervals without skin or oral lesions. Erythema multiforme affects the lips with considerable severity. Biopsy studies can differentiate oral lesions of pemphigus from those of erythema multiforme, because each has a characteristic histopathology.

Mucous membrane pemphigoid may resemble pemphigus when it is confined to the mouth. Biopsy studies will demonstrate subepithelial vesiculation, with "lifting off" of the epithelium from the underlying corium, instead of the acantholytic lesion characteristic of pemphigus.

Bullous lichen planus must also be considered in the differential diagnosis. The primary lesion of pemphigus may be of a bullous character, followed by erosion with associated pain and discomfort. In lichen planus, however, the characteristic dendritic lesions are invariably found associated with the bullae. Biopsy studies are usually sufficient to differentiate this condition from pemphigus, with its acantholytic changes.

Therapy. Therapy for pemphigus involves the use of systemic corticosteroids, usually in a moderate to high dosage. If the patient responds well to the corticosteroid agent, the dosage can be gradually reduced, but a low maintenance level of the drug is usually necessary to prevent the recurrence of lesions. In some patients the steroid can be withdrawn completely. In patients who do not respond to corticosteroids or who gradually adapt to them, antimetabolites such as methotrexate or azathioprine are

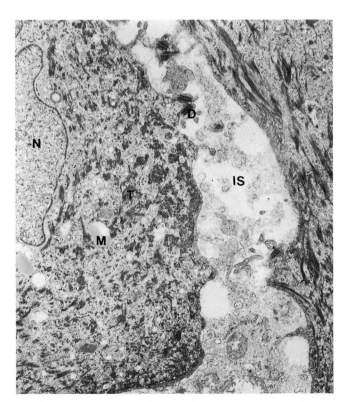

FIGURE 20–13. Oral pemphigus. Electron micrograph of acantholytic cells showing the disappearance of desmosomes (D) and the separation of cells by widening of the intercellular space (IS). Tonofibrils (T) show clumping, and mitochondria (M) are degenerating. The nucleus (N) demonstrates on intact membrane.

used. In general, oral lesions of pemphigus are more resistant to therapy than are skin lesions.

Minimization of irritation in the mouth is important in patients with oral pemphigus. Optimal oral hygiene is essential, because there is usually widespread involvement of the marginal and attached gingivae as well as other areas of the mouth, and the gingival disease represents an exaggerated response to local irritation. Periodontal care is an important part of the overall management of patients with pemphigus. Attention should be given to the fit and design of removable prosthetic appliances, as even slight irritation from these prostheses can result in severe inflammation with vesiculation and ulceration.

Local medication for oral pemphigus may include corticosteroid ointments or creams to reduce the painful symptomatology. Topical anesthetics, such as dyclonine hydrochloride (Dyclone) diluted 50% with water, may be used as a mouth rinse several times daily. The anesthetic effect may last for 40 minutes or longer.

Bullous Pemphigoid

Bullous pemphigoid is a chronic vesiculobullous dermatosis with oral involvement in a small percentage of cases.[73] The skin lesions resemble those of pemphigus clinically, but the microscopic picture is quite distinct from that of pemphigus. There is no evidence of acantholysis, and the developing vesicles are subepithelial rather than intraepithelial. The epithelium separates from the underlying connective tissue at the basement membrane zone. Electron microscopic studies show an actual horizontal splitting or replication of the basal lamina. The separating epithelium remains relatively intact, and the basal layer is present and appears to be regular.

Bullous pemphigoid is also considered to be an autoimmune disease. Antibodies can be demonstrated by immunofluorescent techniques and are seen in the basement membrane area.

Oral Lesions. Oral lesions are seen in about 10% of cases. There is an erosive or desquamative gingivitis and occasional vesicular or bullous lesions.[73]

Therapy. Therapy involves the systemic use of corticosteroids in moderate dosage.

Mucous Membrane Pemphigoid

Mucous membrane pemphigoid (benign mucous membrane pemphigoid) is an unusual chronic vesiculobullous disease with involvement of the oral mucosa and other mucosal tissues. The skin is usually not affected. The oral mucous membrane is usually involved, and other sites of predilection are the conjunctiva, nasal mucosa, vaginal mucosa, rectal mucosa, and urethra. The ocular lesions can be severe and may result in scarring and eventual blindness. Gallagher and Shklar,[25] in a study of 120 cases, found gingival lesions in all patients and other mucosal involvement in 82.5% of patients, with the conjunctiva and genitalia the most common extraoral sites. Females are affected much more frequently than males. It most commonly occurs between 40 and 70 years of age.

Oral Lesions. The most characteristic feature of oral involvement is an erosive or desquamative gingivitis (Fig.

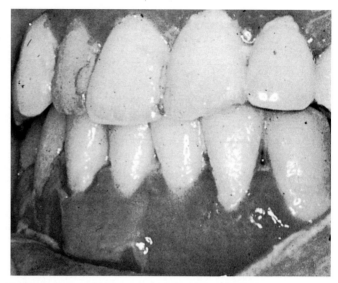

FIGURE 20–14. Benign mucous membrane pemphigoid. Note the remnant of a ruptured bullous lesion in lower left area.

20–14), with areas of desquamation, ulceration, and vesiculation, and often with erythema of the attached gingiva.[71] Vesiculobullous lesions may occur elsewhere in the mouth. The bullae tend to have a relatively thick roof (Fig. 20–15A) and rupture in 2 to 3 days, leaving irregularly shaped areas of ulceration. Healing of the lesions may take up to 3 weeks.

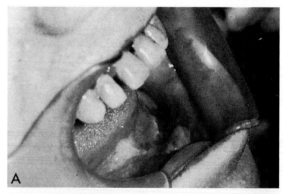

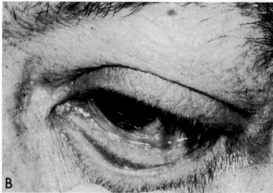

FIGURE 20–15. *A,* Bullae on the floor of the mouth and edentulous mucosa in mucous membrane pemphigoid. *B,* Conjunctivitis with symblepharon in mucous membrane pemphigoid.

Histopathology. The microscopic appearance of the oral lesions, although not completely diagnostic for mucous membrane pemphigoid, is sufficiently distinctive that a tentative diagnosis can be considered. There is a striking subepithelial vesiculation, with the epithelium lifting off from the underlying corium, leaving an intact basal layer (Fig. 20–16). The separation of the epithelium and the connective tissue is at the basement membrane zone, and electron microscopic studies have shown a split in the basal lamina.[81] Various amounts of chronic inflammatory infiltration are found in the connective tissue. The epithelium remains intact until the bulla ruptures and then degenerates. The desquamative or erosive gingivitis presents a thin epithelium with some evidence of degeneration and occasional ulceration. Inflammatory infiltration may be notable.

Immunofluorescence. Positive immunofluorescence in the basement membrane area has been reported with both direct and indirect techniques.[19,37,39]

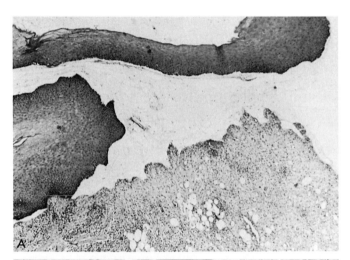

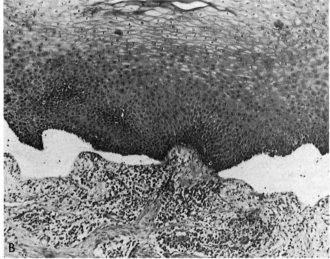

FIGURE 20–16. Biopsy specimen from an oral lesion of mucous membrane pemphigoid. *A,* A low-power view shows clean separation of the epithelium from underlying connective tissue. *B,* A high-power view shows intact basal layer as the epithelium separates from connective tissue at the basement membrane zone. Inflammatory infiltration is also present.

Ocular Lesions. The eyes are affected in many cases of mucous membrane pemphigoid. There is conjunctivitis with the development of fibrous adhesions between the palpebral and bulbar conjunctivae (Fig. 20–15B). There may be adhesions of eyelid to eyeball (symblepharon). Adhesions at the edges of the eyelids (ankyloblepharon) may result in narrowing of the palpebral fissure. Small vesicular lesions may develop on the conjunctiva. Eventually the conjunctival involvement may lead to scarring, corneal damage, and blindness.

Differential Diagnosis. In the differential diagnosis, other vesiculobullous diseases, such as pemphigus, erythema multiforme, and bullous lichen planus, must be considered. Pemphigus may be confined to the oral cavity in its early stage, and the vesicular and ulcerative lesions may resemble those of mucous membrane pemphigoid. An erosive or desquamative gingivitis may also be seen in pemphigus as a rare manifestation. Biopsy studies can quickly rule out pemphigus by revealing the absence of acantholytic changes. In erythema multiforme, there are obvious vesiculobullous lesions, but the onset is usually acute rather than chronic, labial involvement is severe, and the gingivae are usually not affected. A desquamative gingivitis is not seen in erythema multiforme, although occasional vesicular lesions may develop. A biopsy study of an oral lesion will reveal an unusual degeneration of the upper stratum spinosum, characteristically seen in oral erythema multiforme lesions.

Therapy. Mucous membrane pemphigoid can be treated with systemic corticosteroids in a moderate daily or every-other-day dose, with the dosage gradually lowered to a very small maintenance dose (5 to 10 mg of prednisone or comparable doses of other corticosteroids). Topical corticosteroids have limited value, but occasionally applications of corticosteroid ointment may ameliorate severe desquamative gingivitis and help to promote healing. Optimal oral hygiene is essential, as local irritants on the tooth surface will result in an exaggerated gingival inflammatory response. A soft toothbrush and oxidizing mouthwashes are helpful in maintaining good oral hygiene. If the disease is not severe and symptoms are mild, systemic corticosteroids may be omitted. If ocular involvement exists, systemic corticosteroids are indicated.

Erythema Multiforme

Erythema multiforme is an acute inflammatory eruptive disease involving the skin and oral cavity. More than 80% of patients with skin involvement present with oral lesions,[49] and in rare instances erythema multiforme may be confined to the mouth.[46] The pathognomonic skin lesions are of a target or iris variety, with a central vesicle or bulla surrounded by an urticarial zone.

Erythema multiforme is usually a recurrent disease. It may be ushered in with fever preceded by a chill, and the average episode lasts from 10 days to several weeks. The frequency of involvement varies from three or more attacks per year to a single attack every few years.

Erythema multiforme is probably not an etiologic entity, but rather a symptom complex or reaction pattern representing many possible causative factors, such as drugs, emotional stress, or systemic disease.

Oral Lesions. The oral lesions consist of purplish red macules or papules with interspersed bullous lesions. The tongue often is severely involved, with erosion of the bullae followed by ulceration. The lesions are so painful that chewing and swallowing are impaired.

The lips are invariably involved, usually with considerable severity, such that extensive bullous and ulcerative lesions are present on the mucosal surface, and secondary crusting occurs on the dry skin surface. The extensive labial lesions are often helpful in arriving at a clinical diagnosis.

Histopathology. Microscopically, there is liquefaction degeneration of the upper epithelium and the development of intraepithelial vesicles, but without the acantholysis that occurs in pemphigus.[73] Degenerative changes also occur in the basement membrane.

Treatment. There is no specific treatment. Systemic steroid therapy suppresses the symptoms while the disease runs its course.

Lupus Erythematosus

Lupus erythematosus was initially thought to be one of the so-called collagen diseases[24] but is currently considered an autoimmune disease.[70] It has two forms: a chronic discoid type and an acute systemic type. The incidence of oral involvement in lupus erythematosus varies depending on the acuteness of the disease. Although not more than 10% of patients with the chronic discoid type present with oral lesions, as many as 75% of patients with the acute systemic type have some oral manifestation before death. The characteristic "butterfly" distribution of the lesions on the face is a diagnostic aid in this disease (Fig. 20–17). In extremely rare instances, lupus erythematosus may occur on the oral mucous membrane without skin lesions.

Chronic Discoid Type. In the oral cavity, the disease appears as well-defined, slightly elevated, and infiltrated white lesions with an erythematous periphery. The lesions are usually localized and are seen most often on the buccal mucosa.[9] At the border of the lesion, there may be numerous dilated blood vessels in a radial arrangement extending into the surrounding tissue, coupled with whitish, pinhead papules. In the early stages the center of the lesion is slightly depressed and eroded and is covered with a bluish-red epithelial surface showing scarring. In older lesions the erythematous border becomes less elevated and is transformed into a whitish or bluish white peripheral zone of thickened epithelium. The dilated vessels are replaced by white lines with the same diverging radial arrangement. On the tongue the disease occurs as circumscribed, smooth, reddened areas in which the papillae are lost or as patches with a whitish sheen resembling leukoplakia.

On the lip the lesions are somewhat similar to those in the mouth, and in most cases the lip is involved by direct extension from perioral skin lesions. Localized patches may be present, or the entire lip may be involved. Early in the disease the lip is swollen, bluish red, and often everted. The lip lesions may be covered with adherent scales and crusts, which remain localized and are rarely diffuse (see Fig. 20–17). At the margins of the patches, dilated capillaries or fine, branching radial lines may be seen. The lip is tender and sensitive, and on removal of the adherent scales, bleeding from the raw surface is noted. Depressed scars may follow healing of the deeper lesions.

Periods of activity and quiescence occur. The lesions enlarge by peripheral extension and are accompanied by fresh erosions and superficial ulcerations, followed by atrophic changes. Some burning sensation occurs in the erosions and deeper ulcerations.

Microscopically, the epithelial changes in the chronic discoid type consist of keratinization, keratotic plugging, acanthosis, atrophy, pseudocarcinomatous hyperplasia, and liquefaction degeneration of the basal cell layer.[6] The histopathology of the oral lesions is characteristic and consists of hyperkeratosis or parakeratosis, hydropic degeneration of the basal layer of the epithelium, collagen degeneration in the corium, and a perivascular infiltration of lymphocytes.[68] The collagen degeneration shows up clearly with a periodic acid–Schiff stain for mucopolysaccharides.[68]

Acute Systemic Type. In the systemic variety, the oral lesions are more acute, and greater destruction occurs. The lesions are characterized by soft, irregular, superficial, or moderately deep erosions, usually covered with a necrotic, grayish pseudomembrane.

Differential Diagnosis. Diagnosis usually depends on the identification of the accompanying skin lesions. The diagnosis of discoid lupus erythematosus confined to the oral cavity is very difficult to make, but microscopic studies usually reveal the characteristic histopathology.[6] The acute systemic variety may present a variety of oral lesions that are essentially nonspecific and erosive in nature. Erythema multiforme and pemphigus may sometimes look quite similar. Biopsy studies will aid in differentiating between lupus erythematosus and other erosive diseases.

Treatment. The treatment of lupus erythematosus is nonspecific. Systemic bismuth and gold have been used in the past. Adrenocorticotropic hormone (ACTH, or corticotropin) and corticosteroids are used currently for sys-

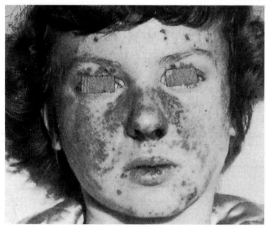
FIGURE 20–17. Lupus erythematosus showing "butterfly" distribution of lesions on the face and crusting of the lips.

temic disease. The antimalarial drugs are very successful in controlling the chronic discoid variety, but in systemic lupus erythematosus these drugs have no effect.

Scleroderma

Scleroderma is characterized by a primary induration and edema of the skin in localized patches or diffuse areas and later by atrophy and pigmentation. There are three distinct forms: diffuse scleroderma, acrosclerosis, and circumscribed scleroderma (morphea).[55,61] The etiology is obscure, although scleroderma is considered by many investigators to be of autoimmune origin. In all types of the disease, the first sign is usually a moderate induration of the skin, gradually followed by the atrophic stage, which results in permanent disfiguration. Ulceration can occur but is rare and is seen only in advanced cases. Hemiatrophy is fairly common in cases of facial involvement and is sometimes accompanied by false ankylosis of the temporomandibular joint.

Oral Lesions. The diffuse and acrosclerotic types frequently involve the oral cavity.[61] Although the entire mucous membrane may be involved, it is the tongue that most commonly shows pathologic changes, followed in frequency by the buccal mucosa and the gingiva. There may be painful induration of the tongue and gingiva.[61] The usual symptom is a minor speech defect as a result of impaired mobility of the tongue. Scleroderma of the mucous membrane is chronic, and its progress is reportedly more rapid than that of the skin lesions.

In the acrosclerotic variety, the lips become thin and rigid, and their movements are greatly restricted. The opening of the oral cavity is usually markedly reduced. Difficulty in eating and talking may follow. Obliterative endarteritis may result in avascularity, with increased susceptibility to infection.[36]

In acrosclerosis and diffuse scleroderma, Stafne and Austin[78] have described a characteristic roentgenographic picture consisting of an increase in the width of the periodontal space. Not all of the teeth may be affected, and the posterior teeth are involved more often than the anterior teeth. Radiographically, the periodontal space in relation to the entire root is widened to an almost uniform thickness.[78] The increase in width of the periodontal spaces occurs at the expense of the alveolar bone. The lamina dura is obliterated. Clinically, the teeth are firm.

Microscopically, the continuity of the periodontal fibers from the cementum to the alveolar bone is broken near the cementum.

Treatment. There is no effective treatment; however, use of an immunosuppressive agent (azathioprine) has been described.[36]

CHRONIC BACTERIAL INFECTIONS

Oral lesions can occur in bacterial infections such as syphilis and tuberculosis (Figs. 20–18 and 20–19).[51,62] The oral lesions in both of these infective diseases are relatively

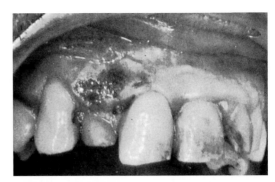

FIGURE 20–18. Primary stage of syphilis. Chancre of the gingiva.

rare and present as chronic ulcers (chancre of primary stage of syphilis, mucous patch of secondary stage, gumma of tertiary syphilis, tuberculous ulcer) or raised, granulomatous lesions with superficial ulceration (tuberculous granuloma, syphilitic gumma) or atrophic interstitial reactions (atrophic glossitis of tertiary syphilis). In very rare instances there may be erosive, ulcerative, or desquamative lesions of the attached gingiva. Diagnosis is made by biopsy, followed by appropriate immunologic and bacteriologic studies. Because the oral lesions represent one manifestation of a generalized systemic disease, appropriate antibacterial therapy is indicated. Results of current therapeutic approaches are invariably successful.

DRUG ERUPTIONS

An increase in the incidence of skin and oral manifestations of hypersensitivity to drugs has been noted since the advent of the sulfonamides, barbiturates, and various antibiotics. *The eruptive skin and oral lesions are attributed to the fact that the drug acts as an allergen, either alone or in combination, sensitizing the tissues and then causing the allergic reaction.*

Eruptions in the oral cavity resulting from sensitivity to drugs that have been taken by mouth or parenterally are termed *stomatitis medicamentosa*. The local reaction from the use of a medicament in the oral cavity (e.g., an aspirin burn or the stomatitis resulting from topical penicillin) is referred to as *stomatitis venenata* or *contact stomatitis*. Such changes may result either from the irritating local action of the drug or from drug sensitivity. In many cases skin eruptions may accompany the oral lesions.

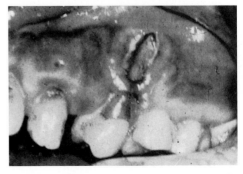

FIGURE 20–19. Ulcerative tuberculous lesion on the gingiva. (Courtesy of Dr. Irving Meyer.)

272

In general, drug eruptions in the oral cavity are multiform. Vesicular and bullous lesions occur most commonly, but pigmented or nonpigmented macular lesions are also frequently observed. Erosions, often followed by deep ulceration with purpuric lesions, may also occur. The lesions are seen in different areas of the oral cavity, with the gingiva frequently affected.[26]

Hundreds of drugs are capable of producing skin eruptions with or without mouth lesions. Constitutional symptoms may be severe or entirely absent. Only a few of the important and most commonly used drugs that may be associated with skin and oral eruptions will be considered here.

Agranulocytosis characterized by necrotic oral lesions, sore throat, and leukopenia may follow the use of gold salts, arsphenamine, aminopyrine, sulfonamides, and antibiotics. The barbiturates[41] and salicylates[16] (Fig. 20–20) occasionally produce vesicular or bullous lesions, followed by erosions in the oral cavity. Phenolphthalein, found in many proprietary laxatives, may produce bullous lesions, followed by erosions (usually confined to a single lesion) on the skin and in the oral cavity.

Iodides and bromides may give rise to bullous and hemorrhagic eruptions in the oral cavity and to acne, urticaria, or suppurating and vegetating lesions on the skin. The sulfonamides are responsible for a variety of skin and oral lesions, including vesicles, bullae, and ulcerations. Sulfonamide ointment has been a factor in producing sensitization in a large percentage of cases.[80] A so-called fixed eruption of mucous membrane and skin caused by sulfadiazine[17] has been reported. Quinacrine hydrochloride (Atabrine), used in the prevention and treatment of malaria in World War II, produced a skin eruption called *atypical lichenoid dermatitis* that was characterized by lesions resembling those of lichen planus on the skin and oral mucosa.

Skin and oral eruptions and acute candidal infection have been associated with the widespread use of antibiotics such as penicillin (Fig. 20–21).

Cancer chemotherapeutic agents are currently responsible for a significant number of cases of oral ulcerative lesions.[14,31]

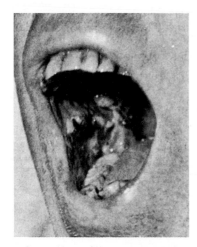

FIGURE 20–20. Stomatitis medicamentosa resulting from bismuth salicylate, causing necrosis of the buccal mucosa with pigmentation.

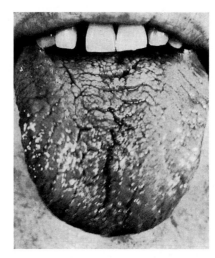

FIGURE 20–21. Prominent papillae and discoloration of the tongue associated with local use of penicillin.

MYCOTIC DISEASES

Although mycotic disease of the oral cavity is relatively uncommon, several conditions are occasionally seen.

Acute Candidiasis (Moniliasis, Thrush)

Acute candidiasis is the most common mycotic infection of the oral mucosa. It is seen in three types of individuals: debilitated or immunosuppressed adults, infants, and adults who have been on antibiotic therapy for some time. The causative organism is *Candida albicans,* an organism commonly found in the mouth that is normally nonpathogenic. In the severely debilitated adult with significantly lowered tissue resistance, the organism may become invasive and destructive, penetrating the oral mucosa and producing necrosis of the epithelium. Candidiasis is seen in immunosuppressed patients and is becoming increasingly frequent in cancer patients who have been treated with high doses of radiation or chemotherapeutic drugs. Candidiasis is also an early and major oral manifestation of acquired immunodeficiency syndrome (AIDS) (see Chapter 15). In fact, AIDS should always be ruled out in a patient with acute candidiasis, particularly if there is any suspicion that the individual may be in a high-risk category for this infection.

Infants are born with a sterile mouth, and the normal oral bacterial-mycotic flora develops gradually. During this early stage, while the flora is becoming established, candidal organisms may proliferate and produce disease. *C. albicans* may proliferate and invade the oral tissues if the normal bacterial components of the oral flora are removed by the use of antibiotics. However, the development of candidiasis as a complication of antibiotic therapy has been overemphasized. It usually requires the use of several different antibiotics over a period of several weeks or months, and affected patients tend to be debilitated by the conditions requiring the antibacterial therapy. An increased incidence of candidiasis is also seen in certain metabolic disorders such as diabetes and the hypothyroid–adrenocortical insufficiency syndrome. Women developing oral candidiasis may also develop vaginal candidiasis, because the organism

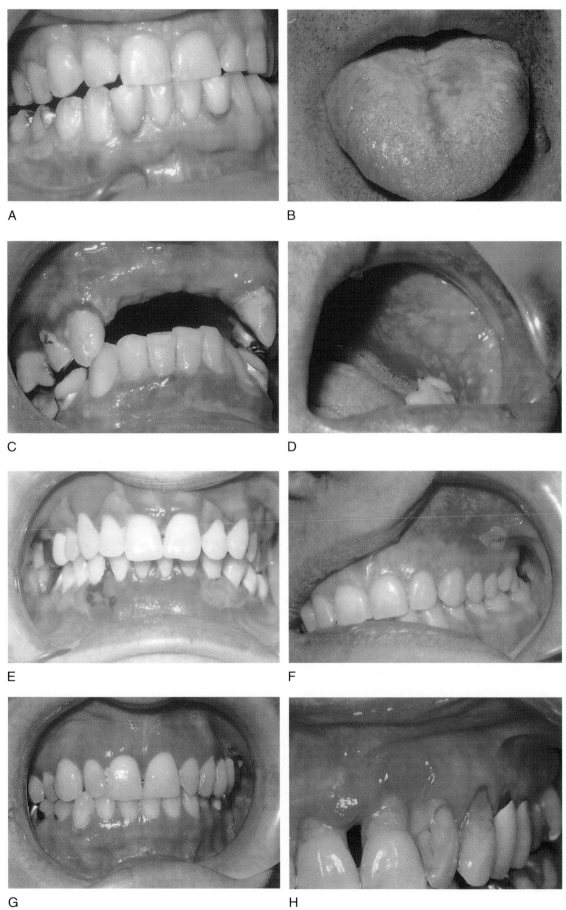

PLATE X. Desquamative lesions. *A,* Lichen planus. *B,* Lichen planus. *C,* Lichen planus. *D,* Lichen planus. *E,* Pemphigus. *F,* Pemphigus. *G,* Mucous membrane pemphigoid. *H,* Carcinoma.

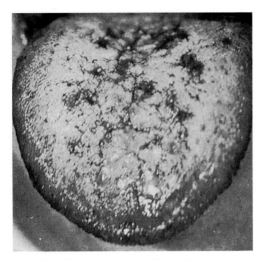

FIGURE 20-22. Acute moniliasis of the tongue.

is also a common inhabitant of the vaginal tract. Pregnancy and the use of contraceptive steroids tend to predispose the female to the development of both oral and vaginal candidiasis.

Microscopic examination of oral lesions of candidiasis reveals the invading mycelia of the organisms within epithelium that is undergoing necrosis.

Biopsy studies are not necessary for diagnostic purposes, because a smear can adequately demonstrate the organisms. Culture of the organisms is unnecessary and misleading, as *C. albicans* is usually present in normal mouths as part of the bacterial-mycotic flora. Candidiasis is not contagious because the organisms are normally present, and some predisposing loss of tissue resistance or depression of the immune response is required.

Oral Lesions. The oral lesions may appear anywhere on the mucosal surface as a simple patch, but usually the lesions are multiple. The characteristic lesions are creamy white, resembling coagulated milk; they are adherent and, when forcibly removed, give rise to bleeding points (Figs. 20–22 and 20–23). Intertriginous maceration at the labial commissures in both children and adults may reveal *C. albicans.*

Fotos and associates,[23] in a study of 100 cases of oral candidiasis, found a wide diversity of presenting symptoms and clinical manifestations, including mucosal erythema

(60%), mucosal white plaque (36%), hyperkeratotic mucosal areas (24%), intraoral ulcerations (20%), papillary atrophy (17%), angular cheilitis (12%), and xerostomia (11%). They defined four clinical types of the disease. In the *pseudomembranous* types there are white, curd-like plaques overlying mucosal erythema and ulceration; large numbers of hyphae and spores are also present at the mucosal surface, with invasion of the epithelium. The *atrophic* type is usually seen on the dorsum of the tongue, with erythema and papillary atrophy. In the *hyperplastic* type there is hyperkeratosis of the epithelium with white plaques that are difficult to scrape off. The *epidermal-and-perioral* type shows scaling patches at the corners of the lips. Patients with prosthetic appliances have a predisposition to candidal infection, and the appliances may act as reservoirs for reinfection if not disinfected with an agent such as chlorhexidine or benzalkonium.

Diagnosis. The diagnosis is based on the patient history, the clinical appearance of the lesions, and the microscopic study of smears or scrapings from them. The smears, when stained with gentian violet or methylene blue, will show spores and mycelia of *C. albicans* (Fig. 20–24).

Clinically, thrush may simulate diphtheria, macerated epithelium of the buccal mucosa from chronic irritation (biting habit), leukoplakia, and possibly lichen planus. However, these conditions are readily ruled out by smears of the necrotic white lesions.

Treatment. Current treatment of acute oral candidiasis favors the use of the antimycotic agent *clotrimazole* (Mycelex) in the form of oral troches. Troches are prescribed for use every 3 hours, for a total of six per day for 7 to 10 days. In immunosuppressed patients, the therapy should be extended to 14 days. Troches are held in the mouth until dissolved. Another antimycotic agent that can be used is nystatin (Mycostatin). Painting the lesions with 1% gentian violet is an older but effective treatment if the clinician can paint all lesions every day for 7 days.

Chronic Candidiasis

Chronic candidiasis is a rare type of *C. albicans* infection resulting in a granulomatous lesion that begins in infancy or early childhood and may persist for several years.[42] The oral lesions are often accompanied by involvement of the nails and skin (Figs. 20–25 to 20–27). In contrast to the mild, superficial acute forms of monilial infection, monilial granuloma is manifested by a deep inflammatory reaction with the production of granulation

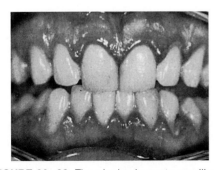

FIGURE 20-23. The gingiva in acute moniliasis.

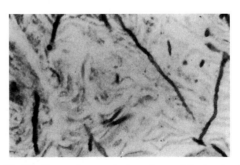

FIGURE 20-24. Smear from a lesion of candidiasis showing proliferating mycelia of *Candida albicans.*

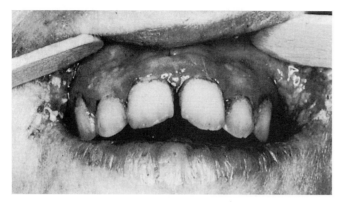

FIGURE 20–25. Chronic candidiasis involving the gingiva in an 18-year-old woman.

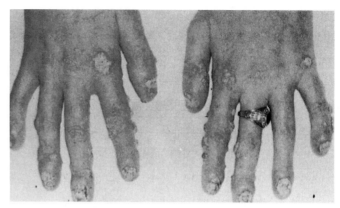

FIGURE 20–27. Lesions of chronic candidiasis on the skin of the hands and on fingernails.

tissue. Ultimate involvement of the lungs with multiple abscesses, often associated with kidney lesions, results in death in many cases.

Diagnosis. As for acute candidiasis, the diagnosis is confirmed by laboratory studies.

Treatment. In chronic or systemic candidiasis, treatment involves the systemic use of *amphotericin B,* a potent but relatively toxic antimycotic agent. Newer antimycotic agents for systemic use are currently being tested.

Other Chronic Mycotic Diseases

Other chronic mycotic lesions of the oral cavity are extremely rare but, when they do occur, present as granulomatous and ulcerative lesions. Oral mucosal lesions of actinomycosis, histoplasmosis,[52,86] coccidiodomycosis, blastomycosis, and mucormycosis have been described. Diagnosis is made by biopsy and the use of special stains to locate the spores and/or mycelia of the fungus within the tissues. Recognition of morphology usually results in a specific diagnosis.

REFERENCES

1. Ahmed AR. Cellular immunity and HLA studies in pemphigus. Clin Dermatol *1:*92, 1983.
2. Ahmed AR, Wagner R, Khatri K, et al. Major histocompatibility complex haplo-
3. types and class 11 genes in non-Jewish patients with pemphigus vulgaris. Proc Natl Acad Sci USA *88:*5056, 1991.
3. Ahmed AR, Workman S. Anti-intercellular substance antibodies. Arch Dermatol *119:*17, 1983.
4. Ahmed AR, Yunis EJ, Alper CA. Complotypes in pemphigus vulgaris differences between Jewish and non-Jewish patients. Hum Immunol *27:*296, 1990.
5. Ahmed AR, Yunis EJ, Khatri K, et al. Major histocompatibility complex haplotype studies in Ashkenazi Jewish patients with pemphigus vulgaris. Proc Natl Acad Sci USA *87:*7658, 1990.
6. Andreasen JO, Poulsen HE. Oral manifestations in discoid and systemic lupus erythematosus. Histologic investigation. Acta Odontol Scand *22:*389, 1964.
7. Andreasen JO. Oral lichen planus. A clinical evaluation of 115 cases. Oral Surg *25:*31, 1968.
8. Anhalt GJ, Labib RS, Voorhees JJ, et al. Induction of pemphigus in neonatal mice by passive transfer of IgG from patients with the disease. N Engl J Med *306:*1189, 1982.
9. Archard HO, Roebuck NF, Stanley HR. Oral manifestations of chronic discoid lupus erythematosus. Oral Surg *16:*696, 1963.
10. Baudet-Pommel M, Janin-Mercier A, Souteyrand P. Sequential immunopathologic study of oral lichen planus treated with tretinoin and etretinate. Oral Surg *71:*197, 1991.
11. Bennett DE. Histoplasmosis of the oral cavity and larynx. Arch Intern Med *120:*417, 1967.
12. Beutner EH, Jordan RE, Chorzelski TP et al. The immunopathology of pemphigus and bullous pemphigoid. J Invest Dermatol *51:*63, 1968.
13. Blank H, Burgoon CF. Abnormal cytology of epithelial cells in pemphigus vulgaris: A diagnostic aid. J Invest Dermatol *18:*213, 1952.
14. Bottomley WK, Perlin E, Ross GR. Antineoplastic agents and their oral manifestations. Oral Surg *44:*527, 1977.
15. Brusati R, Bracchetti A. Electron microscopic study of chronic desquamative gingivitis. J Periodontol *40:*388, 1969.
16. Claman HN. Mouth ulcers associated with prolonged chewing of gum containing aspirin. JAMA *202:*651, 1967.
17. Cole LW. Fixed eruption of mucous membrane and skin caused by sulfadiazine. Arch Dermatol Syph *54:*675, 1946.
18. Combes FL, Canizares O. Pemphigus vulgaris, a clinicopathological study of one hundred cases. Arch Dermatol Syph *62:*786, 1950.
19. Dabelsteen E, Ullman S, Thomson K, et al. Demonstration of basement membrane autoantibodies in patients with benign mucous membrane pemphigoid. Acta Dermatol Venereol (Stockh) *54:*189, 1974.
20. Eisen D, Ellis CN, Duell GA, et al. Effect of topical cyclosporin rinse on oral lichen planus. N Engl J Med *323:*290, 1990.
21. Engel M, Ray HG, Orban B. The pathogenesis of desquamative gingivitis. J Dent Res *29:*410, 1950.
22. Foss CL, Grupe HE, Orban B. Gingivosis. J Periodontol *24:*207, 1953.
23. Fotos PG, Vincent SD, Hellstein JW. Oral candidosis: Clinical, historical and therapeutic features of 100 cases. Oral Surg *74:*41, 1992.
24. Gahan E. Lupus erythematosus. Clinical observations in 443 cases. Arch Dermatol Syph *45:*685, 1942.
25. Gallagher G, Shklar G. Oral involvement in mucous membrane pemphigoid. Clin Dermatol *5:*19, 1987.
26. Gallagher GT. Oral mucous membrane reactions to drugs and chemicals. Curr Opin Dent *1:*777, 1991.
27. Glickman I, Smulow JB. Chronic desquamative gingivitis: Its nature and treatment. J Periodontol *35:*397, 1964.
28. Glickman I, Smulow JB. Histopathology and histochemistry of chronic desquamative gingivitis. Oral Surg *21:*325, 1966.
29. Goadby K. Diseases of the Gums and Oral Mucous Membrane. London, Henry Froude and Hodder and Staughton, 1923, p 22.
30. Goldman HM, Ruben MP. Desquamative gingivitis and its response to topical triamcinolone therapy. Oral Surg *21:*579, 1966.

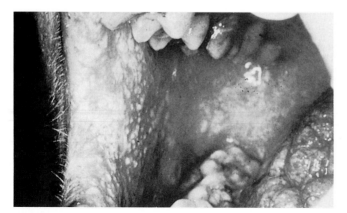

FIGURE 20–26. Lesions of chronic candidiasis on the buccal mucosa.

31. Guggenheimer J, Verbin RS, Appel BN, et al. Clinicopathological effects of cancer chemotherapeutic agents on human buccal mucosa. Oral Surg *44:*58, 1977.
32. Hashimoto K, Dibella R, Shklar G, Lever W. Electron microscopic studies of oral lichen planus. G Ital Dermatol *107:*765, 1966.
33. Hashimoto K. Electron microscopy and histochemistry of pemphigus and pemphigoid. Oral Surg *33:*206, 1972.
34. Ishii T. Immunohistochemical demonstration of T cell subsets and accessory cells in oral lichen planus. J Oral Pathol *15:*268, 1987.
35. Jandinski J, Shklar G. Lichen planus of the gingiva. J Periodontol *47:*724, 1976.
36. Jansen GT, Barraza DF, Ballard JL, et al. Generalized scleroderma. Treatment with immunosuppressive agents. Arch Dermatol *97:*690, 1968.
37. Komori A, Welton NA, Kelln EE. The behavior of the basement membrane of skin and oral lesions in patients with lichen planus, erythema multiforme, lupus erythematosus, pemphigus vulgaris, pemphigoid and epidermolysis bullosa. Oral Surg *22:*752, 1966.
38. Lamey PJ, Rees TD, Binnie WH, Rankin KV. Mucous membrane pemphigoid: Treatment experience at two institutions. Oral Surg *74:*50, 1992.
39. Laskaris G, Angelopoulos A. Cicatricial pemphigoid: Direct and indirect immunofluorescent studies. Oral Surg *51:*48, 1981.
40. Laskaris G, Demetrou N, Angelopoulos A. Immunofluorescent studies in desquamative gingivitis. J Oral Pathol *10:*398, 1981.
41. Lawson BF. Severe stomatitis associated with barbiturate ingestion. J Oral Med *24:*13, 1969.
42. Lehner T. Chronic candidiasis. Br Dent J *116:*539, 1964.
43. Leonard JN, Wright P, Williams DM, et al. The relationship between linear IgA disease and benign mucous membrane pemphigoid. Br J Dermatol *110:*307, 1984.
44. Levell NJ, McLeod RI, Marks JM. Lack of effect of cyclosporin mouthwash in oral lichen planus. Lancet *337:*796, 1991.
45. Lever WF. Pemphigus. Medicine *32:*1, 1953.
46. Lozada F, Silverman S. Erythema multiforme: Clinical characteristics and natural history in fifty patients. Oral Surg *46:*628, 1978.
47. Malmstrom M, Kontinnen YT, Jungell P, et al. Lymphocyte activation in oral lichen planus in situ. Am J Clin Pathol *89:*329, 1988.
48. McCarthy FP, McCarthy PL, Shklar G. Chronic desquamative gingivitis: A reconsideration. Oral Surg *13:*1300, 1960.
49. McCarthy PL, Shklar G. Diseases of the Oral Mucosa. 2nd ed. Philadelphia, Lea & Febiger, 1980.
50. Merritt AH. Chronic desquamative gingivitis. J Periodontol *4:*30, 1933.
51. Meyer I, Shklar G. The oral manifestations of acquired syphilis. Oral Surg *23:*45, 1967.
52. Miller HE, Keddie FM, Johnson HG, et al. Histoplasmosis, cutaneous and mucomembranous lesions. Arch Dermatol Syph *56:*715, 1947.
53. Nikai H, Rose G, Cattoni M. Electron microscopic study of chronic desquamative gingivitis. J Periodont Res 6(suppl):1, 1971.
54. Nisengard RJ, Neiders M. Desquamative lesions of the gingiva. J Periodontol *52:*500, 1981.
55. O'Leary PA, Nomland R. A clinical study of one hundred and three cases of scleroderma. Am J Med Sci *180:*85, 1930.
56. Porter SR, Scully C, Midda M, Eveson JW. Adult linear immunoglobulin A disease manifesting as desquamative gingivitis. Oral Surg *70:*450, 1990.
57. Prinz H. Chronic diffuse desquamative gingivitis. Dent Cosmos *74:*331, 1932.
58. Pullon PA. Ultrastructure of oral lichen planus. Oral Surg *28:*365, 1969.
59. Rogers RS, Sheridan PJ, Jordon RC. Desquamative gingivitis: Clinical, histopathologic and immunopathologic investigations. Oral Surg *42:*316, 1976.
60. Schour I, Massler M. Gingival disease in postwar Italy: Gingivosis in hospitalized children in Naples. Am J Orthod *33:*756, 1947.
61. Scopp IW, Schlagel E. Scleroderma: Its orofacial manifestations. Oral Surg *15:*1510, 1962.
62. Shengold MA, Sheingold H. Oral tuberculosis. Oral Surg *20:*29, 1951.
63. Shklar G, Cataldo E. Histopathology and cytology of oral pemphigus vulgaris. Arch Dermatol *101:*36, 1970.
64. Shklar G. Lichen planus as an oral ulcerative disease. Oral Surg *33:*376, 1972.
65. Shklar G. Oral lesions of erythema multiforme: Histologic and histochemical observations. Arch Dermatol *92:*495, 1965.
66. Shklar G, Flynn E, Szabo G. Basement membrane changes in oral lichen planus. J Invest Dermatol *70:*45, 1978.
67. Shklar G, Frim S, Flynn E. Gingival lesions of pemphigus. J Periodontol *49:*428, 1978.
68. Shklar G, McCarthy PL. Histopathology of oral lesions of chronic discoid lupus erythematous. Arch Dermatol *114:*1031, 1978.
69. Shklar G, McCarthy PL. Oral lesions of mucous membrane pemphigoid. A study of 85 cases. Arch Otolaryngol *93:*354, 1971.
70. Shklar G, McCarthy PL. The Oral Manifestations of Systemic Disease. Boston, Butterworth, 1976.
71. Shklar G, McCarthy PL. The oral lesions of mucous membrane pemphigoid. A study of 85 cases. Arch Otolaryngol *93:*354, 1971.
72. Shklar G, Meyer I. The histopathology and histochemistry of dermatologic lesions in the mouth. Oral Surg *14:*1069, 1961.
73. Shklar G, Meyer I, Zacarian S. Oral lesions in bullous pemphigoid. Arch Dermatol *99:*663, 1969.
74. Silverman S. Lichen planus. Curr Opin Dent *1:*769, 1991.
75. Sklavounou A, Laskaris G. Frequency of desquamative gingivitis in skin disease. *56:*141, 1983.
76. Sognnaes RF, Weisberger D, Albright JT. Pathologic desquamation of oral epithelium examined by electron microscopy and histochemistry. J Natl Cancer Inst *17:*329, 1956.
77. Sorrin S. Chronic desquamative gingivitis. J Am Dent Assoc *27:*250, 1940.
78. Stafne EC, Austin LT. A characteristic dental finding in acrosclerosis and diffuse scleroderma. Am J Orthod Oral Surg *30:*25, 1944.
79. Sugerman PB, Rollason PA, Savage NW, Seymour GJ. Suppressor cell function in oral lichen planus. J Dent Res *71:*1916, 1992.
80. Sulzberger MB, Kanof A, Baer RL, Lowenberg C. Sensitization by topical application of sulfonamides. J Allergy *18:*92, 1947.
81. Susi FR, Shklar G. Histochemistry and fine structure of oral lesions of mucous membrane pemphigoid. Arch Dermatol *104:*244, 1971.
82. Tomes J, Tomes C. Dental Surgery. 4th ed. London, J & A Churchill, 1894.
83. Walsh LJ, Savage NW, Ishii T, Seymour GJ. Immunopathogenesis of oral lichen planus. J Oral Pathol Med *19:*389, 1990.
84. Whitten JB. Intraoral lichen planus simplex: An ultrastructural study. J Periodontol *41:*261, 1970.
85. Whitten JB. The fine structure of desquamative stomatitis. J Periodontol *39:*75, 1968.
86. Young LL, Dolan CT, Sheridan PJ, et al: Oral manifestations of histoplasmosis. Oral Surg Oral Med Oral Pathol *33:*191, 1972.
87. Zegarelli DJ, Zegarelli EV. Intraoral pemphigus vulgaris. Oral Surg *44:*384, 1977.
88. Ziskin D, Silvers HF. Report of a case of desquamative gingivitis and lichen planus. J Periodontol *16:*7, 1945.
89. Ziskin D, Zegarelli EV. Chronic desquamative gingivitis. Am J Orthod *33:*756, 1947.

21

Gingival Disease in Childhood

FERMIN A. CARRANZA, JR.

The effects of periodontal disease observed in adults have their inception earlier in life. Gingival disease in the child may progress to jeopardize the periodontium of the adult.

The developing dentition and certain systemic metabolic patterns are peculiar to childhood. There are also gingival and periodontal disturbances that occur more frequently in childhood and are therefore identified with this period. Consequently, some degree of coherence is provided by considering gingival and periodontal problems in childhood and in adolescence separately. This chapter will cover gingival diseases; juvenile forms of periodontitis are covered in Chapter 27.

THE PERIODONTIUM OF THE DECIDUOUS DENTITION

The gingiva of the deciduous dentition is pale pink and firm and may be either smooth or stippled (stippling is found in 35% of children between 5 and 13 years of age[27]) (Fig. 21–1). The interdental gingiva is broad faciolingually and tends to be relatively narrow mesiodistally, in conformity with the contour of the approximal tooth surfaces. Its structure is comparable to that of the adult in that it consists of a facial papilla and a lingual papilla with an intervening depression, or *col*.

The mean gingival sulcus depth for the primary dentition is 2.1 mm ± 0.2 mm.[25] The width of the attached gingiva is greater in the incisor area, decreases over the cuspids, and increases again over premolars (primary molars) and permanent molars.[28] The attached gingiva increases in width with age.

Microscopically, the stratified squamous epithelium of the gingiva presents well-differentiated rete pegs with a parakeratinized (Fig. 21–2) or keratinized surface, the latter correlated with stippling. The connective tissue is predominantly fibrillar, but the well-differentiated collagen bundles seen in the adult are not present in childhood. The epithelium covering the col is a few cells thick and nonkeratinized.

The periodontal ligament of the deciduous teeth is wider than that of the permanent dentition. During eruption the principal fibers are parallel to the long axis of the teeth; the bundle arrangement seen in the adult dentition occurs when the teeth encounter their functional antagonists.

Radiographically, the alveolar bone in relation to the deciduous dentition shows a prominent lamina dura, both in the crypt stage and during eruption. The trabeculae of the alveolar bone are fewer but thicker than in the adult, and the marrow spaces tend to be larger. The crests of the interdental septa are flat.[6]

In beagle dogs, the juvenile gingiva shows a thicker keratinized layer of oral epithelium than does the gingiva of the adult. In addition, the juvenile junctional epithelium structurally resembles the oral epithelium, and there is a cuticular structure at the surface of the junctional epithelium.[18] These differences might explain the reduced inflammatory response to plaque accumulation in juvenile dogs.

Oral flora and dental plaque in childhood are discussed in Chapter 6.

PHYSIOLOGIC GINGIVAL CHANGES ASSOCIATED WITH TOOTH ERUPTION

During the transition period in the development of the dentition, changes associated with eruption of the permanent teeth occur in the gingiva. It is important to recognize these physiologic changes and to differentiate them from the gingival disease that often accompanies tooth eruption.

Pre-eruption Bulge. Before the crown appears in the oral cavity, the gingiva presents a bulge that is firm, may be slightly blanched, and conforms to the contour of the underlying crown.

Formation of the Gingival Margin. The marginal gingiva and sulcus develop as the crown penetrates the oral mucosa. In the course of eruption the gingival margin is usually edematous, rounded, and slightly reddened (Fig. 21–3).

Normal Prominence of the Gingival Margin. During the period of mixed dentition it is normal for the marginal gingiva around the permanent teeth to be quite prominent,

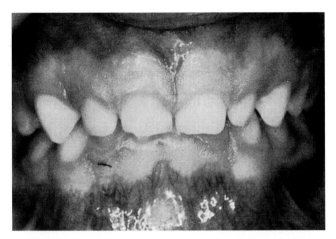

FIGURE 21–1. Deciduous dentition with stippled gingiva.

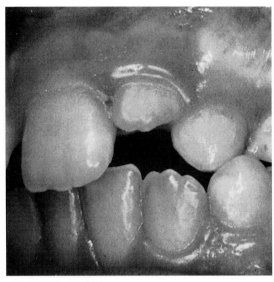

FIGURE 21–3. Gingivitis associated with tooth eruption. Note the prominent rolled gingival margin, which is slightly inflamed and edematous around the erupting maxillary lateral incisor.

particularly in the maxillary anterior region. At this stage in tooth eruption the gingiva is still attached to the crown, and it appears prominent when superimposed on the bulk of the underlying enamel (Fig. 21–4).

TYPES OF GINGIVAL DISEASE

Chronic Marginal Gingivitis

Chronic marginal gingivitis is the most prevalent type of gingival change in childhood. The gingiva exhibits all the changes in color, size, consistency, and surface texture characteristic of chronic inflammation. A fiery red surface discoloration is often superimposed on underlying chronic changes. Gingival color change and swelling appear to be

more common expressions of gingivitis in children than are bleeding and increased pocket depth.[5]

Etiology. In children, as in adults, *the cause of gingivitis is plaque;* local conditions such as materia alba and poor oral hygiene favor its accumulation (Fig. 21–5). In preschool children, however, the gingival response to bacterial plaque has been found to be markedly less than that in adults.[16,17] Dental plaque appears to form more rapidly in children age 8 to 12 years than in adults.

Calculus is uncommon in infants; it occurs in approximately 9% of children 4 to 6 years old, in 18% of those 7 to 9 years old, and in 33% to 43% of those 10 to 15 years old. In children with cystic fibrosis, calculus formation is more common (occurring in 77% of those 7 to 9 years old and in 90% of those 10 to 15 years old) and more severe; this is probably related to increased concentrations of phosphate, calcium, and protein in the saliva.[21]

Gingivitis associated with tooth eruption is frequent and has given rise to the term *eruption gingivitis.* However, tooth eruption per se does not cause gingivitis. The inflam-

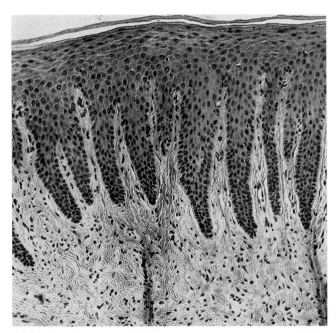

FIGURE 21–2. Normal gingiva in a 4-year-old patient showing stratified squamous epithelium with rete pegs and surface keratinization. The papillary arrangement of the underlying connective tissue can also be seen.

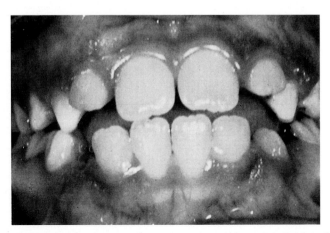

FIGURE 21–4. Prominent marginal gingiva on the cervical third of partially erupted maxillary anterior teeth.

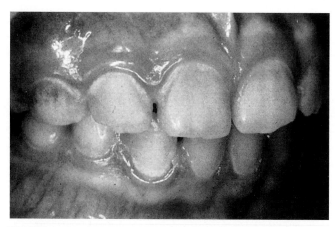

FIGURE 21–5. Chronic marginal gingivitis associated with plaque and materia alba.

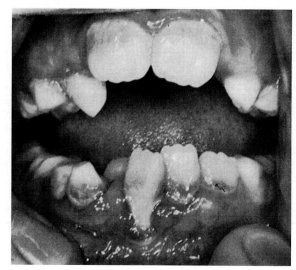

FIGURE 21–7. Severe gingivitis associated with accumulation of plaque around malposed teeth.

mation results from plaque accumulation around erupting teeth. The initiation of gingivitis appears to be related to plaque accumulation rather than to tissue remodeling associated with eruption.[10] Plaque retention around deciduous teeth facilitates plaque formation around juxtaposed permanent teeth.[10] The inflammatory changes accentuate the normal prominence of the gingival margin and create the impression of a marked gingival enlargement (Fig. 21–6).

Partially exfoliated, loose deciduous teeth frequently cause gingivitis. The eroded margin of partially resorbed teeth favors plaque accumulation, which causes gingival changes varying from slight discoloration and edema to abscess formation with suppuration. Other factors favoring plaque buildup are food impaction and materia alba accumulation around teeth partially destroyed by caries. Children frequently develop unilateral chewing habits to avoid loose or carious teeth, aggravating the accumulation of plaque on the nonchewing side.

Gingivitis occurs more frequently and with greater severity around *malposed teeth* because of their in-

creased tendency to accumulate plaque and materia alba. Severe changes include gingival enlargement, bluish red discoloration, ulceration (Fig. 21–7), and the formation of deep pockets from which pus can be expressed. Gingival health and contour are restored by correction of the malposition (Figs. 21–8 and 21–9); plaque elimination; and, when necessary, surgical removal of the enlarged gingiva.

Gingivitis is increased in children with *excessive overbite and overjet, nasal obstruction,* and *mouth breathing habit.*

According to Maynard and Wilson,[19] mucogingival problems start in the primary dentition as a consequence of developmental aberrations in eruption and deficiencies in the thickness of the periodontium. If there is also inadequate plaque control or excessive toothbrushing trauma, a mucogingival problem develops. However, the width of the attached gingiva increases with age, and these problems may resolve.

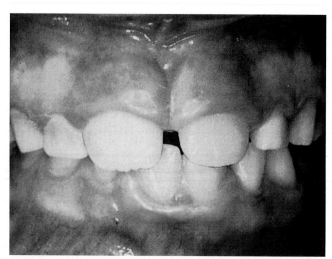

FIGURE 21–6. Developmental gingival enlargement caused by inflammation superimposed on the normal prominence of the teeth at this stage of tooth eruption.

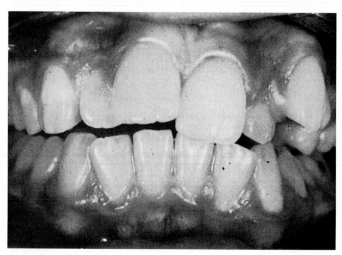

FIGURE 21–8. Gingival enlargement in relation to malposed maxillary lateral and canine teeth (*left side*).

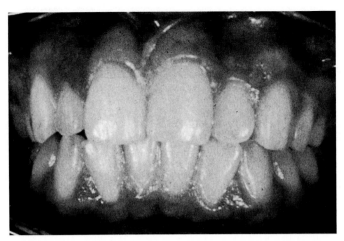

FIGURE 21–9. Disappearance of the gingival enlargement shown in Figure 21–8 after orthodontic correction of the malposed teeth.

Histopathology. Chronic gingivitis in children[13,14] is characterized by loss of collagen in the area around the junctional epithelium, an important vascular component, and an infiltrate consisting mostly of lymphocytes and small numbers of polymorphonuclear leukocytes, plasma cells, monocytes, mast cells, fibroblasts, and endothelial cells.

The composition of the inflammatory infiltrate in gingivitis in children has given rise to controversy. According to Gillett and colleagues,[8] the inflammatory infiltrate is composed mostly of untransformed B lymphocytes, and the resulting clinical lesions are nondestructive and nonprogressive. This may also characterize the composition of the infiltrate in quiescent lesions in adults. According to Longhurst et al.[13,14] and Seymour et al.,[26] the infiltrate is predominantly composed of T cells that shift to B cells (plasma cells) when the lesion becomes destructive.

A higher prevalence and severity of gingivitis and gingival enlargement is found in the circumpubertal period; this form of gingivitis has been termed *pubertal gingivitis.* The most frequent manifestation is a significant increase in bleeding interdental sites.[20] This inflammatory lesion may include a gingival enlargement as a result of hormonal changes that magnify the tissue response to local irritants. It occurs in males and females and resolves partially after puberty (see also Chapters 14 and 18).

Localized Gingival Recession

Gingival recession around individual teeth or groups of teeth is a common source of concern. The gingiva may be inflamed or free of disease, depending on the presence or absence of local irritants. There are many causes of gingival recession (see Chapter 17), but in children the position of the tooth in the arch is the most important.[23] Gingival recession occurs on teeth in labial version (Fig. 21–10) and on those that are tilted or rotated so that the roots project labially. Anterior open bite increases the prevalence of gingival recession.[15] The recession may be a transitional phase

in tooth eruption and may correct itself when the teeth attain proper alignment, or it may be necessary to realign the teeth orthodontically.[3]

Acute Gingival Infections

Acute Herpetic Gingivostomatitis. This is the most common type of acute gingival infection in childhood and often occurs as a sequela of upper respiratory tract infection. (For a detailed discussion, see Chapter 19.)

Candidiasis. This is a mycotic infection of the oral cavity caused by the fungus *Candida albicans.* For a complete discussion, see Chapters 15 and 20.

Acute Necrotizing Ulcerative Gingivitis. The incidence of acute necrotizing ulcerative gingivitis (ANUG) in childhood is low. (For a detailed discussion, see Chapter 19.) In children living in areas where chronic malnutrition is common and in children with Down syndrome, the incidence and severity of ANUG gingivitis are increased.[11,24] Acute herpetic gingivostomatitis, which is more common in childhood, is occasionally erroneously diagnosed as ANUG.

TRAUMATIC CHANGES IN THE PERIODONTIUM

Traumatic changes may occur in the periodontal tissues of deciduous teeth under several conditions. In the process of shedding deciduous teeth, resorption of teeth and bone weakens the periodontal support, so that the existing functional forces are injurious to the remaining supporting tissues.[4] Excessive occlusal forces may be produced by malalignment, mutilation, loss or extraction of teeth, or dental restorations. In the mixed dentition stage, the periodontium of the permanent teeth may be traumatized, because the permanent teeth bear an increased occlusal load when the adjacent deciduous teeth are shed. The periodontal ligament of an erupting permanent tooth may be injured by occlusal forces transmitted through the deciduous tooth it is replacing.[9]

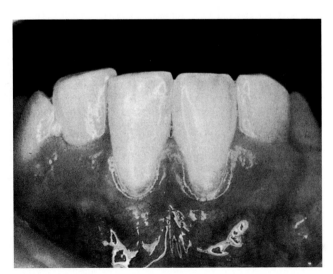

FIGURE 21–10. Gingival recession on labially positioned mandibular central incisors.

Microscopically,[12,22] the least severe traumatic changes involve compression, ischemia, and hyalinization of the periodontal ligament. With severe injury there is crushing and necrosis of the periodontal ligament (see Chapter 24).

In most instances the injuries are repaired, and tooth loss does not result. However, traumatized teeth may be sore or loose. Repair may result in ankylosis of the tooth to the bone, fixing the tooth in situ. When the permanent dentition erupts, ankylosed deciduous teeth appear to be submerged.

THE ORAL MUCOUS MEMBRANE IN CHILDHOOD DISEASES

Some childhood diseases present specific alterations in the oral mucosa, including the gingival tissues. Among these are the communicable diseases, such as varicella (chickenpox), rubeola (measles), scarlatina (scarlet fever), and diphtheria. For a more thorough discussion of this topic, the reader is referred to books in oral and pediatric pathology.

REFERENCES

1. Alcoforado GA, Kristoffersen T, Johannessen AC, Nilsen R. The composition of gingival inflammatory cell infiltrates in children studied by enzyme histochemistry. J Clin Periodontol 17:335, 1990.
2. Andlin-Sobocki A, Marcusson A, Persson M. 3-year observations on gingival recession in mandibular incisors in children. J Clin Periodontol 18:155, 1991.
3. Baer PN, Benjamin SD. Periodontal Disease in Children and Adolescents. Philadelphia, JB Lippincott, 1974.
4. Bernick S, Freedman N. Microscopic studies of the periodontium of the primary dentitions of monkeys. II. Posterior teeth during the mixed dentitional period. Oral Surg Oral Med Oral Pathol 7:322, 1954.
5. Bimstein E, Lustmann J, Soskolne WA. A clinical and histometric study of gingivitis associated with the human deciduous dentition. J Periodontol 56:293, 1985.
6. Brauer JC, Highley LB, Massler M, Schour I. Dentistry for Children. 2nd ed. Philadelphia, Blakiston, 1947.
7. Everett FG, Tuchler H, Lu KH. Occurrence of calculus in grade school children in Portland, Oregon. J Periodontol 34:54, 1963.
8. Gillett R, Cruckley A, Johnson NW. The nature of the inflammatory infiltrates in childhood gingivitis, juvenile periodontitis and adult periodontitis: Immunocytochemical studies using a monoclonal antibody to HLA Dr. J Clin Periodontol 13:281, 1986.
9. Grimmer EA. Trauma in an erupting premolar. J Dent Res 18:267, 1939.
10. Hock J. A clinical study of gingivitis of deciduous and succedaneous permanent teeth in dogs. J Periodont Res 13:68, 1978.
11. Jimenez M, Ramos J, Garrington G, Baer PN. The familial occurrence of acute necrotizing gingivitis in Colombia. J Periodontol 40:414, 1969.
12. Kronfeld R, Weinmann J. Traumatic changes in the periodontal tissues of deciduous teeth. J Dent Res 19:441, 1940.
13. Longhurst P, Gillett R, Johnson NW. Electron microscope quantitation of inflammatory infiltrates in childhood gingivitis. J Periodont Res 15:255, 1980.
14. Longhurst P, Johnson NW, Hopps RM. Differences in lymphocyte and plasma cell densities in inflamed gingiva from adults and young children. J Periodontol 48:705, 1977.
15. Machtei EE, Zubery Y, Bimstein E, Becker A. Anterior open bite and gingival recession in children and adolescents. Int Dent J 40:369, 1990.
16. Mackler SB, Crawford JJ. Plaque development in the primary dentition. J Periodontol 44:18, 1973.
17. Mattson L. Development of gingivitis in preschool children and young adults. A comparative experimental study. J Clin Periodontol 5:24, 1978.
18. Mattson L, Attstrom R. Histologic characteristics of experimental gingivitis in the juvenile and adult beagle dog. J Clin Periodontol 6:334, 1979.
19. Maynard JG, Wilson RD. Diagnosis and management of mucogingival problems in children. Dent Clin North Am 24:683, 1980.
20. Mombelli R, Gusberti FR, van Oosten MA, Lang NP. Gingival health and gingivitis development during puberty. A 4-year longitudinal study. J Clin Periodontol 16:451, 1989.
21. Notman S, Mandel ID, Mercadante J. Calculus in normal children and children with cystic fibrosis. International Association for Dental Research Program and Abstracts, 48th General Meeting, 1970, p 64.
22. Orban B, Weinmann J. Signs of traumatic occlusion in average human jaws. J Dent Res 13:216, 1933.
23. Parfitt GJ, Mjor IA. A clinical evaluation of local gingival recession in children. J Dent Child 31:257, 1964.
24. Pindborg JJ, Bhat M, Devanath KR, et al. Occurrence of acute necrotizing gingivitis in South India children. J Periodontol 37:14, 1966.
25. Rosenblum FN. Clinical study of the depth of the gingival sulcus in the primary dentition. J Dent Child 5:289, 1966.
26. Seymour GJ, Crouch MS, Powell RN, et al. The identification of lymphoid cell subpopulations in sections of human lymphoid tissue and gingivitis in children using monoclonal antibodies. J Periodont Res 17:247, 1982.
27. Soni NN, Silberkweit M, Hayes RL. Histological characteristics of stippling in children. J Periodontol 34:31, 1963.
28. Srivastava B, Chandra S, Jaiswal JS, et al. Cross-sectional study to evaluate variations in attached gingiva and gingival sulcus in the three periods of dentition. J Clin Pediatr Dent 15:17, 1990.

22

The Periodontal Pocket

FERMIN A. CARRANZA, JR.

[handwritten margin notes: FALSE = swollen tissue; TRUE = epi. attachment migrates apically]

The periodontal pocket, defined as a pathologically deepened gingival sulcus, is one of the important clinical features of periodontal disease.

CLASSIFICATION

Deepening of the gingival sulcus may occur by coronal movement of the gingival margin, apical displacement of the gingival attachment, or a combination of the two processes (Fig. 22–1). Pockets can be classified as follows:

Gingival Pocket (Relative or False): This type of pocket is formed by gingival enlargement without destruction of the underlying periodontal tissues. The sulcus is deepened because of the increased bulk of the gingiva (Fig. 22–2A). Gingival pockets are discussed in Chapter 18.

Periodontal Pocket (Absolute or True): This type of pocket occurs with destruction of the supporting periodontal tissues. Progressive pocket deepening leads to destruction of the supporting periodontal tissues and loosening and exfoliation of the teeth. The remainder of this chapter refers to this type of pocket.

There are two types of periodontal pockets:

Suprabony (supracrestal or supra-alveolar), in which the bottom of the pocket is coronal to the underlying alveolar bone (Fig. 22–2B).

Infrabony (intrabony, subcrestal, or intra-alveolar), in which the bottom of the pocket is apical to the level of the adjacent alveolar bone. In this second type, the lateral pocket wall lies between the tooth surface and the alveolar bone (Fig. 22–2C).

Pockets can involve one, two, or more tooth surfaces and can be of different depths and types on different sur-

faces of the same tooth and on approximating surfaces of the same interdental space. Pockets can also be spiral (i.e., originating on one tooth surface and twisting around the tooth to involve one or more additional surfaces) (see Fig. 22–3). These types of pockets are most common in furcation areas.

CLINICAL FEATURES

Clinical signs such as bluish red, thickened marginal gingiva, a bluish red vertical zone from the gingival margin to the alveolar mucosa, gingival bleeding and/or suppuration, tooth mobility, and diastema formation and symptoms such as localized pain or pain deep "in the bone" are suggestive of the presence of periodontal pockets. The only reliable method of locating periodontal pockets and determining their extent is careful probing of the gingival margin along each tooth surface (Fig. 22–4 and Table 22–1). For a more detailed discussion of the clinical aspects of periodontal pockets, see Chapter 28.

PATHOGENESIS *[handwritten: mechanism by which disease develops]*

Periodontal pockets are caused by microorganisms and their products, which produce pathologic tissue changes that lead to deepening of the gingival sulcus. On the basis of depth alone, it is sometimes difficult to differentiate a deep normal sulcus from a shallow periodontal pocket. In

[handwritten margin notes at bottom: other terms: simple, compound, complex; amount depends on immune system]

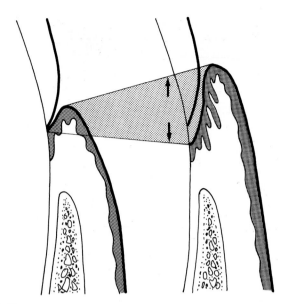

FIGURE 22–1. Illustration of pocket formation indicating expansion in two directions (*arrows*) from the normal gingival sulcus (*left*) to the periodontal pocket (*right*).

such borderline cases, pathologic changes in the gingiva distinguish the two conditions.

Changes involved in the transition from the normal gingival sulcus to the pathologic periodontal pocket are associated with different proportions of bacterial cells in dental plaque. Healthy gingiva is associated with few microorganisms, mostly coccoid cells and straight rods. Diseased gingiva is associated with increased numbers of spirochetes and motile rods.[33–35]

Pocket formation starts as an inflammatory change in the connective tissue wall of the gingival sulcus caused by bacterial plaque. The cellular and fluid inflammatory exudate causes degeneration of the surrounding connective tissue, including the gingival fibers.

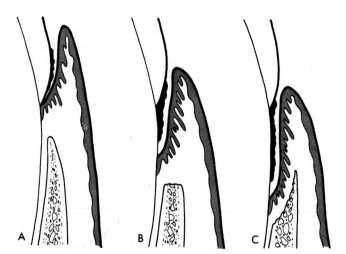

FIGURE 22–2. Different types of periodontal pockets. *A*, Gingival pocket. There is no destruction of the supporting periodontal tissues. *B*, Suprabony pocket. The base of the pocket is coronal to the level of the underlying bone. Bone loss is horizontal. *C*, Infrabony pocket. The base of the pocket is apical to the level of the adjacent bone. Bone loss is vertical.

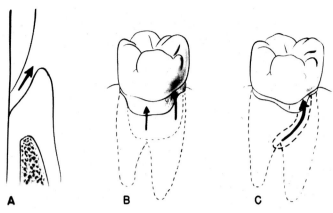

FIGURE 22–3. Classification of pockets according to involved tooth surfaces. *A*, Simple pocket. *B*, Compound pocket. *C*, Complex pocket.

Just apical to the junctional epithelium, an area of destroyed collagen fibers develops[15,50] and becomes occupied by inflammatory cells and edema. Immediately apical to this is a zone of partial destruction and then an area of normal attachment.

Two hypotheses have been advanced regarding the mechanism of collagen loss: (1) collagenases and other lysosomal enzymes from polymorphonuclear leukocytes[61] and macrophages[44] become extracellular and destroy collagen; and (2) fibroblasts phagocytize collagen fibers by extending cytoplasmic processes to the ligament–cementum interface and by resorbing the inserted collagen fibrils and the fibrils of the cementum matrix.[15,17]

As a consequence of the loss of collagen, the apical portion of the junctional epithelium proliferates along the root, extending finger-like projections two or three cells in thickness.

The coronal portion of the junctional epithelium detaches from the root as the apical portion migrates. As a result of inflammation, polymorphonuclear neutrophils (PMNs) invade the coronal end of the junctional epithelium in increasing numbers. The PMNs are not joined to one another or to the remaining epithelial cells by desmosomes. When the relative volume of PMNs reaches approximately 60% or more of the junctional epithelium, the tissue loses cohesiveness and detaches from the tooth surface. Thus, the sulcus bottom shifts apically, and the oral sulcular epithelium occupies a gradually increasing portion of the sulcular (pocket) lining.[52]

The initial deepening of the pocket has been described as occurring between the junctional epithelium and the tooth[26,51] or within the junctional epithelium.[8,19,34] According to Takada and Donath,[62] in the early lesion (stage II gingivitis) degenerative changes occur first in the second or third layer from the innermost cell layer of the most coronal part of the junctional epithelium, which faces the microbial plaque. Consequently, an intraepithelial cleavage is formed, followed by degeneration of the cells lining the cleavage, resulting in a deep crevice formation.

Extension of the junctional epithelium along the root requires the presence of healthy epithelial cells. Marked degeneration or necrosis of the junctional epithelium retards rather than accelerates pocket formation. Degenerative

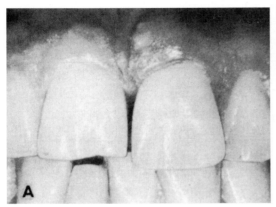 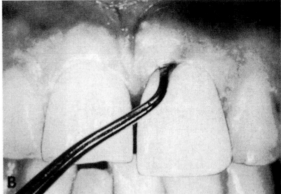

FIGURE 22–4. *A,* Extrusion of the central incisor and diastema associated with the periodontal pocket. *B,* The entire length of the periodontal probe inserted to the base of the periodontal pocket in the central incisor.

changes seen in the junctional epithelium at the base of periodontal pockets are usually less severe than those in the epithelium of the lateral pocket wall. Because migration of the junctional epithelium requires healthy, viable cells, it is reasonable to assume that the degenerative changes seen in this area occur after the junctional epithelium reaches its position on the cementum.

The degree of leukocyte infiltration of the junctional epithelium is independent of the volume of inflamed connective tissue, and thus this process may occur in gingiva with only slight signs of clinical inflammation.[50]

With continued inflammation, the gingiva increases in bulk, and the crest of the gingival margin extends toward the crown. The junctional epithelium continues to migrate along the root and separate from it. The epithelium of the lateral wall of the pocket proliferates to form bulbous, cord-like extensions into the inflamed connective tissue. Leukocytes and edema from the inflamed connective tissue infiltrate the epithelium lining the

pocket, resulting in various degrees of degeneration and necrosis.

The transformation of a gingival sulcus into a periodontal pocket creates an area where plaque removal becomes impossible, and the following feedback mechanism is established:

Plaque → Gingival inflammation → Pocket formation → More plaque formation

The rationale for pocket reduction is based on the need to eliminate areas of plaque accumulation.

HISTOPATHOLOGY

Changes occurring in the initial stages of gingival inflammation are presented in Chapter 16. Once the pocket is formed, several microscopic features are present, as discussed in the following sections.

Table 22–1. CORRELATION OF CLINICAL AND HISTOPATHOLOGIC FEATURES OF THE PERIODONTAL POCKET

Clinical Features	Histopathologic Features
1. The gingival wall of the periodontal pocket presents various degrees of bluish red discoloration; flaccidity; a smooth, shiny surface; and pitting on pressure.	1. The discoloration is caused by circulatory stagnation; the flaccidity, by destruction of the gingival fibers and surrounding tissues; the smooth, shiny surface, by the atrophy of the epithelium and edema; the pitting on pressure, by edema and degeneration.
2. Less frequently, the gingival wall may be pink and firm.	2. In such cases fibrotic changes predominate over exudation and degeneration, particularly in relation to the outer surface of the pocket wall. However, despite the external appearance of health, the inner wall of the pocket invariably presents some degeneration and is often ulcerated (see Fig. 22–13).
3. Bleeding is elicited by gently probing the soft tissue wall of the pocket.	3. Ease of bleeding results from increased vascularity, thinning and degeneration of the epithelium, and the proximity of the engorged vessels to the inner surface.
4. When explored with a probe, the inner aspect of the periodontal pocket is generally painful.	4. Pain on tactile stimulation is due to ulceration of the inner aspect of the pocket wall.
5. In many cases pus may be expressed by applying digital pressure.	5. Pus occurs in pockets with suppurative inflammation of the inner wall.

Soft Tissue Wall

The connective tissue is edematous and densely infiltrated with plasma cells (approximately 80%)[68] and lymphocytes and a scattering of PMNs. The blood vessels are increased in number, dilated, and engorged. The connective tissue exhibits varying degrees of degeneration. Single or multiple necrotic foci are occasionally present.[43] In addition to exudative and degenerative changes, the connective tissue shows proliferation of the endothelial cells, with newly formed capillaries, fibroblasts, and collagen fibers (Fig. 22–5).

The junctional epithelium at the base of the pocket is usually much shorter than that of a normal sulcus. Although marked variations are found as to length, width, and condition of the epithelial cells, usually the coronoapical length of the junctional epithelium is reduced to only 50 to 100 μm.[11] The cells may be well formed and in good condition or may exhibit slight to marked degeneration (Fig. 22–6).

The most severe degenerative changes in the periodontal pocket occur along the lateral wall (Fig. 22–7). The epithelium of the lateral wall of the pocket presents striking proliferative and degenerative changes. Epithelial buds or interlacing cords of epithelial cells project from the lateral wall into the adjacent inflamed connective tissue and frequently extend farther apically than the junctional epithelium. These epithelial projections, as well as the remainder of the lateral epithelium, are densely infiltrated by leukocytes and edema from the inflamed connective tissue. The cells undergo vacuolar degeneration and rupture to form vesicles. Progressive degeneration and necrosis of the epithelium lead to ulceration of the lateral wall, exposure of the underlying markedly inflamed connective tissue, and suppuration. In some cases acute inflammation is superimposed on the underlying chronic changes.

The severity of the degenerative changes is not necessarily related to pocket depth. Ulceration of the lateral wall may occur in shallow pockets, and deep pockets are occasionally observed in which the lateral epithelium is relatively intact and shows only slight degeneration.

The epithelium at the gingival crest of a periodontal pocket is generally intact and thickened, with prominent rete pegs.

A detailed electron microscopic study of the pocket epithelium in experimentally induced pockets in dogs has been performed by Muller-Glauser and Schroeder.[40]

Bacterial Invasion. Bacterial invasion of the apical and lateral areas of the pocket wall may occur in human chronic periodontitis. Filaments, rods, and coccoid organisms with predominant gram-negative cell walls have been found in intercellular spaces of the epithelium.[22,23] Bacteria invade the intercellular space initially under exfoliating epithelial cells, but they are also found between deeper epithelial cells and accumulating on the basement lamina. Some bacteria traverse the basement lamina and invade the subepithelial connective tissue[49] (Figs. 22–8 and 22–9). The significance, if any, of bacterial invasion in the patho-

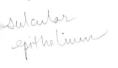

sulcular epithelium

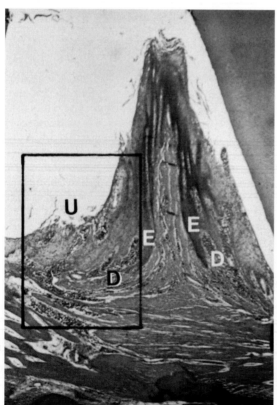

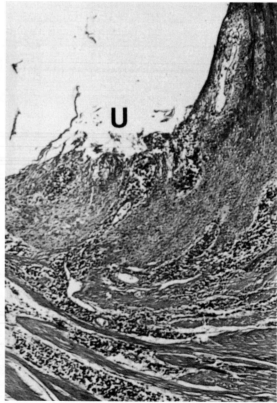

FIGURE 22–5. *Left,* Interdental papilla with suprabony pockets on proximal tooth surfaces. D, Densely inflamed connective tissue; E, proliferating pocket epithelium; U, ulcerated pocket epithelium. *Right,* Magnification of the rectangular area on the left. Note the ulcerated area (U) and the infiltrate between the collagen fibers.

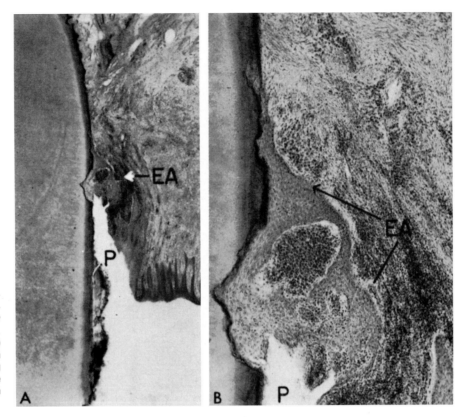

FIGURE 22–6. *A,* Low-power section of periodontal pocket (P). The location of the junctional epithelium is indicated by the arrow (EA). The lateral epithelial wall is ulcerated. *B,* Detailed study of junctional epithelium (EA) at the base of the pocket (P). Note extension of well-formed epithelial cells (*arrow*) along the resorbed root surface. There is a dense accumulation of leukocytes enclosed within the epithelium.

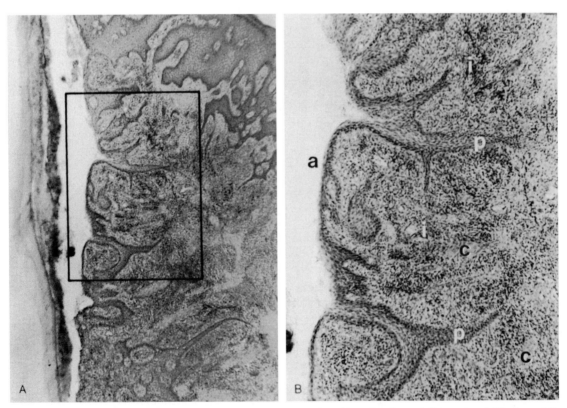

FIGURE 22–7. *A,* Low-power view of the lateral wall of a periodontal pocket. Note the dense inflammatory infiltrate and the proliferating epithelium. *B,* High-power view of the rectangular area in *A.* Note the areas of atrophic epithelium (a) and epithelial proliferation (p). The connective tissue is densely infiltrated (i); some remnants of collagen fibers (c) can be seen.

Also: think of site specificity

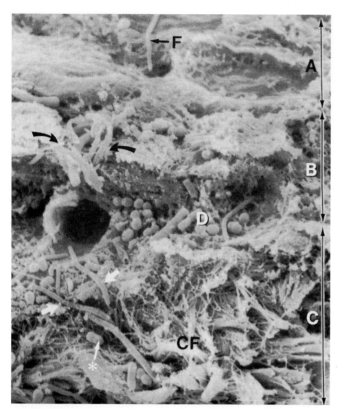

FIGURE 22–8. Electron micrograph of a section of pocket wall in advanced periodontitis in a human specimen, showing bacterial penetration into the epithelium and connective tissue. Scanning electron microscope view of surface of pocket wall (A), sectioned epithelium (B), and sectioned connective tissue (C). Curved arrows point to areas of bacterial penetration into the epithelium. Thick white arrows point to bacterial penetration into the connective tissue through a break in the continuity of the basal lamina. CF, Connective tissue fibers; D, accumulation of bacteria (rods, cocci, filaments) on basal lamina; F, filamentous organism on surface of epithelium. Asterisk points to coccobacillus in connective tissue.

genesis of periodontal disease has not, however, been clarified.[13,32]

Microtopography of the Gingival Wall of the Pocket

Scanning electron microscopy has permitted the description of several areas in the soft tissue wall of the pocket where different types of activity take place.[46] These areas are irregularly oval or elongated and adjacent to one another and measure about 50 to 200 μm. These findings suggest that the pocket wall is constantly changing as a result of the interaction between the host and the bacteria. The following areas have been noted:

1. *Areas of relative quiescence,* showing a relatively flat surface with minor depressions and mounds and occasional shedding of cells ("A" in Fig. 22–10).
2. *Areas of bacterial accumulation,* which appear as depressions on the epithelial surface, with abundant debris and bacterial clumps penetrating into the enlarged intercellular spaces. These bacteria are mainly cocci, rods, and filaments, with a few spirochetes ("B" in Fig. 22–10).
3. *Areas of emergence of leukocytes,* where leukocytes appear

in the pocket wall through holes located in the intercellular spaces (Fig. 22–11).

4. *Areas of leukocyte–bacteria interaction,* where numerous leukocytes are present and covered with bacteria in an apparent process of phagocytosis. Bacterial plaque associated with the epithelium is seen either as an organized matrix covered by a fibrin-like material in contact with the surface of cells or as bacteria penetrating into the intercellular spaces ("C" in Fig. 22–10).
5. *Areas of intense epithelial desquamation,* which consist of semiattached and folded epithelial squames, sometimes partially covered with bacteria ("D" in Fig. 22–10).
6. *Areas of ulceration,* with exposed connective tissue (Fig. 22–12).
7. *Areas of hemorrhage,* with numerous erythrocytes.

The transition from one area to another could be postulated as follows: bacteria accumulate in previously quiescent areas, triggering the emergence of leukocytes and the leukocyte–bacteria interaction. This would lead to intense epithelial desquamation and, finally, to ulceration and hemorrhage.

Periodontal Pockets as Healing Lesions

Periodontal pockets are chronic inflammatory lesions and as such are constantly undergoing repair. *The condition of the soft tissue wall of the periodontal pocket results from the interplay of destructive and constructive tissue changes.*

The *destructive changes* are characterized by the fluid and cellular inflammatory exudate and by the associated degenerative changes initiated by plaque bacteria. The *constructive changes* consist of the formation of blood vessels in an effort to repair the tissue damage caused by inflammation.

Complete healing does not occur because of the persis-

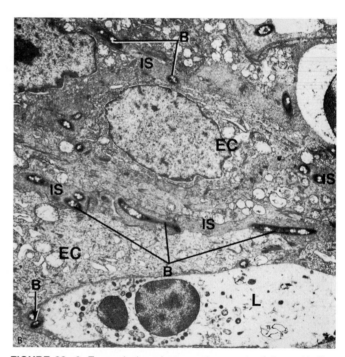

FIGURE 22–9. Transmission electron micrograph of the epithelium in the periodontal pocket wall showing bacteria in the intercellular spaces. B, Bacteria; EC, epithelial cell; IS, intercellular space; L, leukocyte about to engulf bacteria. ×8000.

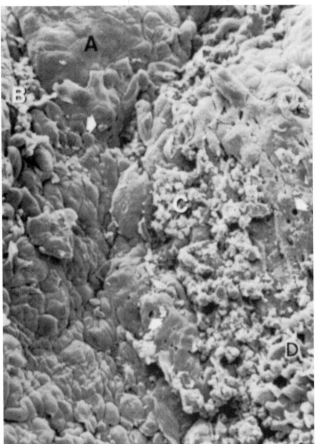

FIGURE 22-10. Scanning electron frontal micrograph of the periodontal pocket wall. Different areas can be seen in the pocket wall surface. A, Area of quiescence; B, bacterial accumulation; C, bacterial-leukocyte interaction; D, intense cellular desquamation. Arrows point to emerging leukocytes and holes left by them in the pocket wall. ×800.

pocket are walled off by fibrous tissue on the outer aspect (Fig. 22-13). Outwardly the pocket appears pink and fibrotic, despite the inflammatory changes occurring within.

Pocket Contents

Periodontal pockets contain debris consisting principally of microorganisms and their products (enzymes, endotoxins, and other metabolic products), gingival fluid, food remnants, salivary mucin, desquamated epithelial cells, and leukocytes. Plaque-covered calculus usually projects from the tooth surface (Fig. 22-14). Purulent exudate, if present, consists of living, degenerated, and necrotic leukocytes; living and dead bacteria; serum; and a scant amount of fibrin.[38] The contents of periodontal pockets filtered free of organisms and debris have been demonstrated to be toxic when injected subcutaneously into experimental animals.[27]

Significance of Pus Formation. There is a tendency to overemphasize the importance of the purulent exudate and to equate it with severity of periodontal disease. Because it is a dramatic clinical finding, early observers assumed that it was responsible for the loosening and exfoliation of the teeth. *Pus is a common feature of periodontal disease, but it is only a secondary sign.* The presence of pus or the ease with which it can be expressed from the pocket merely reflects the nature of the inflammatory changes in the pocket wall. It is not an indication of the depth of the pocket or

tence of local irritants. These irritants continue to stimulate fluid and cellular exudate, which in turn causes degeneration of the new tissue elements formed in the continuous effort at repair.

The balance between destructive and constructive changes determines clinical features such as color, consistency, and surface texture of the pocket wall. If the inflammatory fluid and cellular exudate predominate, the pocket wall is bluish red, soft, spongy, and friable, with a smooth, shiny surface. If there is a relative predominance of newly formed connective tissue cells and fibers, the pocket wall is more firm and pink. At the clinical level, the former condition is generally referred to as an *edematous pocket wall* and the latter as a *fibrotic pocket wall* (see Chapter 28).

Edematous and fibrotic pockets represent opposite extremes of the same pathologic process, not different disease entities. They are subject to constant modification, depending on the relative predominance of exudative and constructive changes.

Fibrotic pocket walls may be misleading, because they do not necessarily reflect what is taking place throughout the pocket wall. The most severe degenerative changes in periodontal pockets occur along the inner aspect. In some cases inflammation and ulceration on the inside of the

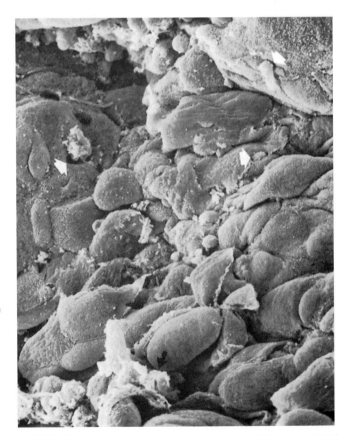

FIGURE 22-11. Scanning electron micrograph of the periodontal pocket wall, frontal view, in a case of advanced periodontitis in a human. Note the desquamating epithelial cells and leukocytes (*white arrows*) emerging onto the pocket space. Scattered bacteria can also be seen (*black arrow*). ×150.

Most of the time: fibrotic pockets are generalized.

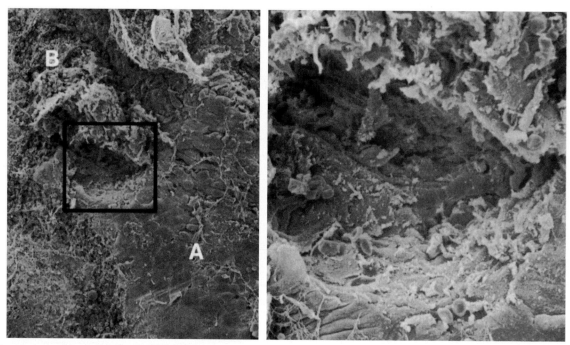

FIGURE 22–12. *Left,* Area of ulceration in the lateral wall of a deep periodontal pocket in a human specimen. A, Surface of pocket epithelium in a quiescent state; B, area of hemorrhage. ×800. *Right,* Magnification of the square area on the left. Connective tissue fibers and cells can be seen in the bottom of the ulcer. Scanning electron microscopy. ×3000.

the severity of the destruction of the supporting tissues. Extensive pus formation may occur in shallow pockets, whereas deep pockets may exhibit little or no pus.

Localized accumulation of pus constitutes an abscess, which will be discussed later in this chapter.

Root Surface Wall

The root surface wall of periodontal pockets often undergoes changes that are significant because they may perpetu-

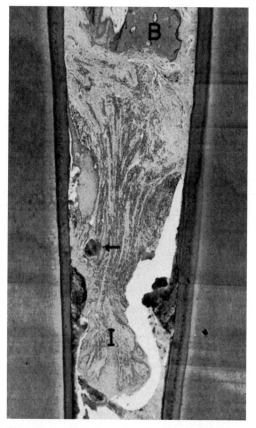

FIGURE 22–14. Interdental papilla (I) with ulcerated suprabony periodontal pockets on its mesial and distal aspects. Calculus is present on the approximal tooth surfaces and within the gingiva (*arrow*). The bone is shown at B.

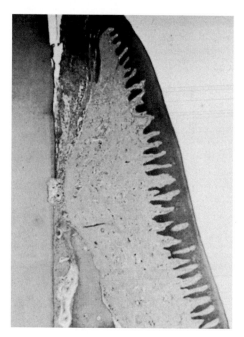

FIGURE 22–13. Periodontal pocket wall. The inner half is inflamed and ulcerated; the outer half is densely collagenous.

ate the periodontal infection, cause pain, and complicate periodontal treatment. The root cementum suffers structural, chemical, and cytotoxic changes.

Structural Changes. The following structural changes in cementum are seen:

1. *Presence of pathologic granules,*[7] which have been observed with optical and electron microscopy[5] and may represent areas of collagen degeneration or areas where collagen fibrils have not been fully mineralized initially.

2. *Areas of increased mineralization,*[54] probably a result of an exchange, on exposure to the oral cavity, of minerals and organic components at the cementum–saliva interface. The hypermineralized zones are detectable by electron microscopy and are associated with increased perfection of the crystal structure and organic changes suggestive of a subsurface cuticle.[54] These zones have also been seen in microradiographic studies[56] as a layer 10 to 20 μm thick, with areas as thick as 50 μm. No decrease in mineralization was found in deeper areas, thereby indicating that increased mineralization does not come from adjacent areas. A loss of or reduction in the cross-banding of collagen near the cementum surface[24,25] and a subsurface condensation of organic material of exogenous origin[54] have also been reported.

3. *Areas of demineralization,* commonly related to root caries. Exposure to oral fluid and bacterial plaque results in proteolysis of the embedded remnants of Sharpey's fibers; the cementum may be softened and may undergo fragmentation and cavitation.[29] Unlike enamel caries, root surface caries tend to progress around rather than into the tooth.[39] Active root caries lesions appear as well-defined yellowish or light brown areas, are frequently covered by plaque, and have a softened or leathery consistency on probing.[21] Inactive lesions are well-defined darker lesions with a smooth surface and a harder consistency on probing.[21]

Involvement of the cementum is followed by bacterial penetration of the dentinal tubules, resulting in destruction of the dentin (Fig. 22–15). In severe cases large sections of necrotic cementum become detached from the tooth and separated from it by masses of bacteria (Fig. 22–16).

The dominant microorganism in root surface caries is *Actinomyces viscosus,*[60] although its specific responsibility in the development of the lesion has not been established.[21]

The tooth may not be painful, but exploration of the root surface reveals the presence of a defect, and penetration of the involved area with a probe causes pain.

A prevalence rate study of root caries in 20- to 64-year-old individuals revealed that 42% had one or more root caries lesions and that these lesions tended to increase with age.[31]

Caries of the root may lead to *pulpitis,* sensitivity to sweets and thermal changes, or severe pain. Pathologic exposure of the pulp occurs in severe cases. Root caries may be the cause of toothache in patients with periodontal disease and no evidence of coronal decay.

Caries of the cementum requires special attention when the pocket is treated. The necrotic cementum must be removed by scaling and root planing until firm tooth surface is reached, even if this entails extension into the dentin.

Areas of cellular resorption of cementum and dentin are common in roots unexposed by periodontal disease (see Fig. 2–20).[57] These areas are of no particular significance because they are symptom free, and as long as the root is covered by the periodontal ligament, they are apt to un-

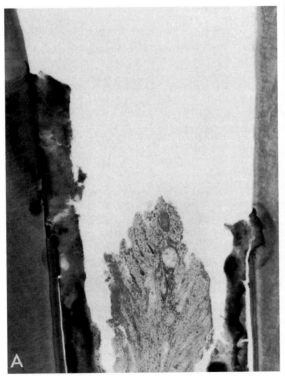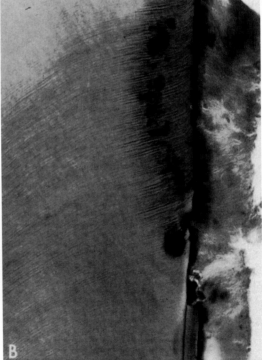

FIGURE 22–15. Caries on root surfaces exposed by periodontal disease. *A,* Interdental space, showing inflamed gingiva and caries on proximal tooth surfaces. *B,* Caries of cementum and dentin, showing bacterial invasion of dentinal tubules. Note the filamentous structure of the dental plaque and darker staining of calculus adherent to the root.

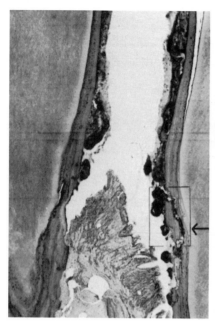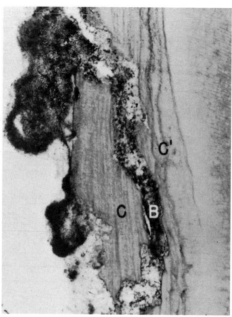

FIGURE 22–16. *Left,* Mesiodistal section through an interdental space in a patient with extensive periodontal destruction. An area of cementum necrosis is enclosed within the rectangle designated by the arrow. *Right,* Detailed section of the rectangular area showing a necrotic fragment of cementum (C) separated from lamellated cementum (C') by clumps of bacteria (B).

dergo repair. However, if the root is exposed by progressive pocket formation before repair of such areas occurs, these appear as isolated cavitations that penetrate into the dentin. These areas can be differentiated from caries of the cementum by their clear-cut outline and hard surface. They may be sources of considerable pain, requiring the placement of a restoration.

Chemical Changes. The mineral content of exposed cementum is increased.[53] The following minerals are increased in diseased root surfaces: calcium,[56] magnesium,[41,56] phosphorus,[41] and fluoride.[41] Microhardness, however, remains unchanged.[45,67]

Exposed cementum may absorb calcium, phosphorus, and fluoride from its local environment, making possible the development of a highly calcified layer that is resistant to decay.[2] This ability of cementum to absorb substances from its environment may be harmful if the absorbed materials are toxic.

Cytotoxic Changes. Bacterial penetration into the cementum can be found as deep as the cementodentinal junction.[14,69] In addition, bacterial products such as endotoxins[3,4] have also been detected in the cementum wall of periodontal pockets.

When root fragments from teeth with periodontal disease are placed in tissue culture, they induce irreversible morphologic changes in the cells of the culture. Such changes are not produced by normal roots.[28] Diseased root fragments also prevent the in vitro attachment of human gingival fibroblasts, whereas normal root surfaces allow the cells to attach freely.[3,4] When reimplanted in the oral mucosa of the patient, diseased root fragments induce an inflammatory response even if autoclaved.[36]

The surface morphology of the tooth wall of periodontal pockets has been studied by several authors.[6,9,30,47,48,64] The following zones can be found in the bottom of a periodontal pocket (Fig. 22–17):

1. *Cementum covered by calculus,* where all the changes described in the preceding paragraphs can be found.

2. *Attached plaque,* which covers calculus and extends apically from it to a variable degree, probably 100 to 500 μm.

3. *The zone of unattached plaque* that surrounds attached plaque and extends apically to it.

4. *The zone where the junctional epithelium is attached to the tooth.* The extension of this zone, which in normal sulci is more than 500 μm, is usually reduced in periodontal pockets to less than 100 μm.[11]

5. Apical to the junctional epithelium, there may be a *zone of semidestroyed connective tissue fibers* (see "Pathogenesis").

Areas 3, 4, and 5 compose the so-called *plaque-free zone* seen in extracted teeth. The total width of the plaque-free zone varies according to the type of tooth (it is wider in molars than in incisors) and the depth of the pocket (it is narrower in deeper pockets).[47]

PERIODONTAL DISEASE ACTIVITY

For many years the loss of attachment produced by periodontal disease was thought to be a slow but continuously progressive phenomenon. More recently, and as a result of studies on the specificity of plaque bacteria, the concept of periodontal disease activity has evolved.

According to this concept, periodontal pockets go through periods of quiescence and exacerbation. *Periods of quiescence* are characterized by a reduced inflammatory response and little or no loss of bone and connective tissue attachment. A buildup of unattached plaque, with its gram-negative, motile, and anaerobic bacteria (see Chapter 6), starts a *period of exacerbation* in which bone and connective tissue attachment are lost and the pocket deepens. This period may last for days, weeks, or months and is eventually followed by a period of remission or quiescence in which gram-positive bacteria proliferate and a more stable condition is established. Based on a study of I 125 absorptiometry, McHenry and colleagues have confirmed that bone loss in untreated periodontal disease occurs in an episodic manner.[37]

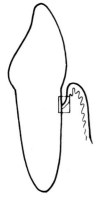

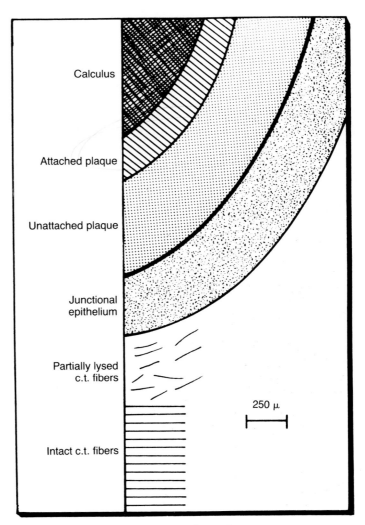

Calculus

Attached plaque

Unattached plaque

Junctional epithelium

Partially lysed c.t. fibers

250 μ

Intact c.t. fibers

FIGURE 22-17. Illustration of the area at the bottom of a pocket.

These periods of quiescence and exacerbation are also known as *periods of activity and inactivity.* Clinically, active periods show bleeding, either spontaneously or with probing, and greater amounts of gingival exudate. Histologically, the pocket epithelium appears thin and ulcerated, and an infiltrate composed predominantly of plasma cells[16] and/or polymorphonuclear leukocytes[44] is seen; bacterial samples from the pocket lumen, analyzed with darkfield microscopy, show high proportions of motile organisms and spirochetes.[35] Over a period of time, loss of bone should be detected radiographically.

Methods to detect periods of activity or inactivity are currently being investigated (see Chapter 30).

SITE SPECIFICITY

Periodontal destruction does not occur in all parts of the mouth at the same time, but rather on a few teeth at a time or even on only some aspects of some teeth at any given time. This is referred to as the *site specificity* of periodontal disease. It is very common to find sites of periodontal destruction next to sites with little or no destruction. *There-*

fore, the severity of periodontitis increases by (1) the development of new disease sites and/or (2) the increased breakdown of existing sites.

PULP CHANGES ASSOCIATED WITH PERIODONTAL POCKETS

The spread of infection from periodontal pockets may cause pathologic changes in the pulp. Such changes may give rise to painful symptoms or adversely affect the response of the pulp to restorative procedures. Involvement of the pulp in periodontal disease occurs through either the apical foramen or the lateral canals in the root after infection spreads from the pocket through the periodontal ligament. Atrophic and inflammatory pulpal changes occur in such cases (see also Chapter 58).

RELATION OF LOSS OF ATTACHMENT AND BONE LOSS TO POCKET DEPTH

Pocket formation causes loss of attachment of the gingiva and denudation of the root surface. The severity of the

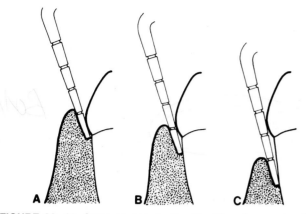

FIGURE 22–18. Same pocket depth with different amounts of recession. *A,* Gingival pocket with no recession. *B,* Periodontal pocket of similar depth as in *A,* but with some degree of recession. *C,* Pocket depth same as in *A* and *B,* but with still more recession.

attachment loss is generally, but not always, correlated with the depth of the pocket. This is because the degree of attachment loss (recession) depends on the location of the base of the pocket on the root surface, whereas the depth is the distance between the base of the pocket and the crest of the gingiva. Pockets of the same depth may be associated with different degrees of attachment loss (Fig. 22–18), and pockets of different depths may be associated with the same amount of attachment loss (Fig. 22–19).

Severity of bone loss is generally correlated with pocket depth, but not always. Extensive bone loss may be associated with shallow pockets, and slight bone loss can occur with deep pockets.

AREA BETWEEN THE BASE OF THE POCKET AND THE ALVEOLAR BONE

Normally the distance between the junctional epithelium and the alveolar bone is relatively constant. The distance

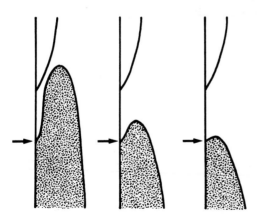

FIGURE 22–19. Different pocket depths with the same amount of recession. *Arrows* point to bottom of the pocket. The distance between the arrow and the cemento-enamel junctions remains the same, in spite of different pocket depths.

between the bottom of the calculus and the alveolar crest in human periodontal pockets is most constant, having a mean length of 1.97 mm ± 33.16%.[59,63]

The distance from attached plaque to bone is never less than 0.5 mm and never more than 2.7 mm.[64,65] These findings suggest that the bone-resorbing activity induced by the bacteria is exerted within these distances. However, the finding of isolated bacteria and/or clumps of bacteria in the connective tissue[49] and on the bone surface[23] may modify these considerations.

RELATIONSHIP OF THE PERIODONTAL POCKET TO BONE

In infrabony pockets the base is apical to the level of the alveolar bone, and the pocket wall lies between the tooth and the bone. Infrabony pockets most often occur interproximally but may be located on the facial and lingual tooth surfaces. Most often the pocket spreads from the surface on which it originated to one or more contiguous surfaces. The suprabony pocket has its base coronal to the crest of the bone.

The inflammatory, proliferative, and degenerative changes in infrabony and suprabony pockets are the same, and both lead to destruction of the supporting periodontal tissues.

Differences Between Infrabony and Suprabony Pockets

The principal differences between infrabony and suprabony pockets are the relationship of the soft tissue wall of the pocket to the alveolar bone, the pattern of bone destruction, and the direction of the transseptal fibers of the periodontal ligament[12] (Figs. 22–20 to 22–22).

In suprabony pockets the alveolar crest and the fibrous apparatus attached to it gradually attain a more apical position in relation to the tooth but retain their general morphology and architecture, whereas in infrabony pockets the morphology of the alveolar crest changes completely. This may have an effect on the function of the area.[10]

The distinguishing features of suprabony and infrabony pockets are summarized in Table 22–2. The morphologic features of the infrabony pocket are important because they necessitate modification in treatment techniques (see Chapters 56 and 57).

The classification of infrabony pockets is discussed in Chapter 23.

PERIODONTAL ABSCESS

A periodontal abscess is a localized purulent inflammation in the periodontal tissues (Fig. 22–23). It is also known as a *lateral* or *parietal abscess.* Abscesses localized in the gingiva and not extruding into the supporting structures are called gingival abscesses. They originate with injury to the outer surface of the gingiva and may occur in the absence of a periodontal pocket.

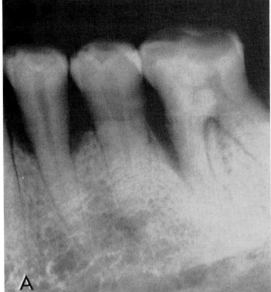

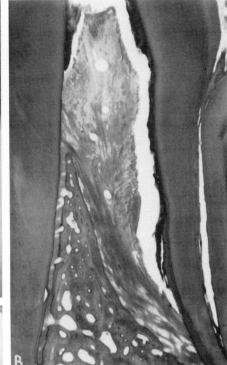

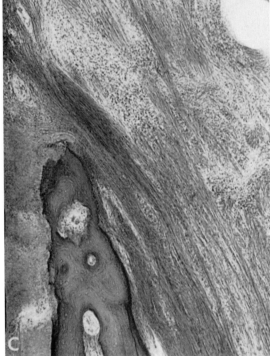

FIGURE 22–20. Infrabony pocket on the mesial surface of a molar. *A,* Radiograph showing a deep angular defect on the mesial surface of the first molar. The bifurcation is also involved. Note the calculus on the mesial surface of the molar. *B,* Interdental space between the second premolar with a suprabony pocket (*left*) and the first molar with an infrabony pocket. Note the transseptal fibers that extend from the base of the infrabony pocket along the bone to the root of the premolar, the relationship of the epithelial lining of the pocket to the transseptal fibers, and the calculus on the root. *C,* Transseptal fibers extending from the distal surface of the premolar over the crest of the bone into the infrabony pocket. Note the leukocytic infiltration of the transseptal fibers.

Periodontal abscess formation may occur in the following ways:

1. Extension of infection from a periodontal pocket deeply into the supporting periodontal tissues and localization of the suppurative inflammatory process along the lateral aspect of the root.
2. Lateral extension of inflammation from the inner surface of a periodontal pocket into the connective tissue of the pocket wall. Localization of the abscess results when drainage into the pocket space is impaired (Fig. 22–24).
3. In a pocket that describes a tortuous course around the root, a periodontal abscess may form in the cul-de-sac, the deep end of which is shut off from the surface.
4. Incomplete removal of calculus during treatment of a periodontal pocket. In this instance, the gingival wall shrinks, occluding the pocket orifice, and a periodontal abscess occurs in the sealed-off portion of the pocket.
5. A periodontal abscess may occur in the absence of periodontal disease after trauma to the tooth or perforation of the lateral wall of the root in endodontic therapy.

Periodontal abscesses are classified according to location as follows:

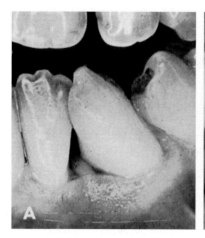 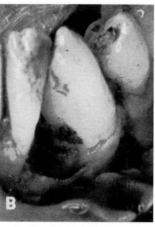

FIGURE 22–21. Infrabony pocket on the mesial surface of the mandibular canine. *A,* Rolled gingival margin and space between gingiva and canine suggest the presence of a periodontal pocket. *B,* Flap reflected to show calculus on the root and a three-wall bone defect.

1. *Abscess in the supporting periodontal tissues* along the lateral aspect of the root. In this condition there is generally a sinus in the bone that extends laterally from the abscess to the external surface.
2. *Abscess in the soft tissue wall of a deep periodontal pocket.*

Microscopically, an abscess is a localized accumulation of viable and necrotic PMNs within the periodontal pocket wall. The dead leukocytes liberate enzymes that digest the cells and other tissue structures, forming the liquid product known as pus, which constitutes the center of the abscess. An acute inflammatory reaction surrounds the purulent area, and the overlying epithelium exhibits intracellular and extracellular edema and invasion of leukocytes (Fig. 22–25).

The localized acute abscess becomes a chronic abscess when its purulent content drains through a fistula into the outer gingival surface or into the periodontal pocket.

Bacterial invasion of tissues has been reported in abscesses; the invading organisms were identified as gram-negative cocci, diplococci, fusiforms, and spirochetes.[18] Invasive fungi were also found and were interpreted as being opportunistic invaders.[18] Microorganisms that colonize the periodontal abscess have been reported to be primarily gram-negative anaerobic rods.[42]

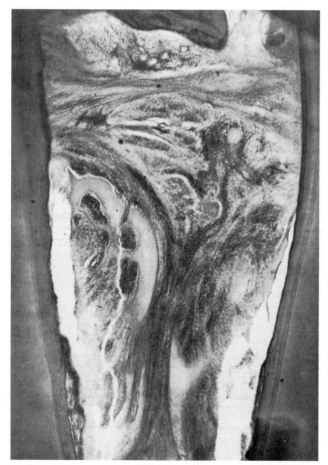

FIGURE 22–22. Two suprabony pockets in an interdental space between the maxillary cuspid and the lateral incisor. Note the normal horizontal arrangement of the transseptal fibers.

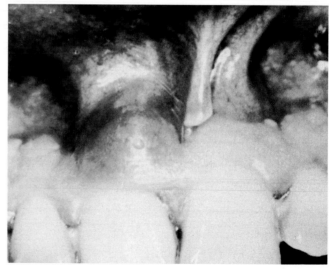

FIGURE 22–23. Periodontal abscess on an upper central incisor.

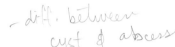

Table 22-2. DISTINGUISHING FEATURES OF THE SUPRABONY AND INFRABONY POCKETS

Suprabony Pocket	Infrabony Pocket
1. The base of the pocket is coronal to the level of the alveolar bone.	1. The base of the pocket is apical to the crest of the alveolar bone, so that the bone is adjacent to the soft tissue wall (see Fig. 22-2).
2. The pattern of destruction of the underlying bone is horizontal.	2. The bone destructive pattern is vertical (angular) (see Figs. 22-20 and 22-21).
3. Interproximally, the transseptal fibers that are restored during progressive periodontal disease are arranged horizontally in the space between the base of the pocket and the alveolar bone (see Fig. 22-22).	3. Interproximally, the transseptal fibers are oblique rather than horizontal. They extend from the cementum beneath the base of the pocket along the bone and over the crest to the cementum of the adjacent tooth (see Fig. 22-20).
4. On the facial and lingual surfaces, the periodontal ligament fibers beneath the pocket follow their normal horizontal-oblique course between the tooth and the bone.	4. On the facial and lingual surfaces, the periodontal ligament fibers follow the angular pattern of the adjacent bone. They extend from the cementum beneath the base of the pocket along the bone and over the crest to join with the outer periosteum.

PERIODONTAL CYST — *diff. between cyst & abscess*

The periodontal cyst is an uncommon lesion that produces localized destruction of the periodontal tissues along a lateral root surface, most often in the mandibular canine-premolar area.[20,58]

The following possible etiologies have been suggested:

1. Odontogenic cyst caused by proliferation of the epithelial rests of Malassez; the stimulus initiating the cellular activity is not known.
2. Lateral dentigerous cyst retained in the jaw after tooth eruption.
3. Primordial cyst of supernumerary tooth germ.
4. Stimulation of epithelial rests of the periodontal ligament by infection from a periodontal abscess or from the pulp through an accessory root canal.

A periodontal cyst is usually asymptomatic and without grossly detectable changes, but it may present as a localized tender swelling. Radiographically, an interproximal periodontal cyst appears on the side of the root as a radiolucent area bordered by a radiopaque line. Its radiographic appearance cannot be differentiated from that of a periodontal abscess.

Microscopically, the cystic lining may be (1) a loosely arranged, nonkeratinized, thickened, proliferating epithelium; (2) a thin, nonkeratinized epithelium; or (3) an odontogenic keratocyst.[20]

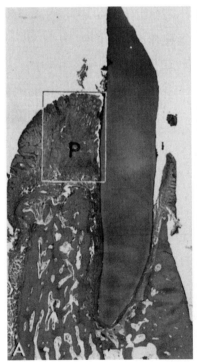
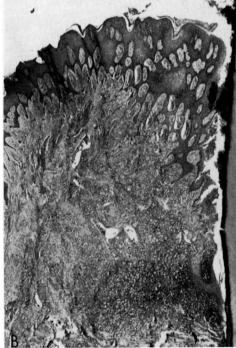

FIGURE 22-24. *A,* Periodontal abscess (P, enclosed in rectangle) on the lingual surface of the mandibular incisor. *B,* Detailed view of a periodontal abscess showing dense leukocytic infiltration and suppuration.

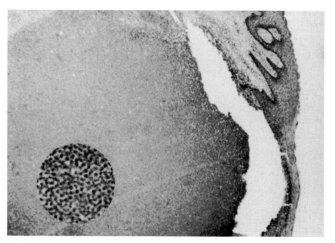

FIGURE 22–25. Microscopic view of a periodontal abscess showing dense accumulation of polymorphonuclear neutrophils covered by stratified squamous epithelium. *Inset,* Magnification of PMNs.

REFERENCES

1. Adriaens PA, DeBoever JA, Loesche WJ. Bacterial invasion in root cementum and radicular dentin of periodontally diseased teeth in humans. A reservoir of periodontopathic bacteria. J Periodontol 59:222, 1988.
2. Aleo JJ, Vandersall DC. Cementum. Recent concepts related to periodontal disease therapy. Dent Clin North Am 24:627, 1980.
3. Aleo JJ, DeRenzis FA, Farber PA. In vitro attachment of human gingival fibroblasts to root surfaces. J Periodontol 46:639, 1975.
4. Aleo JJ, DeRenzis FA, Farber PA, Varboncoeur AP. The presence and biologic activity of cementum bound endotoxin. J Periodontol 45:672, 1974.
5. Armitage GC, Christie TM. Structural changes in exposed cementum. I. Light microscopic observations. J Periodont Res 8:343, 1973; II. Electronmicroscopic observations. J Periodont Res 8:356, 1973.
6. Bass CC. A demonstrable line on extracted teeth indicating the location of the outer border of the epithelial attachment. J Dent Res 25:401, 1946.
7. Bass CC. A previously undescribed demonstrable pathologic condition in exposed cementum and the underlying dentine. Oral Surg 4:641, 1951.
8. Becks H. Normal and pathologic pocket formation. J Am Dent Assoc 16:2167, 1929.
9. Brady JM. A plaque-free zone on human teeth: Scanning and transmission electron microscopy. J Periodontol 44:416, 1973.
10. Carranza FA, Carranza FA Jr. The management of alveolar bone in the treatment of the periodontal pocket. J Periodontol 27:29, 1956.
11. Carranza FA Jr. Histometric evaluation of periodontal pathology. A review of recent studies. J Periodontol 38:741, 1967.
12. Carranza FA Jr, Glickman I. Some observations on the microscopic features of the infrabony pockets. J Periodontol 28:33, 1957.
13. Coons DB, Charbeneau TD, Rivera-Hidalgo F. Quantification of bacterial penetration in spontaneous periodontal disease in beagle dogs. J Periodontol 60:23, 1989.
14. Daly CG, Seymour GJ, Kieser JB, Corbet EF. Histological assessment of periodontally involved cementum. J Clin Periodontol 9:266, 1982.
15. Davenport RH Jr, Simpson DM, Hassell TM. Histometric comparison of active and inactive lesions of advanced periodontitis. J Periodontol 53:285, 1982.
16. Deporter DA, Brown DJ. Fine structural observations on the mechanisms of loss of attachment during experimental periodontal disease in the rat. J Periodont Res 15:304, 1980.
17. Deporter DA, Ten Cate AR. Collagen resorption by periodontal ligament fibroblasts at the hard tissue–ligament interfaces of the mouse molar periodontium. J Periodontol 51:429, 1980.
18. DeWitt GV, Cobb CM, Killoy WJ. The acute periodontal abscess: Microbial penetration of the soft tissue wall. Int J Periodont Restor Dent 5:39, 1985.
19. Euler H. Der Epithelansatz in neuere Beleuchtung. Vjschr Zahnheilk 29:103, 1923.
20. Fantasia JE. Lateral periodontal cyst. An analysis of 46 cases. Oral Surg Oral Med Oral Pathol 48:237, 1979.
21. Fejerskov O, Nyvad B. Pathology and treatment of dental caries in the aging individual. In Holm-Pedersen P, Loe H, eds. Geriatric Dentistry. Copenhagen, Munksgaard, 1986.
22. Frank RM. Bacterial penetration in the apical wall of advanced human periodontitis. J Periodont Res 15:563, 1980.
23. Frank RM, Voegel RC. Bacterial bone resorption in advanced cases of human periodontitis. J Periodont Res 13:251, 1978.
24. Furseth R. Further observations on the fine structure of orally exposed carious human dental cementum. Arch Oral Biol 16:71, 1971.
25. Furseth R, Johanson E. The mineral phase of sound and carious human dental cementum studies by electron microscopy. Acta Odontol Scand 28:305, 1970.
26. Gottlieb B. Der Epithelansatz am Zahne. Dtsch Monatsschr Zahnheilk 39:142, 1921.
27. Graham JW. Toxicity of sterile filtrate from parodontal pockets. Proc R Soc Med 30:1165, 1937.
28. Hatfield CG, Baumhammers A. Cytotoxic effects of periodontally involved surfaces of human teeth. Arch Oral Biol 16:465, 1971.
29. Herting HC. Electron microscope studies of the cementum surface structures of periodontally healthy and diseased teeth. J Dent Res 46(suppl):1247, 1967.
30. Hoffman ID, Gold W. Distances between plaque and remnants of attached periodontal tissues on extracted teeth. J Periodontol 42:29, 1971.
31. Katz RV, Hazen SP, Chilton NW, Mumma RD Jr. Prevalence and intraoral distribution of root caries in an adult population. Caries Res 16:265, 1982.
32. Liakoni H, Barber P, Newman HN. Bacterial penetration of pocket soft tissues in chronic adult and juvenile periodontitis cases. An ultrastructural study. J Clin Periodontol 14:22, 1987.
33. Lindhe J, Liljenberg B, Listgarten MA. Some microbiological and histopathological features of periodontal disease in man. J Periodontol 52:264, 1980.
34. Listgarten MA. Structure of the microbial flora associated with periodontal health and disease in man. J Periodontol 47:1, 1976.
35. Listgarten MA, Hellden L. Relative distributions of bacteria at clinically healthy and periodontally diseased sites in humans. J Clin Periodontol 5:665, 1978.
36. Lopez NJ, Belvederessi M, de la Sotta R. Inflammatory effects of periodontally diseased cementum studied by autogenous dental root implants in humans. J Periodontol 51:582, 1980.
37. McHenry KR, Hausman E, Genco RJ, Slots J. 125I absorptiometry: Alveolar bone mass measurements in untreated periodontal disease. Abstract. J Dent Res 60(suppl A):387, 1981.
38. McMillan L, Burrill DY, Fosdick LS. An electron microscope study of particulates in periodontal exudate. Abstract. J Dent Res 37:51, 1958.
39. Mount GJ. Root surface caries: A recurrent dilemma. Austr Dent J 31:288, 1986.
40. Muller-Glauser W, Schroder HE. The pocket epithelium: A light and electronmicroscopic study. J Periodontol 53:133, 1982.
41. Nakata T, Stepnick R, Zipkin I. Chemistry of human dental cementum. The effect of age and exposure on the concentration of F, Ca, P and Mg. J Periodontol 43:115, 1972.
42. Newman MG, Sims TN. The predominant cultivable microbiota of the periodontal abscess. J Periodontol 50:350, 1979.
43. Orban B, Ray AG. Deep necrotic foci in the gingiva. J Periodontol 19:91, 1948.
44. Page RC, Schroeder HH. Structure and pathogenesis. In Schluger S, Youdelis R, Page R, eds. Periodontal Disease. Philadelphia, Lea & Febiger, 1977.
45. Rautiola CA, Craig RG. The micro hardness of cementum and underlying dentin of normal teeth and teeth exposed to periodontal disease. J Periodontol 32:113, 1961.
46. Saglie FR, Carranza FA Jr, Newman MG, Pattison GL. Scanning electron microscopy of the gingival wall of deep periodontal pockets in humans. J Periodont Res 17:284, 1982.
47. Saglie FR, Johansen JR, Flotra L. The zone of completely and partially destroyed periodontal fibers in pathologic pockets. J Clin Periodontol 2:198, 1975.
48. Saglie FR, Johansen JR, Tollefsen T. Plaque-free zones on human teeth in periodontitis. J Clin Periodontol 2:190, 1975.
49. Saglie FR, Newman MG, Carranza FA Jr, Pattison GL. Bacterial invasion of gingiva in advanced periodontitis in humans. J Periodontol 53:217, 1982.
50. Schroeder HE. Quantitative parameters of early human gingival inflammation. Arch Oral Biol 15:383, 1970.
51. Schroeder HE, Attstrom R. The Borderland between Caries and Periodontal Disease. Vol 2. London, Grune & Stratton, 1980, pp 99–123.
52. Schroeder HE, Listgarten MA. Fine Structure of the Developing Epithelial Attachment of Human Teeth. Monographs in Developmental Biology. Vol 2. Basel, S Karger, 1977.
53. Selvig KA. Ultrastructural changes in cementum and adjacent connective tissue in periodontal disease. Acta Odontol Scand 24:459, 1966.
54. Selvig KA. Biological changes at the tooth-saliva interface in periodontal disease. J Dent Res 48(suppl):846, 1969.
55. Selvig KA, Hals E. Periodontally diseased cementum studied by correlated microradiography, electron probe analysis and electron microscopy. J Periodont Res 12:419, 1977.
56. Selvig KA, Zander HA. Chemical analysis and microradiography of cementum and dentin from periodontally diseased human teeth. J Periodontol 33:303, 1962.
57. Sottosanti JS. A possible relationship between occlusion, root resorption, and the progression of periodontal disease. J West Soc Periodontol 25:69, 1977.
58. Standish SN, Shafer WG. The lateral periodontal cyst. J Periodontol 29:27, 1958.
59. Stanley HR. The cyclic phenomenon of periodontitis. Oral Surg Oral Med Oral Pathol 8:598, 1955.
60. Syed SA, Loesche WJ, Pape HL, Grenier E. Predominant cultivable flora isolated from human root surface caries plaque. Infect Immunol 11:727, 1975.
61. Taichman N. Potential mechanisms of tissue destruction in periodontal disease. J Dent Res 47:928, 1968.
62. Takada T, Donath K. The mechanism of pocket formation. A light microscopic study of undecalcified human material. J Periodontol 59:215, 1988.
63. Wade AB. The relation between the pocket base, the epithelial attachment and

the alveolar process. In Les Parodontopathies. 16th ARPA Congress, Vienna, 1960.
64. Waerhaug J. The gingival pocket. Odont Tidsk *60*(suppl 1), 1952.
65. Waerhaug J. The angular bone defect and its relationship to trauma from occlusion and downgrowth of subgingival plaque. J Clin Periodontol *6:*61, 1979.
66. Waerhaug J. The infrabony pocket and its relationship to trauma from occlusion and subgingival plaque. J Periodontol *50:*355, 1979.

67. Warren EB, Hanse NM, Swartz ML, Phillips RW. Effects of periodontal disease and of calculus solvents on microhardness of cementum. J Periodontol *35:*505, 1964.
68. Wittwer JW, Dickler EH, Toto PD. Comparative frequencies of plasma cells and lymphocytes in gingivitis. J Periodontol *40:*274, 1969.
69. Zander HA. The attachment of calculus to root surfaces. J Periodontol *24:*16,

23

Bone Loss and Patterns of Bone Destruction

FERMIN A. CARRANZA, JR.

**Bone Destruction Caused by Extension of
    Gingival Inflammation**
**Bone Destruction Caused by Trauma From
    Occlusion**
Bone Destruction Caused by Systemic Disorders

**Factors Determining Bone Morphology in
    Periodontal Disease**
**Bone Destruction Patterns in Periodontal
    Disease**

Although periodontitis is an infectious disease of the gingival tissue, changes that occur in bone are crucial because it is the destruction of bone that is responsible for tooth loss.

The height of the alveolar bone is normally maintained by an equilibrium, regulated by local and systemic influences,[14,18] between bone formation and bone resorption. When resorption exceeds formation, bone height is reduced. It has been claimed that a reduction in the height of the alveolar bone, termed *physiologic* or *senile atrophy,* occurs with aging.[23] This concept has not been proved (see Chapter 3).

Bone destruction in periodontal disease is caused by local factors. These local factors fall into two groups: those that cause gingival inflammation and those that cause trauma from occlusion. Acting singly or together, inflammation and trauma from occlusion are responsible for bone destruction in periodontal disease and determine its severity and pattern. Bone loss caused by extension of gingival inflammation is responsible for reduction in the height of the alveolar bone, whereas trauma from occlusion causes bone loss lateral to the root surface.

The level of bone is the consequence of past pathologic experiences, whereas changes in the soft tissue of the pocket wall reflect the present inflammatory condition. Therefore, the degree of bone loss is not necessarily correlated with the depth of periodontal pockets, the severity of ulceration of the pocket wall, or the presence or absence of pus.

BONE DESTRUCTION CAUSED BY EXTENSION OF GINGIVAL INFLAMMATION

Chronic inflammation is the most common cause of bone destruction in periodontal disease, as it results in the extension of the inflammatory process to the bone. The extension of inflammation from the marginal gingiva into the supporting periodontal tissues marks the transition from gingivitis to periodontitis.

Periodontitis is always preceded by gingivitis, but not all gingivitis progresses to periodontitis. Some cases of gingivitis will apparently never become periodontitis, and others go through a brief gingivitis phase and rapidly develop into periodontitis. The factors that are responsible for the extension of inflammation to the supporting structures and that bring about the conversion of gingivitis to periodontitis are not known.

The transition from gingivitis to periodontitis is associated with changes in the composition of bacterial plaque. In advanced stages of disease, the number of motile organisms and spirochetes increases, whereas the number of coccoid rods and straight rods decreases.[40]

The cellular composition of the infiltrated connective tissue also changes with increasing severity of the lesion (see Chapter 16). Fibroblasts and lymphocytes predominate in stage I gingivitis, whereas the number of plasma cells and blast cells increases gradually as the disease progresses. Seymour and associates[68,69] have postulated a stage of "contained" gingivitis in which T lymphocytes are preponderant; they believe that as the lesion becomes a B-lymphocyte lesion, it becomes progressively destructive.

Heijl and coworkers[28] were able to convert a confined, naturally occurring chronic gingivitis into a progressive periodontitis in experimental animals. They placed a silk ligature into the sulcus and tied it around the neck of the tooth. This induced ulceration of the sulcular epithelium, a shift in the connective tissue population from predominantly plasma cells to predominantly polymorphonuclear leukocytes, and osteoclastic resorption of the alveolar crest. The recurrence of episodes of acute destruction over a period of time may be one mechanism leading to progressive bone loss in marginal periodontitis.

The extension of inflammation to the supporting structures of a tooth may be modified by the pathogenic potential of plaque or by the resistance of the host. The latter includes immunologic activity (see Chapter 9) and other tissue-related mechanisms, such as the degree of fibrosis of the gingiva, probably the width of the attached gingiva, and the reactive fibrogenesis and osteogenesis that occur peripheral to the inflammatory lesion. A fibrin-fibrinolytic system has been mentioned as "walling off" the advancing lesion.[63] *The pathway of the spread of inflammation is critical, because it affects the pattern of bone destruction in periodontal disease.* Considerable controversy has existed about the possible changes in the pathway of gingival inflammation caused by trauma from occlusion. The suggested change in the pathway of inflammation, going toward the periodontal ligament rather than to the bone,[15] has not been confirmed.[8,70]

Histopathology. Gingival inflammation extends along the collagen fiber bundles and follows the course of the blood vessels through the loosely arranged tissues around them into the alveolar bone[77] (Fig. 23–1). Although the inflammatory infiltrate is concentrated in the marginal periodontium, the reaction is a much more diffuse one, often reaching the bone and eliciting a response before there is evidence of crestal resorption or loss of attachment.[51] In the upper molar region, inflammation can extend to the maxillary sinus, resulting in thickening of the sinus mucosa.[50]

Interproximally, inflammation spreads in the loose connective tissue around the blood vessels, through the transseptal fibers, and then into the bone through vessel channels that perforate the crest of the interdental septum. *The site at which the inflammation enters the bone depends on the location of the vessel channels.* It may enter the interdental septum at the center of the crest (Fig. 23–2), toward the side of the crest (Fig. 23–3), or at the angle of the septum, and it may enter the bone through more than one channel. After reaching the marrow spaces, the inflammation may return from the bone into the periodontal ligament. Less frequently, the inflammation spreads from the gingiva directly into the periodontal ligament and from there into the interdental septum (Fig. 23–4).[1]

Facially and lingually, inflammation from the gingiva spreads along the outer periosteal surface of the bone (see Fig. 23–4) and penetrates into the marrow spaces through vessel channels in the outer cortex. Along its course from the gingiva to the bone, the inflammation destroys the gingival and transseptal fibers, reducing them to disorganized

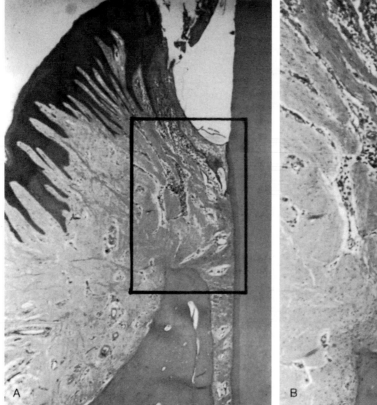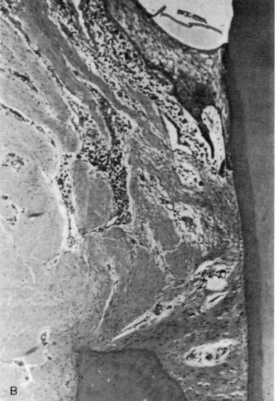

FIGURE 23–1. *A,* Area of inflammation extending from the gingiva into the suprabony area. *B,* Detailed view of rectangular area in *A,* showing extension of inflammation along blood vessels in between collagen bundles.

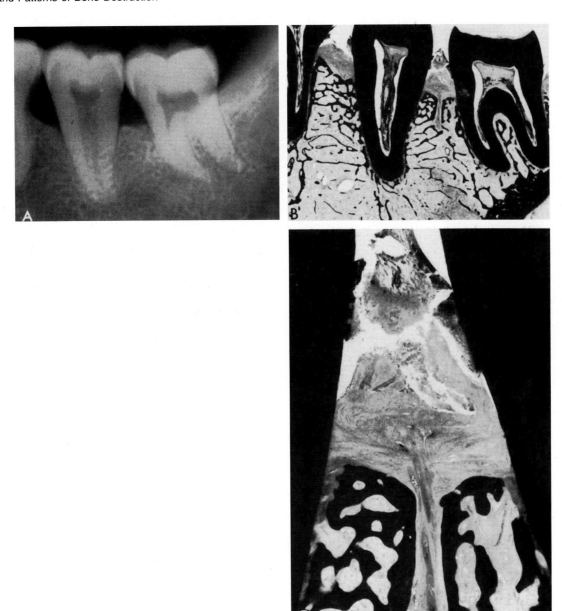

FIGURE 23–2. Extension of inflammation into the center of the interdental septum. *A,* Molar region showing periodontal bone loss. *B,* Survey section of the second and third molars. *C,* Inflammation from the gingiva penetrates the transseptal fibers and enters the bone around blood vessel in the center of the septum.

granular fragments interspersed among the inflammatory cells and edema (Fig. 23–5).[55] However, there is a continuous tendency to recreate transseptal fibers across the crest of the interdental septum farther along the root as the bone destruction progresses. As a result, transseptal fibers are present, even in cases of extreme periodontal bone loss (Fig. 23–6).

The dense transseptal fibers are of clinical importance when surgical procedures are used to eradicate periodontal pockets. They form a firm covering over the bone, which is encountered after the superficial granulation tissue is removed.

After inflammation reaches the bone by extension from the gingiva, it spreads into the marrow spaces and replaces the marrow with a leukocytic and fluid exudate, new blood vessels, and proliferating fibroblasts (Fig. 23–7). Multinuclear osteoclasts and mononuclear phagocytes are increased in number, and the bone surfaces are lined with cove-like resorption lacunae (Fig. 23–8).

In the marrow spaces, resorption proceeds from within, causing first a thinning of the surrounding bony trabeculae and enlargement of the marrow spaces, followed by destruction of the bone and a reduction in bone height. Normally fatty bone marrow is partially or totally replaced by a fibrous type of marrow in the vicinity of the resorption.

Bone destruction in periodontal disease is not a process of bone necrosis.[33] It involves the activity of living cells along viable bone. When tissue necrosis and pus are present in periodontal disease, they occur in the soft tissue

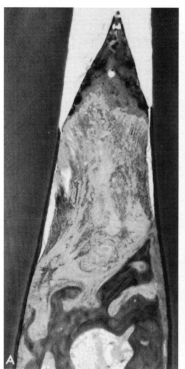
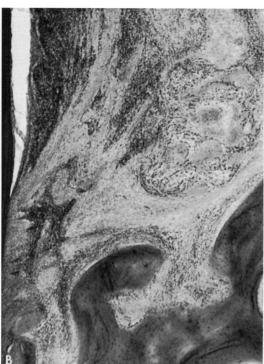

FIGURE 23-3. Inflammation enters the interdental septum at the center of the crest and near the crestal angle. *A,* Interdental periodontal pockets with inflammation extending into the bone. *B,* Inflammation enters the crest of the interdental bone at two areas. Note the granular necrosis of the collagen fibers in the inflamed area above the bone.

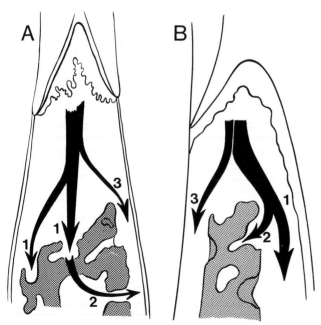

FIGURE 23-4. Pathways of inflammation from the gingiva into the supporting periodontal tissues in periodontitis. *A,* Interproximally, from the gingiva into the bone (1), from the bone into the periodontal ligament (2), and from the gingiva into the periodontal ligament (3). *B,* Facially and lingually, from the gingiva along the outer periosteum (1), from the periosteum into the bone (2), and from the gingiva into the periodontal ligament (3).

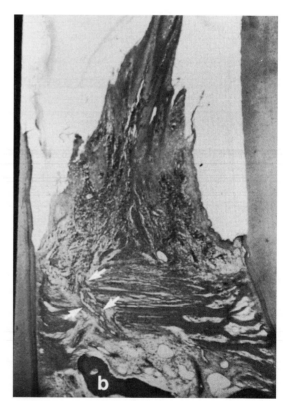

FIGURE 23-5. Interruption and/or destruction of transseptal fibers (*arrows*) as inflammation extends to the bone (b) around blood vessels.

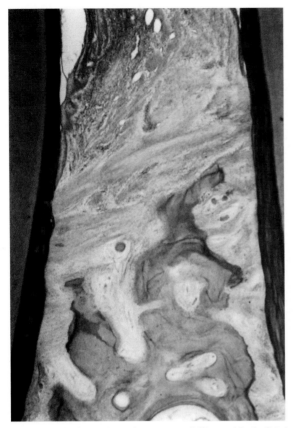

FIGURE 23–6. Reformation of transseptal fibers. Mesiodistal section through interdental septum showing gingival inflammation and bone loss. Re-created transseptal fibers can be seen above the bone margin, partially infiltrated by the inflammatory process.

walls of periodontal pockets, not along the resorbing margin of the underlying bone.

It has been hypothesized that two cell types are involved in bone resorption: the *osteoclast,* which removes the mineral portion of the bone, and the *mononuclear cell,* which plays a role in organic matrix degradation.[27] Both kinds of cells have been found in resorbing bone surfaces in experimentally induced periodontitis in animals.

The amount of inflammatory infiltrate correlates with the degree of bone loss but not with the number of osteoclasts. However, the distance from the apical border of the inflammatory infiltrate to the alveolar bone crest correlates with both the number of osteoclasts on the alveolar crest and the total number of osteoclasts.[62] Similar findings have been reported in experimentally induced periodontitis in animals.[38]

Radius of Action. Garant and Cho[12] suggested that locally produced bone resorption factors may have to be present in the proximity of the bone surface to be able to exert their action. Page and Schroeder,[57] on the basis of Waerhaug's measurements made on human autopsy specimens,[73,75] postulated that there is a range of effectiveness of about 1.5 to 2.5 mm within which bacterial plaque can induce loss of bone. Beyond 2.5 mm there is no effect; interproximal angular defects can appear only in spaces wider than 2.5 mm, because narrower spaces would be destroyed entirely. Tal[71] corroborated this with measurements in human patients.

Large defects far exceeding 2.5 mm from the tooth surface (as described in localized juvenile periodontitis, rapidly progressing periodontitis, and Papillon-Lefèvre syndrome) may be caused by the presence of bacteria in the tissues.[6,10,65]

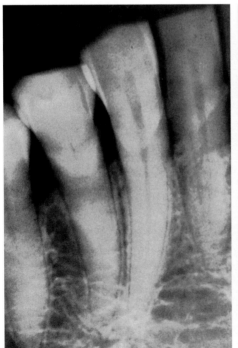
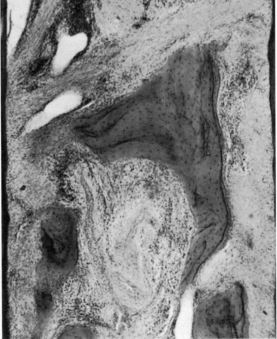

FIGURE 23–7. Early periodontal bone destruction. *A,* Early bone loss in the canine and premolar areas. *B,* Interdental septum beneath the periodontal pockets between the canine and the first premolar. The inflammation has invaded the marrow space, and there is lacunar resorption of the surrounding bone surface. Note the inflammation in the periodontal ligament in the right side.

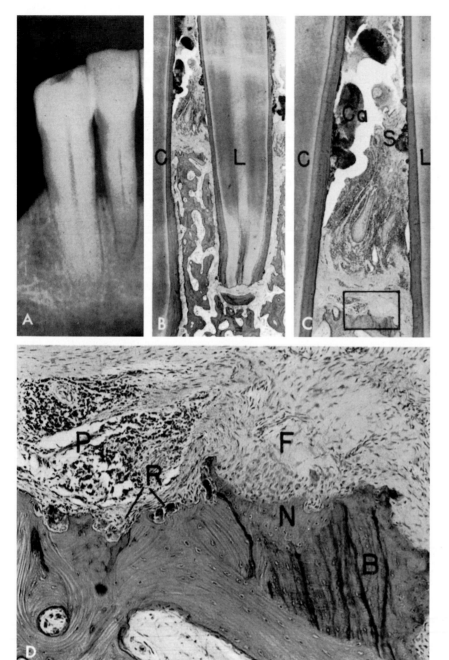

FIGURE 23-8. Bone resorption and formation in periodontal disease. *A,* Lateral incisor and canine with bone loss. *B,* Survey section of lateral incisor (L) and canine (C). *C,* Interdental space between lateral incisor (L) and canine (C), showing calculus (Ca) and periodontal pockets with suppuration (S). *D,* A detailed view of the bone margin within the rectangle showing bone margin beneath the periodontal pockets. Note the osteoclastic resorption (R) beneath the inflammation (P) and newly formed bone (N) with a thin surface layer of osteoid and osteoblasts adjacent to the resorption. The new bone is separated from the lamellated bone (B) by an irregular resorption line. An area of fibrosis is shown at F.

Rate of Bone Loss. In a study of Sri Lankan tea laborers with no oral hygiene and no dental care, Löe and associates found the rate of bone loss to average about 0.2 mm a year for facial surfaces and about 0.3 mm a year for proximal surfaces when periodontal disease was allowed to progress untreated.[41] However, the rate of bone loss may vary, depending on the type of disease present. Löe and coworkers[42] identified three subgroups of patients with periodontal disease based on interproximal loss of attachment* and tooth mortality:

1. Eight percent of persons had rapid progression of periodontal disease, characterized by a yearly loss of attachment of 0.1 to 1 mm.
2. Eighty-one percent of individuals had moderately progressive periodontal disease, with a yearly loss of attachment of 0.05 to 0.5 mm.
3. The remaining 11% persons had minimal or no progression of destructive disease (0.05 to 0.09 mm yearly).

Periods of Destruction. *Periodontal destruction occurs in an episodic, intermittent fashion, with periods of inactivity or quiescence.* The destructive periods result in loss of collagen and alveolar bone with deepening of the periodontal pocket. The reasons for the onset of destructive periods have not been totally elucidated, although the following theories have been offered:

1. Bursts of destructive activity are associated with subgingival

* Loss of attachment can be equated with loss of bone, although the former precedes the latter by about 6 to 8 months.[21]

ulceration and an acute inflammatory reaction, resulting in rapid loss of alveolar bone.[57,66]

2. Bursts of destructive activity coincide with the conversion of a predominately T-lymphocyte lesion to one with a predominance of B lymphocyte–plasma cell infiltrate.[69]

3. Periods of exacerbation are associated with an increase of the loose, unattached, motile, gram-negative, anaerobic pocket flora, and periods of remission coincide with the formation of a dense, unattached, nonmotile, gram-positive flora with a tendency to mineralize.[53]

4. Tissue invasion by one or several bacterial species is followed by an advanced local host defense that controls the attack.[65]

Mechanisms of Bone Destruction. Many investigations have been conducted and many explanations considered, but the mechanism or mechanisms by which inflammation and/or plaque-derived products destroy bone in inflammatory periodontal disease have not yet been determined. The following possible pathways by which plaque products could cause alveolar bone loss in periodontal disease have been listed by Hausmann:[25]

1. Direct action of plaque products on bone progenitor cells induces the differentiation of these cells into osteoclasts.

2. Plaque products act directly on bone, destroying it through a noncellular mechanism.

3. Plaque products stimulate gingival cells, causing them to release mediators, which in turn induce bone progenitor cells to differentiate into osteoclasts.

4. Plaque products cause gingival cells to release agents that can act as cofactors in bone resorption.

5. Plaque products cause gingival cells to release agents that destroy bone by direct chemical action, without osteoclasts.

In an experiment with gnotobiotic rats monoinfected with *Actinomyces naeslundii, Actinomyces viscosus,* or *Streptococcus mutans,* and in another experiment with conventional rats superinfected with *A. naeslundii,* Irving[30] found that bone loss was not accompanied by osteoclasts and seemed to be more a result of gradual cessation of bone formation than of active resorption.

A histomorphometric study of bone loss in ligature-induced periodontitis in rats by Ubios and coworkers showed an increase in the number of osteoclasts that peaked 72 hours after initiation of the experiment in spite of the length of erosive areas and presence of granulation tissue in the area remaining constant.[72] Notably, in bone resorption induced by tooth movement, the increase in resorptive areas precedes the increase in the number of osteoclasts.[44] This may point to different mechanisms of bone resorption.

Pharmacologic Agents and Bone Resorption. Several local agents that are capable of inducing bone resorption in vitro can play a role in periodontal disease (for a review, see Goldhaber and Rabadjija[19]). These include prostaglandins and their precursors and osteoclast-activating factor, all of which are present in inflamed gingiva, and endotoxins produced by plaque bacteria. Endotoxin from black-pigmented *Bacteroides* organisms stimulates osteoclastic bone resorption[26,61]; lipoteichoic acid acts in a similar way.[26]

Prostaglandins are a group of naturally occurring lipids that participate in the inflammatory process and have hormone-like effects.[22] When injected intradermally, they induce the vascular changes seen in inflammation. When injected over a bone surface, they induce bone resorption[32] in

the absence of inflammatory cells and with few multinucleated osteoclasts.[22] Complement may enhance the synthesis of prostaglandins by the bone and therefore induce bone resorption.[59]

Prostaglandin formation from fatty acid precursors, such as arachidonic acid, is controlled by cyclooxygenase (prostaglandin synthetase), which converts the fatty acid prostaglandin precursors to cyclic endoperoxidases.[19] *Flurbiprofen,* a nonsteroidal anti-inflammatory drug, is a potent inhibitor of the cyclooxygenase pathway of arachidonic acid metabolism. Flurbiprofen slows bone loss in naturally occurring periodontal disease in beagle dogs and in humans; this effect occurs without changes in gingival inflammation and rebounds 6 months after cessation of administration of the drug.[31,78]

Bone resorption can also be induced by supernatants of leukocyte cultures stimulated by antigens from dental plaque.[29] Horton and coworkers hypothesized that lymphocytes produce an *osteoclast-activating factor* that induces osteoclast formation and activity.[29]

Proteolytic enzymes produced in the periodontal tissue or by plaque bacteria may also participate in bone resorption.[32] *Collagenase* is present in the normal periodontium and is increased in inflamed gingiva; it is also produced by oral bacteria. Collagenolytic activity is produced in resorbing bone in vitro, but the collagen content is not correlated with the severity of bone loss.[11] By breaking down the bone matrix ground substance, *hyaluronidase* produced by oral bacteria may influence the resorptive process.

Bone Formation in Periodontal Disease. Areas of bone formation are also found immediately adjacent to sites of active bone resorption (Fig. 23–9) and along trabecular surfaces at a distance from the inflammation in an apparent effort to reinforce the remaining bone (buttressing bone formation). This osteogenic response is clearly found in experimentally produced periodontal bone loss in animals.[7] In humans it is less obvious but has been confirmed by histometric[4,5] and histologic studies.[16]

The response of alveolar bone to inflammation includes bone formation as well as resorption; thus, *bone loss in periodontal disease is not simply a destructive process but results from the predominance of resorption over formation.* New bone formation retards the rate of bone loss, compensating in some degree for the bone destroyed by inflammation.

Autopsy specimens from individuals with untreated disease occasionally show areas where bone resorption has ceased and new bone is being formed on the previously eroded bone margin. This indicates that *bone resorption in periodontal disease may be an intermittent process, with periods of remission and exacerbation.* This is consistent with the varied rates of progression observed clinically in untreated periodontal disease.

These periods of remission and exacerbation (or inactivity and activity, respectively) appear to coincide with the quiescence or exacerbation of gingival inflammation, manifested by changes in the extent of bleeding, the amount of exudate, and the composition of bacterial plaque (see Chapter 22).

The presence of bone formation in response to inflammation, even in active periodontal disease, has a bearing on

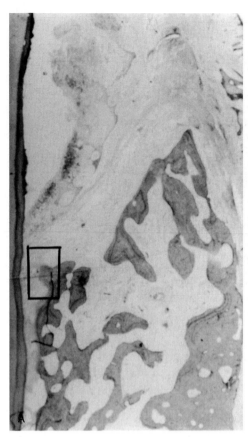
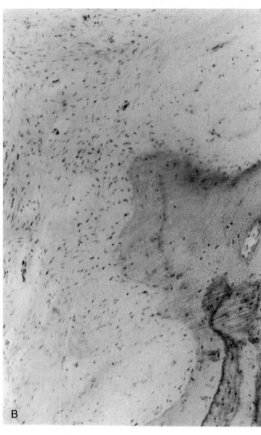

FIGURE 23–9. Bone formation in untreated periodontal disease. *A,* Section showing an infrabony pocket with deep angular bone loss. *B,* Magnification of the rectangular area in *A,* showing newly formed bone at bottom of defect.

the outcome of treatment. The basic aim of periodontal therapy is the elimination of inflammation to remove the stimulus for bone resorption and therefore allow the inherent constructive tendencies to predominate.

BONE DESTRUCTION CAUSED BY TRAUMA FROM OCCLUSION

The second cause of periodontal destruction is trauma from occlusion. Trauma from occlusion can produce bone destruction in the absence or presence of inflammation (see Chapter 24).

Trauma in the Absence of Inflammation. In the absence of inflammation, the changes caused by trauma from occlusion vary from increased compression and tension of the periodontal ligament and increased osteoclasis of alveolar bone[44] to necrosis of the periodontal ligament and bone and resorption of bone and tooth structure. These changes are reversible in that they can be repaired if the offending forces are removed. However, persistent trauma from occlusion results in funnel-shaped widening of the crestal portion of the periodontal ligament, with resorption of the adjacent bone.[39] These changes, which may cause the bony crest to have an angular shape, represent adaptation of the periodontal tissues aimed at "cushioning" increased occlusal forces, but the modified bone shape may weaken tooth support and cause tooth mobility.

Trauma Combined With Inflammation. When com-bined with inflammation, trauma from occlusion aggravates the bone destruction caused by the inflammation[39] and causes bizarre bone patterns.

BONE DESTRUCTION CAUSED BY SYSTEMIC DISORDERS

Local and systemic factors regulate the physiologic equilibrium of bone.[14] When there is a generalized tendency toward bone resorption, bone loss initiated by local inflammatory processes may be magnified. This systemic influence on the response of alveolar bone has been termed the *bone factor* in periodontal disease.[14]

The bone factor concept, developed by Irving Glickman[14] in the early 1950s, envisioned a systemic component in all cases of periodontal disease. In addition to the amount and virulence of plaque bacteria, the nature of the systemic component, not its presence or absence, influences the severity of periodontal destruction. Although the term *bone factor* is not in current use, the concept of a role played by systemic defense mechanisms has been validated, particularly by studies of immune deficiencies in severely destructive types of periodontitis, such as the juvenile forms of the disease.

Periodontal bone loss may also occur in generalized skeletal disturbances (such as hyperparathyroidism, leukemia, and Hand-Schüller-Christian disease) by mechanisms that may be totally unrelated to the usual periodontal problem.

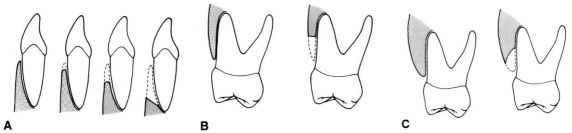

FIGURE 23–10. *A,* A lower incisor with thin labial bone. Bone loss can become vertical only when it reaches thicker bone in apical areas. *B,* Upper molars with thin facial bone, where only horizontal bone loss can occur. *C,* Upper molar with a thick facial bone, allowing for vertical bone loss.

FACTORS DETERMINING BONE MORPHOLOGY IN PERIODONTAL DISEASE

Normal Variation in Alveolar Bone. There is considerable normal variation in the morphologic features of alveolar bone (see Chapter 2), which affect the osseous contours produced by periodontal disease. The bone features that substantially affect the bone destructive pattern in periodontal disease include the following:

The thickness, width, and crestal angulation of the interdental septa.

The thickness of the facial and lingual alveolar plates.

The presence of fenestrations and/or dehiscences.

The increased thickness of the alveolar bone margins to accommodate functional demands.

The alignment of the teeth.

For example, angular osseous defects cannot form in thin facial or lingual alveolar plates, which have little or no cancellous bone between the outer and inner cortical layers. In such instances the entire crest of the plate is destroyed, and the height of the bone is reduced (Fig. 23–10).

Exostoses. Exostoses are outgrowths of bone of varied size and shape. Palatal exostoses have been found in 40% of human skulls.[52] They can occur as small nodules, large nodules, sharp ridges, spike-like projections, or any combination of these (see Fig. 23–20). Exostoses have been described in rare cases as developing after the placement of free gingival grafts.[56]

Trauma From Occlusion. Trauma from occlusion may be a factor in determining the dimension and shape of bone deformities. It may cause a thickening of the cervical margin of alveolar bone or a change in the morphology of the bone (e.g., angular defects and buttressing bone [see fol-

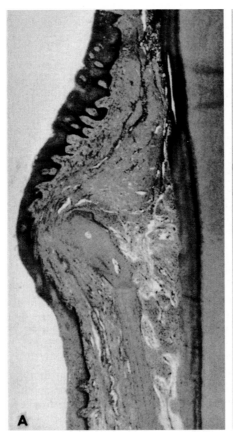
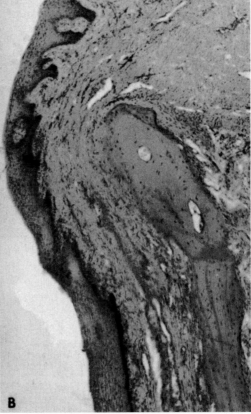

FIGURE 23–11. Lipping of facial bone. *A,* Peripheral buttressing bone formation along the external surface of the facial bony plate and at the crest. Note the deformity in the bone produced by the buttressing bone formation and the bulging of the mucosa. *B,* Detailed view showing lipping and deformity produced by buttressing bone formation.

lowing discussion]) on which inflammatory changes will later be superimposed.

Buttressing Bone Formation (Lipping). Bone formation sometimes occurs in an attempt to buttress bony trabeculae weakened by resorption. When it occurs within the jaw, it is termed *central buttressing bone formation.*[16] When it occurs on the external surface, it is referred to as *peripheral buttressing bone formation.* The latter may cause bulging of the bone contour, termed *lipping,* which sometimes accompanies the production of osseous craters and angular defects (Fig. 23–11).

Food Impaction. Interdental bone defects often occur where proximal contact is abnormal or absent. Pressure and irritation from food impaction contribute to the inverted bone architecture. In some instances the poor proximal relationship may be the result of a shift in tooth position because of extensive bone destruction that preceded food im-

paction. In such cases food impaction is a complicating factor rather than the cause of the bone defect.

Juvenile Periodontitis. A vertical or angular pattern of alveolar bone destruction is found around the first molars in juvenile periodontitis. The cause of the localized bone destruction in this type of periodontal disease is unknown (see Chapter 27).

BONE DESTRUCTION PATTERNS IN PERIODONTAL DISEASE

Periodontal disease alters the morphologic features of the bone, in addition to reducing bone height. An understanding of the nature and pathogenesis of these alterations is essential for effective diagnosis and treatment.

Horizontal Bone Loss. This is the most common pattern

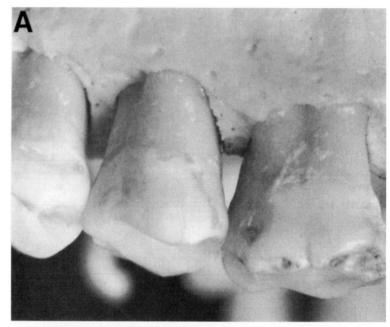
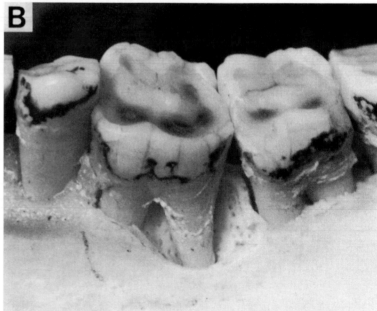

FIGURE 23–12. *A,* Horizontal bone loss. Note the reduction in height of the marginal bone, exposing cancellous bone and reaching the furca of the second molar. *B,* Vertical (angular) bone loss on the distal root of the first molar.

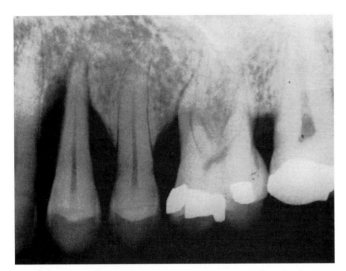

FIGURE 23–13. Angular (vertical) defects of different depths.

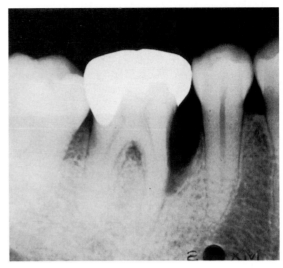

FIGURE 23–14. Angular defect on the mesial surface of the first molar. Note also the furcation involvement.

of bone loss in periodontal disease. The bone is reduced in height, but the bone margin remains roughly perpendicular to the tooth surface. The interdental septa and the facial and lingual plates are affected, but not necessarily to an equal degree around the same tooth (Fig. 23–12A).

Bone Deformities (Osseous Defects). Different types of bone deformities can result from periodontal disease. These usually occur in adults and have been reported in human skulls with deciduous dentitions.[34] Their presence may be suggested on radiographs, but careful probing and surgical exposure of the areas are required to determine their exact conformation and dimensions.

Vertical or Angular Defects. Vertical or angular defects are those that occur in an oblique direction, leaving a hollowed-out trough in the bone alongside the root; the base of the defect is located apical to the surrounding bone

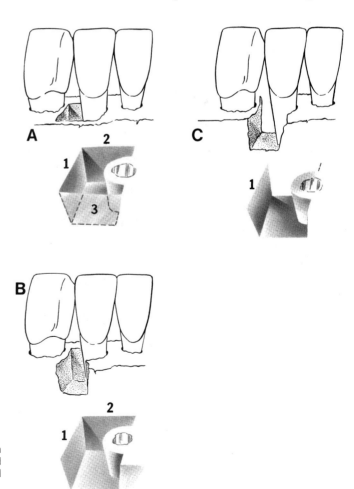

FIGURE 23–15. One-, two-, and three-walled vertical defects on right lateral incisor. *A,* Three bony walls: distal (1), lingual (2), and facial (3). *B,* Two-wall defect: distal (1) and lingual (2). *C,* One-wall defect: distal wall only (1).

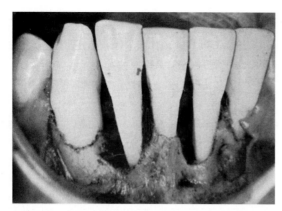

FIGURE 23–16. One-wall vertical defect on the mesial surface of the left lateral incisor and 1½-wall defect (distal wall and half of the labial wall) on the distal surface of the right lateral incisor.

(Figs. 23–12*B*, 23–13, and 23–14). In most instances angular defects have accompanying infrabony pockets; such pockets always have an underlying angular defect.

Angular defects are classified on the basis of the number of osseous walls.[20] Angular defects may have one, two, or three walls (Figs. 23–15 to 23–17). The number of walls in the apical portion of the defect may be greater than that in its occlusal portion; in these cases the term *combined osseous defect* is used (Fig. 23–18).

Vertical defects occurring interdentally can generally be seen on the radiograph, although sometimes thick, bony plates may obscure them. Angular defects can also appear on facial and lingual or palatal surfaces, but these defects are not seen on radiographs. Surgical exposure is the only sure way to determine the presence and configuration of vertical osseous defects.

Vertical defects increase with age.[54] Approximately 60% of persons with interdental angular defects have only a single defect.[54] Vertical defects found radiographically are most common on the distal surfaces of molar teeth.[54] Three-wall defects, however, are more frequent on the mesial surfaces of upper and lower molars.[35]

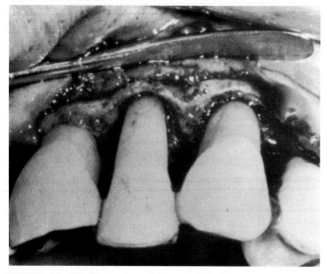

FIGURE 23–17. Circumferential vertical defect in relation to the upper lateral incisor and canine.

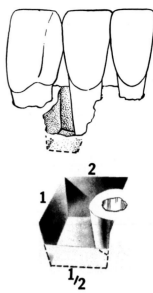

FIGURE 23–18. Combined type of osseous defect. Because the facial wall is half the height of the distal (1) and lingual (2) walls, this is an osseous defect with three walls in its apical half and two walls in the occlusal half.

The three-wall vertical defect has also been called an *intrabony defect.* This defect appears most frequently on the mesial aspects of second and third maxillary and mandibular molars. The one-wall vertical defect is also called a *hemiseptum.*

Osseous Craters. Osseous craters are concavities in the crest of the interdental bone confined within the facial and lingual walls (Fig. 23–19). *Craters have been found to make up about one third (35.2%) of all defects and about two thirds (62%) of all mandibular defects.* They are twice as common in posterior segments as in anterior segments.[48,49]

The heights of the facial and lingual crests of a crater have been found to be identical in 85% of cases, with the remaining 15% being nearly equally divided between higher facial crests and higher lingual crests.[64] The following reasons for the high frequency of interdental craters have been suggested:

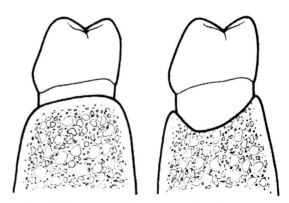

FIGURE 23–19. Diagrammatic representation of an osseous crater in a faciolingual section between two lower molars. *Left,* Normal bone contour. *Right,* Osseous crater.

The interdental area collects plaque and is difficult to clean.

The normal flat or even concave faciolingual shape of the interdental septum in lower molars may favor crater formation.

Vascular patterns from the gingiva to the center of the crest may provide a pathway for inflammation.[46,47,64]

Bulbous Bone Contours. These are bony enlargements caused by exostoses, adaptation to function, or buttressing bone formation (Fig. 23–20). They are found more frequently in the maxilla than in the mandible.

Reversed Architecture. These defects are produced by loss of interdental bone, including the facial and/or lingual plates, without concomitant loss of radicular bone, thereby reversing the normal architecture (Fig. 23–21). Such defects are more common in the maxilla.[54]

Ledges. Ledges are plateau-like bone margins caused by resorption of thickened bony plates (Fig. 23–22).

Furcation Involvements. The term *furcation involvement* refers to the invasion of the bifurcation and trifurcation of multirooted teeth by periodontal disease.[13] The mandibular first molars are the most common sites, and the maxillary premolars are the least common; the number of furcation involvements increases with age.[36,37]

The denuded furcation may be visible clinically or covered by the wall of the pocket. The extent of involvement is determined by exploration with a blunt probe, along with a simultaneous blast of warm air to facilitate visualization (Figs. 23–23 and 23–24).

Furcation involvements have been classified as grades I, II, III, and IV according to the amount of tissue destruction. Grade I is incipient bone loss, grade II is partial bone loss (cul-de-sac), and grade III is total bone loss with through-and-through opening of the furcation. Grade IV is similar to grade III, but with gingival recession exposing the furcation to view.

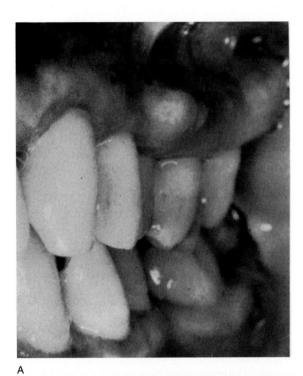

A

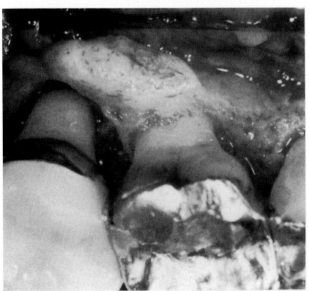

B

FIGURE 23–20. *A,* Exostosis in the facial aspect. *B,* Exostosis in the palatal aspect. Note also the circumferential defect in the second molar.

Microscopically, furcation involvement presents no unique pathologic features. It is simply a phase in the rootward extension of the periodontal pocket. In its early stages, there is a widening of the periodontal space, with cellular and fluid inflammatory exudation (Fig. 23–25), followed by epithelial proliferation into the furcation area from an adjoining periodontal pocket (Fig. 23–26). Extension of the inflammation into the bone leads to resorption and reduction in bone height (Fig. 23–27). The bone destructive pattern may produce horizontal loss, or there may be angular osseous defects associated with infrabony pockets (Figs. 23–28 and 23–29). Plaque, calculus, and bacterial debris occupy the denuded furcation space.

The destructive pattern in a furcation involvement varies in different cases and with the degree of involvement. Bone loss around each individual root may be horizontal or angular, and very frequently a crater develops in the interradicular area. Probing to determine the presence of these destructive patterns must be done horizontally as well as vertically around each involved root and in the crater area to establish the depth of the vertical component.

Furcation involvement is a stage of progressive periodontal disease and has the same etiology. The difficulty, and sometimes the impossibility,[2,3] of controlling plaque in furcations is responsible for the presence of extensive lesions in this area.[76]

The role of trauma from occlusion in the etiology of furcation lesions is controversial. Some assign a key role to trauma, believing that furcation areas are most sensitive to injury from excessive occlusal forces.[17] Others deny the initiating effect of trauma and consider that inflammation and edema caused by plaque in the furcation area tend to extrude the tooth, which then becomes traumatized and sensitive.[76]

Trauma from occlusion should be particularly suspected as a contributing etiologic factor in cases of furcation in-

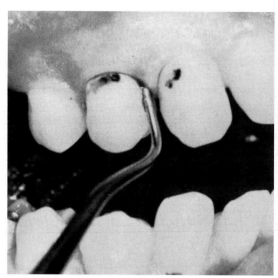
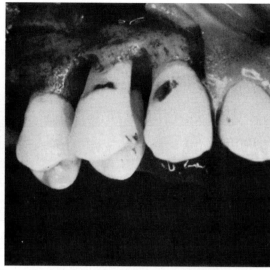

FIGURE 23–21. Reversed architecture. *Left,* Probe in the deep infrabony pocket on the mesial surface of maxillary premolar. *Right,* Elevated flap shows irregular bone margin with notching of interdental bone.

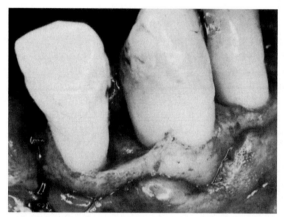

FIGURE 23–22. Labial ledge produced by interproximal resorption.

volvement with crater-like or angular deformities in the bone and especially when bone destruction is localized to one of the roots.

Other factors that may play a role are the presence of enamel projections into the furcation,[48] which occurs in about 13% of multirooted teeth, and the proximity of the furcation to the cemento-enamel junction, which occurs in about 75% of cases of furcation involvement.[37]

The presence of accessory pulpal canals in the furcation area may extend pulpal inflammation to the furcation[24]; this possibility should be carefully explored, particularly when mesial and distal bone retain their normal height. Accessory canals connecting the pulp chamber floor to the furcation have been found in 36% of maxillary first molars, 12% of maxillary second molars, 32% of mandibular first molars, and 24% of mandibular second molars.[73]

The diagnosis of furcation involvement is made by clinical examination and careful probing with one of the specially designed probes (see Chapter 28). Radiographic examination of the area is helpful, but lesions can be

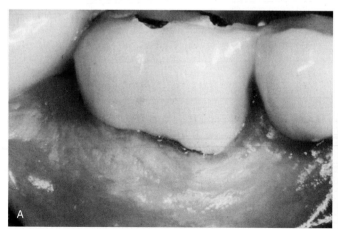
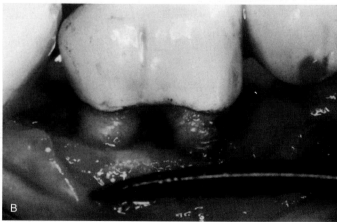

FIGURE 23–23. *A,* Partially stippled gingiva covering the furcation area of the lower first molar. *B,* Flap elevation reveals furcation involvement.

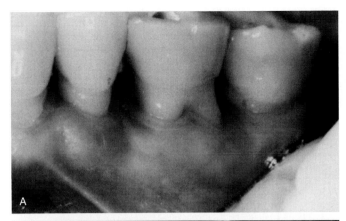

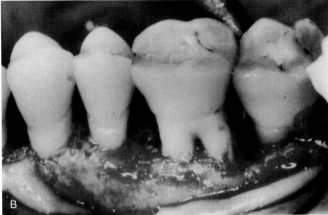

FIGURE 23–24. *A*, Furcation area barely covered by gingival tissue. *B*, Flap elevation reveals partial furcation involvement.

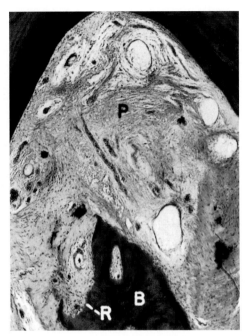

FIGURE 23–25. Furcation area in a mandibular molar. The periodontal space is widened. There is edema, slight leukocytic infiltration of the periodontal ligament (P), and an area of resorption (R) at the margin of the bone (B).

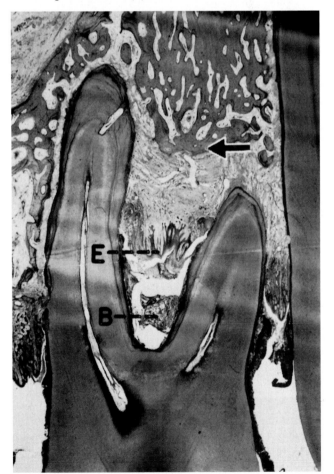

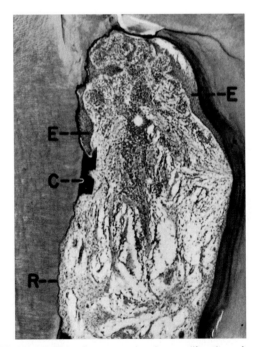

FIGURE 23–26. Furcation area showing proliferation of epithelium (E), edema and degeneration of connective tissue, bone loss, and destruction of cementum (C) and dentin with irregularly hollowed-out lacunae along the dentinal surface (R).

FIGURE 23–27. Furcation involvement. Maxillary first molar showing pronounced bone loss, inflammation, and epithelial proliferation (E). Bacterial debris is shown at B. Note the different height of bone between the mesial surface *(left)* and the furcation area *(arrow)*.

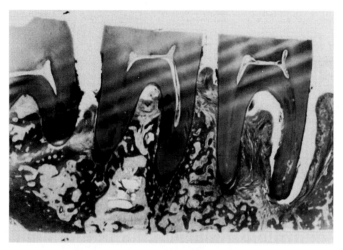

FIGURE 23–28. Different degrees of furcation involvement in a human autopsy specimen. Moderate involvement is found in the third molar; a more advanced lesion in the second molar; and a very severe lesion in the first molar, exposing almost the entire mesial root.

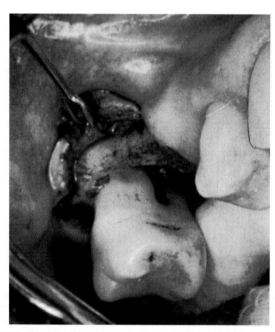

FIGURE 23–29. Crater-like osseous defect in trifurcation of a molar.

obscured by angulation of the beam and the radiopacity of neighboring structures (see Chapter 29).

For more detailed clinical considerations in the diagnosis and treatment of furcation involvements, see Chapters 28 and 56.

REFERENCES

1. Akiyoshi M, Mori K. Marginal periodontitis: A histological study of the incipient stage. J Periodontol 38:45, 1967.
2. Bower RC. Furcation morphology relative to periodontal treatment. Furcation entrance architecture. J Periodontol 50:23, 1979.
3. Bower RC. Furcation morphology relative to periodontal treatment. Furcation root surface anatomy. J Periodontol 50:366, 1979.
4. Carranza FA Jr. Histometric evaluation of periodontal pathology. A review of recent studies. J Periodontol 38:741, 1967.
5. Carranza FA Jr, Cabrini RL. Histometric studies of periodontal tissues. Periodontics 5:308, 1967.
6. Carranza FA Jr, Saglie R, Newman MG. Scanning and transmission electron microscopy study of tissue invading microorganisms in juvenile periodontitis. J Periodontol 54:598, 1983.
7. Carranza FA Jr, Simes RJ, Mayo J, Cabrini RL. Histometric evaluation of periodontal bone loss in rats. J Periodont Res 6:65, 1971.
8. Comar MD, Kollar JD, Gargiulo AW. Local irritation and occlusal trauma as cofactors in the periodontal disease process. J Periodontol 40:193, 1969.
9. Easley JR, Drennan GA. Morphological classification of the furca. J Can Dent Assoc 35:104, 1969.
10. Frank RM, Voegel JC. Bacterial bone resorption in advanced cases of human periodontitis. J Periodont Res 13:251, 1978.
11. Fullmer HM, et al. Collagenase and gingival disease. Proceedings of the First Pan-Pacific Congress of Dental Research, 1970, p 167.
12. Garant PR, Cho MJ. Histopathogenesis of spontaneous periodontal disease in conventional rats. I. Histometric and histologic study. J Periodont Res 14:297, 1979.
13. Glickman I. Bifurcation involvement in periodontal disease. J Am Dent Assoc 40:528, 1950.
14. Glickman I. The experimental basis for the "bone factor" concept in periodontal disease. J Periodontol 20:7, 1951.
15. Glickman I, Smulow JB. Alterations in the pathway of gingival inflammation into the underlying tissues induced by excessive occlusal forces. J Periodontol 33:7, 1962.
16. Glickman I, Smulow J. Buttressing bone formation in the periodontium. J Periodontol 36:365, 1965.
17. Glickman I, Stein RS, Smulow JB. The effects of increased functional forces upon the periodontium of splinted and nonsplinted teeth. J Periodontol 32:290, 1961.
18. Glickman I, Wood H. Bone histology in periodontal disease. J Dent Res 21:35, 1942.
19. Goldhaber P, Rabadjija L. Influence of pharmacological agents on bone resorption. In Genco RJ, Mergenhagen SE, eds. Host-Parasite Interactions in Periodontal Disease. Washington, DC, American Society for Microbiology, 1982.
20. Goldman HM, Cohen DW. The intrabony pocket: Classification and treatment. J Periodontol 29:272, 1958.
21. Goodson JM, Haffajee AD, Socransky SS. The relationship between attachment level loss and alveolar bone loss. J Clin Periodontol 11:348, 1984.
22. Goodson JM, McClatchy K, Revell C. Prostaglandin-induced resorption of the adult calvarium. J Dent Res 53:670, 1974.
23. Gottlieb B, Orban BJ. Biology and Pathology of the Tooth and Its Supporting Mechanism. New York, Macmillan, 1938.
24. Gutman JL. Prevalence, location and patency of accessory canals in the furcation region of permanent molars. J Periodontol 49:21, 1978.
25. Hausmann E. Potential pathways for bone resorption in human periodontal disease. J Periodontol 45:338, 1974.
26. Hausmann E, Raisz LG, Miller WA. Endotoxin: Stimulation of bone resorption in tissue culture. Science 168:793, 1970.
27. Heersche JNM. Mechanism of osteoclastic bone resorption: A new hypothesis. Calcif Tissue Res 26:81, 1978.
28. Heijl L, Rifkin BR, Zander HA. Conversion of chronic gingivitis to periodontitis in squirrel monkeys. J Periodontol 47:710, 1976.
29. Horton JE, Raisz LG, Simmons HA, et al. Bone resorbing activity in supernatant fluid from cultured human peripheral blood leukocytes. Science 177:793, 1972.
30. Irving JT. Factors concerning bone loss associated with periodontal disease. J Dent Res 49:262, 1970.
31. Jeffcoat MK, Williams RC, Wachter WJ, et al. Flurbiprofen treatment of periodontal disease in beagles. J Periodont Res 21:624, 1986.
32. Klein DC, Raisz LG. Prostaglandins: Stimulation of bone resorption in tissue culture. Endocrinology 86:1436, 1970.
33. Kronfeld R. Condition of alveolar bone underlying periodontal pockets. J Periodontol 6:22, 1935.
34. Larato DC. Periodontal bone defects in the juvenile skull. J Periodontol 41:473, 1970.
35. Larato DC. Intrabony defects in the dry human skull. J Periodontol 41:496, 1970.
36. Larato DC. Furcation involvements: Incidence of distribution. J Periodontol 41:499, 1970.
37. Larato DC. Some anatomical factors related to furcation involvements. J Periodontol 46:608, 1975.
38. Lindhe J, Ericsson I. Effect of ligature placement and dental plaque on periodontal tissue breakdown in the dog. J Periodontol 49:343, 1978.
39. Lindhe J, Svanberg G. Influence of trauma from occlusion on progression of experimental periodontitis in beagle dogs. J Clin Periodontol 1:3, 1974.
40. Lindhe J, Liljenberg B, Listgarten MA. Some microbiological and histopathological features of periodontal disease in man. J Periodontol 51:264, 1980.
41. Löe H, Anerud A, Boysen H, Morrison E. Natural history of periodontal disease in man. Rapid, moderate and no loss of attachment in Sri Lankan laborers 14 to 46 years of age. J Clin Periodontol 13:431, 1986.
42. Löe H, Anerud A, Boysen H, Smith MR: The natural history of periodontal disease in man. The rate of periodontal destruction before 40 years of age. J Periodontol 49:607, 1978.
43. Löe H, Anerud A, Boysen H, Smith MR. The natural history of periodontal dis-

ease in man. The rate of periodontal destruction before 40 years of age. J Periodontol *49:*607, 1978.

44. Lopez-Otero R, Parodi RJ, Ubios AM, et al. Histologic and histometric study of bone resorption after tooth movement in rats. J Periodont Res *8:*327, 1973.
45. Macapanpan LC, Weinmann JP. The influence of injury to the periodontal membrane on the spread of gingival inflammation. J Dent Res *33:*263, 1954.
46. Manson JD, Nicholson K. The distribution of bone defects in chronic periodontitis. J Periodontol *45:*88, 1974.
47. Manson JD. Bone morphology and bone loss in periodontal disease. J Clin Periodontol *3:*14, 1976.
48. Masters DH, Hoskins SW. Projection of cervical enamel into molar furcations. J Periodontol *35:*49, 1963.
49. Melcher AH, Eastoe JE. Biology of the Periodontium. New York, Academic Press, 1969, p 315.
50. Moskow BS. A histomorphologic study of the effects of periodontal inflammation on the maxillary sinus mucosa. J Periodontol *63:*674, 1992.
51. Moskow BS, Polson AM. Histologic studies on the extension of the inflammatory infiltrate in human periodontitis. J Clin Periodontol *18:*534, 1991.
52. Nery EB, Corn H, Eisenstein IL. Palatal exostoses in the molar region. J Periodontol *48:*663, 1977.
53. Newman MG. The role of *Bacteroides melaninogenicus* and other anaerobes in periodontal infections. Rev Infect Dis *1:*313, 1979.
54. Nielsen JI, Glavind L, Karring T. Interproximal periodontal intrabony defects. Prevalence, localization and etiological factors. J Clin Periodontol *7:*187, 1980.
55. Ooya K, Yamamoto H. A scanning electron microscopic study of the destruction of human alveolar crest in periodontal disease. J Periodont Res *13:*498, 1978.
56. Pack ARC, Gaudie WM, Jennings AM. Bony exostosis as a sequela to free gingival grafting: Two case reports. J Periodontol *62:*269, 1991.
57. Page RC, Schroeder HE. Periodontitis in Man and Other Animals. A Comparative Review. Basel, Karger, 1982.
58. Prichard JF. Periodontal Surgery, Practical Dental Monographs. Chicago, Year Book Medical, 1961, p 16.
59. Raisz LG, Sandberg AL, Goodson JM, et al. Complement-dependent stimulation of prostaglandin synthesis and bone resorption. Science *185:*789, 1974.
60. Rifkin BR, Heijl L. The occurrence of mononuclear cells at sites of osteoclastic bone resorption in experimental periodontitis. J Periodontol *50:*636, 1979.
61. Rizzo AA, Mergenhagen SE. Histopathologic effects of endotoxin injected into rabbit oral mucosa. Arch Oral Biol *9:*659, 1964.

62. Rowe DJ, Bradley LS. Quantitative analyses of osteoclasts, bone loss and inflammation in human periodontal disease. J Periodont Res *16:*13, 1981.
63. Ruben M, Cooper SJ. Tissue factors modifying the spread of periodontal inflammation: A perspective. Contin Educ Dent *2:*387, 1981.
64. Saari JT, Hurt WC, Briggs NL. Periodontal bony defects on the dry skull. J Periodontol *39:*278, 1968.
65. Saglie RF, Rezende M, Pertuiset J, et al. Bacterial invasion during disease activity as determined by significant loss of attachment. Abstract. J Periodontol *58:*336, 1987.
66. Schroeder HE, Lindhe J. Conditions and pathological features of rapidly destructive experimental periodontitis in dogs. J Periodontol *51:*6, 1980.
67. Schroeder HE. Discussion: Pathogenesis of periodontitis. J Clin Periodontol *13:*426, 1986.
68. Seymour GJ, Dockrell HM, Greenspan JS. Enzyme differentiation of lymphocyte subpopulations in sections of human lymph nodes, tonsils, and periodontal disease. Clin Exp Immunol *32:*169, 1978.
69. Seymour GJ, Powell RN, Davies WJR. Conversion of a stable T cell lesion to a progressive B cell lesion in the pathogenesis of chronic inflammatory periodontal disease: A hypothesis. J Clin Periodontol *6:*267, 1979.
70. Stahl SS. The response of the periodontium to combined gingival inflammation and occlusofunctional stresses in four surgical specimens. Periodontics *6:*14, 1968.
71. Tal H. Relationship between interproximal distance of roots and the prevalence of intrabony pockets. J Periodontol *55:*604, 1984.
72. Ubios AM, Costa OR, Cabrini RL. Early steps in bone resorption in experimental periodontitis. A histomorphometric study. Acta Odont Lat-Am *7:*45, 1993.
73. Vertucci FJ, Anthony RL. An SEM investigation of accessory foramina in the furcation and pulp chamber floor of molar teeth. Oral Surg *62:*319, 1986.
74. Waerhaug J. The angular bone defect and its relationship to trauma from occlusion and downgrowth of subgingival plaque. J Clin Periodontol *6:*61, 1979.
75. Waerhaug J. The furcation problem. Etiology, pathogenesis, diagnosis, therapy and prognosis. J Clin Periodontol *7:*73, 1980.
76. Waerhaug J. The infrabony pocket and its relationship to trauma from occlusion and subgingival plaque. J Periodontol *50:*355, 1979.
77. Weinmann JP. Progress of gingival inflammation into the supporting structures of the teeth. J Periodontol *12:*71, 1941.
78. Williams RC, Jeffcoat MK, Kaplan ML, et al. Flurbiprofen: A potent inhibitor of alveolar bone resorption in beagles. Science *227:*640, 1985.

24

Periodontal Response to External Forces

FERMIN A. CARRANZA, JR.

PHYSIOLOGIC ADAPTIVE CAPACITY OF THE PERIODONTIUM TO OCCLUSAL FORCES

The periodontium tries to accommodate to the forces exerted on the crown. This adaptive capacity varies in differ-

ent persons and in the same person at different times. The effect of occlusal forces on the periodontium is influenced by their magnitude, direction, duration, and frequency.

When the *magnitude* of occlusal forces is increased, the periodontium responds with a thickening of the periodontal ligament, an increase in the number and width of periodon-

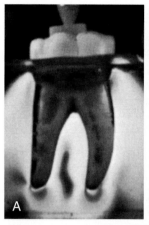 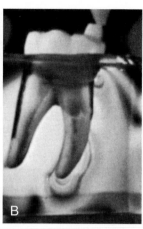

FIGURE 24–1. Stress patterns around the roots changed by shifting the direction of occlusal forces (experimental model using photoelastic analysis). *A,* Buccal view of an ivorine molar subjected to an axial force. The shaded fringes indicate that the internal stresses are at the root apices. *B,* Buccal view of ivorine molar subjected to a mesial tilting force. The shaded fringes indicate that the internal stresses are along the mesial surface and at the apex of the mesial root. (From Glickman I, Roeber F, Brion M, Pameijer J. Photoelastic analysis of internal stresses in the periodontium created by occlusal forces. J Periodontol *41:*30, 1970.)

tal ligament fibers, and an increase in the density of alveolar bone.

Changing the *direction* of occlusal forces causes a reorientation of the stresses and strains within the periodontium[21] (Fig. 24–1). The principal fibers of the periodontal ligament are arranged so that they best accommodate occlusal forces along the long axis of the tooth. Lateral (horizontal) forces and torque (rotational) forces are more likely to injure the periodontium.

The response of alveolar bone is also affected by the *duration* and *frequency* of occlusal forces. Constant pressure on the bone is more injurious than intermittent forces. The more frequent the application of an intermittent force, the more injurious the force to the periodontium.

TRAUMA FROM OCCLUSION

An inherent "margin of safety" common to all tissues permits some variation in occlusion without adversely affecting the periodontium. However, *when occlusal forces exceed the adaptive capacity of the tissues, tissue injury results.*[3,5,11,24,32,34,46,47] The resultant injury is termed *trauma from occlusion.**

Thus, *trauma from occlusion refers to the tissue injury, not the occlusal force.* An occlusion that produces such injury is called a *traumatic occlusion.*[2] Excessive occlusal forces may also disrupt the function of the masticatory musculature and cause painful spasms, injure the temporomandibular joints, or produce excessive tooth wear, but the term *trauma from occlusion* is generally used in connection with injury in the periodontium.

Acute and Chronic Trauma

Trauma from occlusion may be acute or chronic. *Acute trauma from occlusion* results from an abrupt change in occlusal force, such as that produced by biting on a hard object (e.g., an olive pit). In addition, restorations or prosthetic appliances that interfere with or alter the direction of occlusal forces on the teeth may induce acute trauma. The results are tooth pain, sensitivity to percussion, and increased tooth mobility. If the force is dissipated by a shift in the position of the tooth or by wearing away or correction of the restoration, the injury heals and the symptoms subside. Otherwise, periodontal injury may worsen and develop into necrosis accompanied by periodontal abscess formation or persist as a symptom-free chronic condition. Acute trauma can also produce cementum tears (see Chapter 2).

Chronic trauma from occlusion is more common than the acute form and is of greater clinical significance. It most often develops from gradual changes in occlusion produced by tooth wear, drifting movement, and extrusion of teeth, combined with parafunctional habits such as bruxism and clenching, rather than as a sequela of acute periodontal trauma (see Chapter 28). The features of chronic trauma from occlusion and their significance are discussed in the text that follows.

The criterion that determines whether an occlusion is traumatic is whether it produces periodontal injury, not how the teeth occlude. Any occlusion that produces periodontal injury is traumatic. Malocclusion is not necessary to produce trauma; periodontal injury may occur when the occlusion appears normal. The dentition may be anatomically and aesthetically acceptable but functionally injurious. Similarly, not all malocclusions are necessarily injurious to the periodontium. Traumatic occlusal relationships are referred to by such terms as *occlusal disharmony, functional imbalance,* and *occlusal dystrophy.* These terms refer to the occlusion's effect on the periodontium, not to the position of the teeth. Because trauma from occlusion refers to the tissue injury rather than to the occlusion, an increased occlusal force is not traumatic if the periodontium can accommodate it.

Primary and Secondary Trauma From Occlusion

Trauma from occlusion may be caused by alterations in occlusal forces and/or reduced capacity of the periodontium to withstand occlusal forces. When trauma from occlusion is the result of alterations in occlusal forces, it is called *primary trauma from occlusion.* When it results from reduced ability of the tissues to resist the occlusal forces, it is known as *secondary trauma from occlusion.*

Primary trauma from occlusion occurs if trauma from occlusion is considered the primary etiologic factor in periodontal destruction and if the only local alteration to which a tooth is subjected is from occlusion. Examples are periodontal injury produced around teeth with a previously healthy periodontium following (1) the insertion of a "high filling," (2) the insertion of a prosthetic replacement that creates excessive forces on abutment and antagonistic teeth, (3) the drifting movement or extrusion of teeth into spaces created by unreplaced missing teeth, or (4) the orthodontic

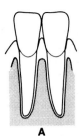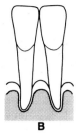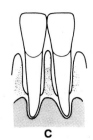

A   **B**   **C**

FIGURE 24–2. Traumatic forces can occur on *A*, normal periodontium with normal height of bone; *B*, normal periodontium with reduced height of bone; or *C*, marginal periodontitis with reduced height of bone.

movement of teeth into functionally unacceptable positions. Most studies on experimental animals of the effect of trauma from occlusion have examined the primary type of trauma. Changes produced by primary trauma do not alter the level of connective tissue attachment and do not initiate pocket formation. This is probably because the supracrestal gingival fibers are not affected and therefore prevent apical migration of the junctional epithelium.[50]

Secondary trauma from occlusion occurs when the adaptive capacity of the tissues to withstand occlusal forces is impaired by bone loss resulting from marginal inflammation. This reduces the periodontal attachment area and alters the leverage on the remaining tissues. The periodontium becomes more vulnerable to injury, and previously well-tolerated occlusal forces become traumatic.

Figure 24–2 depicts three different situations on which excessive occlusal forces can be superimposed:

1. Normal periodontium with normal height of bone.
2. Normal periodontium with reduced height of bone.
3. Marginal periodontitis with reduced height of bone.

The first case is an example of primary trauma from occlusion, whereas the last two represent secondary trauma from occlusion. The effects of trauma from occlusion in these different situations will be analyzed in the following discussion.

It has been found in experimental animals that systemic disorders can reduce tissue resistance and that previously tolerable forces may become excessive.[27,54,65] This could theoretically represent another mechanism by which tissue resistance to increased forces is lowered, resulting in secondary trauma from occlusion.

TISSUE RESPONSE TO INCREASED OCCLUSAL FORCES

Stages of Tissue Response

Tissue response occurs in three stages:[7,14] injury, repair, and adaptive remodeling of the periodontium.

Stage I: Injury. Tissue injury is produced by excessive occlusal forces. The body then attempts to repair the injury and restore the periodontium. This can occur if the forces are diminished or if the tooth drifts away from them. However, if the offending force is chronic, the periodontium is remodeled to cushion its impact. The ligament is widened at the expense of the bone, resulting in angular bone defects without periodontal pockets, and the tooth becomes loose.

Under the forces of occlusion, a tooth rotates around a

fulcrum or axis of rotation, which is located, in single-rooted teeth, in the junction between the middle third and the apical third of the clinical root (see Fig. 2–12). This creates areas of pressure and tension on opposite sides of the fulcrum. Different lesions are produced by different degrees of pressure and tension; if jiggling forces are exerted, these different lesions may coexist in the same area.

Slightly excessive pressure stimulates resorption of the alveolar bone, with a resultant widening of the periodontal ligament space. *Slightly excessive tension* causes elongation of the periodontal ligament fibers and apposition of alveolar bone. In areas of increased pressure, the blood vessels are numerous and reduced in size; in areas of increased tension, they are enlarged.[71]

Greater pressure produces a gradation of changes in the periodontal ligament, starting with compression of the fibers, which produces areas of hyalinization.[57,58] Subsequent injury to the fibroblasts and other connective tissue cells leads to necrosis of areas of the ligament.[55,59] Vascular changes are also produced: within 30 minutes, retardation and stasis of blood flow occur; at 2 to 3 hours, blood vessels appear to be packed with erythrocytes, which start to fragment; and between 1 and 7 days, there is disintegration of the blood vessel walls and release of the contents into the surrounding tissue.[56] In addition, increased resorption of alveolar bone and resorption of the tooth surface occur[34,38] (Figs. 24–3 and 24–4).

Severe tension causes widening of the periodontal ligament, thrombosis, hemorrhage, tearing of the periodontal ligament, and resorption of alveolar bone.

Pressure severe enough to force the root against bone causes necrosis of the periodontal ligament and bone. The bone is resorbed from viable periodontal ligament adjacent to necrotic areas and from marrow spaces, a process called undermining resorption.[31,46]

The areas of the periodontium most susceptible to injury from excessive occlusal forces are the furcations.[28]

Injury to the periodontium produces a temporary depression in mitotic activity and the rate of proliferation and differentiation of fibroblasts,[66] in collagen formation, and in bone formation.[34,61,66] These return to normal levels after dissipation of the forces.

Stage II: Repair. Repair is constantly occurring in the normal periodontium, and trauma from occlusion stimulates increased reparative activity.

The damaged tissues are removed, and new connective tissue cells and fibers, bone, and cementum are formed in an attempt to restore the injured periodontium (Fig. 24–5). Forces remain traumatic only as long as the damage produced exceeds the reparative capacity of the tissues.

When bone is resorbed by excessive occlusal forces, the body attempts to reinforce the thinned bony trabeculae with new bone (Fig. 24–6). This attempt to compensate for lost bone is called *buttressing bone formation* and is an important feature of the reparative process associated with trauma from occlusion.[25] It also occurs when bone is destroyed by inflammation or osteolytic tumors.

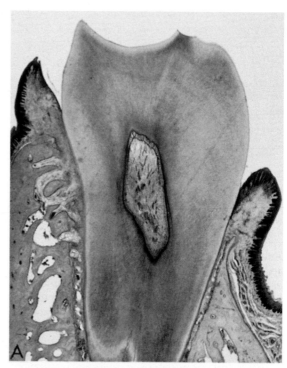

FIGURE 24–3. Periodontal accommodation to lateral forces. *A,* Mandibular premolar. *B,* Lingual surface, showing new bone formation in response to tension on the periodontal ligament. Note the pale-staining osteoid bordered by osteoblasts and the incremental lines indicative of previous additions to the bone. *C,* Facial surface shows compression of the periodontal ligament and osteoclastic resorption of the bony plate. Note the new bone formed on the external surface. This is peripheral buttressing bone, which reinforces the resorbing facial plate. Note, too, that the buttressing bone has produced a bulge in the bony contour.

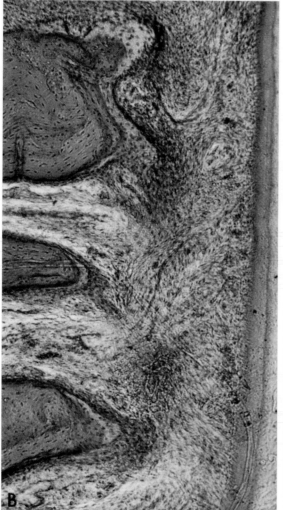

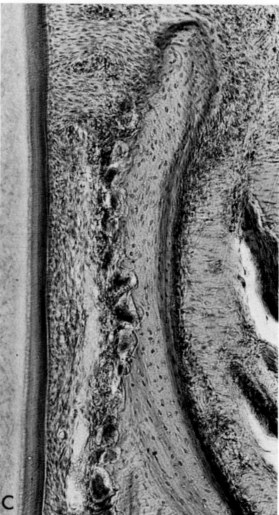

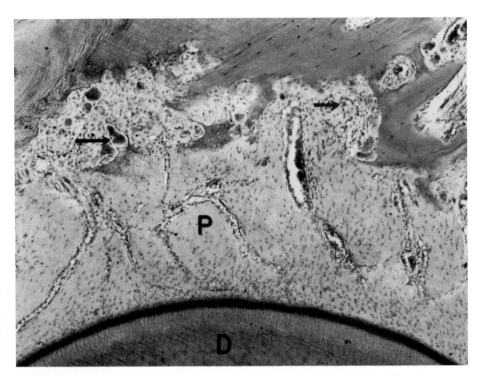

FIGURE 24-4. Trauma from occlusion at the root apex. Note bone resorption with prominent osteoclasts *(arrows)*. The periodontal ligament (P) is widened as the result of bone resorption, and the blood vessels are engorged. The root is shown at D.

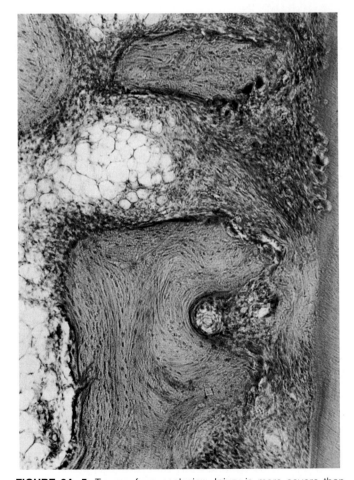

FIGURE 24-5. Trauma from occlusion. Injury is more severe than that shown in Figure 24-4. The cementum *(right)* is undergoing resorption, the periodontal ligament is compressed and necrotic, and the bone is undergoing resorption. Note the osteoblasts and new bone (central buttressing bone formation) on the trabecular margins adjacent to the marrow.

Buttressing bone formation occurs within the jaw (*central buttressing*) and on the bone surface (*peripheral buttressing*). In central buttressing the endosteal cells deposit new bone, which restores the bony trabeculae and reduces the size of the marrow spaces (see Fig. 24–6). Peripheral buttressing occurs on the facial and lingual surfaces of the alveolar plate. Depending on its severity, peripheral buttressing may produce a shelf-like thickening of the alveolar margin, referred to as *lipping* (Fig. 24–7; see also Fig. 24–3), or a pronounced bulge in the contour of the facial and lingual bone[14,22] (see Chapter 23).

Cartilage-like material sometimes develops in the periodontal ligament space as an aftermath of the trauma.[19] Formation of crystals from erythrocytes has also been shown.[60]

Stage III: Adaptive Remodeling of the Periodontium. If the repair process cannot keep pace with the destruction caused by the occlusion, the periodontium is remodeled in an effort to create a structural relationship in which the forces are no longer injurious to the tissues. *This results in a thickened periodontal ligament, which is funnel shaped at the crest, and angular defects in the bone, with no pocket formation. The involved teeth become loose.*[70] *Increased vascularization has also been reported.*[13]

The three stages in the evolution of traumatic lesions have been differentiated histometrically by means of the relative amounts of periodontal bone surface undergoing resorption or formation[8,14] (Fig. 24–8). The injury phase shows an increase in areas of resorption and a decrease in bone formation, whereas the repair phase demonstrates decreased resorption and increased bone formation. After adaptive remodeling of the periodontium, resorption and formation return to normal.

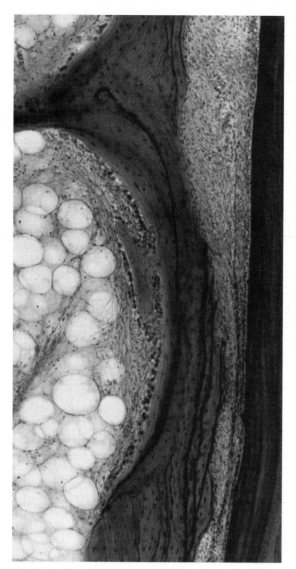

FIGURE 24–6. Central buttressing bone. New bone formation on the marrow side of alveolar bone that is undergoing resorption on the side of the periodontal ligament.

EFFECTS OF INSUFFICIENT OCCLUSAL FORCE

Insufficient occlusal force may also be injurious to the supporting periodontal tissues.[9,40] Insufficient stimulation causes thinning of the periodontal ligament, atrophy of the fibers, osteoporosis of the alveolar bone, and reduction in bone height. Hypofunction can result from an open-bite relationship, an absence of functional antagonists, or unilateral chewing habits that neglect one side of the mouth.

REVERSIBILITY OF TRAUMATIC LESIONS

Trauma from occlusion is reversible. When trauma is artificially induced in experimental animals, the teeth move away or intrude into the jaw. When the impact of the artificially created force is relieved, the tissues undergo repair. Although trauma from occlusion is reversible under such conditions, it does not always correct itself, nor is it therefore always temporary and of limited clinical significance. The injurious force must be relieved for repair to occur.[28,51] If conditions in humans do not permit the teeth to escape from or adapt to excessive occlusal force, periodontal damage persists[11] and worsens.

The presence in the periodontium of inflammation as a result of plaque accumulation may impair the reversibility of traumatic lesions.[35,51]

EFFECTS OF EXCESSIVE OCCLUSAL FORCES ON DENTAL PULP

The effects of excessive occlusal forces on the dental pulp have not been established. Some clinicians report the disappearance of pulpal symptoms after correction of excessive occlusal forces. Pulpal reactions have been noted in animals subjected to increased occlusal forces[12,39] but did not occur when the forces were minimal and occurred over short periods.[39]

INFLUENCE OF TRAUMA FROM OCCLUSION ON PROGRESSION OF MARGINAL PERIODONTITIS

Numerous studies have been performed to clarify the role of trauma from occlusion in the etiology of periodontal disease. Initial studies involved the placement of high crowns or restorations on the teeth of dogs or monkeys, resulting in a continuous or intermittent force in one direction.[2,32] These investigations provided an orthodontic type of force and gave clear descriptions of changes occurring in pressure zones and tension zones. These procedures usually resulted in tooth displacement and consolidation in a new, nontraumatized position.

Trauma from occlusion in humans, however, occurs as a result of forces that act alternately in opposing directions. These were analyzed in experimental animals with jiggling forces, usually produced by means of a high crown combined with an orthodontic appliance that would bring the traumatized tooth back to its original position when the force was dissipated by separating the teeth. In another method the teeth were separated by wooden or elastic material wedged interproximally to displace a tooth toward the opposite proximal side; after 48 hours the wedge was removed, and the procedure was repeated on the opposite side.

The procedures in these studies resulted in a combination of changes produced by pressure and tension on both sides of the tooth, with an increase in the width of the ligament and increased tooth mobility. None of these methods caused gingival inflammation or pocket formation, and the results essentially represented different degrees of functional adaptation to increased forces.[50,71]

To more closely mimic the problem in humans, studies were conducted on the effect produced by jiggling trauma and simultaneous plaque-induced gingival inflammation.

The local irritants that initiate gingivitis and periodontal pockets affect the marginal gingiva, but trauma from occlusion occurs in the supporting tissues and does not affect

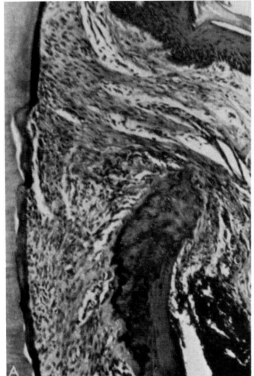
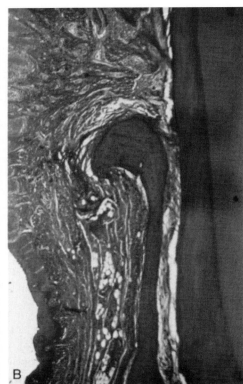

FIGURE 24–7. *A,* Widening of the periodontal ligament space in cervical area and a change in the shape of marginal alveolar bone as a result of chronic prolonged trauma from occlusion in rats. *B,* A comparable change in shape of marginal bone found in a human autopsy case.

the gingiva (Fig. 24–9). The marginal gingiva is unaffected by trauma from occlusion because its blood supply is sufficient to maintain it, even when the vessels of the periodontal ligament are obliterated by excessive occlusal forces.[30] Trauma from occlusion does not cause pockets or gingivitis,[2,29,34,53,69,70,72] nor does it have any influence on bacterial repopulation of pockets after scaling and root planing.[36]*

---

* Of historical interest are references 4 and 67, which describe periodontal pocket formation in animals as a result of trauma from occlusion.

As long as inflammation is confined to the gingiva, the inflammatory process is not affected by occlusal forces.[37] When inflammation extends from the gingiva into the supporting periodontal tissues (i.e., when gingivitis becomes periodontitis), plaque-induced inflammation enters the zone influenced by occlusion. Two groups have studied this topic extensively, with conflicting results, probably owing to the different methods used. The Eastman Dental Center group in Rochester, NY, used squirrel monkeys, induced trauma by repetitive interdental wedging, and induced mild to

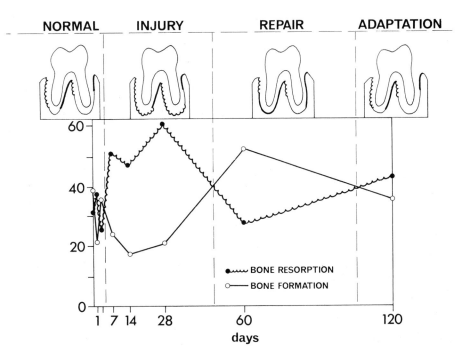

FIGURE 24–8. Evolution of traumatic lesions as depicted experimentally in rats by variations in relative amounts of areas of bone formation and bone resorption in periodontal bone surfaces. Horizontal axis: days after initiation of traumatic interference. Vertical axis: percentage of bone surface undergoing resorption or formation. The stages in the evolution of the lesions are represented in the top drawings, which show the average amount of bone activity for each group. See references 7 and 14.

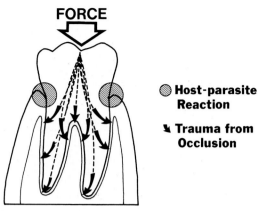

FORCE

⊘ **Host-parasite Reaction**

↘ **Trauma from Occlusion**

FIGURE 24–9. The reaction between dental plaque and the host takes place in the gingival sulcus region. Trauma from occlusion appears in the tissues supporting the tooth.

moderate gingival inflammation; experimental times were up to 10 weeks. They reported that the presence of trauma did not increase the loss of attachment induced by periodontitis.[45,48,49,52] The University of Gothenburg group in Sweden used beagle dogs, induced trauma by placing cap splints and orthodontic appliances, and induced severe gingival inflammation; experimental times were up to 1 year. This group found that occlusal stresses increase the periodontal destruction induced by periodontitis.[16,17,43]

When trauma from occlusion is eliminated, a substantial reversal of bone loss occurs, except in the presence of periodontitis. This indicates that inflammation inhibits the potential for bone regeneration.[35,42,50,51] *Thus, it is important to eliminate the marginal inflammatory component in cases of trauma from occlusion, because the presence or absence of inflammation affects bone regeneration after the removal of the traumatizing contacts.*[35] It has also been shown in experimental animals that trauma from occlusion does not induce progressive destruction of the periodontal tissues in regions kept healthy after the elimination of pre-existent periodontitis.[16]

Trauma from occlusion also tends to change the shape of the alveolar crest. The change in shape consists of a widening of the marginal periodontal ligament space, a narrowing of the interproximal alveolar bone, and a shelf-like thickening of the alveolar margin.[14,43,45] Therefore, although trauma from occlusion does not alter the inflammatory process, it changes the architecture of the area around the inflamed site.[14,43] *Thus, in the absence of inflammation, the response to trauma from occlusion is limited to adaptation to the increased forces. However, in the presence of inflammation, the changes in the shape of the alveolar crest may be conducive to angular bone loss, and existing pockets may become infrabony.*

Other theories that have been proposed to explain the interaction of trauma and inflammation include the following:

1. Trauma from occlusion may alter the pathway of extension of gingival inflammation to the underlying tissues. Inflammation then may proceed to the periodontal ligament rather than to the bone. Resulting bone loss would be angular, and pockets could become infrabony.[1,20,22,24,26,44]

2. Trauma-induced areas of root resorption uncovered by apical migration of the inflamed gingival attachment may offer a favorable environment for the formation and attachment of plaque and calculus and may therefore be responsible for the development of deeper lesions.[62]

3. Supragingival plaque can become subgingival if the tooth is tilted orthodontically or migrates into an edentulous area, resulting in the transformation of a suprabony pocket into an infrabony pocket.[15,18]

The possible combined effect of inflammation and trauma from occlusion does not rule out the possibility that both may be present without resulting in infrabony pockets and angular defects. The inflammation or the trauma may not be severe enough or the anatomy of the tooth or bone may not be conducive to the formation of such pockets or defects. In addition, these periodontal lesions may be produced by etiologic factors other than the combination of inflammation and trauma from occlusion. *Therefore, although not every infrabony pocket develops because of a combination of trauma and inflammation, this possibility should always be considered.*

Clinical and Radiographic Signs of Trauma From Occlusion Alone

The most common clinical sign of trauma to the periodontium is increased tooth mobility. In the injury stage of trauma from occlusion, there is destruction of periodontal fibers, which will increase the mobility of the tooth. In the final stage, the accommodation of the periodontium to increased forces entails a widening of the periodontal ligament, which also leads to increased tooth mobility. Although this tooth mobility is greater than the so-called normal mobility, it cannot be considered pathologic, because it is an adaptation and not a disease process. When it becomes progressively worse, it can be considered pathologic.

Other causes of increased tooth mobility include advanced bone loss, inflammation of the periodontal ligament that is of periodontal or periapical origin, and some systemic causes (e.g., pregnancy). The destruction of surrounding alveolar bone, such as occurs in osteomyelitis or jaw tumors, may also increase tooth mobility (see Chapter 28).

The radiographic signs of trauma from occlusion include (1) increased width of the periodontal space, often with thickening of the lamina dura along the lateral aspect of the root, in the apical region, and in bifurcation areas; (2) a "vertical" rather than "horizontal" destruction of the interdental septum; (3) radiolucence and condensation of the alveolar bone; and (4) root resorption (see Chapter 29).

The widening of the periodontal space and thickening of the lamina dura do not necessarily indicate destructive changes. They may result from thickening and strengthening of the periodontal ligament and alveolar bone, which constitute a favorable response to increased occlusal forces (Fig. 24–10).

In summary, trauma from occlusion does not initiate gingivitis or periodontal pockets, but it may affect the progress and severity of periodontal pockets started by local irritation. An understanding of the effect of trauma from occlu-

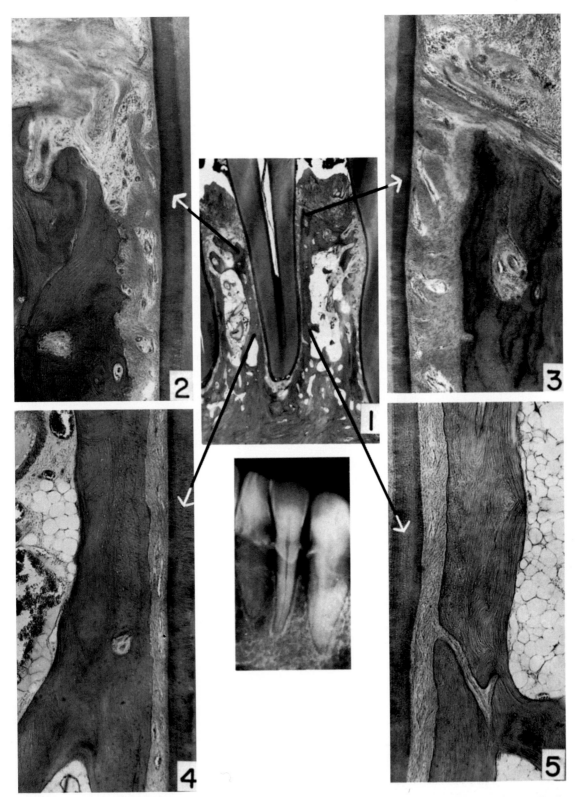

FIGURE 24–10. Widened periodontal space produced by two types of tissue response to increased occlusal forces. Radiograph shows thickening of periodontal space and lamina dura around the lateral incisor. *1,* Survey microscopic section of the lateral incisor. *2,* Mesial surface widening of the periodontal space has resulted from resorption of alveolar bone associated with pressure. *3,* Distal surface widening of the periodontal space has resulted from thickening of the periodontal ligament, which is a favorable response to increased tension. *4* and *5,* Thinned periodontal ligament at axis of rotation, one third the distance from the apex.

sion on the periodontium is useful in the clinical management of periodontal problems.

PATHOLOGIC TOOTH MIGRATION

Pathologic migration refers to tooth displacement that results when the balance among the factors that maintain physiologic tooth position is disturbed by periodontal disease. Pathologic migration is relatively common and may be an early sign of disease, or it may occur in association with gingival inflammation and pocket formation as the disease progresses.

Pathologic migration occurs most frequently in the anterior region, but posterior teeth may also be affected. The teeth may move in any direction, and the migration is usually accompanied by mobility and rotation. Pathologic migration in the occlusal or incisal direction is termed *extrusion.* All degrees of pathologic migration are encountered, and one or more teeth may be affected (Fig. 24–11). It is important to detect it in its early stages and to prevent more serious involvement by eliminating the causative factors. Even in the early stage, some degree of bone loss occurs.

Pathogenesis

Two major factors play a role in maintaining the normal position of the teeth: the health and normal height of the periodontium and the forces exerted on the teeth. The latter includes the forces of occlusion, as well as pressure from the lips, cheeks, and tongue. The following factors are important in relation to the forces of occlusion: tooth morphologic features and cuspal inclination; the presence of a full complement of teeth; a physiologic tendency toward mesial migration; the nature and location of contact point relationships; proximal, incisal, and occlusal attrition; and the axial inclination of the teeth. Alterations in any of these factors start an interrelated sequence of changes in the environment of a single tooth or group of teeth that results in pathologic migration. Thus, pathologic migration occurs under conditions that weaken the periodontal support and/or increase or modify the forces exerted on the teeth.

Weakened Periodontal Support. *The inflammatory destruction of the periodontium in periodontitis creates an imbalance between the forces maintaining the tooth in position and the occlusal and muscular forces it is ordinarily called on to bear.* The tooth with weakened support is unable to maintain its normal position in the arch and moves away from the opposing force, unless it is restrained by proximal contact. The force that moves the weakly supported tooth may be created by factors such as occlusal contacts or pressure from the tongue.

It is important to understand that *the abnormality in pathologic migration rests with the weakened periodontium.* The force itself need not be abnormal. Forces that are acceptable to an intact periodontium become injurious when periodontal support is reduced. An example of this is the tooth with abnormal proximal contacts. Abnormally located proximal contacts convert the normal anterior component of force to a wedging force that moves the tooth occlusally or

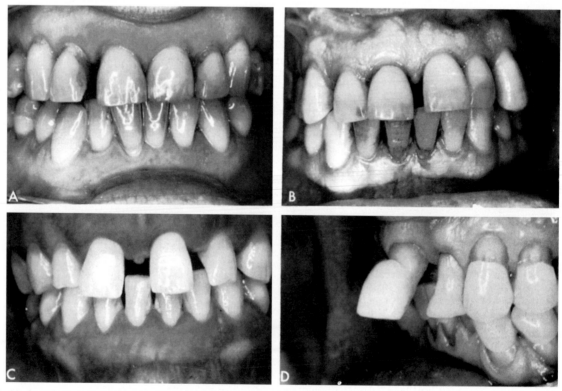

FIGURE 24–11. Stages in pathologic migration. *A,* Migration of the right maxillary lateral incisor. *B,* Labial migration of maxillary central incisors and left canine, and mesial migration of the right lateral incisor. *C,* Migration and extrusion of maxillary and mandibular incisors. *D,* Severe migration of the maxillary central incisor.

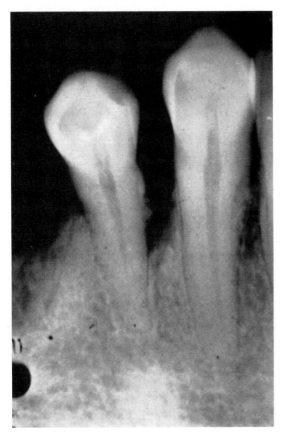

FIGURE 24–12. Calculus and bone loss on the mesial surface of a canine that has drifted distally.

incisally. The wedging force, which can be withstood by the intact periodontium, causes the tooth to extrude when the periodontal support is weakened by disease. *As its position changes, the tooth is subjected to abnormal occlusal forces, which aggravate the periodontal destruction and the tooth migration.*

Pathologic migration may continue after a tooth no longer contacts its antagonist. Pressures from the tongue,

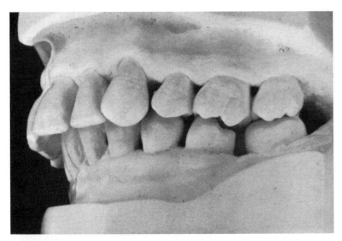

FIGURE 24–13. Maxillary first molar tilted and extruded into the space created by a missing mandibular tooth.

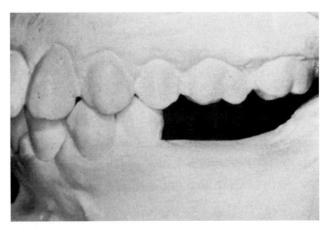

FIGURE 24–14. No drifting or extrusion despite 4 years' absence of mandibular teeth.

from the food bolus during mastication, and from proliferating granulation tissue provide the force.

Pathologic migration is also an early sign of localized juvenile periodontitis. Weakened by loss of periodontal support, the maxillary and mandibular anterior incisors drift labially and extrude, creating diastemata between the teeth (see Chapter 27).

Changes in the Forces Exerted on the Teeth. Changes in the magnitude, direction, or frequency of the forces exerted on the teeth can induce pathologic migration of a tooth or group of teeth. These forces do not have to be abnormal to cause migration if the periodontium is sufficiently weakened. Changes in the forces may occur as a result of unreplaced missing teeth, failure to replace first molars, or other causes.

Unreplaced Missing Teeth. Drifting of teeth into the spaces created by unreplaced missing teeth often occurs. Drifting differs from pathologic migration in that it does not result from destruction of the periodontal tissues. However, it usually creates conditions that lead to periodontal disease, and thus the initial tooth movement is aggravated by loss of periodontal support (Fig. 24–12).

Drifting generally occurs in a mesial direction, combined with tilting or extrusion beyond the occlusal plane. The premolars frequently drift distally (Fig. 24–13). Although drifting is a common sequela when missing teeth are not replaced, it does not always occur (Fig. 24–14).

Failure to Replace First Molars. The pattern of changes that may follow failure to replace missing first molars is characteristic. In extreme cases it consists of the following:

1. The second and third molars tilt, resulting in a decrease in vertical dimension (Fig. 24–15).
2. The premolars move distally, and the mandibular incisors tilt or drift lingually. The mandibular premolars, while drifting distally, lose their intercuspating relationship with the maxillary teeth and may tilt distally.
3. Anterior overbite is increased. The mandibular incisors strike the maxillary incisors near the gingiva or traumatize the gingiva.
4. The maxillary incisors are pushed labially and laterally (Fig. 24–16).

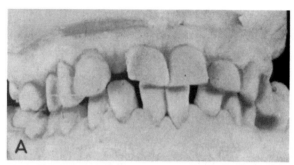

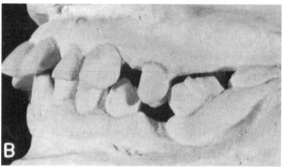
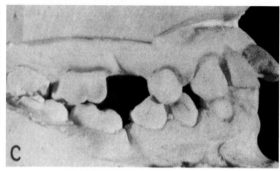

FIGURE 24–15. *A–C,* Mutilation of occlusion associated with unreplaced missing teeth. Note pronounced pathologic migration, disturbed proximal contacts, and functional relationships with closing of the bite.

5. The anterior teeth extrude because the incisal apposition has largely disappeared.
6. Diastemata are created by the separation of the anterior teeth (see Fig. 24–15).

The disturbed proximal contact relationships lead to food impaction, gingival inflammation, and pocket formation, followed by bone loss and tooth mobility. Occlusal disharmonies created by the altered tooth positions traumatize the supporting tissues of the periodontium and aggravate the destruction caused by the inflammation. Reduction in periodontal support leads to further migration of the teeth and mutilation of the occlusion.

Other Causes. *Trauma from occlusion* may cause a shift in tooth position either by itself or in combination with inflammatory periodontal disease. The direction of movement depends on the occlusal force.

Pressure from the tongue may cause drifting of the teeth in the absence of periodontal disease or may contribute to pathologic migration of teeth with reduced periodontal support (Fig. 24–17).

In tooth support weakened by periodontal destruction, *pressure from the granulation tissue of periodontal pockets* has been mentioned as contributing to pathologic migration.[33] The teeth may return to their original positions after the pockets are eliminated, but if there has been more destruction on one side of a tooth than on the other, the healing tissues tend to pull in the direction of the lesser destruction.

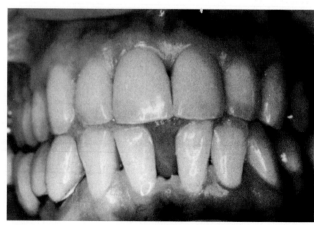

FIGURE 24–16. Maxillary incisors pushed labially in patient with bilateral unreplaced mandibular molars. Note extrusion of the maxillary molars.

FIGURE 24–17. Pathologic migration associated with tongue pressure.

REFERENCES

1. Ballbe R, Carranza FA, Erausquin R. Los paradencios del caso ocho. Rev Odont (Buenos Aires) 26:606, 1938.
2. Bhaskar SN, Orban B. Experimental occlusal trauma. J Periodontol 26:270, 1955.
3. Box HK. Traumatic occlusion and traumatogenic occlusion. Oral Health 20:642, 1930.
4. Box HK. Experimental traumatogenic occlusion in sheep. Oral Health 25:9, 1935.
5. Box HK. Twelve Periodontal Studies. Toronto, University of Toronto Press, 1940, p 55.
6. Budtz-Jorgensen E. Bruxism and trauma from occlusion. J Clin Periodontol 7:149, 1980.
7. Carranza FA Jr. Histometric evaluation of periodontal pathology. J Periodontol 38:741, 1970.
8. Carranza FA Jr, Cabrini RL. Histometric studies of periodontal tissues. Periodontics 5:308, 1967.
9. Cohn SA. Disuse atrophy of the periodontium in molar teeth of mice. J Dent Res 40:707, 1961.
10. Comar MD, Kollar JA, Gargiulo AW. Local irritation and occlusal trauma as cofactors in the periodontal disease process. J Periodontol 40:193, 1969.
11. Coolidge ED. Traumatic and functional injuries occurring in the supporting tissues on human teeth. J Am Dent Assoc 25:343, 1938.
12. Cooper MB, Landay MA, Seltzer S. The effects of excessive occlusal forces on the pulp. II. Heavier and longer term forces. J Periodontol 42:353, 1971.
13. Dotto CA, Carranza FA Jr, Cabrini RL, Itoiz ME. Vascular changes in experimental trauma from occlusion. J Periodontol 38:183, 1967.
14. Dotto CA, Carranza FA Jr, Itoiz ME. Efectos mediatos del trauma experimental en ratas. Rev Asoc Odontol Argent 54:48, 1966.
15. Ericsson I. The combined effects of plaque and physical stress on periodontal tissues. J Clin Periodontol 13:918, 1986.
16. Ericsson I, Lindhe J. Lack of effect of trauma from occlusion on the recurrence of experimental periodontitis. J Clin Periodontol 4:115, 1977.
17. Ericsson I, Lindhe J. Effect of longstanding jiggling on experimental marginal periodontitis in the beagle dog. J Clin Periodontol 9:497, 1982.
18. Ericsson I, Thilander B, Lindhe J, Okamoto H. The effect of orthodontic tilting movements on the periodontal tissues of infected and noninfected dentitions in dogs. J Clin Periodontol 4:278, 1977.
19. Everett FG, Bruckner RJ. Cartilage in the periodontal ligament space. J Periodontol 41:165, 1970.
20. Glickman I. Occlusion and the periodontium. J Dent Res 46(suppl 53):53, 1967.
21. Glickman I, Roeber F, Brion M, Pameijer J. Photoelastic analysis of internal stresses in the periodontium created by occlusal forces. J Periodontol 41:30, 1970.
22. Glickman I, Smulow JB. Alterations in the pathway of gingival inflammation into the underlying tissues induced by excessive occlusal forces. J Periodontol 33:7, 1962.
23. Glickman I, Smulow JB. Buttressing bone formation in the periodontium. J Periodontol 36:365, 1965.
24. Glickman I, Smulow JB. Effect of excessive occlusal forces upon the pathway of gingival inflammation in humans. J Periodontol 36:141, 1965.
25. Glickman I, Smulow JB. Adaptive alterations in the periodontium of the rhesus monkey in chronic trauma from occlusion. J Periodontol 39:101, 1968.
26. Glickman I, Smulow JB. The combined effects of inflammation and trauma from occlusion to periodontitis. Int Dent J 19:393, 1969.
27. Glickman I, Smulow JB, Moreau J. Effect of alloxan diabetes upon the periodontal response to excessive occlusal forces. J Periodontol 37:146, 1966.
28. Glickman I, Stein RS, Smulow JB. The effects of increased functional forces upon the periodontium of splinted and nonsplinted teeth. J Periodontol 32:290, 1961.
29. Glickman I, Weiss L. Role of trauma from occlusion in initiation of periodontal pocket formation in experimental animals. J Periodontol 26:14, 1955.
30. Goldman H. Gingival vascular supply in induced occlusal traumatism. Oral Surg Oral Med Oral Pathol 9:939, 1956.
31. Gottlieb B, Orban B. Changes in the Tissue due to Excessive Force upon the Teeth. Leipzig, G Thieme, 1931.
32. Gottlieb B, Orban B. Tissue changes in experimental traumatic occlusion with special reference to age and constitution. J Dent Res 11:505, 1931.
33. Hirschfeld I. The dynamic relationship between pathologically migrating teeth and inflammatory tissue in periodontal pockets: A clinical study. J Periodontol 4:35, 1933.
34. Itoiz ME, Carranza FA Jr, Cabrini RL. Histologic and histometric study of experimental occlusal trauma in rats. J Periodontol 34:305, 1963.
35. Kantor M, Polson AN, Zander HA. Alveolar bone regeneration after removal of inflammatory and traumatic factors. J Periodontol 46:687, 1976.
36. Kaufman H, Carranza FA Jr, Enders B, et al. The influence of trauma from occlusion on the bacterial repopulation of periodontal pockets in dogs. J Periodontol 55:86, 1984.
37. Kenney EB. A histopathologic study of incisal dysfunction and gingival inflammation in the rhesus monkey. J Periodontol 42:3, 1971.
38. Kvam E. Scanning electron microscopy of tissue changes on the pressure surface of human premolars following tooth movement. Scand J Dent Res 80:357, 1972.
39. Landay MA, Nazimov H, Seltzer S. The effects of excessive occlusal forces on the pulp. J Periodontol 41:3, 1970.
40. Levy G, Mailland ML. Etude quantitative des effets de l'hypofonction occlusale sur la largeur desmodontale et la resorption osteoclastique alveolaire chez le rat. J Biol Buccale 8:17, 1980.
41. Lindhe J, Ericsson I. The influence of trauma from occlusion on reduced but healthy periodontal tissues in dogs. J Clin Periodontol 3:110, 1976.
42. Lindhe J, Ericsson I. The effect of elimination of jiggling forces on periodontally exposed teeth in the dog. J Periodontol 53:562, 1982.
43. Lindhe J, Svanberg G. Influence of trauma from occlusion on progression of experimental periodontitis in the beagle dog. J Clin Periodontol 1:3, 1974.
44. Macapanpan LC, Weinmann JP. The influence of injury to the periodontal membrane on the spread of gingival inflammation. J Dent Res 33:263, 1954.
45. Meitner S. Co-destructive factors of marginal periodontitis and repetitive mechanical injury. J Dent Res 54:C78, 1975.
46. Orban B. Tissue changes in traumatic occlusion. J Am Dent Assoc 15:2090, 1928.
47. Orban B, Weinmann JP. Signs of traumatic occlusion in average human jaws. J Dent Res 13:216, 1933.
48. Polson AM. Trauma and progression of marginal periodontitis in squirrel monkeys. II. Codestructive factors of periodontitis and mechanically produced injury. J Periodontol Res 9:108, 1974.
49. Polson AM. The relative importance of plaque and occlusion in periodontal disease. J Clin Periodontol 13:923, 1986.
50. Polson AM, Meitner SW, Zander HA. Trauma and progression of marginal periodontitis in squirrel monkeys. III. Adaption of interproximal alveolar bone to repetitive injury. J Periodont Res 11:279, 1976.
51. Polson AM, Meitner SW, Zander HA. Trauma and progression of marginal periodontitis in squirrel monkeys. IV. Reversibility of bone loss due to trauma alone and trauma superimposed upon periodontitis. J Periodont Res 11:290, 1976.
52. Polson AM, Zander HA. Effect of periodontal trauma upon intrabony pockets. J Periodontol 54:586, 1983.
53. Ramfjord SP, Kohler CA. Periodontal reaction to functional occlusal stress. J Periodontol 30:95, 1959.
54. Rothblatt JM, Waldo CM. Tissue response to tooth movement in normal and abnormal metabolic states. J Dent Res 32:678, 1953.
55. Rygh P. Ultrastructural cellular reactions in pressure zones of rat molar periodontium incident to orthodontic movement. Acta Odontol Scand 30:575, 1972.
56. Rygh P. Ultrastructural vascular changes in pressure zones of rat molar periodontium incident to orthodontic movement. Scand J Dent Res 80:307, 1972.
57. Rygh P. Ultrastructural changes in pressure zones of human periodontium incident to orthodontic tooth movement. Acta Odontol Scand 31:109, 1973.
58. Rygh P. Ultrastructural changes of the periodontal fibers and their attachment in rat molar periodontium incident to orthodontic tooth movement. Scand J Dent Res 81:467, 1973.
59. Rygh P. Elimination of hyalinized periodontal tissues associated with orthodontic tooth movement. Scand J Dent Res 82:57, 1974.
60. Rygh P, Selvig KA. Erythrocytic crystallization in rat molar periodontium incident to tooth movement. Scand J Dent Res 81:62, 1973.
61. Solt CW, Glickman I. A histologic and radioautographic study of healing following wedging interdental injury in mice. J Periodontol 39:249, 1968.
62. Sottosanti JS. A possible relationship between occlusion, root resorption and the progression of periodontal disease. J West Soc Periodont 25:69, 1977.
63. Stahl SS. The responses of the periodontium to combined gingival inflammation and occlusofunctional stresses in four human surgical specimens. Periodontics 6:14, 1968.
64. Stahl SS. Accommodation of the periodontium to occlusal trauma and inflammatory periodontal disease. Dent Clin North Am 19:531, 1975.
65. Stahl SS, Miller SC, Goldsmith ED. The effects of vertical occlusal trauma on the periodontium of protein deprived young adult rats. J Periodontol 28:87, 1957.
66. Stallard RE. The effect of occlusal alterations on collagen formation within the periodontium. Periodontics 2:49, 1964.
67. Stones HH. An experimental investigation into the association of traumatic occlusion with paradontal disease. Proc Soc Med 31:479, 1938.
68. Svanberg G, Lindhe J. Vascular reactions to the periodontal ligament incident to trauma from occlusion. J Clin Periodontol 1:58, 1974.
69. Waerhaug J, Hansen ER. Periodontal changes incidental to prolonged occlusal overload in monkeys. Acta Odontol Scand 24:91, 1966.
70. Wentz FM, Jarabak J, Orban B. Experimental occlusal trauma imitating cuspal interferences. J Periodontol 29:117, 1958.
71. Zaki AE, Van Huysen G. Histology of the periodontium following tooth movement. J Dent Res 42:1373, 1963.
72. Zander HA, Muhlemann HR. The effect of stresses on the periodontal structures. Oral Surg Oral Med Oral Pathol 9:380, 1956

25

Slowly Progressive Periodontitis

FERMIN A. CARRANZA, JR., DONALD F. ADAMS, and
MICHAEL. G. NEWMAN

Clinical Features	**Prevalence**
Etiology	**Progression**
Symptoms	**Types**

Periodontitis is the most common type of periodontal disease. It results from extension of the inflammatory process initiated in the gingiva to the supporting structures of the tooth. Various classifications of periodontitis have been developed since the second or third decade of the 20th century, when "modern" analysis techniques began to be used to study its microscopic and clinical characteristics. The classification adopted in this book and presented in Chapter 4 is summarized in Table 25–1.

CLINICAL FEATURES

The characteristic findings in slowly progressive periodontitis (SPP) are gingival inflammation, which results from the accumulation of plaque, and loss of periodontal attachment and alveolar bone, which results in the formation of a pocket (Fig. 25–1). In many patients gingival inflammation is not visible on inspection and can be detected only by examination with a periodontal probe. Because SPP often takes many years to progress, it has often been called *chronic adult periodontitis* or *chronic inflammatory periodontitis.*

The disease is usually generalized, although some areas may be more deeply involved than others. Areas of more advanced involvement are usually associated with poorer plaque control and can be found in relatively inaccessible sites such as furcation areas or malposed teeth. However, there is no consistent pattern of distribution of periodontitis lesions, except for the distinction that the lesions are usually not isolated to one or two sites. Isolated localized lesions of periodontitis that occur in adults are most often associated with exacerbating local etiologic factors and occur after active periodontitis treatment. These localized sites that do not respond to mechanical periodontal maintenance therapy are often called *refractory sites,* and the patient is called a *refractory periodontitis patient.*

The gingivae will ordinarily be slightly to moderately swollen and exhibit alterations in color ranging from a pale red to magenta. Loss of stippling and changes in the surface topography may include blunted or rolled gingival margins and flattened or cratered papillae. In some cases, probably as a result of long-standing low-grade inflammation, thickened, fibrotic marginal tissues may obscure the underlying inflammatory changes. As previously mentioned, a periodontal probe must be used to detect the periodontitis lesion.

Gingival bleeding, either spontaneous or easily provoked, is frequent, and inflammation-related exudate and suppuration from the pocket may also be found. When the pocket is sealed off, pus cannot drain, and an abscess may form. These localized areas of acute inflammation do not develop very often, but when they do, they may require emergency care.

Pocket depths are variable, and both horizontal and angular bone loss can be found. Tooth mobility often appears in advanced cases when bone loss has been considerable.

Therefore, SPP can be diagnosed clinically by the detection of chronic inflammatory changes in the marginal gingiva and the presence of periodontal pockets; it is diagnosed radiographically by evidence of bone loss. These findings may be similar to those seen in rapidly progressive disease; the differential diagnosis is based on the patient's history and/or responsiveness to therapy.

When trauma from occlusion coexists, a higher incidence of infrabony pockets, angular bone loss, widening of the periodontal ligament, and earlier and more severe tooth mobility are found.

ETIOLOGY

SPP is always associated with the presence of plaque. Plaque is found in abundance in areas where clinical changes are more extensive; calculus, both supragingival and subgingival, is also found in abundance. Thus, SPP is closely related to poor oral hygiene.

Although immunocompetency can vary, SPP apparently is not associated with unusual systemic immunologic defects, as no serum, neutrophil, or monocyte abnormalities have been identified[4] (see Chapter 9).

Intercurrent development of systemic diseases (e.g., diabetes), hormonal alterations, or immunologic defects may alter the host response to existing plaque, accelerating the progression of periodontitis and exacerbating the severity and extent of the resultant tissue destruction. Patients with

Table 25–1. CLASSIFICATION OF PERIODONTITIS

Classification	Abbreviation	Common Synonym
Slowly progressive periodontitis	SPP	Adult periodontitis
Rapidly progressive periodontitis		
Adult onset (age >20 yr)	RPP	Rapidly progressive periodontitis
Pubertal and adolescent onset (age between 11 and 19 yr)	JP	Juvenile periodontitis, localized juvenile periodontitis
Prepubertal onset (age <11 yr)	PPP	Prepubertal periodontitis
Necrotizing ulcerative periodontitis	NUP	Necrotizing periodontitis
Refractory periodontitis	RP	Refractory periodontitis, nonresponsive periodontitis

contributory systemic diseases should always be considered as if their disease is in the process of converting from slowly progressive disease to rapidly progressive periodontal disease.

SYMPTOMS

SPP is usually painless. This fact is considered a major obstacle in convincing patients to seek treatment. In addition, a negative response to questions such as "Are you in pain?" is not sufficient to eliminate suspicion of SPP. Occasionally, exposed roots may be sensitive to heat and/or cold in the absence of caries. Areas of localized dull pain, sometimes radiating deep into the jaw, have been associated with SPP. The presence of areas of food impaction may add to the patient's discomfort. Gingival tenderness or "itchiness" can also be found.

Acute pain may result from the formation of a periodontal abscess, and root caries or recurrent caries may result in pulpal symptoms.

PREVALENCE

The incidence and prevalence of SPP vary throughout the world and are discussed in detail in Chapter 5. Periodontitis increases in prevalence and severity with age, generally affecting both sexes equally. In the Sri Lanka studies conducted by Löe and coworkers,[3] 81% of the individuals who had never received dental treatment had slowly or moderately progressive disease characterized by a yearly loss of attachment of 0.05 to 0.5 mm.

PROGRESSION

Adults appear to have the same susceptibility to SPP throughout their lives. Onset of this form of periodontitis can occur at any time, but the first signs can often be detected during adolescence. Because of its slow rate of progression, SPP becomes clinically significant in the mid-thirties or later. In patients who are untreated or undertreated, it reaches advanced stages in the forties or fifties. Its rate of progress is quite variable.

SPP does not progress at an equal rate in all affected sites throughout the mouth. Some involved areas may remain static for long periods of time,[1] whereas others may progress more rapidly. More rapidly progressive lesions oc-

cur most frequently in interproximal areas[2] and are usually associated with areas of greater plaque accumulation and inaccessibility to plaque control measures (e.g., furcation areas, overhanging margins, sites of malposed teeth, or areas of food impaction).

For those sites that do exhibit breakdown, a common impression is that the disease extends slowly and inexorably to tooth loss. Intervals between periodontal maintenance appointments are often based on the belief that the disease will continue to progress.

Several models have been proposed to describe the rate of disease progression.[5] In these models progression is measured by determining how much attachment is lost over a given period of time and throughout many periods. The *continuous model,* the *random* or *episodic burst model,* and the *asynchronous multiple burst model* are described in Chapter 9.

Periodontitis is the result of a complex, multifactorial interaction between host and infective agents, and the entire pathogenic relationship, as well as the mechanism of progression, is still unclear. The progression of periodontitis results from a lack of balance between the microbial insult to the attachment apparatus and the competency of the host's defense mechanisms. Local host defense factors appear to play an important role in the particular pattern and severity of disease at the local site. In SPP, systemic disease does not cause the pathologic changes.

The microbiology of the associated plaque has been described in Chapter 6. In general *attached* subgingival plaque usually contains *Actinomyces* species and a flora consisting of gram-positive and gram-negative filaments; spirochetes and gram-negative motile and nonmotile rods dominate subgingival *unattached* plaque.

TYPES

Mild periodontitis is usually characterized by probing attachment loss of 2 to 4 mm, minimal furcation invasions, and little tooth mobility. Supra- and subgingival plaque are present, along with various amounts of calculus. Bleeding on gentle probing is commonly seen. Radiographic evidence of bone loss is minimal (usually less than 20% of the total attachment). This stage of involvement can be localized to several teeth or generalized to many areas throughout the mouth.

Patients with *moderate periodontitis* exhibit 4 to 7 mm of probing attachment loss, early to moderate furcation invasions, and slight to moderate tooth mobility. Radiographi-

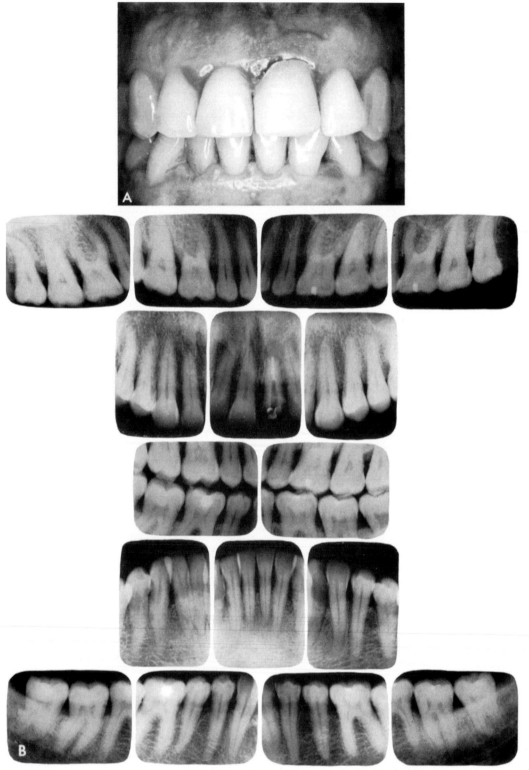

FIGURE 25–1. Marginal periodontitis in a 47-year-old female. *A,* Clinical view showing generalized gingival inflammation and periodontal pocket formation. *B,* Radiographs showing generalized horizontal bone loss that varies in severity in different areas.

cally evident bone loss is usually horizontal and may consist of up to 40% of the total possible periodontal attachment on the tooth. Furcation radiolucencies may be evident. Bleeding on probing is a frequent finding, and purulence may be seen.

Patients with *severe periodontitis* have a probing at-

tachment loss of 7 mm or more with significant furcation invasions, often through and through. Excessive tooth mobility is commonly found. Radiographic bone loss exceeds 40%, and angular bony defects are seen. Purulent exudate can be present, along with bleeding on probing.

REFERENCES

1. Lindhe J, Okamoto H, Yoneyama T, et al. Longitudinal changes in periodontal disease in untreated subjects. J Clin Periodontol *16:*662, 1989.
2. Lindhe J, Okamoto H, Yoneyama T, et al. Periodontal loser sites in untreated adult subjects. J Clin Periodontol *16:*671, 1989.
3. Löe H, Ånerud Å, Boysen H, Morrison E. Natural history of periodontal disease in man: Rapid, moderate and no loss of attachment in Sri Lanka laborers 14 to 46 years of age. J Clin Periodontol *13:*431, 1986.
4. Page RC, Schroeder HE. Periodontitis in Man and Other Animals. New York, Karger, 1982.
5. Socransky SS, Haffajee AD, Goodson JM, Lindhe J. New concepts of destructive periodontal disease. J Clin Periodontol *11:*21, 1984.

26

Rapidly Progressive Periodontitis, Necrotizing Ulcerative Periodontitis, and Refractory Periodontitis

FERMIN A. CARRANZA, JR., DONALD F. ADAMS, and
MICHAEL G. NEWMAN

Rapidly Progressive Periodontitis—Adult Onset
Necrotizing Ulcerative Periodontitis
Non-AIDS Type Necrotizing Ulcerative Periodontitis

AIDS-Associated Necrotizing Ulcerative Periodontitis
Refractory Periodontitis

This chapter will cover rapidly progressive periodontitis of adult onset, necrotizing ulcerative periodontitis (NUP), and the refractory forms of periodontitis.

When rapidly progressive periodontitis (RPP) occurs in adults, it is often referred to as *adult onset RPP*. The disease also affects juveniles and is referred to as *juvenile onset RPP*. Juveniles (generally considered to be anyone younger than 20 years old) can be further differentiated as either *prepubertal* or *postpubertal*. The pattern of involvement can be generalized or localized. Juvenile onset forms of RPP are discussed in Chapter 27.

RAPIDLY PROGRESSIVE PERIODONTITIS—ADULT ONSET

Clinical Findings. Differentiating between slowly progressive periodontitis (SPP) (see Chapter 25) and RPP, which is a more aggressive lesion, is often difficult, because their clinical features often overlap. A patient with SPP might develop one or several sites that deteriorate much more rapidly than other spots. In periodontal maintenance patients, multiple sites often break down between periodontal maintenance treatments. These patients are often not diagnosed as having RPP, because (1) there are relatively few sites involved at any one time, (2) "normal"

maintenance treatment is usually sufficient to re-establish health, and (3) attachment loss is very minimal, if present at all.

A rapidly progressive lesion can be determined only by evaluating the rate of destruction over a period of time. Therefore, the diagnosis of RPP depends on careful analysis and documentation of the periodontal condition over a minimum of two time periods. The interval between evaluations can be as short as a few weeks.

Two gingival tissue responses can be found in cases of RPP. One is a severe, acutely inflamed tissue, often proliferating, ulcerated, and fiery red (Figs. 26–1 and 26–2; Plate XI*A, B*). Bleeding may occur spontaneously or with slight stimulation. Suppuration may be an important feature. This tissue response is considered to occur in the destructive stage, in which attachment and bone are actively lost.

In other cases the gingival tissues may appear pink, free of inflammation, and occasionally with some degree of stippling, although the last feature may be absent (Figs. 26–3 and 26–4; Plate XI*C–E*). However, in spite of the apparently mild clinical appearance, deep pockets can be revealed by probing. This tissue response has been considered by Page and Schroeder[16] to coincide with periods of quiescence in which the bone level remains stationary. Radiographs will often show bone loss that has progressed since the previous evaluation.

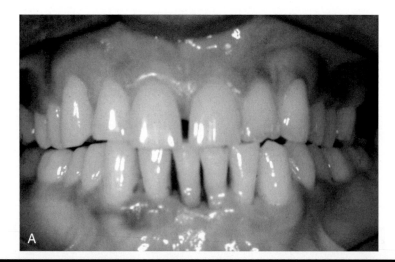

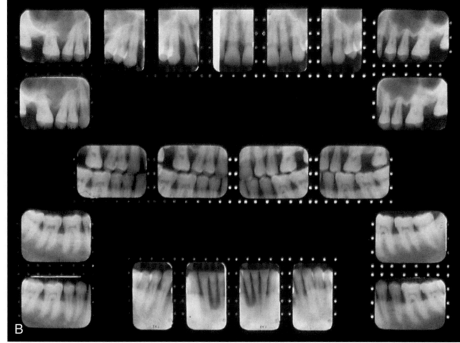

FIGURE 26–1. *A,* Rapidly progressive periodontitis in a 38-year-old Indian patient. Note the intense generalized diffuse reddening of the tissue as well as the lack of stippling. *B,* Radiographs showing advanced bone loss in upper premolar and molar areas and in lower anterior areas.

Some patients with RPP may have systemic manifestations such as weight loss, mental depression, and general malaise.[16] All patients with a presumptive diagnosis of RPP must have their medical history updated and reviewed. These patients should receive a medical evaluation to rule out possible systemic involvement.

Distribution of Lesions. In contrast to localized juvenile periodontitis (LJP), the lesions of adult onset RPP are more generalized. All or most teeth can be affected without any definite pattern of distribution. Furcated teeth, however, may present with deeper lesions because of the difficulty with performing effective oral hygiene in these areas.

Progression. RPP can follow an episodic pattern in its progression, with periods of advanced destruction followed by stages of quiescence of variable length (weeks to months or years). The possibility for rapid periodontal destruction differentiates this form of periodontitis from the more typical SPP.

Page and coworkers[15] described sites in RPP patients that demonstrated osseous destruction of 25% to 60% during a 9-week period. Despite this extreme loss, other sites in the same patient showed no bone loss. Obviously, not all patients will exhibit this extremely rapid bone loss, but advanced loss is usually found before 30 years of age.

Age and Sex. The age at onset of this disease ranges from the middle to late teens and to 30 years old. By 30 to 35 years of age, cases of RPP will have progressed to advanced bone loss.

Cases of RPP may be arrested spontaneously or after therapy, while others may continue to progress inexorably to tooth loss, despite intervention with conventional treatment. The latter type of disease is considered refractory periodontitis.

Sex differences have not been mentioned in the literature for RPP.

Etiology. The microbial populations in RPP include *Actinobacillus actinomycetemcomitans, Porphyromonas gingivalis, Prevotella intermedia, Bacteroides forsythus, Bac-*

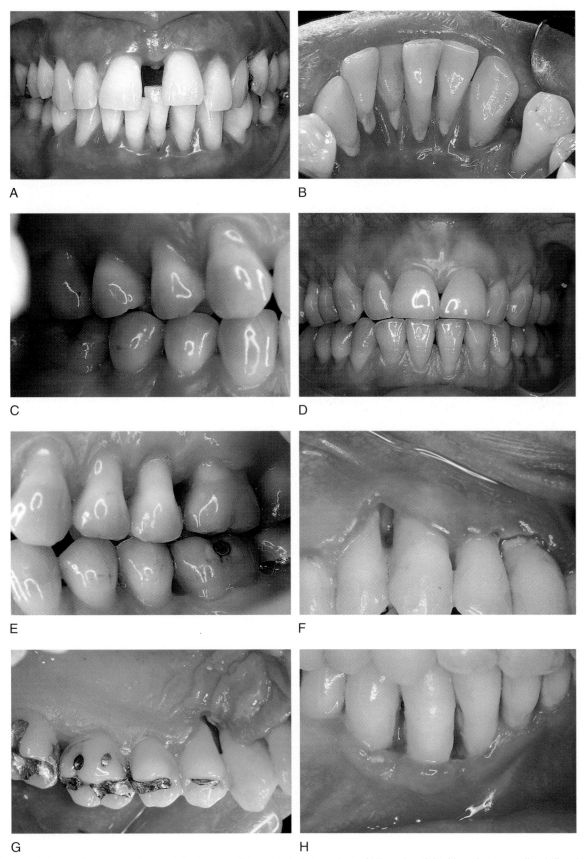

PLATE XI. *A* and *B,* Rapidly progressive periodontitis in a 30-year-old white patient of Hispanic origin. Note the generalized discoloration and smooth surface of the gingival tissues. Radiographs of this patient are shown in Fig. 26–2. *C–E,* Rapidly progressive periodontitis in a 32-year-old white female. Note the apparently normal color and surface texture of the gingival tissues. Radiographs of this patient taken 4 years apart (1988 and 1992) are shown in Fig. 26–4. Clinical pictures were taken at the later date. *F–H,* Necrotizing ulcerative periodontitis in a 45-year-old white male, HIV-negative. Note the deep craters associated with bone loss. (*A–E* courtesy of Dr. Philip Melnick, Los Angeles, CA.)

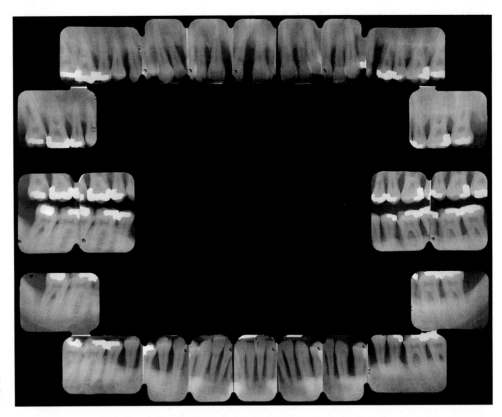

FIGURE 26–2. Radiographs of the patient shown in Plate XI*A, B*. Note the advanced generalized bone loss.

teroides capillus, Eikenella corrodens, Eubacterium brachy, Eubacterium nodatum, Eubacterium timidum, Fusobacterium nucleatum, Lactobacillus minutus, and *Campylobacter rectus*. Gram-negative organisms and spirochetes adhere loosely to the pocket epithelium and are found at the apical extent of the pocket.

An altered chemotactic response in neutrophils has been reported in most RPP patients.[15,16] Van Dyke et al.[23] have reported that treatment of an aggressive periodontitis resulted in a return to normal neutrophil function and that chemokinesis was normal in the untreated case. Serum antibodies to several of the gram-negative species previously mentioned are elevated.

Autoimmunity has been considered to have a role in RPP by Anusaksathien and Dolby,[2] who found host antibodies to collagen, DNA, and immunoglobulin G (IgG). Possible immune mechanisms include an increase in the expression of type II major histocompatibility complex (MHC) molecules, altered helper or suppressor T-cell function, polyclonal activation of B cells by microbial plaque, and genetic predisposition. (See Chapters 8 and 10 for a detailed description of the immunology of RPP patients.)

Prevalence. Long-term follow-up studies performed in periodontal private practices have reported an incidence of 4%[7] to 8%[13] of cases that do not respond to treatment and continue to worsen, based on the number of teeth lost over periods of many years. These cases may be classified as RPP or as refractory periodontitis (see later discussion).

In the Sri Lanka study conducted by Löe and colleagues,[9] 8% of the population had rapid progression of periodontal disease characterized by a yearly loss of attachment of 0.1 to 1.0 mm.

NECROTIZING ULCERATIVE PERIODONTITIS

Two types of NUP have been described according to their relationship with acquired immunodeficiency syndrome (AIDS).

Non-AIDS Type Necrotizing Ulcerative Periodontitis

Clinical Features. This type of periodontitis occurs after repeated long-term episodes of acute necrotizing ulcerative gingivitis (ANUG). ANUG is characterized by areas of ulceration and necrosis of the gingival margin that become covered by a whitish-yellowish soft material known as a *pseudomembrane*. The ulcerated margin is surrounded by an erythematous halo. The lesions are painful and bleed often, giving rise to localized lymphadenopathy and even fever and malaise. Microscopically, ANUG lesions are a nonspecific necrotizing inflammation presenting a predominantly polymorphonuclear neutrophil (PMN) infiltrate in the ulcerated areas with an abundant chronic component (lymphocytes and plasma cells) in the peripheral and deeper areas.

The inflammatory infiltrate in lesions of ANUG, especially in long-standing cases, can extend to the underlying bone, resulting in deep, crater-like osseous lesions, most often located in interdental areas. These cases are diagnosed as NUP.

Lesions resembling this description and progressing to become *gangrenous stomatitis*, or *noma*, have been described in children with severe malnutrition in underdeveloped countries. Jimenez and Baer[8] described ANUG in

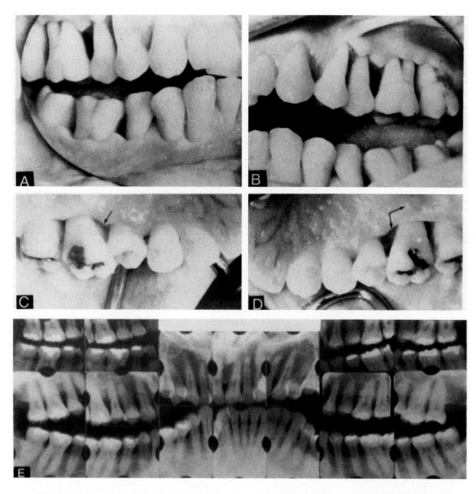

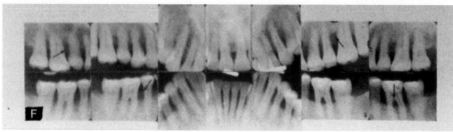

FIGURE 26–3. Rapidly progressive periodontitis. *A* to *D,* Clinical pictures showing advanced destructive lesions in premolar and molar areas in a 36-year-old white female. *E,* Radiographs taken in April 1980 show mild to moderate generalized horizontal bone loss. *F,* Radiographs taken 9 weeks later (June 1980) demonstrate extreme bone loss around molars and premolars. (From Page RC, Altman LC, Ebersole JL, et al. Rapidly progressive periodontitis: A clinical entity. J Periodontol *54*:196, 1983.)

children and adolescents ages 2 to 14 with malnutrition in Colombia; in advanced stages, ANUG extended from the gingiva to other areas of the oral cavity, becoming gangrenous stomatitis or noma and causing exposure, necrosis, and sequestration of the alveolar bone. Experimentally, noma-like lesions have been produced in rats by administering cortisone and causing mechanical injury to the gingiva[20] and in hamsters by total body irradiation.[12]

NUP is characterized by deep interdental osseous craters (Fig. 26–5; Plate XI*F–H*), but deep "conventional" pockets are not found, because the ulcerative and necrotizing character of the gingival lesion destroys the junctional epithelium, removing the mechanism of pocket deepening (see Chapter 22).

Superficial lesions compatible with a diagnosis of ANUG may be found, although very often signs and symptoms are subdued, and the necrotizing lesion can be considered to be in a chronic stage. Lesions of NUP can lead to advanced bone loss, tooth mobility, and tooth loss.

Etiology. The etiologic agents of NUP have not been studied, but they can be assumed to be similar to those present in ANUG, which has been extensively investigated. However, this similarity has not been established. The mechanisms by which cases of ANUG may become NUP have also not been investigated. Cutler et al.[4] have described impaired bactericidal activity of PMNs in two children with acute necrotizing ulcerative periodontitis (ANUP).

AIDS-Associated Necrotizing Ulcerative Periodontitis

Clinical Features. Gingival and periodontal lesions are frequently found in patients with AIDS. These gingival and periodontal lesions in human immunodeficiency

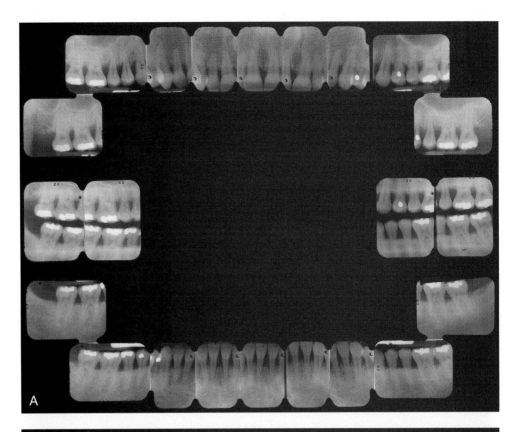

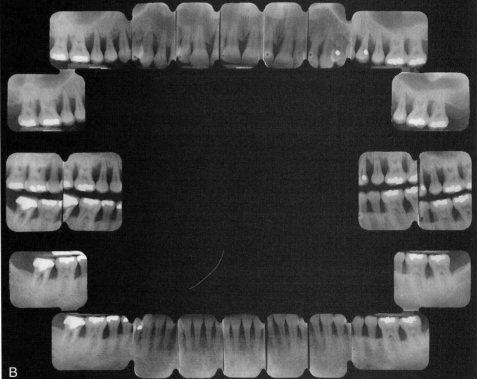

FIGURE 26–4. Radiographs of the patient shown in Plate XI*C–E. A,* Radiographs taken in 1988. In spite of repeated aggressive treatment, the patient's condition continued to deteriorate. *B,* Radiographs taken in 1992. (Courtesy of Dr. Philip Melnick, Los Angeles, CA.)

virus (HIV)–positive patients appear to be similar to those seen in NUP in HIV-negative patients but frequently result in complications that are extremely rare in non-AIDS patients. These complications consist of large areas of soft tissue necrosis with exposure of bone and sequestration of bone fragments, sometimes extending to the vestibular area and/or the palate and becoming necrotizing stomatitis.

Progression. Bone loss associated with HIV-positive NUP may be extremely rapid. Winkler and colleagues[25] mention cases in which 10 mm of bone were lost in 3 months.

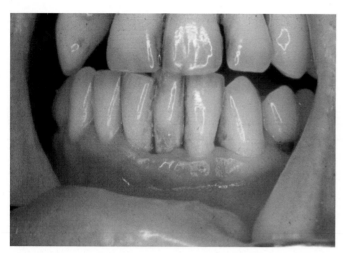

FIGURE 26–5. Necrotizing ulcerative periodontitis in a 42-year-old HIV-negative white male.

Etiology. AIDS favors the occurrence of opportunistic infections leading to ANUG, atypical gingivitis, RPP, and NUP.

Murray and coworkers[14] have reported that cases of NUP in AIDS patients demonstrate greater numbers of the opportunistic fungus *Candida albicans* and higher prevalence of *A. actinomycetemcomitans, P. intermedia, P. gingivalis, F. nucleatum,* and *Campylobacter* spp. They also observed that the destructive periodontal lesions seen in AIDS patients differ substantially from ANUG lesions; particularly noteworthy is the low or variable level of spirochetes, which is inconsistent with the ANUG flora. The flora found in NUP in AIDS patients is more in line with that of classic slowly progressive periodontitis.

For a more detailed description of these diseases, see Chapters 15 and 19; treatment is discussed in Chapters 39 and 46.

REFRACTORY PERIODONTITIS

Cases that, for unknown reasons, do not respond to therapy and/or recur soon after adequate treatment have been referred to as refractory periodontitis. Refractory periodontitis should be distinguished from recurrent disease, in which a complete remission occurs after therapy, followed by recurrence of the disease as a result of reformation of the irritational infective factors, plaque, and calculus. To classify cases as refractory (or unresponsive), the clinician must clearly differentiate them from "maltreated" or incompletely treated cases. In such patients the irritants were never completely removed, and the disease may temporarily have become less severe but never disappeared.

The incorporation of refractory periodontitis into the classification of periodontal diseases may be a reflection of our ignorance with respect to the factors that result in unresponsiveness to therapy. This classification is undoubtedly a "mixed bag" of diseases and conditions that do not readily "fit" into other classifications. It is hoped that cases will be reclassified as our knowledge increases.

An example of this happened with so-called localized juvenile periodontitis (LJP). Most cases of this disease were refractory to therapy until some of the key organisms involved were identified and their susceptibility to tetracycline or other antibiotics was determined, and it was discovered that bacteria penetrated the tissues, therefore requiring systemic administration of the antibiotic. This new knowledge resulted in successful treatment of the disease.

Because of the lack of clear guidelines and parameters for the diagnosis and classification of patients as having refractory periodontitis, two different opinions have been expressed in the literature:

1. Refractory periodontitis is a distinct entity, different from other types of periodontitis.[3,24] Refractory periodontitis results from different bacterial agents, specific alterations of the host response, or a combination of these factors. According to this view, there may be multiple categories or subtypes of refractory patients. Until more information is known, these patients are grouped together into the default designation of refractory periodontitis.

2. Refractory periodontitis is not a distinct entity, and all cases of refractory periodontitis can fall into some of the other categories of periodontitis.[1] Obviously, very advanced cases of any type with a "hopeless" prognosis could be considered to belong in this category. In general, however, and excluding such cases, refractory periodontitis consists of few cases of SPP, many cases of RPP, and practically all cases of prepubertal periodontitis.

Clinical Features. Pretreatment clinical findings and severity are not diagnostic of refractory periodontitis. After the initial treatment, Magnusson et al. reported no difference in the amount of plaque in sites that were gaining or losing attachment, but losing sites had persistent bleeding on probing and suppuration.[11]

Deterioration in cases of refractory periodontitis occurs either by new involvement of additional teeth or by increased bone and attachment loss in previously treated areas.

Etiology. Refractory periodontitis may be due to abnormal host response, resistant organisms, untreatable morphologic problems, or a combination of any of these. Plaque accumulation and smoking have been consistently associated with the lack of clinical responsiveness.

Two types of refractory periodontitis have been considered. The first type consists of patients with adult periodontitis in whom anatomic conditions (e.g., furcations, irregular root surfaces) prevent complete removal of plaque. In general, these would be refractory "sites" rather than refractory "cases." Refractory sites probably harbor the same flora seen in nonrefractory sites, although topographic conditions may favor the proliferation of some microorganisms, resulting in rapidly destructive lesions. The relationship of invading microorganisms to this group awaits further elucidation. This type of refractory periodontitis is probably the most common and can be successfully treated if diagnosed and treated early and adequately maintained.

The second type of refractory periodontitis includes cases of RPP, both adult and early onset, but particularly cases of early onset periodontitis, such as the prepubertal and circumpubertal forms of periodontitis associated with agranulocytosis, Chédiak-Higashi disease, and Papillon-Lefèvre syndrome. In these cases, the existence of severe PMN defects or other immunologic problems accounts for the refractoriness of the disease (see Chapter 10). Adequate treatment methods for these cases have not yet been developed.

A high proportion of *A. actinomycetemcomitans* and *P. intermedia* has been reported in refractory periodontitis.[19] Rodenburg et al. noted that the total number of bacteria in the pockets of refractory patients was lower than that in untreated patients, but *A. actinomycetemcomitans* made up a larger proportion of the subgingival microflora than in untreated patients.[19] This has been explained (1) by the assumption that *A. actinomycetemcomitans* is more difficult to eradicate from the subgingival area than are other bacteria because of its invasive capability[17] and (2) by reinfection from other sites of the mouth.[18]

Slots and Rams[21] have noted the following microorganisms and their incidence in adult refractory periodontitis: *F. nucleatum* (75% of patients/sites), *P. intermedia* (40%), *A. actinomycetemcomitans* (30%), *Peptostreptococcus micros* (30%), *Staphylococcus* sp. (30%), *B. forsythus* (25%), *C. rectus* (25%), *P. gingivalis* (15%), *Candida* sp. (15%), and *Enterobacteriaceae/Pseudomonadacea* spp. (10%).

Haffajee et al.[5] identified three major microbial complexes in patients with refractory periodontitis: (1) *B. forsythus*, *F. nucleatum*, and *C. rectus*; (2) *S. intermedius*, *B. gingivalis*, and *P. micros*; and (3) *S. intermedius* and *F. nucleatum*.

Walker et al.[24] have indicated that at least two patterns or rates of attachment loss may be associated with refractory periodontitis and that each pattern may be indicative of a different flora: The pattern associated with a relatively rapid loss of attachment was characterized by a gram-negative flora that contained spirochetes, *P. intermedia,* and *Fusobacterium* species. A slow, continuous rate was associated with a predominantly gram-negative flora containing a high proportion of *S. intermedius* or *S. intermedius*-like organisms.

MacFarlane et al.[10] have described impaired PMN phagocytosis in cases of refractory periodontitis and reduction of PMN chemotaxis. They also found a high percentage of smokers in the group of refractory cases. Hernichel-Gorbach et al.[6] have evaluated the host responses of patients with generalized refractory periodontitis and reported that a majority of these patients may have some alteration in the mononuclear cell–cytokine system.

Frequency. Cases of refractory periodontitis may be similar to cases identified by Hirschfeld and Wasserman[7] as "extreme downhill," which constituted 4.2% of the 600 patients studied and followed for 22 years. In McFall's study of 100 patients followed for 19 years, 8% were identified as "extreme downhill."[13]

REFERENCES

1. Adams DF. Diagnosis and treatment of refractory periodontitis. Curr Opin Dent 2:33, 1992.
2. Anusaksathien O, Dolby AE. Autoimmunity in periodontal disease. J Oral Pathol Med 20:101, 1991.
3. Cram S, Rasheed A, Meador H, et al. Objective parameters of refractory periodontitis. Abstract 1428. J Dent Res 68(special issue):360, 1989.
4. Cutler CW, Wasfy MO, Ghaffar K, et al. Impaired bactericidal activity of PMN from two brothers with necrotizing ulcerative gingivo-periodontitis. J Periodontol 65:357, 1994.
5. Haffajee AD, Socransky SS, Dzink JL, et al. Clinical, microbiological and immunological features of subjects with refractory periodontal diseases. J Clin Periodontol 15:390, 1988.
6. Hernichel-Gorbach E, Kornman KS, Holt SC, et al. Host responses in patients with generalized refractory periodontitis. J Periodontol 65:8, 1994.
7. Hirschfeld L, Wasserman B. A long-term survey of tooth loss in 600 treated periodontal patients. J Periodontol 49:225, 1978.
8. Jimenez M, Baer PN. Necrotizing ulcerative gingivitis in children: A 9 year clinical study. J Periodontol 46:715, 1975.
9. Löe H, Anerud A, Boysen H, Morrison E. Natural history of periodontal disease in man. Rapid, moderate and no loss of attachment in Sri Lankan laborers 14 to 46 years of age. J Clin Periodontol 13:431, 1986.
10. MacFarlane GD, Herzberg MC, Wolff LF, Hardie NA. Refractory periodontitis associated with abnormal PMN leukocyte phagocytosis and cigarette smoking. J Periodontol 63:908, 1993.
11. Magnusson I, Marks RG, Clark WB, et al. Clinical, microbiological and immunological characteristics of subjects with "refractory" periodontal disease. J Clin Periodontol 18:291, 1991.
12. Mayo J, Carranza FA Jr, Epper CE, Cabrini RL. The effect of total body irradiation on the oral tissues of the Syrian hamster. Oral Surg Med Pathol 15:739, 1962.
13. McFall WT Jr. Tooth loss in 100 treated patients with periodontal disease. A long-term study. J Periodontol 53:539, 1982.
14. Murray PA, Holt SC. Microbiology of HIV-associated gingivitis and periodontitis. In Robertson PB, Greenspan JS, eds. Perspectives on Oral Manifestations of AIDS. Littleton, MA, PSG Publishing, 1988.
15. Page RC, Altman LC, Ebersole JL, et al. Rapidly progressive periodontitis. A distinct clinical condition. J Periodontol 54:197, 1983.
16. Page RC, Schroeder HE. Periodontitis in Man and Other Animals. A Comparative Review. Basel, Karger, 1982.
17. Pertuiset JH, Saglie FR, Lofthus J, et al. Recurrent periodontal disease and bacterial presence in the gingiva. J Periodontol 58:553, 1987.
18. Renvert S, Wikström M, Dahlen G, et al. On the inability of root debridement and periodontal surgery to eliminate *Actinobacillus actinomycetemcomitans* from periodontal pockets. J Clin Periodontol 17:351, 1990.
19. Rodenburg JP, Winkelhoff AJ, Winkel EG, et al. Occurrence of *Bacteroides gingivalis, Bacteroides intermedius* and *Actinobacillus actinomycetemcomitans* in severe periodontitis in relation to age and treatment history. J Clin Periodontol 17:392, 1990.
20. Selye H. Effect of cortisone and somatotrophic hormone upon the development of a noma-like condition in the rat. Oral Surg Med Pathol 6:557, 1953.
21. Slots J, Rams T. New views on periodontal microbiota in special patient categories. J Clin Periodontol 18:411, 1991.
22. Van Dyke TE, Lester MA, Shapira L. The role of the host response in periodontal disease progression: Implications for future treatment strategies. J Periodontol 64:792, 1993.
23. Van Dyke TE, Offenbacher S, Place D, et al. Refractory periodontitis: Mixed infection with *Bacteroides gingivalis* and other unusual *Bacteroides* species (case report). J Periodontol 59:184, 1988.
24. Walker CB, Gordon JM, Magnusson I, Clark WB. A role for antibiotics in the treatment of refractory periodontitis. J Periodontol 64:772, 1993.
25. Winkler JR, Grassi M, Murray PA. Clinical description and etiology of HIV-associated periodontal diseases. In Robertson PB, Greenspan JS, eds. Perspectives on Oral Manifestations of AIDS. Littleton, MA, PSG Publishing, 1988.

27

Prepubertal and Juvenile Periodontitis

FERMIN A. CARRANZA, JR.

Prepubertal Periodontitis
Juvenile Periodontitis

Although the term *juvenile periodontitis* is generally used to refer to the localized periodontitis that appears at puberty, in reality it should be used to refer to all diseases of the periodontium in the preadult years. Severe, rapid periodontal destruction and tooth loss occur infrequently in children and teenagers and can be classified in two groups according to the age of onset: *prepubertal forms,* which occur before 11 years of age, although they may extend beyond this period, and the *pubertal and adolescent forms,* which are seen approximately between 11 and 19 years of age. The term *juvenile periodontitis* is used in this book to refer to the second group.

Cases of prepubertal periodontitis are commonly associated with systemic diseases such as Papillon-Lefèvre syndrome, hypophosphatasia, and blood dyscrasias. The form of periodontitis that occurs in the circumpubertal and adolescent period is known as *juvenile periodontitis* and occurs commonly in otherwise healthy individuals. Both prepubertal and pubertal forms have been subclassified into localized and generalized forms, depending on their distribution in the mouth.

PREPUBERTAL PERIODONTITIS

Prepubertal periodontitis has its onset before 11 years of age in the primary or mixed dentition, and it frequently persists after puberty. Prepubertal periodontitis is usually associated with systemic diseases; published cases not associated with systemic disturbances are questionable owing to insufficient data presented.[82] Prepubertal periodontitis appears in Papillon-Lefèvre syndrome, Down syndrome, neutropenias, Chédiak-Higashi syndrome, hypophosphatasia, acute and subacute leukemia, and leukocyte adhesion deficiency. A localized form has also been described.

Papillon-Lefèvre Syndrome. This syndrome is characterized by hyperkeratotic skin lesions, severe destruction of the periodontium, and, in some cases, calcification of the dura.[2,14,26,33,52,63] The cutaneous and periodontal changes usually appear together before the age of 4 years. The skin lesions consist of hyperkeratosis and ichthyosis of localized areas on palms, soles, knees, and elbows (Figs. 27–1 and 27–2).

Periodontal involvement consists of early inflammatory changes that lead to bone loss and exfoliation of teeth. Primary teeth are lost by 5 or 6 years of age. The permanent dentition then erupts normally, but within a few years the permanent teeth are lost owing to destructive periodontal disease. By the age of 15 years, patients are usually edentulous except for the third molars. These, too, are lost a few years after they erupt. Tooth extraction sites heal uneventfully.[25]

The microscopic changes reported include marked chronic inflammation of the lateral wall of the pocket, with a predominantly plasma cell infiltrate, considerable osteoclastic activity and apparent lack of osteoblastic activity, and an extremely thin cementum.[52]

Bacterial flora studies of plaque in a case of Papillon-Lefèvre syndrome revealed a similarity to bacterial flora in adult periodontitis.[57] Spirochete-rich zones in the apical portion of the pockets, as well as spirochete adherence to the cementum and microcolony formation of *Mycoplasma,* have been reported in Papillon-Lefèvre syndrome.[40] Gram-negative cocci and rods appear at the apical border of plaque.[79] No significant alterations have been found in peripheral blood lymphocytes[15] and polymorphonuclear neutrophils (PMNs).[74]

Papillon-Lefèvre syndrome is inherited and appears to follow an autosomal recessive pattern.[30] Parents are not affected, and both must carry the autosomal genes for the syndrome to appear in the offspring. It may occur in siblings; males and females are equally affected. The estimated frequency is one to four cases per million.[30]

Rare cases of adult onset of this syndrome, albeit with mild periodontal lesions, have also been described.[9]

Down Syndrome. Down syndrome (mongolism, trisomy 21) is a congenital disease caused by a chromosomal abnormality and characterized by mental deficiency and growth retardation. The prevalence of periodontal disease in Down syndrome is high (occurring in almost 100% of patients younger than 30 years[67]). Although plaque, calculus, and local irritants (e.g., diastemata, crowding of teeth,

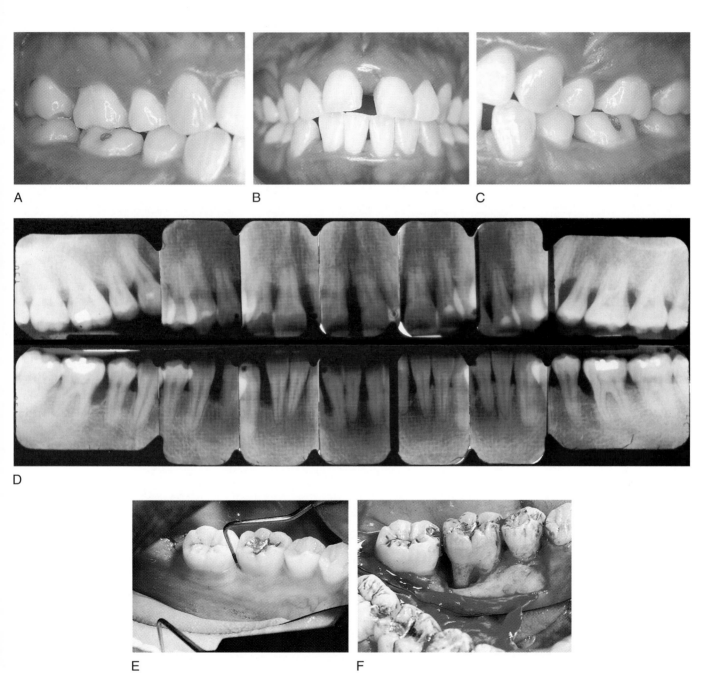

PLATE XII. Juvenile periodontitis. *A–C*, Clinical views of a case of juvenile periodontitis in a 19-year-old female. Note the migration of upper anterior teeth, lack of calculus, and scant clinical inflammation. *D*, Radiographs of the same case showing typical molar-incisor lesions. (Courtesy of Dr. Philip Melnick.) *E*. Lingual view of the left mandibular molar area in a patient with juvenile periodontitis. Note the apparently normal gingival tissue and the presence of a deep pocket, as denoted by the probe. *F*. The same area after elevation of the flap. Note the advanced bone loss localized to the first molar. (Courtesy of Dr. Terry Fiori.)

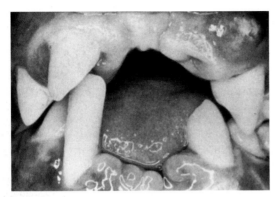

FIGURE 27–1. Dentition of a 17-year-old boy with Papillon-Lefèvre syndrome. The missing teeth were exfoliated.

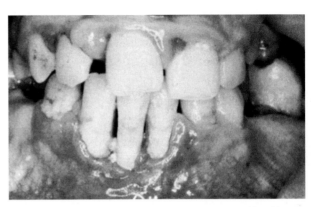

FIGURE 27–3. Down syndrome patient, 14 years old, with severe periodontal destruction.

high frenum attachments, and malocclusion) are present and oral hygiene is poor, the severity of periodontal destruction exceeds that explainable by local factors alone.[21,39,67,77]

Periodontal disease in Down syndrome is characterized by formation of deep periodontal pockets associated with a substantial plaque accumulation and moderate gingivitis (Fig. 27–3). These findings are usually generalized, although they tend to be more severe in the lower anterior region; marked recession is also sometimes seen in this region, apparently associated with high frenum attachment. The disease progresses rapidly. Acute necrotizing lesions are a frequent finding.

Two factors have been proposed to explain the high prevalence and increased severity of periodontal destruction associated with Down syndrome: a reduced resistance to in-

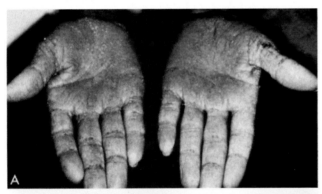

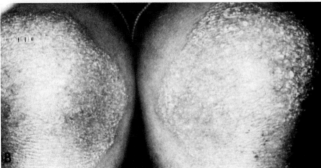

FIGURE 27–2. Palms *(A)* and knees *(B)* of the patient in Figure 27–1. Note the hyperkeratotic scaly lesions.

fections because of poor circulation, especially in areas of terminal vascularization such as the gingival tissue,[4,24] and a defect in T-cell maturation and in polymorphonuclear leukocyte chemotaxis.[38,67] Increased numbers of *Prevotella melaninogenica* have been reported in the mouths of children with Down syndrome.[48]

Neutropenias. Destructive generalized periodontal lesions have been described in children with neutropenia.[63] For further information, see Chapter 14.

Chédiak-Higashi Syndrome. This rare syndrome, which is characterized by recurrent bacterial infections including rapidly destructive periodontitis, is discussed in Chapters 10 and 14.

Hypophosphatasia. This is a rare familial skeletal disease characterized by rickets, poor cranial bone formation, craniostenosis, and premature loss of primary teeth, particularly the incisors. Patients have a low level of serum alkaline phosphatase, and phosphoethanolamine is present in serum and urine.[82]

Teeth are lost with no clinical evidence of gingival inflammation and show reduced cementum formation.[6] In patients with minimal bone abnormalities, premature loss of deciduous teeth may be the only symptom of hypophosphatasia. In adolescents, this disease resembles localized juvenile periodontitis.[84]

Acute and Subacute Leukemia. These diseases in children may be accompanied by severe periodontal changes (see Chapters 10 and 14).

Leukocyte Adhesion Deficiency. These cases are rare and begin during or immediately after eruption of the primary teeth. Extremely acute inflammation and proliferation of the gingival tissues, with rapid destruction of bone, are found. Profound defects in peripheral blood neutrophils and monocytes and an absence of neutrophils in the gingival tissues have been noted in patients with leukocyte adhesion deficiency (LAD)[61,62]; these patients also have frequent respiratory tract infections and sometimes otitis media. All primary teeth are affected, but the permanent dentition may not be affected.[62]

Localized Prepubertal Periodontitis. Localized prepubertal periodontitis has been described by Page and coworkers.[61] This form of periodontitis involves only a few teeth and is characterized by minor inflammation and slower bone loss. Mild defects in neutrophils or monocytes, but not both, are found.

JUVENILE PERIODONTITIS

Historical Background. In 1923 Gottlieb[31] reported on a patient with a fatal case of epidemic influenza and a disease that he called *diffuse atrophy of the alveolar bone* and described as being different from marginal atrophy. This disease was characterized by a loss of collagen fibers in the periodontal ligament and their replacement by loose connective tissue and extensive bone resorption, resulting in a widened periodontal ligament space. The gingiva was apparently not involved. In 1928 Gottlieb[32] attributed this condition to the inhibition of continuous cementum formation, which he considered essential for maintenance of the periodontal ligament fibers; he then termed the disease *deep cementopathia.* Gottlieb hypothesized that deep cementopathia was a "disease of eruption." Senescent cementum initiated a foreign body response, and the host attempted to exfoliate the tooth, resulting in bone resorption and pocket formation.[32]

In 1938 Wannenmacher[81] described incisor–first molar involvement and called the disease *parodontitis marginalis progressiva.* Unlike others at that time, Wannenmacher considered this disease an inflammatory process.

In 1940 Thoma and Goldman[78] used the term *paradontosis* to refer to this disease; the initial abnormality was located in the alveolar bone rather than in the cementum and consisted of vascular resorption and halisteresis rather than lacunar resorption. In 1947 Goldman[29] described vascular resorption and halisteresis in a spider monkey as being due to a degenerative noninflammatory disease of the supporting structures.

In 1942 Orban and Weinmann[59] introduced the term *periodontosis* and, on the basis of one autopsy case studied in detail, described three stages in the development of the disease. *Stage 1* involves the degeneration of the principal fibers of the periodontal ligament, which induces cessation of cementum formation and resorption of the alveolar bone. In this stage, tooth migration occurs without detectable inflammatory involvement. In *Stage 2* the lack of periodontal fibers results in rapid proliferation of the junctional epithelium along the root, and the earliest signs of inflammation appear. *Stage 3* is characterized by progressive inflammation and the development of deep, infrabony periodontal pockets.

Most of these mentioned studies considered "periodontosis" a degenerative disease caused by unknown systemic factors. In 1952 Glickman[28] wrote that the conditions described in these studies did not represent a different periodontal disease, but instead were extreme variants of destructive processes common to all periodontal disease.

Other investigators denied the existence of a degenerative type of periodontal disease and attributed the changes observed to trauma from occlusion.[12,55,65] In 1966 the World Workshop in Periodontics[66] concluded that the concept of periodontosis as a degenerative entity was unsubstantiated and that the term should be eliminated from periodontal nomenclature. The committee did recognize that a clinical entity different from adult periodontitis might occur in adolescents and young adults.

The term *juvenile periodontitis* was introduced by Chaput and colleagues in 1967 and by Butler[10] in 1969. In 1971 Baer[2] defined it as "a disease of the periodontium occurring in an otherwise healthy adolescent which is characterized by a rapid loss of alveolar bone about more than one tooth of the permanent dentition. . . . The amount of destruction manifested is not commensurate with the amounts of local irritants."

Prevalence. Two independent radiographic studies on 16-year-old adolescents, one in Finland[71] and the other in Switzerland,[42] followed the strict diagnostic criteria delineated by Baer and reported a prevalence rate of 0.1%. A clinical and radiographic study of 7266 English adolescents 15 to 19 years old also showed a prevalence rate of 0.1%.[69] A study conducted in 2500 adolescents 15 to 19 years old in Santiago, Chile, reported an overall prevalence rate of juvenile periodontitis of 0.32%.[50]

In the United States, a study of 11,007 adolescents age 14 to 17 reported that 0.66% had juvenile periodontitis (0.53% had the localized type, and 0.13% had the generalized form).[11] Bial and Mellonig[7] radiographically screened 49,380 U.S. naval recruits 17 to 32 years of age and found 182 cases of localized juvenile periodontitis, for a prevalence rate of 0.37%. A clinical and radiographic study by Melvin et al. on 5013 recruits found an overall prevalence rate of 0.76%.[54]

Several studies found the highest prevalence rate of juvenile periodontitis among black males,[11,47,54,69] followed in descending order by black females, white females, and white males.[54]

Age and Sex Distribution. Juvenile periodontitis affects both males and females and is seen most frequently in the period between puberty and 20 years of age. Some studies show a predilection for female patients, particularly in the youngest age groups,[37] whereas others report no male–female differences in incidence.[34,47] Among blacks, males are affected more than females.[54]

Distribution of Lesions. Three types of bone loss localization have been defined by Hormand and Frandsen:[37] (1) first molars and/or incisors; (2) first molars, incisors, and some additional teeth (total of fewer than 14 teeth); and (3) generalized involvement. There is an increase in the number of affected teeth with advancing age, which has led to the widely accepted assumption that the disease starts with localized lesions and at later stages becomes generalized.

The localized form has received a lot of attention and is referred to as *localized juvenile periodontitis* (LJP). The distribution of lesions in LJP is characteristic and as yet unexplained. *The classic distribution is in the region of the first molars and incisors, with the least destruction in the cuspid-premolar area* (Figs. 27–4 to 27–6 and Plate XIIA–D).

Frequently, bilaterally symmetric patterns of bone loss occur. In a series of 28 patients, Manson and Lehner[51] classified the typical pattern of bone loss (first molar–incisor) according to symmetric and asymmetric distribution; they found 15 symmetric and 13 asymmetric cases.

The following possible reasons for the limitation of periodontal destruction to certain teeth have been suggested:

1. After initial colonization of the first permanent teeth to erupt (the first molars and incisors), *Actinobacillus actinomycetemcomitans* evades the host defenses by different mechanisms, including production of polymorphonuclear leukocyte chemotaxis-inhibiting factors, endotoxins, collagenases, leukotoxins, and other factors that allow bacteria to invade and destroy the tissues. After this initial attack, adequate immune defenses are stimulated to produce opsonizing

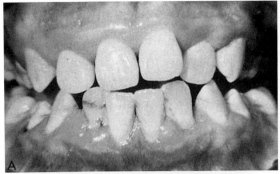

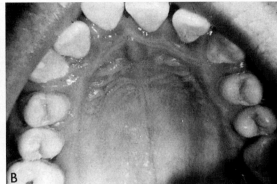

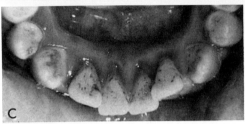

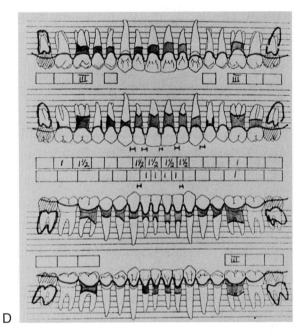

FIGURE 27–4. Juvenile periodontitis in a 14-year-old boy. *A–C,* Clinical picture showing gingival inflammation and migration of teeth with diastema formation. *D,* Diagram depicting pocket depth (shaded areas on teeth), tooth mobility (in boxes between upper and lower teeth), and furcation involvements (in boxes with Roman numerals adjacent to molars and first upper premolars).

antibodies to enhance phagocytosis of invading bacteria and neutralize destructive factors. In this manner colonization of other sites may be prevented.[85]

2. Bacteria antagonistic to *A. actinomycetemcomitans* may develop, thereby decreasing the destructiveness of the lesions and reducing the number of colonization sites.[36]

3. *A. actinomycetemcomitans* may lose its leukotoxin-producing ability for unknown reasons.[76] When this happens, the progress of the disease may become arrested or retarded and new colonization sites averted.

4. The possibility that a defect in cementum formation may be responsible for the localization of the lesions has been suggested.[60] Root surfaces of teeth extracted from patients with juvenile periodontitis have been found to have hypoplastic or aplastic cementum.[46] This was true not only of root surfaces exposed to periodontal pockets, but also of roots still surrounded by their periodontium.

Clinical Findings. *The most striking feature of early juvenile periodontitis is the lack of clinical inflammation, despite the presence of deep periodontal pockets* (Plate XIIE,F). Early descriptions of initial bone loss without pocket formation[59] have not been substantiated.

Clinically, *there is a small amount of plaque, which forms a thin film on the tooth and rarely mineralizes to become calculus.*[80] The most common initial symptoms are

mobility and migration of the first molars and the incisors.

Classically, the clinician sees *a distolabial migration of the maxillary incisors, with diastema formation.* The lower incisors seem to have less propensity to migrate than the upper ones. Occlusal patterns and tongue pressure can modify the amount and type of migration noted. Along with anterior tooth migration, an apparent increase in the size of the clinical crown, accumulation of plaque and calculus, and clinical inflammation appear.

As the disease progresses, other symptoms may arise. Denuded root surfaces become sensitive to thermal and tactile stimuli. Deep, dull, radiating pain may occur with mastication, probably because of irritation of the supporting structures by mobile teeth and impacted food. Periodontal abscesses may form at this stage, and regional lymph node enlargement may occur.[51]

Radiographic Findings. Vertical loss of alveolar bone around the first molars and incisors in otherwise healthy teenagers is a diagnostic sign of classic juvenile periodontitis. Radiographic findings include an "arc-shaped loss of alveolar bone extending from the distal surface of the second premolar to the mesial surface of the second molar."[56] There is evidence that the bone loss is not the result of any developmental or congenital absence or defect. Alveolar

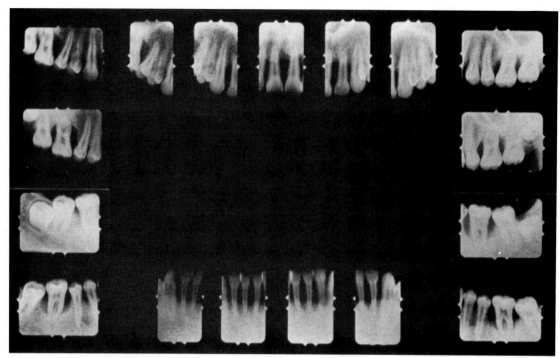

FIGURE 27–5. Radiographs of the patient in Figure 27–4 demonstrating the typical first molar–incisor distribution of bone loss. Note the higher bone level in canines and premolars and in second molars.

bone in patients in this age group develops normally with tooth eruption, and only subsequently does it undergo resorptive changes.

Clinical Course. Juvenile periodontitis progresses rapidly. There is evidence that *the rate of bone loss is about three to four times faster than in typical periodontitis.*[2,3] In affected persons, bone resorption progresses until the teeth are treated, exfoliated, or extracted. There is no consistent or reliable evidence that the disease process per se spreads to unaffected areas. However, it has been reported that in later stages of the disease, other teeth are involved with a form of periodontitis accompanied by the usual inflammatory changes (see Fig. 27–6).

Heredity. Several authors have described a familial pattern of alveolar bone loss and have implicated (without substantial evidence) a genetic factor in localized juvenile periodontitis.[10,19,49] Benjamin and Baer,[5] in the most comprehensive study on familial patterns, described the disease in identical twins, siblings, and first cousins, as well as in parents and offspring. The familial pattern has suggested the possibility of a transmissible microbiologic component in the pathogenesis of the disease.[58]

Several investigators have concluded that juvenile periodontitis is inherited as an autosomal recessive trait,[35] whereas others consider it to be transmitted as an X-linked dominant disease.[53]

Histopathology. A thin, frequently ulcerated pocket epithelium, infiltrated by numerous leukocytes, covers large areas of inflammatory cell accumulation composed mainly of plasma cells and blast cells, with lymphocytes and macrophages present in small numbers.[44] Collagen and other tissue components constitute only a small proportion of the diseased site, unlike the situation in adult periodontitis.[44]

Electron microscopy studies of juvenile periodontitis have revealed bacterial invasion of connective tissue[27] that reaches the bone surface.[13] The invading flora has been described as morphologically mixed but composed mainly of gram-negative bacteria, including cocci, rods, filaments, and spirochetes.[27] Using different methods, including immunocytochemistry and electromicroscopy, several tissue-invading microorganisms have been identified in juvenile periodontitis: *A. actinomycetemcomitans, Capnocytophaga sputigena, Mycoplasma,* and spirochetes.[68]

Subgingival plaque in juvenile periodontitis remains relatively thin (20 to 200 μm in depth) and does not tend to mineralize.[80] Scanning electron microscopy studies of root surfaces in juvenile periodontitis showed scattered clumps of rods, cocci, and filaments, with the apical 400 μm occupied by large numbers of rods with uniform morphologic features on the cemental and soft tissue surfaces.[1] Bacterial morphotypes differed from those seen in adult periodontitis only in the middle and apical portions of the pockets, where cocci, bacilli, coccobacilli, and various sizes of spirochetes were found.[23]

Bacteriology. The relationship between lesions of juvenile periodontitis and a bacterial flora different from that seen in adult periodontitis has been described. This flora consists mainly of gram-negative anaerobic rods, along with a minimal amount of attached plaque with a larger unattached component. The two types of bacteria considered to be pathogens in juvenile periodontitis are *A. actino-*

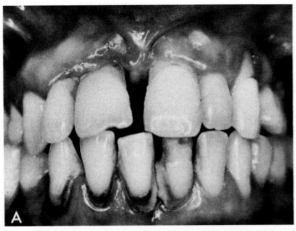

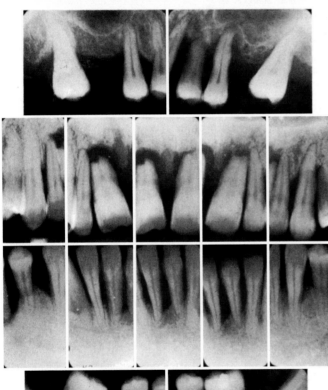

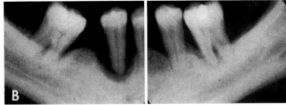

FIGURE 27–6. Advanced postjuvenile periodontitis in a 27-year-old woman. *A,* Gingival inflammation, heavy calculus deposits, and anterior open bite with diastema formation associated with tongue-thrusting habit. *B,* Severe generalized bone destruction obscures the limitation of bone loss to the anterior and molar regions seen in early juvenile periodontitis.

mycetemcomitans[75,76] and *Capnocytophaga*[58] (see Chapters 6 and 9).

Immunology. Some immune defects have been implicated in the pathogenesis of juvenile periodontitis. Several investigators[17,18,43] showed that patients with juvenile periodontitis display functional defects of PMNs and/or monocytes. These defects can impair either the chemotactic at-

traction of the PMN to the site or its ability to phagocytose and digest the microorganisms. These defects may be induced by the invading bacteria.

Lindhe and Slots[45] listed the following possible destructive mechanisms that may be used by microorganisms in juvenile periodontitis:

1. *A. actinomycetemcomitans* can produce substances that can kill PMNs and monocytes, thereby compromising the patient's ability to fight invading bacteria or their products. This leukotoxin may be counteracted by the development of serum antibodies.
2. Inhibition of PMN chemotaxis may be induced by some gram-negative bacteria.
3. Endotoxins from *A. actinomycetemcomitans* can induce Shwartzman's reaction, macrophage toxicity, platelet aggregation, complement activation, and bone resorption.
4. *A. actinomycetemcomitans, Capnocytophaga,* and *Bacteroides* can produce potent proteolytic enzymes that can destroy collagen, activate the complement system, or degrade immunoglobulins.
5. *A. actinomycetemcomitans* and *Capnocytophaga* can produce a fibroblast-inhibiting factor that impairs the defense mechanisms (i.e., fibroblast cytotoxicity).
6. Polyclonal B-lymphocyte activation by periodontal bacteria may result in production of antibodies unrelated to the activating agent.

In addition, areas of loss of collagen have been found around invading bacteria, which may suggest a direct lytic action. One or more of these mechanisms may cause tissue destruction in localized juvenile periodontitis.

Treatment. Treatment options consist of local therapy plus a systemic antibacterial regimen. See Chapter 46 for further details.

REFERENCES

1. Allen AL, Brady JM. Periodontosis: A case report with SEM observations. J Periodontol *49:*415, 1978.
2. Baer PN. The case for periodontosis as a clinical entity. J Periodontol *42:*516, 1971.
3. Baer PN, Benjamin SD. Periodontal Disease in Children and Adolescents. Philadelphia, JB Lippincott, 1974.
4. Benda CE. Mongolism and cretinism. London, Heinemann, 1947.
5. Benjamin SD, Baer PN. Familial patterns of advanced alveolar bone loss in adolescence (periodontosis). Periodontics *5:*82, 1967.
6. Beumer J III, Trowbridge HO, Silverman S Jr, Eisenberg E. Childhood hypophosphatasia and the premature loss of teeth. Oral Surg Oral Med Oral Pathol *35:*631, 1973.
7. Bial JJ, Mellonig JT. Radiographic evaluation of juvenile periodontitis (periodontosis). J Periodontol *58:*321, 1987.
8. Brown RS, Hays GL, Flaitz CM, et al. A possible late onset variation of Papillon-Lefèvre syndrome: A report of 3 cases. J Periodontol *64:*379, 1993.
9. Bullon P, Pascual A, Fernandez-Novoa MC, et al. Late onset Papillon-Lefèvre syndrome? J Clin Periodontol *20:*662, 1993.
10. Butler JH. A familial pattern of juvenile periodontitis (periodontosis). J Periodontol *40:*115, 1969.
11. Burmeister JA, Best AM, Palcanis KG, et al. Localized juvenile periodontitis and generalized severe periodontitis: Clinical findings. J Clin Periodontol *11:*181, 1984.
12. Carranza FA Sr, Carranza FA Jr. A suggested classification of common periodontal disease. J Periodontol *30:*140, 1959.
13. Carranza FA Jr, Saglie R, Newman MG. Scanning and transmission electron microscopy study of tissue invading microorganisms in localized juvenile periodontitis. J Periodontol *54:*598, 1983.
14. Carvel RI. Palmar-plantar hyperkeratosis and premature periodontal destruction. J Oral Med *24:*73, 1969.
15. Celenligil H, Kansu E, Ruacan S, Eratalat K. Papillon-Lefèvre syndrome. Characterization of peripheral blood and gingival lymphocytes with monoclonal antibodies. J Clin Periodontol *19:*392, 1992.
16. Christersson LA, Albini B, Zambon J, et al. Demonstration of *Actinobacillus actinomycetemcomitans* in gingiva in localized juvenile periodontitis in humans. Abstract. J Dent Res *62:*255, 1983.
17. Cianciola LJ, Genco RJ, Ratters MR, et al. Defective polymorphonuclear leukocyte function in a human periodontal disease. Nature *265:*445, 1977.

18. Clark RA, Page RC, Wilde G. Defective neutrophil chemotaxis in juvenile periodontitis. Infect Immun *18:*694, 1977.

19. Cohen DW, Goldman HM. Periodontal disease in children. Pract Dent Monog July 1962, p 3.

20. Cohen DW, Goldman HM. Clinical observations on the modification of human oral tissue metabolism by local intraoral factors. Ann NY Acad Sci *85:*68, 1960.

21. Cohen MM, Winer RA, Schwartz S, Shklar G. Oral aspects of mongolism. Part I. Periodontal disease in mongolism. Oral Surg Oral Med Oral Pathol *14:*92, 1961.

22. Cooley TB, Witwer ER, Lee P. Anemia in children with splenomegaly and peculiar changes in bones. Am J Dis Child *34:*347, 1927.

23. Douglass KD, Cobb CM, Berkstein S, Killow WJ. Microscopic characterization of root-surface associated microbial plaque in localized juvenile periodontitis. J Periodontol *61:*475, 1990.

24. Dow RS. Preliminary study of periodontoclasia in mongoloid children at Polk State School. Am J Ment Defic *55:*535, 1951.

25. Farzim I, Edalat M. Periodontitis with hyperkeratosis palmaris et plantaris (Papillon-Lefèvre syndrome). J Periodontol *45:*316, 1974.

26. Galanter DR, Bradford S. Hyperkeratosis palmoplantaris and periodontosis: The Papillon-Lefèvre syndrome. J Periodontol *40:*40, 1969.

27. Gillett R, Johnson NW. Bacterial invasion of the periodontium in a case of juvenile periodontitis. J Clin Periodontol *9:*93, 1982.

28. Glickman I. Periodontosis: A critical evaluation. J Am Dent Assoc *44:*706, 1952.

29. Goldman HM. Similar condition to periodontosis in two spider monkeys. Am J Orthod *33:*749, 1947.

30. Gorlin RJ, Sedano H, Anderson VE. The syndrome of palmar-plantar hyperkeratosis and premature periodontal destruction of the teeth. J Pediatr *65:*895, 1964.

31. Gottlieb B. Die diffuse Atrophy des Alveolarknochens. Z Stomatol *21:*195, 1923.

32. Gottlieb B. The formation of the pocket: Diffuse atrophy of alveolar bone. J Am Dent Assoc *15:*462, 1928.

33. Haneke E. The Papillon-Lefèvre syndrome; keratosis palmoplantaris with periodontopathy. Hum Genet *51:*1, 1979.

34. Hart TC, Marazita ML, Schenkein HA, et al. No female preponderance in juvenile periodontitis after correction of ascertainment bias. J Periodontol *62:*745, 1991.

35. Hart TC, Marazita ML, Schenkein HA, Diehl SR. Reinterpretation of the evidence for X-linked dominant inheritance in juvenile periodontitis. J Periodontol *63:*169, 1992.

36. Hillman JD, Socransky SS. Bacterial interference in the oral ecology of *Actinobacillus actinomycetemcomitans* and its relationship to human periodontosis. Arch Oral Biol *27:*75, 1982.

37. Hormand J, Frandsen A. Juvenile periodontitis. Localization of bone loss in relation to age, sex, and teeth. J Clin Periodontol *6:*407, 1979.

38. Izumi Y, Sugiyama S, Shinozuka O, et al. Defective neutrophil chemotaxis in Down's syndrome patients and its relationship to periodontal disease. J Periodontol *60:*238, 1989.

39. Johnson NP, Young MA. Periodontal disease in Mongols. J Periodontol *34:*41, 1963.

40. Jung JR, Carranza FA Jr, Newman MG. Scanning electronmicroscopy of plaque in Papillon-Lefèvre syndrome. J Periodontol *52:*442, 1981.

41. Kaslick RS, Chasens AI. Periodontosis with periodontitis: A study involving young adult males. Oral Surg Oral Med Oral Pathol *25:*327, 1968.

42. Kronauer E, Borsa G, Lang NP. Prevalence of incipient juvenile periodontitis at age 16 years in Switzerland. J Clin Periodontol *13:*103, 1986.

43. Lavine WS, Maderazo EG, Stolman J, et al. Impaired neutrophil chemotaxis in patients with juvenile and rapidly progressing periodontitis. J Periodont Res *14:*10, 1979.

44. Liljenberg B, Lindhe J. Juvenile periodontitis. Some microbiological, histopathological and clinical characteristics. J Clin Periodontol *7:*48, 1980.

45. Lindhe J, Slots J. Juvenile periodontitis. In Lindhe J, ed. Textbook of Clinical Periodontology. Copenhagen, Munksgaard, 1983.

46. Lindskog S, Blomlof L. Cementum hypoplasia in teeth affected by juvenile periodontitis. J Clin Periodontol *10:*443, 1983.

47. Löe H, Brown LJ. Early onset periodontitis in the United States of America. J Periodontol *62:*608, 1991.

48. Loesche WJ, Hockett RN, Syed SA. The predominant cultivable flora of tooth surface plaque removed from institutionalized subjects. Arch Oral Biol *17:*1311, 1972.

49. Lopez NJ. Clinical, laboratory and immunological studies of a family with a high prevalence of generalized prepubertal and juvenile periodontitis. J Periodontol *63:*457, 1992.

50. Lopez NJ, Rios V, Pareja MA, Fernandez O. Prevalence of juvenile periodontitis in Chile. J Clin Periodontol *18:*529, 1991.

51. Manson JD, Lehner T. Clinical features of juvenile periodontitis (periodontosis). J Periodontol *45:*636, 1974.

52. Martinez Lalis RR, Lopez Otero R, Carranza FA Jr. A case of Papillon-Lefèvre syndrome. Periodontics *3:*292, 1965.

53. Melnick M, Shields ED, Bixler D. Periodontosis: A phenotypic and genetic analysis. Oral Surg Oral Med Oral Pathol *42:*32, 1976.

54. Melvin WL, Sandifer JB, Gray JL. The prevalence and sex ratio of juvenile periodontitis in a young racially mixed population. J Periodontol *62:*330, 1991.

55. Mezl Z. Contribution a l'histologie pathologique du paradentium. Paradentologie *2:*60, 1948.

56. Miller SC. Precocious advanced alveolar atrophy. J Periodontol *19:*146, 1948.

57. Newman MG, Angel I, Karge H, et al. Bacterial studies of the Papillon-Lefèvre syndrome. J Dent Res *56:*545, 1977.

58. Newman MG, Socransky SS. Predominant cultivable microbiota in periodontosis. J Periodont Res *12:*120, 1977.

59. Orban B, Weinmann JP. Diffuse atrophy of alveolar bone. J Periodontol *13:*31, 1942.

60. Page RC, Baab DA. A new look at the etiology and pathogenesis of early-onset periodontitis. Cementopathia revisited. J Periodontol *56:*748, 1985.

61. Page RC, Bowen T, Altman L, et al. Prepubertal periodontitis. I. Definition of a clinical disease entity. J Periodontol *54:*257, 1983.

62. Page RC, Schroeder HE. Periodontitis in Man and Other Animals. Basel, S Karger, 1982.

63. Papillon MM, Lefèvre P. Deux cas de keratodermie palmaire et plantaire symetrique familiale (maladie de Meleda) chez le frere et la soeur. Coexistance dans les deux cas d'alterations dentaires graves. Soc Franc Derm Syph *31:*82, 1924.

64. Prichard JF, Ferguson DM, Windmiller J, Hurt WC. Prepubertal periodontitis affecting the deciduous and permanent dentition in a patient with cyclic neutropenia. J Periodontol *55:*114, 1984.

65. Ramfjord SP. Effect of acute febrile diseases on the periodontium of rhesus monkeys with reference to poliomyelitis. J Dent Res *30:*615, 1951.

66. Ramfjord SP, Ash MM, Kerr DA, eds. World Workshop in Periodontics. Ann Arbor, University of Michigan, 1966.

67. Renland-Bosma W, van Dijk J. Periodontal disease in Down's syndrome: A review. J Clin Periodontol *13:*64, 1986.

68. Saglie FR, Carranza FA Jr, Newman MG, et al. Identification of tissue invading bacteria in juvenile periodontitis. J Periodont Res *17:*452, 1982.

69. Saxby MS. Juvenile periodontitis: An epidemiologic study in the West Midlands of the United Kingdom. J Clin Periodontol *14:*594, 1987.

70. Saxen L. Juvenile periodontitis. J Clin Periodontol *7:*1, 1980.

71. Saxen L. Prevalence of juvenile periodontitis in Finland. J Clin Periodontol *7:*177, 1980.

72. Saxen L. Heredity of juvenile periodontitis. J Clin Periodontol *7:*276, 1980.

73. Saxen L, Aula S, Westermarck T. Periodontal disease associated with Down's syndrome: An orthopantomographic evaluation. J Periodontol *48:*337, 1977.

74. Schroeder HE, Seger RA, Keller HU, Rateitschak-Pluss EM. Behavior of neutrophilic granulocytes in a case of Papillon-Lefèvre syndrome. J Clin Periodontol *10:*618, 1983.

75. Slots J, Reynolds HS, Genco RJ. *Actinobacillus actinomycetemcomitans* in human periodontal disease: A cross-sectional microbiological investigation. Infect Immun *29:*1013, 1980.

76. Slots J, Zambon JJ, Rosling BC, et al. *Actinobacillus actinomycetemcomitans* in human periodontal disease. Association, serology, leukotoxicity, and treatment. J Periodont Res *17:*447, 1982.

77. Sznajder N, Carraro JJ, Otero E, Carranza FA Jr. Clinical periodontal finding in trisomy 21 (mongolism). J Periodont Res *3:*1, 1968.

78. Thoma KH, Goldman HM. Wandering and elongation of the teeth and pocket formation in paradontosis. J Am Dent Assoc *27:*335, 1940.

79. Vrahopoulos TP, Barber P, Liakoni H, Newman HN. Ultrastructure of the periodontal lesion in a case of Papillon-Lefèvre syndrome (PLS). J Clin Periodontol *15:*17, 1988.

80. Waerhaug J. Subgingival plaque and loss of attachment in periodontosis as well as observed in autopsy material. J Periodontol *47:*636, 1976.

81. Wannenmacher E. Ursachen auf dem Gebiet der Paradentopathien. Zbl Gesant Zahn Mund Kieferheilk *3:*81, 1938.

82. Watanabe K. Prepubertal periodontitis: A review of diagnostic criteria, pathogenesis and differential diagnosis. J Periodont Res *25:*31, 1990.

83. Watanabe K, Umeda M, Seki T, Ishikawa I. Clinical and laboratory studies of severe periodontal disease in an adolescent associated with hypophosphatasia. A case report. J Periodontol *64:*174, 1993.

84. Yendt ER. The parathyroids and calcium metabolism. In Volpe R, ed. Clinical Medicine. Vol 8: Endocrinology. Philadelphia, Harper & Row, 1986.

85. Zambon JJ, Christersson LA, Slots J. *Actinobacillus actinomycetemcomitans* in human periodontal disease. Prevalence in patient groups and distribution of biotypes and serotypes within families. J Periodontol *54:*707, 1983.

Section Five

Treatment of Periodontal Disease

Periodontal treatment requires an interrelationship between the care of the periodontium and other phases of dentistry. The concept of *total treatment* is based on the elimination of gingival inflammation and the factors that lead to it (e.g., plaque accumulation favored by calculus and pocket formation, inadequate restorations, and areas of food impaction).

In some cases total treatment will require consideration of *systemic aspects*—systemic adjuncts to local treatment and special precautions in patient management necessitated by systemic conditions. It may also entail consideration of *functional aspects*—establishment of optimal occlusal relationships for the entire dentition.

All of these aspects are embodied in a *master plan,* which consists of a rational sequence of dental procedures that includes periodontal and other measures necessary to create a well-functioning dentition in a healthy periodontal environment.

28

Clinical Diagnosis

FERMIN A. CARRANZA, JR.

First Visit
Overall Appraisal of the Patient
Medical History
Dental History
Intraoral Radiographic Survey
Casts
Clinical Photographs

Review of the Initial Examination
Second Visit
Oral Examination
Examination of the Teeth
Examination of the Periodontium
The Periodontal Screening and Recording System

Proper diagnosis is essential to intelligent treatment. *Periodontal diagnosis should first determine whether disease is present; then identify its type, extent, distribution, and severity; and finally provide an understanding of the underlying pathologic processes and their cause.* Sections IV and V of this book provide a detailed description of the different diseases that can afflict the periodontium. In general, they fall into three broad categories.

1. The gingival diseases (Table 28–1)
2. The various types of periodontitis (Table 28–2)
3. The periodontal manifestations of systemic diseases

Periodontal diagnosis is determined after careful analysis of the case history and evaluation of the clinical signs and symptoms as well as the results of various tests (e.g., probing mobility assessment, radiographs, blood tests, and biopsies).

The interest should be in the patient who has the disease and not simply in the disease itself. Diagnosis must therefore include a general evaluation of the patient as well as consideration of the oral cavity.

Diagnostic procedures must be systematic and organized for specific purposes. It is not enough to assemble facts. The findings must be pieced together so that they provide a meaningful explanation of the patient's periodontal problem.

The following is a recommended sequence of procedures for the diagnosis of periodontal diseases.

FIRST VISIT

Overall Appraisal of the Patient

From the first meeting, the clinician should attempt an overall appraisal of the patient. This includes consideration of the patient's mental and emotional status, temperament, attitude, and physiologic age.

Medical History

Most of the medical history is obtained at the first visit and can be supplemented by pertinent questioning at subsequent visits. The health history can be obtained verbally by questioning the patient and recording his or her responses on a blank piece of paper or by means of a printed questionnaire that the patient fills out.

The importance of the medical history should be explained to the patient, because patients often omit information that they cannot relate to their dental problem. The medical history will aid the clinician in (1) the diagnosis of oral manifestations of systemic disease and (2) the detection of systemic conditions that may be affecting the periodontal tissue response to local factors or that require special precautions and/or modifications in treatment procedures. For a detailed discussion of conditions requiring special precautions, see Chapter 34.

The medical history should include reference to the following:

1. Whether the patient is under the care of a physician and, if so, the nature and duration of the problem and the therapy. The name, address, and telephone number of the physician should be recorded, as direct communication with him or her may be necessary.
2. Hospitalization and operations, including diagnosis, kind of operation, and untoward events such as anesthetic, hemorrhagic, or infectious complications.
3. All medications being taken, whether prescribed or obtained over the counter. All the possible effects of these medications should be carefully analyzed to determine their effect, if any, on the oral tissues and also to avoid administering medications that would interact adversely with them. Special inquiry should be made regarding the dosage

Table 28–1. GINGIVAL DISEASES

Chronic marginal gingivitis
Acute necrotizing ulcerative gingivitis
Acute herpetic gingivostomatitis
Allergic gingivitis
Gingivitis associated with skin diseases
Gingivitis associated with endocrine-metabolic disturbances
Gingivitis associated with hematologic-immunologic disturbances
Gingival enlargement associated with medications
Gingival tumors

and duration of therapy with anticoagulants and corticosteroids.

4. History of all medical problems (cardiovascular, hematologic, endocrine, etc.), including infectious diseases and sexually transmitted diseases and high-risk behavior for human immunodeficiency virus (HIV) infection.
5. Possibility of occupational disease.
6. Abnormal bleeding tendencies, such as nose bleeds, prolonged bleeding from minor cuts, spontaneous ecchymoses, tendency toward excessive bruising, and excessive menstrual bleeding.
7. History of allergy, including hay fever, asthma, sensitivity to foods, or sensitivity to drugs such as aspirin, codeine, barbiturates, sulfonamides, antibiotics, procaine, and laxatives or to dental materials such as eugenol or acrylic resins.
8. Information regarding the onset of puberty and, for females, menopause, menstrual disorders, hysterectomy, pregnancies, miscarriages.
9. Family medical history, including bleeding disorders and diabetes.

Dental History

Current Illness. Some patients may be unaware of any problems but many may report bleeding gums; loose teeth; spreading of the teeth with the appearance of spaces where none existed before; foul taste in the mouth; and an itchy feeling in the gums, relieved by digging with a toothpick. There may also be pain of varied types and duration, including constant, dull, gnawing pain; dull pain after eating; deep radiating pains in the jaws; acute throbbing pain; sensitivity when chewing; sensitivity to heat and cold; burning sensation in the gums; and extreme sensitivity to inhaled air.

A preliminary oral examination is done to explore the source of the patient's chief complaint and to determine whether immediate emergency care is required. If this is the case, the problem is addressed after consideration of the medical history (see Chapter 34).

The dental history should include reference to the following:

1. Visits to the dentist: frequency; date of the most recent visit; nature of the treatment; and oral prophylaxis or cleaning by a dentist or hygienist, including frequency and date of most recent cleaning.
2. Toothbrushing: frequency, time of day, method, type of toothbrush and dentifrice, and interval at which brushes are replaced. The clinician should also ask about other methods for mouth care, such as mouthwashes, finger massage, interdental stimulation, water irrigation, and dental floss.
3. Orthodontic treatment: duration and approximate date of termination.
4. Pain in the teeth or in the gums: the manner in which the pain is provoked, its nature and duration, and the manner in which it is relieved.
5. Bleeding gums: when first noted; whether it occurs spontaneously, on brushing or eating, at night, or with regular periodicity; whether it is associated with the menstrual period or other specific factors; and the duration of the bleeding and the manner in which it is stopped.
6. Bad taste in the mouth and areas of food impaction.
7. Tooth mobility: Do the teeth feel "loose" or insecure? Is there difficulty in chewing?
8. Habits: grinding the teeth or clenching the teeth during the

Table 28–2. FEATURES OF TYPES OF PERIODONTITIS

Parameter	SPP	RPP	PPP	JP	NUP
Age (years)	35+	20–35	< 11	11–19	15–35
Calculus	Moderate to abundant	Scanty to moderate	Scanty	Scanty	Scanty
Disease progression	Slow	Rapid	Rapid	Rapid	Rapid
Distribution	Generalized; associated with etiologic factors	Generalized; no consistent pattern	Generalized; no consistent pattern	Localized to first molar and incisors; may become generalized	?
Prevalence	US: >50% Sri Lanka: 81%	US: 4–5% (?) Sri Lanka: 11%	?	LJP: 0.53%* GJP: 0.13%*	?
Racial predilection	No	No	No	More common in blacks	No
Familial tendency	No	?	Yes	Yes	?
Sex distribution	More severe in males	?	?	?	?
Predominant pathogens †	A	B	C	D	E
PMN/macrophage defects	No	Yes	Yes	Yes	Yes
Association with systemic problems	No	Some cases	Yes	Yes	Yes
Response to therapy	Very good	Variable	Poor	Good	Variable

SPP, Slowly progressive periodontitis; RPP, rapidly progressive periodontitis; PPP, prepubertal periodontitis; JP, juvenile periodontitis; NUP, necrotizing ulcerative periodontitis; LJP, localized juvenile periodontitis; GJP, generalized juvenile periodontitis.

* Prevalence in adolescents 14–17 years of age in the United States.

† Suspected major bacteria; others may be found in individual cases. A, *Porphyromonas gingivalis, Prevotella intermedia, Actinobacillus actinomycetemcomitans, Campylobacter rectus, Bacteroides forsythus,* spirochetes, *Fusobacterium nucleatum, Eikenella corrodens;* B, *Porphyromonas gingivalis, Prevotella intermedia,* small spirochetes; C, *Fusobacterium, Selenomonas, Campylobacter, Capnocytophaga,* black-pigmented bacilli; D, *Actinobacillus actinomycetemcomitans* in the localized type. *Porphyromonas gingivalis* plus *Eikenella corrodens, Prevotella intermedia, Capnocytophaga,* and *Neisseria* in the generalized form; E, Same as A, plus probably abundant *P. intermedia* and intermediate-sized spirochetes.

day or at night. Do the teeth or muscles feel "sore" in the morning? Are there other habits, such as tobacco smoking or chewing, nail biting, or biting on foreign objects?

9. History of previous periodontal problems: the nature of the condition and, if previously treated, the type of treatment received (surgical or nonsurgical), and approximate period of termination of previous treatment. If, in the opinion of the patient, the present problem is a recurrence of previous disease, what does he or she think caused it?

Intraoral Radiographic Survey

The radiographic survey should consist of a minimum of 14 intraoral films and four posterior bite-wing films (Fig. 28–1).

Panoramic radiographs are a simple and convenient method of obtaining a survey view of the dental arch and surrounding structures (see Fig. 28–1). They are helpful for the detection of developmental anomalies, pathologic le-sions of the teeth and jaws, and fractures (Fig. 28–2) and for dental screening examinations of large groups. They provide an informative overall radiographic picture of the distribution and severity of bone destruction in periodontal disease, but *a complete intraoral series is required for peri-odontal diagnosis and treatment planning.* Chapter 29 gives a detailed description of radiographic interpretation in peri-odontics.

Casts

Casts from dental impressions are extremely useful ad-juncts in the oral examination. They indicate the position of the gingival margins and the position and inclination of the teeth, proximal contact relationships, and food impaction areas. In addition, they provide a view of lingual-cuspal re-lationships. They are important records of the dentition be-fore it is altered by treatment. Finally, casts also serve as

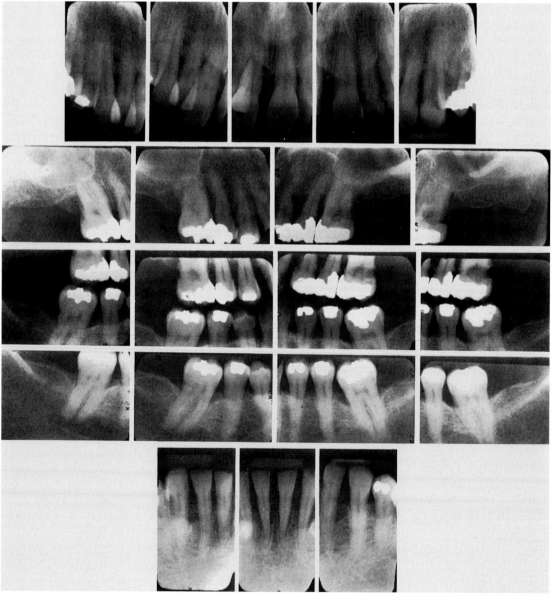

FIGURE 28–1. Full-mouth intraoral radiographic series (16 periapical films and four bite-wing films) used as an adjunct in periodontal di-agnosis.

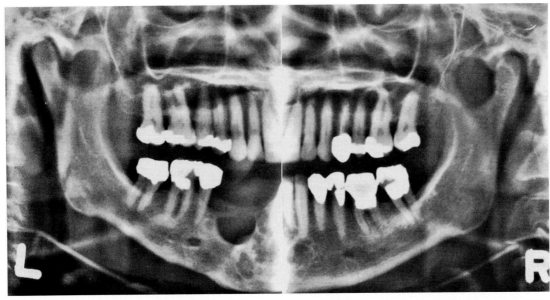

FIGURE 28–2. Panoramic radiograph showing temporomandibular joints and "cystic" spaces in the jaw. Areas of periodontal bone loss are not seen in detail. (Compare with Fig. 28–1.)

visual aids in discussions with the patient and are useful for pre- and post-treatment comparisons, as well as for reference at checkup visits.

Clinical Photographs

Color photographs are not essential, but they are useful for recording the appearance of the tissue before and after treatment. Photographs cannot always be relied on for comparing subtle color changes in the gingiva, but they do depict gingival morphologic changes.

Review of the Initial Examination

If no emergency care is required, the patient is dismissed and instructed as to when to report for the second visit. Before this visit, a correlated examination is made of the radiographs and casts to relate the radiographic changes to unfavorable conditions represented on the casts. The casts are checked for evidence of abnormal wear, plunger cusps, uneven marginal ridges, malposed or extruded teeth, crossbite relationships, or other conditions that could cause occlusal disharmony or food impaction. Such areas are marked on the casts to serve as a reference during the detailed examination of the oral cavity. The radiographs and casts are valuable diagnostic aids; however, it is the clinical findings in the oral cavity that constitute the basis for diagnosis.

SECOND VISIT

Oral Examination

Oral Hygiene. The cleanliness of the oral cavity is appraised in terms of the extent of accumulated food debris, plaque, materia alba, and tooth surface stains (Fig. 28–3). Disclosing solution may be used to detect plaque that would otherwise be unnoticed. The amount of plaque detected, however, is not necessarily related to the severity of the disease present. For example, juvenile periodontitis is a destructive type of periodontitis in which plaque is scanty. Qualitative assessments of plaque are more meaningful, and their value in diagnosis is discussed in Chapter 30.

Mouth Odors. Halitosis, also termed *fetor ex ore* or *fetor oris,* is foul or offensive odor emanating from the oral cavity. Mouth odors may be of diagnostic significance, and their origin may be either oral or extraoral (remote). The term *oral malodor* has been suggested for the former type.

Local sources of mouth odors include the retention of odoriferous food particles on and between the teeth, coated tongue, acute necrotizing ulcerative gingivitis (ANUG), dehydration states, caries, artificial dentures, smoker's breath, and healing surgical or extraction wounds. *The fetid odor characteristic of ANUG is easily identified.* Chronic peri-

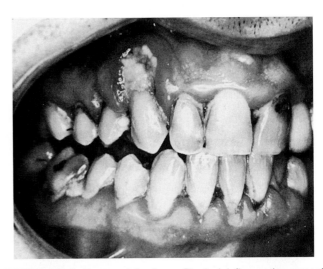

FIGURE 28–3. Poor oral hygiene. Gingival inflammation associated with plaque, materia alba, and calculus in a patient with hemophilia.

odontitis with pocket formation may also cause unpleasant mouth odor from accumulated debris and the increased rate of putrefaction of the saliva.[7]

Extraoral sources of mouth odors include infections or lesions of the respiratory tract (bronchitis, pneumonia, bronchiectasis, or others) and odors excreted through the lungs from aromatic substances in the blood stream, such as metabolites from ingested foods or excretory products of cell metabolism. Alcoholic breath, the acetone odor of diabetes, and the uremic breath that accompanies kidney dysfunction are examples of the last group.

Examination of the Oral Cavity. *The entire oral cavity should be carefully examined.* The examination should include the lips, the floor of the mouth, the tongue, the palate, and the oropharyngeal region and the quality and quantity of saliva. Although findings may not be related to the periodontal problem, they should enable the dentist to detect any pathologic changes present in the mouth. Textbooks in oral medicine and oral diagnosis cover these topics in detail.

Examination of Lymph Nodes. Because periodontal, periapical, and other oral diseases may result in lymph node changes, the diagnostician should routinely examine and evaluate head and neck lymph nodes. Lymph nodes can become enlarged and/or indurated as a result of an infectious episode, malignant metastases, or residual fibrotic changes.

Inflammatory nodes become enlarged, palpable, tender, and fairly immobile. The overlying skin may be red and warm. Patients are frequently aware of the presence of "swollen glands." Acute herpetic gingivostomatitis, ANUG, and acute periodontal abscesses may produce lymph node enlargement. After successful therapy, lymph nodes return to normal in a matter of days or a few weeks.

Examination of the Teeth

The teeth are examined for caries, developmental defects, anomalies of tooth form, wasting, hypersensitivity, and proximal contact relationships.

Wasting Disease of the Teeth. *Wasting is defined as any gradual loss of tooth substance characterized by the formation of smooth, polished surfaces, without regard to the possible mechanism of this loss.* The forms of wasting are erosion, abrasion, and attrition.

Erosion (cuneiform defect) is a sharply defined wedge-shaped depression in the cervical area of the facial tooth surface.[47] The long axis of the eroded area is perpendicular to the vertical axis of the tooth (Fig. 28–4). The surfaces

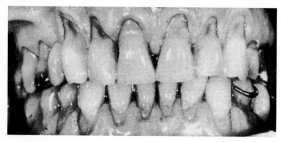

FIGURE 28–4. Erosion involving the enamel, cementum, and dentin.

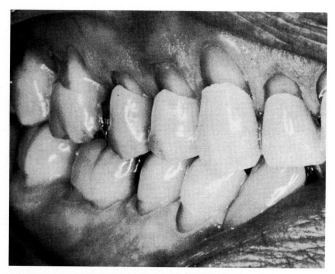

FIGURE 28–5. Abrasion attributed to aggressive toothbrushing. Involvement of the roots is followed by undermining of the enamel.

are smooth, hard, and polished. Erosion generally affects a group of teeth. In the early stages, it may be confined to the enamel, but it generally extends to involve the underlying dentin as well as the cementum.

The etiology of erosion is not known. Decalcification by acid beverages[29] or citrus fruits and the combined effect of acid salivary secretion and friction[31] are suggested causes. Sognnaes[54] refers to these lesions as *dentoalveolar ablations* and attributes them to forceful frictional actions between the oral soft tissues and the adjacent hard tissues. In patients with erosion, the salivary pH, buffering capacity, and calcium and phosphorus content have been reported as normal, with the mucin level elevated.[28]

Abrasion refers to the loss of tooth substance induced by mechanical wear other than that of mastication. Abrasion results in saucer-shaped or wedge-shaped indentations with a smooth, shiny surface. Abrasion starts on exposed cementum surfaces rather than on the enamel and extends to involve the dentin of the root. Continued exposure to the abrasive agent, combined with decalcification of the enamel by locally formed acids, may result in loss of enamel, followed by loss of the dentin of the crown (Fig. 28–5).

Toothbrushing[19] with an abrasive dentifrice and the action of clasps are common causes of abrasion; the former is by far the more prevalent. The degree of tooth wear from toothbrushing depends on the abrasive effect of the dentifrice and the angle of brushing.[26,27] Horizontal brushing at right angles to the vertical axis of the teeth results in the severest loss of tooth substance. Occasionally, abrasion of the incisal edges occurs as a result of habits such as holding objects (e.g., a bobby pin or tacks) between the teeth.

Attrition is occlusal wear resulting from functional contacts with opposing teeth. It is described in Chapter 13.

Dental Stains. These are pigmented deposits on the teeth. They should be carefully examined to determine their origin (see Chapter 12).

Hypersensitivity. Root surfaces exposed by gingival recession may be hypersensitive to thermal changes or tactile stimulation. Patients often direct the operator to the sensitive areas. These may be located by gentle exploration with a probe or cold air.

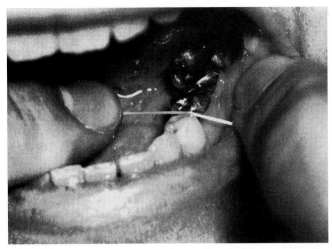

FIGURE 28-6. Tightness of contact points checked with dental floss.

Proximal Contact Relations. Slightly open contacts permit food impaction. The tightness of contacts should be checked by means of clinical observation and with dental floss (Fig. 28-6). Abnormal contact relationships may also initiate occlusal changes, such as a shift in the median line between the central incisors, labial version of the maxillary canine, buccal or lingual displacement of the posterior teeth, and an uneven relationship of the marginal ridges.

Tooth Mobility. All teeth have a slight degree of physiologic mobility, which varies for different teeth and at different times of the day.[37] It is greatest on arising in the morning and progressively decreases. The increased mobility in the morning is attributed to slight extrusion of the tooth because of limited occlusal contact during sleep. During the waking hours, mobility is reduced by chewing and swallowing forces, which intrude the teeth in the sockets. These 24-hour variations are less marked in persons with a healthy periodontium than in persons with occlusal habits such as bruxism and clenching.

Single-rooted teeth have more mobility than multirooted teeth, with incisors having the most. Mobility is principally in a horizontal direction, although some axial mobility occurs, to a much lesser degree.[39]

Tooth mobility occurs in two stages:

1. The *initial* or *intrasocket stage*, in which the tooth moves within the confines of the periodontal ligament. This is associated with viscoelastic distortion of the ligament and redistribution of the periodontal fluids, interbundle content, and fibers.[20] This initial movement occurs with forces of about 100 lb and is of the order of 0.05 to 0.10 mm (50 to 100 μm).[32]

2. The *secondary stage*, which occurs gradually and entails elastic deformation of the alveolar bone in response to increased horizontal forces.[34] When a force of 500 lb is applied to the crown, the resulting displacement is about 100 to 200 μm for incisors, 50 to 90 μm for canines, 8 to 10 μm for premolars, and 40 to 80 μm for molars.[32]

When a force such as that applied to teeth in occlusion is discontinued, the teeth return to their original position in two stages: the first is an immediate, spring-like elastic recoil; the second is a slow, asymptomatic recovery movement. The recovery movement is pulsating and is apparently associated with the normal pulsation of the periodontal vessels, which occurs in synchrony with the cardiac cycle.[33]

Many attempts have been made to develop mechanical or electronic devices for the precise measurement of tooth mobility.[33,38,40,52] Even though standardization of the grading of mobility would be helpful in diagnosing periodontal disease and in evaluating the outcome of treatment, these devices are not widely used. As a general rule, mobility is graded clinically with a simple method such as the following: The tooth is held firmly between the handles of two metallic instruments or with one metallic instrument and one finger (Fig. 28-7), and an effort is made to move it in all directions; abnormal mobility most often occurs faciolingually. Mobility is graded according to the ease and extent of tooth movement as follows:

Normal mobility.
Grade I: Slightly more than normal.
Grade II: Moderately more than normal.
Grade III: Severe mobility faciolingually and/or mesiodistally, combined with vertical displacement.

Mobility beyond the physiologic range is termed *abnormal* or *pathologic*. It is pathologic in that it exceeds the limits of normal mobility values; the periodontium is not necessarily diseased at the time of examination. Increased mobility is caused by one or more of the following factors:

1. *Loss of tooth support (bone loss)* can result in mobility. The amount of mobility depends on the severity and distribution of bone loss at individual root surfaces, the length and shape of the roots, and the root size compared with that of the crown.[42] A tooth with short, tapered roots is more likely to loosen than one with normal-size or bulbous roots with the same amount of bone loss. Because bone loss usually results from a combination of factors and does not occur as an isolated finding, the severity of tooth mobility does not necessarily correspond to the amount of bone loss.

2. *Trauma from occlusion* (i.e., injury produced by excessive occlusal forces or incurred because of abnormal occlusal habits such as bruxism and clenching) is a common cause of tooth mobility. Mobility is also increased by hypofunction. Mobility produced by trauma from occlusion occurs initially

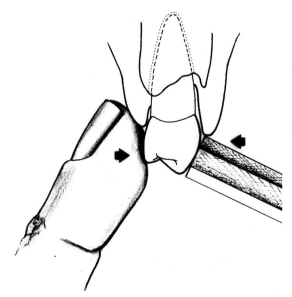

FIGURE 28-7. Tooth mobility checked with one metal instrument and one finger.

as a result of resorption of the cortical layer of bone, leading to reduced fiber support, and later as an adaptation phenomenon resulting in a widened periodontal space.

3. *Extension of inflammation from the gingiva or from the periapex* into the periodontal ligament results in changes that increase mobility. The spread of inflammation from an acute periapical abscess may increase tooth mobility in the absence of periodontal disease.

4. *Periodontal surgery* temporarily increases tooth mobility for a short period.[43-46]

5. *Tooth mobility is increased in pregnancy and is sometimes associated with the menstrual cycle or the use of hormonal contraceptives.* It occurs in patients with or without periodontal disease, presumably because of physicochemical changes in the periodontal tissues.

6. *Pathologic processes of the jaws that destroy the alveolar bone and/or the roots of the teeth* can also result in mobility. Osteomyelitis and tumors of the jaws belong in this category.

Trauma From Occlusion. Trauma from occlusion refers to tissue injury produced by occlusal forces, not to the occlusal forces themselves (see Chapter 24). The criterion that determines whether an occlusal force is injurious is whether it causes damage in the periodontal tissues; therefore, the diagnosis of trauma from occlusion is made from the condition of the periodontal tissues. The periodontal findings are then used as a guide for locating the responsible occlusal relationships.

Periodontal findings that suggest the presence of trauma from occlusion include excessive tooth mobility, particularly in teeth showing radiographic evidence of a widened periodontal space (see Chapter 29); vertical or angular bone destruction; infrabony pockets; and pathologic migration, especially of the anterior teeth (see following discussion).

Pathologic Migration of the Teeth. Alterations in tooth position should be carefully noted, particularly with a view toward identifying abnormal forces, a tongue-thrusting habit, or other habits that may be contributing factors (see Chapter 24). Premature tooth contacts in the posterior region that deflect the mandible anteriorly contribute to destruction of the periodontium of the maxillary anterior teeth and to pathologic migration (Fig. 28-8). Pathologic migration of anterior teeth in young persons may be a sign of juvenile periodontitis.

Sensitivity to Percussion. Sensitivity to percussion is a feature of acute inflammation of the periodontal ligament. Gentle percussion of a tooth at different angles to the long axis often aids in localizing the site of the inflammatory involvement.

Dentition with the Jaws Closed. Examination of the dentition with the jaws closed can detect conditions such as irregularly aligned teeth, extruded teeth, improper proximal contacts, and areas of food impaction, all of which may favor plaque accumulation.

Excessive overbite, seen most frequently in the anterior region, may cause impingement of the teeth on the gingiva and food impaction, followed by gingival inflammation, gingival enlargement, and pocket formation. The real significance of excessive overbite for gingival health, however, is controversial.[2]

In *open bite* relationships, abnormal vertical spaces exist between the maxillary and mandibular teeth. The condition occurs most often in the anterior region, although posterior open bite is occasionally seen. Reduced mechanical cleansing by the passage of food may lead to accumulation of debris, calculus formation, and extrusion of teeth.

In *crossbite,* the normal relationship of the mandibular teeth to the maxillary teeth is reversed, with the maxillary teeth being lingual to the mandibular teeth. Crossbite may be bilateral or unilateral or affect only a pair of antagonists. Trauma from occlusion, food impaction, spreading of the mandibular teeth, and associated gingival and periodontal disturbances may be caused by crossbite.

Functional Occlusal Relationships. Examination of functional occlusal relationships is an important part of the diagnostic procedure. Dentitions that appear normal when the jaws are closed may present marked functional abnormalities. Systematic procedures for the detection and correction of functional abnormalities are presented in Chapter 47.

Examination of the Periodontium

The periodontal examination should be systematic, starting in the molar region in either the maxilla or the mandible and proceeding around the arch. This will avoid overemphasis of spectacular findings at the expense of other conditions, which, although less striking, may be equally important. *It is important to detect the earliest signs of gingival and periodontal disease.*

Charts to record the periodontal and associated findings provide a guide for a thorough examination and record of the patient's condition (Fig. 28-9). They are also used for evaluating the response to treatment and for comparison at recall visits. However, excessively complicated mouth charting may lead to identification of a frustrating maze of minutiae rather than clarification of the patient's problem. Computerized dental examination systems using high-resolution graphics and voice-activated technology permit easy retrieval and comparison of data.[6]

A method for periodontal screening and recording (PSR) has been developed jointly by the American Academy of Periodontology and the American Dental Association, with the support of the Procter & Gamble Company.[41] This method is designed for the general dental practitioner, and its purpose is to identify patients requiring periodontal care and to determine, in general terms, the type of care required. This method will be presented at the end of this chapter.

Plaque and Calculus. There are many methods for assessing plaque and calculus accumulation.[10] The presence of supragingival plaque and calculus can be directly observed and the amount measured with a calibrated probe. For the detection of subgingival calculus, each tooth surface is carefully checked to the level of the gingival attachment with a sharp no. 17 or no. 3A explorer (Fig. 28-10). Warm air may be used to deflect the gingiva and aid in visualization of the calculus.

Although the radiograph may sometimes reveal heavy calculus deposits interproximally (see Chapter 29) and even on the facial and lingual surfaces, *it cannot be relied on for the thorough detection of calculus.*

Gingiva. The gingiva must be dried before accurate observations can be made (Fig. 28-11). Light reflection from

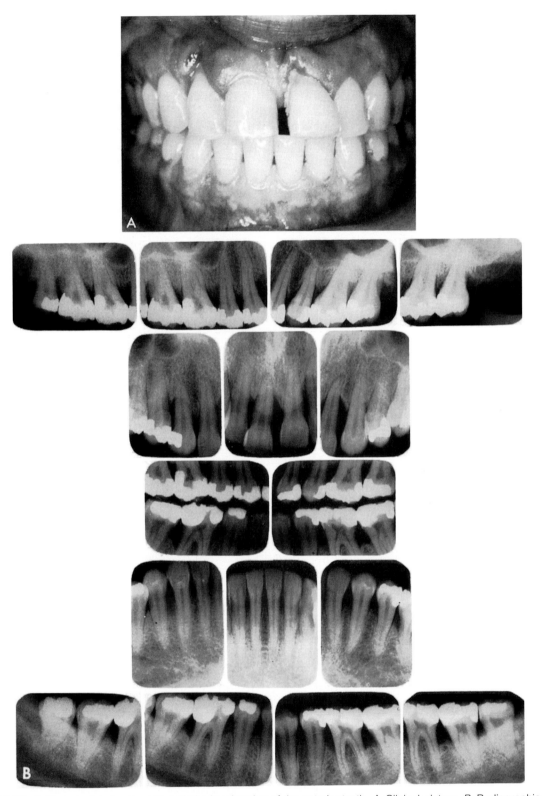

FIGURE 28–8. Periodontal disease with pathologic migration of the anterior teeth. *A,* Clinical picture. *B,* Radiographic view.

moist gingiva obscures detail. In addition to visual examination and exploration with instruments, firm but gentle palpation should be used for detecting pathologic alterations in normal resilience, as well as for locating areas of pus formation.

Each of the following features of the gingiva should be considered: color, size, contour, consistency, surface texture, position, ease of bleeding, and pain (see Chapters 17 and 18). No deviation from the normal should be overlooked. The distribution of gingival disease and its acuteness or chronicity should also be noted.

From a clinical point of view, gingival inflammation can

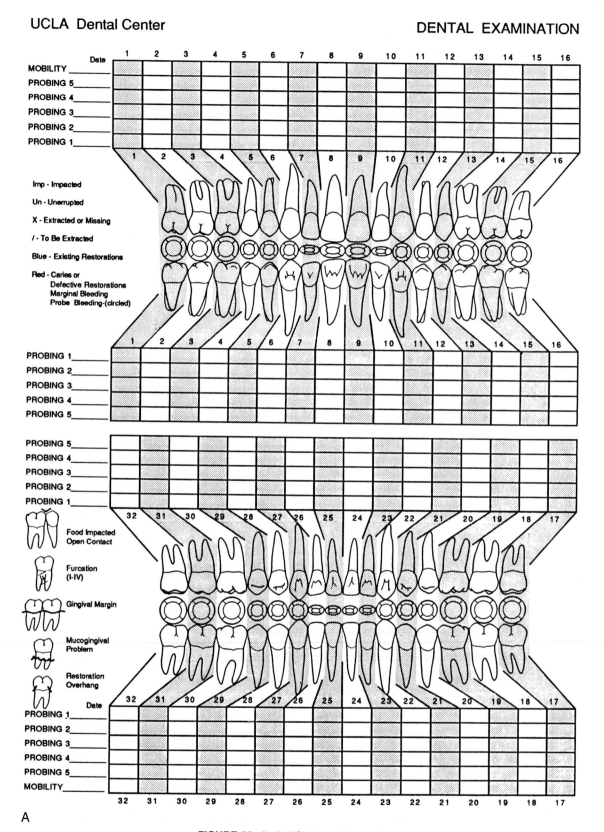

FIGURE 28–9. *A,* UCLA periodontal chart.

produce two basic types of tissue response: edematous and fibrotic. *Edematous tissue response* is characterized by a smooth, glossy, soft, red gingiva. In the *fibrotic tissue response,* some of the characteristics of normalcy persist; the gingiva is more firm, stippled, and opaque, although it is usually thicker, and its margin appears rounded (Plate XIII).

Use of Clinical Indices in Dental Practice. There has been a tendency to extend the use of indices originally designed for epidemiologic studies into dental practice. A de-

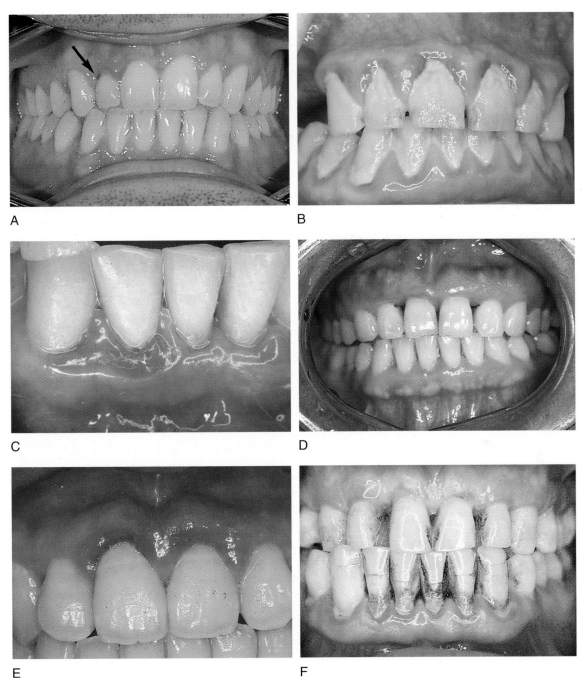

PLATE XIII. *A,* Incipient marginal gingivitis. Note the slight puffiness and bleeding *(arrow)* around the upper right lateral incisor. *B,* Edematous type of gingival inflammation. Note the loss of stippling, increase in size, abundant plaque and materia alba, and change in color. *C,* close-up view of edematous type of gingival inflammation. Note the red, shiny. smooth gingiva. *D,* Fibrotic type of gingival inflammation. Pockets of moderate depth are present, but the gingiva retains its stippling in some areas. *E,* Severe generalized gingival inflammation and inflammatory gingival enlargement. *F,* Fibrotic gingival inflammation. Note the abundant calculus and the gingival recession. The patient has pockets of moderate to severe depth in the mandibular anterior teeth and shallower pockets in the maxillary teeth.

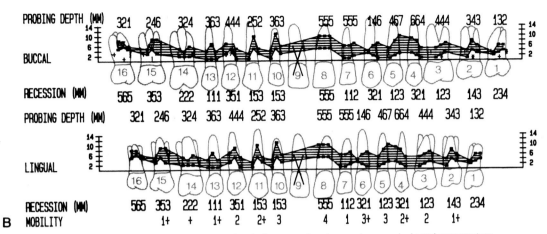

PROBING DEPTH (MM)	321	246	324	363	444	252	363		555	555	146	467	664	444		343	132
BUCCAL																	
tooth #	16	15	14	13	12	11	10	9	8	7	6	5	4	3	2	1	
RECESSION (MM)	565	353	222	111	351	153	153		555	112	321	123	321	123		143	234
PROBING DEPTH (MM)	321	246	324	363	444	252	363		555	555	146	467	664	444		343	132
LINGUAL																	
tooth #	16	15	14	13	12	11	10	9	8	7	6	5	4	3	2	1	
RECESSION (MM)	565	353	222	111	351	153	153		555	112	321	123	321	123		143	234
B MOBILITY	1+	+	1+	2	2+	3			4	1	3+	3	2+	2		1+	

FIGURE 28–9 *Continued B,* Computerized diagram showing various periodontal parameters.

tailed description of these indices can be found in Chapter 5. Of all the indices that have been proposed, the Gingival Index and the Sulcus Bleeding Index appear to be the most useful and most easily transferred to clinical practice.

The *Gingival Index* (Löe and Silness) provides an assessment of gingival inflammatory status that can be used in practice to compare gingival health before and after Phase I therapy or before and after surgical therapy; it can also be used to compare gingival status at recall visits. It is important that good intra- and interexaminer calibration be attained in the dental office.

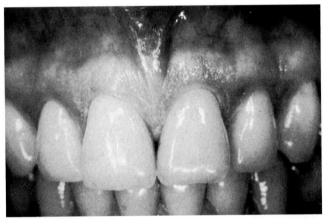

FIGURE 28–11. Normal gingiva. Normal surface features are revealed by drying the gingiva.

The *Sulcus Bleeding Index* (Mühlemann and Son) provides an objective, easily reproducible assessment of the gingival status. It is extremely useful for detecting early inflammatory changes and the presence of inflammatory lesions located at the base of the periodontal pocket, an area inaccessible to visual examination. Because it is easily un-

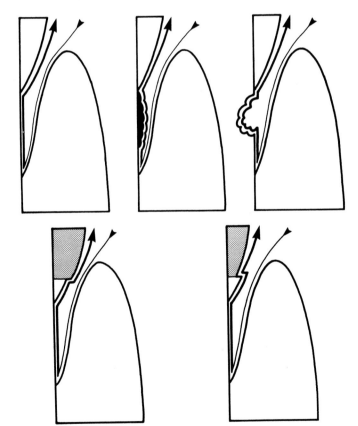

FIGURE 28–10. *Top left,* Detection of smoothness or various irregularities on the root surface with outward motion of a probe or explorer. *Top center,* Calculus. *Top right,* Caries. *Bottom left and right,* Irregular margins of restorations.

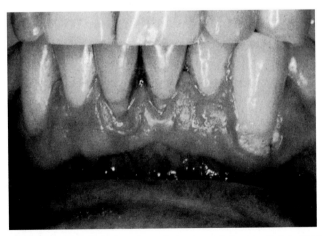

FIGURE 28–12. Periodontal pockets around the central incisors and left canine, showing rolled margins and separation from the tooth surface. Note the materia alba on the canine.

derstood by the patient, the Sulcus Bleeding Index can be used to enhance the patient's motivation for plaque control.

Periodontal Pockets. Examination for periodontal pockets must include consideration of the following: the presence and distribution on each tooth surface, the pocket depth, the level of attachment on the root, and the type of pocket (suprabony or infrabony).

Signs and Symptoms. Although probing is the only reliable method of detecting pockets, clinical signs such as color changes (bluish-red marginal gingiva, bluish-red vertical zone extending from the gingival margin to the attached gingiva); a "rolled" edge separating the gingival margin from the tooth surface; or an enlarged, edematous gingiva may suggest their presence. The presence of bleeding, suppuration, and loose, extruded teeth may also denote the presence of a pocket (Figs. 28–12 to 28–16 and Plate XIII).

Periodontal pockets are generally painless but may give rise to symptoms such as localized or sometimes radiating pain or sensation of pressure after eating, which gradually diminishes. A foul taste in localized areas, sensitivity to hot and cold, and toothache in the absence of caries is also sometimes present.

Detection of Pockets. The only accurate method of detecting and measuring periodontal pockets is careful exploration with a periodontal probe. Pockets are not detected by radiographic examination. The periodontal pocket is a soft tissue change. Radiographs indicate areas of bone loss where pockets may be suspected; they do not show pocket presence or depth, and consequently they show no difference before or after pocket elimination unless bone has been modified.

Gutta percha points or calibrated silver points[18] can be used with the radiograph to assist in determining the level of attachment of periodontal pockets (Fig. 28–17). They may be used effectively for individual pockets or in clinical research, but their routine use throughout the mouth would

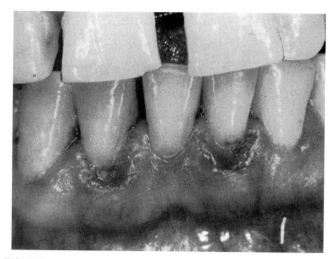

FIGURE 28–14. Periodontal pocket with puffy, discolored gingiva and exposed root surfaces.

be rather cumbersome. Clinical examination and probing are more direct and efficient.

Pocket Probing. There are two different pocket depths: the biologic or histologic depth and the clinical or probing depth[21] (Fig. 28–18) (see Chapter 1). The *biologic depth* is the distance between the gingival margin and the base of the pocket (the coronal end of the junctional epithelium). This can be measured only in carefully prepared and adequately oriented histologic sections. The *probing depth* is the distance to which an ad hoc instrument (probe) penetrates into the pocket. The depth of penetration of a probe in a pocket depends on factors such as the size of the probe, the force with which it is introduced, the direction of penetration, the resistance of the tissues, and the convexity of the crown.

Several studies have been made to determine the depth of penetration of a probe in a sulcus or pocket. Armitage and colleagues[4] used beagle dogs to evaluate the penetration of a probe using a standardized force of 25 ponds.*

---

* One pond is equal to 1 gm of absolute force.

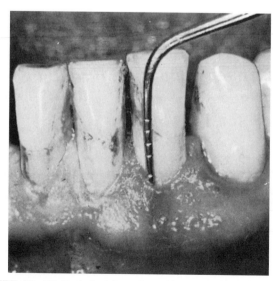

FIGURE 28–13. Periodontal pocket with vertical discolored zone extending to the alveolar mucosa.

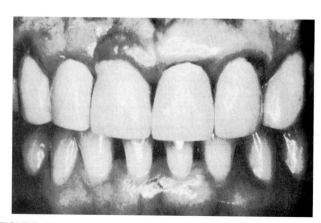

FIGURE 28–15. Purulent exudate from the periodontal pocket on the maxillary left central incisor.

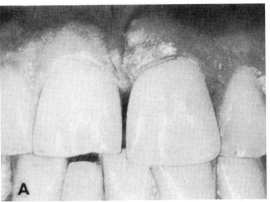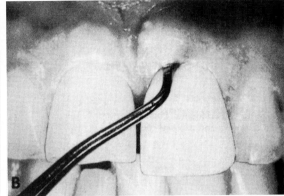

FIGURE 28–16. *A,* Extrusion of the maxillary left central incisor and diastema associated with a periodontal pocket. *B,* Deep periodontal pocket revealed by probing. The probe has penetrated to its entire length.

They reported that in healthy specimens, the probe penetrated the epithelium to about two thirds of its length; in gingivitis specimens, it stopped 0.1 mm short of its apical end; and in periodontitis specimens, the probe tip consistently went past the most apical cells of the junctional epithelium (Fig. 28–19).

In humans, the probe tip penetrates to the most coronal intact fibers of the connective tissue attachment.[23,52] The depth of penetration of the probe in the connective tissue apical to the junctional epithelium in a periodontal pocket is about 0.3 mm.[23,49,55] This is important in evaluating differences in probing depth before and after treatment, as the reduction in probe penetration may be a result of reduced inflammatory response rather than gain in attachment.[21,24]

The probing forces have been explored by several investigators[11,59]; forces of 0.75 N have been found to be well tolerated and accurate.[58] Interexaminer error (depth discrepancies between examiners) was reported to be as much as 2.1 mm, with an average of 1.5 mm, in the same areas.[17]

Probing Technique. The probe should be inserted parallel to the vertical axis of the tooth and "walked" circumferentially around each surface of each tooth to detect the areas of deepest penetration (Fig. 28–20).

In addition, special attention should be directed to detecting the presence of interdental craters and furcation involvements. To detect an *interdental crater,* the probe should be placed obliquely from both the facial and lingual surfaces so as to explore the deepest point of the pocket located beneath the contact point (Fig. 28–21). In multirooted teeth the possibility of furcation involvement should be carefully explored. The use of specially designed probes (e.g., Nabers probe) allows an easier and more accurate exploration of the horizontal component of furcation lesions (Fig. 28–22).

Level of Attachment Versus Pocket Depth. Pocket depth is the distance between the base of the pocket and the gingival margin. It may change from time to time even in untreated periodontal disease owing to changes in the position of the gingival margin, and therefore it is unrelated to the existing attachment of the tooth.

The level of attachment, on the other hand, is the distance between the base of the pocket and a fixed point on the crown, such as the cemento-enamel junction. Changes in the level of attachment can be due only to gain or loss of attachment and afford a better indication of the degree of periodontal destruction. *Shallow pockets attached at the*

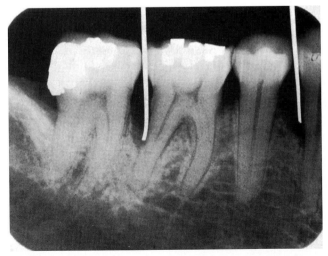

FIGURE 28–17. Blunted silver points assist in locating the base of pockets.

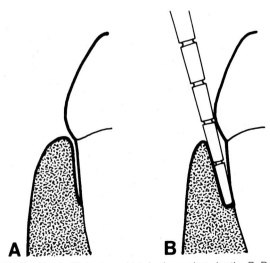

FIGURE 28–18. *A,* Biologic or histologic pocket depth. *B,* Probing or clinical pocket depth.

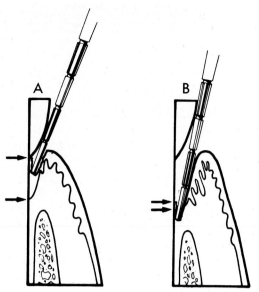

FIGURE 28–19. *A,* In a normal sulcus with a long junctional epithelium *(between arrows),* the probe penetrates about one third to one half the length of the junctional epithelium. *B,* In a periodontal pocket with a short junctional epithelium *(between arrows),* the probe penetrates beyond the apical end of the junctional epithelium.

level of the apical third of the root connote more severe destruction than deep pockets attached at the coronal third of the roots (see Chapter 22 and Figs. 22–19 and 22–20).

Determining the Level of Attachment. When the *gingival margin is located on the anatomic crown,* the level of attachment is determined by subtracting from the depth of the pocket the distance from the gingival margin to the cemento-enamel junction. If both are the same, the loss of attachment is 0.

When the *gingival margin coincides with the cemento-enamel junction,* the loss of attachment equals the pocket depth.

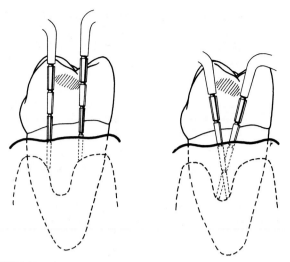

FIGURE 28–21. Vertical insertion of the probe *(left)* may not detect interdental craters; oblique positioning of the probe *(right)* reaches the depth of the crater.

When the *gingival margin is located apical to the cemento-enamel junction,* the loss of attachment will be greater than the pocket depth, and therefore the distance between the cemento-enamel junction and the gingival margin should be added to the pocket depth. Drawing the gingival margin on the chart where pocket depths are entered will help clarify this important point.

Bleeding on Probing. The insertion of a probe to the bottom of the pocket will elicit bleeding if the gingiva is inflamed and the pocket epithelium is atrophic or ulcerated. Noninflamed sites will rarely bleed. In most cases, bleeding on probing is an earlier sign of inflammation than gingival color changes[30] (see Chapter 17). However, sometimes color changes are found with no bleeding on probing.[14]

To test for bleeding after probing, the probe is carefully introduced to the bottom of the pocket and gently moved

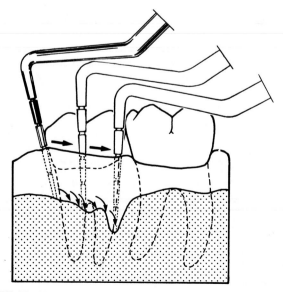

FIGURE 28–20. "Walking" the probe to explore the entire pocket.

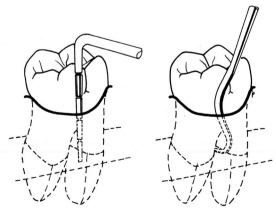

FIGURE 28–22. Exploring with a periodontal probe *(left)* may not detect furcation involvement; specially designed instruments (Nabers probe) *(right)* can enter the furcation area.

laterally along the pocket wall. Sometimes bleeding will appear immediately after removal of the probe; other times it may be delayed a few seconds. Therefore, the clinician should recheck for bleeding 30 to 60 seconds after probing.

Insertion of a soft wooden interdental stimulator in the interdental space produces a similar bleeding response[3] and can be used by the patient to self-examine his or her tissues for the presence of inflammation.[8]

Depending on the severity of inflammation, bleeding can vary from a tenuous red line along the gingival sulcus to profuse bleeding.[1] After successful treatment, bleeding on probing ceases.[3]

Determination of Disease Activity. The determination of pocket depth or attachment levels does not provide information on whether the lesion is in an active or inactive state. Currently there is no sure method to determine activity or inactivity of a lesion. *Inactive lesions* may show little or no bleeding on probing and minimal amounts of gingival fluid; the bacterial flora as revealed by darkfield microscopy consists mostly of coccoid cells. *Active lesions* bleed more readily on probing and have large amounts of fluid and exudate; their bacterial flora shows a greater number of spirochetes and motile bacteria.[15] In patients with juvenile periodontitis, progressing and nonprogressing sites may show no differences in bleeding on probing.[25]

The precise determination of disease activity will have a direct influence on diagnosis, prognosis, and therapy. The goals of therapy may change, depending on the state of the periodontal lesion. Chapter 30 describes in more detail the current state of knowledge in this important area.

Amount of Attached Gingiva. It is important to establish the relation between the bottom of the pocket and the mucogingival line. *The width of the attached gingiva is the distance between the mucogingival junction and the projec-*

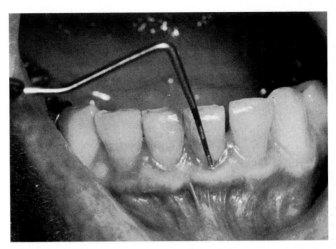

FIGURE 28–24. To determine the width of the attached gingiva, the pocket is probed at the same time that the lip (or cheek) is extended to demarcate the mucogingival line.

tion on the external surface of the bottom of the gingival sulcus or the periodontal pocket. It should not be confused with the width of the keratinized gingiva, because the latter also includes the marginal gingiva (Fig. 28–23).

The width of the attached gingiva is determined by subtracting the sulcus or pocket depth from the total width of the gingiva (gingival margin to mucogingival line). This is done by stretching the lip or cheek to demarcate the mucogingival line while the pocket is being probed (Fig. 28–24). The amount of attached gingiva is generally considered to be insufficient when stretching of the lip or cheek induces movement of the free gingival margin.

Other methods used to determine the amount of attached gingiva include pushing the adjacent mucosa coronally with a dull instrument or painting the mucosa with Schiller's potassium iodide solution, which stains keratin.

Alveolar Bone Loss. Alveolar bone levels are evaluated by clinical and radiographic examination. Probing is helpful for determining (1) the height and contour of the facial and lingual bones obscured on the radiograph by the dense roots and (2) the architecture of the interdental bone. Transgingival probing, performed after the area is anesthetized, is a more accurate method of evaluation and provides additional information on bone architecture[13,57] (see Chapter 56).

Palpation. Palpating the oral mucosa in the lateral and apical areas of the tooth may help locate the origin of radiating pain that the patient cannot localize. Infection deep in the periodontal tissues and the early stages of a periodontal abscess may also be detected by palpation.

Suppuration. To determine whether pus is present in a periodontal pocket, the ball of the index finger is placed along the lateral aspect of the marginal gingiva, and pressure is applied in a rolling motion toward the crown (Fig. 28–25). Visual examination without digital pressure is not enough. The purulent exudate is formed in the inner pocket wall, and therefore the external appearance may give no indication of its presence. Pus formation does not occur in all periodontal pockets, but digital pressure often

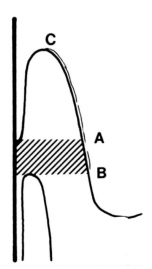

FIGURE 28–23. The shaded area shows the attached gingiva, which extends between the projection on the external surface of the bottom of the pocket (A) and the mucogingival junction (B). The keratinized gingiva may extend from the mucogingival junction (B) to the gingival margin (C).

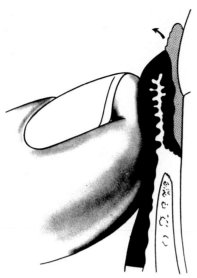

FIGURE 28-25. Purulent exudate expressed from a periodontal pocket by digital pressure.

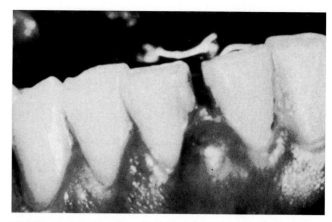

FIGURE 28-27. Acute periodontal abscess between the lower central incisors.

reveals it in pockets where its presence is not suspected (Fig. 28-26).

Periodontal Abscess. A periodontal abscess is a localized accumulation of pus within the gingival wall of a periodontal pocket (see Chapter 22). Periodontal abscesses may be acute or chronic.

The *acute periodontal abscess* appears as an ovoid elevation of the gingiva along the lateral aspect of the root (Figs. 28-27 to 28-29). The gingiva is edematous and red, with a smooth, shiny surface. The shape and consistency of the elevated area vary; the area may be dome-like and relatively firm, or pointed and soft. In most cases, pus may be expressed from the gingival margin with gentle digital pressure.

The acute periodontal abscess is accompanied by symptoms such as throbbing, radiating pain; exquisite tenderness of the gingiva to palpation; sensitivity of the tooth to palpation; tooth mobility; lymphadenitis; and, less frequently, systemic effects such as fever, leukocytosis, and malaise. Occasionally, the patient may have symptoms of an acute

periodontal abscess without any notable clinical lesion or radiographic changes.

The *chronic periodontal abscess* usually presents a sinus that opens onto the gingival mucosa somewhere along the length of the root. There may be a history of intermittent exudation. The orifice of the sinus may appear as a difficult-to-detect pinpoint opening, which, when probed, reveals a sinus tract deep in the periodontium (Fig. 28-30). The sinus may be covered by a small, pink, bead-like mass of granulation tissue (Fig. 28-31). The chronic periodontal abscess is usually asymptomatic. However, the patient may report episodes of dull, gnawing pain; slight elevation of the tooth; and a desire to bite down on and grind the tooth. The chronic periodontal abscess often undergoes acute exacerbations, with all the associated symptoms.

Diagnosis of the periodontal abscess requires correlation of the history and clinical and radiographic findings. The suspected area should be probed carefully along the gingival margin in relation to each tooth surface to detect a channel from the marginal area to the deeper periodontal tissues. Continuity of the lesion with the gingival margin is clinical evidence that the abscess is periodontal.

The abscess is not necessarily located on the same sur-

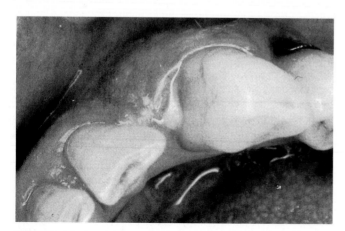

FIGURE 28-26. Pus formation on the mesial surface of the mandibular canine.

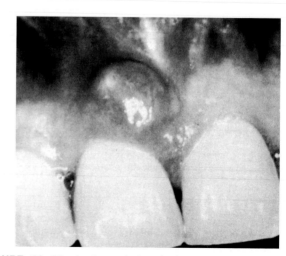

FIGURE 28-28. Acute periodontal abscess associated with a deep periodontal pocket facial and mesial of upper central incisor.

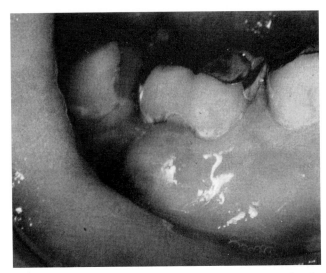

FIGURE 28–29. Chronic periodontal abscess in the wall of a deep pocket.

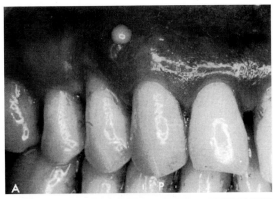

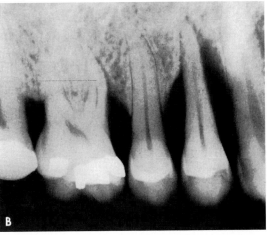

FIGURE 28–30. Suppuration from a chronic periodontal abscess. *A,* Suppurative draining sinus between the canine and first premolar. *B,* Radiograph showing extensive bone destruction in the area of the draining sinus.

face of the root as the pocket from which it is formed. A pocket at the facial surface may give rise to a periodontal abscess interproximally. It is common for a periodontal abscess to be located at a root surface other than that along which the pocket originated, because drainage is more likely to be impaired when a pocket follows a tortuous course.

In children a sinus orifice along the lateral aspect of a root is usually the result of periapical infection of a deciduous tooth. In the permanent dentition such an orifice may be caused by a periodontal abscess as well as by apical involvement. The orifice may be patent and draining, or it may be closed and appear as a red, nodular mass (Fig. 28–32). Exploration of such masses with a probe usually reveals a pinpoint orifice that communicates with an underlying sinus.

Periodontal Abscess and Gingival Abscess. The principal differences between the periodontal abscess and the gingival abscess are the location and history (see Chapters 18 and 22). The gingival abscess is confined to the marginal gingiva, and it often occurs in previously disease-free areas (Fig. 28–33). It is usually an acute inflammatory response to forcing of foreign material into the gingiva. The periodontal abscess involves the supporting periodontal structures and generally occurs in the course of chronic destructive periodontitis.

Periodontal Abscess and Periapical Abscess. Several characteristics can be used as guidelines in differentiating a periodontal abscess from a periapical abscess. If the tooth is nonvital, the lesion is most likely periapical. However, a

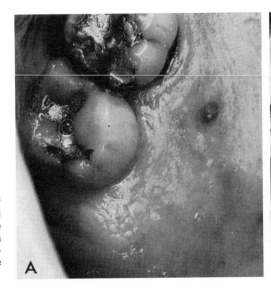

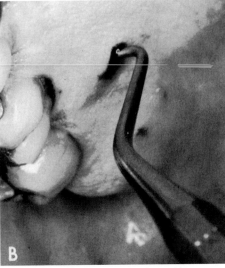

FIGURE 28–31. Pinpoint orifice of a sinus from a palatal periodontal abscess. *A,* Pinpoint orifice on the palate indicative of a sinus from a periodontal abscess. *B,* Probe extends into the abscess deep in the periodontium.

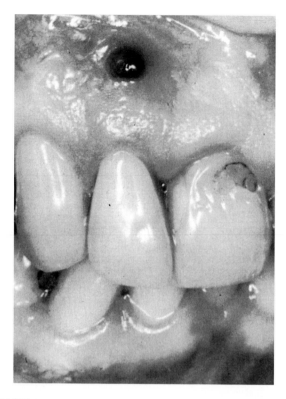

FIGURE 28–32. Nodular mass at the orifice of a draining sinus.

the presence of a periodontal abscess, whereas apical rarefaction suggests a periapical abscess. However, acute periodontal abscesses that show no radiographic changes frequently cause symptoms in teeth with long-standing, radiographically detectable periapical lesions that are not contributing to the patient's complaint. Clinical findings, such as the presence of extensive caries, pocket formation, lack of tooth vitality, and the existence of continuity between the gingival margin and the abscess area, often prove to be of greater diagnostic value than radiographic appearance.

A draining sinus on the lateral aspect of the root suggests periodontal rather than apical involvement; a sinus from a periapical lesion is more likely to be located further apically. However, sinus location is not conclusive. In many instances, particularly in children, the sinus from a periapical lesion drains on the side of the root rather than at the apex (see Chapter 58).

THE PERIODONTAL SCREENING & RECORDING SYSTEM*

The Periodontal Screening & Recording™ (PSR®) system is designed for easier and faster screening and recording of the periodontal status of a patient by a general practitioner or a dental hygienist.[41] It uses a specially designed

*Periodontal Screening & Recording™ and PSR® are service marks and trademarks of the American Dental Association.

previously nonvital tooth can have a deep periodontal pocket that can abscess. Moreover, a deep periodontal pocket can extend to the apex and cause pulpal involvement and necrosis.

An apical abscess may spread along the lateral aspect of the root to the gingival margin, but when the apex and lateral surface of a root are involved by a single lesion that can be probed directly from the gingival margin, the lesion is more likely to have originated in a periodontal abscess.

Radiographic findings are sometimes helpful in differentiating between a periodontal and a periapical lesion (see Chapter 29). Early acute periodontal and periapical abscesses present no radiographic changes. Ordinarily, a radiolucent area along the lateral surface of the root suggests

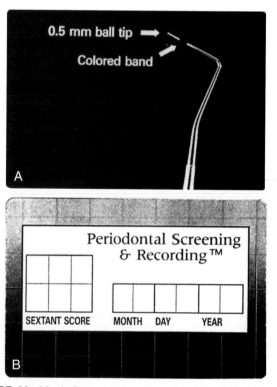

FIGURE 28–34. *A,* Periodontal probe especially designed for the PSR system. Note the ball tip and the color coding, 3.5 to 5.5 mm from the probe tip. *B,* Special sticker to be placed in the patient's chart with the code for each sextant. (From the American Dental Association and the American Academy of Periodontology. Periodontal Screening & Recording™ Training Manual, 1992. Reprinted with permission from the American Dental Association.)

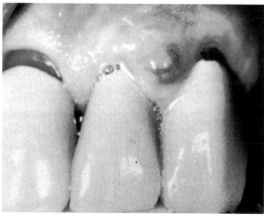

FIGURE 28–33. Gingival abscess between upper lateral incisor and canine. The area is essentially free of gingivitis.

probe that has a 0.5-mm ball tip and is color coded from 3.5 to 5.5 mm (Fig. 28–34*A*).

The patient's mouth is divided into six sextants (maxillary right, anterior and left; mandibular left, anterior and right), and each tooth is probed, with the clinician walking the probe around the entire tooth to examine at least six points around each tooth: mesiofacial, midfacial, distofacial, and the corresponding lingual/palatal areas. The deepest finding is recorded in each sextant, along with other findings, according to the following code:

Code 0: In the deepest sulcus of the sextant, the probe's colored band remains completely visible. Gingival tissue is healthy and does not bleed on gentle probing. No calculus or defective margins are found. These patients require only appropriate preventive care.

Code 1: The colored band of the probe remains completely visible in the deepest sulcus of the sextant; no calculus or defective margins are found, but some bleeding after gentle probing is detected. Treatment for these patients consists of subgingival plaque removal and appropriate oral hygiene instructions.

Code 2: The probe's colored band is still completely visible, but there is bleeding on probing, and supragingival or subgingival calculus and/or defective margins are found. Treatment should include plaque and calculus removal, correction of plaque-retentive margins of restorations, and oral hygiene instruction.

Code 3: The colored band is partially submerged. This indicates the need for a comprehensive periodontal examination and charting of the affected sextant to determine the necessary treatment plan. If two or more sextants score Code 3, a comprehensive full-mouth examination and charting is indicated.

Code 4: The colored band completely disappears in the pocket, indicating a depth greater than 5.5 mm. In this case a comprehensive full-mouth periodontal examination, charting, and treatment planning are needed.

Code *: When any of the following abnormalities are seen, an asterisk (*) is entered, in addition to the code number: furcation involvement, tooth mobility, mucogingival problem, or gingival recession extending to the colored band of the probe (3.5 mm or greater).

The code finding for each sextant and the date are entered on a sticker (Fig. 28–34*B*), which is placed on the patient's record.

REFERENCES

1. Abrams K, Caton J, Polson AM. Histologic comparisons of interproximal gingival tissues related to the presence or absence of bleeding. J Periodontol 55:629, 1984.
2. Alexander AG, Tipnis AK. The effect of irregularity of teeth and the degree of overbite and overjet on the gingival health. Br Dent J 128:539, 1970.
3. Amato R, Caton J, Polson A, Espeland M. Interproximal gingival inflammation related to the conversion of a bleeding to a non-bleeding state. J Periodontol 57:63, 1986.
4. Armitage GC, Svanberg GK, Löe H. Microscopic evaluation of clinical measurements of connective tissue attachment levels. J Clin Periodontol 4:173, 1977.
5. Bailey BL. Malpractice and periodontal disease. J Am Dent Assoc 115:845, 1987.
6. Baumgartner HS. A voice-input computerized dental examination system using high resolution graphics. Compend Contin Educ Dent 9:446, 1988.
7. Berg M, Burrill DY, Fosdick LS. Chemical studies in periodontal disease. IV. Putrefactive rate as index of periodontal disease. J Dent Res 26:67, 1947.
8. Caton J, Polson A. The interdental bleeding index: A simplified procedure to monitor gingival health. Compend Contin Educ Dent 6:89, 1985.
9. Dombrowski JC, Schachterle GR, Livne JK, White DK. A rapid chairside test for the severity of periodontal disease using gingival fluid. J Periodontol 49:391, 1978.
10. Fischman SL, Picozzi A. Review of the literature: The methodology of clinical calculus evaluation. J Periodontol 40:607, 1969.
11. Gabathuler H, Hassel TM. A pressure sensitive periodontal probe. Helv Odontol Acta 15:114, 1971.
12. Golub LM, Kaplan R, Mulvihill JE, Ramanurthy NS. Collagenolytic activity of crevicular fluid and of adjacent gingival tissue. J Dent Res 58:2132, 1979.
13. Greenberg J, Laster L, Listgarten MA. Transgingival probing as a potential estimator of alveolar bone level. J Periodontol 47:514, 1976.
14. Greenstein G. The role of bleeding upon probing in the diagnosis of periodontal disease. A literature review. J Periodontol 55:684, 1984.
15. Greenstein G, Caton J, Polson AM. Histologic characteristics associated with bleeding after probing and visual signs of inflammation. J Periodontol 52:420, 1981.
16. Hancock EB. Determination of periodontal disease activity. J Periodontol 52:492, 1981.
17. Hassel TM, German MA, Saxer UP. Periodontal probing: Interinvestigator discrepancies and correlations between probing force and recorded depth. Helv Odontol Acta 17:38, 1973.
18. Hirschfeld L. A calibrated silver point for periodontal diagnosis and recording. J Periodontol 24:94, 1953.
19. Kitchen PC. The prevalence of tooth root exposure and the relation of the extent of such exposure to the degree of abrasion in differing age classes. J Dent Res 20:565, 1941.
20. Kurashima K. Viscoelastic properties of periodontal tissue. Bull Tokyo Med Dent Univ 12:240, 1965.
21. Listgarten MA. Periodontal probing: What does it mean? J Clin Periodontol 7:165, 1980.
22. Listgarten MA, Hellden L. Relative distribution of bacteria at clinically healthy and periodontally diseased sites in humans. J Clin Periodontol 5:115, 1978.
23. Listgarten MA, Mao R, Robinson PJ. Periodontal probing: The relationship of the probe tip to periodontal tissues. J Periodontol 47:511, 1976.
24. Magnusson I, Listgarten MA. Histological evaluation of probing depth following periodontal treatment. J Clin Periodontol 7:26, 1980.
25. Mandell RL, Ebersole JL, Socransky SS. Clinical, immunologic and microbiologic features of active disease sites in juvenile periodontitis. J Clin Periodontol 14:534, 1987.
26. Manly RS. Abrasion of cementum and dentin by modern dentifrices. J Dent Res 20:583, 1941.
27. Manly RS. Factors influencing tests on the abrasion of dentin by brushing with dentifrices. J Dent Res 23:59, 1944.
28. Mannerberg F. Saliva factors in cases of erosion. Odont Rev 14:156, 1963.
29. McCay CM, Wills L. Erosion of molar teeth by acid beverages. J Nutr 39:313, 1949.
30. Meitner SW, Zander HA, Iker HP, Polson AM. Identification of inflamed gingival surfaces. J Clin Periodontol 6:93, 1979.
31. Miller WD. Experiments and observations on the wasting of tooth tissue variously designated as erosion, abrasion, chemical abrasion, denudation, etc. D Cosmos 49:1, 1907.
32. Muhlemann HR. Ten years of tooth mobility measurements. J Periodontol 31:110, 1960.
33. Muhlemann HR. Tooth mobility: A review of clinical aspects and research findings. J Periodontol 38:686, 1967.
34. Muhlemann HR, Savdir S, Rateitschak KH. Tooth mobility—its causes and significance. J Periodontol 36:148, 1965.
35. Mukherjee S. The temperature of the gingival sulcus. J Periodontol 49:580, 1978.
36. Ng GC, Compton FH, Walker TW. Measurement of human gingival sulcus temperature. J Periodont Res 13:295, 1978.
37. O'Leary TJ. Tooth mobility. Dent Clin North Am 3:567, 1969.
38. O'Leary TJ, Rudd KD. An instrument for measuring horizontal mobility. Periodontics 1:249, 1963.
39. Parfitt GJ. Measurement of the physiologic mobility of individual teeth in an axial direction. J Dent Res 39:608, 1960.
40. Parfitt GJ. The dynamics of a tooth in function. J Periodontol 32:102, 1961.
41. Periodontal Screening and Recording. Training Program. From the American Academy of Periodontology and the American Dental Association, sponsored by Procter & Gamble, 1992.
42. Perlitsch MJ. A systematic approach to the interpretation of tooth mobility and clinical implications. Dent Clin North Am 24:177, 1980.
43. Persson R. Assessment of tooth mobility using small loads. II. Effect of oral hygiene procedures. J Clin Periodontol 7:506, 1980.
44. Persson R. Assessment of tooth mobility using small loads. III. Effect of periodontal treatment including a gingivectomy procedure. J Clin Periodontol 8:4, 1981.
45. Persson R. Assessment of tooth mobility using small loads. IV. The effect of periodontal treatment including gingivectomy and flap procedures. J Clin Periodontol 8:88, 1981.
46. Persson R, Svensson A. Assessment of tooth mobility using small loads. I. Technical devices and calculations of tooth mobility in periodontal health and disease. J Clin Periodontol 7:259, 1980.
47. Robinson HBG. Abrasion, attrition and erosion of teeth. Health Center J Ohio State Univ 3:21, 1949.
48. Rudin HJ, Overdiek HF, Rateitschak KH. Correlation between sulcus fluid rate and clinical histological inflammation of the marginal gingiva. Helv Odontol Acta 14:21, 1970.
49. Saglie R, Johanson JR, Flotra L. The zone of completely and partially destructed periodontal fibers in pathological pockets. J Clin Periodontol 2:198, 1975.

50. Shapiro A, Goldman H, Bloom A. Sulcular exudate flow in gingival inflammation. J Periodontol *50:*301, 1979.
51. Shapiro L, Novaes AB Jr., Fillios L, Sulcular exudate protein levels as an indicator of the clinical inflammatory response. J Periodontol *51:*86, 1980.
52. Schulte W, D'Hoedt B, Scholz F, et al. Periotest—neues Messverfahren der Funktion des Parodontiums. Zahnarztl Mitt *73:*1229, 1983.
53. Sivertson JF, Burgett FG. Probing of pockets related to the attachment level. J Periodontol *47:*281, 1976.
54. Sognnaes RF. Periodontal significance of intraoral frictional ablation. J West Soc Periodontol *25:*112, 1977.
55. Spray JR, Garnick JJ, Doles LR, Klawitter JJ. Microscopic demonstration of the position of periodontal probes. J Periodontol *49:*148, 1978.
56. Tenuovo J, Anttonen T. Application of a dehydrated test strip. Hemastix for the assessment of gingivitis. J Clin Periodontol *5:*206, 1978.
57. Tibbetts LS. Use of diagnostic probes for detection of periodontal disease. J Am Dent Assoc *78:*549, 1969.
58. Van der Velden U. Probing force and the relationship of the probe tip to the periodontal tissues. J Clin Periodontol *6:*106, 1979.
59. Van der Velden U, De Vries JH. Introduction of a new periodontal probe. The pressure probe. J Clin Periodontol *5:*188, 1978.

29

Radiographic and Other Aids in the Diagnosis of Periodontal Disease

FERMIN A. CARRANZA, JR.

RADIOGRAPHS IN THE DIAGNOSIS OF PERIODONTAL DISEASE

The radiograph is a valuable aid in the diagnosis of periodontal disease, the determination of patient prognosis, and the evaluation of the outcome of treatment. However, *it is an adjunct to the clinical examination, not a substitute for it.*

The radiograph reveals alterations in calcified tissue; it does not reveal current cellular activity but shows the effects of past cellular events on the bone and roots. Special techniques that are not yet in routine clinical usage are required to show changes in the soft tissues of the periodontium.

Normal Interdental Septa

Radiographic evaluation of bone changes in periodontal disease is based mainly on the appearance of the interdental septa, because the relatively dense root structure obscures the facial and lingual bony plates. The interdental septum normally presents a thin, radiopaque border adjacent to and

at the crest of the periodontal ligament; this border is referred to as the *lamina dura* (Fig. 29–1). This appears radiographically as a continuous white line, but in reality it is perforated by numerous small foramina and traversed by blood vessels, lymphatics, and nerves, which pass between the periodontal ligament and the bone. *Because the lamina dura represents the bone surface lining the tooth socket, the shape and position of the root and changes in the angulation of the x-ray beam produce considerable variations in its appearance.*[14]

The width and shape of the interdental septum and the angle of the crest normally vary according to the convexity of the proximal surfaces of the teeth and the level of the cemento-enamel junctions of the approximating teeth.[25] The interdental space, and therefore the interdental septum, between teeth with prominently convex proximal crown surfaces is wider anteroposteriorly than that between teeth with relatively flat proximal crown surfaces. The faciolingual diameter of the bone is related to the width of the proximal root surface. The angulation of the crest of the interdental septum is generally parallel to a line between the cemento-enamel junctions of the approximating teeth (see

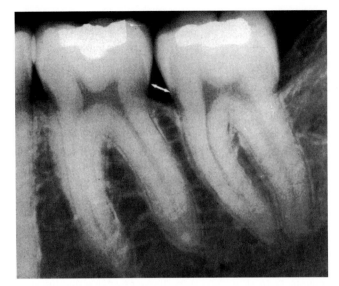

FIGURE 29-1. Crest of interdental septum normally parallel to a line drawn between the cemento-enamel junction of adjacent teeth *(arrow)*. Note the radiopaque lamina dura around the roots and interdental septum.

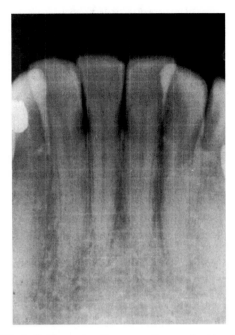

FIGURE 29-2. Radiograph with a superimposed grid calibrated in millimeters.

Fig. 29-1). When there is a difference in the levels of the cemento-enamel junctions, the crest of the interdental bone appears angulated rather than horizontal.

Distortions Produced by Variations in Radiographic Technique

Variations in technique produce artifacts that limit the diagnostic value of the radiograph. *The bone level; the pattern of bone destruction; the width of the periodontal ligament space[37]; and the radiodensity, trabecular pattern, and marginal contour of the interdental septum are modified by altering the exposure and development time, the type of film, and the x-ray angulation.*[16] Standardized, reproducible techniques are required to obtain reliable radiographs for pre- and post-treatment comparisons.[15,21,27] A grid calibrated in millimeters, superimposed on the finished film, is helpful for comparing bone levels in radiographs taken under similar conditions[6] (Fig. 29-2).

The following are useful facts regarding the effects of angulation: The long cone–paralleling technique projects the most realistic image of the level of the alveolar bone[8] (Fig. 29-3). The bisection-of-the-angle technique increases the projection and makes the bone margin appear closer to the crown; the level of the facial bone margin is distorted more than that of the lingual margin (see Fig. 29-3). Shifting the cone mesially or distally without changing the horizontal plane projects the x-rays obliquely and changes the shape of the interdental bone on the radiograph, the radiographic width of the periodontal ligament space, and the appearance of the lamina dura and may distort the extent of furcation involvement (Fig. 29-4).

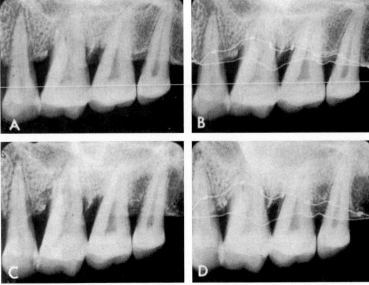

FIGURE 29-3. Long cone–paralleling technique and bisection-of-the-angle technique compared. *A,* Long-cone technique: radiograph of dried specimen. *B,* Long-cone technique, same specimen. The smooth wire is on the margin of the facial plate, and the knotted wire is on the lingual plate to show their relative positions. *C,* Bisection-of-the-angle technique, same specimen. *D,* Bisection-of-the-angle technique, same specimen. Both bone margins are shifted toward the crown. The facial margin (smooth wire) has shifted more than the lingual margin (knotted wire), creating the illusion that the lingual bone margin has shifted apically. (Courtesy of Dr. Benjamin Patur.)

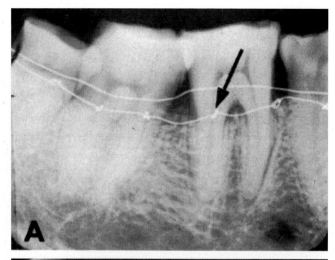

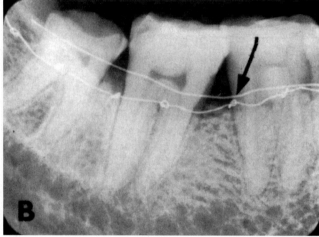

FIGURE 29–4. Distortion by oblique projection. *A,* Long-cone technique. The smooth wire is on the facial bony plate, the knotted wire is on the lingual. Note the knot *(arrow)* near the center of the distal root of the first molar, which shows bifurcation involvement. *B,* Long-cone technique. The cone is placed distally, projecting the rays mesially and obliquely. The oblique projection shifts the image of all structures mesially. *The structures closest to the cone shift the most.* This creates the illusion that the knot *(arrow)* has moved distally. Note that the bifurcation involvement shown in *A* is obliterated in *B.*

Prichard[20] established the following four criteria to determine adequate angulation of periapical radiographs:

1. The radiograph should show the tips of molar cusps with little or none of the occlusal surface showing.
2. Enamel caps and pulp chambers should be distinct.
3. Interproximal spaces should be open.
4. Proximal contacts should not overlap unless teeth are out of line anatomically.

Bone Destruction in Periodontal Disease

The radiograph does not reveal minor destructive changes in bone[2,3,22]; therefore, slight radiographic changes in the periodontal tissues mean that the disease has progressed beyond its earliest stages. Therefore, *the earliest signs of periodontal disease must be detected clinically.*

The radiographic image tends to show less severe bone loss than is actually present.[35] The difference between the actual alveolar crest height and the height as it appears on the radiograph ranges from 0 to 1.6 mm,[23] most of which can be accounted for by x-ray angulation.

Amount of Bone Loss. The radiograph is an indirect method for determining the amount of bone loss in periodontal disease; it shows the amount of bone remaining rather than the amount lost. The amount of bone lost is estimated to be the difference between the physiologic bone level of the patient and the height of the remaining bone.

Distribution of Bone Loss. The distribution of bone loss is an important diagnostic sign, as it indicates the location of destructive local factors in different areas of the mouth and in relation to different surfaces of the same tooth.

Pattern of Bone Destruction. *In periodontal disease, the interdental septa undergo changes that affect the lamina dura, the crestal radiodensity, the size and shape of the medullary spaces, and the height and contour of the bone.* The interdental septa may be reduced in height, with the crest horizontal and perpendicular to the long axis of the adjacent teeth (Fig. 29–5), or they may have angular or arcuate defects (Fig. 29–6). The former condition is called *horizontal bone loss;* the latter is known as *angular* or *vertical bone loss* (see Chapter 23).

Radiographs do not reveal the extent of involvement on the facial and lingual surfaces or the presence of fenestrations or dehiscences, because facial and lingual surface bone destruction is obscured by the dense root structure. Similarly, bone destruction on the mesial and distal root surfaces may be partially hidden by a dense mylohyoid ridge (Fig. 29–7).

Dense cortical plates on the facial and lingual surfaces of the interdental septa obscure destruction that occurs in the intervening cancellous bone. Thus, it is possible to have a deep crater in the bone between the facial and lingual plates without any radiographic indication of its presence. For destruction of the interproximal cancellous bone to be recorded radiographically, the cortical bone must be involved. A reduction of only 0.5 or 1.0 mm in the thickness of the cortical plate is sufficient to permit radiographic visualization of destruction of the inner cancellous trabeculae.[18]

Gutta-percha can be packed around the teeth to help determine the morphology of osseous craters and involvement of the facial and lingual surfaces (Fig. 29–8). However, this is a cumbersome technique and is seldom performed. Surgical exposure and visual examination provide the most definitive information regarding the bone architecture produced by periodontal destruction.[19]

Radiographic Changes in Periodontitis

The sequence of radiographic changes in periodontitis and the tissue changes that produce them is as follows:

1. *Fuzziness and a break in the continuity of the lamina dura* at the mesial or distal aspect of the crest of the interdental septum have been described as the earliest radiographic changes in periodontitis (Fig. 29–9). These result from extension of inflammation from the gingiva into the bone, along with associated widening of the vessel channels and a reduction in calcified tissue at the septal margin. No correlation has been found, however, between crestal lamina dura in radiographs and the presence or absence of clinical inflammation, bleeding on probing, periodontal pockets, or loss of attachment.[11]

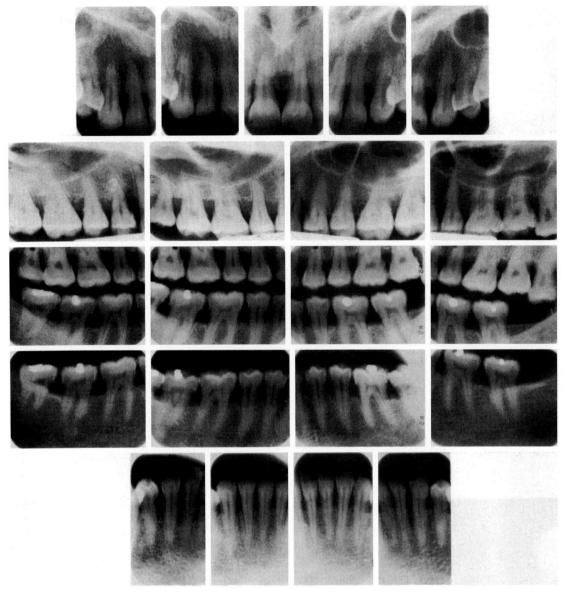

FIGURE 29–5. Generalized horizontal bone loss.

2. *A wedge-shaped radiolucent area* is formed at the mesial or distal aspect of the crest of the septal bone (Fig. 29–9B). The apex of the area is pointed in the direction of the root. This is produced by resorption of the bone at the lateral aspect of the interdental septum, with an associated widening of the periodontal space.
3. The destructive process extends across the crest of the interdental septum and *the height is reduced.* Finger-like radiolucent projections extend from the crest into the septum (Fig. 29–9C). The radiolucent projections into the interdental septum are the result of the deeper extension of the inflammation into the bone. Inflammatory cells and fluid, proliferation of connective tissue cells, and increased osteoclasis cause increased bone resorption along the endosteal margins of the medullary spaces. The radiopaque projections separating the radiolucent spaces are the composite images of the partially eroded bony trabeculae.
4. The height of the interdental septum (Fig. 29–9D) is progressively reduced by the extension of inflammation and the resorption of bone.

Radiographic Appearance of Interdental Craters

Interdental craters are seen as irregular areas of reduced radiopacity on the alveolar bone crests[24]; they are generally not sharply demarcated from the rest of the bone, with which they blend gradually. Radiographs do not accurately depict the morphology or depth of interdental craters, which sometimes appear as vertical defects.

Radiographic Appearance of Furcation Involvements

Definitive diagnosis of furcation involvement is made by clinical examination, which includes careful probing with a specially designed probe (Nabers probe). Radiographs are helpful but show artifacts that make it possible for furcation involvement to be present without detectable radiographic changes.

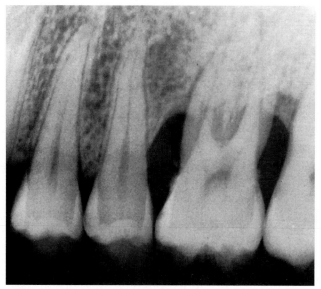

FIGURE 29–6. Angular bone loss on the first molar with involvement of the trifurcation.

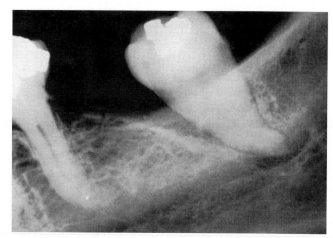

FIGURE 29–7. Angular bone loss on mandibular molar partially obscured by a dense mylohyoid ridge.

As a general rule, *bone loss is always greater than it appears on the radiograph.* Variations in the radiographic technique may obscure the presence and extent of furcation involvement. A tooth may present marked furcation involvement in one film (Fig. 29–10A) but appear to be uninvolved in another (Fig. 29–10B). Radiographs should be taken at different angles to reduce the risk of missing furcation involvement.

The recognition of large, clearly defined radiolucency in the furcation area presents no problem (Fig. 29–10A), but less clearly defined radiographic changes in the furcation are often overlooked. To assist in the radiographic detection of furcation involvement, the following three diagnostic criteria are suggested:

1. The slightest radiographic change in the furcation area should be investigated clinically, especially if there is bone loss on adjacent roots (Fig. 29–11).
2. Diminished radiodensity in the furcation area in which outlines of bony trabeculae are visible (Fig. 29–12) suggests furcation involvement.
3. Whenever there is marked bone loss in relation to a single molar root, it may be assumed that the furcation is also involved (Figs. 29–13 and 29–14).

Radiographic Appearance of Periodontal Abscesses

The typical radiographic appearance of the periodontal abscess is that of a discrete area of radiolucency along the

lateral aspect of the root (Figs. 29–15 and 29–16). However, *the radiographic picture is often not typical* (Fig. 29–17) as a result of any of the following variables:

1. The stage of the lesion. In the early stages the acute periodontal abscess is extremely painful but presents no radiographic changes.
2. The extent of bone destruction and the morphologic changes of the bone.
3. The location of the abscess. Lesions in the soft tissue wall of a periodontal pocket are less likely to produce radiographic changes than those deep in the supporting tissues. Abscesses on the facial or lingual surface are obscured by the radiopacity of the root; interproximal lesions are more likely to be visualized radiographically.

Therefore, *the radiograph alone cannot be relied on for the diagnosis of a periodontal abscess.*

Radiographic Changes in Juvenile Periodontitis

Juvenile periodontitis is characterized by a combination of the following radiographic features:

1. Bone loss occurs initially in the maxillary and mandibular incisor and first molar areas, usually bilaterally, and results in vertical, arc-like destructive patterns (Fig. 29–18).
2. Loss of alveolar bone tends to become generalized as the disease progresses but remains less pronounced in the premolar areas.

Radiographic Changes in Trauma From Occlusion

Trauma from occlusion can produce radiographically detectable changes in the lamina dura, in the morphology of

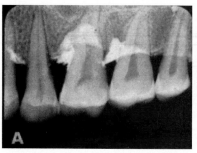
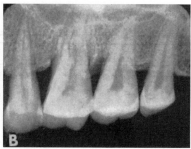

FIGURE 29–8. Gutta-percha aids in detecting bone defects. *A*, Gutta-percha packed around teeth shows interproximal and facial and lingual bone loss. *B*, Same area without gutta-percha gives little indication of the extent of bone involvement.

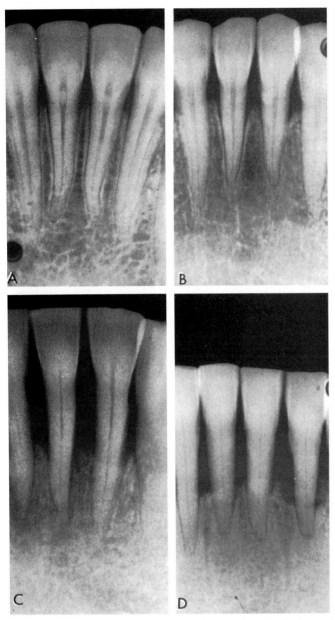

The *injury phase* of trauma from occlusion produces a loss of the lamina dura that may be noted in apices, furcations, and/or marginal areas. This loss of lamina dura will result in widening of the periodontal ligament space (Fig. 29–19). This change, particularly when incipient or circumscribed, may easily be confused with technical variations caused by x-ray angulation or malposition of the tooth; it can be diagnosed with certainty only in radiographs of the highest quality.

The *repair phase* of trauma from occlusion will result in an attempt by the body to strengthen the periodontal structures to better support the increased loads. Radiographically this is manifested by a widening of the periodontal ligament space, which may be generalized or localized.

Although microscopic measurements have determined

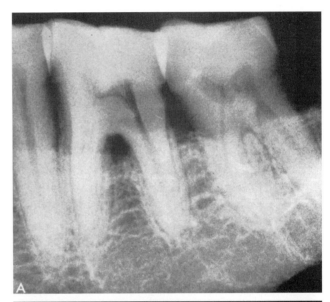

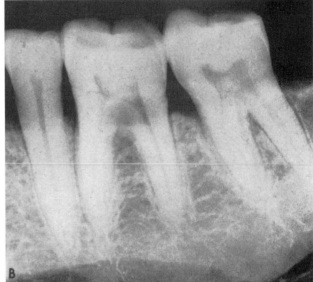

FIGURE 29–9. Radiographic changes in periodontitis. *A,* Normal appearance of interdental septa. *B,* Fuzziness and a break in the continuity of the lamina dura at the crest of the bone distal to the central incisor *(left).* There are wedge-shaped radiolucent areas at the crests of the other interdental septa. *C,* Radiolucent projections from the crest into the interdental septum indicate extension of destructive processes. *D,* Severe bone loss.

the alveolar crest, in the width of the periodontal space, and in the density of the surrounding cancellous bone.

Traumatic lesions manifest themselves more clearly in faciolingual aspects, because mesiodistally the tooth has the added stability provided by the contact areas with adjacent teeth. Therefore, slight variations in the proximal surfaces may indicate greater changes in the facial and lingual aspects. *The radiographic changes discussed in the following paragraphs are not pathognomonic of trauma from occlusion and must be interpreted in combination with clinical findings,* particularly tooth mobility, presence of wear facets, pocket depth, and analysis of occlusal contacts and habits.

FIGURE 29–10. *A,* Furcation involvement indicated by triangular radiolucency in the furcation area of a mandibular first molar. The second molar shows only a slight thickening of the periodontal space in the furcation area. *B,* Same area, different angulation. The triangular radiolucency in the furcation of the first molar is obliterated, and involvement of the second molar is apparent.

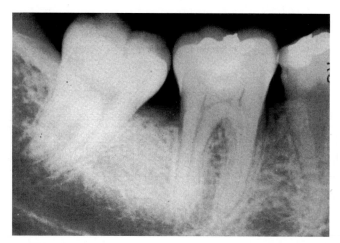

FIGURE 29–11. Early furcation involvement suggested by fuzziness in the bifurcation of the mandibular first molar, particularly when associated with bone loss on the roots.

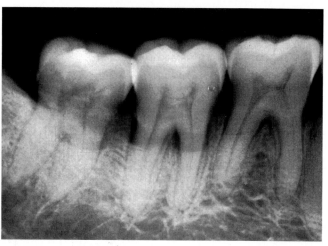

FIGURE 29–12. Furcation involvement of the mandibular first and second molars indicated by thickening of periodontal space in bifurcation area. The furcation of the third molar is also involved, but the thickening of the periodontal space is partially obscured by the external oblique line.

that there are normal variations in the width of the periodontal space in the different regions of the root, these are not generally detected in radiographs. When variations in width between the marginal area and the mid-root or between the mid-root and the apex are detected, it indicates that the tooth is being subjected to increased forces. Successful attempts to reinforce the periodontal structures by widening of the periodontal space will be accompanied by increased width of the lamina dura and sometimes by condensation of the perialveolar cancellous bone.

More advanced traumatic lesions may result in deep angular bone loss, which, when combined with marginal inflammation, may lead to infrabony pocket formation. In terminal stages these lesions extend around the root apex, producing a wide radiolucent periapical image (cavernous lesions).

Root resorption may also occur as a result of excessive forces on the periodontium, particularly those caused by orthodontic appliances. Although trauma from occlusion produces many root resorption areas, they are usually of insufficient magnitude to be detected radiographically.

Additional Radiographic Criteria in the Diagnosis of Periodontal Disease

The following radiographic criteria can be used to aid in the diagnosis of periodontal disease:

Radiopaque horizontal line across the roots. This line demarcates the portion of the root where the labial and/or lingual bony plate has been partially or completely destroyed from the remaining bone-supported portion (Fig. 29–20).

Vessel canals in the alveolar bone. Hirschfeld[13] described linear and circular radiolucent areas produced by interdental canals and their foramina, respectively (Fig. 29–21). These canals indicate the course of the vascular supply of the bone and are normal radiographic findings. The radiographic image of the canals is frequently so prominent, particularly in the anterior region of the mandible, that the canals may be confused with radiolucency resulting from periodontal disease.

Differentiation between treated and untreated periodontal

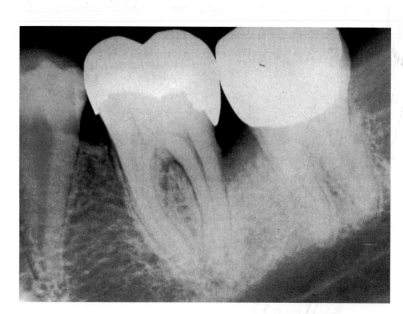

FIGURE 29–13. Furcation involvement of the first molar, associated with bone loss on the distal root.

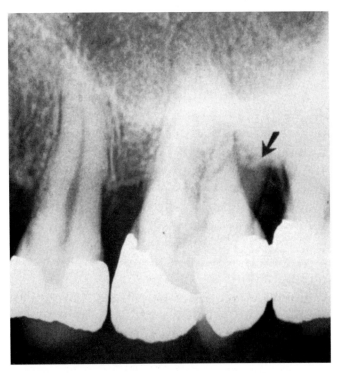

FIGURE 29–14. Furcation involvement of the first molar partially obscured by the radiopaque lingual root. The horizontal line across the distobuccal root demarcates the apical portion *(arrow)*, which is covered by bone, from the remainder of the root, where the bone has been destroyed.

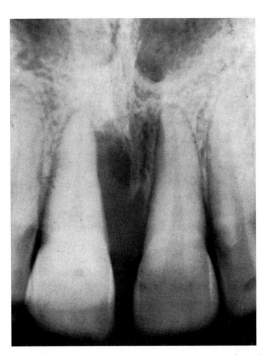

FIGURE 29–16. Typical radiographic appearance of periodontal abscess on the right central incisor.

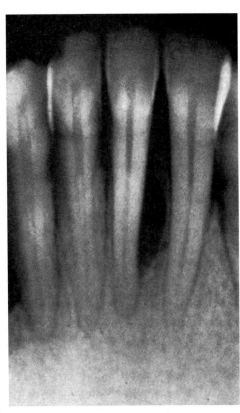

FIGURE 29–15. Radiolucent area on the lateral aspect of the root with chronic periodontal abscess.

disease. It is sometimes necessary to determine whether the reduced bone level is the result of periodontal disease that is no longer destructive (usually after treatment and proper maintenance) or whether destructive periodontal disease is present. Clinical examination is the basic determinant. However, radiographically detectable alterations in the normal clear-cut peripheral outline of the septa are corroborating evidence of destructive periodontal disease.

Skeletal Disturbances Manifested in the Jaws

Skeletal disturbances may produce changes in the jaws that affect the interpretation of radiographs from the periodontal perspective. Destruction of tooth-supporting bone may occur in the following diseases:

Osteitis fibrosa cystica (Recklinghausen's disease of bone) develops in advanced primary or secondary hyperparathyroidism and causes osteoclastic resorption of bone with fibrous replacement (brown tumor) (see Figs. 14–1 and 14–2). Frequently the first manifestation is a cystic lesion of the jaw. This disease results in a diffuse granular mottling, scattered cyst-like radiolucent areas throughout the jaws, and a generalized disappearance of the lamina dura.[26,32] Correction of the parathyroid hyperfunction usually results in rapid reversion of the bone to normal.

In *Paget's disease,* the radiographic appearance of the jaws varies. The normal trabecular pattern may be replaced by a hazy, diffuse meshwork of closely knit, fine trabecular markings, with the lamina dura absent (Fig. 29–22), or there may be scattered radiolucent areas containing irregularly shaped radiopaque zones.[10]

Fibrous dysplasia may appear as a small radiolucent area at a root apex or as an extensive radiolucent area with irregularly arranged trabecular markings.[9] There may be enlargement of the cancellous spaces, with distortion of the

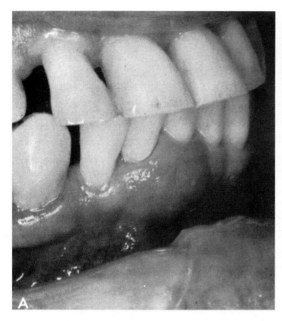
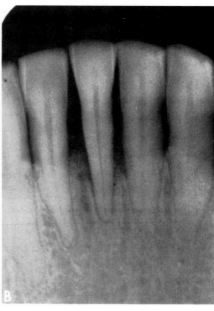

FIGURE 29–17. Chronic periodontal abscess. *A,* Periodontal abscess in the right central and lateral incisor area. *B,* Extensive bone destruction and thickening of the periodontal ligament space around the right central incisor.

normal trabecular pattern and obliteration of the lamina dura (Fig. 29–23).

In *Hand-Schüller-Christian disease,* the radiographic appearance is one of single or multiple areas of radiolucency. Mobility of the teeth results from loss of bony support. *Letterer-Siwe disease* and *Gaucher's disease* may have comparable changes (Fig. 29–24).

Eosinophilic granuloma[28,34] appears as single or multiple radiolucent areas, which may be unrelated to the teeth or entail destruction of the tooth-supporting bone. These lesions may simulate severe localized periodontitis.[15]

Numerous radiolucent areas occur when the jaws are involved by *multiple myeloma.*

In *osteopetrosis* (marble bone disease, Albers-Schönberg dis-

ease),[7] the outlines of the roots may be obscured by diffuse radiopacity of the jaws. In less severe cases, the increased density is confined to the bone in relation to the nutrient canals and the lamina dura.

In *scleroderma* (see Chapter 20), the periodontal ligament is uniformly widened at the expense of the surrounding alveolar bone[1] (Fig. 29–25).

LABORATORY AIDS IN DIAGNOSIS

Biopsy

The gingival biopsy may be important in the diagnosis of some gingival disturbances, particularly if neoplastic

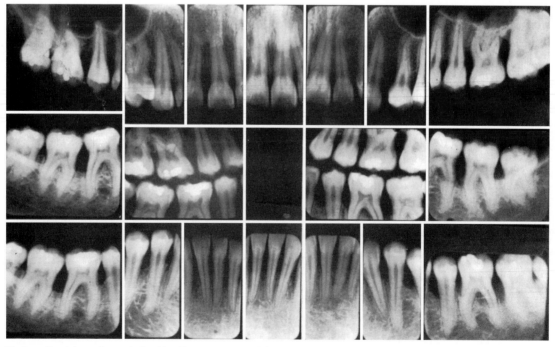

FIGURE 29–18. Localized juvenile periodontitis. The accentuated bone destruction in the anterior and first molar areas is considered to be characteristic of this disease.

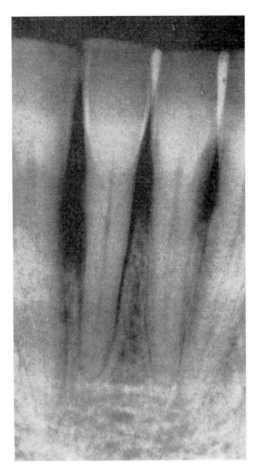

FIGURE 29–19. Widened periodontal space caused by trauma from occlusion. Note the increased density of the surrounding bone caused by new bone formation in response to increased occlusal forces.

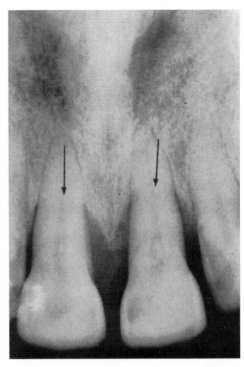

FIGURE 29–20. Horizontal lines across the roots of the central incisors (arrows). The area of the roots below the horizontal lines is partially or completely denuded of the facial and/or lingual bony plates.

changes are suspected. (The reader is referred to books on oral pathology for an in-depth analysis of such changes.) Microscopic study of gingival biopsy specimens is sometimes the only method of detecting local and systemic interrelationships that cannot be discerned by clinical examination. For example, amyloid is present in the gingiva of patients with amyloidosis, many of whom have no clinical gingival changes.[31]

Tissues from the marginal and attached gingivae should be included in the biopsy specimen (Fig. 29–26). Inflammatory changes in the gingival margin tend to obscure any alterations that may be produced by a systemic disturbance. Inclusion of the attached gingiva, in which the effect of local irritants is less likely to be present, offers an opportunity to investigate tissue changes that may be produced by systemic disturbances.

In addition to diagnosing malignancies, the biopsy is useful in differentiating among different types of gingival enlargement and when the presence of diseases such as desquamative gingivitis, benign mucous membrane pemphigoid, pemphigus, or lichen planus is suspected. In these cases, exfoliative cytology also may be helpful.[29,32]

OTHER AIDS USED IN THE DIAGNOSIS OF ORAL MANIFESTATIONS OF SYSTEMIC DISEASE

When unusual gingival or periodontal problems are present and cannot be explained by local causes, the possibility of contributing systemic factors must be explored. Chapter 30 presents the microbiologic, immunologic, and biochemical tests used to determine the pathogenic mechanisms that play a role in periodontitis. In addition, the dentist must understand the oral manifestations of systemic diseases so that he or she can question the patient's physician regarding the type of systemic disturbance that may be involved in individual cases.

Numerous laboratory tests aid in the diagnosis of systemic diseases. Descriptions of the manner in which they are performed and the interpretation of findings are provided in standard texts on the subject.[36] Tests pertinent to the diagnosis of disturbances often manifested in the oral cavity are discussed briefly here.

Nutritional Status Evaluation

If, when examining a patient, it is the dentist's impression that a nutritional deficiency exists, *this suspicion must be corroborated by a medical evaluation of the patient's nutritional status.* Nutritional therapy in the treatment of periodontal disturbances *must be based on a demonstrated need,* which is best determined by a nutritionist.

Certain signs and symptoms have been identified with

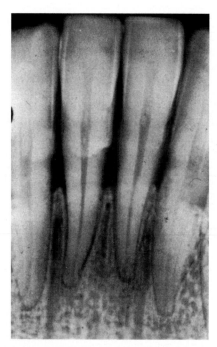

FIGURE 29–21. Prominent vessel canals in the mandible.

various nutritional deficiencies. However, many patients with nutritional disease do not exhibit classic signs of deficiency disorders, and different types of deficiency produce similar clinical findings. Clinical findings are suggestive, but definitive diagnosis of nutritional deficiencies and their

nature requires the combined information revealed by the history, clinical and laboratory findings, and therapeutic trial. Clinical findings identified with specific nutritional deficiencies and the oral manifestations of nutritional disorders are described in Chapter 14.

Patients on Special Diets for Medical Reasons

Patients on low-residue, nondetergent diets may develop gingivitis because the prescribed foods lack cleansing action, and the tendency for plaque and food debris to accumulate on the teeth is increased. Because fibrous foods are contraindicated, special effort is made to compensate for the soft diet by emphasizing the patient's oral hygiene procedures. Patients on salt-free diets should not be given saline mouthwashes, nor should they be treated with saline preparations without consulting their physician. Diabetes, gallbladder disease, and hypertension are examples of conditions in which particular care should be taken to avoid the prescription of contraindicated foodstuffs.

Hemogram

Analyses of blood smears, red and white blood cell counts, white blood cell differential counts, and erythrocyte sedimentation rates are used to evaluate the presence of blood dyscrasias and generalized infections. These analyses may be useful aids in the differential diagnosis of certain types of periodontal diseases; the reader is referred to books on hematology[36] for a consideration of this subject.

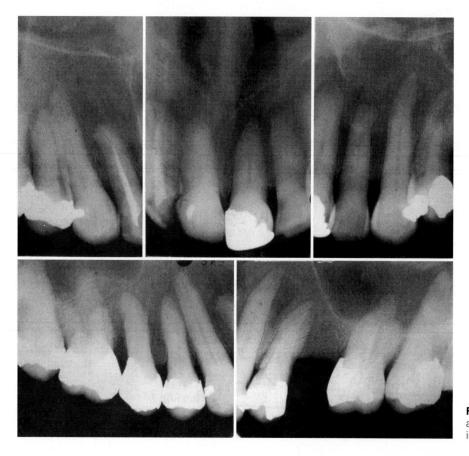

FIGURE 29–22. Altered trabecular pattern and diminution in the prominence of the lamina dura in Paget's disease.

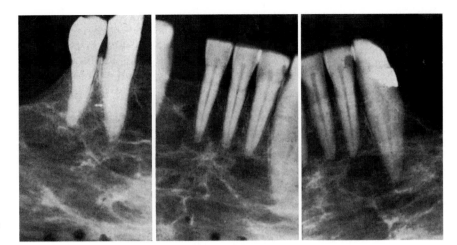

FIGURE 29-23. Osteoporosis and altered trabecular arrangement in fibrous dysplasia.

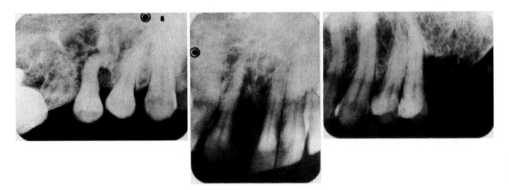

FIGURE 29-24. Osteoporosis in Gaucher's disease.

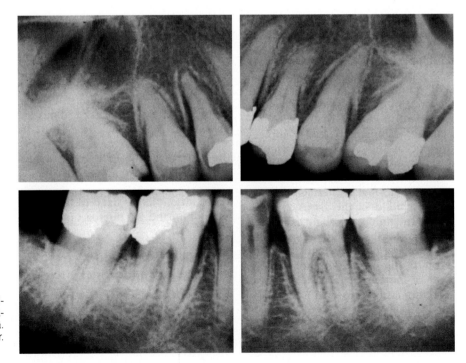

FIGURE 29-25. Scleroderma, showing typical uniform widening of the periodontal ligament and thickening of the lamina dura. (Courtesy of Dr. David F. Mitchell and Dr. Anand P. Chaudhry.)

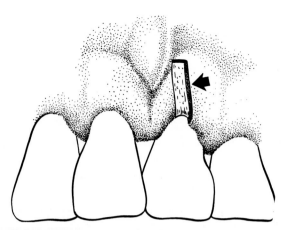

FIGURE 29–26. Diagram of a rectangular gingival biopsy specimen *(arrow)* that includes marginal and attached gingiva.

Laboratory Tests for Determining the Etiology of Spontaneous or Excessive Bleeding

Determinations of coagulation time, bleeding time, clot retraction time, and prothrombin time; a capillary fragility test; and bone marrow studies may, at times, be required. Discussions of their indications and the interpretation of their results can be found in books on clinical and laboratory diagnosis. Chapter 34 describes the use of these tests for the evaluation and management of medically compromised patients.

REFERENCES

1. Alexandridis C, White SC. Periodontal ligament changes in patients with progressive systemic sclerosis. Oral Surg Oral Med Oral Pathol 58:113, 1984.
2. Bender IB, Seltzer S. Roentgenographic and direct observation of experimental lesions in bone. I. J Am Dent Assoc 62:152, 1961.
3. Bender IB, Seltzer S. Roentgenographic and direct observation of experimental lesions in bone. II. J Am Dent Assoc 62:708, 1961.
4. Bjorn H, Holmberg K. Radiographic determination of periodontal bone destruction in epidemiological research. Odont Rev 17:232, 1966.
5. Easley J. Methods of determining alveolar osseous form. J Periodontol 38:112, 1967.
6. Everett FG, Fixott HC. Use of an incorporated grid in the diagnosis of oral roentgenograms. Oral Surg Oral Med Oral Pathol 16:1061, 1963.
7. Fairbank HAT. Osteopetrosis. J Bone Joint Surg 30:339, 1948.
8. Fitzgerald GM. Dental radiography. IV. The voltage factor (k.p.). J Am Dent Assoc 41:19, 1950.
9. Glickman I. Fibrous dysplasia in alveolar bone. Oral Surg Oral Med Oral Pathol 1:895, 1948.
10. Glickman I, Glidden S. Paget's disease of the maxillae and mandible. Clinical analysis and case reports. J Am Dent Assoc 29:2144, 1942.
11. Greenstein G, Polson A, Iker H, Meitner S. Associations between crestal lamina dura and periodontal status. J Periodontol 52:362, 1981.
12. Henry JB. Todd-Sanford-Davidsohn Clinical Diagnosis and Management by Laboratory Methods. 17th ed. Philadelphia, WB Saunders, 1984.
13. Hirschfeld I. Interdental canals. J Am Dent Assoc 14:617, 1927.
14. Manson JD. Lamina dura. Oral Surg Oral Med Oral Pathol 16:432, 1963.
15. Nicopoulou-Karayianni K, Mombelli A, Lang NP. Diagnostic problems of periodontitis-like lesions caused by eosinophilic granuloma. J Clin Periodontol 16:505, 1989.
16. Parfitt GJ. An investigation of the normal variations in alveolar bone trabeculations. Oral Surg 15:1453, 1962.
17. Patur B, Glickman I. Roentgenographic evaluation of alveolar bone changes in periodontal disease. Dent Clin North Am 4:47, 1960.
18. Pauls V, Trott JR. A radiological study of experimentally produced lesions in bone. Dent Pract 16:254, 1966.
19. Prichard JF. Role of the roentgenogram in the diagnosis and prognosis of periodontal disease. Oral Med 14:182, 1961.
20. Prichard JF. Advanced Periodontal Disease. Surgical and Prosthetic Management. 2nd ed. Philadelphia, WB Saunders, 1972.
21. Puckett J. A device for comparing roentgenograms of the same mouth. J Periodontol 39:38, 1968.
22. Ramadan ABE, Mitchell DF. A roentgenographic study of experimental bone destruction. Oral Surg Oral Med Oral Pathol 15:934, 1962.
23. Regan JE, Mitchell DF. Roentgenographic and dissection measurements of alveolar crest height. J Am Dent Assoc 66:356, 1963.
24. Rees TD, Biggs NL, Collings CK. Radiographic interpretation of periodontal osseous lesions. Oral Surg Oral Med Oral Pathol 32:141, 1971.
25. Ritchey B, Orban B. The crests of the interdental septa. J Periodontol 24:75, 1953.
26. Rosenberg EH, Guralnick WC. Hyperparathyroidism. Oral Surg Oral Med Oral Pathol 15(suppl 2):84, 1962.
27. Rosling B, Hollender L, Nyman S, Olsson G. A radiographic method for assessing changes in alveolar bone height following periodontal therapy. J Clin Periodontol 2:211, 1975.
28. Salman I, Darlington CG. Eosinophilic granuloma. Am J Orthodont 31:89, 1945.
29. Sandler HC, Stahl SS, Cahn LR, Freund HR. Exfoliative cytology for the detection of early mouth cancer. Oral Surg Oral Med Oral Pathol 13:994, 1960.
31. Selikoff I, Robitzek E. Gingival biopsy for the diagnosis of generalized amyloidosis. Am J Pathol 23:1099, 1947.
32. Shklar G, Cataldo E, Meyer I. Reliability of cytologic smear in diagnosis of oral cancer. A controlled study. Arch Otolaryngol 91:158, 1970.
33. Silverman S Jr, Gordan G, Grant T, et al. Dental structures in primary hyperparathyroidism: Studies in forty-two consecutive patients. Oral Surg Oral Med Oral Pathol 15:426, 1962.
34. Sleeper E. Eosinophilic granuloma of bone. Oral Surg 4:896, 1951.
35. Theilade J. An evaluation of the reliability of radiographs in the measurement of bone loss in periodontal disease. J Periodontol 31:143, 1960.
36. Thorup OA Jr, ed. Leavell and Thorup's Fundamentals of Clinical Hematology. 5th ed. Philadelphia, WB Saunders, 1987.
37. Van der Linden LWJ, Van Aken J. The periodontal ligament in the roentgenogram. J Periodontol 41:243, 1970.

30

Advanced Diagnostic Techniques

MICHAEL G. NEWMAN and MARIANO SANZ

Knowledge about the microbiologic and immunologic factors responsible for the pathogenesis of periodontal diseases has greatly advanced in the last few years (see Chapters 6 and 10), improving our understanding of the disease process and leading to the development of certain indicators for the identification of persons and/or sites with higher susceptibility to periodontal breakdown. Recognition and assessment of this susceptibility enhance the predictability and outcome of periodontal therapy.

Traditionally used methods of diagnosis are presented in Chapters 28 and 29. This chapter reviews advanced methods in various stages of development. In the future some of these may be incorporated into clinical practice; others may remain in the realm of clinical research.

PRINCIPLES OF DIAGNOSIS

The diagnostic process is not a perfect procedure that always relates the result of the test to the true clinical situation; instead, it is a procedure that results in different degrees of certainty depending on the accuracy of the given diagnostic test. This certainty is measured by a mathematic relationship between the properties of a test and the true clinical situation. The test is considered to be either *positive* or *negative,* and the disease or clinical situation is either *present* or *absent.* The test has given the correct answer when it is positive in the presence of disease and when it is negative in the absence of disease. However, if the test is positive in the absence of disease *(false positive)* or negative in the presence of disease *(false negative),* then the diagnostic tool is misleading.

Diagnostic tests are usually assessed in terms of their sensitivity and specificity.[80] *Specificity* refers to the ability of a test or observation to clearly differentiate one disease from another. It is defined as the percentage or proportion of subjects (or sites) with truly absent disease who have a negative test. A specific test is one in which a positive re-

sult indicates that the disease is likely (i.e., lack of false-positive results).

Sensitivity refers to the ability of a test or observation to detect the disease whenever it is present. It is defined as the percentage or proportion of subjects (or sites) with truly present disease who have a positive test. A sensitive test is one in which a negative result means that the disease is unlikely (i.e., lack of false-negative outcomes).

The sensitivity and specificity of a test should be considered when a decision has to be made as to whether the test should be performed. Once the test has been done, the clinician has to make a therapeutic decision. For this objective, the predictive value of a test is of special interest.

Predictive value refers to the probability that the test result (i.e., the proportion of true-positive results and true-negative results combined) agrees with the disease status. The positive predictive value determines the probability of disease in a subject or site with positive test results. The negative predictive value determines the probability of a healthy clinical situation in the presence of negative test results.

CLINICAL DIAGNOSIS

Differentiation of Periodontal Diseases

Periodontal disease includes inflammatory conditions ranging from marginal gingivitis to the most advanced destructive periodontitis. Until relatively recently, it was thought that inflammatory periodontal disease was a single entity caused predominantly by accumulation of dental plaque and starting from a marginal gingivitis, which, unless effective oral hygiene was implemented, progressed slowly to destructive periodontitis. However, direct attempts to document the conversion of gingivitis to periodontitis have shown that the number of these conversions is small; that is, only a small proportion of sites with gingivitis develop periodontitis.[90] In some patients, gingivitis does not inevitably lead to periodontitis, even in the presence of poor oral hygiene.[4]

There are, therefore, different forms of periodontal disease with different rates of progression, reflecting differences in etiologic factors and host susceptibilities. Differential clinical diagnosis is difficult, because all infections of the periodontium result in inflammation of the periodontal tissues, and all clinical and laboratory tests to detect ongoing pathologic abnormality have shortcomings. Since the mid-1980s, a better understanding of the disease process has challenged some basic assumptions regarding the usefulness of traditional clinical and radiographic measurements and has prompted a revised interpretation of clinical parameters. The development of clinical diagnostic indicators has been directed toward identifying the various disease processes by analyzing the degree of gingival inflammation in the different types of gingivitis and the degree of connective tissue destruction in the different forms of periodontitis.

Clinical Evaluation of Gingival Inflammation

Clinical evaluation of the degree of gingival inflammation includes assessment of the redness and swelling of the gingiva along with assessment of gingival bleeding. Although the earliest clinical signs of gingivitis consist of color and texture changes, there may be underlying structural alterations without corresponding clinical symptoms. Several studies have shown that gingival bleeding is a more sensitive clinical indicator of early gingival inflammation.[100] Moreover, the use of gingival bleeding as an indicator has the clinical advantage of being more objective, because color changes require a subjective estimation. It has also been shown that gingival bleeding is a good indicator of the presence of an inflammatory lesion in the connective tissue at the base of the sulcus and that the severity of bleeding increases with the increase in size of the inflammatory infiltrate.[23,29,42] Therefore, there is a tendency to evaluate gingivitis by gingival bleeding alone,[124] by means of either a periodontal probe or a wooden interdental cleaner,[2] instead of using visual signs of both inflammation and bleeding.[93,105]

Another method of assessing the degree of gingival inflammation is by measurement of the gingival crevicular fluid flow. Different studies have demonstrated a high correlation between clinical and histologic signs of gingivitis and increased amounts of gingival fluid flow.[20,22,73] Crevicular fluid has been collected by using calibrated microcapillary tubes and by placing filter paper strips at the entrance of the crevice and measuring the amount of fluid absorbed by the filter paper. In the latter case this measurement can be done by the Ninhydrin area method (NAM) or by an electronic device, the Periotron 6000 (Harco Electronics, Winnipeg, Manitoba, Canada) (see Chapter 7). Researchers comparing these techniques have established that the Periotron 6000 achieves the easiest and quickest measurement and shows high correlation with other clinical gingival indices.[60,151]

Instruments that measure the temperature in the gingival tissues have also been developed; Kung et al. claim that these thermal probes are sensitive diagnostic devices for measuring early inflammatory changes in the gingival tissues.[74] Studies demonstrate that periodontal disease activity can create measurable elevations in sulcular temperature. One system, the PerioTemp probe (Abiodent, Inc., Danvers, MA), has been developed to test these temperature changes. This probe detects pocket temperature differences of 0.1°C from a referenced subgingival temperature. A naturally occurring temperature gradient exists between maxillary and mandibular teeth and between posterior and anterior teeth. Individual temperature differences are compared with those expected for each tooth, and higher-temperature pockets are signaled with a red-emitting diode. Haffajee et al.[52] used this probe to assess its predictability in identifying loss of attachment, concluding that sites with a red temperature indication had more than twice the risk for future attachment loss than did those with a green indication. However, the influence of pocket depth on temperature is still not clear, and further studies are needed to demonstrate the accuracy of this device.

Clinical Evaluation of Connective Tissue Destruction

The most widely used diagnostic tool for the clinical assessment of connective tissue destruction in periodontitis is the periodontal probe. Increased probing depth and loss of clinical attachment are pathognomonic for periodontal disease. Therefore, pocket probing is a crucial procedure in diagnosis of the periodontium and evaluation of periodontal therapy (see Chapter 28). Reduction of probing depth and gain of clinical attachment are the major clinical criteria used to determine success of treatment.

However, use of the periodontal probe in its classic conception presents many problems in terms of sensitivity and reproducibility of results. Measurements of clinical pocket depth obtained with the periodontal probe do not normally coincide with the histologic pocket depth, because the probe normally penetrates the coronal level of the junctional epithelium,[6,123] and the precise location of the probe tip depends on the degree of inflammation of the underlying connective tissue. If the tissue is inflamed, it offers less resistance to probe penetration, and the probe tip either coincides with or is apical to the coronal level of connective tissue attachment.[89] Conversely, healed gingiva following subgingival instrumentation demonstrates an increased resistance to periodontal probing.[31,87,97]

The disparity between measurements also depends on the probing technique, probing force, size of the probe, angle of insertion of the probe, and precision of the probe calibration.[89] All of these variables contribute to the large standard deviations (0.5 to 1.3 mm) in clinical probing results, which makes detection of small changes difficult.[51]

Since the mid-1980s, different probe prototypes have been developed and tested to overcome these variables. One of the main problems in reproducibility has been the variation in probing force. It was shown that the penetration of the probe was positively correlated with probing force.[101,154] This has been solved with the development of pressure-sensitive probes, which have a standardized controlled insertion pressure[67,153] (Fig. 30–1). Different studies have been undertaken to define the ideal probing pressure. With forces of up to 30 gm the tip of the probe seems to remain within the junctional epithelium,[6,123,129] and forces

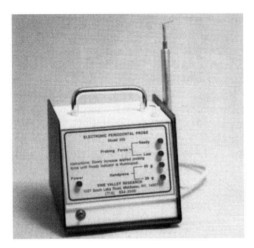

FIGURE 30-1. Electronic periodontal probe with standardized insertion pressures of 25 and 50 gm.

of up to 50 gm are necessary to diagnose periodontal osseous defects.[67] Standardization of probe tips (less than 1 mm) and use of registration stents to maintain reproducible probing angulation have also been tried to overcome sources of error.[7] However, fabrication of stents is time consuming and impractical for clinical diagnosis. In addition, current techniques for data readout and storage are inaccurate and time consuming. This has resulted in the development of new periodontal probing systems.

After a National Institute of Dental Research (NIDR) workshop on the quantitative evaluation of periodontal diseases by physical measurement techniques,[119] there was a proposal to develop and clinically evaluate an improved periodontal pocket depth–attachment level measurement system that would meet the following nine criteria:

1. A precision of 0.1 mm
2. A range of 10 mm
3. A constant probing force
4. Noninvasive, lightweight, and comfortable to use
5. Able to access any location around all teeth
6. A guidance system to ensure probe angulation
7. Complete sterilization of all portions entering the mouth
8. No biohazard from material or electrical shock
9. Digital output

Automated probing systems have been developed and tested in accordance with these strict criteria. These automated probes offer many solutions to the problems of conventional probing but also introduce problems of their own. The probing elements lack tactile sensitivity, mostly because of their independent movement, which forces the operator to predetermine an insertion point and angle. In addition, the use of a fixed-force setting throughout the mouth, regardless of the site or inflammatory status, may generate inaccurate measurements or patient discomfort.[101]

The computerized periodontal probe (Florida probe[36]) system consists of a probe handpiece, a digital readout, a foot switch, a computer interface, and a computer (Fig. 30-2). The end of the probe tip is 0.4 mm in diameter. This probe tip reciprocates through a sleeve, and the edge of the sleeve provides a reference by which measurements are made. These measurements are made electronically and transferred automatically to the computer when the foot switch is pressed. Constant probing force is provided by

coil springs inside the probe handpiece and digital readout. In this system, a fixed reference is needed for attachment level measurements.

Studies of the Florida probe system[95,96] showed a high degree of accuracy and reproducibility for probing depth and attachment level measurements, with standard deviations of 0.5 to 0.6 mm from repeated measurements. These deviations are significantly smaller than those previously reported (0.8 to 0.9 mm) using conventional pressure-sensitive probes.[1,7]

Other probes have also been introduced. Agudio and colleagues[5] described a force-sensitive probe and computer software to chart the data; however, no electronic measurement was provided, and the data had to be entered through the keyboard. An instrument reported by Mombelli and Graf[101] measures probing force and probe tip position electronically but does not provide control of probing force and electronic measurements. Jeffcoat and associates[61–63] described a probe (the Foster-Miller probe) capable of coupling pocket depth measurement with detection of the cemento-enamel junction, from which the clinical attachment level is automatically detected. The probe extends a thin metal fiber along the tooth surface into the sulcus and detects a slight accelerational increase when encountering the cemento-enamel junction, and then undergoes final extension, under constant force, on reaching the base of the pocket.

Researchers at the University of Toronto have described a probe (the Toronto Automated probe) that, like the Florida probe, uses the occlusal-incisal surface to measure clinical attachment levels.[99] The sulcus is probed with a 0.5-mm nickel-titanium wire that is extended under air pressure. It controls angular discrepancies by means of a mercury tilt sensor that limits angulation within ±30°, but it requires reproducible positioning of the patient's head and cannot easily measure second or third molars.

Assessment of Disease Progression (Disease Activity)

The most practical method of determining that disease is progressing (active) is the demonstration that a significant loss of attachment has occurred over time. The measurement of true periodontal pockets has traditionally been used in the diagnosis of periodontal disease. Longitudinal changes in probing depth may result from alteration in the gingival margin level and/or from influences at the pocket base. Changes in the pocket base are the true indicator of progression and/or remission of the disease process, and therefore, probing attachment levels recorded longitudinally from a fixed point on the tooth are the true indicator of previous disease activity. Sequential measurements to disclose sites with loss of attachment are subject to considerable problems of measurement reproducibility and must be interpreted in light of failure of the probe to disclose connective tissue levels accurately. In addition, attachment level measurements are not commonly used in clinical practice, mainly because of the time-consuming nature of these recordings. Instead, clinical signs of the condition of the gingival tissues are used to monitor disease progression and, most frequently, the outcome of therapy. In periodontal patients, clinicians often record changes in the presence of dental plaque, probing depths, and bleeding and suppura-

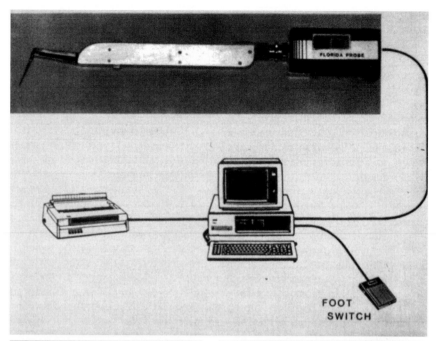

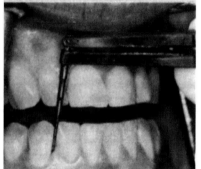
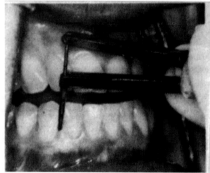

FIGURE 30–2. The Florida probe. *Top,* The probe handpiece, a displacement transducer with digital readout, a computer record-keeping system, and a foot switch. *Bottom,* Probe tip placed in sulcus (*right*) and a reference sleeve in contact with the gingival margin for pocket depth measurement. (From Gibbs CH, Hirschfeld JW, Lee JG, et al. Description and clinical evaluation of a new computerized probe—the Florida probe. J Clin Periodontol *15:*137, 1988. © 1988, Munksgaard International Publishers Ltd., Copenhagen, Denmark.)

tion on probing at several sites during the therapeutic phase and subsequently during the maintenance phase to find indicators of disease progression and thereby prevent further attachment loss.

Gingival bleeding has universally been considered an indicator of gingival inflammation and, by some investigators, an indicator of disease activity[53,122]; *however, its relationship to disease progression is unclear.* Lang and colleagues,[78] in a retrospective study, reported that sites that bled on probing at several visits had a higher probability of losing attachment than those that bled at one visit or did not bleed. However, well-controlled longitudinal studies[8,9,50] investigated the predictive values of such clinical signs, trying to correlate them with attachment loss, but failed to demonstrate a significant correlation between bleeding on probing and other clinical signs and subsequent loss of attachment.[8,9] A further limitation of the use of bleeding as an inflammatory parameter is the possibility that healthy sites may bleed on probing. Lang et al.[79] demonstrated that any force greater than 0.25 N may evoke bleeding in healthy sites with an intact periodontium.

To detect progression of periodontal disease over a short period of time, the clinician must overcome the probing reproducibility sources of error to assess for true changes of the connective tissue level at the base of the pocket. Vari-

ous methods have been used to overcome these errors; these include regression analysis of measurements over time, running medians, the tolerance method, end-point analysis, and the cumulative sum method.[3,7,51] Haffajee and coworkers[47,50,51] recommended the tolerance method. In this method, the difference between replicate attachment level measurements was used to calculate a standard deviation for all measurements made by an individual. The subject threshold for attachment loss in an individual site was considered to be three standard deviations. Therefore, the threshold value for attachment loss was about 3 mm. Although such a procedure has a high specificity, it has a low sensitivity. Thus, a considerable loss of attachment is needed to determine the progression of the disease, and it is likely that the majority of sites losing attachment at a slower rate are missed when the measurement error is excluded.[48] This subject threshold for attachment loss can be decreased with a higher degree of standardization. The development of electronic and automated probes (described in the preceding section) will probably allow more sensitive clinical assessments of disease progression in the near future. The tolerance method is based on the theory that periodontal disease progresses by sudden bursts, as defined by Socransky et al.[140] One study[66] using automated probing systems demonstrated that sites can also lose attachment by slow gradual progression instead of by sudden bursts. In this case the regression method would be more suitable for identifying disease activity.[160]

Another problem in the relationship of attachment level change and disease progression is the change of the probe tip penetration, which may vary from 1.0 to 1.5 mm, depending on the state of inflammation.[31] Therefore, substantial losses and gains of probing attachment may occur only as a consequence of spontaneous exacerbation or resolution of inflammation, without any change in functional connective tissue attachment. Again, these problems will be lessened with the development of pressure-sensitive probes with more accurate limits of detection.

As a result of these limitations of current probing methods, probing attachment measurements may still be the best tool to measure periodontal attachment,[48] but it is not clear whether they are useful or practical to assess rates of disease progression.

RADIOGRAPHIC DIAGNOSIS

Methods to Assess Bone Destruction

Dental radiographs are the traditional method used to assess the destruction of alveolar bone associated with periodontitis. Although radiographs cannot accurately reflect the bony morphology buccally and lingually, they provide useful information on interproximal bone levels. However, even at this level, the exact topography of defects cannot be assessed accurately from radiographs.

It is well known that substantial volumes of alveolar bone must be destroyed before the loss is detectable in radiographs; more than 30% of the bone mass at the alveolar crest must be lost for a change in bone height to be recognized on radiographs.[115] Therefore, radiographs will seldom reveal bone loss when sufficient loss has not taken place. Thus, *radiographs are not sensitive, but they may be specific.* This low degree of sensitivity is mainly due to the subjectivity of the radiographic assessment; the different variables affecting the classic radiographic technique, such as the quality of the x-ray film, x-ray angulation, the direction of the beam, the x-ray source, and the exposure and developing time; and the presence of anatomic calcified structures projected onto the same film in which changes in the bony pattern are simultaneously shown.

These influences can be reduced by the use of well-standardized techniques. To standardize radiographic assessment, radiographs should be obtained in a constant and reproducible plane using film holders with a template containing some kind of impression material, which is placed in a constant position on a group of teeth, and an extension arm that can be precisely attached to both the film holder and the x-ray tube[130] and used to standardize the technique (Fig. 30–3) so that the bone mass can be measured. Such standardization in radiographic techniques has been shown to be valid in evaluating bone changes in longitudinal studies[131] and clinical trials.[68]

Alternative diagnostic methods for imaging marginal alveolar bone structure have been developed and compared with conventional dental radiographs. Orthopantomographs, when compared with intraoral full-mouth radiographs,

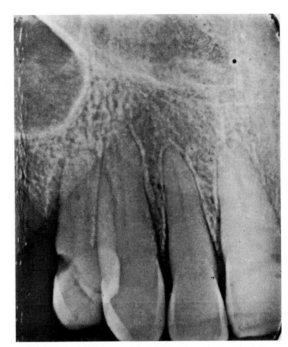

FIGURE 30–3. Xeroradiograph. (Courtesy of Dr. Barton Gratt.)

showed a tendency to underestimate minor bone changes, although there was overall agreement between the two techniques for more than 50% of the teeth.[45]

Xeroradiography is an x-ray imaging system that uses the xerographic copying process to record x-ray images. When compared with intraoral radiography, it has demonstrated better images (Fig. 30–4), mainly in fine structures, such as bony trabeculae, and areas of subtle density differ-

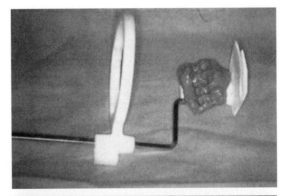

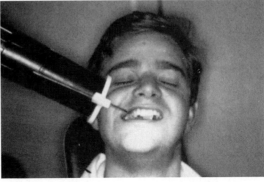

FIGURE 30–4. Positioning device for standardized radiographs.

ences, such as the soft tissues.[41] This system has the additional advantage of a much lower radiation exposure.

Methods to Assess Disease Progression

Conventional dental radiographs provide two-dimensional images of three-dimensional objects and reflect the anatomy of bone at that instant. They do not indicate whether bone loss is progressing or has occurred previously. To obtain a dynamic view of the alveolar bone loss process, replicate measurements must be performed on standardized radiographs. Analysis of the differences in the radiographic images can thus provide a measure of the rate of destruction.

As mentioned in the preceding discussion, the most practical clinical method to determine whether the disease is active remains the demonstration that a significant loss of attachment has occurred over time. Trying to correlate probing attachment loss with radiographic bone loss, Goodson and colleagues[39] monitored 22 untreated subjects for 1 year and quantitatively studied the possible predictability of bone loss on the basis of attachment loss measured clinically. They showed that loss of probing attachment preceded bone loss (as evidenced radiographically) by 6 to 8 months. Therefore, conventional radiographic techniques, even well-standardized ones, have a low predictive value for detecting disease progression.

Radiographic and nuclear medicine techniques have been developed to obtain a higher degree of sensitivity to minor bone changes. *I 125 absorptiometry,* a nonradio-graphic method introduced by Henrikson,[58] is the most sensitive technique for analyzing periodontal bone mass changes. It is based on the absorption by bone of a low-energy gamma beam, originating from a radioactive source of I 125. This method has been shown to measure bone mass with a high degree of accuracy and precision[15,55] and has been used as a standard for comparing the sensitivity of other techniques.[56] Technical considerations limit the use of this system in posterior sites, and the nature of the beam of I 125 makes precise alignment even more critical than with other techniques.

To improve the study of posterior areas, mainly furcations, a *photodensitometric analysis technique* has been developed and tested.[120,121] It is based on absorption of a beam of light by the radiographic film, which also shows the image of an aluminum scale, and transformation of the density readings into millimeters of aluminum equivalents. This is accomplished by a microdensitometer linked to a microcomputer. This technique requires a parallelization technique to obtain accurate superimposable radiographs. It enables the clinician not only to detect and recognize variations that cannot be detected by visual inspection but also to quantify bone changes.

Subtraction radiography, a well-established technique in medicine, has been introduced as a technique in periodontal diagnosis.[44] This technique relies on the conversion of serial radiographs into digital images. The images can then be superimposed and the resultant composite viewed on a video screen. Changes in the density and/or volume of bone can be detected as lighter areas (bone gain) or dark areas (bone loss). Quantitative changes in comparison with the baseline images can be detected using an algorithm

for gray scale levels. This is accomplished by means of a computer (i.e., *computer-assisted subtraction radiography*). This technique requires a parallelization technique to obtain a standardized geometry and accurate superimposable radiographs. Radiographs taken with identical exposure geometry can be scanned using a microphotometer that determines a gray-level value for each picture point. After superimposition of two subsequent radiographs, this technique can show differences in relative densities.

Studies using this technique have shown (1) a high degree of correlation between changes in alveolar bone determined by subtraction radiography and attachment level changes in periodontal patients after therapy[54] and (2) increased detectability of small osseous lesions compared with the conventional radiographs from which the subtraction images are produced.[128] Grondahl and colleagues,[46] using subtraction analysis, showed nearly perfect accuracy at a lesion depth corresponding to 0.49 mm of compact bone, whereas a lesion must be at least three times larger to be detectable with a conventional radiology technique. Subtraction radiography has also shown a degree of sensitivity similar to that for I 125 absorptiometry.[46,114] It can detect a change in bone mass of as little as 5%.[114]

Subtraction radiography has been applied to longitudinal clinical studies. Hausmann et al. detected differences in crestal bone height of 0.87 mm with reliability.[57] Jeffcoat et al.[63] have shown a strong relationship between probing attachment loss detected using sequential measurements made with an automated periodontal probe and bone loss detected with digital subtraction radiography. *This method has great diagnostic potential, even in clinical practice, because of the development of personal computers with capability for digitizing and image processing.*

Another technique that has been introduced is a video-based *computer-assisted densitometric image analysis system* (CADIA).[14] In this system, a video camera measures the light transmitted through a radiograph, and the signals from the camera are converted into gray levels. The camera is interfaced with an image processor and a computer that allow the storage and mathematical manipulation of the images (Fig. 30–5). This system appears to offer an objective method for following alveolar bone density changes quantitatively over time, and, when compared with I 125 absorptiometry and digital subtraction analysis, it has shown a higher sensitivity and a high degree of reproducibility and accuracy.[14]

This technique has also been applied to longitudinal clinical studies. Deas et al.,[24] using replicate measurements of clinical attachment levels and CADIA, demonstrated that the prevalence of progressing lesions in periodontitis (38% of sites per patient), as detected by this radiographic method, may be much higher than previously thought.

One of the most recent advances in the assessment of bone changes involves the use of nuclear medicine to detect changes in bone metabolism that may precede architectural changes. Therefore, this technique has the potential to detect the earliest stage of bone loss. *Nuclear medicine techniques* for the study of bone metabolism use a bone-seeking radiopharmaceutical, such as diphosphonate compound, which is labeled with a radionuclide, Tc 99m. This compound is injected intravenously, and after a waiting pe-

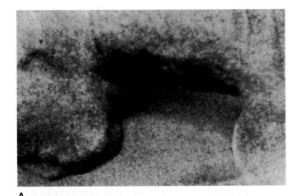

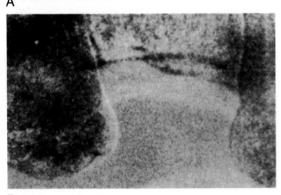

FIGURE 30–5. Digitized dental radiographs: digital subtraction images. *A,* Surgically induced bone and tissue loss after wedge excision and ostectomy/osteoplasty. This image was obtained by subtracting the preoperative from the immediate postoperative radiographs. *B,* Crestal resorption after subtracting the immediate postoperative radiograph from the 6 weeks' postoperative radiograph. Subcrestal increase in bone density and soft tissue healing (*brighter areas against background*) are less clearly visible. (From Brägger U, Pasquali L, Rylander H, et al. Computer assisted densitometric image analysis in periodontal radiography. A methodological study. J Clin Periodontol *15:*27, 1988. © 1988, Munksgaard International Publishers Ltd., Copenhagen, Denmark.)

riod to allow for bony uptake and clearance of the radiopharmaceutical, uptake by the bone is measured with a miniaturized semiconductor probe radiation detector. This semiconductor probe is placed directly buccal to a tooth. Because bone resorption is usually coupled with formation behind the resorbing front, this technique is used to detect alterations in bone metabolism in diseases of bone resorption as well as in diseases of bone formation. In periodontal diseases, measurement of bone-seeking radiopharmaceutical uptake may be indicative of the rate of bone loss. Jeffcoat and colleagues[64,65] reported that low uptake ratios are associated with little or no progression of alveolar bone loss, and high uptake ratios are associated with subsequent bone loss. This technique has exhibited a specificity of 87%, with a total predictive value of 84%.[64] Therefore, it appears to be fairly accurate in predicting subsequent bone changes. Because bone-seeking radiopharmaceutical uptake measurement is performed in a single visit, the technique has the potential to provide an immediate measure of disease activity. Progressive disease can be identified before bone loss is evident on conventional radiographs.[65]

MICROBIOLOGIC DIAGNOSIS

Microbial Differentiation of Periodontal Diseases

Based on the concept of bacterial specificity, which states that the various forms of periodontal disease are caused by a small number of specific pathogens, studies have been carried out to develop means of detecting and enumerating these pathogens in the subgingival microflora of patients with disease. These microbiologic tests may have the potential not only to diagnose various forms of periodontal disease, depending on the bacterial profile, but also to determine which periodontal sites in these patients are at higher risk of undergoing active destruction. These microbial tests could also monitor periodontal therapy directed at the suppression or eradication of periodontopathic organisms. However, even cultural bacteriology, which is considered the standard microbiologic diagnostic method, is not very predictable. Results from many studies carried out since the 1970s (see Chapter 6) have shown that cultural microbiologic results from cases with similar clinical presentation are not predictable. Moore[103] reviewed these results and noted that, of the localized juvenile periodontitis sites sampled microbiologically and reported during a 2-year period, only one third of the sites had *Actinobacillus actinomycetemcomitans* levels greater than 1%. Similar results have been reported for pathogens such as *Porphyromona gingivalis* associated with severe adult periodontitis and rapidly advancing periodontitis.

This apparent inconsistency in microbiologic results might be due to three different reasons, reviewed by Socransky and coworkers:[140] (1) technical difficulties in the procedure, from sample taking to dispersion, cultivation, and characterization and identification of the isolates (see Chapter 6); (2) conceptual problems, both those associated with the complexity of the periodontal microbiota and those related to the nature of periodontal diseases (disease activity, inability to properly differentiate between diseases, and so forth); and (3) problems associated with the adequate analysis of the microbiologic data.

Another explanation proposed by Williams and associates[157] and by Moore[103] is that episodes of periodontal destruction may consist of one assault after another by different species; when the host develops resistance to one species, another comes along and causes additional damage. Further research is needed to establish the exact role of the different pathogens and thus establish the real validity of microbiologic diagnostic tests.

A method has been proposed that uses a combination of clinical and microbiologic parameters to predictably recommend specific therapy[72,109]; this is termed the *predictive treatment model*. Kornman and Newman have shown that refractory periodontitis patients can be separated into "clusters" or groups, as determined by similarity of clinical and microbiologic characteristics. This approach may become important in identifying patients at risk and suggesting specific therapy.

Microbiology and Disease Progression

Because bacteria are the causative agents in periodontal diseases, it makes sense to look for specific bacteria as indicators of disease initiation and progression (i.e., disease activity). The association of specific microorganisms with disease activity involves the problem of clinically assessing disease activity. As mentioned in the preceding discussion, there are no good clinical or radiologic indicators of disease activity, and there is always a discrepancy between the time of initiation of disease and the time of the clinical or radiologic detection of the change. Therefore, there is not a clearly defined time to do the microbiologic sampling. Attempts to associate specific microorganisms with disease activity have used three basic approaches:[69] studies of the microflora in animal models, longitudinal studies, and monitoring of bacterial products in gingival crevicular fluid.

Studies of the Microflora in Animal Models. Kornman and associates[70] and Slots and coworkers[137] induced disease in primates, which developed clinical signs of disease in 2 to 3 months. With a radiographic imaging system, these investigators were able to associate disease progression with the isolated species. Both studies showed increased levels of *P. gingivalis* associated with attachment loss.

Longitudinal Studies. Longitudinal studies determined the pathogens associated with sites undergoing disease activity compared with other sites in the same persons that did not experience attachment loss. In juvenile periodontitis, Mandell[98] found a mean level of 2% *A. actinomycetemcomitans* in active sites and 0.02% in control sites in the same patients; however, other species, such as *P. intermedia, Capnocytophaga* species, and *Fusobacterium nucleatum* showed no significant differences between active and control sites. Dzink and colleagues[26] showed similar results, with a clear association of *A. actinomycetemcomitans* with active sites.

In untreated adult periodontitis, Tanner and associates[145] assessed radiologic changes and Dzink and colleagues[26,26a] assessed critical probing changes and showed that certain species, including *Campylobacter rectus, B. intermedius, Bacteroides forsythus,* and *P. gingivalis,* were found in higher levels at active sites, whereas other species, such as *Streptococcus sanguis, Actinomyces* species, and *Veillonella parvula,* were found in higher levels at inactive sites. Slots and colleagues[136] also associated *A. actinomycetemcomitans, P. gingivalis,* and *P. intermedia* with progressing

periodontitis sites. However, Ranney and associates,[126] assessing longitudinally active periodontitis sites, did not find significant differences in the composition of the microflora between active and control sites in the same individuals.

These limited studies suggest that disease progression in untreated cases of periodontitis may be associated with the specific subset of the subgingival microflora that has shown the greatest pathogenic potential and virulence.[137] Socransky reviewed current knowledge on the bacterial etiology of periodontal disease, defining a limited number of possible pathogens on the basis of their association with disease, animal pathogenicity, virulence factors, the immunologic response of the host to a species, and the relation of successful therapy to the elimination of the species. The interpretation of diagnostic tests for the detection of subgingival species must be dependent on knowledge of the microbial etiology, and therefore, only those species having the aforementioned characteristics should be sought. In addition, current data suggest that pathogens are necessary but not sufficient for disease activity to occur. Other factors, such as the susceptibility of the individual host and the presence of interacting bacterial species, may facilitate or impede disease progression.[141]

Darkfield or phase contrast microscopy is an inexpensive chairside method to detect bacterial morphotypes, determine motility, and identify spirochetes. However, it is unable to differentiate between species with similar shapes. It has been widely used and has been successful in differentiating population groups with and without periodontitis, based on assessment of the percentage of motile bacteria and spirochetes.[83] However, it is unable to discriminate putative periodontal pathogens from those of lesser relevance (Fig. 30–6). Listgarten and coworkers[87] demonstrated that after therapy, patients manifested a flora associated with health—namely, few motile forms and increased coccoid cells. Therefore, it was assumed that ongoing pathosis could be detected by inspecting for motile forms and spirochetes.[88] Using this technique, these authors compared sites with recent evidence of attachment loss with unaffected sites and showed insignificant differences in the percentage of motile bacteria and spirochetes between both. Therefore, this technique was not able to identify the microflora asso-

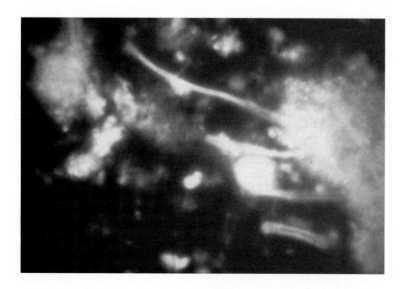

FIGURE 30–6. Darkfield micrograph showing different bacterial morphotypes (cocci, rods, and filaments).

ciated with active periodontal disease, and the presence of high spirochetal counts was more closely related to pocket depth than to disease activity.[91]

Monitoring of Bacterial Products in Gingival Crevicular Fluid. Bacterial products in gingival crevicular fluid have been monitored as a means of detecting periodontal disease initiation and/or progression.[30]

Several studies have shown a positive correlation between gingival inflammation and endotoxin, hydrogen sulfide, butyrate, and propionate.[12,135,142,152] These products have been found in high concentrations in the subgingival plaque of patients with gingivitis, periodontitis, and juvenile periodontitis, and their levels were decreased after treatment and resolution of the inflammation.[30] Although they can be markers of a pathogenic flora, there are no studies showing their association with disease activity.

The polyamines putrescine, spermidine, and spermine are metabolic products of both plaque bacteria and host cells. Cadaverin, however, is produced only by bacterial cells, and therefore, it can be assessed in gingival crevicular fluid as a marker of increased plaque metabolic activity.[30]

Because enzymes can be released by both bacteria and host tissue cells, only those specific substrates that can be differentiated from substrates derived from host cells can be used as direct markers of bacterial activity.[21] Bacterial collagenases in crevicular fluid can be separated by analysis of the breakdown products, because bacterial collagenase cleaves collagen at multiple sites and tissue collagenase cleaves it only at one location.[38] The quantitation of bacterial collagenases has been correlated with *P. gingivalis* activity.[30] However, most of the collagenase in crevicular fluid is of host origin.[38] Lactate dehydrogenase (LDH) is another product of both bacteria and host cells. Studies have shown an association between increased LDH levels in crevicular fluid and increased levels of periodontal disease.[76]

Microbiology to Predict and Monitor Response to Therapy

Several studies have examined the effect of different periodontal therapies on the composition of the subgingival microflora, and several microbial patterns have been associated with therapy success or failure. Since the 1980s there has been an emphasis on the use of microbial markers to predict and monitor the response to periodontal therapy in individuals with systemic diseases or other conditions that predispose them to higher susceptibility to periodontal breakdown.

Listgarten and coworkers,[88] using darkfield microscopy, tried to structure the intervals of maintenance visits by assessing the percentages of motile rods and/or spirochetes in plaque samples. They showed that, compared with scheduled biannual maintenance prophylaxis, an increased length of recall intervals was possible using darkfield bacterial monitoring, but the technique failed to predict the subjects or teeth affected by recurrence of disease.[91] These data suggest that this technique may allow customization of recall intervals in a maintenance program, but it is not a good predictor of the future course of the disease.

In localized juvenile periodontitis (LJP), several investigators[18,71] demonstrated that the persistence of *A. actinomycetemcomitans* in previously treated sites makes those sites nonresponsive to therapy and likely to show recurrence of disease and attachment loss. These data suggest that *A. actinomycetemcomitans* may be a good indicator for monitoring and predicting response to therapy in these LJP patients.

A similar approach has been used to correlate specific microbial findings with clinical findings after treatment of adult periodontitis. Haffajee and associates[47] showed that sites that lost attachment after therapy had higher levels of *A. actinomycetemcomitans, B. forsythus, P. gingivalis, Bacteroides intermedius, Peptostreptococcus micros, Streptococcus intermedius,* and *C. rectus,* whereas sites that did not change or that gained attachment after therapy had higher levels of *Actinomyces* species, *Capnocytophaga ochracea, Streptococcus mitis, S. sanguis,* and *V. parvula.* These data are in agreement with other studies that associate these pathogenic species with active periodontal sites in untreated periodontal patients. Haffajee and colleagues[47] suggested that monitoring these pathogenic bacteria or the "beneficial species" might be useful in evaluating the response to therapy and in predicting recurrence of disease. *Although the facts seem rather clear for LJP cases, extensive additional work is needed before using these microbial diagnostic tests in targeting therapy for advanced destructive, refractory, or rapidly progressing cases of adult periodontitis.*

Rapid Methods of Diagnostic Microbiology

As mentioned in the preceding discussion, only cumbersome anaerobic cultural analysis is able to give predominant cultivable microbiota assessments. However, it has been well established that the various forms of periodontal disease are caused by a small number of specific pathogens, and multiple studies have been carried out to detect and enumerate these pathogens in the subgingival microflora of patients with disease (see Chapter 6). An attempt has been made to develop rapid microbiologic diagnostic methods that are able to detect and quantify these specific periodontopathogens. These methods should be quick and easy in order to be implemented into clinical practice.

Darkfield Microscopy

Darkfield or *phase contrast microscopy* has been suggested as an alternative to culture methods[85] on the basis of its ability to assess motile bacteria and spirochetes. It has been used to indicate periodontal disease status and to structure maintenance programs. However, most of the main putative periodontopathogens, including *A. actinomycetemcomitans, P. gingivalis, B. intermedius, Eikenella corrodens,* and *Eubacterium* species, are nonmotile, and therefore, this technique is unable to identify these species. It is also unable to differentiate among the various species of *Treponema.* Therefore, darkfield microscopy seems an unlikely candidate as a diagnostic test of destructive periodontal diseases.

Immunologic Assays

Immunologic assays for specific periodontal pathogens also have been used. These methods involve the use of monoclonal or polyclonal antibodies directed against specific bacterial antigens or microbial virulence factors and therefore react only with the "target" bacterial species, excluding the rest of the bacteria present in the plaque sample. Several immunologic assays have been used clinically to identify microorganisms in clinical specimens.

Immunofluorescence Microscopy. Immunofluorescence microscopy includes two types of immunofluorescence assays for the identification of specific bacteria in clinical samples: direct and indirect immunofluorescence. In *direct immunofluorescence,* antiserum to a microorganism is conjugated to fluorescein. When the conjugate is incubated on a clinical smear containing the microorganism and then washed off, the antigen–antibody reaction takes place, and the organism is visualized by its fluorescent outline when observed in a fluorescence microscope (Fig. 30–7). If the organism is not present, the smear will appear dark with no fluorescence.

Indirect immunofluorescence is a two-step procedure. Antiserum to the microorganism is incubated on the clinical smear of plaque. It is washed off, and then a conjugate of a fluorescent dye and an antiserum to the first antiserum are incubated on the smear and then washed off.

Both direct and indirect immunofluorescence assays are able not only to identify the pathogen but also to quantify the percentage of the pathogen in the plaque smear. This is accomplished by dividing the total number of specific fluorescent bacteria by the total number of bacteria counted with phase contrast microscopy or counterstain.

Immunofluorescence microscopy has been used mainly to detect *A. actinomycetemcomitans*[12] and *P. gingivalis.*[163] Zambon and associates[162] showed that this technique is comparable to bacterial culture in its ability to identify these pathogens in subgingival dental plaque samples. In fact, immunofluorescence microscopy may be even more likely to detect them in clinical samples because it does not require viable bacterial cells. Comparative studies indicate that the sensitivity of these assays ranges from 82% to 100% for detection of *A. actinomycetemcomitans* and from 91% to 100% for detection of *P. gingivalis,* with specificity

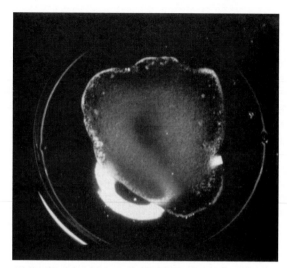

FIGURE 30–8. Latex agglutination test for plaque sample showing positive agglutination to *Actinobacillus actinomycetemcomitans* from a localized juvenile periodontitis site.

values of 88% to 92% and 87% to 89%, respectively.[37,162,163]

Latex Agglutination. Latex agglutination is an immunologic assay based on the binding of protein to latex. Latex beads are coated with the species-specific antibody, and when these beads come in contact with the microbial cell surface antigens or antigen extracts, cross-linking occurs; its agglutination or clumping is then visible usually in 2 to 5 minutes. Because of their simplicity and rapidity, these assays have great potential for widespread use in the clinical detection of periodontal pathogens, and their use is one of the most rapidly growing areas of diagnostic microbiology.

There are two types of latex agglutination tests: the indirect assay and the inhibition assay. The *indirect assay* is the most common latex agglutination test for bacteria. The antibody is bound to latex. When a suspension of the plaque sample is mixed with the sensitized latex and gently agitated for 3 to 5 minutes, resulting agglutination or clumping is indicative of a positive result for the bacteria being tested (Fig. 30–8). The latex *inhibition assay* is based on the principle of inhibiting the expected agglutination reaction between known antigen and known antibody as a result of competition.

Although latex agglutination tests for medical diagnosis are commercially available and their use is becoming standard, there are few reports of their use to detect periodontal pathogens; such use is currently in a developmental stage.

Flow Cytometry. Flow cytometry[59] for the rapid identification of oral bacteria involves labeling bacterial cells from a patient plaque sample with both species-specific antibody and a second fluorescein-conjugated antibody. The suspension is then introduced into the flow cytometer, which separates the bacterial cells into an almost single-cell suspension by means of a laminar flow through a narrow tube. After incubation, the cells are passed through a focused laser beam. The cells then scatter the light at low and wide angles, and the fluorescent emission can be measured by appropriate detectors.

Although this technique has been used to measure bacte-

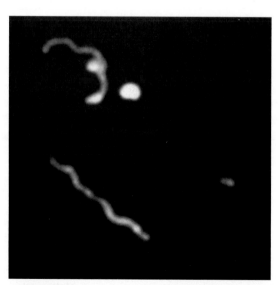

FIGURE 30–7. Immunofluorescence micrograph.

ria in clinical medicine,[13] there are few data regarding its use with dental plaque samples. Many technical questions must be solved to demonstrate efficacy for identification of specific bacteria in plaque. This is likely due to the difficulties inherent in transforming a bacterial plaque composed mainly of bacterial clumps into a single-cell suspension suitable for using this technique.[10]

Enzyme-linked Immunosorbent Assay. Enzyme-linked immunosorbent assay (ELISA) is similar in principle to other radioimmunoassays, but an enzymatically derived color reaction is substituted as the label in place of the radioisotope. ELISA detects either antigens or antibodies. Antigens are incubated in wells in a plastic plate to allow absorption and binding of the material. After washing to remove free antigen, samples containing suspected antigens are incubated with known antibodies to bind to the antigen on the surface of the well. After washing to remove nonbound components, antisera to the immunoglobulin conjugated to either alkaline phosphatase or horseradish peroxidase are then incubated in the wells. A positive reaction is visualized when the addition of a chromogen changes the solution from colorless to colored. The intensity of the color depends on the concentration of the antigen and is usually read photometrically for optimal quantitation.[108] ELISA has been used primarily to detect serum antibodies to periodontopathogens.

Enzymatic Methods of Bacterial Identification

With the accumulated information regarding the enzymatic profiles of plaque bacteria, enzyme diagnostic kits have been developed for the identification of pure cultures of plaque isolates.[82,146] These enzyme assays have permitted rapid and reliable species identification of the black-pigmented bacteria (BPB), because only *P. gingivalis* of the human BPB gives a positive trypsin-like reaction.[94] Enzyme assays can also be used to distinguish *A. actinomycetemcomitans* from other closely related species; *B. forsythus* can also be distinguished from other gram-negative anaerobic rods owing to its specific enzymatic profile. *B. forsythus, P. gingivalis,* the small spirochete *Treponema denticola,* and *Capnocytophaga* species have in common a trypsin-like enzyme. The activity of this enzyme is measured with the hydrolysis of the colorless substrate *N*-benzoyl-DL-arginine-2-naphthylamide (BANA). When the hydrolysis takes place, it releases the chromophore β-naphthylamide, which turns orange red when a drop of fast garnet is added to the solution. Loesche[94] proposed the use of this BANA reaction in subgingival plaque samples to detect the presence of any of these periodontal pathogens and thus serve as a marker of disease activity. Using probing depths as a measure of periodontal morbidity, Loesche showed that shallow pockets exhibited only 10% positive BANA reactions, whereas deep pockets (7 mm) exhibited 80% to 90% positive BANA reactions.[13,93] Beck et al.[11] used the BANA test as a risk indicator for periodontal attachment loss. Taken collectively, results using this diagnostic method suggest that positive BANA findings are a good indication that *T. denticola, P. gingivalis,* or both are present at sampled sites.

Other Assays for Bacterial Identification: DNA Probes

The use of bacteria-specific DNA fragments via DNA:DNA hybridization technology to detect specific microorganisms has become the subject of much interest and has progressed from a research technique to a practical clinical laboratory assay.

The *DNA probe* identifies species-specific sequences of nucleic acids that make up DNA, thereby permitting identification of organisms. The technique is based on the concept that DNA is a double helix consisting of two complementary strands of paired bases. When the double strand is split, separation occurs between the base pairs. If renatured, they bind again (hybridize).

To prepare the probe, specific pathogens used as marker organisms are lysed to remove their DNA. Their double helix is denatured, creating single strands that are individually labeled with a radioactive isotope. Subsequently, when a plaque sample is sent for analysis, it undergoes lysis and denaturation. Single strands are chemically treated, attached to a special filter paper, and then exposed to the DNA library. If complementary base pairs hybridize (cross-link), the radiolabeled strands will also be fixed to the filter paper. After the filter is washed to remove any unhybridized strands, it is covered with a radiographic plate. The radioactive labels create spots on the film, which are read with a densitometer. The darkness and size of the spots indicate the concentration of the organisms present in the given plaque sample.[42,107,124]

The DNA library includes probes for *A. actinomycetemcomitans, P. gingivalis, B. intermedius, C. rectus, E. corrodens, F. nucleatum,* and *T. denticola.* These probes are able to detect as few as 10^2 to 10^4 cells of these periodontal pathogens. The sensitivity and specificity of these tests have proved optimal, as the tests are not affected by the presence of unrelated bacteria in mixed culture samples.[32,132]

Another method of DNA analysis of putative periodontal pathogens is *restriction endonuclease analysis.* Restriction endonucleases recognize and cleave double-stranded DNA at specific base pair sequences. The DNA fragments generated are separated by electrophoresis, stained with ethidium bromide, and visualized with ultraviolet light. The genetic heterogeneity and homogeneity of strains can then be evaluated by comparing the number and size (electrophoretic pattern) of the DNA fragments obtained. These DNA fragment patterns constitute a specific "fingerprint" to characterize each strain. Restriction endonuclease analysis is thus a powerful tool for determining the distribution of a specific pathogenic strain throughout a population.[35]

Drawbacks

The main drawback of these specifically targeted bacterial assays is that they are available for only a few putative pathogens. It is quite possible that *A. actinomycetemcomitans, P. gingivalis, B. intermedius, C. rectus, E. corrodens, F. nucleatum,* and *T. denticola* are not present in high levels in all forms of periodontitis. This may be the case in patients with refractory periodontitis who have not responded to mechanical therapy combined with systemic antibiotics.

Periodontal lesions in such patients can become superinfected with yeasts, enteric rods, and pseudomonads. In addition, the DNA probes do not provide any information about the antibiotic sensitivities of the infecting bacteria. At present, the only known way to determine antibiotic susceptibilities of suspected pathogens is by cultural analysis of the subgingival flora.

IMMUNOLOGIC DIAGNOSIS

Immunologic Differentiation of Periodontal Diseases

The association of specific bacteria with the different forms of periodontal disease has also generated considerable information regarding serum antibody levels. Since the mid-1980s there has been an enormous increase in the number of studies showing correlations between specific disease categories and elevated antibody titers to the pathogen suspected of initiating that form of periodontal disease. For LJP, different investigators have shown elevated serum antibody titers to antigenic determinants of *A. actinomycetemcomitans*.[27,86] These investigators showed that almost all patients with LJP had elevated serum antibodies to this organism, whereas few healthy or adult periodontitis subjects had detectable titers. Serum antibodies to *P. gingivalis* have been shown to be elevated in patients with adult periodontitis and rapidly progressing periodontitis,[104,149] and antibodies to *B. intermedius* and intermediate-size spirochetes have been found to be elevated in patients with acute necrotizing ulcerative gingivitis (ANUG).[19]

With this positive correlation among specific bacteria, elevated serum antibody titers, and specific clinical conditions, it may be reasonable to use serum antibody titers as an adjunct in the diagnosis of some periodontal diseases. Genco and coworkers[34] calculated the diagnostic value of *A. actinomycetemcomitans* serum antibody determination for LJP and reported a sensitivity of 71%, a specificity of 89%, and a positive predictive value of 86%. These researchers also reported a strong correlation between serum antibody titers and local gingival fluid antibody titers. Other investigators have shown a correlation among the microorganism, local crevicular fluid antibody titers, and the clinical disease status of the affected site.[28]

Dysfunction of the neutrophil and/or monocyte white blood cells has been associated with LJP, rapidly progressing periodontitis, and prepubertal periodontitis.[155] These abnormalities, which are reported to be genetically transmitted, have been identified by their chemotaxis, motility, and adherence capability.[116]

Immunology and Disease Progression

In general, the studies showing associations between high antibody titers against specific microorganisms and the different forms of periodontal disease used cross-sectional data. However, with the relatively recent conceptual change to progression of disease through "bursts" of disease activity, it is presumed that the dynamics of the immune response follow a similar pattern. Studies have shown that 80% of the samples from active sites contained detectable

levels of the microorganism to which the individual exhibited an elevated antibody response.[147] In contrast, only 20% of the inactive sites sampled at the same time showed a similar pattern. Based on these data, it appears that systemic antibody titers are a reflection of the host response to an infection associated with an episode of disease activity. Therefore, antibody titer changes together with microbial changes could be used as diagnostic markers for disease activity. Because multiple sites may be undergoing challenge, local antibody titer monitoring may be more relevant in studies of disease activity.

In animal experiments in which periodontitis lesions were induced by implanting specific microorganisms, peak antibody responses preceded the major periods of periodontal tissue destruction.[147] These results also demonstrate that antibody response to specific organisms is associated with periods of active periodontal destruction.

Immunology and Response to Therapy

Studies have attempted to monitor antibody levels after therapy, both in juvenile periodontitis[50] and in adult periodontitis patients.[150] These studies tend to reflect the antigen exposure and antigen challenge (colonization of a periodontal site) that cause a boost in the humoral response. Successful elimination of the antigen by means of therapy causes a decrease in the antigenic load and a subsequent decrease in antibody levels. However, the diagnostic value of this approach in determining long-term success of therapy remains to be determined.

BIOCHEMICAL DIAGNOSIS

Traditional periodontal diagnostic procedures cannot distinguish between active and inactive sites at a given point in time, nor can they identify susceptible individuals. Thus, a problem central to periodontology is our inability to detect actively deteriorating sites and highly susceptible patients other than by longitudinal observations of attachment level or alveolar bone status.

A large research effort is underway to identify potential diagnostic tests based on host-derived factors that would enable the clinician to identify active sites or susceptible individuals. Such tests could be performed using saliva, gingival crevicular fluid (GCF), blood serum, blood cells, or urine. Information concerning the components of saliva and their relationship to disease susceptibility or disease activity is meager. Likewise, analysis of urine shows little promise except for its use in differential diagnosis of tooth loss related to hypophosphatasia in young children, in whom the presence of phosphoethanolamine in urine is diagnostic for the disease. Most efforts to date have been based on the use of components of GCF and, to a lesser extent, blood serum, identifying serum antibody levels against pathogenic bacteria.[117]

More than 40 components of GCF have been studied (see Chapter 7). They can be divided into three main groups: host-derived enzymes, tissue breakdown products, and inflammatory mediators.

Host-Derived Enzymes. Various enzymes are released from host cells during the development and progression of periodontal infections. The enzymes that have received the most attention as possible markers of active periodontal lesions are aspartate aminotransferase (AST), collagenase, β-glucuronidase, lactate dehydrogenase, arylsulfatase, and elastase. Some of these enzymes are released from dead and dying cells of the periodontium; some come from polymorphonuclear neutrophils; and other are produced by inflammatory, epithelial, and connective tissue cells of affected sites.

AST is an enzyme released from dead cells from a variety of tissues throughout the body, including the heart (after myocardial infarction) and the liver (during hepatitis). Several studies evaluating the association between elevated AST levels in GCF and periodontal disease have demonstrated a marked elevation in AST levels in GCF samples from sites with severe gingival inflammation[16] and from sites with a recent history of progressive attachment loss. A rapid chairside test kit for AST has been developed. The test involves collection of GCF with a filter paper strip, which is then placed in tromethamine hydrochloride buffer. A substrate reaction mixture containing L-aspartic and α-ketoglutaric acids is added and allowed to react for 10 minutes. In the presence of AST, the aspartate and α-glutarate are catalyzed to oxalacetate and glutamate. The addition of a dye, such as fast red, results in a color product, the intensity of which is proportional to the AST activity in the GCF sample. A potential problem with the AST test is its strong relationship to the presence of severe gingival inflammation, defined as the tendency to bleed on probing, because not all sites that bleed on probing are progressively losing attachment. It remains to be demonstrated whether this test offers some advantage over existing clinical indicators of disease.

A variety of lysosomal enzymes capable of lysing components of the extracellular matrix have been preliminarily examined as possible markers for periodontal destruction. Those appearing to be the most promising include collagenases, β-glucuronidase,[75–77] arylsulfatase,[76,77] and elastase.[161] Further studies are warranted on all of these enzymes, because they appear to have a distinct relationship to the progression of periodontitis.

Tissue Breakdown Products. One of the major features of periodontitis is the destruction of the extracellular matrix (collagen and glycosaminoglycans). Analysis of GCF obtained from sites with periodontitis clearly shows elevated levels of hydroxiproline and glycosaminoglycans.[81] However, the research on these potential activity markers is very meager.

Inflammatory Mediators. A variety of inflammatory mediators are produced by tissues afflicted by gingivitis and periodontitis. Some of these mediators have been investigated for their potential use as markers for progressing periodontal lesions.

Tumor necrosis factor α[132] and interleukin-1β[143] are two cytokines produced by macrophages at diseased sites. Both are potent immunoregulatory molecules with a variety of biologic effects, including fibroblast stimulation and bone resorption. The amounts of the two substances recoverable from GCF are sufficient to play a potentially important role in the pathogenesis of periodontitis, although their concentrations are very low in samples harvested from healthy or slightly inflamed sites.

Prostaglandin E_2 is a product of the cyclooxygenase pathway of the metabolism of arachidonic acid. It is a potent mediator of inflammation and bone resorption. In cases of untreated periodontitis, the concentration of prostaglandin E_2 found in GCF dramatically increased during active phases of periodontal destruction.[111–113]

Although clear correlations have been demonstrated between some components of the GCF and progressing periodontal lesions, the database is still small, and additional clinical studies are needed to document claims of diagnostic or therapeutic value. As a consequence, although most GCF components show promise, we do not yet know their potential as a basis for diagnostic tests.

REFERENCES

1. Abbas F, Hart AAM, Oosting J, Van der Velden U. Effect of training and probing force on the reproducibility of pocket depth measurements. J Periodont Res *17:*226, 1982.
2. Abrams K, Caton J, Polson A. Histologic comparisons of interproximal gingival tissues related to the presence or absence of bleeding. J Periodontol *55:*629, 1984.
3. Aeppli DM, Philstrom BL. Detection of longitudinal changes in periodontitis. J Periodont Res *24:*329, 1989.
4. Africa CW, Parker JR, Reddy J. Bacteriological studies of subgingival plaque in a periodontitis resistant population. Darkfield microscopic studies. J Periodont Res *20:*1, 1985.
5. Agudio G, Prato GP, Bartolucci C. Computerized charting of probing depths. J Periodontol *56:*766, 1985.
6. Armitage GC, Svanberg GK, Löe H. Microscopic evaluation of clinical measurements of connective tissue attachment levels. J Clin Periodontol *4:*173, 1977.
7. Badersten A, Nilveus R, Egelberg J. Reproducibility of probing attachment level measurements. J Clin Periodontol *11:*475, 1984.
8. Badersten A, Nilveus R, Egelberg J. Effect of non-surgical periodontal therapy. VII. Bleeding, suppuration and probing depth in sites with probing attachment loss. J Clin Periodontol *12:*432, 1985.
9. Badersten A, Nilveus R, Egelberg J. Effect of non-surgical periodontal therapy. VIII. Probing attachment changes related to clinical characteristics. J Clin Periodontol *14:*425, 1987.
10. Barnett JM, Cuchens MA, Buchanan W. Automated immunofluorescent specification of oral bacteria using flow cytometry. J Dent Res *63:*1040, 1984.
11. Beck JD, Koch GG, Rozier RG, Tudor GE. Prevalence and risk indicators for periodontal attachment loss in a population of older community-dwelling blacks and whites. J Periodontol *61:*521, 1990.
12. Bonta Y, Zambon JJ, Neiders M, Genco RJ. Rapid identification of a periodontal pathogen in subgingival dental plaque: A comparison of indirect immunoflorescence microscopy with bacterial culture for the detection of *Actinobacillus actinomycetemcomitans.* J Dent Res *64:*693, 1985.
13. Boye E, Steen HB, Skarstad K. Flow cytometry: A promising tool in experimental and clinical microbiology. J Gen Microbiol *129:*973, 1983.
14. Bragger U, Pasquali L, Rylander H, et al. Computer assisted densitometric image analysis in periodontal radiography. A methodological study. J Clin Periodontol *15:*27, 1988.
15. Cameron JR, Mazess RB, Sorenson JA. Precision and accuracy of bone mineral determination by direct photon absorptiometry. Invest Radiol *3:*141, 1968.
16. Chambers DA, Crawford JM, Mukherjee S, Cohen RL. Aspartate aminotransferase increases in crevicular fluid during experimental periodontitis in beagle dogs. J Periodontol *55:*236, 1984.
17. Chambers DA, Imrey PB, Cohen R, et al. A longitudinal study of aspartate aminotransferase in human gingival crevicular fluid. J Periodont Res *26:*65, 1991.
18. Christersson LA, Slots J, Rosling BG, Genco RJ. Microbiological and clinical effects of surgical treatment of localized juvenile periodontitis. J Clin Periodontol *12:*465, 1985.
19. Chung CP, Nisengard R, Slots J, Genco RJ. Bacterial IgG and IgM antibody titers in acute necrotizing ulcerative gingivitis. J Periodontol *54:*557, 1983.
20. Cimasoni G. Crevicular fluid updated. In Ureyers HM, ed. Monographs in Oral Science. Basel, Karger, 1983.
21. Clark WB, Yang MCK, Magnusson I. Measuring clinical attachment: Reproducibility and relative measurements with an electronic probe. J Periodontol *63:*831, 1992.
22. Daneshmann H, Wade AB. Correlation between gingival fluid measurements and macroscopic and microscopic characteristics of gingival tissue. J Periodont Res *11:*35, 1976.
23. Davenport RH, Simpson DM, Hassell TM. Histometric comparison of active and inactive lesions of advanced periodontitis. J Periodontol *53:*285, 1982.
24. Deas D, Pasquali LA, Yuan CH, Kornman KS. The relationship between prob-

ing attachment loss and computerized radiographic analysis in monitoring the progression of periodontitis. J Periodontol 62:135, 1991.

25. Dzink JL, Socransky SS, Haffajee AD. The predominant cultivable microbiota of active and inactive lesions of destructive periodontal diseases. J Clin Periodontol 15:316, 1988.

26. Dzink JL, Tanner ACR, Haffajee AD, Socransky SS. Gram negative species associated with active destructive periodontal lesions. J Clin Periodontol 12:648, 1985.

26a. Ebersole JL, Frey DE, Taubman MA, et al. Dynamics of systemic antibody responses in periodontal disease. J Periodont Res 22:184, 1987.

27. Ebersole JL, Taubman MA, Smith DJ, et al. Human immune responses to oral organisms. I. Association of localized juvenile periodontitis with serum antibody responses to *Actinobacillus actinomycetemcomitans*. Clin Exp Immunol 46:43, 1982.

28. Ebersole JL, Taubman MA, Smith DJ. Local antibody responses in periodontal diseases. J Periodontol 56(suppl II):51, 1985.

29. Engelberger T, Hefti A, Kallenberger A, Rateitschak KH. Correlations among Papilla Bleeding Index, other clinical indexes and histologically determined inflammation of gingival papilla. J Clin Periodontol 10:579, 1983.

30. Fine DH, Mandel ID. Indicators of periodontal disease activity: An evaluation. J Clin Periodontol 13:533, 1986.

31. Fowler C, Garret S, Crigger M, Egelberg J. Histologic probe position in treated and untreated human periodontal tissues. J Clin Periodontol 9:373, 1982.

32. French CK, Savitt ED, Simon SL, et al. DNA detection of periodontal pathogens. Oral Microbiol Immunol 1:58, 1986.

33. Gangbar S, Overall CM, McCuloch GAG, Sodek J. Identification of polymorphonuclear leukocyte collagenase and gelatinase activities in mouthrinse samples. Correlation with periodontal disease activity in adult and juvenile periodontitis. J Periodont Res 25:257, 1990.

34. Genco RJ, Zambon JJ, Murray PA. Serum and gingival fluid antibodies as adjuncts in the diagnosis of *Actinobacillus actinomycetemcomitans*–associated periodontal disease. J Periodontol 56(suppl 11):41, 1985.

35. Genco RJ, Loos BG. The use of genomic DNA fingerprinting in studies of the epidemiology of bacteria in periodontitis. J Clin Periodontol 18:396, 1991.

36. Gibbs CH, Hirschfeld JW, Lee JG, et al. Description and clinical evaluation of a new computerized periodontal probe—the Florida probe. J Clin Periodontol 15:137, 1988.

37. Gmur R, Guggenheim B. Monoclonal antibodies for the detection of periodontopathic bacteria. Arch Oral Biol 35(suppl):145, 1990.

38. Golub LM, Siegel K, Ramamurthy NS, Mandel ID. Some characteristics of collagenase activity in gingival crevicular fluid and its relationship to gingival disease in humans. J Dent Res 55:1049, 1976.

39. Goodson JM, Haffajee AD, Socransky SS. The relationship between attachment level loss and alveolar bone loss. J Clin Periodontol 11:348, 1984.

40. Goodson JM, Tanner ACR, Haffajee AD, et al. Patterns of progression and regression of advanced destructive periodontal disease. J Clin Periodontol 9:472, 1982.

41. Gratt BM, Sickles EA, Armitage GC. Use of dental xeroradiographs in periodontics. Comparison with conventional radiographs. J Periodontol 51:1, 1980.

42. Greenstein G, Caton J, Polson AM. Histologic characteristics associated with bleeding after probing and visual signs of inflammation. J Periodontol 52:420, 1981.

42a. Greenstein G, Caton J. Periodontal disease activity: A critical assessment. J Periodontol 61:543, 1990.

43. Greenstein G. Advances in periodontal diagnosis. Int J Periodont Prost Dent 10:351, 1990.

44. Grondahl HG, Grondahl K. Subtraction radiography for the diagnosis of periodontal bone lesions. Oral Surg 55:208, 1983.

45. Grondahl HG, Johnson E, Lindahl B. Diagnosis of marginal bone destruction with orthopantomography and intraoral full mouth radiography. Tandlak Tidskr 6:435, 1971.

46. Grondahl K, Kullendorff B, Strid H-G, et al. Detectability of artificial marginal bone lesions as a function of lesion depth. J Clin Periodontol 15:156, 1988.

47. Haffajee AD, Dzink JL, Socransky SS. Effect of modified Widman flap surgery and systemic tetracycline on the subgingival microbiota of periodontal lesions. J Clin Periodontol 15:255, 1988.

48. Haffajee AD, Socransky SS. Attachment level changes in destructive periodontal diseases. J Clin Periodontol 13:461, 1986.

49. Haffajee AD, Socransky SS, Ebersole JL, Smith DJ. Clinical, microbiological and immunological features associated with the treatment of active periodontosis lesions. J Clin Periodontol 9:600, 1984.

50. Haffajee AD, Socransky SS, Goodson JM. Clinical parameters as predictors of destructive periodontal activity. J Clin Periodontol 10:257, 1983.

51. Haffajee AD, Socransky SS, Goodson JM. Comparisons of different data analysis for detecting changes in attachment level. J Clin Periodontol 10:298, 1983.

52. Haffajee AD, Socransky SS, Goodson JM. Subgingival temperature. Relation to future periodontal attachment loss. J Clin Periodontol 19:409, 1992.

53. Hancock EB. Determination of periodontal disease activity. J Periodontol 52:492, 1981.

54. Hausmann E, Christersson L, Dunford R, et al. Usefulness of subtraction radiography in the evaluation of periodontal therapy. J Periodontol 56(suppl 11):4, 1985.

55. Hausmann E, McHenry K, Christersson L, et al. Techniques for assessing alveolar bone mass changes in periodontal disease with emphasis on ^{125}I absorptiometry. J Clin Periodontol 10:455, 1983.

56. Hausmann E, Ortman LF, McHenry K, Fallon J. Relationship between alveolar bone measured by ^{125}I absorptiometry with analysis of standardized radiographs. J Periodontol 53:307, 1982.

57. Hausmann E, Allen K, Carpio L, et al. Computerized methodology for detection of alveolar crestal bone loss from serial intraoral radiographs. J Periodontol 63:657, 1992.

58. Henrikson CO. Iodine as a source for odontological roentgenology. Acta Radiol 13:377, 1967.

59. Hernichel E, Newman MG, Nachnani S, Rodriquez A. Validation of a latex agglutination test for periodontal pathogens. Abstract. J Dent Res 68:900, 1989.

60. Hinrichs JE, Brandt CL, Smith JA. Relative error associated with an improved instrument for measuring GCF. J Periodontol 55:294, 1984.

61. Jeffcoat MK, Jeffcoat RL, Jens SC, Captain K. A new periodontal probe with automated cemento-enamel junction detection. J Clin Periodontol 13:276, 1986.

62. Jeffcoat MK. Diagnosing periodontal disease: New tools to solve old problems. J Am Dent Assoc 122:54, 1991.

63. Jeffcoat MK. Radiographic methods for the detection of progressive alveolar bone loss. J Periodontol 63:367, 1992.

64. Jeffcoat MK, Williams RC, Kaplan ML, Goldhaber P. Nuclear medicine: An indicator of active alveolar bone loss in beagle dogs treated with a non-steroidal anti-inflammatory drug. J Periodontol 56(suppl 11):8, 1985.

65. Jeffcoat MK, Williams RC, Kaplan ML, Goldhaber P. Nuclear medicine techniques for the detection of active alveolar bone loss. Adv Dent Res 1:80, 1987.

66. Jeffcoat MK, Reddy M. Progression of probing attachment loss in adult periodontitis. J Periodontol 62:185, 1991.

67. Kalkwarf KL, Kahldal WD, Patil KD. Comparison of manual and pressure controlled periodontal probing. J Periodontol 57:467, 1986.

68. Kelly GP, Cain RJ, Knowles JW, et al. Radiographs in clinical periodontal trials. J Periodontol 46:381, 1975.

69. Kornman KS. Nature of periodontal diseases: Assessment and diagnosis. J Periodont Res 22:192, 1987.

70. Kornman KS, Holt SC, Robertson PB. The microbiology of ligature-induced periodontitis in the cynomolgus monkey. J Periodont Res 16:363, 1981.

71. Kornman KS, Robertson PB. Clinical and microbiological evaluation of therapy for juvenile periodontitis. J Periodontol 56:443, 1985.

72. Kornman KS, Newman MG, Flemmig T, et al. Treatment of refractory periodontitis with metronidazole plus amoxicillin or Augmentin. Abstract. J Dent Res 68:917, 1989.

73. Kowashi Y, Jaccard F, Cimasoni G. Sulcular polymorphonuclear leukocytes and gingival exudate during experimental gingivitis in man. J Periodont Res 15:151, 1980.

74. Kung RT, Ochs B, Goodson JM. Temperature as a periodontal diagnostic. J Clin Periodontol 17:557, 1990.

75. Lamster IB, Hartley LJ, Vogel RI. Development of a biochemical profile for gingival crevicular fluid. J Periodontol 56(suppl 11):13, 1985.

76. Lamster IB, Vogel RS, Hartley LJ, et al. Lactate dehydrogenase, β-glucuronidase and arylsulfatase activity in gingival crevicular fluid associated with experimental gingivitis. J Periodontol 56:139, 1985.

77. Lamster IB, Oshrain RL, Harper CS, et al. Enzyme activity in crevicular fluid for the detection and prediction of clinical attachment loss in patients with chronic adult periodontitis. J Periodontol 59:516, 1988.

78. Lang NP, Joss A, Orsanic T, et al. Bleeding on probing. A predictor for the progression of periodontal disease? J Clin Periodontol 13:590, 1986.

79. Lang NP, Nyman S, Senn C, Joss A. Bleeding on probing as it relates to probing pressure and gingival health. J Clin Periodontol 18:257, 1991.

80. Lang NP, Brägger U. Periodontal diagnosis in the 1990s. J Clin Periodontol 18:370, 1991.

81. Last KS, Stanbury JB, Embery G. Glycosaminoglycans in human gingival sulcus fluid as indicators of active periodontal disease. Arch Oral Biol 30:275, 1985.

82. Laughon BE, Syed SA, Loesche WJ. API-ZYM system for identification of *Bacteroides* sp., *Capnocytophaga* sp. and spirochetes of oral origin. J Clin Microbiol 15:97, 1982.

83. Listgarten MA. Direct microscopy of periodontal pathogens. Oral Microbiol Immunol 1:31, 1986.

84. Listgarten MA. Periodontal probing: What does it mean? J Clin Periodontol 7:165, 1980.

85. Listgarten MA, Hellden L. Relative distribution of bacteria at clinically healthy and periodontally diseased sites in humans. J Clin Periodontol 5:115, 1978.

86. Listgarten MA, Lai CH, Evian CI. Comparative antibody titers to *Actinobacillus actinomycetemcomitans* in juvenile periodontitis, chronic periodontitis and periodontically healthy subjects. J Clin Periodontol 8:155, 1981.

87. Listgarten MA, Levin S, Schifter C, et al. Comparative differential darkfield microscopy of subgingival bacteria from tooth surfaces with recent evidence of recurring periodontitis and from non-affected sites. J Periodontol 55:398, 1984.

88. Listgarten MA, Levin S, Schifter CC, et al. Comparative longitudinal study of two methods of scheduling maintenance visits; 2 year data. J Clin Periodontol 13:692, 1986.

89. Listgarten MA, Mao R, Robinson PJ. Periodontal probing and the relationship of the probe tip to periodontal tissues. J Periodontol 47:511, 1976.

90. Listgarten MA, Schifter CC, Laster L. 3-year longitudinal study of the periodontal status of an adult population with gingivitis. J Clin Periodontol 12:225, 1985.

91. Listgarten MA, Schifter CC, Sullivan P, et al. Failure of a microbial assay to reliably predict disease recurrence in a treated periodontitis population receiving

regularly scheduled prophylaxis. J Clin Periodontol *13:*768, 1987.

92. Löe H, Anerud A, Boysen H, Smith M. The natural history of periodontal disease in man. J Periodontol *49:*607, 1978.
93. Löe H, Silness J. Periodontal disease in pregnancy. Prevalence and severity. Acta Odont Scand *21:*533, 1963.
94. Loesche WJ. The identification of bacteria associated with periodontal disease and dental caries by enzymatic methods. Oral Microbiol Immunol *1:*65, 1986.
95. Magnusson I, Clark WB, Marks RG, et al. Attachment level measurements with a constant force electronic probe. J Clin Periodontol *15:*185, 1988.
96. Magnusson I, Fuller WW, Heins PJ, et al. Correlation between electronic and visual readings of pocket depths with a newly developed constant force probe. J Clin Periodontol *15:*180, 1988.
97. Magnusson I, Listgarten MA. Histological evaluation of probing depth following periodontal treatment. J Clin Periodontol *7:*26, 1980.
98. Mandell RL. A longitudinal microbiological investigation of *Actinobacillus actinomycetemcomitans* and *Eikenella corrodens* in juvenile periodontitis. Infect Immun *45:*778, 1984.
99. McCulloch CA, Birek P. Automated probe: Futuristic technology for diagnosis of periodontal disease. Univ Toronto Dent J *4:*6, 1991.
100. Meitner SW, Zander HA, Iker HP, Polson AM. Identification of inflamed gingival surfaces. J Clin Periodontol *6:*93, 1979.
101. Mombelli A, Graf H. Depth force patterns in periodontal probing. J Clin Periodontol *13:*126, 1986.
102. Mombelli A, Mukle T, Frigg RJ. Depth-force patterns of periodontal probing attachment gain in relation to probing force. J Clin Periodontol *19:*295, 1992.
103. Moore WEC. Microbiology of periodontal disease. J Periodont Res *22:*335, 1987.
104. Mouton C, Hammond PG, Slots J, Genco RJ. Serum antibodies to oral *Bacteroides asaccharolyticus (Bacteroides gingivalis):* Relationship to age and periodontal disease. Infect Immun *31:*182, 1981.
105. Mühlemann HR, Son S. Gingival sulcus bleeding, a leading symptom of initial gingivitis. Helv Odontol Acta *15:*105, 1971.
106. Nachnani S, Nisengard R, Zelonis L, et al. Latex agglutination for the rapid clinical identification of periodontopathogens. J Dent Res *67*(special issue):159, 1988.
107. Nagahata T, Kiyoshige T, Tomono S, et al. Oral implantation of *Bacteroides asacrolyticus* and *Eikenella corrodens* in conventional hamsters. Infect Immun *36:*304, 1982.
108. Newman MG, Nisengard R. Diagnostic microbiology and immunology. In Newman MG, Nisengard R, eds. Oral Microbiology and Immunology. Philadelphia, WB Saunders, 1988.
109. Newman MG, Kornman KS, Flemmig TF, et al. Treatment of refractory periodontitis with Augmentin. Abstract. J Dent Res *68:*917, 1989.
110. Niekrash CE, Patters MR. Assessment of complement cleavage in gingival fluid in humans with and without periodontal disease. J Periodont Res *21:*233, 1986.
111. Offenbacher S, Farr DH, Goodson JM. Measuring of prostaglandin E in crevicular fluid. J Clin Periodontol *8:*359, 1981.
112. Offenbacher S, Odle BM, Gray RC, Van Dyke TE. Crevicular fluid prostaglandin E levels as a measure of periodontal disease status of adult and juvenile patients. J Periodont Res *19:*1, 1984.
113. Offenbacher S, Odle BM, Van Dyke TE. The use of crevicular fluid prostaglandin E2 levels as predictor of periodontal attachment loss. J Periodont Res *21:*101, 1986.
114. Ortman LF, Dunford R, McHenry K, Haussman E. Subtraction radiography and computer assisted densitometric analyses of standardized radiographs. A comparison study with ^{125}I absorptiometry. J Periodont Res *20:*644, 1985.
115. Ortman LF, McHenry K, Hausmann E. Relationship between alveolar bone measured by ^{125}I absorptiometry with analysis of standardized radiographs. J Periodontol *53:*311, 1982.
116. Page RC, Beatty P, Waldrop TC. Molecular basis for the functional abnormality in neutrophils from patients with generalized prepubertal periodontitis. J Periodontol Res *22:*182, 1987.
117. Page RC. Host response tests for diagnosing periodontal diseases. J Periodontol *63:*356, 1992.
118. Page RC, Schroeder HB. Periodontitis in Man and Other Animals. Basel, Karger, 1982.
119. Parakkal PF. Proceedings of the workshop on quantitative evaluation of periodontal diseases by physical measurement techniques. J Dent Res *58:*547, 1979.
120. Payot P, Bickel M, Cimasoni G. Longitudinal quantitative radiodensitometric study of treated and untreated lower molar furcation involvement. J Clin Periodontol *14:*8, 1987.
121. Payot P, Haroutunian B, Pochon Y, et al. Densitometric analysis of lower molar interradicular areas in superposable radiographs. J Clin Periodontol *14:*1, 1987.
122. Polson AM, Caton JG. Current status of bleeding in the diagnosis of periodontal diseases. J Periodontol *56*(suppl 11):1, 1985.
123. Polson AM, Caton JG, Yeaple RN, Zander H. Histological determination of probe tip penetration into gingival sulcus of humans using an electronic pressure-sensitive probe. J Clin Periodontol *7:*479, 1980.
124. Polson AM, Goodson JM. Periodontol diagnosis. Current status and future needs. J Periodontol *56:*25, 1985.
125. Quivey RG. The use of DNA probes in dental diagnosis and therapy. Adv Dent Res *1:*99, 1987.
126. Ranney PR, Best AM, Breen TJ, et al. Bacterial flora of progressing periodontitis lesions. J Periodont Res *22:*205, 1987.
127. Reddy J, Africa CW, Parker JR. Darkfield microscopy of subgingival plaque of an urban black population with poor oral hygiene. J Clin Periodontol *13:*579, 1986.
128. Rethman M, Ruttimann U, O'Neal R, et al. Diagnosis of bone lesions by subtraction radiography. J Periodontol *56:*324, 1985.
129. Robinson PJ, Vitek RM. The relationship between gingival inflammation and resistance to probe penetration. J Periodont Res *14:*239, 1979.
130. Rosling B, Hollender L, Nyman S, Olsson G. A radiographic method for assessing changes in alveolar height following periodontal therapy. J Clin Periodontol *2:*211, 1975.
131. Rosling B, Nyman S, Lindhe J. The effect of systemic plaque control on bone regeneration of infrabony pockets. J Clin Periodontol *3:*38, 1976.
132. Rossomando EF, Kennedy JE, Hadjimichael J. Tumor necrosis factor alpha in gingival crevicular fluid as a possible indicator of periodontal disease in humans. Arch Oral Biol *35:*431, 1990.
133. Savitt ED, Keville MW, Peros WJ. DNA probes in the diagnosis of periodontal microorganisms. Arch Oral Biol *35*(suppl):153, 1990.
133. Shapiro L, Lodato FM, Courant PR, Stallard RE. Endotoxin determinations in gingival inflammation. J Periodontol *43:*591, 1972.
134. Singer RE, Buckner BA. Butirate and propionate: Important components of toxic dental plaque extracts. Infect Immun *32:*458, 1981.
135. Slots J, Bragd L, Wikstrm M, Dahlen G. The occurrence of *Actinobacillus actinomycetemcomitans, Bacteroides gingivalis* and *Bacteroides intermedius* in destructive periodontal disease in adults. J Clin Periodontol *13:*570, 1986.
136. Slots J, Genco RJ. Microbial pathogenicity. Black pigmented *Bacteroides* species, *Caphocytophaga* species, and *Actinobacillus actinomycetemcomitans* in human periodontal disease. J Dent Res *63:*412, 1984.
137. Slots J, Hafstrom C, Rosling B, Dahlen G. Detection of *Actinobacillus actinomycetemcomitans* and *Bacteroides gingivalis* in subgingival smears by the indirect fluorescent-antibody technique. J Periodont Res *20:*613, 1985.
138. Slots J, Hausmann E. Longitudinal study of experimentally induced periodontal disease in *Macaca arctoides:* Relationship between microflora and alveolar bone loss. Infect Immun *23:*260, 1979.
139. Socransky SS, Haffajee AD, Goodson JM, Lindhe J. New concepts of destructive periodontal disease. J Clin Periodontol *11:*21, 1984.
140. Socransky SS, Haffajee AD, Smith GLE, Dzink JL. Difficulties encountered in the search for the etiologic agents of destructive periodontal diseases. J Clin Periodontol *14:*588, 1987.
141. Socransky SS, Haffajee AD. The bacterial etiology of destructive periodontal disease. J Periodontol *63:*322, 1992.
142. Solis-Gaffar MC, Rustogi KN, Gaffar A. Hydrogen sulfide production from gingival crevicular fluid. J Periodontol *51:*607, 1980.
143. Stashenko P, Fujiyoshi P, Obernesser MS, et al. Levels of interleukin 1β in tissue from sites of active periodontal disease. J Clin Periodontol *18:*548, 1991.
144. Tanner ACR. The identification of bacteria associated with periodontal disease and dental caries by enzymatic methods. Oral Microbiol Immunol *1:*71, 1986.
145. Tanner ACR, Socransky SS, Goodson JM. Microbiota of periodontal pockets losing crestal alveolar bone. J Periodont Res *19:*279, 1984.
146. Tanner ACR, Strzempko MN, Belsky CA, McKinley GA. API-Zym and API-ANADENT reactions of fastidious gram negative species. J Clin Microbiol *22:*333, 1985.
147. Taubman MA, Yoshie H, Wetherell JR, et al. Immune response and periodontal bone loss in germ free rats immunized and infected with *Actinobacillus actinomycetemcomitans*. J Periodont Res *18:*393, 1983.
148. Thurre C, Robert M, Cimasoni G, Baehni P. Gingival sulcular leukocytes in periodontitis and in experimental gingivitis in humans. J Periodont Res *19:*457, 1984.
149. Tolo K, Schenck K. Activity of serum immunoglobulins G, A, and M to six anaerobic oral bacteria in diagnosis of periodontitis. J Periodont Res *20:*113, 1985.
150. Tolo K, Schenck K, Johansen JR. Activity of human serum immunoglobulins to seven anaerobic oral bacteria before and after periodontal treatment. J Periodont Res *17:*481, 1982.
151. Tsuchida K, Hara K. Clinical significance of gingival fluid measurement by Periotron. J Periodontol *52:*599, 1981.
152. Tzamouranis A, Matthys J, Ishikawa I, Cimasoni G. Increase of endotoxin concentration in gingival washings during experimental gingivitis in man. J Periodontol *50:*175, 1979.
153. Van der Velden U, de Vries JH. Introduction of new periodontal probe: The pressure probe. J Clin Periodontol *5:*188, 1978.
154. Van der Velden U. Probing force and the relationship of the probe to the periodontal tissues. J Clin Periodontol *6:*106, 1979.
155. Van Dyke TE, Levine MJ, Genco RJ. Neutrophil dysfunction and oral disease. J Oral Pathol *14:*95, 1985.
156. Villela B, Cogen RB, Bartolucci AA, Birkedal-Hansen H. Crevicular fluid collagenase activity in healthy, gingivitis, chronic adult periodontitis and localized juvenile periodontitis. J Periodont Res *22:*209, 1987.
157. Williams BI, Ebersole JL, Spektor MD, Page RC. Assessment of serum antibody patterns and analysis of subgingival microflora of members of a family with a high prevalence of early onset periodontitis. Infect Immun *49:*742, 1985.
158. Williams RC, Jeffcoat MK. Flurbiprofen—a potent inhibitor of alveolar bone resorption in beagles. Science *227:*640, 1985.
159. Woolweaver DA, Koch GG, Crawford JJ, Lumdblad RL. Relation of the orogranulocytic migration rate to periodontal disease and blood leukocyte count. J Dent Res *51:*929, 1972.

160. Yang MCK, Marks RG, Clark WB, Magnusson I. Predictive power of various models for longitudinal attachment level change. J Clin Periodontol *19:*77, 1992.
161. Zafiropoulos GGK, Flores-de-Jacoby L, Todt G, et al. Gingival crevicular fluid elastase-inhibitor complex: Correlation with clinical indexes and subgingival flora. J Periodont Res *26:*24, 1991.
162. Zambon JJ, Bochacki V, Genco RJ. Immunological assays for putative periodontal pathogens. Oral Microbiol Immunol *1:*39, 1986.
163. Zambon JJ, Reynolds HS, Chen P, Genco RJ. Rapid identification of periodontal pathogens in subgingival dental plaque: Comparison of indirect immunofluorescence microscopy with bacterial culture for detection of *Bacteroides gingivalis.* J Periodontol *56*(suppl 11):32, 1985.

31

Determination of the Prognosis

FERMIN A. CARRANZA, Jr.

Prognosis for Patients With Gingival Disease
Prognosis for Patients With Periodontitis
Overall Prognosis

Prognosis for Individual Teeth
Clinical Application

The *prognosis* is a prediction of the duration, course, and termination of a disease and its response to treatment. It must be determined after the diagnosis is made and before treatment is planned.

Prognosis is often confused with the term *risk*. Risk generally refers to the probability of acquiring the disease before it starts. Many times risk factors and prognosis factors are the same. For example, patients with diabetes are more at risk of acquiring periodontal disease and, once they have it, generally have a worse prognosis.

PROGNOSIS FOR PATIENTS WITH GINGIVAL DISEASE

The prognosis for patients with gingival disease depends on the role of inflammation in the overall disease process. If inflammation is the only pathologic change, the prognosis is favorable, provided all local irritants are eliminated, gingival contours conducive to the preservation of health are attained, and the patient cooperates by maintaining good oral hygiene.

If inflammatory changes are complicated by systemically caused tissue changes (e.g., as in gingival enlargement associated with phenytoin therapy or changes associated with hormonal disorders or systemic diseases), gingival health may be improved temporarily through local therapy alone, but long-term prognosis depends on the control or correction of the systemic factors.

PROGNOSIS FOR PATIENTS WITH PERIODONTITIS

There are two aspects to the determination of prognosis in patients with periodontitis: the overall prognosis and the prognosis for individual teeth.

Overall Prognosis

Overall prognosis is concerned with the dentition as a whole. It answers the questions, "Should treatment be undertaken?", "Is it likely to succeed?" and, when prosthetic replacements are needed, "Are the remaining teeth able to support the added burden of the prosthesis?"

Type of Periodontitis. The overall prognosis should initially take into account the type of periodontitis present. *Slowly progressive periodontitis* is the most common form; onset occurs in the patient's thirties or forties, and the disease progresses slowly (see Chapter 25) (Figs. 31–1 and 31–2). These cases usually respond well to conventional treatment, provided that they are not very severe and that local irritants can be controlled.

In cases of slowly progressing periodontitis, the prognosis of periodontal disease is directly related to the severity of inflammation and to the height of remaining bone. Given two patients with comparable bone destruction, the prognosis may be better for the patient with the greater degree of inflammation, since a larger component of that patient's bone destruction may be attributable to local irritants. In such a patient, removal of local irritants can be expected to be more effective in arresting the bone destruction. For other types of periodontitis, the degree of inflammation may be inversely correlated with prognosis.

With respect to the height of remaining bone, the question to be answered is, "Assuming bone destruction can be arrested, is there enough bone remaining to support the teeth?" The answer is readily apparent in extreme cases, i.e., when there is so little bone loss that tooth support is not in jeopardy (see Figs. 31–1 and 31–2) or when bone loss is so severe that the remaining bone is obviously insufficient for proper tooth support (Fig. 31–3). Most patients, however, do not fit into these extreme categories. The height of the remaining bone is somewhere between, making the bone level alone inconclusive for determining the overall prognosis.

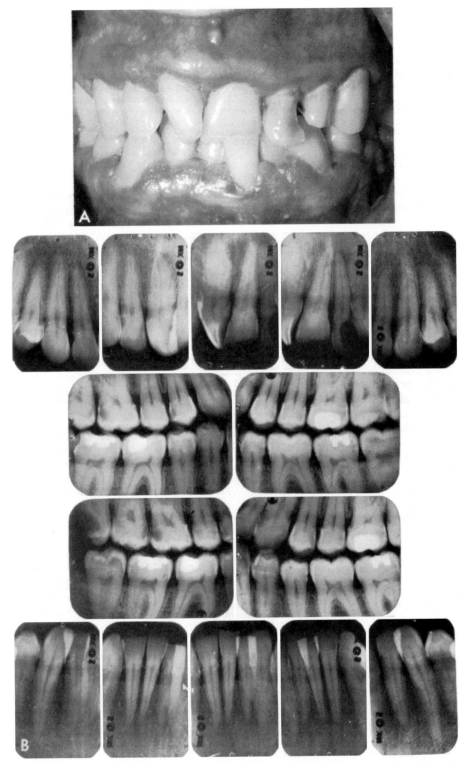

FIGURE 31–1. Adult-type periodontitis, overall prognosis favorable. *A,* A 32-year-old man with generalized chronic marginal gingivitis, periodontal pocket formation, and excessive anterior overbite. *B,* The bone picture is excellent despite unfavorable inflammatory and occlusal factors.

Rapidly progressive periodontitis, on the other hand, is less common; onset is usually in the patient's twenties, and those affected exhibit rapid bone loss (Fig. 31–4). Patients with rapidly destructive periodontitis may show either slight inflammation not at all suggestive of the marked underlying osseous destruction or an excessive inflammatory reaction that may lead to rapid bone loss, with a hopeless prognosis.[18]

These patients may have leukocytic defects and associated systemic diseases (see Chapter 26). Some cases are re-

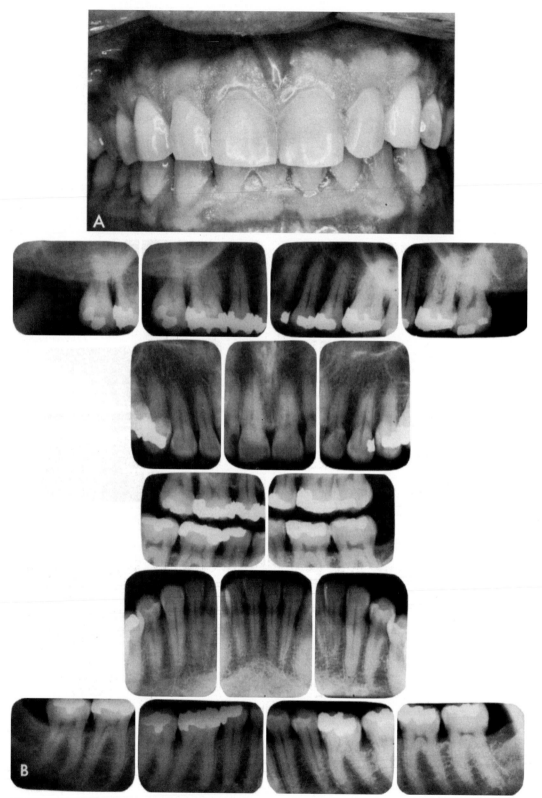

FIGURE 31–2. Adult-type periodontitis in a 42-year-old man. *A,* Gingival inflammation, poor oral hygiene, and pronounced anterior overbite. *B,* Bone loss is slight, considering the age of the patient and the unfavorable local factors.

sponsive to conventional therapy plus antibiotics, whereas others are refractory or resistant to therapy. There are no methods available to predict before therapy whether the response will be favorable.

Patients diagnosed as having *refractory periodontitis,* are, by definition, resistant to treatment. This can be due to impaired defense mechanisms, resistant bacteria, untreatable morphologic problems, or combinations of these factors.

Juvenile periodontitis starts at puberty; is limited, at least initially, to first molars and incisors; and is associated with a specific flora (see Fig. 31–3); patients may also have leukocyte defects (see Chapter 27). Prognosis for these patients used to be poor, but the administration of systemic tetracycline in conjunction with surgical pocket therapy has greatly improved the expected results.

Other types of destructive periodontitis in children, known as *prepubertal periodontitis,* are usually associated with systemic diseases (see Chapter 27), and in most cases patients have a poor prognosis.

Age. Consideration of the prognoses for the different types of periodontitis, as already presented, points to the fact that for two patients with comparable levels of remaining alveolar bone, the prognosis is better in the older of the two. For the younger patient, who may have suffered a more rapid bone destruction than the older patient, the prognosis is not as good because of the shorter period in which the bone loss has occurred. In some cases this may be because the younger patient suffers from a rapidly progressive type of periodontitis. In addition, although the younger patient would ordinarily be expected to have a greater bone reparative capacity, the occurrence of so much bone destruction in a relatively short period of time may reflect unfavorably on the patient's bone reparative capacity.

Systemic Background. The patient's systemic background affects overall prognosis in several ways. In patients with known systemic disorders that could affect the periodontium (e.g., diabetes, nutritional deficiency, hyperthyroidism, or hyperparathyroidism), prognosis improves with correction of the systemic problem.

The prognosis is guarded when surgical periodontal treatment is required but cannot be provided because of the patient's health. Incapacitating conditions that limit the patient's performance of oral hygiene procedures (e.g., Parkinson's disease) also adversely affect the prognosis. Newer "automated" oral hygiene devices such as electric toothbrushes may be helpful for these patients and improve their prognosis.

Malocclusion. Irregularly aligned teeth, malformation of the jaws, and abnormal occlusal relationships may be important factors in the etiology of periodontal disease, as they may interfere with plaque control or produce occlusal interferences. In these cases, orthodontic or prosthetic correction is essential if periodontal treatment is to succeed. The overall prognosis is poorer for patients with occlusal deformities that cannot be corrected.

Assessment of Periodontal Status and Prosthetic Possibilities. Overall prognosis requires a general consideration of bone levels (evaluated radiographically) and pocket depths (determined clinically) to establish whether enough

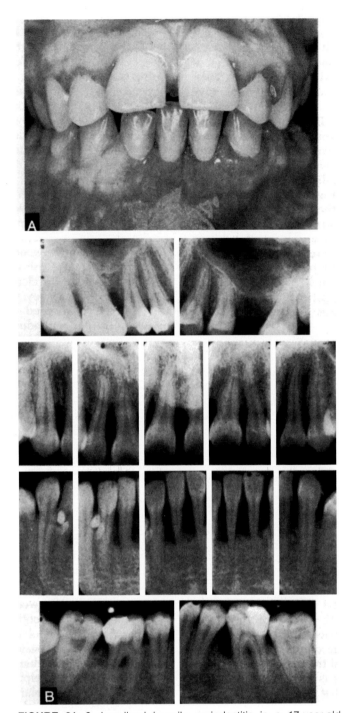

FIGURE 31–3. Localized juvenile periodontitis in a 17-year-old girl. *A,* Gingival inflammation, periodontal pockets, and pathologic migration. *B,* Severe bone destruction.

teeth can be saved either to provide a functional and aesthetic dentition or to serve as abutments for a useful prosthetic replacement of the missing teeth.

At this point, the overall prognosis and the prognosis for individual teeth overlap, because the prognosis for key individual teeth may affect the overall prognosis, particularly relative to prosthetic possibilities. For example, saving or losing a key tooth may determine whether other teeth are saved or extracted or whether the prosthesis used is fixed

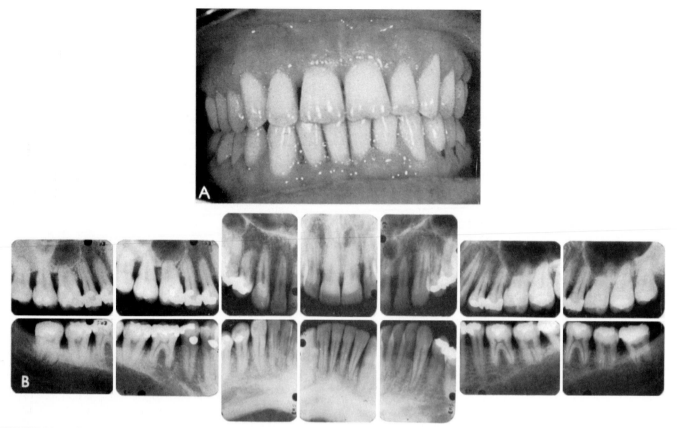

FIGURE 31–4. Rapidly progressive periodontitis, overall prognosis poor. *A,* Clinical picture of a 27-year-old man with generalized chronic gingivitis and periodontal pocket formation. *B,* Radiographic evaluation shows a fairly advanced bone destruction.

or removable. When few teeth remain, the prosthodontic needs become more important, and sometimes periodontally savable teeth may have to be extracted if they are not compatible with the design of the prosthesis.

The possibility of replacing missing teeth with dental implants has added a new dimension to the periodontal prognosis of the remaining natural teeth. When feasible, implants can replace teeth without creating a burden to the natural teeth and offer an attractive prosthetic alternative (see Chapter 63).

Smoking. It should be made clear to the patient that a direct relationship exists between smoking and gingivitis and periodontitis, as well as between smoking and impaired healing. Therefore, cessation of smoking will improve (1) the patient's chances of successful resolution of the periodontal problem and (2) the predictability of treatment (see Chapter 12).

Cooperation of the Patient. The prognosis for patients with gingival and periodontal disease is critically dependent on the patient's attitude, desire to retain the natural teeth, and willingness and ability to maintain good oral hygiene. Without these, treatment will not succeed.

Patients should be clearly informed of the important role they must play for treatment to succeed. If patients are unwilling or unable to perform adequate plaque control and to receive the maintenance checkups and treatments deemed necessary by the dentist, then the dentist can (1) refuse to accept the patient for treatment or (2) extract teeth that have a doubtful prognosis and perform only scaling and root planing in the remaining teeth. The dentist should make it clear to the patient and in the patient's record that further treatment is needed but will not be performed because of a lack of patient cooperation.

Prognosis for Individual Teeth

The prognosis for individual teeth is determined after the overall prognosis and is affected by it.[13] For example, in a patient with a poor overall prognosis, the dentist likely would not attempt to retain a tooth that has a questionable prognosis because of local conditions. When determining the prognosis for individual teeth, one should consider mobility, periodontal pockets, mucogingival problems, furcation involvement, tooth morphology, teeth adjacent to edentulous areas, location of remaining bone in relation to the individual tooth surfaces, relation to adjacent teeth, and caries, nonvital teeth, and tooth resorption.

Mobility. The principal causes of tooth mobility are loss of alveolar bone; inflammatory changes in the periodontal ligament, usually as a consequence of periapical disease; and trauma from occlusion. Tooth mobility caused by inflammation and trauma from occlusion may be correctable.[14] However, tooth mobility resulting from loss of alveolar bone alone is not likely to be corrected. The likelihood of restoring tooth stability is inversely proportional to the extent to which mobility is caused by loss of alveolar bone.

A longitudinal 8-year study of the response to treatment of teeth with different degrees of mobility revealed that pockets on clinically mobile teeth do not respond as well to periodontal therapy as pockets on firm teeth exhibiting the same initial disease severity.[7] Another study, however, in which ideal control of plaque was attained, found similar healing in hypermobile and firm teeth.[19]

Periodontal Pockets. The following variables should be carefully recorded because they are important for determining prognosis: pocket depth, level of attachment, degree of bone loss, and type of pocket. These are determined by probing and radiographic evaluation.

The determination of the level of clinical attachment reveals the approximate extent of root surface that is devoid of periodontal ligament; the radiographic examination shows the amount of root surface still covered by bone. Pocket depth is less important than level of attachment, because it is not necessarily related to bone loss; in general, a tooth with deep pockets and little bone loss has a better prognosis than one with shallow pockets and severe bone loss.

Prognosis is adversely affected if the base of the pocket (level of attachment) is close to the root apex. The presence of apical disease also worsens the prognosis. When the periodontal pocket has extended to involve the apex, the prognosis is poor. However, surprisingly good apical and lateral bone repair can sometimes be obtained by combining endodontic and periodontal therapy (see Chapter 58).

The type of pocket must also be determined. For suprabony pockets, prognosis depends on the height of the existing bone, because it is unlikely that clinically significant bone regeneration will be induced by therapy. In the case of infrabony pockets, if the contour of the existing bone and the number of osseous walls are favorable, there is an excellent chance that appropriate therapy could regenerate bone to approximately the level of the crest[19] (see Chapter 57).

Mucogingival Problems. Mucogingival problems, caused by lack of attached gingiva owing to high frenum attachment or by location of the bottom of the pocket apical to the mucogingival junction, can make pocket therapy and case maintenance very difficult, thereby jeopardizing the prognosis unless corrective procedures are included in treatment (see Chapter 59).

Furcation Involvement. The presence of furcation involvement does not automatically indicate a hopeless prognosis (see Chapter 58). However, when a lesion reaches the furcation, it causes two additional important problems: the first is the difficulty of access to the area, both for scaling and root planing and for performing surgery; the second is the inaccessibility of the area to plaque removal by the patient. If both of these problems can be satisfactorily solved, then the prognosis is similar to, or even better than, that of single-rooted teeth with a similar degree of bone loss.

Maxillary first premolars offer the greatest difficulties, and therefore their prognosis is usually unfavorable when the lesion reaches the furcation. Maxillary molars also offer some degree of difficulty; sometimes their prognosis can be improved by resecting one of the buccal roots (either the mesiobuccal or the distobuccal), thereby improving access to the area. When mandibular first molars or buccal furcations of maxillary molars offer good access to the furcation area, their prognosis is usually better.

Tooth Morphology. Prognosis is poor for teeth with short, tapered roots and relatively large crowns (Fig. 31–5). Because of the disproportionate crown-to-root ratio and the reduced root surface available for periodontal support,[10] the periodontium is more susceptible to injury by occlusal forces.

The *morphology of the tooth root* is an important consideration in therapy.[9] Scaling and planing of the root surfaces are fundamental if successful treatment is to be attained, and anything that decreases the efficiency of this procedure, such as bizarre root morphology, can decrease the prognosis. Good oral hygiene is also fundamental for maintaining the healthy state reached in therapy; this, too, can be made difficult by various root morphologies. The dentist should learn to recognize and evaluate such root forms, as their presence will sometimes play an essential role in treatment planning and prognosis determination. These bizarre root shapes offer no problems as long as they are apical to the epithelial attachment and thus are not exposed to the lumen of the pocket. At this stage there is no need to scale the roots, or to clean them later, because they are part of the attachment apparatus. However, as soon as the disease progresses to uncover these areas, the problems appear.

Root concavities and the morphology of the furcation areas are essential features of interest. *Concavities* can vary from shallow flutings to deep depressions present in the proximal surfaces. They increase the attachment area and produce a root shape that is more resistant to torquing forces. Concavities appear more marked in the maxillary first premolars, the mesiobuccal root of the maxillary first molar, both roots of the mandibular first molars, and the mandibular incisors[1,2] (Figs. 31–6 and 31–7). Any tooth, however, can have a proximal concavity.[8]

Access to the *furcation area* is sometimes difficult to obtain (see Chapter 58). In 58% of upper and lower first molars, the furcation entrance diameter is narrower than the width of conventional periodontal curettes[1] (Fig. 31–8).

The presence of *developmental grooves,* which sometimes appear in the maxillary lateral incisors (palatogingival groove)[23] (Fig. 31–9) or in the lower incisors, also creates an accessibility problem[6,9] and worsens the prognosis.[19] These palatal grooves are found in 5.6% of maxillary lateral incisors and 3.4% of maxillary central incisors.[11]

Enamel projections were described in the 19th century.[16] They extend into the furcation of 28.6% of mandibular molars and 17% of maxillary molars[12] and may favor the development of a pocket.[22] Enamel pearls are less frequent (1.1% to 5.7% of permanent molars; 75% of them appear in maxillary third molars).[17] An intermediate bifurcation ridge has been described in 73% of mandibular first molars,

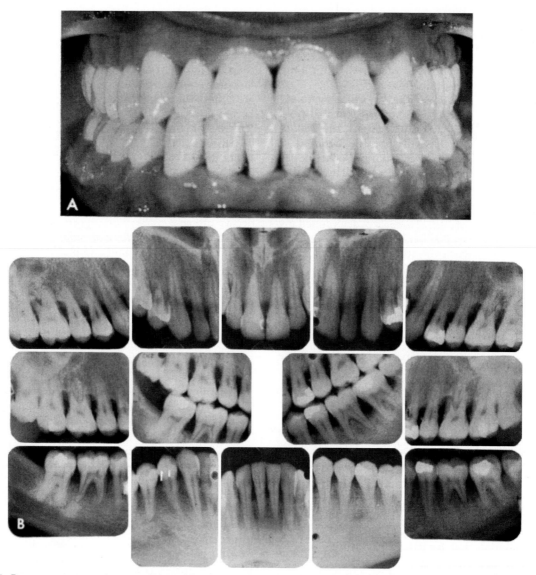

FIGURE 31–5. Poor crown:root ratio, overall prognosis unfavorable. *A,* A 24-year-old patient with generalized gingivitis and periodontal pocket formation. *B,* Severe bone destruction. The contrast between the well-formed crowns and the relatively short, tapered roots worsens the unfavorable prognosis.

crossing from the mesial to the distal root at the midpoint of the bifurcation.[5] These enamel surfaces interfere and prevent regenerative procedures from achieving their maximum potential.

Teeth Adjacent to Edentulous Areas. Teeth that serve as abutments are subjected to increased functional demands. More rigid standards are required when evaluating the prognosis of teeth adjacent to edentulous areas. Also, special oral hygiene measures must be instituted in these areas.

Location of Remaining Bone in Relation to the Individual Tooth Surfaces. When greater bone loss has occurred on one surface of a tooth, the bone height on the less involved surfaces should be taken into consideration when determining the prognosis. Because of the greater height of bone in relation to other surfaces,

the center of rotation of the tooth will be nearer the crown (Fig. 31–10). This will result in a more favorable distribution of forces to the periodontium and less tooth mobility.[21]

Relation to Adjacent Teeth. In dealing with a tooth with a questionable prognosis, the chances of successful treatment should be weighed against any benefits that would accrue to the adjacent teeth if the tooth under consideration were extracted. *Heroic attempts to retain a hopelessly involved tooth may jeopardize the adjacent teeth.* Extraction of the questionable tooth may be followed by partial restoration of the bone support of the adjacent teeth (Fig. 31–11).

Caries, Nonvital Teeth, and Tooth Resorption. In teeth mutilated by extensive caries, the feasibility of adequate restoration and endodontic therapy should be considered

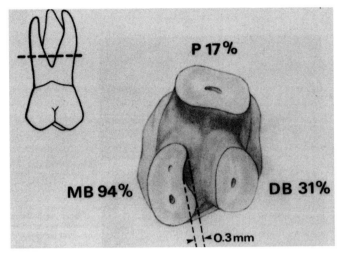

FIGURE 31–6. Root concavities in maxillary first molars sectioned 2 mm apical to the furca. The furcal aspect of the root is concave in 94% of the mesiobuccal (MB) roots, 31% of the distobuccal (DB) roots, and 17% of the palatal (P) roots. The deepest concavity is found in the furcal aspects of the mesiobuccal root (mean concavity, 0.3 mm). The furcal aspect of the buccal roots diverges toward the palate in 97% of teeth (mean divergence, 22 degrees). (Data from Bower RC. Furcation morphology relative to periodontal treatment—furcation root surface anatomy. J Periodontol *50:*366, 1979.)

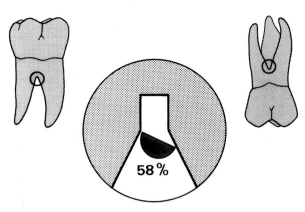

FIGURE 31–8. The furcation entrance is narrower than a standard curette in 58% of first molars. (Data from Bower RC. Furcation morphology relative to periodontal treatment—furcation root surface anatomy. J Periodontol *50:*366, 1979.)

before undertaking periodontal treatment. Extensive idiopathic root resorption jeopardizes the stability of teeth and adversely affects the response to periodontal treatment. The periodontal prognosis of treated nonvital teeth is not different from that of vital teeth. New attachment can occur to the cementum in both nonvital and vital teeth. However, new attachment to exposed root dentin is not likely in nonvital teeth.[15]

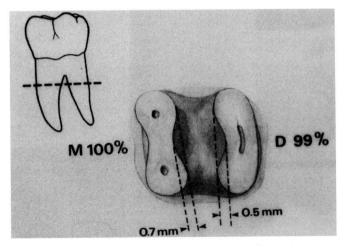

FIGURE 31–7. Root concavities in mandibular first molars sectioned 2 mm apical to the furca. Concavity of the furcal aspect was found in 100% of mesial (M) roots and 99% of distal (D) roots. Deeper concavity was found in the mesial roots (mean concavity, 0.7 mm). (Data from Bower RC. Furcation morphology relative to periodontal treatment—furcation root surface anatomy. J Periodontol *50:*366, 1979.)

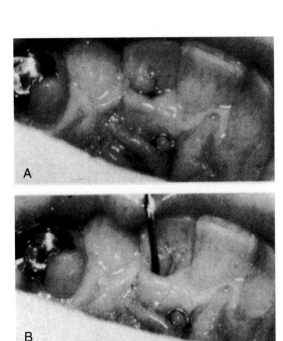

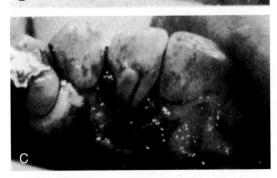

FIGURE 31–9. Palatogingival groove. *A,* Gingival inflammation and exudate in an area palatal to the upper lateral incisor. *B,* Probing shows deep pocket. *C,* The area is flapped, and the presence of a palatogingival groove is confirmed. (Courtesy of Dr. Robert Merin.)

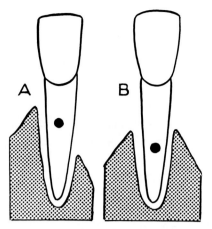

FIGURE 31–10. The prognosis for tooth A is better than that for tooth B, despite the fact that there is less bone on one of the surfaces of A. Because the center of rotation of tooth A is closer to the crown, the distribution of occlusal forces to the periodontium is more favorable than in B.

CLINICAL APPLICATION

The factors to be considered when determining the prognosis of the overall dentition and of the individual teeth have been presented in this chapter. Careful analysis of these factors will allow the clinician in most cases to establish one of the following prognoses:[13]

Excellent prognosis: No bone loss, excellent gingival condition, adequate patient cooperation.

Good prognosis: One or more of the following: adequate remaining bone support; adequate possibilities to control etiologic factors and establish a maintainable dentition; adequate patient cooperation.

Fair prognosis: One or more of the following: less than adequate remaining bone support, some tooth mobility, grade I furcation involvement, adequate maintenance possible, acceptable patient cooperation.

Poor prognosis: One or more of the following: moderate to advanced bone loss, tooth mobility, grade I and II furcation involvements, difficult-to-maintain areas and/or doubtful patient compliance.

Questionable prognosis: One or more of the following: advanced bone loss, grade II and III furcation involvements, tooth mobility, inaccessible areas.

Hopeless prognosis: One or more of the following: advanced bone loss, nonmaintainable areas, extraction(s) indicated.

It should be recognized that excellent, good, and hopeless prognoses are the only prognoses that can be established with a reasonable degree of accuracy. Fair, poor, and even questionable prognoses depend on a large number of factors that can interact in an unpredictable number of ways.[3,4,20] In many of these cases, it may be advisable to establish a *provisional prognosis* until Phase I therapy is completed and evaluated.

The provisional prognosis will allow the clinician to initiate treatment of teeth that have a doubtful outlook in the hope that a very favorable response may tip the balance and allow the tooth to be retained. The re-evaluation step in the treatment sequence allows the clinician to examine the tissue response to scaling and root planing and to the use of any antibacterial agents that may be indicated. The patient's compliance with plaque control measures also can be determined.

A frank reduction in pocket depth and inflammation after Phase I therapy points to a favorable response to treatment and may suggest a better prognosis than previously assumed. If the inflammatory changes present cannot be controlled or reduced by Phase I therapy, the overall prognosis will be unfavorable.

It should also be remembered that progression of periodontitis generally occurs in an episodic manner, alternating periods of quiescence with shorter destructive stages (see Chapter 30). There are no methods available at present to accurately determine whether a given lesion is in a stage of remission or exacerbation.

Advanced lesions, if active, may progress rapidly to a hopeless stage, whereas similar lesions in a quiescent stage may be maintainable for long periods. Phase I therapy will, at least temporarily, transform an active lesion into an inactive one. This is another reason to establish a provisional diagnosis to be reanalyzed after completion of Phase I.

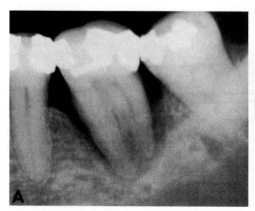
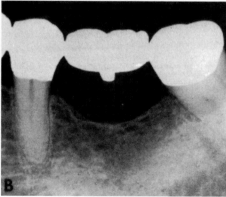

FIGURE 31–11. Extraction of severely involved tooth to preserve bone on adjacent teeth. *A,* Extensive bone destruction around the mandibular first molar. *B,* Radiograph made 8½ years after extraction of the first molar and replacement by a prosthesis. Note the excellent bony support.

REFERENCES

1. Bower RC. Furcation morphology relative to periodontal treatment—furcation entrance architecture. J Periodontol 50:23, 1979.
2. Bower RC. Furcation morphology relative to periodontal treatment—furcation root surface anatomy. J Periodontol 50:366, 1979.
3. Chace R Sr, Low SB. Survival characteristics of periodontally-involved teeth: A 40-year study. J Periodontol 64:701, 1993.
4. Dodson SA, Takei HH, Carranza FA Jr. Significant supracrestal bony repair of a periodontal defect. Report of a case. Submitted for publication, 1994.
5. Everett FG, Jump EB, Holder TD, Williams GC. The intermediate bifurcational ridge: A study of the morphology of the bifurcation of the lower first molar. J Dent Res 37:162, 1958.
6. Everett FG, Kramer GN. The distolingual groove in the maxillary lateral incisor, a periodontal hazard. J Periodontol 43:352, 1972.
7. Fleszar TJ, Knowles JW, Morrison EC, et al. Tooth mobility and periodontal therapy. J Clin Periodontol 7:495, 1980.
8. Fox SC, Bosworth BL. A morphological study of proximal root concavities: A consideration in periodontal therapy. J Am Dent Assoc 114:811, 1987.
9. Gher ME, Vernino AR. Root morphology—clinical significance in pathogenesis and treatment of periodontal disease. J Am Dent Assoc 101:627, 1980.
10. Kay S, Forscher BK, Sackett LM. Tooth root length-volume relationships. An aid to periodontal prognosis. I. Anterior teeth. Oral Surg 7:735, 1954.
11. Kogan SL. The prevalence, location and conformation of palato-radicular grooves in maxillary incisors. J Periodontol 57:2312, 1986.
12. Masters DH, Hoskins SWP. Projection of cervical enamel into molar furcations. J Periodontol 35:49, 1964.
13. McGuire MK. Prognosis versus actual outcome: A long-term survey of 100 treated periodontal patients under maintenance care. J Periodontol 62:51, 1991.
14. Morris ML. The diagnosis, prognosis and treatment of loose tooth. Oral Surg 6:1037, 1953.
15. Morris ML. Healing of human periodontal tissues following surgical detachment and extirpation of vital pulps. J Periodontol 31:23, 1960.
16. Moskow BS, Martinez Canut P. Studies on root enamel. 1. Some historical notes on cervical enamel projections. J Clin Periodontol 17:29, 1990.
17. Moskow BS, Martinez Canut P. Studies on root enamel. 2. Enamel pearls. A review of their morphology, localization, nomenclature, occurrence, classification, histogenesis and incidence. J Clin Periodontol 17:275, 1990.
18. Palcanis KG, Wolfe B, McClung JF, Elzay RP. Rapidly progressive periodontitis, report of a case. J Periodontol 57:378, 1986.
19. Rosling B, Nyman S, Lindhe J. The effect of systematic plaque control on bone regeneration in infrabony pockets. J Clin Periodontol 3:38, 1976.
20. Shapiro N. Retaining periodontally "hopeless" teeth. A case report. J Am Dent Assoc 125:596, 1994.
21. Sorrin S, Burman LR. A study of cases not amenable to periodontal therapy. J Am Dent Assoc 31:204, 1944.
22. Watson AE, Woods EC. Some irregularities of the enamel margin observed in human molars. Br Dent J 48:854, 1926.
23. Withers JA, Brunsvold MA, Killoy WJ, Rahe AJ. The relationship of palato-gingival grooves to localized periodontal disease. J Periodontol 52:41, 1981.

32

The Treatment Plan

FERMIN A. CARRANZA, JR.

**Master Plan for Total Treatment
Sequence of Therapeutic Procedures
Explaining the Treatment Plan to the Patient**

After the diagnosis and prognosis have been established, the treatment is planned. *The treatment plan is the blueprint for case management.* It includes all procedures required for the establishment and maintenance of oral health, such as decisions regarding teeth to be retained or extracted and decisions on techniques to be used for pocket therapy, the need for mucogingival or reconstructive surgical procedures and occlusal correction, the type of restorations to be employed, and which teeth are to be used for abutments.

Unforeseen developments during treatment may necessitate modification of the initial treatment plan. However, *except for emergencies, no treatment should be started until the treatment plan has been established.*

Periodontal treatment requires long-range planning. Its value to the patient is measured in years of healthful functioning of the entire dentition, not by the number of teeth retained at the time of treatment. It is directed toward establishing and maintaining the health of the periodontium throughout the mouth rather than to spectacular efforts to "tighten loose teeth."

The welfare of the dentition should not be jeopardized by a heroic attempt to retain questionable teeth. *The peri-odontal condition of the teeth that are retained is more important than the number of such teeth.* Teeth that can be retained with minimal doubt and a maximal margin of safety provide the basis for the total treatment plan. Teeth on the borderline of hopelessness do not contribute to the overall usefulness of the dentition, even if they can be saved in a somewhat precarious state. Such teeth become sources of recurrent annoyance to the patient and detract from the value of the greater service rendered by the establishment of periodontal health in the remainder of the oral cavity.

MASTER PLAN FOR TOTAL TREATMENT

The aim of the treatment plan is total treatment—that is, coordination of all treatment procedures for the purpose of creating a well-functioning dentition in a healthy periodontal environment. The master plan of periodontal treatment encompasses different therapeutic objectives for each patient according to his or her needs. It is based on the diagnosis, disease severity, and other factors outlined in Chapter

33 and should include a reasoned decision on the techniques to be used for treatment.

The primary goal is elimination of gingival inflammation and correction of the conditions that cause and/or perpetuate it. This will include not only elimination of root irritants, but also pocket elimination and establishment of gingival contour and mucogingival relationships conducive to the preservation of periodontal health; restoration of carious areas; and correction of existing restorations. Consideration of occlusal relationships may be in order and may necessitate occlusal adjustment; restorative, prosthetic, and orthodontic procedures; splinting; and correction of bruxism and clamping and clenching habits.

Systemic conditions should be carefully evaluated, as they may require special precautions during the course of periodontal treatment and may also affect the tissue response to treatment procedures or threaten the preservation of periodontal health after treatment is completed. Such situations should be taken care of in conjunction with the patient's physician.

Supportive periodontal care is also of paramount importance for case maintenance. Such care entails all procedures for maintaining periodontal health after it has been attained. It consists of instruction in oral hygiene and checkups at regular intervals according to the patient's needs to examine the condition of the periodontium and the status of the restoration as it affects the periodontium.

SEQUENCE OF THERAPEUTIC PROCEDURES

Periodontal therapy is an inseparable part of dental therapy. The sequence of procedures presented here includes periodontal procedures (in italics) and other procedures not considered to be within the province of the periodontist.

Preliminary phase
    Treatment of emergencies
        Dental or periapical
        Periodontal
        Other
    Extraction of hopeless teeth and provisional replacement if needed (may be postponed to a more convenient time)
Phase I therapy (etiotropic phase)
    Plaque control
    Diet control (in patients with rampant caries)
    Removal of calculus and root planing
    Correction of restorative and prosthetic irritational factors
    Excavation of caries and restoration (temporary or final, depending on whether a definitive prognosis for the tooth has been arrived at and on the location of caries)
    Antimicrobial therapy (local or systemic)
    Occlusal therapy
    Minor orthodontic movement
    Provisional splinting
Evaluation of response to phase I
    Rechecking
        Pocket depth and gingival inflammation
        Plaque and calculus caries
Phase II therapy (surgical phase)
    Periodontal surgery, including placement of implants
    Root canal therapy
Phase III therapy (restorative phase)
    Final restorations
    Fixed and removable prosthodontics

Evaluation of response to restorative procedures
    Periodontal examination
Phase IV therapy (maintenance phase)
    Periodic recall visits, checking
        Plaque and calculus
        Gingival condition (pockets, inflammation)
        Occlusion, tooth mobility
        Other pathologic changes

EXPLAINING THE TREATMENT PLAN TO THE PATIENT

The following are suggestions for explaining the treatment plan to the patient:

Be specific. Tell the patient, "You have gingivitis," or "You have periodontitis." Then explain exactly what these conditions are, how they are treated, and the future for the patient's mouth after treatment. Avoid vague statements such as, "You have trouble with your gums," or "Something should be done about your gums." Patients do not understand the significance of such statements and disregard them.

Start your discussion on a positive note. Talk about the teeth that can be retained and the long-term service they can be expected to render. Do not start your discussion with the statement: "The following teeth have to be extracted." This creates a negative impression, which adds to the erroneous attitude of hopelessness the patient already may have regarding his or her mouth. Make it clear that every effort will be made to retain as many teeth as possible, but do not dwell on the patient's loose teeth. Emphasize that the important purpose of the treatment is to prevent other teeth from becoming as severely diseased as the loose teeth.

Present the entire treatment plan as a unit. Avoid creating the impression that treatment consists of separate procedures, some or all of which may be selected by the patient. Make it clear that dental restorations and prostheses contribute as much to the health of the gums as elimination of inflammation and periodontal pockets. Do not speak in terms of "having the gums treated and then taking care of the necessary restorations later" as if these were unrelated treatments.

Patients frequently seek guidance from the dentist with such questions as: "Are my teeth worth treating?" "Would you have them treated if you were I?" "Why don't I just go along the way I am until the teeth really bother me, and then have them all extracted?"

If the condition is treatable, make it clear that the best results are obtained by prompt treatment. If the condition is not treatable, the teeth should be extracted. Explain that "doing nothing" or holding onto hopelessly diseased teeth as long as possible is inadvisable for the following reasons:

In periodontal disease, proper mastication of food is impaired because of looseness of the teeth and the discomfort incurred by chewing. This leads to "bolting" of food, which complicates the digestive process and may cause gastrointestinal disturbances. Inability to chew properly leads to food selectivity, with a preference for soft foods, primarily carbohydrates.

Exudate from periodontal pockets spoils the taste of food. In addition, the incorporation of purulent material into the food may irritate the mucosa of the stomach and lead to gastritis. Also, infection in the periodontal area is a potential source of bacteremia.

- It is not feasible to place restorations or bridges on teeth with untreated periodontal disease, because the usefulness of the restoration is limited by the uncertain condition of the supporting structures.
- Failure to eliminate periodontal disease not only results in the loss of teeth that are already involved, but also shortens the life span of other teeth that, with proper treatment, could serve as the foundation for a healthy, functioning dentition.

It is the dentist's responsibility to advise the patient of the importance of periodontal treatment. However, if treatment is to be successful, the patient must be sufficiently interested in retaining the natural teeth to maintain the necessary oral hygiene. Individuals who are not particularly perturbed by the thought of losing their teeth are generally not good candidates for periodontal treatment.

33

Rationale for Periodontal Treatment

FERMIN A. CARRANZA, JR.

What Does Periodontal Therapy Accomplish?
Factors That Affect Healing
Healing After Periodontal Therapy

Regeneration
Repair
New Attachment

WHAT DOES PERIODONTAL THERAPY ACCOMPLISH?*

The effectiveness of periodontal therapy is made possible by the remarkable healing capacity of the periodontal tissues (Fig. 33–1). Periodontal therapy can restore chronically inflamed gingiva such that, from a clinical and structural point of view, it is almost identical with gingiva that has never been exposed to excessive plaque accumulation.[21]

Properly performed, periodontal treatment can be relied on to eliminate pain, eliminate gingival inflammation[29] and gingival bleeding, reduce periodontal pockets and eliminate infection, stop pus formation, arrest the destruction of soft tissue and bone,[30] reduce abnormal tooth mobility,[7] establish optimal occlusal function, restore tissue destroyed by disease (in some instances), re-establish the physiologic gingival contour necessary for the preservation of periodontal health, prevent the recurrence of disease, and reduce tooth loss (Fig. 33–2).[25]

Local Therapy. The cause of periodontitis and gingivitis is bacterial plaque accumulation on the tooth surface in close proximity to the gingival tissue. Plaque accumulation can be favored by a variety of local factors, such as calculus, overhanging margins of restorations, and food impaction. *The removal of plaque and all the factors that favor its accumulation is the primary consideration in local therapy.*

Abnormal forces on the tooth increase tooth mobility. The thorough elimination of plaque and the prevention of new plaque formation, by themselves, are sufficient to maintain periodontal health, even if traumatic forces are allowed to persist.[19,20] However, the elimination of trauma may increase the chances of bone regeneration and gain of attachment.[15] Although this point is not widely accepted,[26] it appears that creating occlusal relations that are more favorable to the periodontal tissues increases the tolerance of the periodontium to minor buildups of plaque, in addition to reducing tooth mobility. It should be remembered that total plaque elimination as obtained in experimental studies may not be possible in all human subjects.

Systemic Therapy. Systemic therapy may be employed as an adjunct to local measures and for specific purposes, such as the control of systemic complications from acute infections, chemotherapy to prevent harmful effects of post-treatment bacteremia, supportive nutritional therapy, and the control of systemic diseases that aggravate the patient's periodontal condition or necessitate special precautions during treatment (see Chapter 34).

Systemic therapy for treatment of the periodontal condition and in conjunction with local therapy is indicated in localized juvenile periodontitis and rapidly progressive periodontitis. In these diseases, systemic antibiotics are used to completely eliminate the bacteria that invade the gingival tissues and can repopulate the pocket after scaling and root planing (see Chapters 44 and 45).

In addition, periodontal manifestations of systemic diseases (see Chapters 10, 14 and 20) are treated primarily by

---

* See Chapter 69 for a more detailed consideration of this topic.

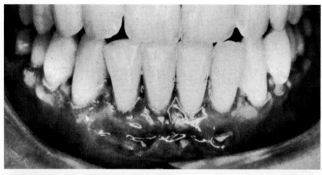

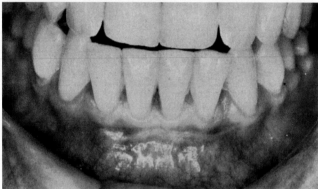

FIGURE 33–1. Excellent healing capacity of the periodontium. *Top,* One week following periodontal surgery, after removal of periodontal dressing. *Bottom,* Result after 7 months, showing healed tissues and restoration of physiologic gingival contour.

methods other than local measures. However, local therapy may still be indicated to reduce or prevent complications of gingival inflammation.

Evidence has been presented that some *nonsteroidal anti-inflammatory drugs* such as flurbiprofen and ibuprofen can slow the development of experimental gingivitis[9] as well as the loss of alveolar bone in periodontitis.[11,36–38] These drugs are propionic acid derivatives and act by inhibiting the cyclooxygenase pathway of arachidonic acid metabolism, thereby reducing prostaglandin formation; they can be administered by mouth[13] or applied topically.[36] This type of therapy is still in experimental stages, and protocols for its clinical use have not been established. However, it shows that future treatment modalities may attempt not only to control the bacterial cause of the disease, but also to suppress the self-destructive components of the host inflammatory response. (For a review on this topic, see Howell and Williams.[11])

Another drug that has a strong inhibitory effect on bone resorption is alendronate, a bisphosphonate that is currently used in humans to treat metabolic diseases (e.g., Paget's disease or hypercalcemia of malignancy) that result in bone resorption. Experimental studies in monkeys have shown that alendronate reduced the bone loss associated with periodontitis.[3,35]

FACTORS THAT AFFECT HEALING

In the periodontium, as elsewhere in the body, healing is affected by local and systemic factors.

Local Factors. Systemic conditions that impair healing may reduce the effectiveness of local periodontal treatment and should be corrected before or during local therapy. However, local factors, particularly plaque microorganisms, are the most common deterrents to healing after periodontal treatment.

Healing is also delayed by excessive tissue manipulation during treatment, trauma to the tissues, the presence of foreign bodies, and repetitive treatment procedures that disrupt the orderly cellular activity in the healing process. An adequate blood supply is needed for the increased cellular activity during healing; if this is impaired or insufficient, areas of necrosis will develop and delay the healing process.

Healing is improved by debridement (the removal of degenerated and necrotic tissue), immobilization of the healing area, and pressure on the wound. The cellular activity in healing entails an increase in oxygen consumption, but healing of the gingiva is not accelerated by artificially increasing the oxygen supply beyond normal requirements.[8]

Systemic Factors. The effects of systemic conditions on healing have been extensively documented in animal experiments but are less clearly defined in humans. Healing capacity diminishes with age,[4,10] probably because of atherosclerotic vascular changes, which are common in aging and result in a reduction in blood circulation. Healing is delayed in patients with generalized infections and in those with diabetes and other debilitating diseases.

Healing is retarded by insufficient food intake; by conditions that interfere with the utilization of nutrients; and by deficiencies in vitamin C,[1,34] proteins,[32] and other nutrients. However, the nutrient requirements of the healing tissues in minor wounds, such as those created by periodontal surgical procedures, are ordinarily satisfied by a well-balanced diet.

Healing is also affected by hormones. Systemically administered glucocorticoids such as cortisone hinder repair by depressing the inflammatory reaction or inhibiting the growth of fibroblasts, the production of collagen, and the formation of endothelial cells. Systemic stress,[31] thyroidectomy, testosterone, adrenocorticotropic hormone (ACTH), and large doses of estrogen suppress the formation of granulation tissue and retard healing.[4] Progesterone increases and accelerates the vascularization of immature granulation tissue[18] and appears to increase the susceptibility of the gingiva to mechanical injury by causing dilation of the marginal vessels.[12]

HEALING AFTER PERIODONTAL THERAPY

The basic healing processes—removal of degenerated tissue debris and replacement of tissues destroyed by disease—are the same after all forms of periodontal therapy. Regeneration, repair, and new attachment are aspects of periodontal healing that have a special bearing on the results obtainable by treatment.

Regeneration

Regeneration is the growth and differentiation of new cells and intercellular substances to form new tissues or parts. Regeneration takes place by growth from the same

RESPONSE TO PERIODONTAL TREATMENT

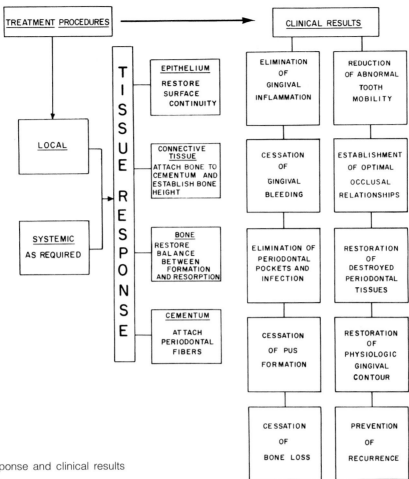

FIGURE 33–2. Tissue response and clinical results after periodontal treatment.

type of tissue that has been destroyed or from its precursor. In the periodontium, gingival epithelium is replaced by epithelium, and the underlying connective tissue and periodontal ligament are derived from connective tissue. Bone and cementum are replaced not by existing bone or cementum but by connective tissue, which is the precursor of both. Undifferentiated connective tissue cells develop into osteoblasts and cementoblasts, which form bone and cementum.

Regeneration of the periodontium is a continuous physiologic process. Under normal conditions new cells and tissues are constantly being formed to replace those that mature and die. This is termed *wear-and-tear repair.*[16] It is manifested by mitotic activity in the epithelium of the gingiva and the connective tissue of the periodontal ligament, by the formation of new bone, and by the continuous deposition of cementum.

Regeneration is also going on during destructive periodontal disease. Most gingival and periodontal diseases are chronic inflammatory conditions and, as such, are healing processes. Regeneration is part of the healing. However, bacteria and bacterial products that perpetuate the disease process and the inflammatory exudate they elicit are injurious to the regenerating cells and tissues and prevent the healing from proceeding to completion.

By removing bacterial plaque and creating the conditions to prevent its new formation, periodontal treatment removes the obstacles to regeneration and enables the patient to benefit from the inherent regenerative capacity of the tissues. There is a brief spurt in regenerative activity immediately after periodontal treatment, but there are no local treatment procedures that promote or accelerate regeneration.

Repair

Repair simply restores the continuity of the diseased marginal gingiva and re-establishes a normal gingival sulcus at the same level on the root as the base of the pre-existing periodontal pocket (Fig. 33–3). This process, called *healing by scar,*[28] arrests bone destruction without necessarily increasing bone height. Restoration of the destroyed periodontium involves mobilization of epithelial and connective tissue cells into the damaged area and increased local mitotic divisions to provide a sufficient number of cells.

New Attachment

New attachment is the embedding of new periodontal ligament fibers into new cementum and attachment of the gingival epithelium to a tooth surface previously denuded by

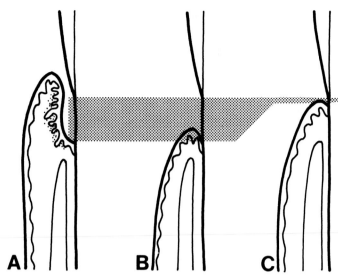

FIGURE 33–3. Two possible outcomes of pocket elimination. *A*, Periodontal pocket before treatment. *B*, Normal sulcus re-established at the level of the base of the pocket. *C*, Periodontium restored on the root surface previously denuded by disease. This is called *new attachment.* Shaded areas show denudation caused by periodontal disease.

disease (see Fig. 33–3). The critical phrase in this definition is "tooth surface previously denuded by disease" (Fig. 33–4). Attachment of the gingiva or the periodontal ligament to areas of the tooth from which it may have been removed in the course of treatment or during the preparation

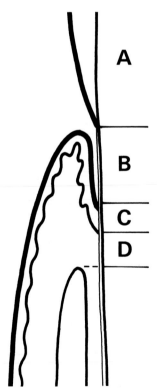

FIGURE 33–4. Zone A, Enamel surface. Zone B, Area of cementum denuded by pocket formation. Zone C, Area of cementum covered by junctional epithelium. Zone D, Area of cementum apical to the junctional epithelium. The term *new attachment* refers to a new junctional epithelium and attached connective tissue fibers formed on zone B.

of teeth for restorations represents *simple healing* or *reattachment* of the periodontium, not new attachment.[14] The term *reattachment* was used in the past to refer to the restoration of the marginal periodontium, but because it is not the existing fibers that reattach but new fibers that are formed and attach to new cementum, the term has been replaced by the term *new attachment.* Reattachment is currently used only to refer to repair in areas of the root not previously exposed to the pocket, such as after surgical detachment of the tissues or after traumatic tears in the cementum, tooth fractures, or treatment of periapical lesions.

Epithelial adaptation differs from new attachment in that it is the close apposition of the gingival epithelium to the tooth surface without complete obliteration of the pocket. The pocket space does not permit passage of a probe (Fig. 33–5). Studies have shown that these deep sulci lined with long, thin epithelium may be as resistant to disease as true connective tissue attachments.[2,22] The absence of bleeding or secretion on probing, the absence of clinically visible inflammation, and the absence of stainable plaque on the root surface when the pocket wall is deflected from the tooth may indicate that the "deep sulcus" persists in an inactive state, causing no further loss of attachment.[5,40] A post-therapy depth of 4 or even 5 mm may be acceptable in these cases.

New attachment and osseous regeneration have been a constant but elusive goal of periodontal therapy for more than a century.[6,17,27,39] Since the 1970s, renewed laboratory and clinical research efforts have resulted in new concepts and techniques that have moved us much closer to attaining this ideal result of therapy. Chapter 57 presents the recommended methods of treatment and their indications and accomplishments.

Melcher pointed out that regeneration of the periodontal ligament is the key to new attachment, because it "provides continuity between the alveolar bone and the cementum and also because it contains cells that can synthesize and remodel the three connective tissues of the alveolar part of the periodontium."[23]

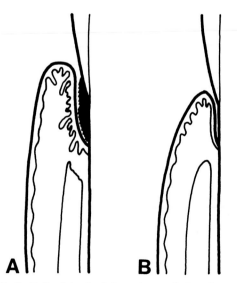

FIGURE 33–5. Epithelial adaptation after periodontal treatment. *A*, Periodontal pocket. *B*, After treatment. The pocket is closely adapted to but not attached to the root.

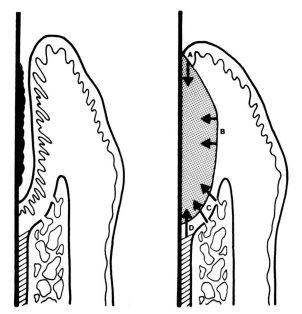

FIGURE 33–6. Sources of regenerating cells in the healing stages of a periodontal pocket. *Left,* Infrabony pocket. *Right,* After therapy, the clot formed is invaded (*arrows*) by cells from the marginal epithelium (A), the gingival connective tissue (B), the bone marrow (C), and the periodontal ligament (D).

During the healing stages of a periodontal pocket, the area is invaded by cells from four different sources (Fig. 33–6): oral epithelium, gingival connective tissue, bone, and periodontal ligament.

The final outcome of periodontal pocket healing depends on the sequence of events during the healing stages.[23] If the epithelium proliferates along the tooth surface before the other tissues reach the area, the result will be a long junctional epithelium. If the cells from the gingival connective tissue are the first to populate the area, the result will be fibers parallel to the tooth surface and remodeling of the alveolar bone, with no attachment to the cementum. If bone cells arrive first, root resorption and ankylosis may occur. Finally, only when cells from the periodontal ligament proliferate coronally is there new formation of cementum and periodontal ligament.[23]

REFERENCES

1. Barr CE. Oral healing in ascorbic acid deficiency. Periodontics *3*:286, 1965.
2. Beaumont RH, O'Leary TJ, Kafrawy AH. Relative resistance of long junctional epithelial adhesions and connective tissue attachments to plaque-induced inflammation. J Periodontol *55*:213, 1984.
3. Brunsvold MA, Chaves ES, Kornman KS, et al. Effects of a bisphosphonate on experimental periodontitis in monkeys. J Periodontol *63*:825, 1992.
4. Butcher EO, Klingsberg J. Age, gonadectomy, and wound healing in the palatal mucosa. J Dent Res *40*:694, 1961.
5. Caffesse RG, Ramfjord SP, Nasjleti CE. Reverse bevel periodontal flaps in monkeys. J Periodontol *39*:219, 1968.
6. Carranza FA Sr. A technique for treating infrabony pockets so as to obtain reattachment. Dent Clin North Am *4*:75, 1960.
7. Ferris RT. Quantitative evaluation of tooth mobility following initial periodontal therapy. J Periodontal *37*:190, 1966.
8. Glickman I, Turesky SS, Manhold J. The oxygen consumption of healing gingiva. J Dent Res *29*:429, 1950.
9. Heasman PA, Seymour RA. The effect of a systemically-administered non-steroidal anti-inflammatory drug (flurbiprofen) on experimental gingivitis in humans. J Clin Periodontol *16*:551, 1989.
10. Holm-Pedersen P, Löe H. Wound healing in the gingiva of young and old individuals. Scand J Dent Res *79*:40, 1971.
11. Howell TH, Williams RC. Nonsteroidal antiinflammatory drugs as inhibitors of periodontal disease progression. Crit Rev Oral Biol Med *4*:177, 1993.
12. Hugoson A. Gingival inflammation and female sex hormones. J Periodont Res Suppl *5*:1, 1970.
13. Jeffcoat MK, Williams RC, Reddy MS, et al. Flurbiprofen treatment of human periodontitis: Effect on alveolar bone height and metabolism. J Periodont Res *23*:381, 1988.
14. Kalkwarf KL. Periodontal new attachment without the placement of osseous potentiating grafts. Periodont Abstr *22*:53, 1974.
15. Kantor M, Polson AM, Zander HA. Alveolar bone regeneration after removal of inflammatory and traumatic factors. J Periodontol *47*:687, 1976.
16. Leblond CP, Walker BE. Renewal of cell populations. Physiol Rev *36*:255, 1956.
17. Leonard HJ. In our opinion—reattachment. J Periodontol 14 (suppl):5, 1943.
18. Lindhe J, Brånemark PI. The effect of sex hormones on vascularization of a granulation tissue. J Periodont Res *3*:6, 1968.
19. Lindhe J, Ericsson I. The influence of trauma from occlusion on reduced but healthy periodontal tissues in dogs. J Clin Periodontol *3*:110, 1976.
20. Lindhe J, Nyman S. The effect of plaque control and surgical pocket elimination on the establishment and maintenance of periodontal health. A longitudinal study of periodontal therapy in cases of advanced periodontal disease. J Clin Periodontol 2:67, 1975.
21. Lindhe J, Parodi R, Liljenberg B, Fornell J. Clinical and structural alterations characterizing healing gingiva. J Periodont Res *13*:410, 1978.
22. Magnusson I, Runstad L, Nyman S, Lindhe J. A long junctional epithelium—a locus minoris resistentiae in plaque infection? J Clin Periodontol *10*:33, 1983.
23. Melcher AH. On the repair potential of periodontal tissues. J Periodontol *47*:256, 1976.
24. Nyman S, Lindhe J, Karring T. Reattachment—new attachment. In Lindhe J, ed. Textbook of Clinical Periodontology. Philadelphia, WB Saunders, 1983.
25. Oliver RC. Tooth loss with and without periodontal therapy. Periodont Abstr *17*:8, 1969.
26. Polson AM. Interrelationship of inflammation and tooth mobility (trauma) in pathogenesis of periodontal disease. J Clin Periodontol *7*:351, 1980.
27. Prichard J. The infrabony technique as a predictable procedure. J Periodontol *28*:202, 1957.
28. Ratcliff PA. An analysis of repair systems in periodontal therapy. Periodont Abstr *14*:57, 1966.
29. Rateitschak K. The therapeutic effect of local treatment on periodontal disease assessed upon evaluation of different diagnostic criteria. 2. Changes in gingival inflammation. J Periodontol *35*:155, 1964.
30. Rateitschak K, Engelberger A, Marthaler TM. The therapeutic effect of local treatment on periodontal disease assessed upon evaluation of different diagnostic criteria. 3. Radiographic changes in appearance of bone. J Periodontol *35*:263, 1964.
31. Stahl SS. Healing gingival injury in normal and systemically stressed young adult male rats. J Periodontol *32*:63, 1961.
32. Stahl SS. The effect of a protein-free diet on the healing of gingival wounds in rats. Arch Oral Biol *7*:551, 1962.
33. Stahl SS. Healing of gingival tissues following various therapeutic regimens—review of histologic studies. J Oral Ther Pharmacol 2:145, 1965.
34. Turesky SS, Glickman I. Histochemical evaluation of gingival healing in experimental animals on adequate and vitamin C deficient diets. J Dent Res *33*:273, 1954.
35. Weinreb M, Quartuccio H, Seedor JG, et al. Histomorphometrical analysis of the effects of the bisphosphonate alendronate on bone loss caused by experimental periodontitis in monkeys. J Periodont Res *29*:35, 1994.
36. Williams RC, Jeffcoat MK, Howell TH, et al. Topical flurbiprofen treatment of periodontitis in beagles. J Periodont Res *23*:166, 1988.
37. Williams RC, Jeffcoat MK, Howell H, et al. Altering the progression of human alveolar bone loss with the non-steroidal anti-inflammatory drug flurbiprofen. J Periodontol *60*:485, 1989.
38. Williams RC, Jeffcoat MK, Kaplan ML, et al. Flurbiprofen: A potent inhibitor of alveolar bone resorption in beagles. Science *227*:640, 1985.
39. Younger W. Pyorrhea alveolaris, from a bacteriological standpoint, with a report of some investigations and remarks on treatment. Int Dent J *20*:413, 1899.
40. Yukna RA. A clinical and histologic study of healing following the excisional new attachment procedure in rhesus monkeys. J Periodontol *47*:701, 1976.

34

Periodontal Treatment of Medically Compromised Patients

JOAN OTOMO-CORGEL

Cardiovascular Diseases
Angina Pectoris
Previous Cardiac Bypass or Myocardial Infarction
Previous Cerebrovascular Accident
Congestive Heart Failure
Hypertension
Presence of Cardiac Pacemakers
Infective Endocarditis
Renal Diseases
Pulmonary Diseases
Immunosuppression and Chemotherapy
Radiation Therapy
Endocrine Disorders
Diabetes
Thyroid Disorders

Parathyroid Disorders
Adrenal Insufficiency
Pregnancy
Hemorrhagic Disorders
Coagulation Disorders
Thrombocytopenic Purpuras
Nonthrombocytopenic Purpuras
Blood Dyscrasias
Leukemia
Agranulocytosis
Infectious Diseases
Hepatitis
Sexually Transmitted Diseases
AIDS
Tuberculosis

Improvements in lifestyles, habits, and medical care have enhanced human longevity. They have also led to the creation of a population with chronic health problems that may require special precautions in dental therapy. The older age of the average periodontal patient increases the likelihood of underlying disease. Therefore, the therapeutic responsibility of the clinician includes identification of the patient's medical problems to formulate proper treatment plans.

Thorough medical histories are paramount. If significant findings are unveiled, consultation with or referral of the patient to an appropriate physician is required. Not only is the patient correctly managed, but also the clinician is covered medicolegally.

This chapter deals with some common medical problems and associated periodontal management. Understanding these problems will enable the clinician to treat the total patient, not merely the periodontal reflection of underlying disease. Because the coverage of the subject in this discussion is necessarily very general, the reader is urged to consult other texts regarding specific diseases.

CARDIOVASCULAR DISEASES

Health histories should be closely scrutinized for cardiovascular problems, as an estimated 60 million Americans are affected by them.[21] Any of several conditions may be detected, and the periodontal treatment plan must be adjusted accordingly. These conditions include angina pectoris, previous cardiac bypass or myocardial infarction, previous cerebrovascular accident, congestive heart failure,

hypertension, presence of cardiac pacemakers, and infective endocarditis.

In most cases the patient's cardiologist should be consulted, and the following precautions should be taken to avoid stress: schedule morning appointments; maintain an open, concerned atmosphere during treatment; and keep appointments short.

Angina Pectoris

Patients with a history of unstable angina pectoris (angina that occurs irregularly or on multiple occasions without predisposing factors) should be treated for emergencies only. Patients with stable angina (angina that occurs infrequently, is associated with exertion or stress, and is easily controlled with medication and rest) can undergo elective dental procedures if the following precautions are taken:

1. Premedication if needed (diazepam [Valium], nitrous oxide–oxygen, or a short-acting barbiturate such as pentobarbital [30 to 60 mg] or secobarbital [60 to 100 mg][7,57])
2. Adequate anesthesia (aspirate frequently and inject slowly)
3. Nitroglycerin premedication sublingually (1/200 grain) 5 minutes before a procedure that the patient feels is stressful

The patient's medication (generally nitroglycerin) should be readily accessible on the dental tray. The expiration date of the patient's nitroglycerin (it expires within a year) should be noted, as well as the expiration date of the nitroglycerin in the office's emergency medical kit. Also, patients may have been prescribed longer-acting nitroglycerins (in tablet or patch form) or calcium channel blockers (also used in the treatment of hypertension). The latter, known generically as nifedipine, verapamil, or diltiazem, can cause gingival hyperplasia (see Chapter 18) and may also have other side effects such as hypotension.

If, during a periodontal procedure, the patient becomes fatigued or uncomfortable or has a sudden change in heart rhythm or rate, the procedure should be discontinued as soon as possible. A patient who has an anginal episode in the dental chair should receive the following emergency medical treatment:

1. Discontinue the periodontal procedure.
2. Administer one tablet (0.3 to 0.6 mg) of nitroglycerin sublingually.
3. Reassure the patient and loosen restrictive garments.
4. Administer oxygen with the patient in a reclining position.
5. If the signs and symptoms cease within 3 minutes, complete the periodontal procedure if possible, making sure that the patient is comfortable. Terminate the procedure at the earliest convenient time.

If the anginal signs and symptoms do not resolve with this treatment within 2 to 3 minutes, administer another dose of nitroglycerin, monitor the patient's vital signs, call his or her physician, and be ready to accompany the patient to the emergency department.

Previous Cardiac Bypass or Myocardial Infarction

Cardiac (aortocoronary) bypass, femoral artery bypass, angioplasty, and thromboendarterectomy have become common surgical procedures. The physician should be consulted prior to elective dental therapy if one of these procedures was performed recently.[40] Although there has not been a statement regarding dental treatment of the bypass or post–myocardial infarction patient, it is advised that elective therapy not be performed until 6 months after bypass or heart attack. Prophylactic antibiotics are not necessary for cardiac bypass and myocardial infarction patients unless the cardiologist recommends it. The cardiologist should inform the dentist regarding the degree of heart damage or arterial occlusive disease, the stability of the patient's condition, and the potential for infective endocarditis or graft rejection. Patients whose bypass procedure involved synthetic patches (e.g., Dacron) have an increased risk of bacterial colonization because of the surface discrepancies between normal arterial intima and the prosthetic pseudointima.[35]

Previous Cerebrovascular Accident

A cerebrovascular accident (CVA), or stroke, occurs as a result of ischemic changes (e.g., cerebral thrombosis owing to an embolus) or hemorrhagic phenomena. Hypertension and arteriosclerosis are predisposing factors to a CVA and should alert the clinician to evaluate the patient's medical history carefully for the possibility of early cerebrovascular insufficiency and to be aware of symptoms of the disease. A physician's referral should precede periodontal therapy if the signs and symptoms of early cerebrovascular insufficiency are evident.

Patients who are seen after a stroke should be treated following these guidelines:

1. No periodontal therapy (unless for an emergency) should be performed for 6 months because of the high risk of recurrence during this period.

2. After 6 months, periodontal therapy may be performed during short (maximum of 60 minutes), atraumatic appointments.
3. Mild sedation should be used only if the patient is extremely excitable or nervous.[38] General anesthetics and oversedation are contraindicated because of the impaired cerebral circulation. Malamed suggests using light levels of nitrous oxide–oxygen to reduce stress.[37]
4. Local anesthetics may be used with caution: aspirate, then inject slowly and carefully (not intravascularly). The 1989 American Academy of Periodontology World Workshop[43] recommended 2 Carpules of lidocaine with epinephrine (1:100,000); others recommend a maximum of 3 to 5 Carpules, depending on the patient's age and weight.
5. Be aware that many poststroke patients have been placed on anticoagulant therapy. If this is the case, (1) check prothrombin time prior to deep scaling or periodontal surgery; (2) consult with the patient's physician to adjust the prothrombin time to not greater than 1.5 times normal; and (3) remember that anticoagulants have known interactions with other drugs, including those used in dental practice.
6. Monitor blood pressure carefully. Recurrence rates for CVAs are high, as are rates of associated functional deficits.
7. Know what to do in case of a recurrent CVA:[37,38]
   - Know the signs and symptoms of a CVA.
   - Terminate the dental treatment.
   - Make the patient comfortable in an upright position, if conscious.
   - Loosen restrictive garments.
   - Give oxygen only if respiratory difficulty develops.
   - Monitor vital signs.
   - Summon medical assistance.
   - If the patient becomes unconscious, perform basic life support procedures, and place the patient in the supine position if cardiopulmonary resuscitation (CPR) is needed; the head should be elevated slightly if CPR is not required.
   - Do not give medicines that elicit depression of the central nervous system.

Congestive Heart Failure

Congestive heart failure (CHF) begins with left ventricular failure caused by a disproportion between the hemodynamic load and the capacity to handle the load.[36] It may be due to a chronic increase in workload (as in hypertension or in aortic, mitral, pulmonary, or tricuspid valvular disease), to direct damage to the myocardium (as in myocardial infarction or rheumatic fever), or to an increase in the body's oxygen requirements (as in anemia, thyrotoxicosis, or pregnancy). Left ventricular failure is related to pulmonary vascular congestion.

Patients with untreated congestive heart failure are *not* candidates for elective dental procedures. For patients with treated congestive heart failure, the clinician should consult with the physician regarding the following:

1. Medications
   - Digitalis
     1. Watch for a tendency toward nausea and/or vomiting
     2. Watch for increased susceptibility to dysrhythmia
   - Diuretics
     1. Watch for susceptibility to orthostatic hypotension
     2. Know the side effects of the prescribed diuretic
   - Dicumarol: Prothrombin time should be 1.5 times normal (adjust with the physician)
   - Analgesics: May increase prothrombin time

2. Degree of control of the medical problem
3. Etiology of the disease process
4. Presence of, or potential for, polycythemia, thrombocytopenia, or leukopenia in compensation for inadequate oxygen in the arterial system
   - Patient may require antibiotic coverage if the white blood cell count is low
   - Potential for bleeding problems
   - Do not allow the patient to dehydrate
   - Procedures should be short
   - Do not place the patient in a flat reclining position
   - Supplemental oxygen administration by nasal cannulas may be used
   - Stress reduction should be emphasized; if the patient becomes fatigued or dyspneic, treatment should not begin or the procedure should be discontinued at the first opportune moment
   - Do not use saline rinses, owing to sodium absorption
   - Understand the treatment steps for active developing CHF
     1. Administer 100% oxygen by full face mask
     2. Position the patient sitting upright
     3. Record vital signs
     4. Apply rotating tourniquets high on the four extremities; this is a bloodless phlebotomy procedure that will reduce the total circulating blood volume; release the tourniquets one at a time for 5 minutes every 30 minutes
     5. Reduce the patient's apprehension through reassurance
     6. Call for medical assistance

Hypertension

Sixty million persons in the United States have hypertensive disease, which is defined as blood pressure elevated to 140/90 mm Hg or greater. Half of this population has not been diagnosed.[53] Hypertension is more prevalent among blacks than whites and increases with age in all groups. Therefore, a patient with hypertensive disease is likely to be seen in a dental practice at least once daily; this likelihood is even greater in a periodontal practice because of the observed increase in blood pressure levels with age.

Hypertension is divided into primary and secondary types. *Primary (essential) hypertension* occurs when no underlying pathologic abnormality can be found to explain the disease.[72] Approximately 95% of all hypertensive patients have primary hypertension. The remaining 5% of hypertensive patients have *secondary hypertension,* in which an underlying etiology can be found and surgical treatment may be possible. Examples of the conditions responsible for secondary hypertension are renal disease, endocrinologic changes, and neurogenic disorders.

The epidemiologic data demonstrate a graded relation between high blood pressure and a person's risk of subsequently developing a CVA, cardiac arrest, blindness, or renal failure. A Veterans Administration cooperative study indicated that, over a 5-year period, major complications from hypertension may be reduced from 55% to 18% by treatment.[68] *The dental office may play a vital role in the detection of hypertension and maintenance care of the patient with hypertensive disease.*

The periodontal recall system is an ideal method for hypertension detection. The first visit should include two blood pressure readings, which are averaged and used as a baseline. Before the clinician refers a patient to a physician because of elevated blood pressure, readings should be taken at a minimum of two appointments, unless the measurements are extremely high (i.e., diastolic pressure greater than 115 mm Hg). Also, to decide whether critical changes in an individual's blood pressure are occurring, that particular patient's baseline levels must already have been established.

Periodontal procedures should not be performed until accurate blood pressure measurements and a history have been taken to identify those patients with significant hypertensive disease. The patient's position, cuff size, and sphygmomanometer calibration must be accurate. Also, normal blood pressure increases from 70/45 mm Hg in infancy to 80/45 in early childhood and 100/75 in adolescence. In one third of the population, a transient increase in blood pressure may occur in early adulthood; an increase is the usual finding after age 60.[57]

The Joint National Committee on Detection, Evaluation and Treatment of High Blood Pressure[50] has recommended the protocol shown in Table 34–1 for evaluation and courses of action, depending on the individual's initial blood pressure measurements. In addition, all adults with systolic blood pressure greater than 160 mm Hg should be advised to have their blood pressure rechecked.

If a patient is currently receiving hypertension therapy, consult his or her physician regarding current medical status, medications, the periodontal treatment plan, and patient management. Many physicians are not knowledgeable about the nature of specific periodontal procedures. It will be up to the dentist to inform the physician regarding the estimated degree of stress, blood loss, length of the procedure, and complexity of the individualized treatment plan. Saline rinses are contraindicated.

No periodontal treatment should be given to a patient who is hypertensive and not under medical management. If the periodontal problem is an emergency, the treatment should be conservative (antibiotics and/or analgesics). Surgical procedures should be avoided because of the potential for excessive bleeding.

Table 34–1. PROTOCOL FOR EVALUATION AND REFERRAL OF HYPERTENSIVE PATIENTS

Condition	Systolic	Diastolic	What to Do
Normal	Less than 130	Less than 85	Recheck in 2 years
High-normal Hypertension	130–139	85–89	Recheck yearly
Stage 1	140–159	90–99	Confirm within 2 months
Stage 2	160–179	100–109	See physician within month
Stage 3	180–209	110–119	See physician within week
Stage 4	210 or higher	120 or higher	See physician immediately

Note: Blood pressure conditions are based on two or more readings taken at two different visits, in addition to the origional screening visit.
From The Fifth Report of the Joint National Committee on Detection, Evaluation and Treatment of High Blood Pressure. Arch Intern Med *153*:6, 1993.

In treating hypertensive patients, the clinician should not use a local anesthetic containing an epinephrine concentration greater than 1:100,000, nor should a vasopressor be used to control local bleeding. Local anesthesia without epinephrine may be used for short procedures (less than 30 minutes). In a patient with hypertensive disease, however, it is important to reduce or eliminate pain with the use of a local anesthetic to avoid an outpouring of endogenous epinephrine. Therefore, dosages should be titrated to be minimal but adequate for pain control and stress minimization.

The clinician should be aware of the many side effects of the various antihypertensive medications. Depression is a common side effect of which many patients are unaware. The frequency of episodes of postural hypertension with or without syncope can be reduced by eliminating sudden positional changes in the dental chair. The chair should be slowly elevated to an upright position prior to the patient's standing up. Nausea may also occur secondary to the use of antihypertensive medications.

Presence of Cardiac Pacemakers

Currently cardiac pacemakers are sustaining life for more than 1 million persons in the United States.[67] Since the first pacemaker was implanted in 1958, it has become apparent that particular attention must be paid to postimplantation patients in the dental environment.

Despite the lack of a definitive protocol for handling the pacemaker patient, there are precautions that should be taken to enhance dental environmental safety. The clinician is medicolegally responsible for recognizing electrophysiologic problems attendant with implantation of electronic circuits.[14] The following guidelines should be used when treating patients with cardiac pacemakers:

1. *Health history:* A question should be included in the patient history regarding pacemaker placement; if an affirmative response is given, the patient's cardiologist should be consulted about the proposed periodontal treatment plan, the associated risks, the precautionary measures that should be taken, and the underlying cardiac reason for pacing.
2. *Positioning:* The patient should be positioned so as to minimize discomfort from strain on the lead wires or on the implant site. Pressure should be minimized over the area of the pacemaker apparatus. Positioning of patients should be determined by their level of comfort.
3. *Devices:* All line-powered devices that come into contact with the patient should be measured for leakage, and all electrically powered dental equipment should be earth grounded.[46]
4. *Limited use of electrical equipment:* Once again, many forms of dental equipment that apply an electrical current directly to the patient may interfere with artificial pacemakers (e.g., ultrasonic and electrosurgical devices). Try to keep all electrical equipment at least 1 foot (30 cm) from the patient.[51] Currently, however, most pacemakers are adequately shielded to prevent these changes.

Infective Endocarditis

Infective endocarditis (IE) is a disease in which microorganisms colonize the damaged endocardium or heart valves. Although the incidence of IE is low, it is a serious disease with a poor prognosis, despite modern therapy.

The term *infective endocarditis* is preferred to the previous term *bacterial endocarditis,* because the disease can also be caused by fungi and viruses. The organisms most commonly encountered in IE are the α-hemolytic streptococci (e.g., *Streptococcus viridans*) (Fig. 34–1).

IE has been divided into acute and subacute forms. The acute form involves virulent organisms, generally nonhemolytic streptococci and strains of staphylococci, which invade normal cardiac tissue, produce septic emboli, and cause infections that run a rapid, generally fatal course. The subacute form, on the other hand, occurs as a result of colony formation on damaged endocardium or heart valves by low-grade pathogenic organisms; the classic example is rheumatic carditis consequent to rheumatic fever.

The most susceptible population consists of persons older than 50,[22] owing to the increased occurrence of arteriosclerotic cardiovascular disease and open heart surgery in older individuals. Those defined as *highly susceptible* have a high risk of contracting IE subsequent to dental treatment, and the consequences of the disease are likely to be serious; this group includes individuals with a history of IE and/or those with prosthetic heart valves.

Those defined as *susceptible* are at risk for IE after dental treatment because they have congenital heart disease, rheumatic or other acquired valvular heart disease, idiopathic hypertrophic subaortic stenosis, a history of prosthetic or vascular repair surgery, a history of luetic heart disease, calcified aortic stenosis, calcified mitral anulus, mitral valve prolapse syndrome with regurgitation, or mitral insufficiency; this group also includes patients with permanent transvenous pacemakers and those addicted to drugs administered intravenously.

The practice of periodontics is intimately concerned with the prevention of IE. The American Heart Association Committee Report of 1990 stated that "patients at risk to develop infective endocarditis should maintain the highest level of oral health to reduce potential sources of bacterial seeding. Even in the absence of dental procedures, poor dental hygiene or other dental diseases such as periodontal or periapical infections may induce bacteremia."[29] The report recommended antibiotic prophylaxis for all dental pro-

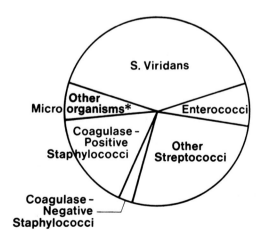

* Mainly enteric gram-negative bacilli, fungi, pneumococci, diphtheroids, and H. influenzae.

FIGURE 34–1. Infective endocarditis: implicated causative microorganisms.

cedures that are likely to cause gingival bleeding, which includes almost all periodontal treatment procedures. To provide adequate preventive measures for IE, periodontists' major concern should be to reduce the microbial population in the oral cavity so as to minimize soft tissue inflammation and bacteremia. Studies have confirmed that bacteremia occurs more frequently and is more severe in patients with periodontal disease than in those without periodontal disease.[30]

Preventive measures to reduce the risk of IE should consist of the following:

1. *Define the susceptible patient.* A careful medical history will disclose the aforementioned susceptible patients. Health questioning should cover rheumatic fever, rheumatic heart disease, cardiac murmurs, congenital heart defects, cardiac surgery, prosthetic heart valves, luetic heart disease, indwelling arteriovenous (AV) shunts, ventriculoatrial shunts, and transvenous pacemakers. If there is any doubt, the patient's physician should be consulted.

2. *Provide oral hygiene instruction.* Oral hygiene should initially be limited to gentle procedures (i.e., oral rinses and gentle toothbrushing with a soft brush). As yet no antibiotic coverage for these procedures has been deemed necessary. Of course, the bacteremia caused by oral hygiene procedures is dependent on the degree of periodontal tissue inflammation. As gingival health improves, more aggressive oral hygiene may be initiated. Because dental irrigation devices have been implicated in association with IE, their use should be discouraged in susceptible individuals.[13,28] Oral hygiene should be practiced with methods that improve gingival health yet minimize bacteremia. Susceptible patients should be encouraged to maintain the highest level of oral hygiene once soft tissue inflammation is controlled.

3. *Currently recommended antibiotic prophylactic regimens should be practiced with all susceptible patients.*[12,17] If there is any doubt regarding susceptibility, the patient's physician should be consulted. Note that in patients who have been re-

ceiving continuous oral penicillin for secondary prevention of rheumatic fever, penicillin-resistant α-hemolytic streptococci are occasionally found in the oral cavity. It is recommended, therefore, that the regular regimen (erythromycin) be followed instead (Table 34–2).

Actinobacillus actinomycetemcomitans has been found with increasing frequency in patients with IE[25] and is present in high numbers in periodontal pockets and tissues of patients with localized juvenile periodontitis (see Chapter 27). This organism is resistant to penicillin and erythromycin but disappears from plaque samples for several weeks after tetracycline therapy (see Chapter 44). Therefore, Slots and coworkers[63] have suggested the following prophylactic regimen for endocarditis-susceptible patients with localized juvenile periodontitis: first, systemic tetracycline, 250 mg four times daily for 14 days, followed by the conventional prophylactic protocol during the time of dental treatment.

4. *Periodontal treatment should be designed for susceptible patients to accommodate their particular degree of periodontal involvement.* The nature of periodontal therapy enhances the problems related to the prophylaxis of subacute IE. Patients are faced with long-term therapy, healing periods that extend beyond a 1-day antibiotic regimen, multiple visits, and procedures that easily elicit gingival bleeding. The following guidelines should aid in the development of periodontal treatment planning for the patient susceptible to IE:

- All periodontal treatment procedures (including probing) require antibiotic prophylaxis; gentle oral hygiene methods are excluded.

- In cases of delayed healing, it is prudent to provide additional doses of antibiotics. Also, periodontal suture removal may be performed more safely by extending antibiotic coverage to the fifth or sixth postoperative day; alternatively, resorbable sutures may be used.

- Little and Falace recommend a concentrated 5- to 7-day oral hygiene–gross debridement program with antibiotic

Table 34–2. RECOMMENDED PROPHYLACTIC REGIMEN FOR PERIODONTAL PROCEDURES IN ADULT PATIENTS WHO ARE AT RISK FOR INFECTIVE ENDOCARDITIS

Standard Regimen

—*Amoxicillin* 3.0 g orally 1 hour before procedure, and 1.5 g 6 hours after initial dose

For Patients Allergic to Amoxicillin/Penicillin

—*Erythromycin ethylsuccinate* 800 mg or *erythromycin stearate* 1.0 g orally 2 hours before procedure, and half the dose 6 hours after initial dose
    or
—*Clindamycin* 300 mg orally 1 hour before procedure, and 150 mg 6 hours after initial dose

Parenteral Administration for Patients Unable to Take Oral Medications

—*Ampicillin* 2.0 g IV or IM 30 minutes before procedure, then *ampicillin* 1.0 g IV or IM or *amoxicillin* 1.5 g orally 6 hours after initial dose

Parenteral Administraiton for Patients Allergic to Penicillin

—*Clindamycin* 300 mg IV 30 minutes before procedure, and 150 mg IV or orally 6 hours after initial dose

IM, Intramuscularly; IV, intravenously.
Adapted from Dajani AS, Bisho AL, Chung KJ, et al. Prevention of bacterial endocarditis: Recommendations by the American Heart Association, Clinical Cardiology. JAMA 264:2919, 1990, Copyright 1990, American Medical Association, and based on recommendations given by the American Heart Association for patients with congenital heart disease, rheumatic heart disease or other valvular heart disease, idiopathic hypertrophic subaortic stenosis, prosthetic heart valve, previous history of endocarditis, surgically constructed systemic-pulmonary shunts or conduits, or mitral valve prolapse with regurgitation.
Reduced dosages are recommended for children weighing less than 30 kg (66 pounds). See reference 12.

coverage.[36] These authors believe that if patients do not seem able or willing to maintain oral hygiene, dentures should be considered. A similar recommendation was made regarding penicillin-allergic patients with diseased heart valves unless such patients are receiving in-hospital dental care. (Note, however, that edentulousness does not eliminate the risk of IE, as ulcerations from ill-fitting dentures have been associated with IE.[42,55]) The severity of periodontal involvement should also influence decisions about edentulation.

- Dental extraction should be avoided in healthy mouths whenever possible. Endodontic therapy is the treatment of choice. Also, single extractions are preferable to multiple extractions.[41]
- Severe periodontal disease and areas of periodontal suppuration or dental focus of infection require elimination.
- Prolonged impingement on the gingival tissues, as with ligatures or tissue retractors, should be avoided, as this increases the opportunity for development of bacteremia.
- One-day antibiotic coverage should be used, with 10 to 14 days elapsing before starting a new coverage period, if one is needed. An equally acceptable alternative would be to rotate different antibiotics to minimize the emergence of resistant strains.
- Prior to surgical procedures, the gingival tissues should be cleansed. Rinsing with 0.12% chlorhexidine mouthwash for 30 seconds is recommended before any periodontal procedure.
- All elective dental procedures should be postponed until the periodontal tissues approximate periodontal health. Rheumatic heart disease patients with recommended antibiotic coverage and no evidence of congestive heart failure may then receive any indicated dental treatment.
- Regular recall appointments, with an emphasis on oral hygiene reinforcement and maintenance of periodontal health, are extremely important in this population.

Until more definitive information is available on prophylaxis of IE, it is better to err on the side of safety.

RENAL DISEASES

The most common causes of renal failure are glomerulonephritis, pyelonephritis, kidney cystic disease, renovascular disease, drug nephropathy, obstructive uropathy, and hypertension.[18,36] Because the dental management of the patient with renal failure is drastically altered, physician consultation is necessary to determine the stage of renal failure and the modality of the medical treatment prescribed and to plan periodontal therapy according to the stage of the disease and the type of associated medical treatment.

The patient in chronic renal failure has a progressive disease that may ultimately require renal transplantation or dialysis. It is preferable to treat a patient before, rather than after, transplant or dialysis.[31] The following treatment modifications should be followed:

1. Consult the patient's physician.
2. Monitor blood pressure (patients in end-stage renal failure are usually hypertensive).[36]
3. Check laboratory values: partial thromboplastin time, prothrombin time, bleeding time, and platelet count; hematocrit; blood urea nitrogen (do not treat if less than 60 mg per 100 ml); and serum creatinine (do not treat if less than 1.5 mg per 100 ml).
4. Eliminate areas of oral infection because of enhanced susceptibility:[9]
   - Oral hygiene should be good.
   - Periodontal treatment should aim at providing easy maintenance. All questionable teeth should be extracted if medical parameters permit.
   - Frequent recall appointments should be scheduled.
5. Drugs that are nephrotoxic or metabolized by the kidney should not be given (e.g., phenacetin, streptomycin, tetracycline). Acetaminophen and acetylsalicylic acid may be used with caution.[71]

The patient who is receiving dialysis requires treatment planning modifications.[70] There are three modes of dialysis: intermittent peritoneal dialysis (IPD), chronic ambulatory peritoneal dialysis (CAPD), and hemodialysis. Only hemodialysis patients require special precautions. Such patients have a high incidence of serum hepatitis, a high incidence of anemia, and a significant incidence of secondary hyperparathyroidism and undergo heparinization during hemodialysis.[4] For these reasons, the following should be added to the recommendations for treating patients with chronic renal disease:

1. Screen for hepatitis B surface antigen (HB$_s$Ag) and antibodies to hepatitis B (HB$_s$Ab) prior to any treatment.
2. Provide antibiotic prophylaxis to prevent endarteritis of the arteriovenous fistula or shunt.
3. Prevent hypoxia.
4. Provide treatment on the day after dialysis, when the effects of heparinization have subsided. Dialysis treatments are generally performed three times a week for 4 hours or twice a week for 5 hours. (Note that IPD and CAPD patients are not systemically heparinized; therefore, they do not usually have the potential bleeding problems associated with hemodialysis.)
5. Establish a long-term maintenance system with frequent recall appointments.
6. Be careful to protect the dialysis shunt or fistula when the patient is in the dental chair. If the shunt or fistula is placed in the arm, do not cramp the limb; blood pressure readings should be taken from the other arm. Do not use the limb for the injection of medication. Patients with leg shunts should avoid sitting with the leg dependent for longer than 1 hour.[4] If appointments last longer, allow the patient to walk about for a few minutes and then resume therapy.
7. Refer the patient to the physician if uremic problems, such as uremic stomatitis, are noted to be developing.

The renal transplant patient's greatest foe is infection. A periodontal abscess is a potentially life-threatening situation. For this reason, a dental team approach should be used before transplantation to determine which teeth can be easily maintained. Teeth with furcation involvements, periodontal abscesses, or extensive surgical requirements should be extracted, leaving an easily maintainable dentition. In addition to the recommendations for patients with chronic renal failure, the following should be considered for the renal transplant patient:

1. HB$_s$Ag screening.
2. Prophylactic antibiotics according to American Heart Association recommendations. Some authors recommend use of an oral antibiotic mouthwash with nystatin (Mycostatin) 1 day before and continuing 2 days after the dental procedure.[4]

PULMONARY DISEASES

The periodontal treatment of a patient with pulmonary disease may require alteration, depending on the nature and the severity of the respiratory problem. Pulmonary diseases range from obstructive lung diseases (e.g., asthma, emphysema, bronchitis, and acute obstruction) to restrictive ventilatory disorders that are due to muscle weakness, scarring, obesity, or any condition that could interfere with effective lung ventilation. Combined restrictive-obstructive lung disease may also develop.[8]

The clinician should be aware of the signs and symptoms of pulmonary disease, such as increased respiratory rate (the normal rate for adults is 12 to 16 breaths/min), central cyanosis, clubbing of the fingers, chronic cough, chest pain, hemoptysis, dyspnea or orthopnea, and wheezing.[36] Patients with these problems should be referred for medical evaluation and treatment. Most patients with chronic lung disease may undergo routine periodontal therapy if they are receiving adequate medical management.

Caution should be taken in relation to the use of ultrasonic instrumentation. Dried, retained secretions that result in partial airway obstruction may, because of their hydrophilic nature, cause complete obstruction when ultrasonic devices are used. Also, use of ultrasonic devices may precipitate bronchospasm owing to the foreign body nature of aerosol droplets.[61] Similar reactions may occur with debris or aerosol from handpieces.

Caution should be practiced in relation to any treatment that may depress respiratory function. Acute respiratory distress may be caused by slight airway obstruction or depression of respiratory function.[5] Because of their limited vital lung capacity, these patients also have a decreased cough effectiveness.[62] They must continually deal with the mental anxiety caused by air hunger and alter their position in attempts to improve their ventilatory efficiency.[23]

The following management should be used during periodontal therapy:

1. Identify and refer patients with signs and symptoms of pulmonary disease.
2. In patients with known pulmonary disease, consult with the physician regarding medications (antibiotics, steroids, chemotherapeutic agents) and the degree and severity of pulmonary disease.
3. Avoid elicitation of respiratory depression or distress:
   - Minimize the stress of a periodontal appointment. The patient with emphysema should be scheduled in the afternoon, several hours after sleep, to allow for airway clearance.
   - Avoid medications that could cause respiratory depression (meperidine, morphine, sedatives, and general anesthetics).
   - Do not give a bilateral mandibular block, which could cause increased airway obstruction.
   - Care should be taken in administering oxygen or nitrous oxide–oxygen and with the use of ultrasonic or rotary devices.
   - Position the patient to allow maximum ventilatory efficiency, be careful to prevent physical airway obstruction, keep the patient's throat clear, and avoid excess periodontal packing.
4. In patients with a history of asthma, make sure the patient's medication is available (e.g., isoproterenol 0.25% aerosol) and avoid complex dental procedures.

5. Patients with active fungal or bacterial diseases should not be treated unless the periodontal procedure is an emergency.

IMMUNOSUPPRESSION AND CHEMOTHERAPY

Immunosuppressed patients possess impaired host defenses as a result of an underlying immunodeficiency or drug administration (primarily related to organ transplantation or cancer chemotherapy).[15,52] Leukopenia, alterations in cellular immunity, disruption of intact integument, and alterations in the inflammatory response may facilitate secondary infection. Also, dose-dependent neutropenia may occur. The oral cavity is an obvious reservoir for potential superinfection microorganisms. *Treatment in these patients should be directed toward the prevention of oral complications that could be life threatening.* The greatest potential for infection occurs during periods of extreme immunosuppression; therefore, treatment should be conservative and palliative.

RADIATION THERAPY

The use of radiotherapy, alone or in conjunction with surgical resection, is common in the treatment of head and neck tumors. The side effects of ionizing radiation include dramatic perioral changes of significant concern to dental health personnel.[3,16,39a] The extent and severity of mucositis, dermatitis, xerostomia, dysphagia, gustatory alteration, radiation caries, vascular changes, trismus, temporomandibular joint degeneration, and periodontal change are dependent on a myriad of radiation factors:[1,16,54] the type of radiation used, the fields of irradiation, the number of ports, the types of tissues in the fields, and the dosage.

Patients scheduled to receive radiation therapy require dental consultation at the earliest possible time to reduce the morbidity of the known perioral side effects. Preirradiation treatment depends on the patient's prognosis, compliance, and residual dentition, in addition to the fields, ports, dose, and immediacy of radiotherapy. The initial visit should include panoramic and intraoral radiographs, a clinical dental examination, periodontal evaluation, and physician consultation. The physician should be asked about the amount of radiation to be administered, the extent and location of the lesion, the nature of any surgical procedures performed or to be performed, the number of radiation ports, the mode of radiation therapy, and the patient's prognosis (i.e., the likelihood of metastasis). Preirradiation treatment should commence immediately after the physician consultation. The first decision that should be made relates to possible extractions, because radiation can cause side effects that interfere with healing.

For head and neck squamous cell carcinomas, the dose is usually 5000 to 7000 rad of cobalt 60 delivered in a fractionated method (150 to 200 rad over a 6- to 7-week course). This is considered full-course radiation treatment, and the degree of perioral side effects will depend on the tissues irradiated. If this dose is administered to the salivary gland tissues, xerostomia will ensue.[59] The parotid is apparently the most radiosensitive of the salivary glands;

saliva may become extremely viscous or nonexistent, depending on the dose delivered to the particular gland. Xerostomia will also cause a decrease in the normal salivary cleansing mechanisms, the buffering capacity of saliva, and the pH of oral fluids. Oral bacterial populations shift to preponderantly cariogenic forms (*Streptococcus mutans, Actinomyces,* and *Lactobacillus*).[6]

Another major concern regarding the decision about extractions involves the radiation dose to be received and the extent of involvement of the body of the mandible. The incidence of osteoradionecrosis of the mandible is directly related to the mandible's apparent lack of vascularity and to the higher incidence of carcinoma in mandibular areas (thus the associated increased frequency of irradiation). Therefore, the greater the glandular involvement and involvement of the body of the mandible, the greater the likelihood that there will be oral complications after radiation therapy.

If the patient is to receive full-course radiation therapy within the aforementioned fields, the required extractions should be performed a minimum of 10 days to 2 weeks prior to the initiation of radiation therapy or should not be performed at all. If the periodontal support is less than half the root length, the teeth are nonrestorable or abscessed, or the patient's oral hygiene and motivation are poor, it is recommended that extractions be performed within the allocated time limit. Beumer believes that all teeth with furcation involvements should be extracted as well.[3] Extractions should be performed in a manner that allows primary closure. Mucoperiosteal flaps should be gently elevated; teeth should be extracted in segments; radical alveolectomy should be performed, allowing no rough osseous spicules to remain; and primary closure should be provided without tension. It is recommended that antibiotic coverage be provided for the initial 7- to 10-day healing period.[19] The first visit should also include instruction in oral hygiene methods for maintenance of the remaining dentition.

During radiation therapy, patients should receive weekly fluoride treatments (i.e., a 1-minute acidulated phosphofluoride rinse [1.23%], followed by a 4-minute stannous fluoride rinse [1.64%]), unless these treatments are irritating to a concurrent mucositis. Patients should be instructed to brush daily with a stannous fluoride gel (0.4%). All remaining teeth should receive thorough debridement (scaling and root planing). The periodontal ligament has been reported to lose much of its cellularity and vascularity after radiation therapy; thus, its healing potential is severely compromised. Pulpal changes may become apparent as well.[1,44] *During the course of radiation therapy, it is important to reinforce the patient's oral hygiene and to perform weekly professional plaque removal.* Simple restorations (alloys) should be placed where required.

Postirradiation morbidity may be manifested as osteoradionecrosis (which occurs in 5% to 10% of patients undergoing irradiation for head or neck carcinoma).[48] Osseous healing may progress slowly or not at all. A decreased vascular supply, along with damaged and diminished numbers of osteocytes and osteoblasts, contributes to this painful, often debilitating pathologic response. Any trauma or infection may lead to osteoradionecrosis. An extraction or periodontal disease that progresses to abscess formation may trigger osteoradionecrosis.[24] In addition, teeth become somewhat brittle after full-course radiation therapy to the head or neck owing to the denaturation of their organic matrices.[20,60] For these reasons, postirradiation periodontal care should be limited to gentle hand instrumentation, oral hygiene reinforcement, and fluoride treatment. Ultrasonic instrumentation is not recommended. Full-thickness flap techniques or periodontal procedures that could expose osseous structures should *not* be performed, especially on the mandible. *Periodontal care should remain conservative for the duration of the patient's life.*

Postirradiation follow-up consists of palliative treatment given as indicated. A 3-month recall interval is ideal. Viscous lidocaine may be prescribed for painful mucositis, or salivary substitutes may be given for xerostomia.[58] Patient monitoring for systemic as well as oral changes is essential.

A final necessity in postirradiation management is a supportive attitude. Many patients undergo severe depression during radiotherapy and experience anxiety after therapy. They should be warned about perioral changes and return or loss of function, and their personal role in decreasing postirradiation morbidity should be emphasized. Understanding and supportive encouragement are essential during this traumatic time.

ENDOCRINE DISORDERS

Diabetes

The diabetic patient requires special precautions prior to periodontal therapy. A full discussion of the role of diabetes in the etiology of periodontal disease is presented in Chapter 14. This section outlines periodontal therapy for the diabetic with respect to the diagnosis of glucose intolerance and the degree of disease control.

If signs of diabetes are noticed in a patient, further investigation via laboratory studies and history taking (e.g., hereditary predisposition) should be performed, because *periodontal treatment in the patient with uncontrolled diabetes is contraindicated.*

If a patient is suspected of being diabetic, the following procedures should be performed:

1. Consult the patient's physician.
2. Analyze laboratory tests (Table 34–3): fasting blood glucose, postprandial blood glucose, glycated hemoglobin,[49] glucose tolerance test, urinary glucose.
3. Rule out acute orofacial infection or severe dental infection; insulin and glucose requirements are altered in the presence of infection; only antibiotic and analgesic care should be administered until a complete physical examination is performed and diabetic control is attained; if there is a periodontal condition that requires immediate care, antibiotic coverage is required prior to incision and drainage; the physician should monitor insulin requirements.
4. Monitor vital signs (especially blood pressure) closely.

If a patient is a "brittle" diabetic (one whose disease is difficult to control), optimal periodontal health is a necessity. Treatment of periodontal disease may reduce insulin requirements.[26] Glucose levels should be continuously monitored, and periodontal treatment should be performed when the disease is in a well-controlled state. Glycated hemoglobin testing reflects glucose levels over the previous 6 to 8

Table 34–3. LABORATORY TESTS FOR DIABETES

Test	Value
Fasting blood glucose	50–100 mg/100 ml normal >100 mg/100 ml suggestive >130 mg/100 ml diagnostic
1- or 2-hour postprandial blood glucose	<170 mg/100 ml 1-hour oral carbohydrate load <120 mg/100 ml 2-hour oral carbohydrate load

Glucose tolerance test
(if pregnant or glucose tolerance is impaired)
    0 hour
    ½ hour
    1 hour
    2 hours
    3 hours
	Glucose load
	
	100 mg/100 ml
	170 mg/100 ml
	170 mg/100 ml
	120 mg/100 ml (diagnostic if >140 mg/100 ml)
	110 mg/100 ml

Glycated hemoglobin (electrophoresis)	% total hemoglobin 4–8 = Normal adult <7.5 = Good control 7.6–8.9 = Fair control 9–20 = Poor control

weeks (or the life of the hemoglobin molecule) and provides information on the degree of diabetic control.[47]

Prophylactic antibiotics, started 2 days preoperatively and continued through the immediate postoperative period, should be administered. Penicillin is the drug of first choice. Periodontal maintenance appointments at frequent intervals are important for stabilization of periodontitis and diabetes. The clinician must also be able to recognize the signs of impending diabetic coma or an insulin reaction.

For the most part, the patient with well-controlled diabetes may be treated as an ordinary patient.[36] However, several guidelines should be followed to ensure diabetes control:

1. The clinician should make certain that the prescribed insulin has been taken, followed by a meal. Morning appointments after breakfast are ideal because of optimal insulin levels.
2. If general anesthesia, intravenous procedures, or surgical procedures are performed that alter the patient's ability to maintain a normal caloric intake, postoperative insulin doses should be altered (Table 34–4). Because there is no agreement on medical management before and after periodontal therapy, individual physician consultation is a prerequisite.

3. Tissues should be handled as atraumatically and as minimally (less than 2 hours) as possible. Anxious patients may require preoperative sedation. The anesthetic should contain epinephrine in concentrations not greater than 1:100,000. Endogenous epinephrine may increase insulin requirements.
4. Diet recommendations should be made to enable the patient to maintain a proper glucose balance. Dietary supplements may be prescribed if deemed necessary.
5. Antibiotic prophylaxis for the prevention of infection is controversial. If therapy is extensive, antibiotic coverage is recommended.
6. Frequent recall appointments and fastidious home oral care should be stressed.

Thyroid Disorders

Periodontal therapy requires minimal alterations in the patient with adequately managed thyroid disease.[34] Patients with thyrotoxicosis and those with inadequate medical management should not receive periodontal therapy until their condition is stabilized. Patients with a history of hyperthyroidism should be carefully evaluated to determine the level of medical management, and they should be treated in a way that limits stress and infection. Medica-

Table 34–4. INSULIN DOSE CHANGES PRIOR TO SURGICAL THERAPY

	Insulin		
	Short-Acting	*Intermediate*	*Long-Acting*
Degree of Dietary Restriction	*Regular (2–4 hr)** *Semilente (2–4 hr)*	*NPH (6–12 hr)* *Lente (6–12 hr)*	*PZI (14–24 hr)* *Ultralente (18–24 hr)*
Minimal	None	None	None
Moderate	Stop A.M. dose	½ A.M. dose, meal given, then other ½ dose	½ A.M. dose
Severe (general anesthesia) No meals for 6 hr	Stop A.M. dose	Stop A.M. dose, followed by surgery in 2 hr	Stop A.M. dose

PZI, Protamine zinc insulin.
* Numbers in parentheses refer to peak activity.

tions such as epinephrine, atropine, and other pressor amines should be given with caution, owing to their overreactive effect in this population; they should not be given to patients with thyrotoxicosis or a poorly controlled thyroid disorder.

Hypothyroid patients require careful administration of sedatives and narcotics because of their diminished inability to tolerate drugs. One source states that only 25% of the dose required for the euthyroid patient is needed for general anesthesia in the hypothyroid patient; also, medical control should be monitored.[34]

Parathyroid Disorders

Once the patient with parathyroid disease has been identified and the proper medical treatment given, routine periodontal therapy may be instituted. However, patients who have not received medical care may have significant renal disease, uremia, and hypertension. Also, if hypercalcemia or hypocalcemia is present, the patient may be more prone to cardiac arrhythmias. Therefore, the dental practitioner must be attuned to the oral and dental changes that occur with hyper- or hypoparathyroidism to provide astute detection and referral.

Adrenal Insufficiency

Acute adrenal insufficiency is associated with significant morbidity and mortality owing to peripheral vascular collapse and cardiac arrest. Therefore, the periodontist should be aware of the clinical manifestations (Table 34–5) and ways of preventing adrenal insufficiency in patients with a history of Addison's disease or in patients with normal adrenal cortices who have been given exogenous glucocorticosteroids.

Most commonly, adrenal insufficiency is seen in persons who have received steroid therapy. Adrenal suppression occurs as a result of adrenocortical atrophy. Sustained hormonal therapy results in a variety of side effects, many of which resemble Cushing's syndrome. In addition, many of these patients cannot tolerate the stress caused by dental anxiety, surgical procedures, trauma, or infection. The degree of suppression depends on the drugs used, the dose, the duration of administration, the length of time elapsed since steroid therapy was terminated, and the route of administration.

Treatment alterations in these patients will differ according to whether they currently take steroids, have previously

Table 34–5. MANIFESTATIONS OF ACUTE ADRENAL INSUFFICIENCY

Mental confusion, fatigue, and weakness
Nausea and/or vomiting
Hypertension
Syncope
Intense abdominal, lower back, and/or leg pain
Loss of consciousness
Coma

Table 34–6. EQUIVALENT DOSES OF CORTICOSTEROIDS

Corticosteroid	Equivalent Dose (mg)
Cortisone	25
Hydrocortisone	20
Prednisone	5
Prednisolone	5
Methylprednisone	5
Methylprednisolone	4
Triamcinolone	4
Dexamethasone	0.75
Betamethasone	0.6

taken steroids, or are in an emergency situation. There is no set protocol for steroid prophylaxis; therefore, endocrine consultation is advised. Medical histories should reveal diseases for which steroids are commonly prescribed and should include the question "Have you ever received steroid therapy?"

For the patient who is currently receiving steroid therapy, the need for corticosteroid prophylaxis depends on the drug used because of the variance in equivalent therapeutic doses (Table 34–6). Most patients with Addison's disease receive a daily oral dose of 25.0 to 37.5 mg of cortisone (equivalent to 5.0 to 7.5 mg of prednisolone). This replaces the normal output of the adrenal cortex, which ranges from 20 to 30 mg per day. Treatment for rheumatoid arthritis, asthma, dermatologic diseases, and so forth may require greater doses, which may readily suppress adrenal function if used for long periods of time. Note that the route of administration is important, because topical corticosteroids may have minimal to no depressant effect.[2] Glucocortico-steroid coverage regimens vary, but most provide a twofold to fourfold increase in coverage, depending on the stress produced by the procedure.

Little and Falace[36] recommend the following:

1. Patients taking low-dose (less than 20 mg) or high-dose (more than 20 mg) cortisol daily for less than 1 month or patients on alternate-day therapy: No supplementation is necessary.
2. Patients taking large doses (more than 20 mg cortisol daily) for extensive and stressful dental procedures: Double or triple the normal maintenance dose the morning of and 1 hour before the procedure; then resume normal dose.
3. Patients on topical steroids: Generally supplementation is not required unless there is prolonged treatment of extensive areas.

For the patient with a past history of steroid therapy, the periodontist should determine the degree of adrenal suppression. Malamed's "rule of twos"—20 mg of cortisone or its equivalent per day, orally or parenterally, given continuously over 2 weeks or longer and within 2 years of dental therapy—should alert the clinician to suspect adrenal suppression.[37] Note that full regeneration of cortical function may occur within 9 to 12 months, but regeneration after 2 years has also been reported. A minimum of 12 months should have passed since the last dose was taken before normal periodontal therapy is performed. Otherwise, steroid prophylaxis may be warranted.

Treatment of the patient in an acute adrenal insufficiency crisis is as follows:

1. Terminate periodontal therapy.
2. Summon medical assistance.
3. Monitor vital signs.
4. Give oxygen.
5. Place the patient in a supine position.
6. Administer 100 mg of hydrocortisone sodium succinate (Solu-Cortef) intravenously over 30 seconds or intramuscularly.

Pregnancy

The aim of periodontal therapy for the pregnant patient is to minimize the potential exaggerated inflammatory response related to pregnancy-associated hormonal alterations. *Meticulous plaque control, scaling, root planing, and polishing should be the only nonemergency periodontal procedures performed.*

The second trimester is the safest time to perform treatment. However, long, stressful appointments, as well as periodontal surgical procedures, should be delayed until the postpartum period.

Owing to the supine hypotensive syndrome of pregnancy that occurs during the third trimester, performing elective periodontal treatment without taking precautions is not advised. Decreasing blood pressure, syncope, and loss of consciousness may occur as a result of uterine pressure on the inferior vena cava. Appointments should be short, and the patient should be allowed to change positions frequently. A fully reclined position should be avoided if possible.

Other precautions during pregnancy relate to the potential toxic or teratogenic effects of therapy on the fetus. Ideally, no medications should be prescribed or radiographs taken unless the situation is an emergency. The patient's obstetrician should be consulted as to whether a drug could cross the placenta or cause fetal respiratory depression.

HEMORRHAGIC DISORDERS

Patients with a history of bleeding problems caused by disease or drugs should be managed so as to minimize risks. Identification of these patients via the health history, clinical examination, and clinical laboratory tests is paramount. Health questioning should cover (1) history of bleeding after previous surgery or trauma, (2) past and present drug history, (3) history of bleeding problems among relatives, and (4) medical history to rule out possible illness associated with bleeding problems.

Clinical examinations should detect the existence of jaundice, ecchymoses, spider telangiectases, hemarthrosis, petechiae, hemorrhagic vesicles, or gingival hyperplasia. Laboratory tests should include methods to measure the hemostatic, coagulation, or lytic phases of the clotting mechanism, depending on clues regarding which phase is involved[10,73] (Table 34–7).

Patients who are severe bleeders should be referred for hematologic evaluation. If the history indicates minor or equivocal bleeding tendencies, simple screening tests, including bleeding time, tourniquet test, complete blood cell count, prothrombin time, partial thromboplastin time, and coagulation time, can be ordered.

Bleeding disorders may be classified as coagulation disorders, thrombocytopenic purpuras, or nonthrombocytopenic purpuras. Of these, the most common disorders are due to acquired, iatrogenic bleeding affecting coagulation.

Coagulation Disorders

Periodontal care for patients on anticoagulation therapy should be altered depending on the medication used to reduce intravascular clotting. Drugs that perform this function include heparin, bishydroxycoumarin (dicumarol), warfarin sodium (Coumadin), phenindione derivatives, cyclocumarol, ethyl biscoumacetate, and aspirin.

Patients on *warfarin therapy* demonstrate an inhibition of prothrombin or of vitamin K–dependent factors (Factors II, VII, IX, and X). Most are outpatients because the drug is administered orally. It is important to note that the duration of action of warfarin is a minimum of 6 days. Periodontal treatment should be altered as follows:

1. Consult the patient's physician to determine the nature of the underlying medical problem and the degree of required anticoagulation. (The general therapeutic range is a prothrombin time between 1.5 and 3.0 times normal.)
2. Periodontal scaling, surgery, and extractions require a prothrombin time less than 1.5 times normal.
   - The physician should be consulted about discontinuing or reducing dicumarol dosage until the desired prothrombin times are achieved.
   - Changes in prothrombin time will not be apparent until 2 to 3 days after changing dosages.
   - A prothrombin time measurement is required on the day of the procedure. If it is greater than 1.5 times normal, cancel the procedure and reschedule for 1 to 3 days later. Remeasure the prothrombin time on the day of surgery.
3. After scaling and curettage, patients should not be dismissed until bleeding has stopped.
4. It is preferable to perform periodontal surgery in a hospital, but small segments of the mouth may be treated in the dental office if these precautions are followed:
   - Minimize trauma.
   - Prophylactic antibiotics are recommended to prevent postoperative infection that may lead to bleeding.[35]
   - Use pressure hemostasis.
   - Attempt to gain closure as close to primary as possible.
   - There are no contraindications to local anesthesia with epinephrine; however, the periodontist should exercise caution with injections (especially blocks), owing to the potential for hematoma formation.
   - Prior to periodontal pack placement, bleeding should be stopped by packing cotton pellets interproximally and applying pressure facially and lingually with a gauze sponge. The periodontal pack may then be placed over the cotton pellets.
5. Do not perform scaling or periodontal surgery if the patient has an acute infection.
6. The patient should return in 3 to 5 days to determine whether healing is normal; if so, the physician may resume the patient's anticoagulation therapy.

Patients on *aspirin therapy* or other nonsteroidal antiinflammatory agents should be screened according to bleeding time and partial thromboplastin time. Salicylates have been known to exert a warfarin-like effect and interfere with normal platelet function. The most severe effects are seen in patients on long-term and/or high-dose therapy. Physicians generally have patients stop aspirin 7 to 14 days prior to periodontal surgery, and they measure

Table 34-7. LABORATORY TESTS FOR COAGULATION AND BLEEDING DISORDERS

	Hemostatic			Lytic
	Vascular	*Platelet*	Coagulation	
Tests	1. Tourniquet test N: 10 petechiae Abn: >10 petechiae 2. Bleeding time N: 1–6 min Abn: >6 min	1. Platelet count N: 150,000–300,000/mm³ Abn: Clinical bleeding occurs at <80,000/mm³ 2. Bleeding time 3. Clot retraction 4. Complete blood cell count	1. Prothrombin time (measures extrinsic and common pathways: Factors I, II, V, VII, and X) N: 11–14 s (depending on laboratory) measured against a control Abn: >1.5–2 times normal 2. Partial thromboplastin time (measures intrinsic and common pathways: Factors III, IX, XI, and low levels of Factors I, II, V, X, and XII) N: 25–40 s (depending on laboratory) measured against a control Abn: >1.5 times normal 3. Clotting (coagulation) time N: 30–40 min Abn: >1 hr	1. Euglobin clot lysis time N: <90 min Abn: >90 min
Clinical disease association	Vascular (capillary) wall defect Rule out: Thrombocytopenia Purpuras Telangiectasia Aspirin therapy Leukemia Renal dialysis	Thrombocytopenia Rule out: Vascular wall defect Acute/chronic leukemia Aplastic anemia Liver disease Renal dialysis	All three tests: Liver disease Warfarin therapy Aspirin therapy Malabsorption syndrome or long-term antibiotic therapy (lack of vitamin K utilization) Prothrombin time: Factor VII deficiency Partial thromboplastin time: Hemophilia, renal dialysis	Increase in fibrinolytic activity

Abn, Abnormal; *N,* normal.

bleeding/platelet times the day of the procedure. *Aspirin should not be prescribed for patients who are receiving anticoagulation therapy or who have illnesses related to bleeding tendencies.*

Heparin therapy is used only in hospital situations because of its parenteral route of administration. Its duration of action is 4 to 8 hours, but it may last up to 24 hours. Refer to the section on renal disease for dental treatment alterations.

Liver disease may affect all phases of blood clotting, as most coagulation factors are synthesized and removed by the liver. A long-term alcohol abuser or a jaundiced individual may have vascular wall alterations and platelet defects secondary to liver damage. Dental treatment planning for patients with liver disease should include the following:

1. Laboratory evaluations: prothrombin time, bleeding time, platelet count, and partial thromboplastin time (in patients in later stages of liver disease).
2. Conservative, nonsurgical periodontal therapy.
3. Evaluation of clinical symptoms such as jaundice in mucous membranes and sclera, clinical bleeding into tissues, fatigue, increased plasma volume, and weight loss.
4. General anesthesia is usually contraindicated because of cardiovascular compromise and impaired ability of the liver to metabolize barbiturates.
5. Look for signs of disease associated with uncontrolled fibrinolysis (e.g., disseminated intravascular coagulation and thrombocytopenia).
6. If planning surgery (in hospital only):
   - Prothrombin time should be no more than 1.5 to 2.0 times normal, and platelet count should exceed 80,000 cells/m^3.[7]
   - If the prothrombin time is greater than 2.0 times normal, vitamin K may be effective in reducing it; if not, only smaller areas of the mouth should be treated in patients with advanced liver disease; daily intravenous doses of vitamin K (150 mg) may be tried, but the administration of fresh whole blood or plasma may also be required.
   - If platelets are low, concentrated platelets may be administered.

Another disorder of coagulation is hereditary *hemophilia.* Periodontal procedures may be performed in hemophiliacs, provided that sufficient precautions are taken.[33,40,64] Conservative therapy and maintenance are preferable to surgery. If surgery is needed, treatment planning should be designed to maximize coordination of blood factor replacement, as determined by the variety of hemophilia and its severity (Table 34–8):

1. Consult with a hematologist.
2. Hospitalize the patient for surgical procedures.
3. Replace coagulation factor (by hematologist).[69]
4. Surgical technique: supply antibiotic coverage; perform as atraumatic a technique as possible, removing all sharp osseous spicules, treating the soft tissues gingerly, and carefully removing all granulation tissue; obtain maximum approximation of the wound edges, avoiding suture strangulation and use of resorbable sutures. Topical hemostatic agents may be applied and a periodontal pack placed after bleeding has been controlled.
5. Postoperative follow-up: bleeding due to clot breakdown usually occurs 3 to 4 days after surgery, and pressure hemostasis should be performed only if there is adequate replacement factor available to prevent subcutaneous bleeding from occurring.
6. Oral hygiene and 3-month maintenance checkups are prerequisites. No aspirin or aspirin products should be prescribed.

Thrombocytopenic Purpuras

Bleeding that is due to a reduced number of platelets (thrombocytopenia) may be seen with idiopathic thrombocytopenic purpuras, radiation therapy, myelosuppressive drug therapy, leukemia, or infections. Normal platelet counts are 250,000 ± 100,000 cells/mm^3. Spontaneous bleeding occurs at levels of 80,000 to 60,000 cells/mm^3. It may result from gingival irritation or inflammation caused by local factors. Periodontal therapy should be directed toward reducing local irritants to avoid the need for more aggressive therapy. Patients who are candidates for periodontal therapy and are suspected of having a platelet abnormality should be managed as follows:

1. Physician referral for a definitive diagnosis and treatment of a platelet disorder.
2. Oral hygiene instruction. If the number of platelets is severely decreased, gentler oral hygiene products should be used (e.g., sponges, chlorhexidine).
3. Prophylactic treatment of potential abscesses. Frequent recall appointments are necessary.
4. No surgical procedures are indicated unless the platelet count is at least 80,000 cells/mm^3. A transfusion of platelets can be given before surgery.
   - Surgical treatment should be as atraumatic as possible.
   - Stents or thrombin-soaked cotton pellets placed interproximally with periodontal dressing should be utilized to aid in clot formation and to prevent clot disruption.
   - Gentle hydrogen peroxide mouthwashes may aid in controlling gingival hemorrhage.
   - Close postsurgical follow-up should ensue.
5. Note that scaling and root planing may be carefully performed at low platelet levels (30,000 cells/mm^3).

Nonthrombocytopenic Purpuras

Nonthrombocytopenic purpuras occur as a result of either vascular wall fragility or platelet dysfunction (thrombasthe-

---

Table 34–8. HEMOPHILIA: TESTS AND TREATMENT

Hemophilia Type	Prolonged	Normal	Treatment
A	Partial thromboplastin time	Prothrombin time Bleeding time	Factor VIII cryoprecipitate, fresh frozen plasma, or fresh whole blood Epsilon-aminocaproic acid
B	Partial thromboplastin time	Prothrombin time Bleeding time	Fresh frozen plasma Lyophilized Factor IX concentrate
von Willebrand's disease	Bleeding time Partial thromboplastin time Variable Factor VIII deficiency	Prothrombin time Platelet count	Cryoprecipitate or plasma

nia). The former occurs from a multitude of causes: hypersensitivity reactions (immunologic connective tissue diseases), scurvy, infections, chemicals (phenacetin and aspirin), dysproteinemia, and several others. Thrombasthenia occurs in uremia, Glanzmann's disease, aspirin ingestion, and von Willebrand's disease.[66] Both kinds of nonthrombocytopenic purpuras may result in "immediate" bleeding after gingival injury. Treatment consists primarily of direct pressure applied for at least 15 minutes. This initial pressure should control the bleeding unless coagulation times are abnormal or reinjury occurs. Surgical therapy should be avoided unless the qualitative and quantitative platelet problems are resolved.

BLOOD DYSCRASIAS

Numerous disorders of red and white blood cells may affect the course of periodontal therapy. Alterations in wound healing, bleeding, tissue appearance, and susceptibility to infection may occur (see Chapter 14). Clinicians should be aware of the clinical signs and symptoms of blood dyscrasias, the availability of screening laboratory tests, and the need for physician referral.

Leukemia

Altered periodontal treatment for leukemic patients is based on such patients' enhanced susceptibility to infections, their bleeding tendency, and the effects of chemotherapy. The treatment plan for these patients is as follows:

1. Refer the patient for medical evaluation and treatment. Close cooperation with the physician is required.
2. Prior to chemotherapy, a complete periodontal plan should be developed with a physician (see the section on treatment for patients receiving chemotherapy).
   - Monitor hematologic laboratory values daily: bleeding time, coagulation time, prothrombin time, and platelet count.
   - Administer antibiotic coverage before any periodontal treatment.
   - Extract all hopeless, nonmaintainable, or potentially infectious teeth a minimum of 10 days before the initiation of chemotherapy, if systemic conditions allow.
   - Periodontal debridement (scaling and root planing) should be performed and thorough oral hygiene instructions given if the patient's condition allows. Twice-daily rinsing with 0.12% chlorhexidine gluconate is recommended after oral hygiene procedures. If there is an irregular bleeding time, careful debridement with cotton pellets soaked in 3% hydrogen peroxide may be performed around the necks of the teeth.
3. During the acute phases of leukemia, patients should receive only emergency periodontal care.
   - Persistent gingival bleeding usually occurs deep in a periodontal pocket and should be treated as follows:
     1. Cleanse the area with 3% hydrogen peroxide or 0.12% chlorhexidine gluconate.
     2. Carefully explore the area and remove any etiologic local factors, making every effort to avoid gingival injury.
     3. Recleanse the area with 3% hydrogen peroxide.
     4. Place a cotton pellet soaked in thrombin against the bleeding point.
     5. Cover with gauze and apply pressure for 15 to 20 minutes.
     6. If oozing persists after the removal of gauze and pressure, replace the cotton pellet (saturated with 3% hydrogen peroxide), hold firmly, and place a periodontal dressing over the area for 24 hours.
   - Acute necrotizing ulcerative gingivitis often complicates the oral picture in acute and subacute leukemia. Treatment should be designed to make the patient comfortable and to eliminate a source of systemic toxicity. Routine treatment procedures for acute necrotizing ulcerative gingivitis should be followed (see Chapter 39).
   - Acute gingival or periodontal abscesses are common sources of pain in these patients and are associated with regional adenopathy and systemic complications. Treatment is as follows:
     1. Systemic antibiotics.
     2. Gentle incision and drainage.
     3. Cleansing with cotton pellets saturated with either 3% hydrogen peroxide or 0.12% chlorhexidine gluconate.
   - Oral ulcerations should be treated with antibiotics and bland mouthrinses.
     1. Topical anesthetic rinses such as viscous lidocaine (Xylocaine) or promethazine hydrochloride syrup may be prescribed.
     2. Topical protective ointments such as Orabase may be applied.
     3. Sharp irritative areas (e.g., bony spicules) or appliances should be removed.
   - Oral moniliasis is common in the leukemic patient and can be treated with nystatin suspensions (100,000 U/ml) or vaginal suppositories.
4. In patients with chronic leukemia and those in remission, scaling and root planing can be performed without complication, but periodontal surgery should be avoided if possible.
   - Bleeding time should be measured on the day of the procedure. If it is low, postpone the appointment and refer the patient to a physician.
   - Plaque control and frequent recall visits should receive particular attention.

Agranulocytosis

Patients with agranulocytosis (cyclic neutropenia and granulocytopenia) are more susceptible to infection than unaffected patients. There is a reduction in total white blood cell count and a reduction in or disappearance of granular leukocytes. The periodontal destruction caused by inflammation is exaggerated, and therefore, treatment should be performed only during periods of remission of the disease. At such times, treatment should be conservative. Oral hygiene instruction should include use of chlorhexidine mouthrinses twice daily. Scaling and root planing should be performed carefully under antibiotic protection. Because aminopyrines, barbiturates, and chloramphenicol have been implicated as potential causes of agranulocytosis, their use should be avoided.

INFECTIOUS DISEASES

Rarely does the periodontist contract or transfer an infectious disease if adequate precautions have been taken.

However, the undiagnosed, untreated patient who provides an incomplete medical history is a potential hazard to the dentist, staff, and other patients. This section provides a discussion of hepatitis, sexually transmitted diseases, acquired immunodeficiency syndrome (AIDS), and tuberculosis in relation to the precautions required in periodontal therapy.

Hepatitis

Hepatitis is divided into three clinically similar diseases (A, B, and non-A, non-B [or C]) that differ in their virology, epidemiology and prophylaxis (Table 34–9).

Because up to 75% of individuals affected with hepatitis are undiagnosed, the clinician must be able to screen for and recognize the symptoms of hepatitis (Table 34–10). The clinician should be aware of high-risk groups, such as renal dialysis patients, hospital (professional) personnel, blood bank personnel, morgue workers, homosexuals, obstetrics and gynecology personnel, immunosuppressed patients, drug users, and institutionalized patients.

Ten to 15 percent of hepatitis B patients may have chronic forms of the disease; therefore, all those who report a past history of hepatitis should be carefully screened. *It is recommended that hepatitis B vaccination be administered to all personnel who come in contact with a patient's blood[11]; also, Occupational Safety and Health Administration guidelines and barrier techniques should be strictly followed.*

The following should be the framework for treating hepatitis patients:

1. If the disease, regardless of type, is active, do not provide periodontal therapy unless the situation is an emergency; in an emergency case, follow the protocol for HB_sAg-positive patients.
2. For patients with a past history of hepatitis, consult the physician to determine type of hepatitis, course and length of the disease, mode of transmission, and required laboratory tests (Table 34–11).
3. For recovered type A hepatitis patients, perform routine periodontal care.
4. For recovered type B patients, consult with the physician and order HB_sAg and anti-HB_s determinations (Fig. 34–2).
   - If HB_sAg and anti-HB_s tests are negative but you suspect that hepatitis B virus is present, order another HB_s determination.
   - Patients who are HB_sAg positive are probably infective; the degree of infectivity is measured via an HB_sAg determination.
   - Patients who are anti-HB_s positive may be treated routinely.
5. If a patient with positive HB_sAg status or active hepatitis requires emergency treatment, use the following precautions:
   - Consult the patient's physician regarding status.
   - If bleeding is likely, measure prothrombin time and bleeding time; alter treatment accordingly.
   - All personnel in clinical contact with the patient should use full barrier technique, including masks, gloves, glasses or eye shield, and disposable gowns.
   - All instruments should be placed on a sheet of aluminum foil.
   - All disposable items (gauze, floss, saliva ejectors, masks, gowns, gloves, and aluminum foil) should be placed in one lined wastebasket.
   - Minimize aerosol production by not using ultrasonic instrumentation, air syringe, or high-speed handpieces; remember that saliva contains a distillate of the virus. Prerinsing with chlorhexidine gluconate for 30 seconds is highly recommended.
   - When the procedure is completed, all equipment should be scrubbed and sterilized. Instruments should be moved while still on the aluminum foil to the sink and rinsed with diluted sodium hypochlorite (1:3) for 10 minutes; next, they should be scrubbed, placed loosely in autoclave bags, and sterilized. Handpieces should also be autoclaved.
   - The dental chair and unit should be wiped down with dilute sodium hypochlorite.
   - Use as many disposable covers as possible; aluminum foil may be used for covering light handles, drawer handles, and bracket trays; headrest covers should also be used.
   - All disposable items should be gathered, bagged in plastic, tied, labeled, and removed for proper disposal.
   - Aseptic technique should be practiced at all time. Remove

Table 34–9. COMPARISON OF HEPATITIS A; B; AND NON-A, NON-B

Features	Type A	Type B	Type Non-A, Non-B
Antigen	A virus (HAV)	B virus (HBV) B surface antigen (HB_sAg) B core antigen (HB_cAg) B e antigen (HB_eAg)	Not specifically identified or characterized
Antibody	Antibody to A virus (anti-HAV)	Antibody to B surface antigen (anti-HB_s) Antibody to B core antigen (anti-HB_c) Antibody to B e antigen (anti-HB_e)	Not specifically identified or characterized
Incubation	15–40 days	50–180 days	15–180 days
Route of transmission	Fecal-oral (may occur parenterally)	Parenteral (has been found in all body fluids, however)	Parenteral
Virus in blood	Early acute and late incubation periods	Acute phase and late incubation phase; may persist for months or years (5%–10% carrier state)	Probably similar to type B
Age group	Children and young adults	All age groups	All age groups

Table 34–10. SIGNS AND SYMPTOMS OF ACUTE VIRAL HEPATITIS

Phase	Signs and Symptoms
Preicteric phase: onset is acute in hepatitis A and insidious in hepatitis B	Fever Fatigue Anorexia Nausea, vomiting Abdominal pain Myalgia
Icteric phase: 4 : 1 anicteric : icteric	Jaundice, biliuria Increased anorexia Increased nausea, vomiting Increased abdominal pain Mental depression Bradycardia Periarteritis
Posticteric phase	Disappearance of signs and symptoms Hepatomegaly may persist

Table 34–11. LABORATORY TESTS FOR HEPATITIS

SGOT and SGPT: determine hepatocellular necrosis (hepatitis A peaks at 40 days; hepatitis B peaks at 80–90 days)
Albumin: determines liver breakdown
Bilirubin: determines extent of liver dysfunction
Prothrombin time: determines clotting factors produced by the liver

SGOT, Serum glutamic-oxaloacetic transaminase; SGPT, serum glutamic-pyruvic transaminase.

rings and arm jewelry, and perform multiple vigorous hand lather and rinse cycles.

6. Patients who are HB$_s$Ag negative may be treated routinely.

For health care personnel exposed to a patient known to be HB$_s$Ag positive the currently available method of secondary prevention is administration of immunoglobulin. Hepatitis B immunoglobulin (0.05–0.07 ml per kilogram of body weight) is administered within 7 days of exposure, and a second dose is given 25 to 30 days later. Immune serum globulin is effective in preventing hepatitis A if given within 2 weeks of exposure. A vaccine of HB$_s$Ag is available for immunization in three doses over a 6-month span. It is believed to be effective over a 5-year period and is recommended for those in high-risk groups.

Sexually Transmitted Diseases

The U.S. Public Health Service has categorized sexually transmitted diseases into four groups: syphilis, gonorrhea, herpes, and AIDS. Those patients with active disease should receive emergency care only. Prophylaxis measures as listed in the section on hepatitis should be adhered to.

Remember that oral lesions of primary and secondary syphilis, gonorrhea, herpes, and AIDS are infectious.

Patients found to be free of disease may receive routine periodontal therapy. If the periodontist finds lesions or symptomatology suggestive of syphilis or gonorrhea, the patient should be referred for medical evaluation. The patient with herpetic lesions may receive treatment when the lesions resolve. However, the periodontist should take precautions if a history of recurrent lesions is given.

AIDS

AIDS was first reported as a specific disease in 1981. Human immunodeficiency virus (HIV) was isolated in 1983 as the causative agent of AIDS and AIDS-related complex (ARC). This retrovirus may take from 6 to 8 weeks from the time of exposure to produce measurable HIV antibodies. Also, clinical symptoms of AIDS and ARC may not become manifest for years. An estimated 1.5 to 3 million individuals are carriers of the virus. A full description of the clinical manifestations is presented in Chapter 15. The management of periodontal disease in AIDS patients is discussed in Chapter 46.

Periodontal treatment for AIDS, ARC, and HIV-positive patients involves close adherence to barrier techniques, care in use of all sharp instruments, and proper sterilization. It has been recommended that clinicians wear a gown if aerosols are to be used; however, the Centers for Disease Control and Prevention (CDC) reports that washing clothing with household bleach in a normal cycle at a high temperature (60°C to 70°C), followed by machine drying

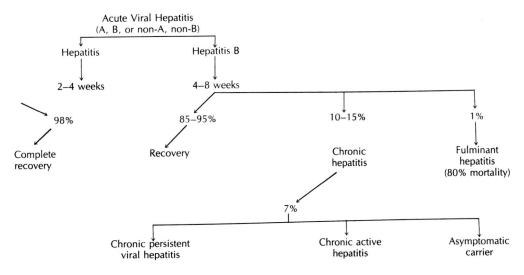

FIGURE 34–2. Clinical courses of hepatitis.

(100°C), will inactivate the AIDS virus. The CDC also recommends sterilization of handpieces; flushing of air-water syringes, Cavitron tips, and handpieces; and thorough removal of blood from surfaces. Areas difficult to disinfect should be wrapped with impervious covering (plastic, waxed or plastic-based papers, or aluminum foil).

Tuberculosis

The patient with tuberculosis should receive emergency care only, following the guidelines listed in the section on hepatitis. If the patient has completed chemotherapy, his or her physician should be consulted regarding infectivity and the results of sputum cultures for *Mycobacterium tuberculosis*. When medical clearance has been given and the sputum culture results are negative, these patients may be treated normally. Any patient who gives a history of poor medical follow-up (e.g., lack of yearly chest radiographs) or shows signs or symptoms indicative of tuberculosis should be referred for evaluation. Note that adequate treatment of tuberculosis requires a minimum of 18 months, and thorough post-treatment follow-up should include chest radiographs, sputum cultures, and a review of the patient's symptoms by the physician at least every 12 months.

REFERENCES

1. Adisman IK. Characteristics of irradiated soft and hard tissues. J Prosthet Dent 35:549, 1976.
2. Bailey GL, ed. Hemodialysis: Principles and Practice. New York, Academic Press, 1972.
3. Beumer J. Maxillofacial Rehabilitation: Prosthodontic and Surgical Considerations. St Louis, CV Mosby, 1979.
4. Bottomley WK, Cioffi RF, Martin AJ. Dental management of the patient treated by renal transplantation: Preoperative and postoperative considerations. J Am Dent Assoc 85:1330, 1972.
5. Brashear RE, Rhodes HL. Chronic Obstructive Lung Disease: Clinical Treatment and Management. St Louis, CV Mosby, 1978.
6. Brown LR, Dreizen S, Daly TE. Interrelations of oral microorganisms, immunoglobulins and dental caries following radiotherapy. J Dent Res 57:882, 1978.
7. Burkett LR. Oral Medicine. 6th ed. Philadelphia, JB Lippincott, 1971.
8. Burton GG, Gee GN, Hodgkin JE, eds. Respiratory Care: A Guide to Clinical Practice. Philadelphia, JB Lippincott, 1977.
9. Butler DL. Team approach to oral health treatment of pre and post renal transplant patients. J Hosp Dent Pract 7:144, 1973.
9a. Carl W: Local radiation and systemic radiotherapy. J Am Dent Assoc 124:119, 1993.
10. Cotran RS, Kumar V, Robbins SL, eds. Robbins Pathologic Basis of Disease. 4th ed. Philadelphia, WB Saunders, 1989.
11. Cottone JA. Recent developments in hepatitis: New virus, vaccine and dosage recommendations. J Am Dent Assoc 120:501, 1990.
12. Dajani AS, Bisho AL, Chung KJ, et al. Prevention of bacterial endocarditis: Recommendations by the American Heart Association, Clinical Cardiology. JAMA 264:2919, 1990.
13. Drapkin MS. Endocarditis after the use of an oral irrigation device. Ann Intern Med 87:455, 1977.
14. Dreifus LS, Cohen D. Implanted pacemakers: Medicolegal implications. Am J Cardiol 36:266, 1975.
15. Reference deleted.
16. Reference deleted.
17. Durack DT. Prophylaxis of infective endocarditis. In Mandell GL, ed. Principles and Practice of Infectious Diseases. 3rd ed. New York, John Wiley & Sons, 1990.
18. Epstein FH, Merrill JP. Chronic renal failure. In Wilson JW, ed. Harrison's Principles of Internal Medicine. 12th ed. New York, McGraw-Hill, 1991.
19. Fine L. Dental care of the irradiated patient. J Hosp Dent Pract 9:127, 1975.
20. Frank RM, et al. Acquired dental defects and salivary gland lesions after irradiation for carcinoma. J Am Dent Assoc 70:168, 1965.
21. Friedewald WT. Epidemiology of cardiovascular disease. In Wyngaarden JB, Smith LH, eds. Cecil Textbook of Medicine. 18th ed. Philadelphia, WB Saunders, 1988.
22. Friedlander AH, Yoshikawa TT. Pathogenesis, management and prevention of infective endocarditis in the elderly dental patient. Oral Surg 69:177, 1990.
23. Frownfelter DL. Chest Physical Therapy and Pulmonary Rehabilitation. 2nd ed. Chicago, Year Book Medical, 1987.
24. Galler C, Epstein JB, Guze KA, et al. The development of osteoradionecrosis from sites of periodontal disease activity: Report of 3 cases. J Periodontol 63:310, 1992.
25. Geraci JE, Wilson WR, Washington JA. Infective endocarditis caused by *Actinobacillus actinomycetemcomitans*. Report of four cases. Mayo Clin Proc 55:415, 1980.
26. Goldman HM, Cohen DW. Periodontal Therapy. 6th ed. St Louis, CV Mosby, 1980.
27. Heard E Jr, Staples AF, Czerwinsku AW. The dental patient with renal disease. Precautions and guidelines. J Am Dent Assoc 96:792, 1978.
28. Kaplan EL, Anderson RC. Infective endocarditis after use of dental irrigation device. Lancet 2:810, 1977.
29. Kaplan EL, Taranta AV, eds. Infective Endocarditis: An American Heart Association Symposium. AHA Monograph Series. 52. Dallas, 1977.
30. Kaye D. Prophylaxis of endocarditis. In Kaplan EL, Taranta AV, eds. Infective Endocarditis. Baltimore, University Park Press, 1976.
31. Kirkpatrick TJ, Morton JB. Factors influencing the dental management of renal transplant and dialysis patients. Br J Oral Surg 9:57, 1971.
32. Kraut RA, Hicks JL. Bacterial endocarditis of dental origin. Report of a case. J Oral Surg 34:1031, 1976.
33. Larson CE, Chang J, Bleyaert AL, Bedger R. Anesthetic considerations for oral surgery patients with hemophilia. J Oral Surg 38:516, 1980.
34. Lenihan J. Considerations of systemic disease. In Steiner RB, Thompson RD, eds. Oral Surgery and Anesthesia. Philadelphia, WB Saunders, 1977.
35. Lindemann RA, Henson JL. The dental management of patients with vascular grafts placed in the treatment of arterial occlusive disease. J Am Dent Assoc 104:625, 1982.
36. Little JW, Falace DA. Dental Management of the Medically Compromised Patient. 3rd ed. St Louis, CV Mosby, 1988.
37. Malamed SF. Medical Emergencies in the Dental Office. St Louis, CV Mosby, 1987.
38. McCarthy FM. Emergencies in Dental Practice. 4th ed. Philadelphia, WB Saunders, 1982.
39. McCarthy FM. Safe treatment of the post heart attack patient. Compend Contin Educ Dent 10:598, 1989.
39a. Mealey BL, Semba SE, Halloran WW. Dentistry and the cancer patient. Part I. Oral manifestation and complications of chemotherapy. Compend Contin Educ Dent 15:142, 1994.
40. Mulkey TF. Outpatient treatment of hemophiliacs for dental extractions. J Oral Surg 34:428, 1976.
41. Munroe CO, Lazarus TL. Predisposing conditions of infective endocarditis. J Can Dent Assoc 42:483, 1976.
42. Neutze JM, Arter WJ. Bacterial endocarditis and the dentist. NZ Dent J 67:79, 1971.
43. Nevins M, Becker W, Kornman K. Proceedings of the World Workshop in Clinical Periodontics. Princeton, NJ, 1989.
44. Nickens GE, Patterson SS, El-Kafrawy AH, et al. Effect of cobalt-60 irradiation on the pulp of restored teeth. J Am Dent Assoc 94:701, 1977.
45. Oparil S. Arterial hypertension. In Wyngaarden JB, Smith LH Jr, Bennett JC, eds. Cecil Textbook of Medicine. 19th ed. Philadelphia, WB Saunders, 1991.
46. Ore DE, Shriner WA. Doctor, don't shut off that pacemaker. CDS Rev 67:22, 1974.
47. Piche JE, Swan RH, Hallman WW. The glycosylated hemoglobin assay for diabetes: Its value to the periodontist. Two case reports. J Periodontol 60:640, 1989.
48. Rankow RW, Weissman B. Osteoradionecrosis of the mandible. Ann Otol Rhinol Laryngol 80:603, 1971.
49. Rees T. The diabetic patient. In Wilson TG, Kornman K, Newman MG, eds. Advances in Periodontics. Chicago, Quintessence Publishing, 1992.
50. Report of the Joint National Committee on Detection, Evaluation and Treatment of High Blood Pressure. Arch Intern Med 153:6, 1993.
51. Rezai FR. Dental treatment of a patient with a cardiac pacemaker: Review of the literature. Oral Surg 44:662, 1977.
52. Rodriguez V. Bacterial infection in immunosuppressed patients. Diagnosis and management. Transplant Proc 5:1249, 1973.
53. Russel RP. Systemic hypertension. In Harvey A, ed. Osler's Principles and Practice of Medicine. 22nd ed. New York, Apple-Century-Crofts, 1988.
54. Santiago A. The role of the dentist in radiotherapy. J Prosthet Dent 30:196, 1973.
55. Santinga JT, Fekety RF Jr, Bottomley WK, et al. Antibiotic prophylaxis for endocarditis in patients with a prosthetic heart valve. J Am Dent Assoc 93:1001, 1976.
56. Schimpff SC, et al. Radiation-related thyroid dysfunction: Implications for the treatment of Hodgkin's disease. Ann Intern Med 92:91, 1980.
57. Scopp IW. An overview of the heart patient in dental practice. NY J Dent 49:48, 1979.
58. Shannon IL, Starcke EN, Wescott WB. Effect of radiotherapy on whole saliva flow. J Dent Res 56:693, 1977.
59. Shannon IL, Wescott WB, Starcke EN, et al. Laboratory study of cobalt-60 irradiated human dental enamel. J Oral Med 33:23, 1978.
60. Shannon IL. A saliva substitute for use by xerostomic patients undergoing radiotherapy to the head and neck. Oral Surg 44:656, 1977.

61. Shapiro BA, et al. Rehabilitation in chronic obstructive pulmonary disease: A two year prospective study. Resp Care *22*:1045, 1977.
62. Shapiro BA. Clinical Application of Respiratory Care. 4th ed. Chicago, Year Book Medical, 1991.
63. Slots J, Rosling BG, Genco RJ. Suppression of penicillin resistant oral *Actinobacillus actinomycetemcomitans* with tetracycline. Considerations in endocarditis prophylaxis. J Periodontol *54*:193, 1983.
64. Steiner RB, Thompson RD, eds. Oral Surgery and Anesthesia. Philadelphia, WB Saunders, 1976.
65. Sugarman JR. Prevalence of diagnosed hypertension among diabetic Navajo Indians. Arch Intern Med *150*:359, 1990.
66. Sydney SB, Ross R. Periodontal surgery in a patient with von Willenbrand's disease. J Am Dent Assoc *102*:660, 1981.
67. Thalen HJ, Meere CC, eds. Fundamentals of Cardiac Pacing. Boston, Nyhoff Publishing, 1979.
68. Veterans Administration Cooperative Study: Effect of treatment on morbidity in hypertension. JAMA *213*:1143, 1970.
69. Wells TJ. A new concept in the control of acute gingival hemorrhage. J Am Dent Assoc *102*:660, 1981.
70. Westbrook SD. Dental management of patients receiving hemodialysis and kidney transplants. J Am Dent Assoc *96*:464, 1978.
71. Whitsett TL. Modification of drug dosages in renal disease. J Okla State Med *65*:129, 1972.
72. Wright AD. Ischaemic heart disease and hypertension. Br Dent J *142*:226, 1977.
73. Wyngaarden JB, Smith LH Jr, Bennett JC, eds. Cecil Textbook of Medicine. 19th ed. Philadelphia, WB Saunders, 1991.

35

Periodontal Treatment of Geriatric Patients

JOAN OTOMO-CORGEL

Demographics
Clinical Assessment of the Geriatric Patient
Treatment of the Geriatric Patient
Intraoral Examination

Oral Hygiene Instruction
Treatment of Periodontal Disease
Root Caries
Xerostomia

Aging is the process by which a person grows old, irrespective of the time required. It includes the complex interactions of biologic, psychologic, and sociologic processes over time.[9] The historically accepted chronologic landmark of old age is 65 years. However, a more useful taxonomy of aging based on function has been established. The geriatric literature refers to the following categories: functionally dependent elderly (with illness or impairment); frail and institutionalized elderly; young old, 65 to 70 years of age (healthy and vigorous); old, 75 to 85 years of age; and old old, 85 years of age and older.[16]

This chapter reviews demographics and periodontal diagnosis and treatment, including alterations and precautions, in the elderly patient. Therapy may depend on the category of the aged patient and the related psychologic and emotional status.

DEMOGRAPHICS

The elderly population has increased in an explosive fashion.[7] In 1900, 3 million people were considered aged. Currently the number is 23 million, or 11.3% of the U.S. population. It is estimated that by 2030, 67 million persons, or 20% of the population, will be 65 years of age or older.[36] The fastest growing segment is the over-85 age group; this group spends more per capita on medical care than any other group.[13]

The National Center for Health Statistics has reported a decrease in edentulousness.[26] The pattern of use of dental services, however, may not have changed dramatically. The American Dental Association has reported an increase in the number of elderly patients seeking restorative and preventive care, yet older people use fewer dental services than younger adults.[15,18] Socioeconomic status seems to play a role,[6,27] as do functional dependence and poorer health status. Studies suggest that 70% of elderly persons require some dental treatment; yet only 25% to 40% perceive this need, and only 20% to 35% actually seek treatment.[2,35] (One survey indicated that 25% of patients in general dental practices are elderly.)

Epidemiologic studies on aging and periodontal disease indicate confusion with regard to prevalence and future trends. There has been a decline in the incidence of edentulousness,[19] but tooth loss in late life is a complex multifaceted problem resulting from cummulative effects on teeth and periodontium. The impact of tooth retention and the potential for increased periodontal disease in the elderly have not been thoroughly researched.

There is evidence of an increase in missing teeth in the elderly compared with the young[5,33]; however, findings of gingivitis[21,31] and advanced periodontal disease[32,34] in the elderly are inconsistent. Ninety-five percent of dentulous individuals older than 65 years have periodontal disease.

According to Douglass and associates, the need for professional periodontal therapy in the elderly will increase for the remainder of the 20th century.[8] After about the year 2010, the proportion of elderly individuals without advanced periodontal disease may begin to decline if younger cohorts in the population maintain improved oral health care status into their older years.[8]

Other investigators, however, believe that the number of elderly individuals requiring periodontal treatment will most likely increase. Findings such as gingival recession, loss of gingival attachment, and decreased number of remaining teeth appear to be significantly correlated with both biologic age and chronologic age, although the correlation is higher with the former.[11] It is apparent that there is a need for further evaluation of the periodontal treatment needs of the elderly as well as of the nature of the disease in this population.

CLINICAL ASSESSMENT OF THE GERIATRIC PATIENT

Physical and Medical Examination. Examination of the patient begins with the first visual encounter. The clinician should assess the patient for posture, gait, color, mobility, and facial characteristics. Medical histories can be enhanced by an astute visual examination. When developing the medical history, the clinician should look at the patient at eye level and speak clearly, not talking down to the patient. The clinician should pace the speed of the examination and be aware that visual and auditory acuity are generally reduced in these patients.

Table 35–1. PHYSICAL MANIFESTATIONS OF AGING

External

Hair—brittle, less abundant, gray

Skin—dehydration, decreased elasticity, thermosensitive (thinner epithelium, senile freckles, keratoses, ash angiomas)

Eyes—diminished vision, enophthalmos, arcus senilis of cornea, presbyopia

Ears—loss of auditory acuity; nerve atrophy of nerve cells in basal coil of cochlea

Nose—diminished sense of smell

Secretory glands—diminished epithelial activity (saliva, tears, gastrointestinal tract, sweat, and sebaceous glands)

Physical stress—impaired homeostasis

Internal

Renal—Decreased renal blood flow leading to water retention and difficulty in removing waste products and drugs. Nocturnal polyuria and prostatic hypertrophy (in men). Increased renal threshold of sugar excretion

Vascular system—Progressive rise in systolic blood pressure. Diastolic pressure should be unaltered

Blood—Red blood cell count and hemoglobin slightly decreased owing to reduced activity of bone marrow and increased fragility of red cells. Anemias are common in women

Gastrointestinal—Constipation and gas accumulation due to hypotonic musculature. Decreased hunger contractions. Decreased gastric activity (hypochlorhydria is common at 50 years, with diminished absorption of calcium and vitamin C)

Gonads—Decrease in estrogen and androgen secretion with disturbances in protein metabolism

Liver—Decreased hepatic function, glycogen content, and bile secretion. Impaired cholesterol metabolism (arteriosclerosis)

Pancreas—Decreased function (susceptibility to diabetes)

Adapted from Freedman KA: Management of the Geriatric Dental Patient. Chicago, Quintessence Publishing, 1979.

Table 35–2. ALTERATIONS IN ORAL MOTOR FUNCTIONS IN AGING

Altered Function	Clinical Implication
Lip posture	Drooling; angular cheilosis
Muscles of mastication	Efficiency of mastication
Tongue function	Speech; dysphagia; traumatic bite injury; snoring; sleep apnea
Swallowing	Dysphagia; regurgitation; choking
Taste	Dysgeusia, ageusia
Salivation	No significant changes in healthy older patients

There is a tendency for the elderly patient to not remember or to deny medical problems. Therefore, medical history taking requires greater time and patience on the part of the practitioner. Eighty-one percent of noninstitutionalized persons older than 65 years of age have one or more chronic diseases. Two of five are categorized as functionally dependent or frail elderly, which indicates that their activities and ability to execute adequate oral hygiene are limited (Table 35–1). The majority are receiving medications (probably more than one) and have altered metabolism and sensitivity to prescription drugs.[1,23] Patients should be advised to bring their medications to the office. Medical histories may be taken from a relative, spouse, or responsible other if the patient is functionally dependent, frail, or an unreliable historian. When eliciting the medical history, it is necessary to assess alterations in motor function to gain insight into potential medical problems[4] (Table 35–2).

Social and Mental Examination. Elderly patients' attitudes toward therapy have a significant impact on the success or failure of periodontal therapy. Freedman[9] has described three commonly encountered behavior types:

1. Overdependent: demanding, urgent, and repetitious.
2. Pseudocooperative: comes on time, pays for service, is friendly and listens to instructions, but somehow never carries them out.
3. Perfectionist: makes unrealistic demands with veiled threats, interprets his or her own symptoms, adjusts own dentures, makes suggestions about the diagnosis or treatment plan, and tries to eat with dentures what he or she could not eat with natural teeth.

Many elderly patients become frustrated easily, especially in the anxiety-provoking dental environment. On the other hand, many geriatric patients may respond well to therapy and be tolerant of long procedures. The dentist must be cognizant of treating individuals who have unique life experiences, expectations, and needs.

TREATMENT OF THE GERIATRIC PATIENT

Intraoral Examination

The oral cavity of an elderly patient often has an altered appearance when compared with that of a youthful patient. There is a decrease in intracellular water content, amount of subcutaneous fat, elasticity, vascularity, muscle tone, and vertical dimension. Nonkeratinized areas may have thinner epithelium with a waxy appearance. Hyperkeratosis exists where keratin is present.

The tongue may have progressive defoliation of the papillae. The dorsum is fissured, whereas lingual surfaces have varicosities. Some investigators[27] say that there is a decrease in or alteration of taste, although other researchers assert that this may not be true.[3] There is a higher occurrence of smooth, glossy, and painful tongues owing to vitamin B_{12} deficiencies, as well as erythema migrans (also known as "geographic tongue") and *Candida* infections.[20] Table 35–3 lists some oral mucous membrane lesions that are common in the elderly.

Aging and periodontal changes are discussed in Chapter 3. According to the data relating to aging and periodontal disease, host response to plaque microorganisms is altered with increasing age. The inflammatory response of the marginal gingiva is more pronounced, which may reflect a local defense mechanism in which the host compensates for a less effective immune response or a decline in the effectiveness of polymorphonuclear leukocytes and monocytes in phagocytosis.[30] No difference in progression of disease in deeper periodontal tissues has been shown between young and elderly individuals, however.

Oral Hygiene Instruction

Before beginning oral hygiene instruction, the practitioner should consider the special needs of the geriatric patient. The clinician should speak clearly, establish good eye contact, not raise his or her voice (especially into a hearing aid), and adapt to the patient. The following should be included in oral hygiene instruction:

1. The patient should establish a daily routine.
2. Fluoride dentifrices should be used.
3. Instruments can be adapted as needed:
   - Toothbrushes can be bent under hot water.
   - Handles can be customized with acrylic coating, a bicycle grip, or a rubber ball to enhance the grip for patients with arthritis or other disorders.
   - The patient can use electrical brushes or interproximal brushes, as needed.

Treatment of Periodontal Disease

Periodontal disease in the elderly can be successfully treated. The clinician, however, must recognize the functional category of the elderly patient being treated by exploring his or her physical as well as psychologic and emotional status. This is necessary to determine prognosis and plan treatment to address the patient's real and perceived needs.

Age is not a contraindication to periodontal surgery.[14] Several considerations should be followed when the elderly patient is a candidate for surgical therapy:[12]

1. Decrease the length of surgical (operative) time (shorter visits).
2. Maintain open communication and establish adequate rapport.
3. Confirm the patient's ability to perform adequate home care.
4. Minimize trauma.
5. Recalculate medication dosages (owing to increased sensitivity in elderly patients).
6. Schedule morning appointments.

Elderly patients categorized as frail, functionally dependent, or emotionally or psychologically not amenable to surgical periodontal therapy may require scaling, root planing, and frequent monitoring, rather than surgical intervention. The treatment plan depends on the goal of therapy and the patient's medical status, attitude, degree of support, and ability to maintain adequate oral hygiene. The range of care options includes palliative therapy, radical therapy (extraction), or tooth retention therapy.

Root Caries

Fluoride treatments should be provided to geriatric patients to counter the increased incidence of caries among the elderly.[6] The majority of dental caries in the older population are root surface caries, which progress slowly, rarely affect the pulp, and are generally painless.[24] Topical fluoride should be provided after preventive maintenance visits in patients who are susceptible to caries.[24]

Studies have shown that meticulous oral hygiene and single topical fluoride treatments with daily use of a fluoride toothpaste can arrest root caries.[29] Recommendations for patients with a high incidence of root caries include (1) daily brushing with a fluoride toothpaste or 0.4% fluoride gel and (2) once-weekly acidulated phosphofluoride rinse, followed immediately by 1.64% stannous fluoride rinse. The patient should be advised to rinse after mechanical

Table 35–3. ORAL MUCOUS MEMBRANE LESIONS IN THE ELDERLY

Problem	Cause	Treatment
Mucositis/glossitis	Systemic disease (e.g., diabetes, hematologic disease/anemia/leukemia, chronic mouth breathing) Nutritional deficiencies (especially vitamin B complexes) Adverse drug reactions (e.g., phenolphthalein, phenacetin, aspirin, antibiotics, contact stomatitis from topical agents)[10]	Complete blood count Vitamin B_{12} evaluation Rule out xerostomia Palliative mouthwash prescription: diphenhydramine (Benadryl)/kaolin (Kaopectate) in equal parts, 1-minute rinse, then expectorate; or lidocaine (Xylocaine viscous) 2%[16]
Infection from immunosuppression Candidiasis	Systemic disease (diabetes, leukemia) Xerostomia Immunosuppression (prolonged steroid use) Antibiotic or antineoplastic medications Ill-fitting prosthesis	Improved oral hygiene Antifungal medications

home care and not to rinse with water, eat, or drink for 30 minutes after fluoride rinsing.

Xerostomia

Saliva has multiple functions in the oral cavity. It is a protective cleanser (with antibacterial activity), a buffer (inhibiting demineralization), a lubricant, a digestive necessity, and a transport medium to taste sensors. When xerostomia ensues, all of these functions are seriously altered. Signs and symptoms include intraoral dryness or burning, alterations in tongue surface, dysphagia, cheilosis, alterations in taste, difficulty with speech, and development of root caries.

Eighty percent of elderly patients receive medications; 90% of these medications can produce xerostomia. More than 200 commonly used drugs have xerostomia as a side effect. In addition, radiation and/or chemotherapy, psychologic conditions, endocrine disorders, and nutritional disorders may contribute to xerostomia.

Treatment of xerostomia should include the following:
1. Scrupulous oral hygiene (with soft toothbrushes).
2. Fluoride rinses and dentifrices.
3. Reduced consumption of alcohol; tobacco; and highly spicy, acidic foods.
4. Frequent water intake (to reduce sugars).
5. Artificial saliva substitutes.
6. Consultation with a physician if mucositis or candidiasis persists.
7. Careful use of home-care products with a high alcohol content.
8. For burning mouth:
   - Rule out other disorders such as candidiasis or pernicious anemia.
   - Treat with any of the following: saliva substitutes, equal-parts elixir of diphenhydramine (Benadryl) and kaolin (Kaopectate), and lidocaine (Xylocaine viscous).

In conclusion, the geriatric population is expanding, and their needs for periodontal services are becoming specialized. The variety of intraoral, medical, social, mental, and physical problems encountered provide unlimited challenges to the clinician. If the needs of the geriatric patient are to be met, clinicians must be willing to care for each individual with patience. The mouth must be viewed as a reflection of the systemic condition, and treatment is approached accordingly.

REFERENCES

1. Baker KA, Levy SH, Chrischilles SA. Medications with dental significance: Usage in a nursing home population. Spec Care Dent *11*:19, 1991.
2. Banting DW. A study of dental care costs, time, and treatment requirements of older persons in the community. Can J Public Health *63*:508, 1972.
3. Baum BJ. The dentistry-gerontology connection. J Am Dent Assoc *109*:899, 1984.
4. Baum BJ, Bodner LJ. Aging and oral motor function: Evidence for altered performance among older persons. J Dent Res *62*:2, 1983.
5. Bossert WA, Marks HH. Prevalence and characteristics of periodontal disease in 12,800 persons under periodic dental observation. J Am Dent Assoc *52*:429, 1956.
6. Chauncey HH, et al. The incidence of coronal caries in normal aging male adults. J Dent Res *57A*:148, 1978.
7. Christensen GJ. The future of dentistry? Treatment shifts to the older adult. J Am Dent Assoc *123*:89, 1992.
8. Douglass C, Gillings D, Sollecito W, Gammon M. The potential for increase in the periodontal diseases of the aged population. J Periodontol *54*:721, 1983.
9. Freedman KA. Management of the Geriatric Dental Patient. Chicago, Quintessence Publishing, 1979.
10. Gandara BK, Truelove EL, Sommers EE. Preventive oral medicine for the geriatric patient: Focus on soft tissue. Calif Dent Assoc J *13*:21, 1985.
11. Hansen GC. An epidemiologic investigation of the effect of biologic aging on the breakdown of periodontal tissue. J Periodontol *44*:269, 1973.
12. Hardin F, ed. Clark's Clinical Dentistry. Vol 3, Section 17. Philadelphia, JB Lippincott, 1991.
13. Health United States. Life expectation at birth according to sex: Selected countries, 1970 and 1976. Washington, DC, US Department of Health, Education and Welfare, DHEW publication no. (PHS) 8-132, 1979, p 95.
14. Holm-Pedersen P. Pathology and treatment of periodontal disease. In Holm-Pedersen P, Löe H. Geriatric Dentistry. St Louis, CV Mosby, 1986.
15. Institute of Medicine. Public Policy Option for Better Dental Health. Publication no. 80-06. Washington, DC, National Academy Press, 1980.
16. Institute of Medicine. The Elderly and Functional Dependency. Washington, DC, June 1977.
17. Kamen S. Current concepts in geriatric dentistry. In Levine N, ed. Current Treatment in Dental Practice. Philadelphia, WB Saunders, 1986, pp 389–398.
18. Kiyik A. Age differences in oral health attitudes and dental service utilization. J Public Health Dept *42*:29, 1982.
19. Lloyd PM, Shag K. The how and why of tooth loss in the elderly. Geriatr Dentist Update VA Med Ctr *2*:1, 1988.
20. Lomax JD. Geriatric Ambulatory and Institutional Care. St Louis, Ishiyaki Euroamerica, 1987.
21. Lovdal A, Waerhaug JA. Incidence of clinical manifestations of periodontal disease in light of oral hygiene and calculus formation. J Am Dent Assoc *56*:21, 1958.
22. Mandel ID. Preventive dentistry for the elderly. Spec Care Dent *4*:157, 1983.
23. Maser MS. Geriatric pharmacology and dental implications. J Gen Dent *40*:215, 1992.
24. Massler M. Geriatric dentistry: Root caries in the elderly. J Prosthet Dent *44*:147, 1980.
25. Meskin LH, Mason LD. Problems in oral health care financing for the elderly. Clin Geriatr Med *8*:685, 1992.
26. National Center for Health Statistics. Edentulous Persons, United States—1971. Department of Health, Education, and Welfare, DHEW publication no. (HRA) 74-1516. Washington, DC, US Government Printing Office, 1974.
27. Narazeh M. Salivary gland hypofunction in elderly patients. Calif Dent Assoc J *22*:62, 1994.
28. Niessen L, Jones J. Dental implications for a grayer America. Calif Dent Assoc J *19*:29, 1991.
29. Nyvad B, Fejerskov G. Active root caries converted into inactive caries as a response to oral hygiene. Scand J Dent Res *94*:281, 1986.
30. Page RC. Periodontal disease in the elderly: A critical evaluation of current information. Gerodontology *3*:63, 1984.
31. Robinson PJ. Periodontal therapy for the aging mouth. Int Dent J *29*:220, 1979.
32. Roper RE, Knerr GW, Gocka EF, et al. Periodontal disease in aged individuals. J Periodontol *43*:304, 1972.
33. Russell AC. Some epidemiologic characteristics of periodontal disease in a series of urban populations. J Periodontol *28*:286, 1957.
34. Russell AC. Epidemiology of periodontal disease. Int Dent J *17*:282, 1967.
35. Smith JM, Sheiham A. Dental treatment needs and demands of an elderly population in England. Community Dent Oral Epidemiol *8*:360, 1980.
36. US Department of Commerce, Bureau of Census. Projections of the Population of the US: 1982 to 2050 (Advanced Report). Series P25, no 922, October 1982, pp 1–15.

36

The Periodontal Instrumentarium

ANNA M. PATTISON, GORDON L. PATTISON, and
HENRY H. TAKEI

Periodontal instruments are designed for specific purposes, such as removing calculus, planing root surfaces, curetting the gingiva, or removing diseased tissue. On first investigation, the variety of instruments available for similar purposes appears confusing. With experience, however, clinicians select a relatively small set that fulfills all requirements.

CLASSIFICATION OF PERIODONTAL INSTRUMENTS

Periodontal instruments are classified according to the purposes they serve, as follows:

1. *Periodontal probes* are used to locate, measure, and mark pockets and determine their course on individual tooth surfaces.
2. *Explorers* are used to locate calculus deposits and caries.
3. *Scaling, root planing, and curettage instruments* are used for removal of calcified deposits from the crown and root of a tooth, removal of altered cementum from the subgingival root surface, and debridement of the soft tissue lining the pocket. Scaling and curettage instruments are classified as follows:
   - *Sickle scalers* are heavy instruments used to remove supragingival calculus.
   - *Curettes* are fine instruments used for subgingival scaling, root planing, and removal of the soft tissue lining the pocket.
   - *Hoe, chisel, and file scalers* are used to remove tenacious

subgingival calculus and altered cementum. Their use is limited compared with that of curettes.
   - *Ultrasonic and sonic instruments* are used for scaling and cleansing tooth surfaces and curetting the soft tissue wall of the periodontal pocket.[3,4,7]
4. *Cleansing and polishing instruments*—rubber cups, brushes, and dental tape—are used to clean and polish tooth surfaces. Also available are air–powder abrasive systems for tooth polishing.

The wearing and cutting qualities of some types of steel used in periodontal instruments have been tested,[8,9] but specifications vary among manufacturers. Stainless steel is used most commonly in instrument manufacture. High-carbon steel instruments are also available and are considered by some clinicians to be superior.

Each group of instruments has characteristic features; individual therapists often develop variations with which they operate most effectively. Small instruments are recommended to fit into pockets without injuring the soft tissues.[12,15,16]

The parts of each instrument, referred to as the blade, shank, and handle, are shown in Figure 36–1.

Periodontal Probes

Periodontal probes are used to measure the depth of pockets and to determine their configuration. The typical probe is a tapered, rod-like instrument calibrated in millimeters, with a blunt, rounded tip (Fig. 36–2). There are

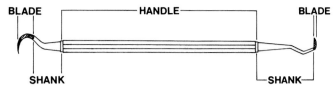

BLADE ——————— HANDLE ——————— BLADE

SHANK   SHANK

FIGURE 36–1. Parts of a typical periodontal instrument.

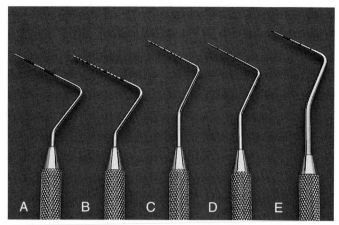

FIGURE 36–3. Types of periodontal probes. *A,* The Marquis color-coded probe. Calibrations are in 3-mm sections. *B,* The UNC-15 probe, a 15-mm-long probe with millimeter markings at each millimeter and color coding at the 5th, 10th, and 15th mm. *C,* The University of Michigan "O" probe, with Williams markings (at 1, 2, 3, 5, 7, 8, 9, and 10 mm). *D,* The Michigan "O" probe with markings at 3, 6, and 8 mm. *E,* The WHO (World Health Organization) probe, which has a 0.5 mm ball at the tip and millimeter markings at 3.5, 8.5, and 11.5 millimeters and color coding from 3.5 to 5.5 mm.

several other designs with various millimeter calibrations. The World Health Organization (WHO) probe has millimeter markings and a small round ball at the tip (Fig. 36–3). Ideally, these probes are thin, and the shank is angled to allow easy insertion into the pocket. Furcation areas can best be evaluated with the curved, blunt Nabers probe (Fig. 36–4).

When measuring a pocket, the probe is inserted with a firm, gentle pressure to the bottom of the pocket. The shank should be aligned with the long axis of the tooth surface to be probed. Several measurements are made to determine the level of attachment along the surface of the tooth.

Explorers

Explorers are used to locate subgingival deposits and carious areas and to check the smoothness of the root surfaces after root planing. Explorers are designed with different shapes and angles for a variety of uses. Some of the most commonly used explorers are shown in Figure 36–5, and their uses and limitations are shown in Figure 36–6. The periodontal probe can also be useful in the detection of subgingival deposits (see Fig. 36–6).

Scaling and Curettage Instruments

Scaling and curettage instruments are illustrated in Figure 36–7.

Sickle Scalers (Supragingival Scalers)

Sickle scalers have a flat surface and two cutting edges that converge in a sharply pointed tip. The arched shape of the instrument makes the tip strong so that it will not break off during use (Fig. 36–8). The sickle is used primarily to remove supragingival calculus (Fig. 36–9). Because of the design of this instrument, it is difficult to insert the blade under the gingiva without damaging the surrounding gingival tissues (Fig. 36–10). The sickle scaler is inserted under ledges of calculus no more than 1 mm below the gingiva. It is used with a pull stroke.

It is important to note that sickle scalers with the same basic design can be obtained with different blade sizes and shank types to adapt to specific uses. The U15/30 (Fig. 36–11) and Ball sickles are large. The Jaquette sickles no.

1, 2, and 3 have medium-sized blades (Fig. 36–12). The Morse sickle has a very small, miniature blade (see Fig. 36–29); it is useful in the mandibular anterior area if there is little interproximal space. The selection of these instruments should be based on the area to be scaled. Sickles with straight shanks are designed for use on anterior teeth and premolars. Sickle scalers with contra-angled shanks adapt to posterior teeth.

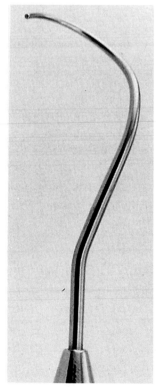

FIGURE 36–4. The curved Nabers probe for detection of furcation areas.

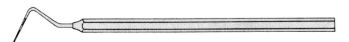

FIGURE 36–2. The periodontal probe is composed of the handle, the shank, and the calibrated working end.

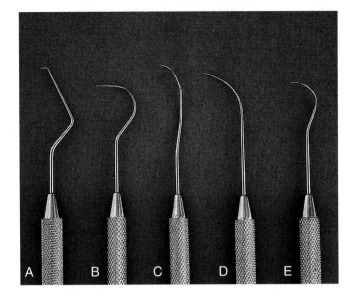

FIGURE 36-5. Five typical explorers. *A,* No. 17. *B,* No. 23. *C,* EXD 11-12 *D,* No. 3. *E,* No. 3CH Pigtail.

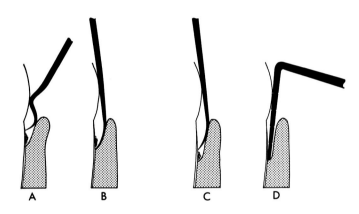

FIGURE 36-6. Insertion of two types of explorers and a probe in a pocket for calculus detection. *A,* The limitations of the pigtail explorer in a deep pocket. *B,* Insertion of the no. 3 explorer. *C,* Limitations of the no. 3 explorer. *D,* Insertion of the probe.

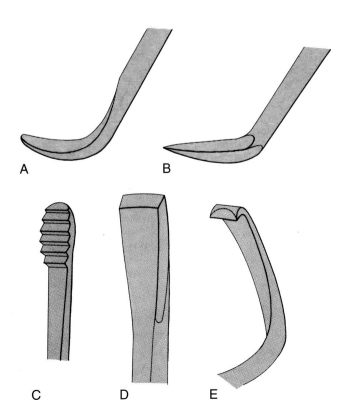

FIGURE 36-7. The five basic scaling instruments. *A,* Curette. *B,* Sickle. *C,* File. *D,* Chisel. *E,* Hoe.

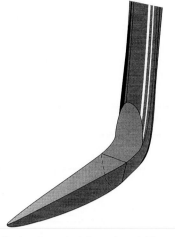

FIGURE 36–8. Basic characteristics of a sickle scaler: triangular shape, double cutting edge, and pointed tip.

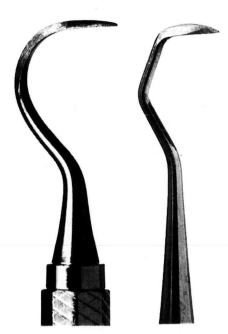

FIGURE 36–11. Both ends of a U15/30 scaler.

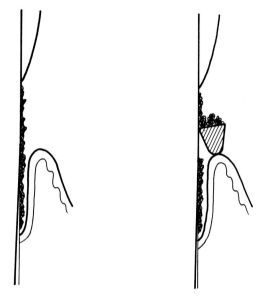

FIGURE 36–9. Use of a sickle scaler for removal of supragingival calculus.

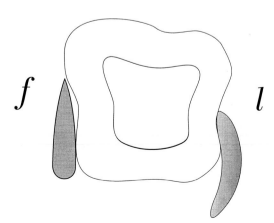

FIGURE 36–10. Subgingival adaptation around the root is better with the curette than with the sickle. f, facial; l, lingual.

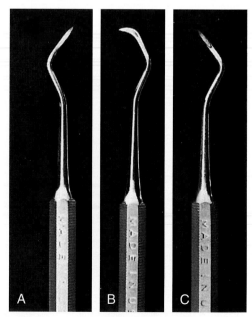

FIGURE 36–12. Jaquette scalers. *A*, No. 2. *B*, No. 1. *C*, No. 3.

Curettes

The curette is the instrument of choice for removing deep subgingival calculus, for root planing altered cementum, and for removing the soft tissue lining the periodontal pocket (Fig. 36–13). Each working end has a cutting edge on both sides of the blade and a rounded toe. The curette is finer than the sickle scalers and does not have any sharp points or corners other than the cutting edges of the blade (Fig. 36–14). Therefore, curettes can be adapted and provide good access to deep pockets, with minimal soft tissue trauma (see Fig. 36–10). In cross section, the blade appears semicircular with a convex base. The lateral border of the convex base forms a cutting edge with the face of the semicircular blade. There are cutting edges on both sides of the blade. Both single- and double-ended curettes may be obtained, depending on the preference of the operator.

As shown in Figure 36–10, the curved blade and rounded toe of the curette allow the blade to adapt better to the root surface, unlike the straight design and pointed end of a sickle scaler, which can cause tissue laceration and trauma. There are two basic types of curettes: universal and area-specific.

Universal Curettes

Universal curettes have cutting edges that may be inserted in most areas of the dentition by altering and adapting the finger rest, fulcrum, and hand position of the operator. The blade size and the angle and length of the shank may vary, but the face of the blade of every universal curette is at a 90-degree angle (perpendicular) to the lower shank when seen in cross section from the tip (Fig. 36–15A). The blade of the universal curette is curved in one direction from the head of the blade to the toe. The Barnhart curettes no. 1–2 and 5–6 and the Columbia curettes no. 13–14, 2R–2L, and 4R–4L (Figs. 36–16 and 36–17) are examples of universal curettes.

Area-Specific Curettes

Gracey Curettes. Gracey curettes are representative of the area-specific curettes, a set of several instruments de-

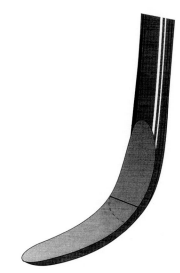

FIGURE 36–14. Basic characteristics of a curette: spoon-shaped blade and rounded tip.

signed and angled to adapt to specific anatomic areas of the dentition (Fig. 36–18). *These curettes and their modifications are probably the best instruments for subgingival scaling and root planing because they provide the best adaptation to complex root anatomy.* Double-ended Gracey curettes are paired in the following manner:

Gracey no. 1–2, Gracey no. 3–4: Anterior teeth
Gracey no. 5–6: Anterior teeth and premolars
Gracey no. 7–8, Gracey no. 9–10: Posterior teeth: facial and lingual
Gracey no. 11–12: Posterior teeth: mesial (Fig. 36–19)
Gracey no. 13–14: Posterior teeth: distal (Fig. 36–20)

Single-ended Gracey curettes can also be obtained; for these curettes, a set comprises 14 instruments. Although these curettes are designed to be used in specific areas described above, an experienced operator can adapt each instrument for use in several different areas by altering the position of his or her hand and the position of the patient.

The Gracey curettes also differ from the universal curettes in that the blade is not at a 90-degree angle to the lower shank. The term *offset blade* is used to describe Gracey curettes, because they are angled approximately 60 to 70 degrees from the lower shank (Fig. 36–15B). This unique angulation allows the blade to be inserted in the precise position necessary for subgingival scaling and root planing, provided that the lower shank is parallel with the long axis of the tooth surface being scaled.

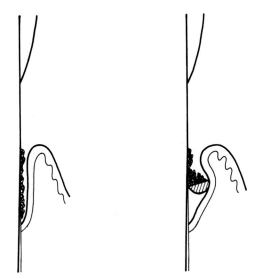

FIGURE 36–13. The curette is the instrument of choice for subgingival scaling and root planing.

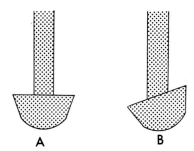

FIGURE 36–15. Principal types of curettes as seen from the toe of the instrument. *A,* Universal curette. *B,* Gracey curette. Note the offset blade angulation of the Gracey curette.

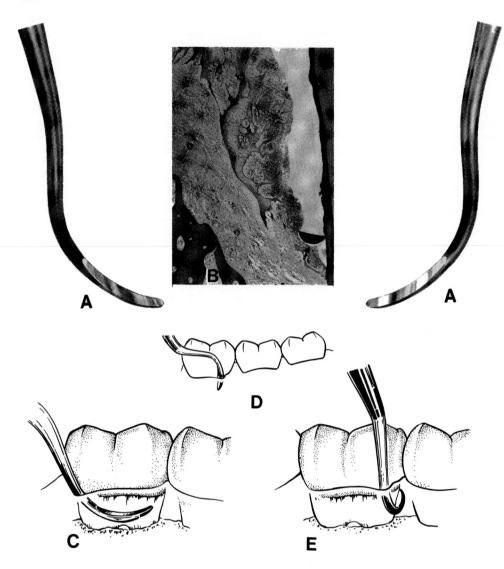

FIGURE 36–16. *A,* Double-ended curette for the removal of subgingival calculus. *B,* Cross section of the curette blade (*arrow*) against the cemental wall of a deep periodontal pocket. *C,* Curette in position at the base of a periodontal pocket on the facial surface of a mandibular molar. *D,* Curette inserted in a pocket with the tip directed apically. *E,* Curette in position at the base of a pocket on the distal surface of the mandibular molar.

Area-specific curettes also have a curved blade. Whereas the blade of the universal curette is curved in one direction, the Gracey blade is curved from head to toe and also along the side of the cutting edge (Fig. 36–21). Thus, only a pull stroke can be utilized. Some of the major differences between Gracey (area-specific) curettes and universal curettes are listed in Table 36–1.

Gracey curettes are available with either a "rigid" or a "finishing" type of shank. The rigid Gracey has a larger, stronger, and less flexible shank and blade than the standard finishing Gracey. The rigid shank makes it possible to remove moderate to heavy calculus without having to employ a separate set of heavy scalers such as sickles and hoes. Although some clinicians prefer the enhanced tactile sensitivity that the flexible shank of the finishing Gracey provides, both types of Graceys are suitable for root planing.

Recent additions to the Gracey curette set have been the

Table 36–1. COMPARISON OF SPECIFIC (GRACEY) AND UNIVERSAL CURETTES

	Gracey Curette	Universal Curette
Area of use	Set of many curettes designed for specific areas and surfaces	One curette designed for all areas and surfaces
Cutting edge		
Use	*One cutting edge used;* work with outer edge only	*Both cutting edges used;* work with either outer or inner edge
Curvature	*Curved in two planes:* blade curves up and to the side	*Curved in one plane:* blade curves up, not to side
Blade angle	*Offset blade:* face of blade beveled at 60 degrees to shank	*Not offset:* face of blade beveled at 90 degrees to shank

Modified from Pattison G, Pattison A. Periodontal Instrumentation. 2nd ed. Norwalk, CT, Appleton & Lange, 1992.

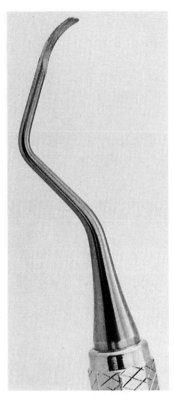

FIGURE 36–17. Columbia 4R–4L universal curette.

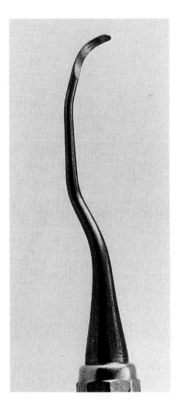

FIGURE 36–19. Gracey 11–12 curette. Note the double turn of the shank.

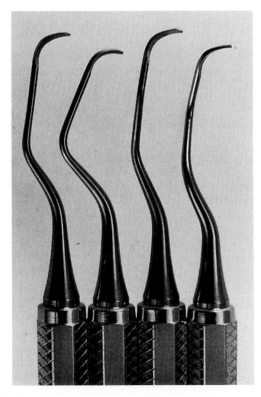

FIGURE 36–18. Reduced set of Gracey curettes. From left, no. 5–6, no. 7–8, no. 11–12, and no. 13–14.

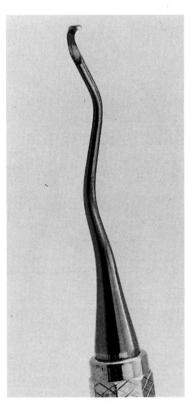

FIGURE 36–20. Gracey no. 13–14 curette. Note the acute turn of the blade.

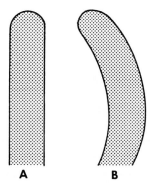

FIGURE 36–21. *A,* Universal curette as seen from the blade. Note that the blade is straight. *B,* Gracey curette as seen from the blade. The blade is curved; only the convex cutting edge is used.

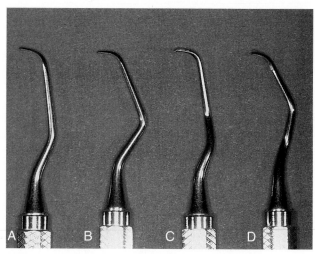

FIGURE 36–23. After Five curette. Note the extra 3 mm in the terminal shank of the After Five curette compared with the standard Gracey curette. *A,* no. 5–6. *B,* no. 7–8. *C,* no. 11–12. *D,* no. 13–14.

Gracey no. 15–16 (Fig. 36–22) and the Gracey no. 17–18. The Gracey no. 15–16 is a modification of the standard Gracey no. 11–12 is designed for the mesial surfaces of posterior teeth. It consists of a Gracey no. 11–12 blade combined with the more acutely angled Gracey no. 13–14 shank. When the clinician is using an intraoral finger rest, it is often difficult to position the lower shank of the Gracey no. 11–12 so that it is parallel with the mesial surfaces of the posterior teeth, especially on the mandibular molars. The new shank angulation of the Gracey no. 15–16 allows better adaptation to posterior mesial surfaces from a front position with intraoral rests. If alternative fulcrums such as extraoral or opposite-arch rests are used, the Gracey no. 11–12 works well, and the new Gracey no. 15–16 is not essential. The Gracey no. 17–18 is a modification of the Gracey no. 13–14. It has a terminal shank elongated by 3 mm and a more accentuated angulation of the shank to provide complete occlusal clearance and better access to all posterior distal surfaces. The hori-

zontal handle position minimizes interference from opposing arches and allows a more relaxed hand position when scaling distal surfaces. In addition, the blade is 1 mm shorter to allow better adaptation of the blade to distal tooth surfaces.

Extended Shank Curettes. Extended shank curettes such as the Hu-Friedy After Five curettes are modifications of the standard Gracey curette design. The terminal shank is 3 mm longer, allowing extension into deeper periodontal pockets of 5 mm or more (Figs. 36–23 and 36–24). Other features include a thinned blade for smoother subgingival insertion and reduced tissue distention and a large-diameter, tapered shank. All of the standard Gracey numbers except for the 9–10 (e.g., 1–2, 3–4, 5–6, 7–8, 11–12, 13–14) are available in the After Five series. The After Five curettes are available in finishing or rigid designs. For heavy or tenacious calculus removal, rigid After Fives should be used. For light scaling or deplaquing in a peri-

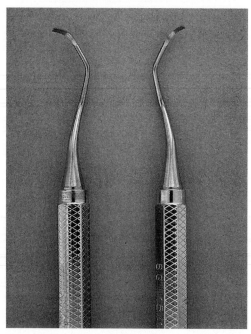

FIGURE 36–22. Gracey no. 15–16. New Gracey curette, designed for mesioposterior surfaces, combines a Gracey no. 11–12 blade with a Gracey no. 13–14 shank.

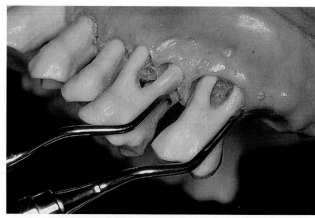

FIGURE 36–24. Comparison of the After Five curette with standard Gracey curette. Rigid Gracey no. 13–14 adapted to the distal surface of the first molar and rigid After Five no. 13–14 adapted to the distal surface of the second molar. Notice the extra long shank of the After Five, which allows deeper insertion and better access.

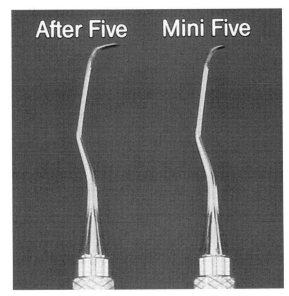

FIGURE 36-25. Comparison of the After Five curette and the Mini Five curette. The shorter Mini Five blade (half the length) allows increased access and reduced tissue trauma.

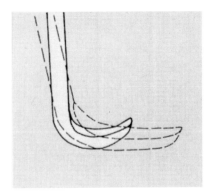

FIGURE 36-27. Gracey Curvette blade. This diagram shows the 50% shorter blade of the Gracey Curvette superimposed on the standard Gracey curette blade (*dotted lines*). Notice the upward curvature of the Curvette blade and blade tip. (From Pattison G, Pattison A, Periodontal Instrumentation. 2nd ed. Norwalk, CT, Appleton & Lange, 1992, p. 414.

odontal maintenance patient, the thinner, finishing After Fives will insert subgingivally more easily.

Mini-bladed Curettes. Mini-bladed curettes such as the Hu-Friedy Mini Five curettes are modifications of the After Five curettes. They feature blades that are half the length of the After Five or standard Gracey curettes (Fig. 36-25). The shorter blade allows easier insertion and adaptation in deep, narrow pockets; furcations; developmental grooves; line angles; and deep, tight, facial, lingual, or palatal pockets. In any area where root morphology or tight tissue prevents full insertion of the standard Gracey or After Five blade, the Mini Five curettes can be used with vertical strokes, with reduced tissue distention and without tissue trauma (Fig. 36-26). In the past, the only solution in most of these areas of difficult access was to use the Gracey curettes with a toe-down horizontal stroke. The Mini Five curettes, along with other short-bladed instruments rela-

tively recently introduced, open a new chapter in the history of root instrumentation by allowing access to areas that previously were extremely difficult or impossible to reach with standard instruments. The Mini Five curettes are available in both the finishing and rigid designs. Rigid Mini Fives are recommended for calculus removal. The more flexible shanked, finishing Mini Fives are appropriate for light scaling and deplaquing in periodontal maintenance patients with tight pockets. As with the After Fives, the Mini Fives are available in all of the standard Gracey numbers except for the 9-10.

The American Gracey Curvettes are another new set of four mini-bladed curettes; the Sub-0 and the 1-2 are used for anteriors and premolars, the 11-12 is used for mesioposterior surfaces, and the 13-14 is used for distoposterior surfaces. The blade length of these instruments is 50% shorter than that of the conventional Gracey curette, and the blade has been curved slightly upward (Fig. 36-27). This curvature allows the American Gracey Curvettes to adapt more closely to the tooth surface than any other curettes, especially on the anterior teeth and on line angles (Fig. 36-28). However, this curvature also carries the po-

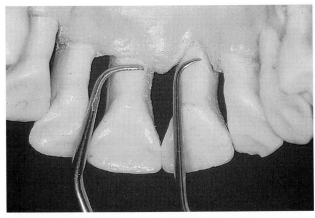

FIGURE 36-26. Comparison of a standard rigid Gracey no. 5-6 with a rigid Mini Five no. 5-6 on the palatal surfaces of the maxillary central incisors. The Mini Five can be inserted to the base of these tight anterior pockets and used with a straight vertical stroke. A standard Gracey or After Five usually cannot be inserted vertically in this area because the blade is too long.

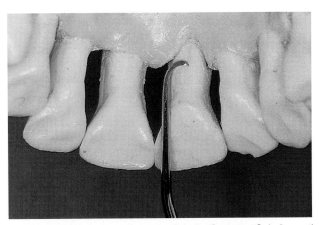

FIGURE 36-28. Gracey Curvette Sub-0. Curvette Sub-0 on the palatal surface of a maxillary central. The long shank and short, curved, and blunted tip make this a superior instrument for deep anterior pockets. This curette provides excellent blade adaptation to the narrow root curvatures of the maxillary and mandibular anterior teeth.

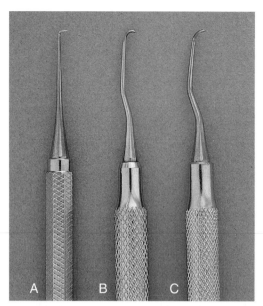

FIGURE 36–29. Comparison of mini-bladed Instruments. Four different mini-bladed instruments designed for use on the maxillary and mandibular anteriors. *A,* Morse sickle scaler, *B,* Gracey Curvette Sub-0, *C,* Mini Five no. 1–2, and *D,* Mini Five no. 5–6.

tential for gouging or grooving into the root surfaces on the proximal surfaces of the posterior teeth when the Curvette no. 11–12 or 13–14 is used. Additional features that represent improvements on the standard Gracey curettes are a precision-balanced blade tip in direct alignment with the handle, a blade tip perpendicular to the handle, and a shank closer to parallel with the handle.

For many years, the Morse scaler, a miniature sickle, was the only mini-bladed instrument available. However, the newly developed mini-bladed curettes have largely replaced this instrument (Fig. 36–29).

Schwartz Periotrievers

The Schwartz Periotrievers are a set of two double-ended, highly magnetized instruments designed for the retrieval of broken instrument tips from the periodontal pocket (Figs. 36–30 and 36–31). They are indispensable

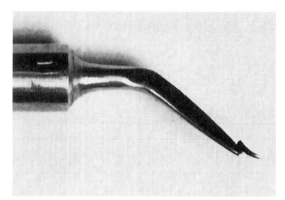

FIGURE 36–31. Broken instrument tip attached to the magnetic tip of the Schwartz Periotriever. (From Pattison G, Pattison A. Periodontal Instrumentation. 2nd ed. Norwalk, CT, Appleton & Lange, 1992, p. 421.)

when the clinician has broken a curette tip in a furcation or deep pocket.

Plastic Instruments for Implants

Several different companies are manufacturing plastic instruments for use on titanium and other implant abutment materials. It is imperative that plastic rather than metal instruments be used to avoid scarring and permanent damage to the implants (Figs. 36–32 and 36–33).

Hoe Scalers

Hoe scalers are used for scaling of ledges or rings of calculus (Fig. 36–34). The blade is bent at a 99-degree angle; the cutting edge is formed by the junction of the flattened terminal surface with the inner aspect of the blade. The cutting edge is beveled at 45 degrees. The blade is slightly bowed so that it can maintain contact at two points on a convex surface. The back of the blade is rounded, and the blade has been reduced to minimal thickness to permit access to the roots without interference from the adjacent tissues.

Hoe scalers are used in the following manner:
1. The blade is inserted to the base of the periodontal pocket

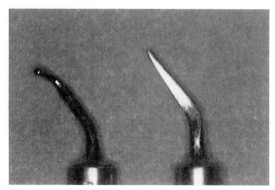

FIGURE 36–30. Schwartz Periotriever tip designs. The long blade is for general use in pockets, and the contra-angled tip is for use in furcations. (From Pattison G, Pattison A. Periodontal Instrumentation. 2nd ed. Norwalk, CT, Appleton & Lange, 1992, p. 421.)

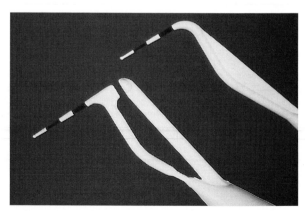

FIGURE 36–32. Plastic probes. Color-coded markings and a pressure indicator are helpful features of these plastic probes from the Pro-Dentec Company, Batesville, AR.

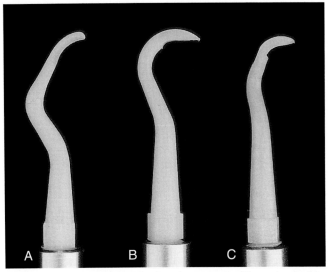

FIGURE 36-33. Implacare implant instruments. These implant instruments from the Hu-Friedy Company have autoclavable stainless steel handles and three different cone-socket plastic tip designs. *A,* The Columbia 4R-4L curette tip. *B,* The H6-H7 sickle scaler tip. *C,* The 204S sickle scaler tip.

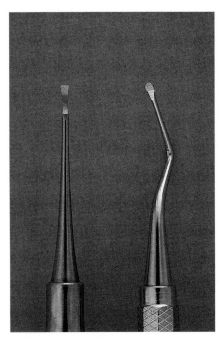

FIGURE 36-35. Chisel and file scaler.

so that it makes two-point contact with the tooth (Fig. 36-34). This stabilizes the instrument and prevents nicking of the root.

2. The instrument is activated with a firm pull stroke toward the crown, with every effort being made to preserve the two-point contact with the tooth.

McCall's hoe scalers no. 3, 4, 5, 6, 7, and 8 are a set of six hoe scalers designed to provide access to all tooth surfaces. Each instrument has a different angle between the shank and handle.

Files

Files were popular at one time but currently are seldom used for scaling and root planing because they gouge and

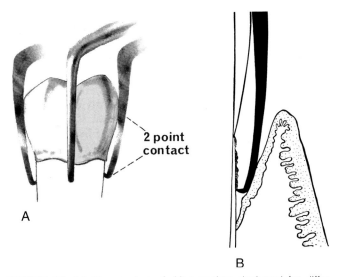

FIGURE 36-34. Hoe scalers. *A,* Hoe scalers designed for different tooth surfaces, showing "two-point" contact. *B,* Hoe scaler in a periodontal pocket. The back of the blade is rounded for easier access. The instrument contacts the tooth at two points for stability.

roughen root surfaces[1] (Fig. 36-35). They are sometimes used for removing overhanging margins of dental restorations.

Chisel Scalers

The chisel scaler, designed for the proximal surfaces of teeth too closely spaced to permit the use of other scalers, is usually used in the anterior part of the mouth. It is a double-ended instrument with a curved shank at one end and a straight shank at the other (Fig. 36-35); the blades are slightly curved and have a straight cutting edge beveled at 45 degrees.

The scaler is inserted from the facial surface. The slight curve of the blade makes it possible to stabilize it against the proximal surface, whereas the cutting edge engages the calculus without nicking the tooth. The instrument is activated with a push motion while the side of the blade is held firmly against the root.

Ultrasonic and Sonic Instruments

Ultrasonic instruments may be used for scaling, curetting, and removing stain.[3,4,7,11,17] Their action is derived from physical vibrations of particles of matter, similar to sound waves, at frequencies ranging from 20,000 to many million cycles per second (also referred to as *Hertz* [Hz]) above the range of human hearing. In periodontal instrumentation, ultrasonic units are composed of an electrical generator that delivers energy in the form of high-frequency (ultrasonic) vibrations to a handpiece into which a variety of specially designed tips may be inserted. There are two types of ultrasonic units: magnetostrictive and piezoelectric.[17] Ultrasonic vibrations at the tip of instruments of both types range from 20,000 to 45,000 cycles per second, depending on the manufacturer. In magnetostrictive units (Fig. 36-36), the pattern of vibration of the tip is el-

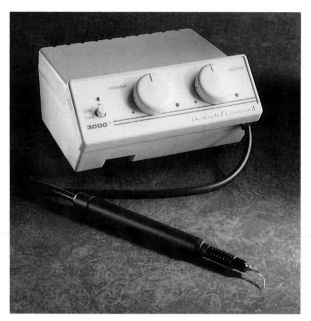

FIGURE 36–36. Magnetostrictive ultrasonic unit. The Cavitron 3000 ultrasonic scaler from Dentsply International Inc., York, PA.

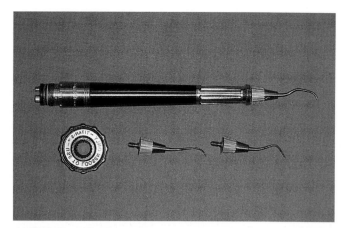

FIGURE 36–38. Sonic scaler. The Titan-S sonic scaler from Star Dental Products, Valley Forge, PA.

liptical, which means that all sides of the tip are active and will work when adapted to the tooth. In piezoelectric units (Fig. 36–37), the pattern of vibration of the tip is linear, or back and forth, meaning that only the two sides of the tip are active and will work when adapted to the tooth.

Sonic units consist of a handpiece that attaches to a compressed air line and uses a variety of specially designed tips (Fig. 36–38). Vibrations at the sonic tip range from 2000 to 6500 cycles per second, which provides less power for calculus removal than ultrasonic units.

A comparison of the three types of power-driven scalers is shown in Table 36–2.

Ultrasonic and sonic tips with different shapes are available for scaling, curetting, root planing, and debriding during periodontal surgery (Fig. 36–39). For many years, only

large, bulky tips designed for supragingival removal of heavy calculus were available. In recent years, however, thinner, more delicate tips designed for subgingival debridement have become available[6] (Fig. 36–40). All tips are designed to operate in a wet field and have attached water outlets. The spray is directed at the end of the tip to dissipate the heat generated by the ultrasonic vibrations. Within the water droplets of this spray mist are tiny vacuum bubbles that quickly collapse, releasing energy in a process known as *cavitation*. The cavitating water spray also serves to flush calculus, plaque, and debris dislodged by the vibrating tip from the pocket. Sonic units do not re-

Table 36–2. COMPARISON OF SONIC AND ULTRASONIC SCALING UNITS

| | Sonic | Ultrasonic | |
		Magnetostrictive	Piezoelectric
Advantages			
Calculus removal	good	excellent	excellent
Treatment time	low	low	low
Tip action	orbital	elliptical	linear
Tip adaptability	fair	fair	fair
Patient comfort	good	good	good
Asepsis	good	good	good
Operator control	good	good	good
Space requirement	low	high	high
Disadvantages			
Enamel abrasion	medium	medium	medium
Tissue abrasion	low	low	low
Cemental roughening	medium	medium	medium
Restoration damage	medium	medium	medium
Heat production	low	high	high
Cost	medium	high	high
Maintenance	medium	high	high
Noise level	high	medium	medium

This table is meant merely as a guide to choosing power-operated instruments. The clinician is advised to investigate the various types and models of sonic and ultrasonic scaling devices, because technical improvements and changes have affected and will continue to affect the way powered instruments are used in dentistry.

From Perry DA, Beemsterboer P, Carranza FA. Techniques and Theory of Periodontal Instrumentation. Philadelphia, WB Saunders, 1990.

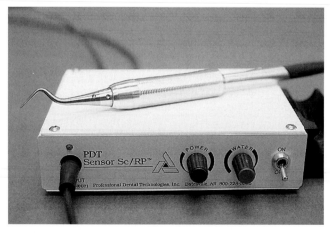

FIGURE 36–37. Piezoelectric ultrasonic unit. The Sensor PDT scaler from the Pro-Dentec Company, Batesville, AR.

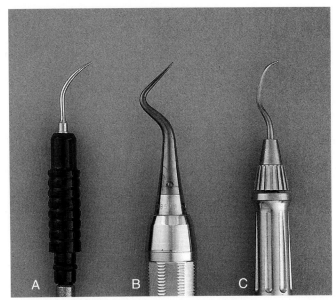

FIGURE 36–39. Ultrasonic and sonic tips. *A*, Ultrasonic inserts for the Cavitron 3000. *B*, Ultrasonic insert for the Sensor PDT scaler. *C*, Sonic inserts for the Titan-S.

lease heat the way ultrasonic units do, but they still have water for cooling and flushing away debris.

The EVA System

Probably the most efficient and least traumatic instruments for correcting overhanging or overcontoured proximal alloy and resin restorations are the motor-driven diamond files of the EVA prophylaxis instrument. These files, which come in symmetric pairs, are made of aluminum in the shape of a wedge protruding from a shaft; one side of the wedge is diamond coated; the other side is smooth. The files can be mounted on a special dental handpiece attachment that generates reciprocating strokes of variable frequency. When the unit is activated interproximally with the diamond-coated side of the file touching the restoration and the smooth side adjacent to the papilla, the oscillating file

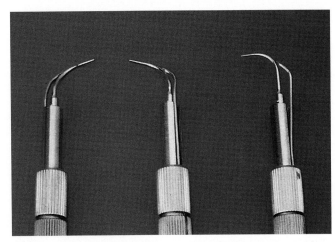

FIGURE 36–40. Cavitron Slim Line ultrasonic tips. New, thin inserts from Dentsply Cavitron allow better insertion into deep periodontal pockets and furcations.

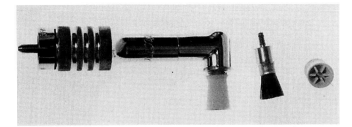

FIGURE 36–41. Prophylaxis handpiece with rubber cup and brush.

swiftly planes the contour of the restoration and reduces it to the desired shape.

Cleansing and Polishing Instruments

Rubber Cups. Rubber cups consist of a rubber shell with or without webbed configurations in the hollow interior (Fig. 36–41). They are used in the handpiece with a special prophylaxis angle. The handpiece, prophylaxis angle, and rubber cup must be sterilized after each patient use, or a disposable plastic prophylaxis angle and rubber cup (Fig. 36–42) may be used and then discarded. A good cleansing and polishing paste that contains fluoride should be used and kept moist to minimize frictional heat as the cup revolves. Polishing pastes are available in fine, medium, or coarse grits and are packaged in small, convenient, single-use containers. Aggressive use of the rubber cup with any abrasive may remove the layer of cementum, which is thin in the cervical area.

Bristle Brushes. Bristle brushes are available in wheel and cup shapes (see Fig. 36–41). The brush is used in the handpiece with a polishing paste. Because the bristles are stiff, use of the brush should be confined to the crown to avoid injuring the cementum and the gingiva.

Dental Tape. Dental tape with polishing paste is used for polishing proximal surfaces that are inaccessible to other polishing instruments. The tape is passed interproximally while being kept at a right angle to the long axis of the tooth and is activated with a firm labiolingual motion. Particular care is taken to avoid injury to the gingiva. The area should be cleansed with warm water to remove all remnants of paste.

Air–Powder Polishing. In the early 1980s, a specially

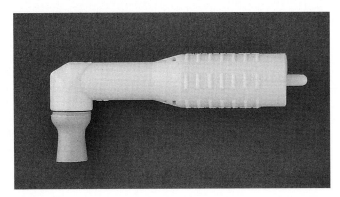

FIGURE 36–42. Disposable plastic prophylaxis angle with rubber cup.

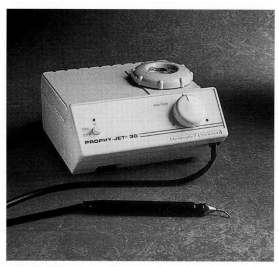

FIGURE 36–43. Prophy-Jet air-powder polishing device from Dentsply Cavitron.

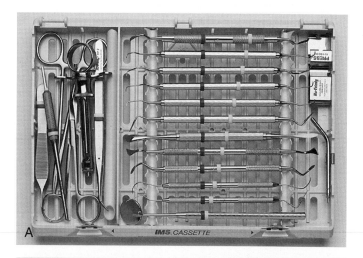

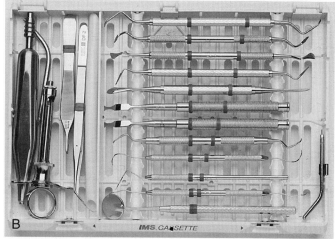

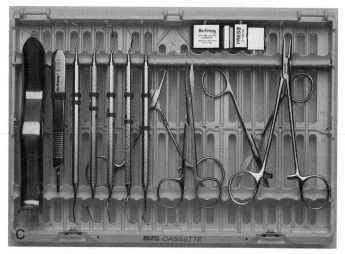

FIGURE 36–44. Instrument cassettes for periodontal surgery. Cassettes shown in *A* and *B* are to be used together for involved cases, while the cassette shown in *C* is a reduced set for simple cases. Additional instruments may be used according to individual preferences and case requirements. *A,* Mirror, explorer, probe, furcation probe, chisels, periosteal elevator, file, knives, surgical curette, dressing pliers, tissue pliers, aspirator tip. *B,* Retractor, scalpel handle, root planing curettes, universal curette, hemostat, scissors, needleholders, suture scissors, scalpel blade remover. *C,* Simplified set: mirror, explorer-probe, furcation probe, knives, periosteal elevator, file, root planing curettes, universal curette, chisel, scalpel handle, dressing pliers, tissue pliers, needleholder, scissors, scalpel blade remover. (Courtesy of Hu-Friedy Instrument Company, Chicago, IL.)

designed handpiece was introduced that delivers an air-powered slurry of warm water and sodium bicarbonate; this instrument is called the *Prophy-Jet* (Fig. 36–43). This system is effective for the removal of extrinsic stains and soft deposits. The slurry removes stains rapidly and efficiently by mechanical abrasion and provides warm water for rinsing and lavage. The flow rate of abrasive cleansing power can be adjusted to increase the amount of powder for heavier stain removal.

The results of studies on the abrasive effect of the air–powder polishing device on cementum and dentin show that tooth substance can be lost. Damage to gingival tissue is transient and insignificant clinically, but composite restorations can be roughened.[10,11]

Patients with medical histories of respiratory illnesses, those with sodium-restricted diets, and individuals on medications affecting the electrolyte balance are not candidates for the use of the air–powder polishing device. Patients with infectious diseases should not be treated with this device because of the large quantity of aerosol created.

SURGICAL INSTRUMENTS

Periodontal surgery is accomplished with numerous instruments; Figure 36–44 shows a typical surgical cassette. Periodontal surgical instruments are classified as follows:
1. Excisional and incisional instruments
2. Surgical curettes and sickles
3. Periosteal elevators
4. Surgical chisels
5. Surgical files
6. Scissors
7. Hemostats and tissue forceps

Excisional and Incisional Instruments

Periodontal Knives (Gingivectomy Knives). The Kirkland knife is representative of knives commonly used for gingivectomy. These knives can be obtained as either double-ended or single-ended instruments. The entire periphery

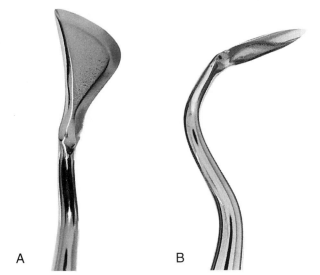

FIGURE 36–45. Gingivectomy knives. *A*, Kirkland knife. *B*, Orban interdental knife.

of these kidney-shaped knives is the cutting edge (Fig. 36–45*A*).

Interdental Knives. The Orban knife no. 1–2 (Fig. 36–45*B*) and the Merrifield knife no. 1, 2, 3, and 4 are examples of knives used for interdental areas. These spear-shaped knives have cutting edges on both sides of the blade and are designed with either double-ended or single-ended blades.

Surgical Blades. Scalpel blades of different shapes and sizes are used in periodontal surgery. The most commonly used blades are nos. 12D, 15, and 15C (Fig. 36–46). The no. 12D blade is a beak-shaped blade with cutting edges on both sides, allowing the operator to engage narrow, restricted areas with both pushing and pulling cutting motions. The no. 15 blade is utilized for thinning flaps and for

all-around use. The no. 15C blade, a narrower version of the no. 15 blade, is useful for making the initial, scalloping type incision. The slim design of this blade allows for incising into the narrow interdental portion of the flap. All of these blades are discarded after one use.

Electrosurgery (Surgical Diathermy) Techniques and Instrumentation. The term *electrosurgery* is currently used to identify surgical techniques performed on soft tissue using controlled high-frequency electrical (radio) currents in the range of 1.5 to 7.5 million cycles per second (Fig. 36–47). There are three classes of active electrodes: single-wire electrodes for incising or excising; loop electrodes for planing tissue; and heavy, bulkier electrodes for coagulation procedures.

There are four basic types of electrosurgical techniques: electrosection, electrocoagulation, electrofulguration, and electrodesiccation.

Electrosection, also referred to as *electrotomy* or *acusection*, is used for incisions, excisions, and tissue planing. Incisions and excisions are performed with single-wire active electrodes that can be bent or adapted to accomplish any type of cutting procedure.

Electrocoagulation provides a wide range of coagulation or hemorrhage control obtained by utilizing the electrocoagulation current. Electrocoagulation can prevent bleeding or hemorrhage at the initial entry into soft tissue, but it cannot stop bleeding after blood is present. All forms of hemorrhage must be stopped first by some form of direct pressure (i.e., air, compress, or hemostat). After bleeding has momentarily stopped, final sealing of the capillaries or large vessels can be accomplished by a short application of the electrocoagulation current. The active electrodes used for coagulation are much bulkier than the fine tungsten wire used for electrosection.

Electrosection and electrocoagulation are the procedures most commonly used in all areas of dentistry. The two monoterminal techniques, electrofulguration and electrodesiccation, are not in general use in dentistry.

The most important basic rule of electrosurgery is: *always keep the tip moving.* Prolonged or repeated application of current to tissue induces heat accumulation and undesired tissue destruction, whereas interrupted application at intervals adequate for tissue cooling (5 to 10 seconds) reduces or eliminates heat buildup. Electrosurgery is not intended to destroy tissue; it is a controllable means of sculp-

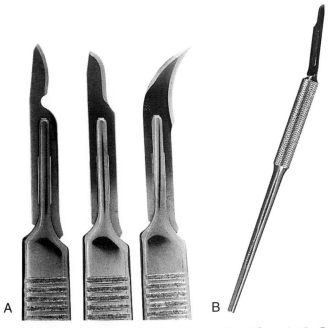

FIGURE 36–46. Surgical blades. *A*, No. 12D, 15C, and 15. *B*, Contra-angled scalpel handle.

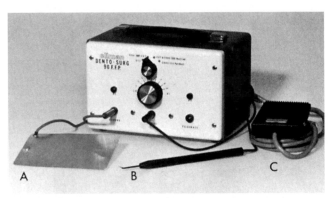

FIGURE 36–47. Electrosurgical unit. *A*, Passive or conductive plate. *B*, Active electrode handle and tip electrode. *C*, Foot switch.

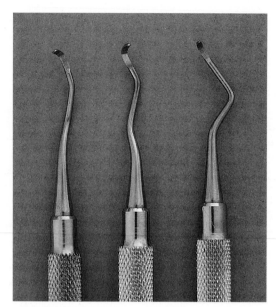

FIGURE 36–48. Kramer heavy surgical curettes no. 1, 2, and 3.

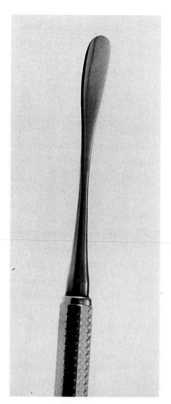

FIGURE 36–49. Glickman periosteal elevator no. 24G.

turing or modifying oral soft tissue with little discomfort and hemorrhage for the patient.

The indications for electrosurgery in periodontal therapy and a description of wound healing after electrosurgery are presented in Chapter 53. Electrosurgery is contraindicated for patients who have noncompatible or poorly shielded cardiac pacemakers.

Surgical Curettes and Sickles

Larger and heavier curettes and sickles are often needed during surgery for the removal of granulation tissue, fibrous interdental tissues, and tenacious subgingival deposits. The Kramer curettes no. 1, 2, and 3 (Fig. 36–48) and the Kirkland surgical instruments are heavy curettes, whereas the Ball scaler no. B2–B3 is a popular heavy sickle. The wider, heavier blades of these instruments make them suitable for surgical procedures.

Periosteal Elevators

These instruments are necessary to reflect and move the flap after the incision has been made for flap surgery. The no. 24G (Fig. 36–49) and the Goldman-Fox no. 14 are well-designed periosteal elevators.

Surgical Chisels and Hoes

Chisels and hoes are used during periodontal surgery for removing and reshaping bone. The hoe shown in Figure 36–50 has a curved shank and blade, whereas the Wiedelstadt and Todd-Gilmore chisels are straight shanked. The surgical hoe has a flattened, fishtail-shaped blade with a pronounced convexity in its terminal portion. The cutting edge is beveled with rounded edges and projects beyond the long axis of the handle to preserve the effectiveness of the instrument when the blade is reduced by sharpening. The surgical hoe is generally used for detaching pocket walls after the gingivectomy incision, but it is also useful

for smoothing root and bone surfaces made accessible by any surgical procedure. The Ochsenbein no. 1–2 (Fig. 36–51A) is a useful chisel with a semicircular indentation on both sides of the shank that allows the instrument to engage around the tooth and into the interdental area. Surgical

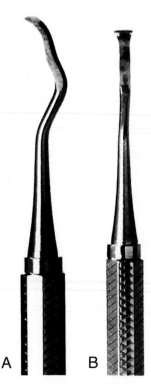

FIGURE 36–50. Lateral (*A*) and frontal (*B*) views of a surgical hoe.

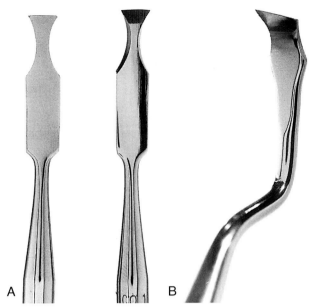

FIGURE 36–51. Surgical chisels. *A,* Ochsenbein chisels. *B,* Rhodes chisel.

hoes are usually used with a pull stroke, whereas chisels are engaged with a push stroke. The Rhodes chisel is shown in Fig. 36–51*B*.

Surgical Files

Periodontal surgical files are used primarily to smooth rough bony ledges and to remove all areas of bone. The

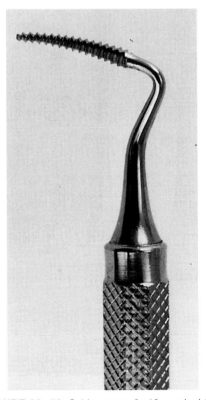

FIGURE 36–52. Schluger no. 9–10 surgical file.

Schluger (Fig. 36–52) and Sugarman files are similar in design and can be used with a push-and-pull stroke, primarily in the interdental areas.

Scissors and Nippers

Scissors and nippers are used in periodontal surgery for such purposes as removing tabs of tissue during gingivectomy, trimming the margins of flaps, enlarging incisions in periodontal abscesses, and removing muscle attachments in mucogingival surgery. There are many types, and the choice is a matter of individual preference. Figure 36–53 shows the Goldman-Fox no. 16 scissors with a curved beveled blade with serrations and the nippers.

Needleholders

Needleholders are used to suture the flap at the desired position after the surgical procedure has been completed.

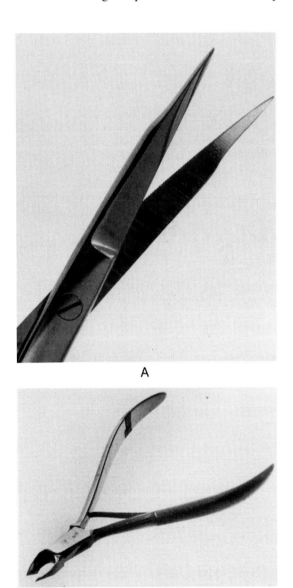

A

B

FIGURE 36–53. *A,* Goldman-Fox no. 16 scissors. *B,* Nippers.

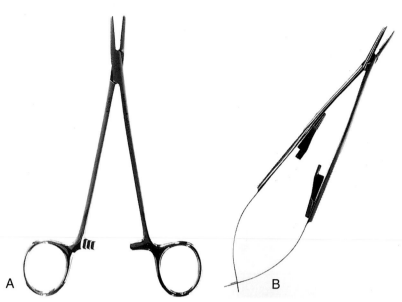

A   B

FIGURE 36–54. *A,* Conventional needleholder. *B,* Castroviejo needleholder.

The regular type of needleholder is illustrated in Figure 36–54*A*, while Figure 36–54*B* shows the Castroviejo needleholder, which is used for delicate, precise techniques requiring quick and easy release and grasp of the suture.

SHARPENING OF PERIODONTAL INSTRUMENTS

It is impossible to carry out periodontal procedures efficiently with dull instruments. A sharp instrument cuts more precisely and quickly than a dull instrument. To do its job at all, a dull instrument must be held more firmly and pressed harder than a sharp instrument. This reduces tactile sensitivity and increases the possibility that the instrument will inadvertently slip. *Therefore, to avoid wasting time and operating haphazardly, clinicians must be thoroughly familiar with the principles of sharpening and able to apply them to produce a keen cutting edge on the instruments they are using.* Development of this skill requires patience and practice, but clinical excellence cannot be attained without it.

Sharpness and How to Evaluate It

The cutting edge of an instrument is formed by the angular junction of two surfaces of its blade. The cutting edges of a curette, for example, are formed where the face of the blade meets the lateral surfaces (Fig. 36–55).

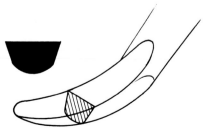

FIGURE 36–55. The cutting edge of a curette is formed by the angular junction of the face and the lateral surfaces of the instrument. When the instrument is sharp, the cutting edge is a fine line.

When the instrument is sharp, this junction is a fine line running the length of the cutting edge. As the instrument is used, metal is worn away at the cutting edge, and the junction of the face and lateral surface becomes rounded or dulled[2,9] (Fig. 36–56). Thus the cutting edge becomes a rounded surface rather than an acute angle. This is why a dull instrument cuts less efficiently and requires more pressure to do its job.[5]

Sharpness can be evaluated by sight and touch in one of the following ways:

1. When a dull instrument is held under a light, the rounded surface of its cutting edge reflects light back to the observer. It appears as a bright line running the length of the cutting edge (Fig. 36–57). The acutely angled cutting edge of a sharp instrument, on the other hand, has no surface area to reflect light. When a sharp instrument is held under a light, no bright line can be observed (see Fig. 36–55).

2. Tactile evaluation of sharpness is performed by drawing the instrument lightly across an acrylic rod known as a *sharpening "test stick."* A dull instrument will slide smoothly, without "biting" into the surface and raising a light shaving as a sharp instrument would.[17]

The Objective of Sharpening

The objective of sharpening is to restore the fine, thin, linear cutting edge of the instrument. This is done by grinding the surfaces of the blade until their junction is once again sharply angular rather than rounded. For any given instrument, several sharpening techniques may produce this result. A technique is acceptable if it produces a sharp cutting edge without unduly wearing the instrument or altering its original design. To maintain the original design, the operator must understand the location and course of the cutting edges and the angles between the surfaces that form them. It is important to restore the cutting edge without

FIGURE 36–56. The cutting edge of a dull curette is rounded.

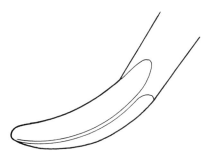

FIGURE 36–57. Light reflected from the rounded cutting edge of a dull instrument appears as a bright line.

distorting the original angles of the instrument. When these angles have been altered, the instrument does not function as it was designed to function, which limits its effectiveness.

Sharpening Stones

Sharpening stones may be quarried from natural mineral deposits or produced artificially. In either case, the surface of the stone is made up of abrasive crystals that are harder than the metal of the instrument to be sharpened. Coarse stones have larger particles and cut more rapidly; they are used on instruments that are dull. Finer stones with smaller crystals cut more slowly and are reserved for final sharpening to produce a finer edge and for sharpening instruments that are only slightly dull. India and Arkansas oilstones are examples of natural abrasive stones. Carborundum, ruby, and ceramic stones are synthetically produced (Fig. 36–58).

Sharpening stones can also be categorized by their method of use.

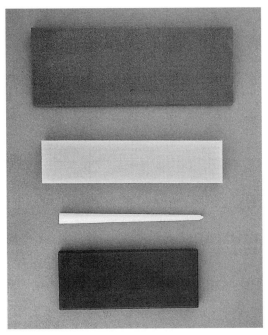

FIGURE 36–58. Sharpening stones. *Top to bottom,* A flat India stone, a flat Arkansas stone, a cone-shaped Arkansas stone, and a ceramic stone.

Mounted Rotary Stones. These stones are mounted on a metal mandrel and used in a motor-driven handpiece. They may be cylindric, conical, or disc shaped. These stones are generally not recommended for routine use, because (1) they are difficult to control precisely and can ruin the shape of the instrument, (2) they tend to wear down the instrument quickly, and (3) they can generate quite a bit of frictional heat, which may affect the temper of the instrument.

Unmounted Stones. These come in a variety of sizes and shapes. Some are rectangular with flat or grooved surfaces, whereas others are cylindric or cone shaped. Unmounted stones may be used in two ways: the instrument may be stabilized and held stationary while the stone is drawn across it, or the stone may be stabilized and held stationary while the instrument is drawn across it.

Principles of Sharpening

1. Choose a stone suitable for the instrument to be sharpened, one that is of an appropriate shape and abrasiveness.
2. Use a sterilized sharpening stone if the instrument to be sharpened will not be resterilized before it is used on a patient.
3. Establish the proper angle between the sharpening stone and the surface of the instrument on the basis of an understanding of its design.
4. Maintain a stable, firm grasp of both the instrument and the sharpening stone. This ensures that the proper angulation is maintained throughout the controlled sharpening stroke. In this manner, the entire surface of the instrument can be reduced evenly, and the cutting edge is not improperly beveled.
5. Avoid excessive pressure. Heavy pressure will cause the stone to grind the surface of the instrument more quickly and may shorten the instrument's life unnecessarily.
6. Avoid the formation of a "wire edge," characterized by minute filamentous projections of metal extending as a roughened ledge from the sharpened cutting edge.[2,5,14,17] When the instrument is used on root surfaces, these projections will produce a grooved surface rather than a smooth surface. A wire edge is produced when the direction of the sharpening stroke is away from, rather than into or toward, the cutting edge.[2,14] When back-and-forth or up-and-down sharpening strokes are used, formation of a wire edge can be avoided by finishing with a down stroke toward the cutting edge.[9]
7. Lubricate the stone during sharpening. This minimizes clogging of the abrasive surface of the sharpening stone with metal particles removed from the instrument.[5,14,17] It also reduces heat produced by friction. Oil should be used for natural stones and water for synthetic stones.
8. Sharpen instruments at the first sign of dullness. A grossly dull instrument is inefficient and requires more pressure when used, which hinders control. Furthermore, sharpening such an instrument requires the removal of a great deal of metal to produce a sharp cutting edge. This shortens the effective life of the instrument.

Sharpening Individual Instruments

Universal Curettes

Several techniques will produce a properly sharpened curette. Regardless of the technique used, the clinician must keep in mind that the angle between the face of the blade and the lateral surface of any curette is 70 to 80 degrees

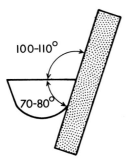

FIGURE 36–59. When the sharpening stone forms a 100- to 110-degree angle with the face of the blade, the 70- to 80-degree angle between the face and the lateral surface is automatically preserved.

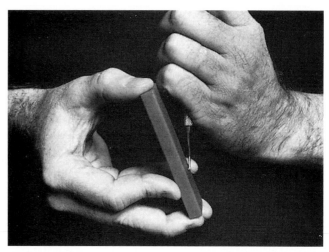

FIGURE 36–61. Using a palm grasp, one holds the universal curette so that the face of the blade is parallel to the floor. The stone makes a 100- to 110-degree angle with the face of the blade.

(Fig. 36–59). This is the most effective design for removing calculus and root planing. Changing this angle distorts the design of the instrument and makes it less effective. A cutting edge of less than 70 degrees is quite sharp but also thin (Fig. 36–60). It wears down quickly and becomes dull. A cutting edge of 90 degrees or more requires heavy lateral pressure to remove deposits. Calculus removal with such an instrument is often incomplete, and root planing cannot be done effectively (see Fig. 36–60).

The following technique is recommended because it enables the clinician to visualize the critical 70- to 80-degree angle easily and thereby consistently restores an effective cutting edge:

Sharpening the Lateral Surface. When a flat, hand-held stone is correctly applied to the lateral surface of a curette to maintain the 70- to 80-degree angle, the angle between the face of the blade and the surface of the stone will be 100 to 110 degrees (see Fig. 36–59). This can best be visualized by holding the curette so that the face of the blade is parallel with the floor. A palm grasp should be used and the upper arm braced against the body for support.

1. Apply the sharpening stone to the lateral surface of the curette so that the angle between the face of the blade and the stone is 100 to 110 degrees (Fig. 36–61; see Fig. 36–59).
2. Beginning at the shank end of the cutting edge and working toward the toe, activate the stone with short up-and-down strokes. Use consistent, light pressure and keep the stone continuously in contact with the blade. Make sure that the 100- to 110-degree angle is constantly maintained (see Fig. 36–61).
3. Check for sharpness as previously described, and continue sharpening as necessary. To prevent the toe of the curette from becoming pointed, sharpen the entire blade from shank end to toe. When approaching the toe, be sure to sharpen around it to preserve its rounded form (Fig. 36–62).
4. As the stone is moved along the cutting edge, finish each section with a down stroke into or toward the cutting edge. This will minimize the formation of a wire edge. Check the cutting edge under a light.
5. Sharpening the curette in this manner tends to flatten the lateral surface. This can be corrected by lightly grinding the lateral surface and the back of the instrument, away from the cutting edge, each time the instrument is sharpened.
6. When one edge has been properly sharpened, the opposite cutting edge can be sharpened in the same manner.

Sharpening the Face of the Blade. This may be done by moving a hand-held cylindric or cone-shaped stone back and forth across the face of the blade. A similar stone mounted in a handpiece may also be used by applying it to the face of the blade with the stone rotating toward the toe. These methods are not recommended for routine use for the following reasons:

1. The angulation between the instrument and the stone is difficult to maintain, and therefore the blade may be improperly beveled[2] (Fig. 36–63).
2. Sharpening the face of the blade narrows the working end from face to back. This weakens the blade and makes it likely to bend or break while in use[2,16,21,25] (see Fig. 36–63).
3. Sharpening the face of the blade with a hand-held stone using a back-and-forth motion produces a wire edge that interferes with the sharpness of the blade.[2]

FIGURE 36–60. At the left is a properly sharpened curette that maintains a 70- to 80-degree angle between its face and lateral surface. The curette in the center has been sharpened so that one of its cutting edges is less than 70 degrees. This fine edge is quite sharp but dulls easily. One of the cutting edges of the curette on the right has been sharpened to 90 degrees. Heavy lateral pressure must be applied to the tooth to remove deposits with such an instrument.

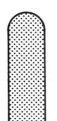 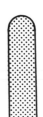 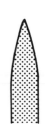

FIGURE 36–62. At the left is a new, unsharpened curette viewed from directly above the face of the blade. The curette in the center has been correctly sharpened to maintain the rounded toe. The curette at the right has been incorrectly sharpened, producing a pointed toe.

FIGURE 36−63. Angulation is difficult to control when sharpening the face of the blade and often results in unwanted beveling, as shown at the left. Sharpening the face also weakens the blade by narrowing it from face to back, as shown at the right.

Area-Specific (Gracey) Curettes

Like a universal curette, a Gracey curette has an angle of 70 to 80 degrees between the face and lateral surface of its blade. Therefore, the technique described for sharpening a universal curette can be used to sharpen a Gracey curette. However, several unique design features that distinguish a Gracey from a universal curette must be understood to avoid distorting the design of the instrument while sharpening (see Gracey Curettes, pp. 431−434).

Gracey curettes have what is known as an *offset* blade (i.e., the face of the blade is not perpendicular to the shank of the instrument, as it is on a universal curette, but is offset at a 70-degree angle) (Fig. 36−64). A Gracey curette is further distinguished by the curvature of its cutting edges. When viewed from directly above the face of the blade, the cutting edges of a universal curette extend in straight lines from shank to toe; both cutting edges can be used for scaling and root planing. The cutting edges of a Gracey curette, on the other hand, curve gently from shank to toe, and only the larger, outer cutting edge is used for scaling and root planing (Fig. 36−65).

With these points in mind, a Gracey curette is sharpened in the following manner:

1. Hold the curette so that the face of the blade is parallel with the floor. Because the blade is offset, the shank of the instrument will not be perpendicular to the floor, as it is with universal curettes (Fig. 36−66).
2. Identify the edge to be sharpened. Remember that only one cutting edge is used, so only that edge must be sharpened. Apply the stone to the lateral surface so that the angle between the face of the blade and the stone is 100 to 110 degrees.
3. Activate short up-and-down strokes, working from the shank end of the blade to the curved toe. Finish with a down stroke.
4. Remember that the cutting edge is curved. Preserve the curve by turning the stone while sharpening from shank to toe. If the stone is kept in one place for too many strokes, the blade will be flattened (Fig. 36−67).
5. Evaluate sharpness as previously described. Continue sharpening as necessary.

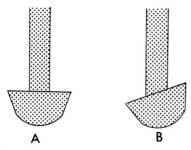

FIGURE 36−64. *A,* The face of a universal curette is at 90 degrees to its shank. *B,* The face of a Gracey curette is offset, forming a 70-degree angle with its shank.

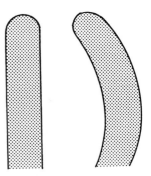

FIGURE 36−65. The cutting edges of a universal curette extend straight from shank to toe. The cutting edges of a Gracey curette gently curve from shank to toe. Only the larger, outer cutting edge at the right is used for scaling and needs to be sharpened.

Extended Shank and Mini-bladed Gracey Curettes

Extended shank Gracey curettes such as the After Fives are sharpened in exactly the same manner as the standard Gracey curettes. Although the terminal shank is 3 mm longer, the blade size and shape are very similar, and therefore, there is no difference in the sharpening technique.

Mini-bladed Gracey curettes such as the Mini Fives or Gracey Curvettes are also sharpened with the same technique. These blades are only half the length of a standard Gracey blade, but the angle between the face and the lateral surface of the blade is still 70 to 80 degrees. However, sharpening too heavily or too often around the toe of a mini-bladed curette should be avoided to prevent excessive shortening of the blade.

Sickle Scalers

There are two types of sickle scalers: the straight sickle and the curved sickle. On a straight sickle, the face of the blade is flat from shank to tip, whereas on a curved sickle, the face of the blade forms a gentle curve (Fig. 36−68). The straight and curved sickles have similar cross-sectional

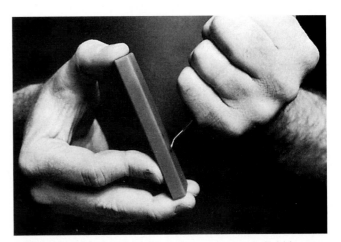

FIGURE 36−66. Note that when a Gracey curette is held in proper sharpening position, its shank is not perpendicular to the floor, owing to its offset blade angle. The stone meets the blade at an angle of 100 to 110 degrees. Compare this position with the sharpening position of a universal curette, as shown in Figure 36−61.

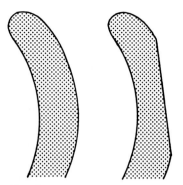

FIGURE 36–67. The Gracey curette on the left has been properly sharpened to maintain a symmetric curve on its outer cutting edge. For the curette on the right, the sharpening stone was activated too long in one place, thereby flattening the blade.

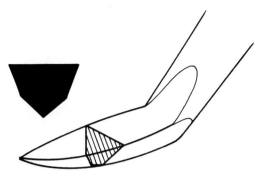

FIGURE 36–69. Like the curette, the sickle has an angle of 70 to 80 degrees between the face of the blade and the lateral surface.

designs, however. As in the curette, the angle between the face of the blade and the lateral surface of a sickle is 70 to 80 degrees (Fig. 36–69). When a sharpening stone is correctly applied to the lateral surface to preserve this angle, the angle between the face of the blade and the surface of the stone is 100 to 110 degrees. With this in mind, the sickle scaler can be sharpened in a manner much like that described for the curette except that the sickle has a sharp, pointed toe that must not be rounded.

A large, flat stone may also be used to sharpen sickles (Fig. 36–70). The stone is stabilized on a table or cabinet with the left hand. The sickle is held in the right hand with a modified pen grasp and applied to the stone so that the angle between the face of the blade and the stone is 100 to 110 degrees. The fourth finger is placed on the right-hand edge of the stone to stabilize and guide the sharpening movement. The right hand then pushes and pulls the sickle across the surface of the stone. To avoid a wire edge, finish with a pull stroke, being sure that the proper angulation is always maintained.

Chisels and Hoes

Chisels have a single, straight cutting edge that is perpendicular to the shank. The face of the blade is continuous with the shank of the instrument, which may be directly in line with the handle or slightly curved. The end of the blade is beveled at 45 degrees to form the cutting edge.

To sharpen a chisel, stabilize a flat sharpening stone on a flat surface. Grasp the instrument with a modified pen grasp. Establish a finger rest with the pads of the third and fourth fingers against the straight edge of the sharpening stone. Apply the flat beveled surface of the chisel to the surface of the stone. If the entire surface of the bevel is contacting the stone, then the 45-degree angle between the beveled surface and the face of the blade will be maintained and the design of the instrument will not be altered (Figs. 36–71 and 36–72).

Using moderate, steady pressure, with the hand and arm acting as a unit and the finger resting on the edge of the stone as a guide, push the instrument across the surface of the sharpening stone. Release pressure slightly and draw the instrument back to its starting point. Repeat the sharpening stroke until a sharp edge has been obtained. Remember to finish with a push stroke to prevent the formation of a wire edge. Check for sharpness as previously described. Examine the instrument carefully to be sure that its design has not been inadvertently altered.

Back-action surgical chisels and hoe scalers are sharpened with exactly the same technique described for chisels except that a pull stroke is used rather than a push stroke.

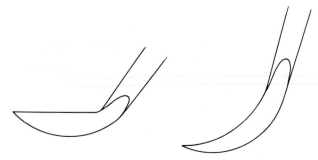

FIGURE 36–68. The face of the blade on a straight sickle is flat from shank to tip, whereas on the curved sickle the blade face forms a gentle arc.

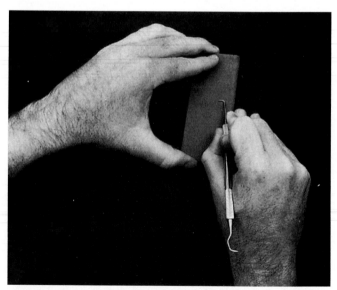

FIGURE 36–70. A large, flat stone may also be used to sharpen the sickle. The stone is stabilized on a flat surface. The fourth finger of the right hand guides the sharpening stroke as the instrument is pulled across the face of the stone toward the operator.

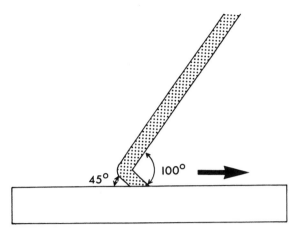

FIGURE 36-71. When the entire bevel on a chisel contacts the sharpening stone, the angle between the instrument and the stone is 45 degrees. The cutting edge will be properly sharpened if this angle is maintained as the instrument is pushed across the stone.

Periodontal Knives

There are two general types of periodontal knives. The first type includes the disposable scalpel blades that come prepackaged. They are presharpened and sterilized by the manufacturer. These are not resharpened when they become dull but are discarded and replaced.

The second type of periodontal knives are reusable and must be sharpened when they become dull. The most commonly used knives in this group are the flat-bladed gingivectomy knives (e.g., the Kirkland knives no. 15K and 16K) and the narrow, pointed interproximal knives.

Flat-Bladed Gingivectomy Knives. These knives have broad, flat blades that are nearly perpendicular to the lower shank of the instrument. The curved cutting edge extends around the entire outer edge of the blade and is formed by bevels on both the front and back surfaces of the blade (Fig. 36-73).

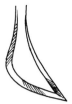

FIGURE 36-73. Flat-bladed gingivectomy knives such as this Kirkland knife have a cutting edge that extends around the entire blade. The entire cutting edge must be sharpened.

When sharpening these instruments, only the bevel on the back surface of the instrument needs be ground. This can be done by drawing the blade across a stationary flat sharpening stone or by holding the instrument stationary and drawing the stone across its blade.

Interproximal Knives. The blades of interproximal knives have two long, straight cutting edges that come together at the sharply pointed tip of the instrument. The cutting edges are formed by bevels on the front and back surfaces of the blade. The entire blade is roughly perpendicular to the lower shank of the instrument (Fig. 36-74).

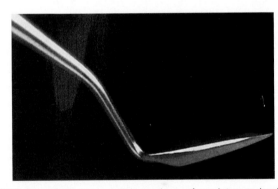

FIGURE 36-74. The two cutting edges of an interproximal knife are formed by bevels on the front and back surfaces of the blade.

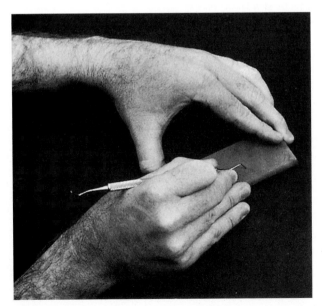

FIGURE 36-72. The chisel is also sharpened on a stationary flat sharpening stone.

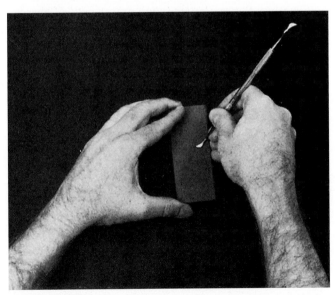

FIGURE 36-75. The gingivectomy knife may be sharpened on a stationary flat stone. The instrument is held with a modified pen grasp. The fourth finger guides the sharpening stroke as the instrument is rolled between the fingers so that all sections of the blade are sharpened.

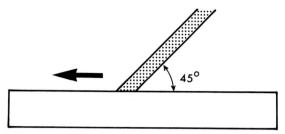

FIGURE 36–76. This cross section of a gingivectomy knife shows the two short bevels that form the cutting edge. The bevel on the back of the blade is applied to the surface of the stone, and the instrument is drawn toward the cutting edge.

As with the flat-bladed gingivectomy knives, only the bevels on the back surface of the interproximal knives need to be sharpened. Again, this can be accomplished by drawing the instrument across a stationary stone or by holding the instrument stationary and moving the stone across it.

Stationary Stone Technique. Stabilize a flat sharpening stone on a flat surface. Grasp the handle of the instrument with a modified pen grasp, and apply the bevel on the back surface of the blade to the flat surface of the sharpening stone. With moderate pressure, pull the instrument toward you (Figs. 36–75, 36–76, and 36–77). Release pressure slightly and return to the starting point. Begin at one end of the cutting edge and continue around the blade by rolling the handle of the instrument slightly between the thumb and the first and second fingers. Finish each section of the blade with a pull stroke to prevent formation of a wire edge. Check for sharpness as described previously.

Stationary Instrument Technique. Grasp the instrument with the palm. Apply the flat surface of a hand-held sharpening stone to the bevel on the back surface of the blade. (Fig. 36–78). Begin at one end of the cutting edge and, with moderate pressure, draw the stone back and forth across the instrument. To prevent the formation of a wire edge, finish each section with a stroke into or toward the cutting edge. Proceed around the entire length of the cutting edge by gradually rotating the instrument and the stone in relation to one another.

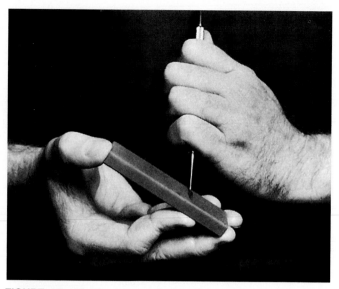

FIGURE 36–78. The interproximal knife may also be sharpened with a hand-held stone. The instrument is held with a palm grasp, and the stone is applied to the entire cutting edge.

REFERENCES

1. Allen EF, Rhoads RH. Effects of high speed periodontal instruments on tooth surface. J Periodontol *34:*352, 1963.
2. Antonini CJ, Brady JM, Levin MP, Garcia WL. Scanning electron microscope study of scalers. J Periodontol *48:*45, 1977.
3. Clark SM. The ultrasonic dental unit: A guide for the clinical application of ultrasonics in dentistry and in dental hygiene. J Periodontol *40:*621, 1969.
4. Ewen SJ, Glickstein C. Ultrasonic Therapy in Periodontics. Springfield, IL, Charles C Thomas, 1968.
5. Green E, Seyer PC. Sharpening Curets and Sickle Scalers. 2nd ed. Berkeley, CA, Praxis Publishing, 1972.
6. Holbrook T, Low S. Power-driven scaling and polishing instruments. In Hardin JF, ed. Clarke's Clinical Dentistry. Philadelphia, JB Lippincott, 1991, pp 1–24.
7. Johnson WN, Wilson JR. The application of the ultrasonic dental units to scaling procedures. J Periodontol *28:*264, 1957.
8. Lindhe J. Evaluation of periodontal scalers. II. Wear following standardized or diagonal cutting tests. Odontol Revy *17:*121, 1966.
9. Lindhe J, Jacobson L. Evaluation of periodontal scalers. I. Wear following clinical use. Odontol Revy *17:*1, 1966.
10. Lubow RM, Cooley RL. Effect of air-powder abrasive instrument on restorative materials. J Prosthet Dent *55:*462, 1986.
11. McCall CM, Szmyd L. Clinical evaluation of ultrasonic scaling. J Am Dent Assoc *61:*559, 1960.
12. Orban B, Manella VB. A macroscopic and microscopic study of instruments designed for root planing. J Periodontol *27:*120, 1956.
13. Orton GS. Clinical use of an air-powder abrasive system. Dent Hyg *75:*513, 1987.
14. Parquette OE, Levin MP. The sharpening of scaling instruments. I. An examination of principles. J Periodontol *48:*163, 1977.
15. Waerhaug J, Arno A, Lovdal A. The dimension of instruments for removal of subgingival calculus. J Periodontol *25:*281, 1954.
16. Wentz FM. Therapeutic root planing. J Periodontol *28:*59, 1957.
17. Wilkins EM. Clinical Practice of the Dental Hygienist. 7th ed. Baltimore, Williams & Wilkins, 1994, pp 494–504.

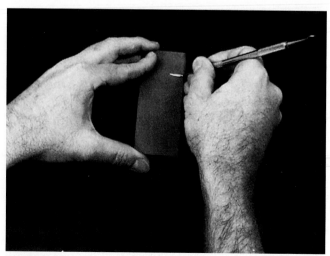

FIGURE 36–77. The interproximal knife may be sharpened on a flat stationary stone. The blade is drawn toward the operator.

37

Principles of Periodontal Instrumentation

GORDON L. PATTISON and ANNA M. PATTISON

GENERAL PRINCIPLES OF INSTRUMENTATION

Effective instrumentation is governed by a number of general principles that are common to all periodontal instruments. Proper position of the patient and the operator, illumination and retraction for optimal visibility, and sharp instruments are fundamental prerequisites. A constant awareness of tooth and root morphologic features and of the condition of the periodontal tissues is also essential. Knowledge of instrument design enables the clinician to efficiently select the proper instrument for the procedure and the area in which it will be performed. In addition to these principles, the basic concepts of grasp, finger rest, adaptation, angulation, and stroke must be understood before clinical instrument-handling skills can be mastered.

Accessibility (Positioning of Patient and Operator)

Accessibility facilitates thoroughness of instrumentation. The position of the patient and operator should provide maximal accessibility to the area of operation. Inadequate accessibility impedes thorough instrumentation, prematurely tires the operator, and diminishes his or her effectiveness.

The clinician should be seated on a comfortable operating stool that has been positioned so that his or her feet are flat on the floor with the thighs parallel to the floor. The clinician should be able to observe the field of operation while keeping the back straight and the head erect.

The patient should be in a supine position and placed so that the mouth is close to the resting elbow of the clinician. For instrumentation of the maxillary arch, the patient should be asked to raise his or her chin slightly to provide

optimal visibility and accessibility. For instrumentation on the mandibular arch, it may be necessary to raise the back of the chair slightly and request that the patient lower his or her chin until the mandible is parallel to the floor. This will especially facilitate work on the lingual surfaces of the mandibular anterior teeth.

Visibility, Illumination, and Retraction

Whenever possible, direct vision with direct illumination from the dental light is most desirable (Fig. 37–1). If this is not possible, indirect vision may be obtained by using the mouth mirror (Fig. 37–2), and indirect illumination may be obtained by using the mirror to reflect light to where it is needed (Fig. 37–3). Indirect vision and indirect illumination are often used simultaneously (Fig. 37–4).

Retraction provides visibility, accessibility, and illumination. Depending on the location of the area of operation, the fingers and/or the mirror are used for retraction. The mirror may be used for retraction of the cheeks or the tongue; the index finger is used for retraction of the lips or cheeks. The following methods are effective for retraction:

1. Use of the mirror to deflect the cheek while the fingers of the nonoperating hand retract the lips and protect the angle of the mouth from irritation by the mirror handle.
2. Use of the mirror alone to retract the lips and cheek (Fig. 37–5).
3. Use of the fingers of the nonoperating hand to retract the lips (Fig. 37–6).
4. Use of the mirror to retract the tongue (Fig. 37–7).
5. Combinations of the preceding methods.

When retracting, care should be taken to avoid irritation to the angles of the mouth. If the lips and skin are dry, softening the lips with petroleum jelly before instrumentation is begun is a helpful precaution against cracking and bleeding. Careful retraction is especially important for patients with a history of recurrent herpes labialis, because these

Material in this chapter was drawn freely from Pattison AM, Pattison GL. Periodontal Instrumentation. 2nd ed. Norwalk, CT, Appleton & Lange, 1992.

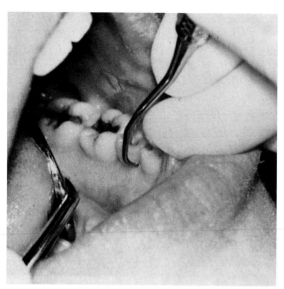

FIGURE 37–1. Direct vision and direct illumination in the mandibular left premolar area.

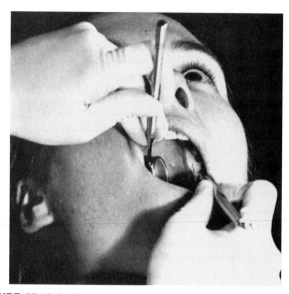

FIGURE 37–3. Indirect illumination using the mirror to reflect light onto the maxillary left posterior lingual region.

patients may easily develop herpetic lesions after instrumentation.

Condition of Instruments (Sharpness)

Prior to any instrumentation, all instruments should be inspected to make sure that they are clean, sterile, and in good condition. The working ends of pointed or bladed instruments must be sharp to be effective. Sharp instruments enhance tactile sensitivity and allow the clinician to work more precisely and efficiently. Dull instruments may lead to incomplete calculus removal and unnecessary trauma because of the excess force usually applied to compensate for their ineffectiveness (see Chapter 36).

Maintaining a Clean Field

Despite good visibility, illumination, and retraction, instrumentation can be hampered if the operative field is obscured by saliva, blood, and debris. The pooling of saliva

interferes with visibility during instrumentation and impedes control, because a firm finger rest cannot be established on wet, slippery tooth surfaces. Adequate suction is essential and can be achieved with a saliva ejector or, if working with an assistant, an aspirator.

Gingival bleeding is an unavoidable consequence of subgingival instrumentation. In areas of inflammation this is not necessarily an indication of trauma from incorrect technique; instead, it indicates ulceration of the pocket epithelium. Blood and debris can be removed from the operative field with suction and by wiping or blotting with gauze squares. The operative field should also be flushed occasionally with water.

Compressed air and gauze squares can be used to facilitate visual inspection of tooth surfaces just below the gingival margin during instrumentation. A jet of air directed into the pocket will deflect a retractable gingival margin. Retractable tissue can also be deflected away from the tooth

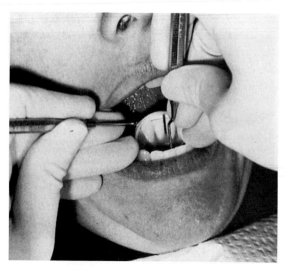

FIGURE 37–2. Indirect vision using the mirror for the lingual surfaces of the mandibular anterior teeth.

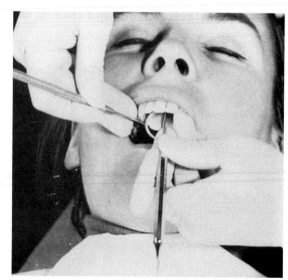

FIGURE 37–4. Combination of indirect illumination and indirect vision for the lingual surfaces of the maxillary anterior teeth.

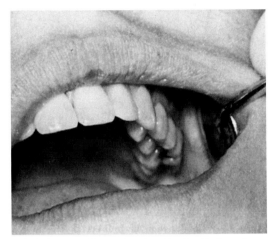

FIGURE 37–5. Retracting the cheek with the mirror.

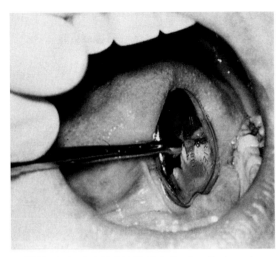

FIGURE 37–7. Retracting the tongue with the mirror.

by gently packing the edge of a gauze square into the pocket with the back of a curette. Immediately after the gauze is removed, the subgingival area should be clean, dry, and clearly visible for a brief interval.

Instrument Stabilization

Stability of the instrument and the hand is the primary requisite for controlled instrumentation. Stability and control are essential for effective instrumentation and avoidance of injury to the patient or the clinician. The two factors of major importance in providing stability are the instrument grasp and the finger rest.

Instrument Grasp. A proper grasp is essential for precise control of movements made during periodontal instrumentation. The most effective and stable grasp for all periodontal instruments is the modified pen grasp (Fig. 37–8). Although other grasps are possible, this modification of the standard pen grasp (Fig. 37–9) ensures the greatest control in performing intraoral procedures. *The thumb, index finger, and middle finger are used to hold the instrument as a pen is held, but the middle finger is positioned so that the side of the pad next to the fingernail is resting on the instrument shank. The index finger is bent at the second joint from the finger tip and is positioned well above the middle finger on the same side of the handle.* The pad of the thumb is placed midway between the middle and index fingers on the opposite side of the handle. This creates a triangle of forces, or a tripod effect, that enhances control because it counteracts the tendency of the instrument to turn uncontrollably between the fingers when scaling force is applied to the tooth. This stable modified pen grasp enhances control because it enables the clinician to roll the instrument in precise degrees with the thumb against the index and middle fingers to adapt the blade to the slightest changes in tooth contour. The modified pen grasp also enhances tactile sensitivity, because slight irregularities on the tooth surface are best perceived when the tactile-sensitive pad of the middle finger is placed on the shank of the instrument.

The palm and thumb grasp (Fig. 37–10) is useful for stabilizing instruments during sharpening and for manipulating air and water syringes, but it is not recommended for periodontal instrumentation. Maneuverability and tactile sensitivity are so inhibited by this grasp that it is unsuitable for the precise and controlled movements necessary during periodontal procedures.

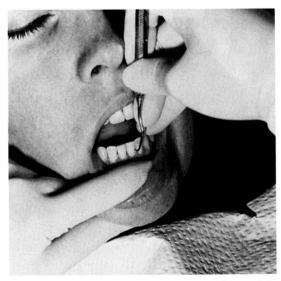

FIGURE 37–6. Retracting the lip with the index finger of the nonoperating hand.

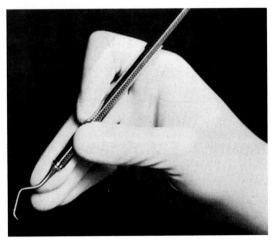

FIGURE 37–8. Modified pen grasp. The pad of the middle finger rests on the shank.

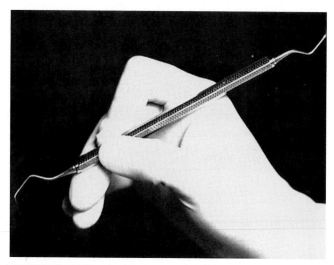

FIGURE 37–9. Standard pen grasp. The side of the middle finger rests on the shank.

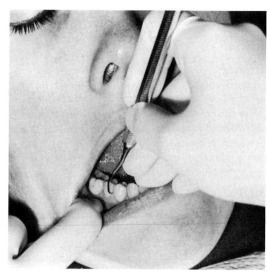

FIGURE 37–11. Intraoral conventional finger rest. The fourth finger rests on the occlusal surfaces of adjacent teeth.

Finger Rest. The finger rest serves to stabilize the hand and the instrument by providing a firm fulcrum as movements are made to activate the instrument. A good finger rest prevents injury and laceration of the gingiva and surrounding tissues by poorly controlled instruments. The fourth (ring) finger is preferred by most clinicians for the finger rest. Although it is possible to use the third (middle) finger for the finger rest, this is not recommended, because it restricts the arc of movement during the activation of strokes and severely curtails the use of the middle finger for both control and tactile sensitivity. Maximal control is achieved when the middle finger is kept between the instrument shank and the fourth finger. This "built-up" fulcrum is an integral part of the wrist-forearm action that activates the powerful working stroke for calculus removal. Whenever possible, these two fingers should be kept together to

work as a one-unit fulcrum during scaling and root planing. Separation of the middle and fourth fingers during scaling strokes results in a loss of power and control because it forces the clinician to rely solely on finger flexing for activation of the instrument.

Finger rests may be generally classified as intraoral finger rests or extraoral fulcrums. Intraoral finger rests on tooth surfaces ideally are established close to the working area. Variations of intraoral finger rests and extraoral fulcrums are utilized whenever good angulation and a sufficient arc of movement cannot be achieved by a finger rest close to the working area. The following examples illustrate the different variations of the intraoral finger rest:

1. *Conventional.* The finger rest is established on tooth surfaces immediately adjacent to the working area (Fig. 37–11).
2. *Cross-arch.* The finger rest is established on tooth surfaces on the other side of the same arch (Fig. 37–12).
3. *Opposite-arch.* The finger rest is established on tooth sur-

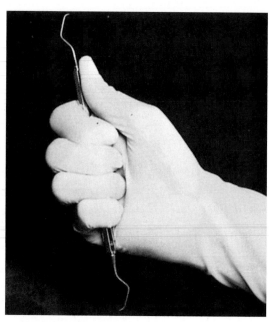

FIGURE 37–10. Palm and thumb grasp, used for stabilizing instruments during sharpening.

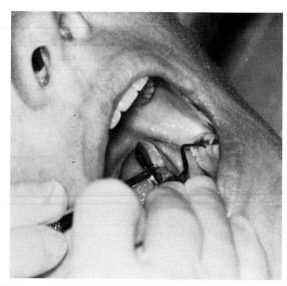

FIGURE 37–12. Intraoral cross-arch finger rest. The fourth finger rests on the incisal surfaces of teeth on the opposite side of the same arch.

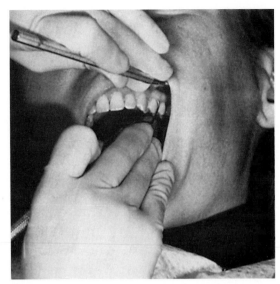

FIGURE 37–13. Intraoral opposite-arch finger rest. The fourth finger rests on the mandibular teeth while the maxillary posterior teeth are instrumented.

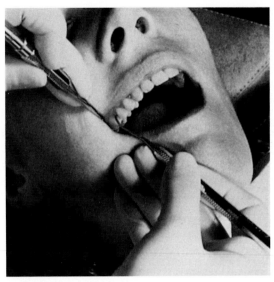

FIGURE 37–15. Extraoral palm-up fulcrum. The backs of the fingers rest on the right lateral aspect of the mandible while the maxillary right posterior teeth are instrumented.

faces on the opposite arch, e.g., mandibular arch finger rest for instrumentation on the maxillary arch (Fig. 37–13).

4. *Finger-on-finger.* The finger rest is established on the index finger or thumb of the nonoperating hand (Fig. 37–14).

Extraoral fulcrums are essential for effective instrumentation of some aspects of the maxillary posterior teeth (see Chapter 38). When properly established, they allow optimal access and angulation while providing adequate stabilization. Extraoral fulcrums are not finger rests in the literal sense, because the tips or pads of the fingers are not used for extraoral fulcrums as they are for intraoral finger rests. Instead, as much of the front or back surface of the fingers as possible is placed on the patient's face to provide the greatest degree of stability. The two most commonly used extraoral fulcrums are as follows:

1. *Palm-up.* The palm-up fulcrum is established by resting the backs of the middle and fourth fingers on the skin overlying

the lateral aspect of the mandible on the right side of the face (Fig. 37–15).

2. *Palm-down.* The palm-down fulcrum is established by resting the front surfaces of the middle and fourth fingers on the skin overlying the lateral aspect of the mandible on the left side of the face (Fig. 37–16).

Both intraoral finger rests and extraoral fulcrums may be reinforced by applying the index finger or thumb of the nonoperating hand to the handle or shank of the instrument for added control and pressure against the tooth. The reinforcing finger is usually employed for opposite-arch or extraoral fulcrums when precise control and pressure are compromised by the longer distance between the fulcrum and the working end of the instrument. Figure 37–17 shows the index finger–reinforced rest, and Figure 37–18 shows the thumb-reinforced rest.

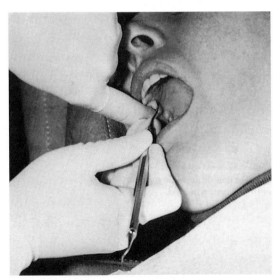

FIGURE 37–14. Intraoral finger-on-finger rest. The fourth finger rests on the index finger of the nonoperating hand.

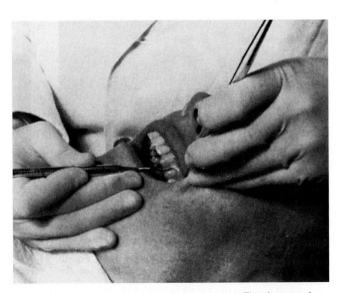

FIGURE 37–16. Extraoral palm-down fulcrum. The front surfaces of the fingers rest on the left lateral aspect of the mandible while the maxillary left posterior teeth are instrumented.

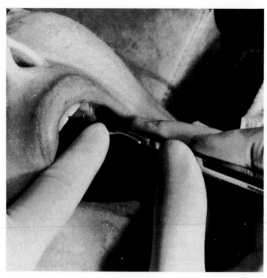

FIGURE 37–17. Index finger–reinforced rest. The index finger is placed on the shank for pressure and control in the maxillary left posterior lingual region.

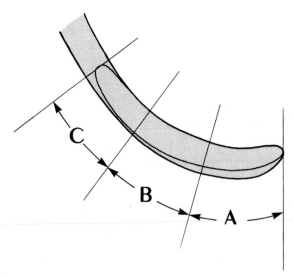

FIGURE 37–19. Gracey curette blade divided into three segments: the lower one third of the blade, consisting of the terminal few millimeters adjacent to the toe (*A*); the middle one third (*B*); and the upper one third, which is adjacent to the shank (*C*).

Instrument Activation

Adaptation. *Adaptation* refers to the manner in which the working end of a periodontal instrument is placed against the surface of a tooth. The objective of adaptation is to make the working end of the instrument conform to the contour of the tooth surface. Precise adaptation must be maintained with all instruments to avoid trauma to the soft tissues and root surfaces and to ensure maximum effectiveness of instrumentation.

Correct adaptation of the probe is quite simple. The tip and side of the probe should be flush against the tooth surface as vertical strokes are activated within the crevice. Bladed instruments such as curettes and sharp-pointed instruments such as explorers are more difficult to adapt. The ends of these instruments are sharp and can lacerate tissue, so adaptation in subgingival areas becomes especially important. The lower third of the working end, which is the

last few millimeters adjacent to the toe or tip, must be kept in constant contact with the tooth while it is moving over varying tooth contours (Fig. 37–19). Precise adaptation is maintained by carefully rolling the handle of the instrument against the index and middle fingers with the thumb. This rotates the instrument in slight degrees so that the toe or tip leads into concavities and around convexities. On convex surfaces such as line angles, it is not possible to adapt more than 1 or 2 mm of the working end against the tooth. Even on what appear to be broader, flatter surfaces, no more than 1 or 2 mm of the working end can be adapted, because the tooth surface, although it may seem flat, is actually slightly curved.

If only the middle third of the working end is adapted on a convex surface so that the blade contacts the tooth at a tangent, the toe or sharp tip will jut out into soft tissue, causing trauma and discomfort (Fig. 37–20). If the instrument is adapted so that only the toe or tip is in contact, the soft tissue can be distended or compressed by the back of

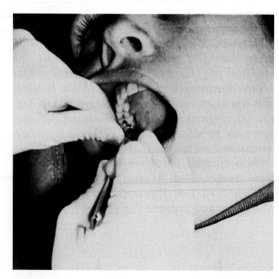

FIGURE 37–18. Thumb-reinforced rest. The thumb is placed on the handle for control in the maxillary right posterior lingual region.

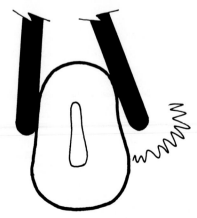

FIGURE 37–20. Blade adaptation. The curette on the left is properly adapted to the root surface. The curette on the right is incorrectly adapted; the toe juts out, lacerating the soft tissues.

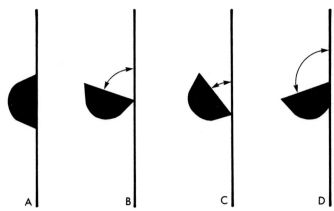

FIGURE 37-21. Blade angulation. *A*, 0 degrees: correct angulation for blade insertion. *B*, 45 to 90 degrees: correct angulation for scaling and root planing. *C*, Less than 45 degrees: incorrect angulation for scaling and root planing. *D*, More than 90 degrees: incorrect angulation for scaling and root planing, correct angulation for gingival curettage.

the working end, also causing trauma and discomfort. A curette that is improperly adapted in this manner can be particularly damaging, because the toe can gouge or groove the root surface.

Angulation. *Angulation* refers to the angle between the face of a bladed instrument and the tooth surface. It may also be called the tooth-blade relationship.

Correct angulation is essential for effective calculus removal. For subgingival insertion of a bladed instrument such as a curette, angulation should be as close to 0 degree as possible (Fig. 37-21). The end of the instrument can be inserted to the base of the pocket more easily with the face of the blade flush against the tooth. During scaling and root planing, optimal angulation is between 45 and 90 degrees (see Fig. 37-21). The exact blade angulation depends on the amount and nature of the calculus, the procedure being performed, and the condition of the tissue. Blade angulation is diminished or closed by tilting the lower shank of the instrument toward the tooth. It is increased or opened by tilting the lower shank away from the tooth. During scaling strokes on heavy, tenacious calculus, angulation should be just less than 90 degrees so that the cutting edge "bites" into the calculus. With angulation of less than 45 degrees, the cutting edge will not bite into or engage the calculus properly (see Fig. 37-21). Instead, it will slide over the calculus, smoothing or "burnishing" it. If angulation is more than 90 degrees, the lateral surface of the blade, rather than the cutting edge, will be against the tooth, and the calculus will not be removed and may become burnished (see Fig. 37-21). After the calculus has been removed, angulation of just less than 90 degrees may be maintained, or the angle may be slightly closed as the root surface is smoothed with light root planing strokes.

When gingival curettage is indicated, angulation greater than 90 degrees is deliberately established so that the cutting edge will engage and remove the pocket lining.

Lateral Pressure. *Lateral pressure* refers to the pressure created when force is applied against the surface of a tooth with the cutting edge of a bladed instrument. The exact amount of pressure applied must be varied according to the nature of the calculus and according to whether the stroke

is intended for initial scaling to remove calculus or for root planing to smooth the root surface.

Lateral pressure may be firm, moderate, or light. When removing calculus, lateral pressure is applied firmly or moderately initially and is progressively diminished until light lateral pressure is applied for the final root planing strokes. When insufficient lateral pressure is applied for the removal of heavy calculus, rough ledges or lumps may be shaved to thin, smooth sheets of burnished calculus that are difficult to detect and remove. This burnishing effect often occurs in areas of developmental depressions and along the cemento-enamel junction.

Although firm lateral pressure is necessary for the thorough removal of calculus, indiscriminate, unwarranted, or uncontrolled application of heavy forces during instrumentation should be avoided. Repeated application of excessively heavy strokes will nick or gouge the root surface.

The careful application of varied and controlled amounts of lateral pressure during instrumentation is an integral part of effective scaling and root planing techniques and is absolutely critical to the success of both of these procedures.

Strokes. Three basic types of strokes are used during instrumentation: the exploratory stroke, the scaling stroke, and the root planing stroke. Any of these basic strokes may be activated by a pull or a push motion in a vertical, oblique, or horizontal direction (Fig. 37-22). Vertical and oblique strokes are used most frequently. Horizontal strokes are used selectively on line angles or deep pockets that cannot be negotiated with vertical or oblique strokes. The direction, length, pressure, and number of strokes necessary for either scaling or root planing are determined by four major factors: gingival position and tone, pocket depth and shape, tooth contour, and the amount and nature of the calculus or roughness.

The *exploratory stroke* is a light, "feeling" stroke that is used with probes and explorers to evaluate the dimensions of the pocket and to detect calculus and irregularities of the tooth surface. With bladed instruments such as the curette, the exploratory stroke is alternated with scaling and root planing strokes for these same purposes of evaluation and detection. The instrument is grasped lightly and adapted with light pressure against the tooth to achieve maximal tactile sensitivity.

The *scaling stroke* is a short, powerful pull stroke that is used with bladed instruments for the removal of both

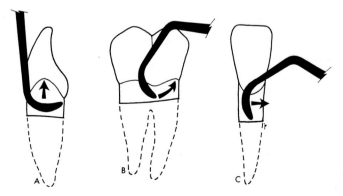

FIGURE 37-22. Three basic stroke directions. *A*, Vertical. *B*, Oblique. *C*, Horizontal.

supragingival and subgingival calculus. The muscles of the fingers and hands are tensed to establish a secure grasp, and lateral pressure is firmly applied against the tooth surface. The cutting edge engages the apical border of the calculus and dislodges it with a firm movement in a coronal direction. The scaling motion should be initiated in the forearm and transmitted from the wrist to the hand with a slight flexing of the fingers. Rotation of the wrist is synchronized with movement of the forearm. The scaling stroke is not initiated in the wrist or fingers, nor is it carried out independently without the use of the forearm.

It is possible to initiate the scaling motion by rotating the wrist and forearm or by flexing the fingers. The use of wrist and forearm action versus finger motion has long been debated among clinicians. Perhaps the strong opinions on both sides should be the most valid indication that there is a time and a place for each. Neither method can be advocated exclusively, because a careful analysis of effective scaling and root planing technique reveals that, indeed, both types of stroke activation are necessary for complete instrumentation. The wrist and forearm motion, pivoting in an arc on the finger rest, produces a more powerful stroke and is therefore preferred for scaling. Finger flexing is indicated for precise control over stroke length in areas such as line angles and when horizontal strokes are used on the lingual or facial aspects of narrow-rooted teeth.

The push scaling motion has been advocated by some clinicians. In the push stroke, the instrument engages the lateral or coronal border of the calculus, and the fingers provide a thrust motion that dislodges the deposit. Because the push stroke may force calculus into the supporting tissues, its use, especially in an apical direction, is not recommended.

The *root planing stroke* is a moderate to light pull stroke that is used for final smoothing and planing of the root surface. Although hoes, files, and ultrasonic instruments have been used for root planing, curettes are widely acknowledged to be the most effective and versatile instruments for this procedure.[8,17,18,25,36,39,46,50] The design of the curette, which allows it to be more easily adapted to subgingival tooth contours, makes curettes particularly suitable for root planing in periodontal patients. With a moderately firm grasp, the curette is kept adapted to the tooth with even, lateral pressure. A continuous series of long, overlapping shaving strokes is activated. As the surface becomes smoother and resistance diminishes, lateral pressure is progressively reduced.

PRINCIPLES OF SCALING AND ROOT PLANING

Definitions and Rationale for Scaling and Root Planing

Scaling is the process by which plaque and calculus are removed from both supragingival and subgingival tooth surfaces. There is no deliberate attempt to remove tooth substance along with the calculus. *Root planing* is the process by which residual embedded calculus and portions of cementum are removed from the roots to produce a smooth, hard, clean surface.

The primary objective of scaling and root planing is to restore gingival health by completely removing from the tooth surface elements that provoke gingival inflammation (i.e., plaque, calculus, and endotoxin). Scaling and root planing are not separate procedures. All the principles of scaling apply equally to root planing. The difference between scaling and root planing is only a matter of degree. The nature of the tooth surface determines the degree to which the surface must be scaled or planed.

On enamel surfaces, plaque and calculus provoke gingival inflammation. Unless they are grooved or pitted, enamel surfaces are relatively smooth and uniform. When plaque and calculus form on enamel, the deposits are usually superficially attached to the surface and are not locked into irregularities. Scaling alone is sufficient to completely remove plaque and calculus from enamel, leaving a smooth, clean surface.

Root surfaces exposed to plaque and calculus pose a different problem. *Deposits of calculus on root surfaces are frequently embedded in cemental irregularities*[32,51]*; therefore, scaling alone is insufficient to remove them, and a portion of the cementum itself must be removed to eliminate these deposits.* Furthermore, when cementum is exposed to plaque and the pocket environment, its surface is contaminated by toxic substances, notably endotoxins.[1,2,20] Recent evidence suggests that these toxic substances are only superficially attached to the root and do not permeate it deeply.[10,11,22,23,31,34,35,41] Removal of extensive amounts of dentin and cementum are not necessary to render the roots free of toxins.[19] However, where cementum is thin, instrumentation may expose dentin. Although this is not the aim of treatment, it may be unavoidable.[39,46]

When the rationale for scaling and root planing is thoroughly understood, it becomes apparent that mastery of these skills is essential to the ultimate success of any course of periodontal therapy. Of all clinical dental procedures, subgingival scaling and root planing in deep pockets are the most difficult and exacting skills to master. It has been argued that such proficiency in instrumentation cannot be attained; therefore, periodontal surgery is necessary to gain access to root surfaces. Others have argued that although proficiency is possible, it need not be developed, because access to the roots can be gained more easily with surgery. However, without mastering subgingival scaling and root planing skills, the clinician will be severely hampered and unable to treat adequately those patients for whom surgery is contraindicated.

Detection Skills

Good visual and tactile detection skills are required for the accurate initial assessment of the extent and nature of deposits and root irregularities before scaling and root planing. Valid evaluation of results of instrumentation depends on these detection skills.

Visual examination of supragingival calculus and of subgingival calculus just below the gingival margin is not difficult with good lighting and a clean field. Light deposits of supragingival calculus are often difficult to see when they are wet with saliva. Compressed air may be used to dry supragingival calculus until it is chalky white and readily visible. Air may also be directed into the pocket in a steady stream to deflect the marginal gingiva away from the tooth so that subgingival deposits near the surface can be seen.

Tactile exploration of the tooth surfaces in subgingival areas of pocket depth, furcations, and developmental depressions is much more difficult than visual examination of supragingival areas and requires the skilled use of a fine-pointed explorer or probe. The explorer or probe is held with a light but stable modified pen grasp. This provides maximal tactile sensitivity for detection of subgingival calculus and other irregularities. The pads of the thumb and fingers, especially the middle finger, should perceive the slight vibrations conducted through the instrument shank and handle as irregularities in the tooth surface are encountered.

After a stable finger rest is established, the tip of the instrument is carefully inserted subgingivally to the base of the pocket. Light exploratory strokes are activated vertically up and down on the root surface. When calculus is encountered, the tip of the instrument should be advanced apically over the deposit until the termination of the calculus on the root is felt. The distance between the apical edge of the calculus and the bottom of the pocket usually ranges from 0.2 to 1.0 mm. The tip is adapted closely to the tooth to ensure the greatest degree of tactile sensitivity and to avoid tissue trauma. When a proximal surface is being explored, strokes must be extended at least halfway across that surface past the contact area to ensure complete detection of interproximal deposits. When an explorer is used at line angles, convexities, and concavities, the handle of the instrument must be rolled slightly between the thumb and fingers to keep the tip constantly adapted to the changes in tooth contour.

Although exploration technique and good tactile sensitivity are important, interpreting various degrees of roughness and making clinical judgments based on these interpretations also require much expertise. The beginning student usually has difficulty detecting fine calculus and altered cementum. Such detection must begin with the recognition of ledges, lumps, or spurs of calculus, then smaller spicules, then slight roughness, and, finally, a slight graininess that feels like a sticky coating or film covering the tooth surface. Overhanging or deficient margins of dental restorations, caries, decalcification, and root roughness caused by previous instrumentation are all commonly found during exploration. These and other irregularities must be recognized and differentiated from subgingival calculus. Because this requires a great deal of experience and a high degree of tactile sensitivity, many clinicians agree that the development of detection skills is as important as the mastery of scaling and root planing technique.

Instruments for Scaling and Root Planing

Universal Curettes. The working ends of the universal curette are designed in pairs so that all surfaces of the teeth can be treated with one double-ended instrument or a matched pair of single-ended instruments.

In any given quadrant, when approaching the tooth from the facial aspect, one end of the universal curette will adapt to the mesial surfaces and the other end will adapt to the distal surfaces. When approaching from the lingual aspect

in the same quadrant, the double-ended universal curette must be turned end for end, because the blades are mirror images. This means that the end that adapts to the mesial surfaces on the facial aspect also adapts to the distal surfaces on the lingual aspect, and vice versa. Both ends of the universal curette are used to instrument the anterior teeth. On posterior teeth, however, owing to the limited access to distal surfaces, a single working end can be used to treat both mesial and distal surfaces by using both of its cutting edges. To do this, the instrument is first adapted to the mesial surface with the handle nearly parallel to the mesial surface. Because the face of the universal curette blade is honed at 90 degrees to the lower shank, if the lower shank is positioned so that it is absolutely parallel to the surface being instrumented, the tooth–blade angulation is 90 degrees. To close this angle and thus obtain proper working angulation, the lower shank must be tilted slightly toward the tooth. The distal surface of the same posterior tooth can be instrumented with the opposite cutting edge of the same blade. This cutting edge can be adapted at proper working angulation by positioning the handle so that it is *perpendicular* to the distal surface (Fig. 37–23).

When adapting the universal curette blade, as much of the cutting edge as possible should be in contact with the tooth surface, except on narrow convex surfaces such as line angles. Although the entire cutting edge should contact the tooth, pressure should be concentrated on the lower third of the blade during scaling strokes. During root planing strokes, however, lateral pressure should be distributed evenly along the cutting edge.

The primary advantage of these curettes is that they are designed to be used universally on all tooth surfaces, in all regions of the mouth. However, universal curettes have limited adaptability for the treatment of deep pockets in which apical migration of the attachment has exposed furcations, root convexities, and developmental depressions. For this reason, the Gracey curettes and the new modifications of Gracey curettes, which are area specific and spe-

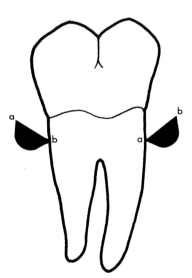

FIGURE 37–23. Adaptation of the universal curette on a posterior tooth. Cross-sectional representations of the same universal curette blade as its cutting edges (a and b) are adapted to the mesial and distal surfaces of a posterior tooth.

cially designed for subgingival scaling and root planing in periodontal patients, are preferred by many clinicians.

Gracey Curettes. Gracey curettes are a set of area-specific instruments that were designed by Dr. Clayton H. Gracey of Michigan in the mid-1930s. Four design features make the Gracey curettes unique: they are area specific, only one cutting edge on each blade is used, the blade is curved in two planes, and the blade is "offset." (These features have been summarized in Table 36–1.) Each of these features directly influences the manner in which the Gracey curettes are used and should be discussed individually.

Area Specificity. There are seven pairs of curettes in the set. The Gracey curettes no. 1–2 and 3–4 are used on anterior teeth. The Gracey no. 5–6 may be used on both anterior and premolar teeth. The facial and lingual surfaces of posterior teeth are instrumented with Gracey curettes no. 7–8 and 9–10. The Gracey no. 11–12 is designed for mesial surfaces of posterior teeth, and the Gracey no. 13–14 adapts to the distal surfaces of posterior teeth. Although these guidelines for areas of use were originally established by Dr. Gracey, it is possible to use a Gracey curette in an area of the mouth other than the one for which it was specifically designed if the general principles regarding these curettes are understood and applied. Gracey curettes need not be reserved exclusively for periodontal patients. In fact, many clinicians prefer Gracey curettes for general scaling because of their excellent adaptability.

Single Cutting Edge Used. Like a universal curette, the Gracey curette has a blade with two cutting edges. Unlike the universal curette, however, the Gracey instrument is designed so that only one cutting edge is used. To determine which of the two is the correct cutting edge to adapt to the tooth, the blade should be held face up and parallel to the floor. When viewed from this angle, the blade can be seen to curve to the side. One cutting edge forms a larger outer curve and the other forms a shorter, small inner curve. The larger outer curve, which has also been described as the inferior cutting edge or as the cutting edge farther away from the handle, is the correct cutting edge (Fig. 37–24).

Blade Curves in Two Planes. Like the toe of the universal curette, the toe of the Gracey curette curves upward. However, the toe of the Gracey curette also curves to the side, as mentioned in the preceding discussion. This unique curvature enhances the blade's adaptation to convexities and concavities as the working end is advanced around the tooth. Only the lower third or half of the Gracey blade is in contact with the tooth during instrumentation. The cutting edge of a universal curette blade, on the other hand, is straight and does not curve to the side. This makes it less adaptable to root concavities.

Offset Blade. Gracey curette blades are honed at an offset angle, which means that the face of the blade is not perpendicular to the lower shank as it is on a universal curette. Instead, Gracey curettes are designed so that the tooth–blade working angulation is 60 to 70 degrees when the lower shank is held parallel to the tooth surface. Gracey curettes were originally designed to be used with push strokes and were beveled to provide a tooth–blade angulation of 40 degrees when the lower shank was parallel to the tooth surface; for many years, Gracey curettes were available only in this form. Currently Gracey curettes are available not only in the original push design, but also in a

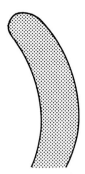

FIGURE 37–24. Determining the correct cutting edge of a Gracey curette. When viewed from directly above the face of the blade, the correct cutting edge is the one forming the larger, outer curve on the right.

modified version to be used with pull strokes. It is important to understand this when purchasing Gracey curettes to avoid obtaining instruments that are not properly designed for pull strokes. If Gracey curettes that are designed to be used with push strokes are used with pull strokes instead, they are likely to burnish calculus rather than completely remove it. The design of the Gracey curette was modified in response to requests from clinicians who liked the shank design and adaptability of the original Gracey instruments but were opposed to the use of push strokes for scaling and root planing. The push stroke is not recommended, especially for the novice clinician, because it is likely to cause undue trauma to the junctional epithelium and to embed fragments of dislodged calculus in the soft tissues.

Principles of Use. The following general principles of use of the Gracey curettes are essentially the same as those for the universal curette; italicized principles apply only to Gracey curettes:

1. *Determine the correct cutting edge.* The correct cutting edge should be determined by visually inspecting the blade and confirmed by lightly adapting the chosen cutting edge to the tooth with the lower shank parallel to the surface of the tooth. With the toe pointed in the direction to be scaled (e.g., mesially with a no. 7–8 curette), only the back of the blade can be seen if the correct cutting edge has been selected (Fig. 37–25). If the wrong cutting edge has been adopted, the flat, shiny face of the blade will be seen instead (Fig. 37–26).

2. *Make sure the lower shank is parallel to the surface to be instrumented.* The lower shank of a Gracey curette is that portion of the shank between the blade and the first bend in the shank. Parallelism of the handle or upper shank is not an acceptable guide with Gracey curettes, because the angulations of the shanks vary. On anterior teeth, the lower shank of the Gracey no. 1–2, 3–4, or 5–6 should be parallel to the mesial, distal, facial, or lingual surfaces of the teeth (Fig. 37–27). On posterior teeth, the lower shank of the no. 7–8 or 9–10 should be parallel to the facial or lingual surfaces of the teeth (Fig. 37–28), the lower shank of the no. 11–12 should be parallel to the mesial surfaces of the teeth (Fig. 37–29), and the lower shank of the no. 13–14 should be parallel to the distal surfaces of the teeth (Fig. 37–30).

3. When using intraoral finger rests, keep the fourth and middle fingers together in a built-up fulcrum for maximum control and wrist–arm action.

4. Use extraoral fulcrums or mandibular finger rests for optimal angulation when working on the maxillary posterior teeth.

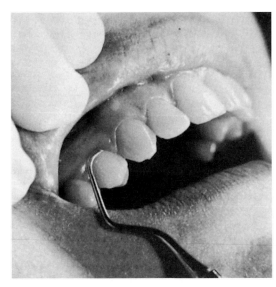

FIGURE 37–25. Correct cutting edge of a Gracey curette adapted to the tooth.

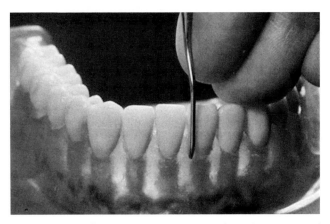

FIGURE 37–27. Gracey no. 5–6 curette adapted to an anterior tooth.

5. *Concentrate on using the lower third of the cutting edge for calculus removal,* especially on line angles or when attempting to remove a calculus ledge by breaking it away in sections, beginning at the lateral edge.
6. Allow the wrist and forearm to carry the burden of the stroke, rather than flexing the fingers.
7. Roll the handle slightly between the thumb and fingers to keep the blade adapted as the working end is advanced around line angles and into concavities.
8. Modulate lateral pressure from firm to moderate to light depending on the nature of the calculus, and reduce pressure as the transition is made from scaling to root planing strokes.

Extended Shank Gracey Curettes. Extended shank Gracey curettes such as the After Five curettes are 3 mm longer in the terminal shank than the standard Gracey curettes but are used with the same technique. They are most useful for deep pockets on maxillary and mandibular posterior teeth, where the longer terminal shank allows better access, especially to deep mesial and distal pockets. Although the longer lower shank makes access easier while using a conventional intraoral finger rest, the use of an extraoral fulcrum will allow better access and adaptation to all of the maxillary posterior teeth. After Five curettes with rigid shanks should be used for scaling of heavy calculus; those with regular, finishing shanks should be used for periodontal maintenance patients with deep residual pockets.

Mini-bladed Gracey Curettes. Mini-bladed Gracey curettes such as the Mini Five curettes and the Gracey Curvettes have a terminal shank that is 3 mm longer than the standard Gracey curettes and a blade that is 50% shorter. These mini-bladed instruments are generally used in the same manner as the Gracey curettes except for the following specific differences:

1. Mini-bladed curettes should not be used routinely in place of standard Gracey or After Five curettes. Instead, they should be used to supplement conventional curettes and ultrasonic instruments in areas of difficult access such as furcations; line angles; and deep, tight, or narrow pockets.
2. Large no. 4 handles are recommended for any mini-bladed instruments, because the larger diameter of the handles allows better control of the small blades.
3. Mini-bladed curettes can be used to scale with the toe directed either mesially or distally. In fact, the Mini Five curettes often adapt more effectively to the root curvatures

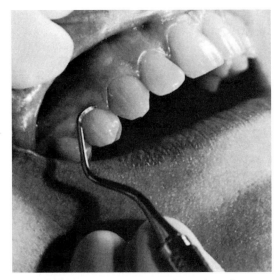

FIGURE 37–26. Incorrect cutting edge of a Gracey curette adapted to the tooth.

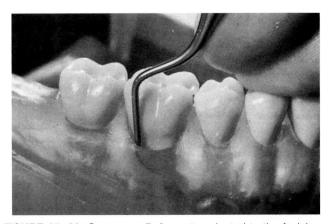

FIGURE 37–28. Gracey no. 7–8 curette adapted to the facial surface of a posterior tooth.

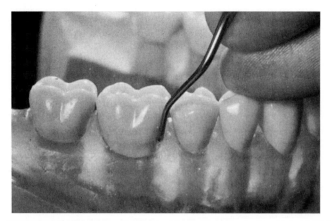

FIGURE 37-29. Gracey no. 11-12 curette adapted to the mesial surface of a posterior tooth.

of many posterior teeth when the blade is inserted with the toe pointed distally and strokes are activated from the mesial toward the distal line angle.

4. Use rigid shank mini-bladed curettes for calculus removal. Use the thinner, standard shank mini-bladed curettes for deplaquing during maintenance.
5. When using mini-bladed curettes for calculus removal, use intraoral finger rests close to the working area. When performing light root planing or deplaquing, either intraoral or extraoral rests may be used. Extraoral rests are usually necessary to gain access to deep pockets on maxillary second and third molars.

Ultrasonic Scaling Instruments. Ultrasonic instruments have been used as a valuable adjunct to conventional hand instrumentation for many years. Until relatively recently, all ultrasonic tips were large and bulky, making them generally suitable only for supragingival scaling or for subgingival scaling where tissue was inflamed and retractable. However, newly designed thin ultrasonic tips have allowed better access to subgingival areas previously accessible only with hand instruments.[21] It is important to understand this historical perspective when attempting to interpret the literature comparing the effects of hand and ultrasonic instruments on root surfaces. Earlier studies using older tip designs generally showed that ultrasonic instruments left a rougher, more damaged surface than curettes.[3,17,18,25,44,46,50] More recent studies, especially those using the newer, thin-

ner tips, show that ultrasonic instruments can produce root surfaces that are as smooth[15,16] or smoother[14-16] than can be produced by curettes. Whether these relative degrees of smoothness are important has not been established.[17,21] It is evident, however, that both methods of instrumentation are able to provide satisfactory clinical results[4-7,19,28,30,37,44,45] as measured by removal of plaque and calculus, reduction of inflammation and pocket depth, and gain in clinical attachment. Ultrasonic instruments have been shown to be more effective than hand instruments at reducing spirochetes and motile rods in class II and III furcations.[29] The selection of either ultrasonic or hand instrumentation should be determined by the clinician's preference and experience and by the needs of each patient. The success of either treatment method is determined by the time devoted to the procedure and the thoroughness of root debridement. In practice, clinicians commonly use a combination of both ultrasonic and hand instrumentation to achieve thorough debridement.

The vibrational energy produced by the ultrasonic instrument makes it useful for removing heavy, tenacious deposits of calculus and stain. Such deposits can be removed more quickly and with less effort ultrasonically than manually. When ultrasonic instruments are properly manipulated, there is less tissue trauma and therefore less postoperative discomfort. This makes ultrasonic instrumentation useful for initial debridement in patients with acute, painful conditions such as necrotizing ulcerative gingivitis. This same quality can be used to advantage with the new, thin ultrasonic tips for subgingival root debridement and deplaquing in maintenance patients with residual pocket depth. Ultrasonic scaling devices have also been used for gingival curettage and to remove overhangs and excess cement after cementing orthodontic appliances. Opinions differ regarding the effectiveness of ultrasonic instruments for removing stain compared with conventional polishing methods.[9,24]

There are some definite contraindications to the use of ultrasonic and sonic scaling devices. No one with a cardiac pacemaker should be exposed to ultrasonic instruments. Patients with known communicable diseases that can be transmitted by aerosols should not be treated with ultrasonic or sonic scaling devices. The water spray creates a contaminated aerosol that fills the operating area, exposing personnel and surfaces.[26,33] Even when treating patients without known communicable diseases, it is especially important that proper infection control measures be observed (i.e., use of protective clothing, eyewear, masks, and gloves) and proper surface decontamination be performed afterward. Prerinsing for 1 minute with an antimicrobial mouthwash such as 0.12% chlorhexidine will significantly reduce the number of bacteria in the aerosol for approximately 1 hour.[47] Patients at risk of respiratory disease should not be treated with ultrasonic or sonic devices; these include patients who are immunosuppressed or suffer from chronic pulmonary disorders. Finally, ultrasonic and sonic instruments are contraindicated for porcelain or bonded restorations, because these can be fractured or removed.

Supragingival Scaling Technique

Supragingival calculus is generally less tenacious and less calcified than subgingival calculus. Because instrumentation is performed coronal to the gingival margin, scaling

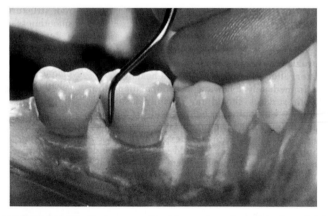

FIGURE 37-30. Gracey no. 13-14 curette adapted to the distal surface of a posterior tooth.

strokes are not confined by the surrounding tissues. This makes adaptation and angulation easier. It also allows direct visibility, as well as a freedom of movement that is not possible during subgingival scaling.

Sickles, curettes, and ultrasonic and sonic instruments are most commonly used for the removal of supragingival calculus. Hoes and chisels are less frequently used. To perform supragingival scaling, the sickle or curette is held with a modified pen grasp, and a firm finger rest is established on the teeth adjacent to the working area. The blade is adapted with an angulation of slightly less than 90 degrees to the surface being scaled. The cutting edge should engage the apical margin of the supragingival calculus while short, powerful, overlapping scaling strokes are activated coronally in a vertical or an oblique direction. The sharply pointed tip of the sickle can easily lacerate marginal tissue or gouge exposed root surfaces, so careful adaptation is especially important when this instrument is being used. The tooth surface is instrumented until it is visually and tactilely free of all supragingival deposits. If the tissue is retractable enough to allow easy insertion of the bulky blade, the sickle may be used slightly below the free gingival margin. If the sickle is used in this manner, final scaling and root planing with the curette should always follow.

Subgingival Scaling and Root Planing Technique

Subgingival scaling and root planing are far more complex and difficult to perform than supragingival scaling. Subgingival calculus is usually harder than supragingival calculus and is often locked into root irregularities, making it more tenacious and therefore more difficult to remove.[32,40,51]

The overlying tissue creates significant problems in subgingival instrumentation. Vision is obscured by the bleeding that inevitably occurs during instrumentation, as well as by the tissue itself. The clinician must rely heavily on tactile sensitivity to detect calculus and irregularities, to guide the instrument blade during scaling and root planing, and to evaluate the results of instrumentation.

In addition, the direction and length of the strokes are limited by the adjacent pocket wall. The confines of the soft tissue make careful adaptation to tooth contours imperative to avoid trauma. Such precise adaptation cannot be accomplished without a thorough knowledge of tooth morphologic features. The clinician must form a mental image of the tooth surface to anticipate variations in contour, continually confirming or modifying the image in response to tactile sensations and visual cues, such as the position of the instrument handle and shank. The clinician must then instantaneously adjust the adaptation and angulation of the working end to the tooth. It is this complex and precise coordination of visual, mental, and manual skills that makes subgingival instrumentation one of the most difficult of all dental skills. *The curette is preferred by most clinicians for subgingival scaling and root planing because of the advantages afforded by its design.* Its curved blade, rounded toe, and curved back allow the curette to be inserted to the base of the pocket and to be adapted to variations in tooth contour with minimal tissue displacement and trauma.

Hoes, files, and ultrasonic instruments are also used for subgingival scaling of heavy calculus. Although some delicate files may be inserted to the base of the pocket to crush or initially fracture tenacious deposits, heavier files, hoes, and standard ultrasonic tips for supragingival use are bulky and cannot easily be inserted into deep pockets or areas where tissue is firm and fibrotic. Hoes and files are not able to produce as smooth a surface as curettes.[8,39] Hoes, files, and standard large ultrasonic tips are all more hazardous than the curette in terms of trauma to the root surface and surrounding tissues.[8,36,39] Thinner ultrasonic tips designed for subgingival scaling of deep pockets and furcations have been made available relatively recently.

Subgingival scaling and root planing are accomplished with either universal or area-specific (Gracey) curettes using the following basic procedure: The curette is held with a modified pen grasp, and a stable finger rest is established. The correct cutting edge is slightly adapted to the tooth, with the lower shank kept parallel to the tooth surface. The lower shank is moved toward the tooth so that the face of the blade is nearly flush with the tooth surface. The blade is then inserted under the gingiva and advanced to the base of the pocket by a light exploratory stroke. When the cutting edge reaches the base of the pocket, a working angulation of between 45 and 90 degrees is established, and pressure is applied laterally against the tooth surface. Calculus is removed by a series of controlled, overlapping, short, powerful strokes primarily utilizing wrist–arm motion (Fig. 37–31). As calculus is removed, resistance to the passage of the cutting edge diminishes until only a slight roughness remains. Longer, lighter root planing strokes are then activated with less lateral pressure until the root surface is completely smooth and hard. The instrument handle must be rolled carefully between the thumb and fingers to keep the blade adapted closely to the tooth surface as line angles, developmental depressions, and other changes in tooth contour are followed. Scaling and root planing strokes should be confined to the portion of the tooth where calculus or altered cementum is found. This zone is known as the *instrumentation zone.* Sweeping the instrument over the

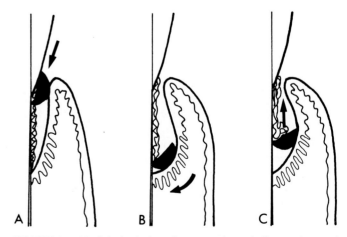

FIGURE 37–31. Subgingival scaling procedure. *A,* Curette inserted with the face of the blade flush against the tooth. *B,* Working angulation (45 to 90 degrees) is established at the base of the pocket. *C,* Lateral pressure is applied, and the scaling stroke is activated in the coronal direction.

crown where it is not needed wastes operating time, dulls the instrument, and causes loss of control.

The amount of lateral pressure applied to the tooth surface depends on the nature of the calculus and on whether the strokes are for initial calculus removal or final root planing. If heavy lateral pressure is continued after the bulk of calculus has been removed and the blade is repeatedly readapted with short, choppy strokes, the result will be a root surface roughened by numerous nicks and gouges, resembling the rippled surface of a washboard.[38] If heavy lateral pressure is continued with long, even strokes, the result will be excessive removal of root structure, producing a smooth but "ditched" or "riffled" root surface. To avoid these hazards of overinstrumentation, a deliberate transition from short, powerful scaling strokes to longer, lighter root planing strokes must be made as soon as the calculus and initial roughness have been eliminated.

When scaling strokes are used to remove calculus, force can be maximized by concentrating the lateral pressure onto the lower third of the blade (see Fig. 37–19). This small section, the terminal few millimeters of the blade, is positioned slightly apical to the lateral edge of the deposit, and a short vertical or oblique stroke is used to split the calculus from the tooth surface. Without withdrawing the instrument from the pocket, the lower third of the blade is advanced laterally and repositioned to engage the next portion of the remaining deposit. Another vertical or oblique stroke is made, slightly overlapping the previous stroke. This process is repeated in a series of powerful scaling strokes until the entire deposit has been removed. The overlapping of these pathways or "channels" of instrumentation[38] ensures that the entire instrumentation zone is covered.

Engaging a large, tenacious ledge or piece of calculus with the entire length of the cutting edge is not recommended, because the force is distributed through a longer section of the cutting edge rather than concentrated. Far more lateral pressure is required to dislodge the entire deposit in one stroke. Although some clinicians may possess the strength to remove calculus completely in this manner, the heavier forces that are required diminish tactile sensitivity and contribute to a loss of control that results in tissue trauma. A single heavy stroke usually is not sufficient to remove calculus entirely. Instead, the blade skips over or skims the surface of the deposit. Subsequent strokes made with the entire cutting edge tend to shave the deposit down layer by layer, and when a series of these repeated whittling strokes is applied, the calculus may be reduced to a thin, smooth, burnished sheet that is difficult to distinguish from the surrounding root surface.

A common error in instrumenting proximal surfaces is failing to reach the mid-proximal region apical to the contact. This area is relatively inaccessible, and the technique requires more skill than does instrumentation of buccal or lingual surfaces. It is extremely important to extend strokes at least halfway across the proximal surface so that no calculus or roughness remains in the interproximal area. With properly designed curettes, this can be accomplished by keeping the lower shank of the curette parallel with the long axis of the tooth (Fig. 37–32). With the lower shank parallel to the long axis, the blade of the curette will reach the base of the pocket and the toe will extend beyond the

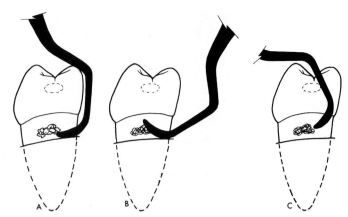

FIGURE 37–32. Shank position for scaling proximal surfaces. *A,* Correct shank position, parallel with the long axis of the tooth. *B,* Incorrect shank position, tilted away from the tooth. *C,* Incorrect shank position, tilted too far toward the tooth.

midline as strokes are advanced across the proximal surface. This extension of strokes beyond the midline ensures thorough exploration and instrumentation of these surfaces. If the lower shank is angled or tilted away from the tooth, the toe will move toward the contact area. Because this prevents the blade from reaching the base of the pocket, calculus apical to the contact will not be detected or removed. Strokes will be hampered because the toe tends to become lodged in the contact. If the instrument is angled or tilted too far toward the tooth, the lower shank will hit the tooth or the contact area, preventing extension of strokes to the mid-proximal region (see Fig. 37–32).

The relationship between the location of the finger rest and the working area is important for two reasons. First, the finger rest or fulcrum must be positioned to allow the lower shank of the instrument to be parallel or nearly parallel to the tooth surface being treated. This parallelism is a fundamental requirement for optimal working angulation. Second, the finger rest must be positioned to enable the operator to use wrist–arm motion to activate strokes. On some aspects of the maxillary posterior teeth, these requirements can be met only with the use of extraoral or opposite-arch fulcrums. When intraoral finger rests are used in other regions of the mouth, the finger rest must be close enough to the working area to fulfill these two requirements. A finger rest that is established too far from the working area forces the clinician to separate the middle finger from the fourth finger in an effort to obtain parallelism and proper angulation. Effective wrist–arm motion is possible only when these two fingers are kept together in a built-up fulcrum. Separation of the fingers commits the clinician to the exclusive use of finger flexing for the activation of strokes.

As instrumentation proceeds from one tooth to the next, the location of the finger rest must be frequently adjusted or changed to allow parallelism and wrist–arm motion.

Ultrasonic Scaling Technique

Ultrasonic instrumentation is accomplished with a light touch and light pressure, keeping the tip constantly in motion. Leaving the tip in one place for too long or using the point of the tip against the tooth can produce gouging and roughening of the root surface or overheating of the tooth. The volume and depth of tooth structure removal may be reduced by using a lower power setting and applying only slight pressure.[13] The working end of the ultrasonic instrument must come in contact with the calculus deposit to fracture and remove it. As with hand instruments, instrument adaptation to the tooth is critical to success. The working tip must contact all aspects of the root surface to throughly remove plaque and toxins. Although as much as 10 mm or more of the length of the ultrasonic tip vibrates, only a small portion of it can be adapted to contact the curved root surface at any one time or at any one point. As with hand instruments, a series of rapid, overlapping strokes must be activated to ensure complete root coverage. However, these rapid, light strokes with a blunt, vibrating working end impair tactile sensitivity, and visibility is hampered by the constant water spray that is necessary for the operation of the instrument. For these reasons, during ultrasonic instrumentation the tooth surface should be frequently examined with an explorer to evaluate the completeness of debridement.

With these points in mind, the ultrasonic device is used in the following manner:

1. The instrument should be properly adjusted to produce a light mist of water at the working tip. Adequate aspiration is necessary to remove this water as it accumulates in the mouth. The power setting should be no higher than necessary to remove calculus. The clinician and the assistant should wear goggles to protect the eyes and masks to minimize inhalation of the contaminated aerosol produced during instrumentation.
2. The instrument is grasped with a light pen or modified pen grasp, and a finger rest or extraoral fulcrum should be established as for hand instrumentation. Extraoral hand rests should be used for the maxillary posterior teeth. For maxillary anterior teeth and the mandibular arch, either intraoral or extraoral fulcrums may be used.
3. The instrument is switched on; short, light, vertical, horizontal, or oblique overlapping strokes are activated; and the working end is passed over the deposit. Heavy lateral pressure is unnecessary, because it is the vibrational energy of the instrument that dislodges the calculus. However, the working end must touch the deposit for this to occur.
4. The working end should be kept in constant motion, and the tip should be kept parallel to the tooth surface or at no more than a 15-degree angle to avoid etching or grooving the tooth surface.[49]
5. The instrument should be switched off periodically to allow for aspiration of water, and the tooth surface should be examined frequently with an explorer.
6. Any remaining irregularities of the root surface may be removed with sharp standard or mini-bladed curettes if necessary.

Evaluation of Scaling and Root Planing

The adequacy of scaling and root planing is evaluated when the procedure is performed and again later, after a period of soft tissue healing.

Immediately after instrumentation, the tooth surfaces should be carefully inspected visually with optimal lighting and the aid of a mouth mirror and compressed air; they should also be examined with a fine explorer or probe. Subgingival surfaces should be hard and smooth. Although complete removal of calculus is definitely necessary for the health of the adjacent soft tissue,[48] there is little documented evidence that root smoothness is necessary.[17,19] Nevertheless, relative smoothness is still the best immediate clinical indication that calculus has been completely removed.[17]

Although smoothness is the criterion by which scaling and root planing are immediately evaluated, the ultimate evaluation is based on tissue response.[48] Clinical evaluation of the soft tissue response to scaling and root planing, including probing, should not be conducted earlier than 2 weeks postoperatively. Re-epithelialization of the wounds created during instrumentation takes from 1 to 2 weeks.[42,43] Until then, gingival bleeding on probing can be expected even when calculus has been completely removed, because the soft tissue wound is not epithelialized. Any gingival bleeding on probing that is noted after this interval is more likely to be due to persistent inflammation produced by residual deposits that were not removed during the initial procedure or to inadequate plaque control. Positive clinical changes after instrumentation often continue for weeks or months. For this reason, a longer period of evaluation may be indicated before deciding whether to intervene with further instrumentation or surgery.[12]

There may be times when the clinician finds that some slight root roughness remains after scaling and root planing. If sound principles of instrumentation have been followed, the roughness may not be calculus. Because calculus removal, not root smoothness per se, has been shown to be necessary for tissue health, it might be more prudent in such a case to stop short of perfect smoothness and re-evaluate the patient's tissue response after 2 to 4 weeks or longer. This avoids overinstrumentation and removal of excessive root structure in the pursuit of smoothness for its own sake. If the tissue is healthy after an interval of 2 to 4 weeks or longer, no further root planing is necessary. If the tissue is inflamed, the clinician must determine to what extent this is due to plaque accumulation or the presence of residual calculus and to what degree further root planing is necessary.

REFERENCES

1. Aleo J, DeRenzis F, Farber P. In vitro attachment of human gingival fibroblasts to root surfaces. J Periodontol *46:*639, 1975.
2. Aleo J, DeRenzis F, Farber P, Varboncoeur A. The presence and biological activity of cementum bound endotoxin. J Periodontol *45:*672, 1974.
3. Allen EF, Rhoads RH. Effects of high speed periodontal instruments on tooth surfaces. J Periodontol *34:*352, 1963.
4. Axelsson P, Lindhe J. Effect of controlled oral hygiene procedures on caries and periodontal disease in adults. Results after 6 years. J Clin Periodontol *8:*239, 1981.
5. Baderstein A, Nilveus R, Egelberg J. Effect of nonsurgical periodontal therapy. I. Moderately advanced periodontitis. J Clin Periodontol *8:*57–72, 1981.
6. Baderstein A, Nilveus R, Egelberg J. 4-year observations of basic periodontal therapy. J Clin Periodontol *14:*438–444, 1987.
7. Baderstein A, Nilveus R, Egelberg J. Scores of plaque, bleeding, suppuration, and probing depth to predict attachment loss. J Clin Periodontol *17:*102–107, 1990.
8. Barnes JE, Schaffer EM. Subgingival root planing: A comparison using files, hoes, and curets. J Periodontol *31:*300, 1960.
9. Burman LR, Alderman NE, Ewen SJ. Clinical application of ultrasonic vibrations for supragingival calculus and stain removal. J Dent Med *13:*156, 1968.
10. Checchi L, Pelliccioni GA. Hand versus ultrasonic instrumentation in the removal of endotoxin from root surface in vitro. J Periodontol *59:*398, 1988.
11. Cheetham WA, Wilson M, Kieser JB. Root surface debridement—an in vitro assessment. J Clin Periodontol *15:*228, 1988.
12. Claffey N. Decision making in periodontal therapy: The reevaluation. J Clin Periodontol *18:*364, 1991.

13. Clark S, Group H, Mabler D. The effect of ultrasonic instrumentation on root surfaces. J Periodontol *39:*125, 1968.
14. Dragoo M. A clinical evaluation of hand and ultrasonic instruments on subgingival debridement. Part I. With unmodified and modified ultrasonic inserts. Int J Periodontol *12:*311–323, 1992.
15. Drisko CL. Scaling and root planing without overinstrumentation: hand versus power-driven scalers. Curr Opin Periodontol 3:78, 1993.
16. Garnick JJ, Dent J. A scanning electron micrographical study of root surfaces and subgingival bacteria after hand scaling and ultrasonic instrumentation. J Periodontol *60:*441–447, 1989.
17. Garrett JS. Root planing: A perspective. J Periodontol *48:*553, 1977.
18. Green E, Ramfjord SR. Tooth roughness after subgingival root planing. J Periodontol *37:*396, 1966.
19. Greenstein G. Periodontal response to mechanical non-surgical therapy: A review. J Periodontol *63:*118–130, 1992.
20. Hatfield CG, Baumhammers A. Cytotoxic effects of periodontally involved surfaces of human teeth. Arch Oral Biol *16:*465, 1971.
21. Holbrook T, Low S. Power-driven scaling and polishing instruments. Clin Dent *3:*1, 1989.
22. Hughes FJ, Smales FC. Immunohistochemical investigation of the presence and distribution of cementum-associated lipopolysaccharides in periodontal disease. J Periodont Res *21:*660, 1986.
23. Hughes FJ, Auger DW, Smales FC. Investigation of the distribution of cementum-associated lipopolysaccharides in periodontal disease with scanning electron microscope immunohistochemistry. J Periodont Res 23:100, 1988.
24. Johnson WN, Wilson JR. The application of the ultrasonic dental units to scaling procedures. J Periodontol 28:264, 1957.
25. Kerry GJ. Roughness of root surfaces after use of ultrasonic instruments and hand curets. J Periodontol *38:*340, 1967.
26. Larato DC, Ruskin PF, Martin A. Effect of an ultrasonic scaler on bacterial counts in air. J Periodontol *38:*550, 1967.
27. Lindhe J, Jacobson L. Evaluation of periodontal scalers. I. Wear following clinical use. Odont Rev *17:*1, 1966.
28. Lindhe J, Nyman S, Karring T. Scaling and root planing in shallow pockets. J Clin Periodontol *9:*415, 1982.
29. Leon LE, Vogel RI. A comparison of the effectiveness of hand scaling and ultrasonic debridement in furcations as evaluated by differential dark-field microscopy. J Periodontol *58:*86, 1987.
30. Lovdahl A, Arno A, Schei O, Waerhaug J. Combined effect of subgingival scaling and controlled oral hygiene on the incidence of gingivitis. Acta Odontol Scand *19:*537, 1961.
31. Moore J, Wilson M, Kieser JB. The distribution of bacterial lipoplysaccharide (endotoxin) in relation to periodontally involved root surfaces, J Clin Periodontol *13:*748, 1986.
32. Moskow BS. Calculus attachment in cemental separations. J Periodontol *40:*125, 1969.
33. Muir KF, Ross PW, MacPhee IT, et al. Reduction of microbial contamination from ultrasonic scalers. Br Dent J *145:*76, 1978.
34. Nakib NM, Bissada NF, Simmelink JW, Goldstein SN. Endotoxin penetration into root cementum of periodontally healthy and diseased human teeth. J Periodontol *53:*368–378, 1982.
35. Nyman S, Westfelt E, Sarhed G, Karring T. Role of "diseased" root cementum in healing following treatment of periodontal disease: A clinical study. J Clin Periodontol *15:*464, 1988.
36. Orban B, Manella V. Macroscopic and microscopic study of instruments designed for root planing. J Periodontol *27:*120, 1956.
37. Oosterwall PJ, Matee MI, Mikx FHM, et al. The effect of subgingival debridement with hand and ultrasonic instruments on subgingival microflora. J Clin Periodontol *14:*528, 1987.
38. Parr R, Green E, Madsen L, Miller S. Subgingival Scaling and Root Planing. Berkeley, CA, Praxis Publishing, 1976.
39. Schaffer EM. Histologic results of root curettage on human teeth. J Periodontol 27:269, 1956.
40. Selvig K. Attachment of plaque and calculus to tooth surfaces. J Periodont Res 5:8, 1970.
41. Smart GJ, Wilson M, Davis EH, Keiser JB. The assessment of ultrasonic root surface debridement by determination of residual endotoxin levels. J Clin Periodontol *17:*174–178, 1990.
42. Stahl SS, Slavkin HC, Yamada L, Levine S. Speculations about gingival repair. J Periodontol *43:*395, 1972.
43. Stahl SS, Weiner JM, Benjamin S, Yamada L. Soft tissue healing following curettage and root planing. J Periodontol *42:*678, 1971.
44. Stende GW, Schaffer EM. A comparison of ultrasonic and hand scaling. J Periodontol *32:*312, 1961.
45. Torfason T, Kiger R, Selvig KA, Egelberg J. Clinical improvement of gingival conditions following ultrasonic versus hand instrumentation of periodontal pockets. J Clin Periodontol 6:165, 1979.
46. Van Volkinburg J, Green E, Armitage G. The nature of root surfaces after curette, cavitron, and alpha-sonic instrumentation. J Periodont Res *11:*374, 1976.
47. Veksler AE, Kayrouz GA, Newman MG. Reduction of salivary bacteria by pre-procedural rinses with chlorhexidine 0.12%. J Periodontol *62:*649, 1991.
48. Waerhaug J. Healing of the dentoepithelial junction following subgingival plaque control. J Periodontol *49:*1, 1978.
49. Wilkins EM. Clinical Practice of the Dental Hygienist. 7th ed. Philadelphia, Williams & Wilkins, 1994, p 518.
50. Wilkinson RF, Maybury J. Scanning electron microscopy of the root surface following instrumentation. J Periodontol *44:*559, 1973.
51. Zander HA. The attachment of calculus to root surfaces. J Periodontol *24:*16, 1953.

38

Instrumentation in Different Areas of the Mouth

GORDON L. PATTISON and ANNA M. PATTISON

Various approaches to instrumentation in different areas of the mouth are illustrated here in atlas form. The examples shown provide maximum efficiency for the clinician and comfort for the patient. For most areas, more than one approach is presented. Other approaches are possible and are acceptable if they provide equal efficiency and comfort.

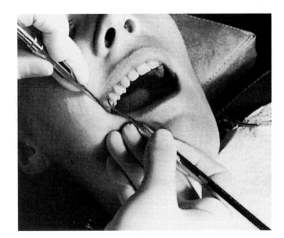

FIGURE 38–1. Maxillary right posterior sextant: facial aspect.
Operator position: Side position.
Illumination: Direct.
Visibility: Direct (indirect for distal surfaces of molars).
Retraction: Mirror or index finger of the nonoperating hand.
Finger rest: Extraoral, palm up. Backs of the middle and fourth fingers on the lateral aspect of the mandible on the right side of the face.

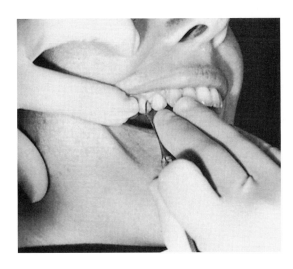

FIGURE 38–2. Maxillary right posterior sextant: facial aspect.
Operator position: Side or front position.
Illumination: Direct.
Visibility: Direct (indirect for distal surfaces of molars).
Retraction: Mirror or index finger of the nonoperating hand.
Finger rest: Intraoral, palm down. Fourth finger on the incisal or facial surfaces of the maxillary anterior teeth or on the occlusal or facial surfaces of the maxillary bicuspid teeth.

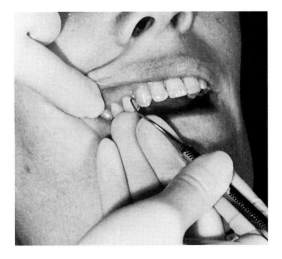

FIGURE 38–3. Maxillary right posterior sextant, premolar region only: facial aspect.
Operator position: Side or back position.
Illumination: Direct.
Visibility: Direct.
Retraction: Mirror or index finger of the nonoperating hand.
Finger rest: Intraoral, palm up. Fourth finger on the occlusal surfaces of the adjacent maxillary posterior teeth.

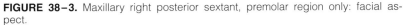

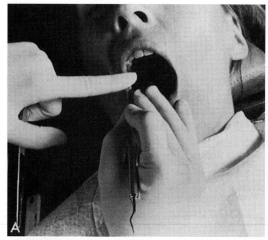
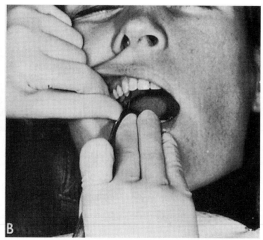
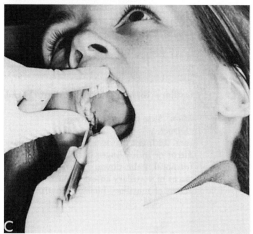

FIGURE 38–4. Maxillary right posterior sextant: lingual aspect.
    Operator position: Front position.
    Illumination: Direct.
    Visibility: Direct.
    Retraction: Index finger of the nonoperating hand (*C*) or no retraction (*A*).
    Finger rest: Intraoral, palm down, opposite arch, reinforced. Fourth finger on incisal edges of mandibular anterior teeth, reinforced with the thumb (*B* and *C*) or index finger (*A*) of the nonoperating hand.

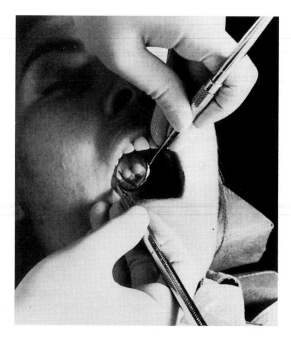

FIGURE 38–5. Maxillary right posterior sextant: lingual aspect.
    Operator position: Side or front position.
    Illumination: Direct and indirect.
    Visibility: Direct or indirect.
    Retraction: None.
    Finger rest: Extraoral, palm up. Backs of the middle and fourth fingers on the lateral aspect of the mandible on the right side of the face.

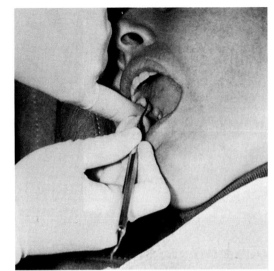

FIGURE 38–6. Maxillary right posterior sextant: lingual aspect.
Operator position: Front position.
Illumination: Direct.
Visibility: Direct.
Retraction: None.
Finger rest: Intraoral, palm up, finger-on-finger. Index finger of the nonoperating hand on the occlusal surfaces of the maxillary right posterior teeth; fourth finger of the operating hand or the index finger of nonoperating hand.

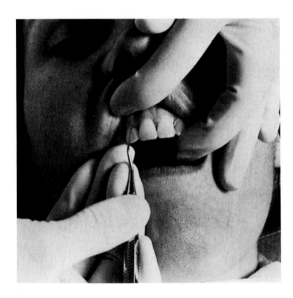

FIGURE 38–7. Maxillary anterior sextant: facial aspect.
Operator position: Back position.
Illumination: Direct.
Visibility: Direct.
Retraction: Index finger of the nonoperating hand.
Finger rest: Intraoral, palm up. Fourth finger on the incisal edges or occlusal surfaces of adjacent maxillary teeth.

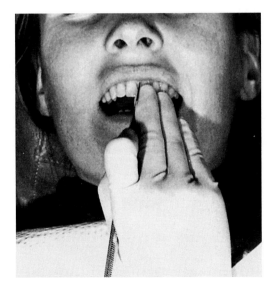

FIGURE 38–8. Maxillary anterior sextant: facial aspect.
Operator position: Front position.
Illumination: Direct.
Visibility: Direct.
Retraction: Index finger of the nonoperating hand.
Finger rest: Intraoral, palm down. Fourth finger on the incisal edges or the occlusal or facial surfaces of adjacent maxillary teeth.

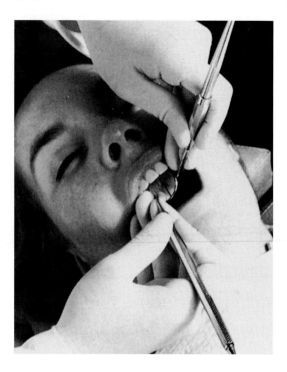

FIGURE 38–9. Maxillary anterior sextant: lingual aspect.
Operator position: Back position.
Illumination: Indirect.
Visibility: Indirect.
Retraction: None.
Finger rest: Intraoral, palm up. Fourth finger on the incisal edges or occlusal surfaces of adjacent maxillary teeth.

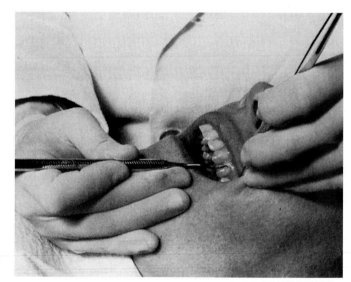

FIGURE 38–10. Maxillary left posterior sextant: facial aspect.
Operator position: Side or back position.
Illumination: Direct or indirect.
Visibility: Direct or indirect.
Retraction: Mirror.
Finger rest: Extraoral, palm down. Front surfaces of the middle and fourth fingers on the lateral aspect of the mandible on the left side of the face.

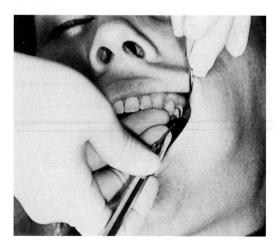

FIGURE 38–11. Maxillary left posterior sextant: facial aspect.
Operator position: Back or side position.
Illumination: Direct or indirect.
Visibility: Direct or indirect.
Retraction: Mirror.
Finger rest: Intraoral, palm up. Fourth finger on the incisal edges or occlusal surfaces of adjacent maxillary teeth.

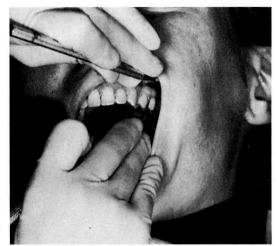

FIGURE 38–12. Maxillary left posterior sextant: facial aspect.
Operator position: Front position.
Illumination: Direct or indirect.
Visibility: Direct or indirect.
Retraction: Mirror.
Finger rest: Intraoral, palm down, opposite arch. Fourth finger on the incisal edges or the occlusal or facial surfaces of the mandibular left teeth.

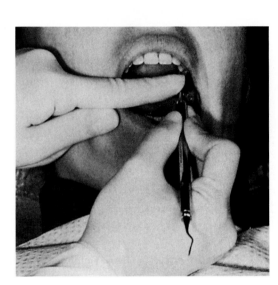

FIGURE 38–13. Maxillary left posterior sextant: lingual aspect.
Operator position: Front position.
Illumination: Direct.
Visibility: Direct.
Retraction: None.
Finger rest: Intraoral, palm down, opposite arch, reinforced. Fourth finger on the incisal edges of the mandibular anterior teeth or the facial surfaces of the mandibular premolars, reinforced with the index finger of the nonoperating hand.

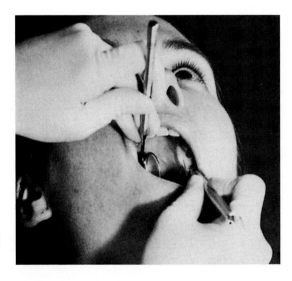

FIGURE 38–14. Maxillary left posterior sextant: lingual aspect.
Operator position: Front position.
Illumination: Direct and indirect.
Visibility: Direct and indirect.
Retraction: None.
Finger rest: Intraoral, palm down, opposite arch. Fourth finger on the incisal edges of the mandibular anterior teeth or the facial surfaces of the mandibular premolars. The nonoperating hand holds the mirror for indirect illumination.

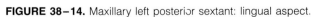

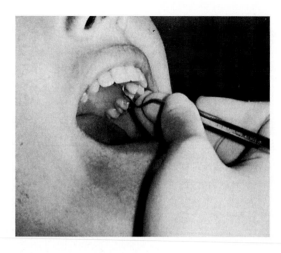

FIGURE 38–15. Maxillary left posterior sextant: lingual aspect.
  Operator position: Side or front position.
  Illumination: Direct.
  Visibility: Direct.
  Retraction: None.
  Finger rest: Intraoral, palm up. Fourth finger on the occlusal surfaces of adjacent maxillary teeth.

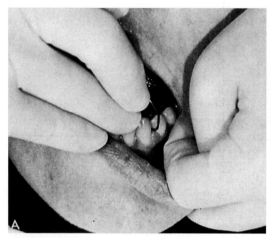 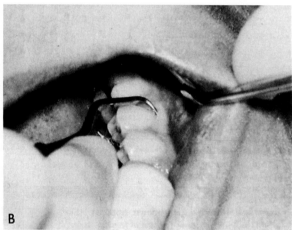

FIGURE 38–16. Mandibular left posterior sextant: facial aspect.
  Operator position: Side or back position.
  Illumination: Direct.
  Visibility: Direct or indirect.
  Retraction: Mirror *(B)* or index finger *(A)* of the nonoperating hand.
  Finger rest: Intraoral, palm down. Fourth finger on the incisal edges or the occlusal or facial surfaces of adjacent mandibular teeth.

FIGURE 38–17. Mandibular left posterior sextant, premolar region only: facial aspect.
  Operator position: Front position.
  Illumination: Direct.
  Visibility: Direct.
  Retraction: Index finger of the nonoperating hand.
  Finger rest: Intraoral, palm down, finger-on-finger. Index finger of the nonoperating hand is placed in the mandibular left vestibule; fourth finger of the operating hand rests on the index finger of the nonoperating hand.

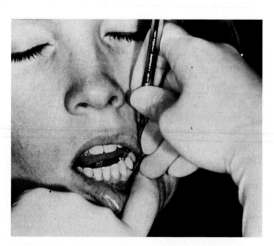

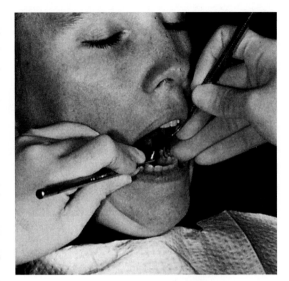

FIGURE 38–18. Mandibular left posterior sextant: lingual aspect.
Operator position: Front or side position.
Illumination: Direct and indirect.
Visibility: Direct.
Retraction: Mirror retracts tongue.
Finger rest: Intraoral, palm down. Fourth finger on the incisal edges or the occlusal surfaces of adjacent mandibular teeth.

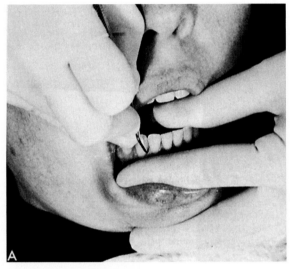
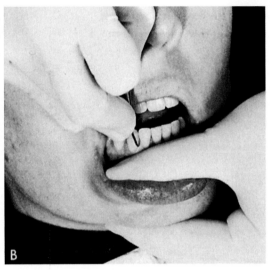

FIGURE 38–19. Mandibular anterior sextant: facial aspect.
Operator position: Back position.
Illumination: Direct.
Visibility: Direct.
Retraction: Index finger *(A)* or thumb *(B)* of the nonoperating hand.
Finger rest: Intraoral, palm down. Fourth finger on the incisal edges or the occlusal surfaces of adjacent mandibular teeth.

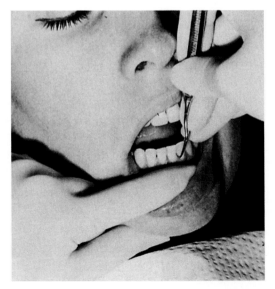

FIGURE 38–20. Mandibular anterior sextant: facial aspect.
Operator position: Front position.
Illumination: Direct.
Visibility: Direct.
Retraction: Index finger of the nonoperating hand.
Finger rest: Intraoral, palm down. Fourth finger on the incisal edges or the occlusal surfaces of adjacent mandibular teeth.

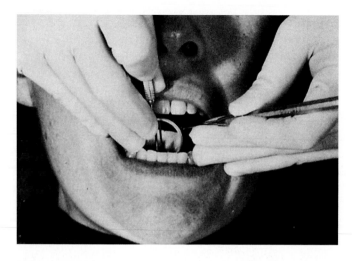

FIGURE 38–21. Mandibular anterior sextant: lingual aspect.
Operator position: Back position.
Illumination: Direct and indirect.
Visibility: Direct and indirect.
Retraction: Mirror retracts tongue.
Finger rest: Intraoral, palm down. Fourth finger on the incisal edges or the occlusal surfaces of adjacent mandibular teeth.

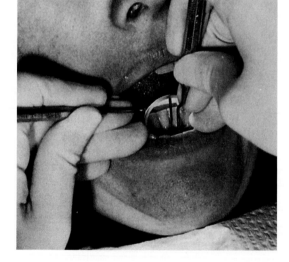

FIGURE 38–22. Mandibular anterior sextant: lingual aspect.
Operator position: Front position.
Illumination: Direct and indirect.
Visibility: Direct and indirect.
Retraction: Mirror retracts tongue.
Finger rest: Intraoral, palm down. Fourth finger on the incisal edges or the occlusal surfaces of adjacent mandibular teeth.

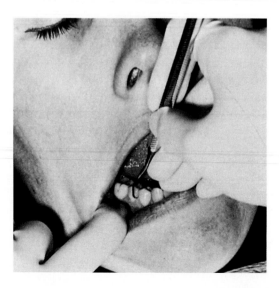

FIGURE 38–23. Mandibular right posterior sextant: facial aspect.
Operator position: Side or front position.
Illumination: Direct.
Visibility: Direct.
Retraction: Mirror or index finger of the nonoperating hand.
Finger rest: Intraoral, palm down. Fourth finger on the incisal edges or the occlusal surfaces of adjacent mandibular teeth.

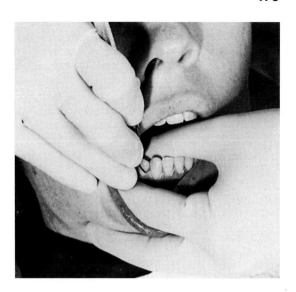

FIGURE 38–24. Mandibular right posterior sextant, premolar region only: facial aspect.

Operator position: Back position.
Illumination: Direct.
Visibility: Direct.
Retraction: Index finger of the nonoperating hand.
Finger rest: Intraoral, palm down, finger-on-finger. Index finger of the nonoperating hand is placed in the mandibular right vestibule; fourth finger of the operating hand rests on the index finger of the nonoperating hand.

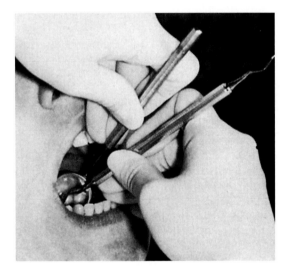

FIGURE 38–25. Mandibular right posterior sextant: lingual aspect.

Operator position: Front position.
Illumination: Direct and indirect.
Visibility: Direct and indirect.
Retraction: Mirror retracts tongue.
Finger rest: Intraoral, palm down. Fourth finger on the incisal edges or the occlusal surfaces of adjacent mandibular teeth.

39

Treatment of Acute Gingival Disease

FERMIN A. CARRANZA, JR.

Treatment of acute gingival disease entails alleviation of the acute symptoms and elimination of all other periodontal disease, chronic as well as acute, throughout the oral cavity. Treatment is not complete as long as periodontal pathologic changes or factors capable of causing them are present.

TREATMENT OF ACUTE NECROTIZING ULCERATIVE GINGIVITIS

Acute necrotizing ulcerative gingivitis (ANUG) can occur in a mouth essentially free of any other gingival involvement, or it can be superimposed on underlying chronic gingival disease. Treatment should include alleviation of the acute symptoms and correction of the underlying chronic gingival disease. The former is the simplest part of the treatment; the latter requires more comprehensive procedures.

The treatment of ANUG consists of (1) alleviation of the acute inflammation plus treatment of chronic disease either underlying the acute involvement or elsewhere in the oral cavity, (2) alleviation of generalized toxic symptoms such as fever and malaise, and (3) correction of systemic conditions that contribute to the initiation or progress of the gingival changes. Chapter 46 provides further information on the management and treatment of ANUG in patients with AIDS.

Treatment of ANUG should follow an orderly sequence, as described in the following paragraphs.

First Visit. At the first visit, the dentist should obtain a general impression of the patient's background, including information regarding recent illness, living conditions, dietary background, type of employment, hours of rest, and mental stress. He or she should observe the patient's general appearance, apparent nutritional status, and responsiveness or lassitude and should take the patient's temperature. The submaxillary and submental areas should be palpated to detect enlarged lymph glands.

The oral cavity is examined for the characteristic lesion of ANUG (see Chapter 19), its distribution, and possible involvement of the oropharyngeal region. Oral hygiene is evaluated, and the presence of pericoronal flaps, periodontal pockets, and local irritants is determined. A bacterial smear may be made from material in the involved areas, but this is merely corroboratory and is not to be relied on for diagnosis.

The patient is questioned regarding the history of the acute disease and its onset and duration. Is it recurrent? Are the recurrences associated with specific factors such as menstruation, particular foods, exhaustion, or mental stress? Has there been any previous treatment? When, and for how long? The clinician should also inquire as to the type of treatment received and the patient's impression regarding its effect.

Treatment during this initial visit is confined to the acutely involved areas, which are isolated with cotton rolls and dried. A topical anesthetic is applied, and after 2 or 3 minutes the areas are gently swabbed with a cotton pellet to remove the pseudomembrane and nonattached surface debris. Each cotton pellet is used in a small area and is then discarded; sweeping motions over large areas with a single pellet are not recommended. After the area is cleansed with warm water, the superficial calculus is removed. Ultrasonic scalers are very useful for this purpose, as they do not elicit pain, and the water jet aids in lavage of the area.

Subgingival scaling and curettage are contraindicated at this time because of the possibility of extending the infection into deeper tissues and also of causing a bacteremia. *Unless an emergency exists, procedures such as extractions or periodontal surgery are postponed until the patient has been symptom free for a period of 4 weeks, to minimize the likelihood of exacerbation of the acute symptoms.*

The patient is also told to rinse the mouth every 2 hours with a glassful of an equal mixture of warm water and 3% hydrogen peroxide. Twice-daily rinses with 0.12% chlorhexidine are also very effective.

Patients with moderate or severe ANUG and local lymphadenopathy or other systemic symptoms are placed on an antibiotic regimen of penicillin, 250 or 500 mg orally every 6 hours. For penicillin-sensitive patients, other antibiotics such as erythromycin (250 or 500 mg every 6 hours) are prescribed. Metronidazole (250 or 500 mg three times daily for 7 days), which is extensively used in Europe, is also effective.

Patients are told to report back to the dentist in 1 to 2 days. The patient should be advised of the extent of total treatment the condition requires and warned that treatment is not complete when the pain stops. He or she should be informed of the presence of chronic gingival and periodontal disease, which must be eliminated to prevent recurrence of the acute symptoms.

Instructions to the Patient. The patient is discharged with the following instructions:

1. Avoid tobacco, alcohol, and condiments.
2. Rinse the mouth with a glassful of an equal mixture of 3% hydrogen peroxide and warm water every 2 hours and/or twice daily with 0.12% chlorhexidine solution.
3. Pursue usual activities, but avoid excessive physical exertion or prolonged exposure to the sun.
4. Confine toothbrushing to the removal of surface debris with

a bland dentifrice; overzealous brushing and the use of dental floss or interdental cleaners will be painful. The chlorhexidine mouthrinses will be also very helpful in controlling plaque throughout the mouth.

Second Visit. At the second visit, 1 to 2 days later, the patient's condition is usually improved, and the pain is diminished or no longer present. The gingival margins of the involved areas are erythematous, but without a superficial pseudomembrane.

Scaling is performed if sensitivity permits. Shrinkage of the gingiva may expose previously covered calculus, which is gently removed. The instructions to the patient are the same as those given previously.

Third Visit. At the next visit, 1 to 2 days after the second, the patient should be essentially symptom free. There may still be some erythema in the involved areas, and the gingiva may be slightly painful on tactile stimulation (Fig. 39–1). Scaling and root planing are repeated. The patient is instructed in plaque control procedures (described in Chapter 42), which are essential for success of the treatment and maintenance of periodontal health. The hydrogen peroxide rinses are discontinued, but chlorhexidine rinses can be maintained for 2 or 3 weeks.

Subsequent Visits. In subsequent visits, the tooth surfaces in the involved areas are scaled and smoothed, and plaque control performed by the patient is checked and corrected if necessary.

Unfortunately, treatment is often stopped at this time because the acute condition has subsided, but this is when comprehensive treatment of the patient's chronic periodontal problem should start. Appointments should be scheduled for treatment of chronic gingivitis, periodontal pockets, and pericoronal flaps and for elimination of all forms of local irritation.

Patients without gingival disease other than the treated acute involvement are dismissed for 1 week. If the condition is satisfactory at that time, the patient is dismissed for 1 month, at which time the schedule for subsequent recall visits is determined according to the patient's needs.

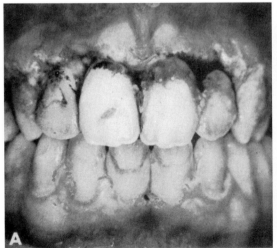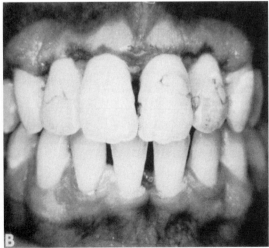

FIGURE 39–1. Initial response to treatment of acute necrotizing ulcerative gingivitis. *A,* Severe acute necrotizing ulcerative gingivitis. *B,* Third day after treatment. There is still some erythema, but the condition is markedly improved.

Gingival Changes With Healing

The characteristic lesion of ANUG undergoes the following changes in the course of healing in response to treatment:

1. Removal of the surface pseudomembrane exposes the underlying red, hemorrhagic, crater-like depressions in the gingiva.
2. In the next stage the bulk and redness of the crater margins are reduced, but the surface remains shiny.
3. This is followed by the early signs of restoration of normal gingival contour and color.
4. In the final stage normal gingival color, consistency, surface texture, and contour are restored. Portions of the root exposed by the acute disease are covered by healthy gingiva (Figs. 39–2 and 39–3). When the menstrual period occurs in the course of treatment, there is a tendency toward exacerbation of the acute signs and symptoms, giving the appearance of a relapse. Patients should be informed of this possibility and spared unnecessary anxiety regarding their oral condition.

Additional Treatment Considerations

Contouring the Gingiva as an Adjunctive Procedure. Even in cases of severe gingival necrosis, healing ordinar-

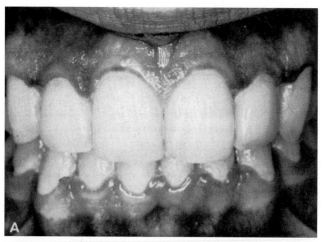
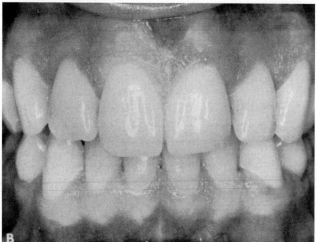

FIGURE 39–2. Treatment of acute necrotizing ulcerative gingivitis. *A,* Before treatment. Note the characteristic interdental lesions. *B,* After treatment. Note the restoration of healthy gingival contour.

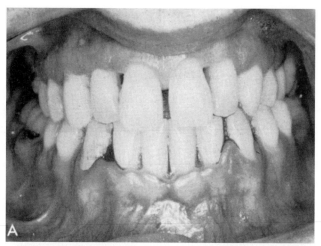
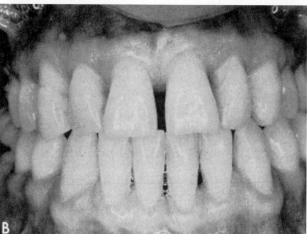

FIGURE 39–3. Physiologic contour and new attachment of gingiva after treatment of acute necrotizing ulcerative gingivitis. *A,* Acute necrotizing ulcerative gingivitis showing the characteristic punched-out eroded gingival margin with surface pseudomembrane. *B,* After treatment. Note the restoration of physiologic gingival contour and reattachment of the gingiva to the surfaces of the mandibular teeth, which had been exposed by the disease.

ily leads to restoration of the normal gingival contour (Fig. 39–4). However, if the teeth are irregularly aligned, healing sometimes results in the formation of a shelf-like gingival margin, which favors retention of food and recurrence of gingival inflammation. This can be corrected by reshaping the gingiva with a periodontal knife or with electrosurgery (Fig. 39–5). Effective plaque control by the patient is particularly important to establish and maintain normal gingival contour in areas of tooth irregularity.

Surgical Procedures. Tooth extraction or periodontal surgery should be postponed until 4 weeks after the acute signs and symptoms of ANUG have subsided. If emergency surgery is required in the presence of acute symptoms, prophylactic chemotherapy with systemic penicillin or other antibiotics is indicated to prevent worsening or spreading of the acute disease.

Role of Drugs. A large variety of drugs, some of which are listed in Table 39–1, have been used for topical treatment of ANUG.[3] Topical drug therapy is only an adjunctive measure; *no drug, when used alone, can be considered complete therapy.*

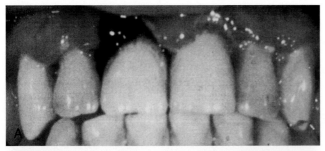

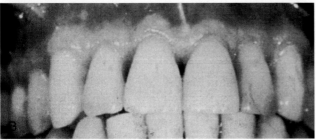

FIGURE 39–4. Gingival healing after treatment. *A,* Before treatment. Severe acute necrotizing ulcerative gingivitis with crater formation. *B,* After treatment. Note the restored gingival contour.

Escharotic drugs such as phenol, silver nitrate, and chromic acid should not be used. They are necrotizing agents that alleviate painful symptoms by destroying the nerve endings in the gingiva. However, they also destroy the young cells necessary for repair and delay healing. Re-

peated use of these agents results in the loss of gingival tissue, which is not restored when the disease subsides.[15]

Systemic Antibiotics. *Antibiotics are administered systemically only in patients with toxic systemic complications or local adenopathy.* They are not recommended for ANUG patients who do not have these complications.

The antibiotic of choice is penicillin (amoxicillin 250 or 500 mg every 6 hours). Patients who are allergic to penicillin should be given erythromycin (250 or 500 mg every 6 hours). Metronidazole (Flagyl) (250 to 500 mg every 8 hours) may also be used.

Antibiotics are continued until the systemic complications or the local lymphadenopathy has subsided. Systemic antibiotics also reduce the oral bacterial flora and alleviate the oral symptoms,[25,26] but they are only an adjunct to the complete local treatment the disease requires. Patients treated with systemic antibiotics alone should be cautioned that the acute painful symptoms may recur after the drug is discontinued.

Supportive Systemic Treatment. In addition to systemic antibiotics, supportive treatment consists of copious fluid consumption and administration of analgesics for relief of pain. Bed rest is necessary for patients with toxic systemic complications such as high fever, malaise, anorexia, and general debility.

Nutritional Supplements. The rationale for nutritional supplements in the treatment of ANUG is based on the following:

1. Lesions resembling those of ANUG have been produced ex-

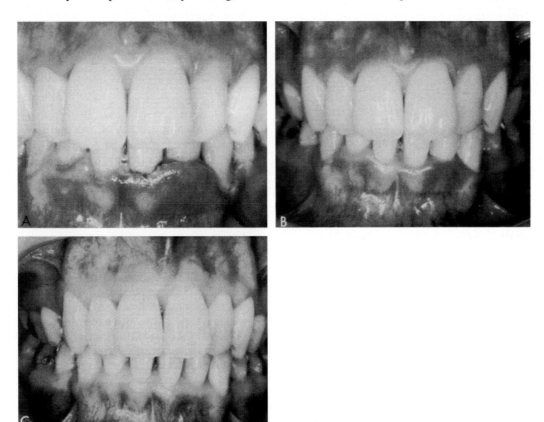

FIGURE 39–5. Reshaping the gingiva in the treatment of acute necrotizing ulcerative gingivitis. *A,* Before treatment. Note the bulbous gingiva and interdental necrosis in the mandibular anterior area. *B,* After treatment. Note that the gingival contours are still undesirable. *C,* Final result, with physiologic contours obtained by reshaping the gingiva.

Table 39–1. TOPICAL MEDICATIONS USED TO TREAT ANUG

Oxygen-liberating agents
  Zinc peroxide
  Hydrogen peroxide
  Sodium perborate
  Potassium chlorate
  Potassium permanganate
  Sodium peroxyborate[27]
Mercurial derivatives
  Tincture nitromersol (Metaphen) 1:200 (untinted)
  Mercuric cyanide 1%
  Thimerosal (Merthiolate) 1:1,000
  Mercuric chloride 1:2,000
Spirocheticides
  Sodium carbonate 10% aqueous
  Arsphenamine 10% aqueous
  Oxophenarsine (Mapharsen)
  Neoarsphenamine
  Stibophen (Fouadin)
Escharotics (caustics)
  Copper sulfate and zinc chloride
  Chromic acid 8%
  Negatan
  Zinc chloride 8%
  Phenol 95%
  Trichloroacetic acid 50%
  Iodine 16.5% and silver nitrate 35%
Aniline dyes
  Viogen (Berwick's solution)
  Acriviolet 1%
  Gentian violet 1%
  Acriflavine 1%
  Methylene blue 1%
Other agents
  Ascoxal[5]
  Copper sulfate, phenol, glycerin, and water
  Metronidazole[7,26]
  Penicillin[8]
  Sulfonamide in paraffin (especially sulfadiazine)
  Surgical pack (zinc oxide–resin, eugenol)
  Vancomycin[6,19]

perimentally in animals with certain nutritional deficiencies (see Chapter 19).

2. It is possible that difficulty in chewing raw fruits and vegetables in a painful condition such as ANUG could lead to the selection of a diet inadequate in vitamins B and C.
3. Isolated clinical studies[17,18] report fewer recurrences when local treatment of ANUG is supplemented with vitamin B or vitamin C.

When the intake of water-soluble vitamins B and C has been severely curtailed because of pain resulting from ANUG, nutritional supplements may be indicated along with local treatment to ward off deficiencies of these vitamins. Under such circumstances the patient may be given a standard multivitamin preparation combined with a therapeutic dose of vitamins B and C.

The patient should be placed on a natural diet with the required detergent action and nutritional content as soon as the oral condition permits. Nutritional supplements may be discontinued after 2 months.

Local procedures are the keystone of treatment of ANUG. Inflammation is a local conditioning factor that impairs the nutrition of the gingiva regardless of the systemic nutritional status. Local irritants should be eliminated to foster normal metabolic and reparative processes in the gingiva. Persistent or recurrent ANUG is more likely to be caused by failure to remove local irritants and by inadequate plaque control than by nutritional deficiency.

Sequelae of Inadequate Treatment

Persistent or "Unresponsive" Cases. If the dentist finds it necessary to change from drug to drug in an effort to relieve a "stubborn" case of ANUG, then something is wrong with the overall treatment regimen that is not likely to be corrected by changing drugs. When confronted with such a problem, the following four steps should be taken:

1. All local drug therapy should be discontinued so that the condition may be studied in an uncomplicated state.
2. Careful differential diagnosis should be undertaken to rule out diseases that resemble ANUG (see Chapter 19).
3. A search should be made for contributing local and systemic etiologic factors that may have been overlooked.
4. Special attention should be given to instructing the patient in plaque control before undertaking comprehensive local treatment.

Recurrent ANUG. Three factors should be explored in patients with recurrent ANUG: inadequate local therapy, pericoronal flap, and anterior overbite. Inadequate plaque control and heavy use of tobacco are also common causes of recurrent disease.

Inadequate Local Therapy. Too frequently, treatment is discontinued when the symptoms have subsided, without eliminating the chronic gingival disease and periodontal pockets that remain after the superficial acute condition is relieved. Persistent chronic inflammation causes degenerative changes that predispose the gingiva to recurrence of acute involvement.

Pericoronal Flap. Recurrent acute involvement in the mandibular anterior area is often associated with persistent pericoronal inflammation arising from difficult eruption of third molars.[12] The anterior involvement is less likely to recur after the third molar situation is corrected.

Anterior Overbite. Marked overbite is often a contributing factor in the recurrence of disease in the anterior region. When the incisal edges of the maxillary teeth impinge on the labial gingival margin or the mandibular teeth strike the palatal gingiva, the resultant tissue injury predisposes the gingiva to recurrent acute disease. Less severe overbite produces food impaction and gingival trauma. Correction of the overbite is necessary for complete treatment of ANUG.

TREATMENT OF ACUTE PERICORONITIS

The treatment of pericoronitis depends on the severity of the inflammation, the systemic complications, and the advisability of retaining the involved tooth. All pericoronal flaps should be viewed with suspicion. Persistent symptom-free pericoronal flaps should be removed as a preventive measure against subsequent acute involvement.

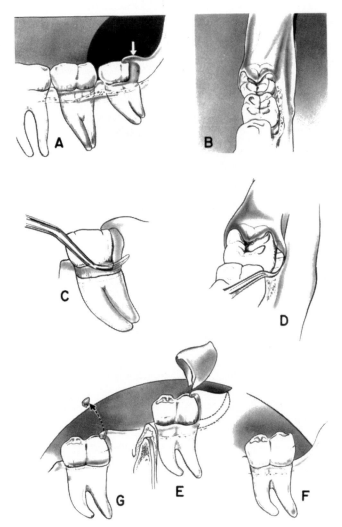

FIGURE 39–6. Treatment of acute pericoronitis. *A,* Inflamed pericoronal flap *(arrow)* in relation to the mandibular third molar. *B,* Anterior view of the third molar and flap. *C,* Lateral view with a scaler in position to gently remove debris under flap. *D,* Anterior view of the scaler in position. *E,* Removal of a section of the gingiva distal to the third molar, after the acute symptoms have subsided. The line of incision is indicated by the broken line. *F,* Appearance of the healed area. *G,* Incorrect removal of the tip of the flap, permitting the deep pocket to remain distal to the molar.

The treatment of acute pericoronitis consists of (1) gently flushing the area with warm water to remove debris and exudate and (2) swabbing with antiseptic after elevating the flap gently from the tooth with a scaler. The underlying debris is removed, and the area is flushed with warm water (Fig. 39–6). Antibiotics can be prescribed in severe cases. If the gingival flap is swollen and fluctuant, an anteroposterior incision to establish drainage is made with a No. 15 Bard-Parker blade.

After the acute symptoms have subsided, a determination is made as to whether the tooth is to be retained or extracted. This decision is governed by the likelihood of further eruption into a good functional position. Bone loss on the distal surface of the second molars is a hazard after the extraction of partially or completely impacted third molars,[2] and the problem is significantly greater if the third molars

are extracted after the roots are formed or in patients older than the early twenties. To reduce the risk of bone loss around second molars, partially or completely impacted third molars should be extracted as early as possible in their development.

If it is decided to retain the tooth, the pericoronal flap is removed using periodontal knives or electrosurgery (see Fig. 39–6). It is necessary to remove the tissue distal to the tooth as well as the flap on the occlusal surface. Incising only the occlusal portion of the flap leaves a deep distal pocket, which invites recurrence of acute pericoronal involvement.

After the tissue is removed, a periodontal pack is applied. The pack may be retained by bringing it forward along the facial and lingual surfaces into the interproximal space between the second and third molars. The pack is removed after 1 week.

Pericoronitis and ANUG

Pericoronal flaps that are chronically inflamed may become sites of ANUG. The disease is treated in the same manner as elsewhere in the mouth; after the acute symptoms have subsided, the flap is removed. Pericoronal flaps are often referred to as *primary incubation zones* in ANUG; their elimination is one of many measures required to minimize the likelihood of recurrent disease.

TREATMENT OF ACUTE HERPETIC GINGIVOSTOMATITIS

Primary herpetic gingivostomatitis occurs primarily, but not exclusively, in children. It runs a 7- to 10-day course and heals without scars. Various medications have been used to treat this condition, with little success; these have included local applications of escharotics, vitamins, radiation, and antibiotics.[1,4,9,10,13,16] Some limited success has been attained with the use of herpesvirus-specific drugs, such as acyclovir ointment.[20]

Treatment consists of palliative measures to make the patient comfortable until the disease runs its course. Plaque, food debris, and superficial calculus are removed to reduce gingival inflammation, which complicates the acute herpetic involvement. Extensive periodontal therapy should be postponed until the acute symptoms subside to avoid the possibility of exacerbation (Fig. 39–7). Herpetic infection of a dentist's finger, referred to as *herpetic whitlow,* can occur if a seronegative clinician becomes infected with a patient's herpetic lesions.[20,23]

Relief of pain to enable the patient to eat comfortably is obtained with topical anesthetic mouthwashes, such as lidocaine hydrochloride viscous solution. Before each meal the patient should swish with one tablespoon of this solution and spit out.

Supportive Treatment. Supportive measures include copious fluid intake and systemic antibiotic therapy for the management of toxic systemic complications. For the relief of pain, systemically administered aspirin is

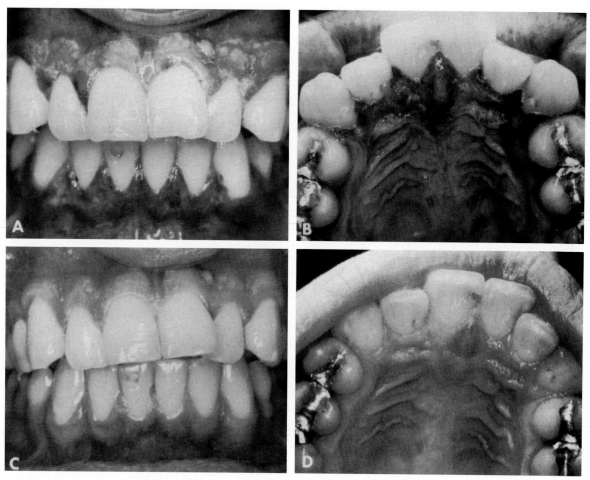

FIGURE 39–7. Treatment of acute herpetic gingivostomatitis. *A,* Before treatment. Note the diffuse erythema and surface vesicles. *B,* Before treatment, lingual view. Note the gingival edema and ruptured vesicle on palate. *C,* One month after treatment. Note restoration of the normal gingival contour and stippling. *D,* One month after treatment, lingual view.

usually sufficient. A dosage of 10 grains every 3 hours may be prescribed for adults, with smaller doses used for children.

REFERENCES

1. Arnold HL, Domzalski CA, Austin ER. Aureomycin mouthwash for herpetic stomatitis. Proc Staff Meet Honolulu *15:*85, 1949.
2. Ash MM Jr, Costich ER, Hayward JR. A study of periodontal hazards of third molars. J Periodontol *33:*209, 1962.
3. Burket LW. Oral Medicine. 3rd ed. Philadelphia, JB Lippincott, 1946, p 53.
4. Burket LW, Hickman GC. Oral herpes (simplex) manifestations: Treatment with vitamin B complex. J Am Dent Assoc *29:*411, 1942.
5. Clausen FP. Local treatment of acute necrotizing ulcerative gingivitis with ascoxal: Clinical experiences from treatment of military personnel. Tandlaegebladet *70:*1009, 1966.
6. Collins J, Hood HM. Topical antibiotic treatment of acute necrotizing ulcerative gingivitis. J Oral Med *22:*59, 1967.
7. Duckworth R, Waterhouse JP, Britton DER, et al. Acute ulcerative gingivitis: A double-blind controlled clinical trial of metronidazole. Br Dent J *120:*599, 1966.
8. Emslie R. Treatment of acute ulcerative gingivitis. A clinical trial using chewing gum containing metronidazole or penicillin. Br Dent J *122:*307, 1967.
9. Everett FG. Aureomycin in the therapy of herpes simplex labialis and recurrent oral aphthae. J Am Dent Assoc *40:*555, 1950.
10. Fisher AA. Treatment of herpes simplex with moccasin snake venom. Arch Dermatol Syph *43:*444, 1941.
11. Frank SB. Formalized herpes virus therapy and the neutralizing substance in herpes simplex. J Invest Dermatol *1:*267, 1940.
12. Frankl Z. Dentitio difficilis and parodontosis. Paradentologie *1:*107, 1947.
13. Gerstenberger HJ. The etiology and treatment of herpetic (aphthous and aphthoulcerative) stomatitis and herpes labialis. Am J Dis Child *26:*309, 1923.
14. Glickman I. The use of penicillin lozenges in the treatment of Vincent's infection and other acute gingival inflammations. J Am Dent Assoc *34:*406, 1947.
15. Glickman I, Johannessen LB. The effect of a six per cent solution of chromic acid on the gingiva of the albino rat—a correlated gross, biomicroscopic, and histologic study. J Am Dent Assoc *41:*674, 1950.
16. Jacobs HG, Jacobs MH. Aureomycin: Its use in infections of the oral cavity. Oral Surg *2:*1015, 1949.
17. King JD. Nutritional and other factors in "trench mouth" with special reference to the nicotinic acid component of the vitamin B2 complex. Br Dent J *74:*113, 1943.
18. Linghorne WJ, McIntosh WG, Tice JW, et al. The relation of ascorbic acid intake to gingivitis. J Can Dent Assoc *12:*49, 1946.
19. Mitchell DF, Baker BR. Topical antibiotic control of necrotizing gingivitis. J Periodontol *39:*81, 1968.
20. Regezi JA, Sciubba JJ. Oral Pathology. Clinical-Pathologic Correlations. Philadelphia, WB Saunders, 1989.
21. Savitt LE, Ayres S Jr. Persistent multiple herpeslike eruption. Response to repeated intradermal injections of smallpox vaccine. Arch Dermatol Syph *59:*653, 1949.
22. Shinn DLS, Squires S, McFadzean A. The treatment of Vincent's disease with metronidazole. Dent Pract *15:*275, 1965.
23. Snyder ML, Church DH, Rickles NH. Primary herpes infection of right second finger. Oral Surg *27:*598, 1969.
24. Stephen KW, McLatchie MF, Mason DK, et al. Treatment of acute ulcerative gingivitis (Vincent's type). Br Dent J *121:*313, 1966.
25. Wade AB, Blake GC, Manson JD, et al. Treatment of the acute phase of ulcerative gingivitis (Vincent's type). Br Dent J *115:*372, 1963.
26. Wade AB, Blake G, Mirza K. Effectiveness of metronidazole in treating the acute phase of ulcerative gingivitis. Dent Pract *16:*440, 1966.
27. Wade AB, Mirza KB. The relative effectiveness of sodium peroxyborate and hydrogen peroxide in treating acute ulcerative gingivitis. Dent Pract *14:*185, 1964.

40

Treatment of the Periodontal Abscess

FERMIN A. CARRANZA, JR.

The Acute Periodontal Abscess
Drainage Through the Pocket
Drainage Through an External Incision

The Gingival Abscess
The Chronic Periodontal Abscess
Treatment by Flap Operation

Periodontal abscesses may be acute or chronic. Acute abscesses are painful, edematous, red, shiny, ovoid elevations of the gingival margin and/or attached gingiva. After their purulent content is partially exuded, they become chronic. Chronic abscesses may produce a dull pain and may at times become acute (see Chapter 28).

THE ACUTE PERIODONTAL ABSCESS

The purpose of treatment of an acute abscess is to alleviate pain, control the spread of infection, and establish drainage.[1] After the cause is diagnosed, the patient's general systemic response should be evaluated and his or her temperature taken. Drainage can be established through the pocket or by means of an incision from the outer surface; the former is preferable.

Drainage Through the Pocket

After application of a topical anesthetic, a flat instrument or a probe is carefully introduced into the pocket in an attempt to distend the pocket wall. A small curette or a Morse scaler can then be gently used to penetrate the tissue and establish drainage. When drainage cannot be easily established via the pocket or when the abscess can be seen pointing through the gingiva, an external incision is indicated.

Drainage Through an External Incision

The abscess is isolated with gauze sponges and dried and swabbed with an antiseptic solution, followed by a topical anesthetic. The clinician should wait 2 or 3 minutes for the anesthetic to become effective; then the abscess is palpated gently to locate the most fluctuant area.

With a Bard-Parker no. 12 blade, a vertical incision is made through the most fluctuant part of the lesion, extending from the mucogingival fold to the gingival margin (Fig. 40–1). If the swelling is on the lingual surface, the incision

is started just apical to the swelling and extended through the gingival margin. The blade should penetrate to firm tissue to be sure of reaching deep, purulent areas. After the initial extravasation of blood and pus, the clinician should irrigate the area with warm water and gently spread the incision to facilitate drainage.

If the tooth is extruded, it should be ground slightly to avoid contact with its antagonists. The tooth is stabilized with the index finger to reduce vibration and discomfort. It is often preferable to grind the teeth in the opposing jaw to avoid discomfort.

After the drainage stops, the area is dried and painted with an antiseptic. Patients without systemic complications are instructed to rinse hourly with a solution of a teaspoon of salt in a glass of warm water and to return the next day. In addition to the rinses, penicillin or other antibiotics are prescribed for patients with fever. The patient is also instructed to avoid exertion and is put on a copious fluid diet. If necessary, bed rest is recommended. Analgesics are prescribed for pain.

By the next day, the swelling is generally markedly reduced or absent, and the symptoms should have subsided. If acute symptoms persist, the patient is instructed to continue the regimen prescribed the previous day and to return in 24 hours. The symptoms invariably disappear by that time, and the lesion is ready for the usual treatment of a chronic periodontal abscess.

THE GINGIVAL ABSCESS

In contrast to the periodontal abscess, which involves the supporting tissues, the gingival abscess is a lesion of the marginal or interdental gingiva that is usually produced by an impacted foreign object.

After topical anesthesia is applied, the fluctuant area of the lesion is incised with a Bard-Parker blade, and the incision is gently widened to permit drainage. The area is cleansed with warm water and covered with a gauze pad. After bleeding stops, the patient is dismissed for 24 hours and instructed to rinse every 2 hours with a glassful of warm water.

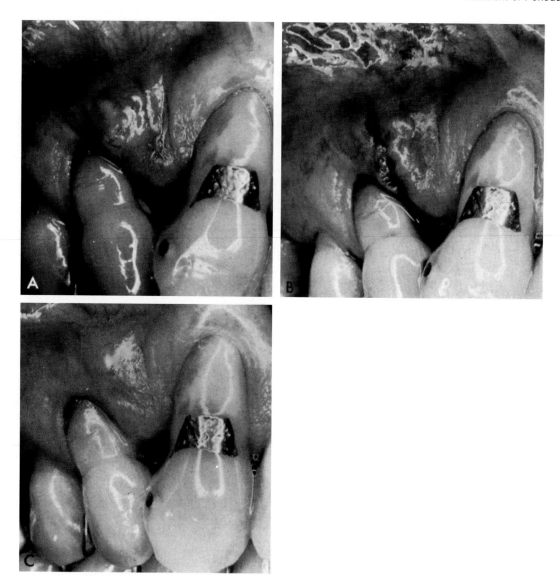

FIGURE 40–1. Incision of acute periodontal abscess. *A,* Fluctuant acute periodontal abscess. *B,* Abscess incised. *C,* After acute signs subside.

When the patient returns, the lesion is generally reduced in size and symptom free. A topical anesthetic is applied, and the area is scaled. If the residual size of the lesion is too great, the lesion is removed surgically.

THE CHRONIC PERIODONTAL ABSCESS

Treatment by Flap Operation*

The first requirement is to determine the relative facial or lingual location of the purulent focus of the abscess. Lingual abscesses may produce swelling on the facial surface, and facial abscesses may produce swelling on the lingual surface. To locate the abscess area, the dentist should probe around the gingival margin, following tortuous pockets to their termination. If a sinus is present, the abscess may be probed through it. Because it offers better accessi-

visibility, the facial approach is preferred and is used unless the abscess is close to the lingual surface.

After the approach is decided on and the area is anes-

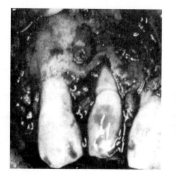 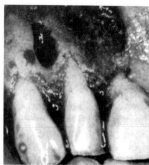

FIGURE 40–2. Full-thickness flap operation for periodontal abscess. *Left,* Full-thickness flap elevated, showing granulation tissue at the gingival margin and sinus opening filled with spongy, purulent tissue. *Right,* Sinus curetted. Note the narrow marginal bridge of bone, which is usually infected and is removed to facilitate healing.

---

* General principles of periodontal surgery are presented in Chapter 50, and the flap technique is discussed in detail in Chapter 54.

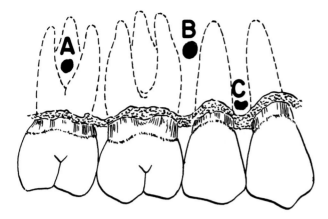

FIGURE 40–3. Various levels at which the sinus from a periodontal abscess may be located. In the case of C, the narrow marginal bridge of bone is removed during treatment.

thetized, the superficial calculus is removed, and two vertical incisions are made from the gingival margin to the mucobuccal fold, outlining the field of operation (Fig. 40–2A). If the lingual approach is used, the incisions are made from the gingival margin to the level of the root apices. The operative field should be large enough to allow unhampered visibility and accessibility. A flap that is too narrow or too short jeopardizes the outcome of the treatment.

After the vertical incisions are made, a mesiodistal incision is made across the interdental papilla with a knife to facilitate detachment of the flap. A full-thickness flap is raised with a periosteal elevator and held in position with a retractor.

A flap on either the facial or lingual surface usually suffices. In the case of an abscess that was initially acute, the edges of the incision made the previous day are usually united so that the flap can be raised in one piece. Elevation of the flap reveals some or all of the following conditions (see Fig. 40–2A):

1. Granulation tissue at the gingival margin.
2. Calculus on the root surface.

4. A sinus opening on the external bone, which can be probed inwardly to the tooth.
5. Purulent spongy tissue in the orifice of the sinus.

After the field is carefully surveyed, the granulation tissue is removed with curettes to provide a clear view of the root. All deposits are scaled from the teeth, and the root surfaces are planed with hoe scalers and smoothed with curettes. If a sinus is present, it is explored and curetted (Fig. 40–2B).

The location of the sinus determines the manner in which the bone is managed. The bone is not disturbed except in cases in which only a thin rim of bone separates the sinus from the crest of the alveolar bone (Fig. 40–3). Thin marginal bridges of bone are removed because they are usually pathologically involved and act as foreign bodies that impair healing.

The facial and lingual surfaces are covered with a piece of gauze shaped into a U, which is held in position until the bleeding stops. The gauze is then removed, and the flap is sutured and covered with a periodontal pack.

The patient is instructed not to rinse until the next day, when a pleasant-tasting mouthwash diluted 1:3 in warm water is used every 2 hours. The area should be cleansed gently with a soft toothbrush and water irrigation under medium pressure. The patient is told to return in 1 week, at which time the pack and sutures are removed and the patient is instructed in plaque control. Repacking is usually not necessary.

The appearance of the gingiva returns to normal within 6 to 8 weeks; repair of the bone requires approximately 9 months. The prospects for bone repair and fill are better for osseous defects produced by rapidly destructive acute periodontal disease than for slowly progressing chronic lesions.[2]

REFERENCES

1. Manson JD. Periodontics. 3rd ed. Philadelphia, Lea & Febiger, 1975.
2. Nabers JM, Meador HL, Nabers CL. Chronology, an important factor in the repair of osseous defects. Periodontics 2:304, 1964.

The initial phase of periodontal therapy is directed at (1) removing all local irritants that may cause gingival inflammation and (2) instructing and motivating the patient in plaque control. It is the etiotropic treatment phase, because its goal is to eliminate the etiologic factor of periodontal disease. The terms *Phase I, initial phase,* and *hygienic phase* are commonly used to refer to this stage of therapy.

41

Preparation of the Tooth Surface

MAX O. SCHMID

Rationale
Procedure
Step 1: Limited Plaque Control Instruction
Step 2: Supragingival Removal of Calculus
Step 3: Recontouring Defective Restorations and Crowns

Step 4: Obturation of Carious Lesions
Step 5: Comprehensive Plaque Control Instruction
Step 6: Subgingival Root Treatment
Step 7: Tissue Re-evaluation

RATIONALE

Phase I therapy is the first step in the chronologic sequence of procedures that constitute periodontal treatment. The objective of Phase I therapy is the reduction or elimination of gingival inflammation (Plate XIV); this is achieved by complete removal of calculus, correction of defective restorations, obturation of carious lesions, and institution of a comprehensive plaque control regimen.[3,10,23,24,46] This first phase of therapy is administered to patients with periodontal pockets who will later be re-evaluated for possible surgical treatment, as well as to patients with chronic gingivitis or mild periodontitis without a foreseeable need for periodontal surgery. Procedures included in Phase I therapy may therefore constitute the only therapy needed to solve the patient's periodontal problems, or they may be the preparatory phase for surgical therapy.

Data from clinical research indicate that the long-term success of periodontal treatment is dependent predominantly on maintaining the results achieved with Phase I therapy and much less on a specific surgical procedure.[25,32,39] In addition, Phase I therapy provides an opportunity for the periodontist to evaluate tissue response and the patient's attitude toward periodontal care, both of which are crucial to the prognosis of periodontal conditions.

The objectives of Phase I therapy are (1) to reduce or eliminate gingival inflammation, (2) to eliminate periodontal pockets produced by the edematous enlargement of inflamed gingiva, (3) to achieve surgical manageability of the gingiva (i.e., firm consistency and minimal bleeding), and (4) to improve healing after periodontal surgery.

Based on the concept that microbial plaque harbors the primary pathogens of gingival inflammation, the specific aim of Phase I therapy is effective plaque control by eliminating rough and irregular contours from the tooth surfaces and establishing a suitable plaque control regimen. Effective plaque control by the patient is a key objective of every therapeutic periodontal procedure. However, effective control can be expected only if the tooth surfaces are free of rough deposits or irregular contours and are readily accessible to oral hygiene aids.

After careful analysis of a case, the number of appointments needed to complete this phase of treatment is estimated. Patients with small amounts of calculus and relatively healthy tissues can be treated in one appointment. Most other patients require several treatment sessions. The dentist should estimate the number of appointments needed on the basis of the number of teeth in the mouth, the severity of inflammation, the amount and location of calculus, the depth and activity of pockets, the presence of furcation involvements, and the patient's comprehension of and compliance with oral hygiene instructions.

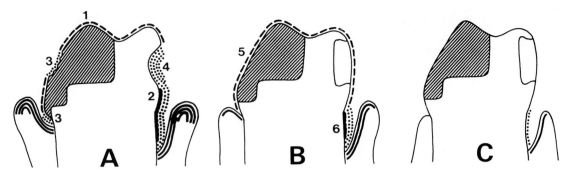

FIGURE 41–1. Steps in Phase I therapy. *A,* Before starting therapy. Dashed line (1) shows areas that can be cleaned by the patient. Dotted lines are areas that must be corrected by the dentist before the patient can clean them. 2, Calculus. 3, Rough surfaces and overhanging margins of restorations. 4, Caries. Parallel lines in the gingiva denote the presence and degree of inflammation. *B,* After removal of supragingival calculus, correction of restorations, and temporary sealing of caries, the area amenable to plaque control has been considerably extended (dashed line, 5). Inflammation is reduced (parallel lines in gingiva). 6, Subgingival calculus still not removed. *C,* After removal of subgingival calculus. The pocket is still present, and the plaque accumulated in it cannot be removed by the patient. Surgical pocket elimination may be indicated.

PROCEDURE

Step 1: Limited Plaque Control Instruction

Introducing an oral hygiene program to the patient is of high priority in every periodontal treatment plan (see Chapter 42). Plaque control instructions should begin at the first therapeutic appointment. The patient is taught how to clean all smooth and regular surfaces of the teeth. However, when therapy is initiated, a number of tooth surfaces usually show irregularities such as calculus, defective restorations, carious lesions, or necrotic cementum (Fig. 41–1A). These irregularities prevent sufficient access for oral hygiene aids; the patient cannot be expected to remove plaque from such areas.

The toothbrush is often the only hygiene aid indicated at this stage of therapy. Dental floss should be used on smooth proximal tooth surfaces only, because flossing around sharp edges and coarse surfaces of calculus or overhanging restorations causes the floss to shred and break. This leads to ineffective plaque removal and is often a frustrating, dissuasive experience for the patient.

Step 2: Supragingival Removal of Calculus

Dental calculus by itself is not injurious to the periodontium,[2,52] but it provides a highly retentive surface for the oral microflora. Therefore, calculus must be eliminated entirely to allow for effective plaque control.

When inflamed, friable gingiva is present adjacent to

deep periodontal pockets, calculus is first dislodged from all supragingival tooth surfaces. This leads to a substantial improvement in the condition of the marginal gingiva. Removal of subgingival calculus from these areas prior to the resolution of pronounced marginal gingivitis is not recommended, because it may produce undue laceration of the diseased gingiva and provoke an acute inflammatory tissue response.

Supragingival calculus can be dislodged with ultrasonic scalers, hand scalers, or curettes.[41] Scaling is performed with a pull motion, except on the proximal surfaces of closely spaced anterior teeth, where thin chisel scalers may be used with push strokes. In the pull motion, the instrument engages the apical or lateral edges of a deposit and dislodges the entire accretion or part of it with a firm stroke in the direction of the crown (Fig. 41–2).

The pull motion is initiated in the forearm and transmitted from the wrist to the hand with a slight flexing of the fingers. Rotation of the wrist is synchronized with movement of the forearm. The scaling motion is not initiated in the wrist or fingers, nor is it carried out independently without the use of the forearm.

In the push motion, the fingers activate the instrument. The instrument engages the lateral edge of the calculus, and the fingers provide a thrust motion that dislodges the deposit.

The removal of calculus is not a whittling operation. Calculus is not "pared down" until the tooth surface is reached, but is dislodged in its full thickness with a few de-

FIGURE 41–2. Instrumentation for calculus removal. *A,* Calculus is removed by engaging the apical or lateral edge of the deposit with the cutting edge of a scaler; vertical movement of the instrument will remove the fragment of calculus engaged by the instrument, as seen in the shaded drawing. *B,* The instrument is moved laterally and again engages the edge of calculus, overlapping to some extent the previous stroke; the shaded drawing shows further removal. *C,* The final portion of the deposit is engaged and removed. Note how in an interdental space the operation is performed by entering facially and lingually.

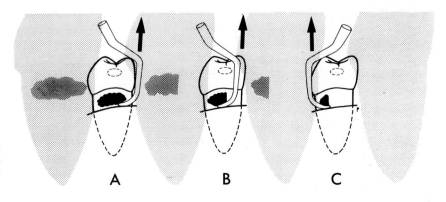

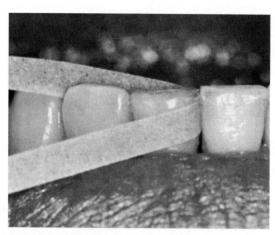

FIGURE 41–3. Finishing strips are effective for removing stains and calculus from proximal tooth surfaces adjacent to tight contact areas and narrow embrasures.

cisive strokes. After calculus is removed from one surface area of the tooth, the instrument is advanced laterally to engage adjacent deposits.

Scaling is confined to a small area of the tooth on both sides of the cemento-enamel junction, where calculus and other deposits are usually located. Sweeping the instrument over the crown where scaling is not needed lengthens operating time, dulls the instrument, and is contrary to the careful attention to detail required for effective instrumentation.

Complete interproximal access for scaling instruments is often difficult, especially between incisor teeth with narrow embrasures. In those areas, sharp-pointed sickle scalers rather than round-ended curettes should be used to reach close to the contact zones. Crowding of anterior teeth fre-

quently results in long, tight contact zones and extremely narrow embrasures. This prevents adequate access even for sharp-pointed sickle scalers. Abrasive finishing strips inserted between the teeth can be used for effective removal of calculus and stain from such areas (Fig. 41–3).

Scaling invariably leaves the treated tooth, especially cementum and dentin, with a rough and scratched surface that favors the quick re-establishment of plaque and calculus. Therefore, after calculus removal, the tooth surface must be planed with suitable scalers or curettes[9,12,13,15,20,30,38,49,53] and polished with an appropriate abrasive paste on a rotary rubber cup or brush. Smooth, polished tooth surfaces are conducive to effective plaque control and resist calculus formation considerably better than do rough surfaces.[50]

Step 3: Recontouring Defective Restorations and Crowns

With few exceptions,[36] rough, overcontoured, overhanging, or smooth but subgingivally located restorations have been found to be associated with pronounced accumulation of periodontally pathogenic organisms,[5,7,51,52] periodontal inflammation[1,4,16,21,22,31,34,35,54] (Fig. 41–4), and loss of alveolar bone and periodontal attachment.[6,8,14,18,29,44,48] Like calculus, such restorations interfere with efficient plaque control and must therefore be corrected or removed. This is as important as the removal of calculus and should preferably be completed at the same time. Adequate plaque control by the patient on teeth with restorations is feasible only if the restorations are well contoured and their surfaces are smooth (Fig. 41–5A,B).

Defective restorations, especially overhanging margins, are detected clinically by running a fine explorer along

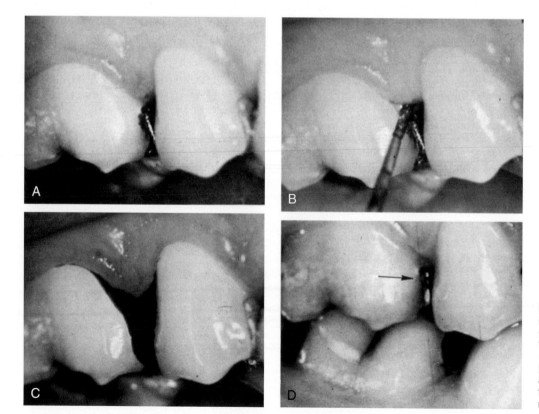

FIGURE 41–4. Effect on the gingiva of an overhanging amalgam restoration mesial on the first molar. *A,* Clinical aspect. *B,* Interproximal probing provokes profuse bleeding from the col area *(C),* a sign of gingival inflammation. *D,* Clinical aspect of recontoured restoration *(arrow).*

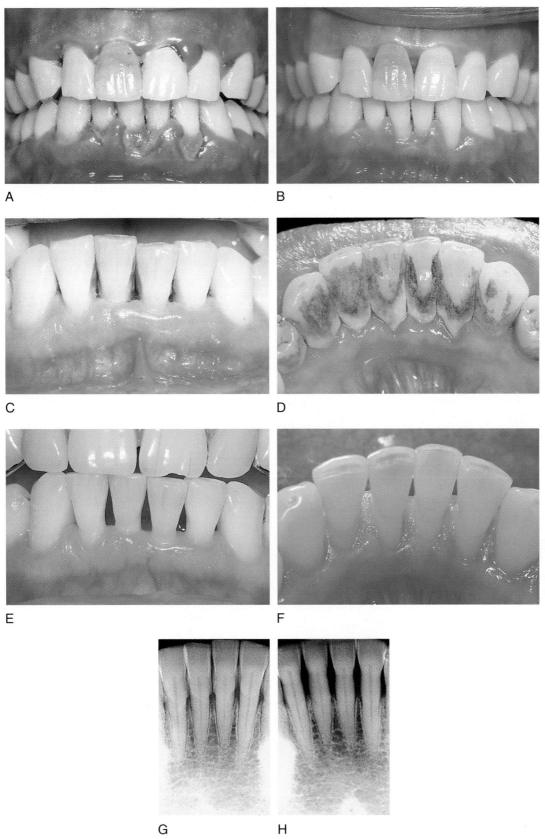

PLATE XIV. Results of Phase I therapy. *A*, Heavy calculus deposits and severe gingival inflammation. *B*, Three weeks after elimination of irritants, gingival healing has resulted. *C–H*, Patient before and 18 months after Phase I therapy. *C* and *D*, Clinical preoperative view. Note edematous gingival enlargement and abundant calculus. *E* and *F*, Clinical postoperative views after Phase I therapy and maintenance visits. Note excellent contour and color of the receded gingiva. *G* and *H*, Radiographs taken before and 1½ years after treatment, respectively. Note presence of calculus in the preoperative radiograph and the clean root surface seen after treatment. Bone height remained unchanged. (*C–H* courtesy of Dr. Steven Levine.)

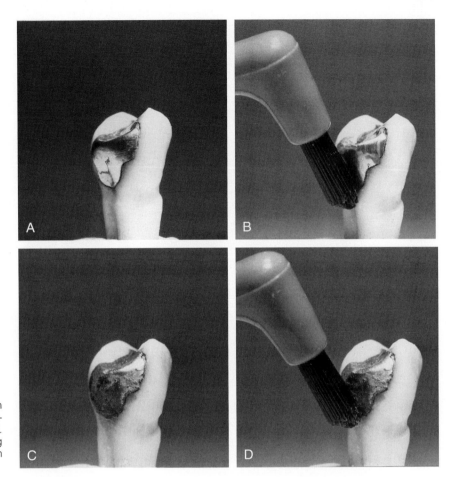

FIGURE 41–5. Effect of restoration contours on plaque control. *A,* Recontoured restoration, providing adequate access for oral hygiene aid *(B).* *C,* Overcontoured amalgam restoration, causing poor accessibility for oral hygiene aid in furcation area *(D).*

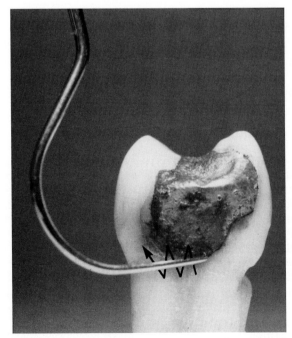

FIGURE 41–6. Identification of defective restorations. Rough surfaces and overhanging margins can be detected with the tip of a fine explorer. Crooked arrow denotes the path of movement of the explorer tip.

their periphery, moving the explorer tip continuously back and forth across the margins of the restoration (Fig. 41–6). In the presence of an overhanging margin, clicking sounds are produced when running the explorer from the restoration to the tooth, and a definitive catch is felt when moving the instrument from the tooth to the restoration. Bite-wing radiographs can be a helpful diagnostic adjunct in determining the approximate mesiodistal and occluso-apical dimension of a proximal overhang.

Restorations on the root surfaces of molars and premolars require special attention. Frequently, such restorations do not follow the concave interradicular depressions found on these teeth. Instead, they exhibit overcontoured surfaces that make it difficult for the patient to reach the subjacent tooth surface with an oral hygiene instrument (Fig. 41–5C,D).

Overhanging margins are eliminated either by replacing the entire restoration or by correcting the contour of the existing restoration. In this phase of therapy, the latter, although often only a temporary measure, is preferred whenever feasible because it involves considerably less time and effort than does replacing an entire restoration.

Overhanging portions of alloy and resin restorations are removed with finishing burs (Fig. 41–7A) or diamond-coated files mounted on a special handpiece attachment that generates reciprocating strokes of high frequency. These motor-driven files have been improved by the addition of a water spray to the handpiece (Fig. 41–7B) and by a wider selection of diamond tips capable of recontouring

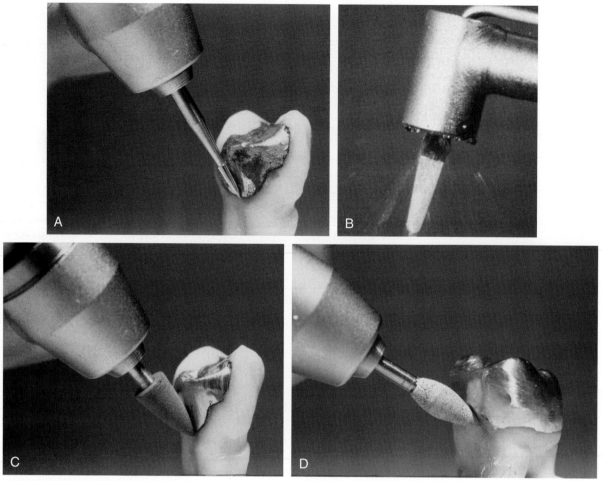

FIGURE 41–7. Instruments for recontouring existing restorations. *A,* Finishing bur. *B,* Diamond file mounted on a special handpiece *with water spray. C,* Rubber cone for final polishing. *D,* Mounted stone.

composite, gold, and porcelain surfaces.[26,28] Small size, high working speed, and water spray enable finishing burs and motor-driven files to efficiently remove large overhangs from all supragingival tooth surfaces, particularly in narrow embrasures, leaving reasonably smooth restoration surfaces.

When a bur is used, the instrument is pressed gently against the restoration and moved across the overhanging ledge to the tooth surface. The procedure is repeated until the overhang is eliminated. The bur should not be guided from the tooth toward the restoration, as this is likely to undermine the restoration and traumatize subjacent tooth structures. Final polishing of the recontoured restoration is accomplished with abrasive discs, finishing strips, or rubber points (Fig. 41–7C).

When a motor-driven diamond file is used, it is centered with a continuous circular burnishing motion over the ledge of the restoration until all excess material has been shaved down. For polishing, the procedure is repeated after replacing the file in the handpiece with a plastic tip of similar shape, coated with polishing paste. Because most polishing pastes tend to roughen restorative materials, especially conventional composites, they should be carefully selected.[40]

Grossly overhanging gold restorations and precious metal and ceramic crowns are corrected best with thin, tapered diamond burs or abrasive stones (Fig. 41–7D). Final pol-

Recontouring in subgingival areas, especially when working with finishing burs, may necessitate reflection of the gingiva to facilitate access and avoid laceration of the soft tissues.

Step 4: Obturation of Carious Lesions

Caries in the vicinity of the gingiva interferes with gingival health, even in the absence of adjacent calculus or defective restorations, because it acts as a large and usually inaccessible reservoir of microorganisms. Therefore, the obturation of carious lesions is an integral part of Phase I therapy. Complete debridement of such lesions and permanent closure of the clean cavities are desirable whenever possible.

Temporary restorations are also acceptable. However, their primary purpose in Phase I periodontal therapy is to eliminate microbial reservoirs that are injurious to the gingiva, not to restore the form and function of the affected teeth. Therefore, temporary restorations should be placed only in cases in which (1) permanent restorative care is not immediately available to the patient, (2) access for final preparation of a subgingival cavity requires prior apical displacement of the gingival margin, or (3) the prognosis and future existence of a decayed tooth depend on the result of periodontal therapy.

Final cavity preparation and placement of a permanent restoration should be performed as soon as periodontal therapy of the affected tooth is completed.

Step 5: Comprehensive Plaque Control Instruction

After removal of supragingival calculus, recontouring of defective restorations, and sealing of carious lesions, the dentition is restored to the point at which a comprehensive plaque control regimen can be instituted. The patient should be able to remove plaque from the entire supragingival surface of all teeth (see Fig. 41–1B). Chapter 42 provides a detailed description of plaque control methods.

Step 6: Subgingival Root Treatment

When the patient has learned to control supragingival plaque and marginal gingivitis, subgingival root treatment is initiated. This consists of removing calculus, eliminating necrotic cementum, and planing the root surface and constitutes the final step in achieving smooth and regular contours on all oral tooth surfaces (see Fig. 41–1C).

Subgingival calculus is removed with curettes. This form of calculus is much harder and more tenacious than supragingival calculus. Its removal requires considerable force and good control of the working instrument. Accidental injury to the soft periodontal tissues adjacent to the root surface being treated is not uncommon. Therefore, inflammation of the marginal gingiva should be under control before subgingival root therapy is initiated; this reduces friability of the gingiva and the risk of tissue laceration during instrumentation.

The extent of subgingival calculus deposits should be appraised before an effort is made to remove them. In the absence of adequate visibility, this entails gently sliding a fine instrument (probe or explorer) over the surface of each deposit in the direction of the apex until the apical margin of the accretion on the root is identified. The distance between the apical ledge of calculus and the bottom of the pocket usually ranges from 0.2 to 1.0 mm. The operator should try to see the entire calculous mass by blowing warm air between the tooth and the gingival margin or by deflecting the gingiva with a probe. Although subgingival calculus is generally brown or dark gray and can be readily distinguished from the tooth, it is difficult to see calculus in deep pockets where the bulk of the soft tissue wall obstructs the view.

Complete removal of subgingival calculus from deep pocket areas requires the development of a delicate sense of touch. With the toe of the curette sliding along the tooth surface, the instrument is gently inserted in the pocket and moved apically beyond the deepest portion of the calculus (Fig. 41–8A). The curette should never be pushed hard in an apical direction, because this may force calculus and other debris into the soft tissue and elicit an acute inflammatory response.

Calculus is dislodged from the tooth and the pocket by firmly pressing the tip of the curette laterally against the root surface and pulling the instrument out of the pocket with a long, swift stroke (Fig. 41–8B). Short, abrupt chipping at the tooth should be avoided because it may result in "nicking" of the root surface, necessitating extensive planing with undue loss of tooth structure.

In the course of the scaling procedure, the smoothness of the root must be checked and rechecked with a fine probe or explorer (see Fig. 41–6). There is often a shallow vertical groove on the proximal root surfaces of posterior teeth. Smooth and feather-edged calculus lodged in these grooves often gives the root a regular contour, conveying the erroneous impression that the root surface is clean. The same phenomenon occurs at cemento-enamel junctions.

It is not enough to eliminate the calculus from the subgingival root surface. Areas in which the root feels softened or rough indicate the presence of necrotic changes in the cementum or scratches from heavy instrumention. The root must be planed until it feels smooth to the explorer or the probe. Where visual inspection is not feasible, smoothness of the root surface is one of the most reliable clinical signs for determining the absence of calculus or necrotic cementum.

Root planing requires the same instruments and procedures that are used for subgingival calculus removal. Initially, pull strokes with firm pressure against the tooth are indicated for efficient removal of necrotic cementum or roughened dentin. As the surface becomes smoother, the pressure is gradually reduced while the length and frequency of the strokes are increased; in addition, vertical strokes are combined with oblique and horizontal strokes. This produces the required smoothness of the root.

Manual scaling and root planing are strenuous procedures. As a result, the application of power-driven root sur-

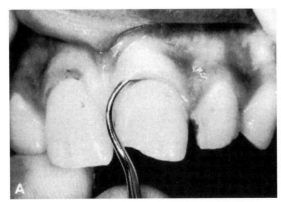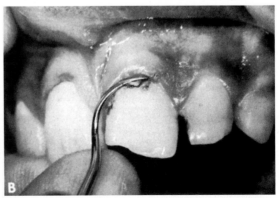

FIGURE 41–8. Removal of subgingival calculus. *A,* Curette inserted below gingival margin. *B,* Flint-like subgingival calculus removed.

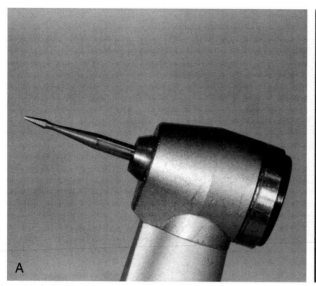
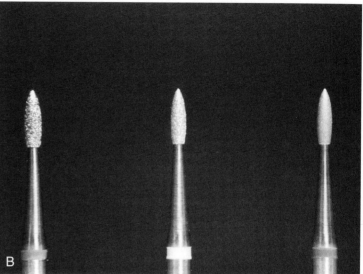

FIGURE 41–9. Rotary scaler and diamond burs for calculus removal and root planing. *A,* Scaler tip inserted in high-speed handpiece. *B, Left to right,* coarse, medium, and fine-grit diamond burs for root shaping and planing.

face instruments to these tasks has gained increasing attention (Fig. 41–9). Comparative studies indicate that ultrasonic scalers, handpiece-mounted curettes,[17] rotary scalers, or fine grit diamond burs[33,42,43] can be used safely and effectively in debriding and planing periodontally diseased root surfaces, although there is a high risk of tissue damage if they are used improperly.[11,27,37,42,43,45,47]

Within 3 to 4 weeks after the removal of subgingival calculus and necrotic cementum, gingival inflammation usually is substantially reduced or eliminated. This healing process is frequently accompanied by transient root hypersensitivity and unsightly recession of the gingival margin (see Plate XIV). The patient must be informed in advance of these therapeutic sequelae to prevent potential distrust and loss of motivation with regard to periodontal therapy.

Step 7: Tissue Re-evaluation

The periodontal tissues are re-examined to determine the need for further therapy. Pockets are reprobed to decide whether surgical treatment is indicated. However, additional improvement of a periodontal condition through surgery can be expected only if Phase I therapy has been successfully completed. Therefore, surgical treatment of periodontal pockets should be attempted only if a patient is exercising effective plaque control and the gingiva is free of overt inflammation.

REFERENCES

1. Alexander AG. Periodontal aspects of conservative dentistry. Br J Dent *124:*111, 1968.
2. Allen DL, Kerr DA. Tissue response in the guinea pig to sterile and nonsterile calculus. J Periodontol *36:*121, 1965.
3. Axelsson P, Lindhe J. The effect of a preventive programme on dental plaque, gingivitis and caries in school children. Results after one and two years. J Clin Periodontol *1:*126, 1974.
4. Bergman B, Hugoson A, Olsson CO. Periodontal and prosthetic conditions in patients treated with removable partial dentures and artificial crowns. A longitudinal study. Acta Odontol Scand *29:*621, 1971.
5. Bjorby A, Löe H. The relative significance of different local factors in the initiation and development of periodontal inflammation. J Periodont Res *2:*76, 1967.
6. Bjorn AL, Bjorn H, Grkovic B. Marginal fit of restorations and its relation to periodontal bone level. I. Metal fillings. Odontol Rev *20:*311, 1969.
7. Brebou M, Mühlemann HR. The role of surface roughness of plastic foils in the collection of early calculus deposits. Helv Odontol Acta *10:*137, 1966.
8. Brunsvold MA, Lane JJ. The prevalence of overhanging dental restorations and their relationship to periodontal disease. J Clin Periodontol *17:*67, 1990.
9. Burke SW, Green E. Effectiveness of periodontal files. J Periodontol *41:*39, 1970.
10. Chawla TN, Nanda RS, Kapoor KK. Dental prophylaxis procedures in control of periodontal disease in Lucknow (rural). Indian J Periodontol *46:*498, 1975.
11. Ellman IA. Safe highspeed periodontal instrument. Dent Surv *36:*759, 1960.
12. Ewen SJ. A photomicrographic study of root scaling. Periodontics *4:*273, 1966.
13. Ewen SJ, Gwinnett AJ. A scanning electron microscopic study of teeth following periodontal instrumentation. J Periodontol *48:*92, 1977.
14. Gilmore N, Sheiham A. Overhanging dental restorations and periodontal disease. J Periodontol *42:*8, 1971.
15. Green E, Ramfjord SP. Tooth roughness after subgingival root planing. J Periodontol *37:*396, 1966.
16. Gullo CA, Powell RN. The effect of placement of cervical margins of class II amalgam restorations on plaque accumulation and gingival health. J Oral Rehabil *6:*317, 1979.
17. Haenggi D, Ritz L, Rateitschak KH. Perioplaner/periopolisher. Schweiz Monatsschr Zahnmed *101:*1535, 1991.
18. Jeffcoat MK, Howell TH. Alveolar bone destruction due to overhanging amalgams in periodontal disease. J Periodontol *51:*599, 1980.
19. Karlsen K. Gingival reactions to dental restorations. Acta Odontol Scand *28:*895, 1970.
20. Kerry GJ. Roughness of root surfaces after use of ultrasonic instruments and hand curettes. J Periodontol *38:*340, 1967.
21. Koivumaa KK, Wennstrom A. A histological investigation of the changes in gingival margins adjacent to gold crowns. Odont Tidskrift *68:*373, 1960.
22. Lang NP, Kiel RA, Anderhalden K. Clinical and microbiological effects of subgingival restorations with overhanging or clinically perfect margins. J Clin Periodontol *10:*563, 1983.
23. Lightner LM, O'Leary TJ, Drake RB, et al. Preventive periodontics treatment procedures: Results over 46 months. J Periodontol *42:*555, 1971.
24. Lindhe J, Koch G. The effect of supervised oral hygiene on the gingiva of children. Progression and inhibition of gingivitis. J Periodont Res *1:*260, 1966.
25. Lindhe J, Nyman S. The effect of plaque control and surgical pocket elimination on the establishment and maintenance of periodontal health. A longitudinal study of periodontal therapy in cases of advanced disease. J Clin Periodontol *2:*67, 1975.
26. Lutz F, Mörmann W. Interdentale Restorationsuberhange—rationelle Entfernung mit neuentwickelten Maschineninstrumenten. Schweiz Monatsschr Zahnheilkd *91:*115, 1981.
27. Meyer K, Lie T. Root surface roughness in response to periodontal instrumentation studied by combined use of microroughness measurements and scanning electron microscopy. J Clin Periodontol *4:*77, 1977.
28. Mörmann W, Lutz F, Curilovic Z. Die Bearbeitung von Gold, Keramik und Amalgam mit Composhape-Diamantschleifern und Proxoshape-Interdentalfeilen. Quintessenz *28:*1575, 1983.
29. Pack ARC, Coxhead LJ, McDonald BW. The prevalence of overhanging margins in posterior amalgam restorations and its periodontal consequences. J Clin Periodontol *17:*145, 1990.

30. Pameijer CH, Stallard RE, Hiep N. Surface characteristics of teeth following periodontal instrumentation: A scanning electron microscope study. J Periodontol *43:*628, 1972.

31. Perel ML. Axial crown contours. J Prosthet Dent *25:*642, 1971.

32. Ramfjord SP, Knowles JW, Nissle RR, et al. Results following three modalities of periodontal therapy. J Periodontol *46:*522, 1975.

33. Rateitschak KH, Rateitschak EM, Wolf HF, Hassell TM. The Perio-set Color Atlas of Dental Medicine. Vol 1. Periodontology. 2nd ed. New York, Thieme, page 172, 1989.

34. Renggli HH. Reaktion der Gingiva auf uberhangende Fullungsrander. Dtsch Zahnarztl Z *27:*322, 1972.

35. Renggli HH. Auswirkungen subgingivaler approximaler Fullungsrander auf den Etzundungsgrad der benachbarten Gingiva. Thesis, Dental Institute, Zurich, Switzerland, 1974.

36. Richter WA, Ueno H. Relationship of crown margin placement to gingival inflammation. J Prosthet Dent *30:*156, 1973.

37. Ritz L, Hefti AF, Rateitschak KH. An in vitro investigation on the loss of root substance in scaling with various instruments. J Clin Periodontol *18:*643, 1991.

38. Rosenberg RM, Ash MM Jr. The effect of root roughness on plaque accumulation and gingival inflammation. J Periodontol *45:*146, 1974.

39. Rosling B, Nyman S, Lindhe J, Jern B. The healing potential of the periodontal tissues following different techniques of periodontal surgery in plaque-free dentitions. A 2-year clinical study. J Clin Periodontol *3:*233, 1976.

40. Roulet JF, Roulet Mehrens TK. The surface roughness of restorative materials and dental tissues after polishing with prophylaxis and polishing pastes. J Periodontol *53:*257, 1982.

41. Schaffer EM. Periodontal instrumentation: Scaling and root planing. Int Dent J *17:*297, 1967.

42. Schwartz JP, Hefti AF, Rateitschak KH. Vergleich der Oberflaechenrauhigkeiten des Wurzeldentins nach Bearbeitung mit Diamantsschleifkoerpern und Handinstrumenten. Schweiz Monatsschr Zahnmed *94:*47, 1984.

43. Schwartz JP, Guggenheim R, Dueggelin M, et al. The effectiveness of root debridement in open flap procedures by means of a comparison between hand instruments and diamond burs. J Clin Periodontol *16:*510, 1989.

44. Silness J. Periodontal conditions in patients treated with dental bridges. III. The relationship between the location of the crown margin and the periodontal condition. J Periodont Res *5:*225, 1970.

45. Stewart JL, Briggs RL, Drisko RR, Jamison HC. Relative calculus and tooth structure loss with use of power-driven scaling instruments. J Am Dent Assoc *83:*840, 1971.

46. Suomi JD, Greene JC, Vermillion JR, et al. The effect of controlled oral hygiene procedures on the progression of periodontal disease in adults: Results after third and final year. J Periodontol *42:*152, 1971.

47. Torfason T, Kiger R, Selvig KA, Egelberg J. Clinical improvement of gingival conditions following ultrasonic versus hand instrumentation of periodontal pockets. J Clin Periodontol *6:*165, 1979.

48. Valderhaug J, Birkeland JM. Periodontal conditions in patients 5 years following insertion of fixed prostheses. I. Pocket depths and loss of attachment. J Oral Rehabil *3:*237, 1967.

49. Van Volkinburg JW, Green E, Armitage GC. The nature of root surfaces after curette, cavitron, and alpha-sonic instrumentation. J Periodont Res *11:*374, 1976.

50. Villa P. Degree of calculus inhibition by habitual tooth brushing. Helv Odontol Acta *12:*31, 1968.

51. Waerhaug J. Tissue reactions around artificial crowns. J Periodontol *24:*172, 1953.

52. Waerhaug J. Effect of rough surfaces upon gingival tissue. J Dent Res *35:*323, 1956.

53. Wilkinson RF, Maybury JE. Scanning electron microscopy of the root surface following instrumentation. J Periodontol *44:*559, 1973.

54. Wright WH. Local factor in periodontal disease. Periodontics *1:*163, 1963.

42

Plaque Control

DOROTHY A. PERRY and MAX O. SCHMID

Toothbrushes
Powered Toothbrushes
Dentifrices
Toothbrushing Methods
The Bass Method
The Modified Stillman Method
The Charters Method
Methods of Cleaning With Powered Brushes
Interdental Cleaning Aids
Dental Floss

Interdental Cleaning Devices
Gingival Massage
Oral Irrigation Devices
Chemical Plaque Control
Disclosing Agents
Frequency of Plaque Removal
Recommendations for Plaque Control Instruction
Motivation
Education
Instruction

Plaque control is the removal of microbial plaque and the prevention of its accumulation on the teeth and adjacent gingival surfaces. Plaque control also retards the formation of calculus.[86] The removal of microbial plaque leads to resolution of gingival inflammation, and cessation of plaque control measures leads to a recurrence of inflammation.[72] Thus, plaque control is an effective way of treating and preventing gingivitis and therefore is a critical part of all the procedures involved in the treatment and prevention of periodontal diseases.[18]

To date, the most dependable mode of plaque control is mechanical cleaning with a toothbrush and other hygiene aids. Chemical inhibitors of plaque and calculus incorporated in mouthwashes or dentifrices have a place as adjunctive agents to mechanical techniques and should be prescribed according to the needs of individual patients. Chemical plaque control is a rapidly growing field and will no doubt become more important in the future.

Plaque control is one of the key elements of the practice of dentistry. It permits each patient to assume responsibility for his or her own oral health. Without it, oral health cannot be attained or preserved. Every patient in every dental practice should be on a plaque control program. Good plaque control facilitates a return to health for patients with gingival and periodontal diseases, as well as the preservation of that health.

TOOTHBRUSHES

The bristle toothbrush appeared about the year 1600 in China, was first patented in America in 1857, and has since undergone little change. Generally, toothbrushes vary in size and design, as well as in length, hardness, and arrangement of the bristles (Fig. 42–1).[92] The American Dental Association has described the range of dimensions of acceptable brushes: these have a brushing surface 1 to 1.25 inches (25.4 to 31.8 mm) long and 5/16 to 3/8 inch (7.9 to 9.5 mm) wide, two to four rows of bristles, and 5 to 12 tufts per row.[2] A toothbrush should be able to reach and efficiently clean most areas of the teeth. The type of brush is a matter of individual preference. Although some products claim superiority of design for such things as minor modification of bristle placement, there is no demonstrated superiority of clinical significance for any one type of toothbrush. Ease of manipulation by the patient is an important factor in brush selection, as is the patient's perception that the brush works well. The effectiveness of and potential injury from different types of brushes depend to a great degree on how the brushes are used.[17]

There are two kinds of bristle material used in toothbrushes: natural bristles from hogs and artificial filaments made predominantly of nylon. Both types remove plaque.[14] However, in terms of homogeneity of the material, uniformity of bristle size, elasticity, resistance to fracture, and repulsion of water and debris, nylon filaments are clearly superior. Natural bristles, because of their tubular form, are significantly more susceptible to fraying, breaking, contamination with diluted microbial debris, softening, and loss of elasticity. Patients accustomed to the softness of an old natural bristle brush can traumatize the gingiva when using a new brush with comparable vigor. It is helpful to point this out when a patient changes from natural to nylon bristles.

Toothbrush bristles are grouped in tufts that are usually arranged in three or four rows. Multitufted toothbrushes contain more bristles and may clean more efficiently than skimpier brushes. Rounded bristle ends cause fewer scratches on the gingiva than flat cut bristles with sharp ends.[92] The question of the most desirable bristle hardness is not settled. Bristle hardness is proportional to the square of the diameter and inversely proportional to the square of bristle length.[47] Diameters of commonly used bristles range from 0.007 inch (0.2 mm) for soft brushes to 0.012 inch (0.3 mm) for medium brushes and 0.014 inch (0.4 mm) for hard brushes.[50] Soft bristle brushes of the type described by Bass[11] have gained wide acceptance. Bass recommended a straight handle and nylon bristles 0.007 inch (0.2 mm) in diameter and 0.406 inch (10.3 mm) long, with rounded ends, arranged in three rows of tufts, six evenly spaced tufts per row, with 80 to 86 bristles per tuft. For children, the brush is smaller, with thinner (0.005 inch or 0.1 mm) and shorter (0.344 inch or 8.7 mm) bristles.

Opinions regarding the merits of hard and soft bristles are based on studies carried out under different conditions; these studies are often inconclusive and contradict one another.[51] Soft bristles are more flexible, clean beneath the gingival margin (sulcus brushing),[12] and reach farther into the proximal tooth surfaces.[36] Use of hard-bristled toothbrushes is associated with more gingival recession, and frequent brushers who use hard bristles have more recession than frequent brushers who use soft bristles.[58] However, the manner in which a brush is used and the abrasiveness of the dentifrice affect the action and abrasion to a greater degree than the bristle hardness itself.[1,74] Bristle hardness does not significantly affect wear on enamel surfaces.[87]

Overzealous brushing can lead to gingival recession; bacteremia, especially in patients with pronounced gingivitis; wedge-shaped defects in the cervical area of root surfaces[35,88]; and painful ulceration of the gingiva.[83] This type of brushing should be identified and discouraged.

To maintain cleaning effectiveness, toothbrushes must be replaced as soon as the bristles begin to fray. Wear patterns differ widely among individuals, but with conscientious, regular use, most brushes wear out in about 3 months. If all the bristles are flattened after 1 week, brushing is probably too vigorous; if the bristles are still straight after 6 months, either the brushing is done very gently or the brush has not been used every day. Unfortunately, there is a tendency to use a brush as long as possible, often long after the bristles have lost their cleaning effectiveness. Brushes with wear reminders (e.g., a blue dye on some of the bristles) are currently available. The dye fades with use and can be helpful in reminding patients to replace their toothbrushes.

The preference of handle characteristics is a matter of individual taste. The handle should fit comfortably in the palm of the hand; it may be straight or angled, but straight handles are more common (see Fig. 42–1). Brushes with modest angulation between the head and the handle are available, and their manufacturers claim these brushes improve access to the lingual surfaces of premolars and molars. The clinical significance of this has not been determined.

For most patients, short-headed brushes with straight-cut, round-ended, soft to medium nylon bristles arranged in three or four rows of tufts are recommended. However, if a patient perceives any benefit from a particular brush design characteristic, use of that brush should be encouraged.

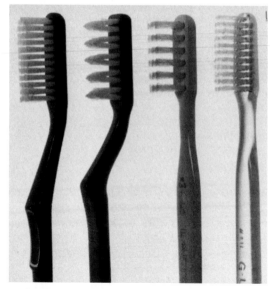

FIGURE 42–1. Types of manual toothbrushes. The two brushes on the left have contra-angle shanks.

POWERED TOOTHBRUSHES

In 1939, electrically powered toothbrushes were invented to make plaque control easier. There are many types of powered toothbrushes, some with reciprocal or back-and-forth motions, some with a combination of both, some with a circular motion, and some with an elliptical motion. Powered brushes with reciprocating bristle tufts are also available (Fig. 42–2). Powered tooth cleaners for home use, resembling a dental prophylaxis handpiece with a rotary rubber cup, are also available, as are powered brushes with shaped tips designed for interproximal cleaning (Fig. 42–3). Regardless of the type of device, best results are obtained when the patient is instructed in its proper use, because the moving bristles have to be placed correctly around the mouth.[6] Patients who can develop the ability to use a toothbrush properly usually do equally well with a manual or a powered brush. Less diligent brushers do better with powered toothbrushes, which generate stroke motions automatically and require less operator effort.[39] Powered brushes are recommended for (1) individuals lacking fine motor skills, (2) small children or handicapped or hospitalized patients who need to have their teeth cleaned by someone else, (3) patients with orthodontic appliances, and (4) patients who prefer them.

Powered toothbrushes are not superior to manual ones.

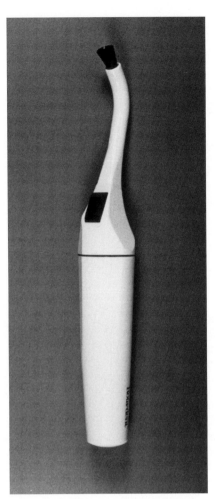

FIGURE 42–3. Powered toothbrush with shaped tips.

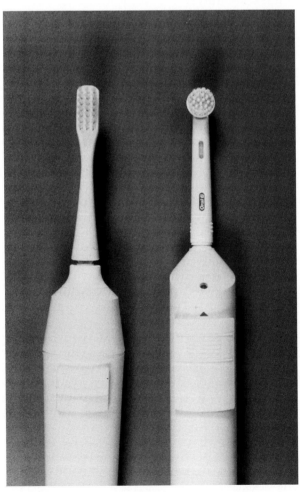

FIGURE 42–2. Types of powered brushes.

Although some researchers report that electrically powered toothbrushes are superior to manual toothbrushes in terms of removing plaque, reducing calculus accumulation, and improving gingival health,[68,73,86] others have shown that manual and powered brushes are equally effective.[9,39,76] Generally, if a powered toothbrush can be helpful to a particular patient, it should be recommended and encouraged.

One interesting new powered brush has double round heads and is designed to brush the buccal and lingual surfaces simultaneously. These have been shown to clean comparably to manual toothbrushes and more conventional powered toothbrushes.[59]

Conclusion. *No specific toothbrush can be singled out as clearly superior for the routine removal of microbial deposits from the teeth.* Brush requirements differ greatly among individuals, and types should be recommended after considering factors such as the morphology of the dentition, periodontal health, and manual dexterity. Because of the wide acceptance of oral hygiene principles first reported by Bass,[11,13] the one brush most commonly recommended by dentists appears to be the four-row, multitufted, soft nylon, hand-held brush. This brush will be adequate in most cases but will not fit the needs of every patient in every practice.

Powered toothbrushes can be valuable replacements for manual brushes if used regularly and properly. They are particularly useful for people with limited dexterity, children who like them, and caregivers of ill patients. Some adult patients simply prefer powered brushes and are more compliant with oral hygiene procedures when using them.

DENTIFRICES

Dentifrices are aids for cleaning and polishing tooth surfaces. They are used mostly in the form of pastes, although tooth powders and gels are also available. Dentifrices are made up of abrasives such as silicon oxides, aluminum oxides, and granular polyvinyl chlorides; water; humectants; soap or detergent; flavoring and sweetening agents; therapeutic agents such as fluorides; and colors and preservatives.[48]

Dentifrices should be sufficiently abrasive for satisfactory cleansing and polishing but should provide a margin of safety to protect the aggressive toothbrusher from wearing away tooth substance and soft restorative materials.[89] Abrasives, commonly in the form of insoluble inorganic salts, make up 20% to 40% of a dentifrice. The proper use of a dentifrice can enhance the abrasive action of a toothbrush as much as 40 times.[74] Tooth powders contain about 95% abrasives and are five times more abrasive than pastes. The abrasive quality of dentifrices affects enamel, but abrasion is more of a concern in patients with exposed roots, because dentin is abraded 25 times faster and cementum 35 times faster than enamel. This can lead to surface abrasion and root sensitivity.[97] Existing literature suggests that hard tissue damage from oral hygiene procedures is mainly due to abrasive dentifrices, whereas gingival lesions can be produced by a toothbrush alone.[83,87]

Abrasions are more prevalent on maxillary than on mandibular teeth and are found more frequently on the left than on the right half of the dental arch.[30] This suggests that access and right- or left-handedness may also contribute to the abrasion. Dentifrices that provide the effectiveness required for plaque control with a minimum of abrasion are preferable.

There is considerable interest in improving dentifrices by using them as vehicles for chemotherapeutic agents to inhibit plaque, calculus, caries, or root hypersensitivity. The pronounced caries-preventive effect of fluorides incorporated in dentifrices has been proved beyond question.[96] To achieve this effect, free fluoride ions must be available in the paste, not bound to the ingredients in the abrasive system. Fluoride dentifrices have been voluntarily evaluated by the American Dental Association (ADA) Council on Dental Therapeutics, and several pastes have been found to have fluoride available in the correct amount (1100 ppm), along with clinical studies documenting their caries reduction effects. These carry the ADA seal of approval for caries control and can be relied on to provide caries protection.

Substances such as chlorhexidine,[29] penicillin, dibasic ammonium phosphate, vaccines, vitamins, chlorophyll, formaldehyde, and strontium chloride have proved to be of little therapeutic value. Tartar control toothpastes with the active ingredient *pyrophosphate* are currently available. This ingredient interferes with crystal formation in calculus and does not affect the fluoride ion in the paste or increase tooth sensitivity. The formation of supragingival calculus has been reduced 29% to 45% by this type of dentifrice.[78] *These pastes are beneficial only for supragingival calculus. They do not affect subgingival calculus formation or gingival inflammation.*

TOOTHBRUSHING METHODS

Many methods of toothbrushing have been described,[13,23,33,52,95,103] but controlled studies evaluating the effectiveness of the most common brushing techniques have shown that no one method is clearly superior. The scrub technique is probably the most common method of brushing, whereas for patients with periodontal disease, the sulcular technique is the one most frequently recommended. The roll technique seems to be the least effective method, perhaps because it generates only intermittent pressure against the teeth compared with the sustained force applied with the sulcular and scrub techniques.[17]

Three methods of toothbrushing are presented in this discussion; any of them, if properly performed, can accomplish excellent plaque control. For each patient, the feasibility of each technique should be considered to recommend a plaque control program that is tailored to the individual.

The Bass Method[13]

Technique. Place the head of a soft brush parallel with the occlusal plane, with the brush head covering three teeth, beginning at the most distal tooth in the arch (Fig. 42–4). Place the bristles at the gingival margin, establishing an angle of 45 degrees to the long axis of the teeth. Exert gentle vibratory pressure, using short back-and-forth motions without dislodging the tips of the bristles. This forces the bristle ends into the gingival sulci (Fig. 42–5) as well as into the interproximal embrasures and should produce perceptible blanching of the gingiva (Fig. 42–6). Complete 20 strokes in the same position. This cleans the tooth surfaces, concentrating on the apical third of the clinical crowns, as well as the adjacent gingival sulci and onto the proximal surfaces as far as the bristles reach. Lift the brush, move it anteriorly, and repeat the process for the next three teeth.

Continue around the arch, buccal and lingual, brushing three teeth at a time. Then move to the mandibular arch

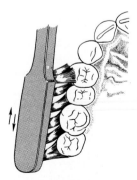

FIGURE 42–4. Bass method. Toothbrush position on facial and facioproximal surfaces of maxillary molars.

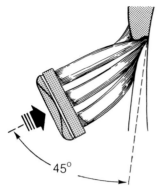

FIGURE 42–5. Bass method. Intrasulcus position of the brush at a 45-degree angle to the long axis of the tooth.

and brush in the same manner until the entire dentition is completed (Figs. 42–7 and 42–8). To help reach the lingual surfaces of the anterior teeth, if the brush seems too large, insert the brush vertically (Figs. 42–9 and 42–10). Press the "heel" of the brush into the gingival sulci and proximal surfaces at a 45-degree angle to the long axis of the teeth. Activate the brush with 20 short vibratory strokes.

To reach the occlusal surfaces, press the bristles firmly into the pits and fissures (Fig. 42–11). Activate the brush with 20 short back-and-forth strokes, advancing section by section until all posterior teeth in all four quadrants are cleaned.

To reach the distal surface of the last tooth in the arch, open the mouth wide and vibrate the tip of the brush against that surface, 20 times for each tooth.

Common Errors. The following errors in the use of the brush often result in unsatisfactory cleaning or soft tissue injury:

1. When the arm holding the brush becomes tired, there is a tendency to relax and let the brush slide down, creating an angle between the occlusal plane and the long axis of the brush. This prevents the main bulk of the bristles from adequately penetrating interproximally and into the gingival sulci. The error is corrected by raising the elbow as far as necessary.
2. The bristles are placed on the attached gingiva rather than into the gingival sulci. When the brush is activated, the gingival margin and the tooth surfaces are neglected, whereas the attached gingiva and the alveolar mucosa may be trau-

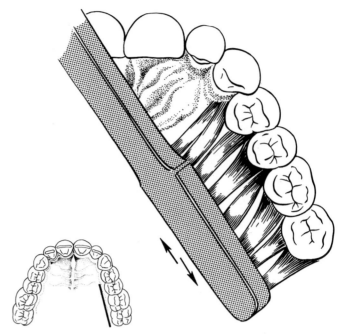

FIGURE 42–7. Bass method. Palatal position on molars and premolars.

matized (Fig. 42–12). The error is corrected by careful positioning of the brush.

3. The bristles are pressed sideways against the teeth rather than directed into the gingival sulci. Activating the brush cleans facial surfaces but misses interproximal surfaces and surfaces along the gingival margin. The error is corrected by proper placement of the brush.
4. The brush is "scrubbed" across the teeth in long horizontal strokes instead of short back-and-forth movements. Correction requires reinforcement of the short vibratory movements of the bristle tips. This can lead to toothbrush trauma recession of the gingiva, and notching of the root surfaces (see Fig 42–12).

Sequence of Positions. The Bass technique requires approximately 40 different toothbrush positions to cover a full dentition. Therefore, the mouth of each patient should be divided into sections and a systematic cleaning sequence individually prescribed (Fig. 42–13).

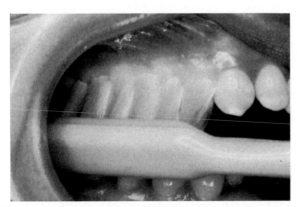

FIGURE 42–6. Bass method. Correct application of the brush should produce perceptible blanching of the gingiva.

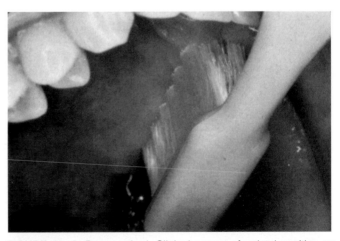

FIGURE 42–8. Bass method. Clinical aspect of palatal position on molars and premolars.

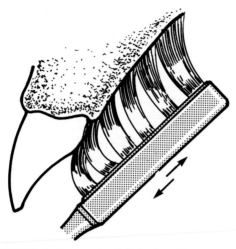

FIGURE 42–9. Bass method. Palatal position on incisors.

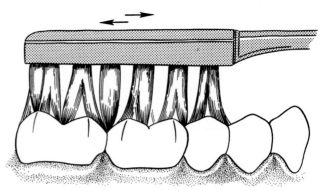

FIGURE 42–11. Brush position on occlusal surfaces used with the Bass, Stillman, or Charters method.

Advantages. The Bass method has the following distinct advantages over other techniques:

1. The short back-and-forth motion is easy to master because it requires the same simple movement familiar to most patients who are accustomed to the commonly used scrub technique.
2. It concentrates the cleaning action on the cervical and interproximal portions of the teeth, where microbial plaque is most detrimental to the gingiva.

The Bass technique can be recommended for the routine patient with or without periodontal involvement.

The Modified Stillman Method[52,95]

A soft or medium, multitufted brush can be used with the modified Stillman method. The brush should be placed with the bristle ends resting partly on the cervical portion of the teeth and partly on the adjacent gingiva, pointing in an apical direction at an oblique angle to the long axis of the teeth (Fig. 42–14). Pressure is applied laterally against the gingival margin to produce a perceptible blanching. The brush is activated with 20 short back-and-forth strokes and is simultaneously moved in a coronal direction along the attached gingiva, the gingival margin, and the tooth surface.

This process is repeated on all tooth surfaces, proceeding systematically around the mouth. To reach the lingual surfaces of the maxillary and mandibular incisors, the handle of the brush is held in a vertical position, engaging the heel of the brush. With this technique, the sides rather than the ends of the bristles are used, and penetration of the bristles into the gingival sulci is avoided.

The occlusal surfaces of molars and premolars are cleaned with the bristles perpendicular to the occlusal plane and penetrating into the grooves and interproximal embrasures (see Fig. 42–11).

The modified Stillman method may be recommended for cleaning in areas with progressing gingival recession and root exposure to prevent abrasive tissue destruction.

The Charters Method[23]

A soft or medium, multitufted brush is placed on the tooth with the bristles pointed toward the crown at a 45-degree angle to the long axis of the teeth (Fig. 42–15). The sides of the bristles are flexed against the gingiva, and the back-and-forth vibratory motion is used to massage the gingiva. The bristle tips should not move across the gingiva. To clean the occlusal surfaces, the bristle tips are placed in the pits and fissures, and the brush is activated with short

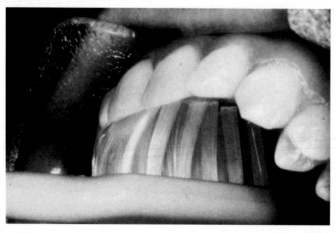

FIGURE 42–10. Bass method. Clinical aspect of palatal position on incisors.

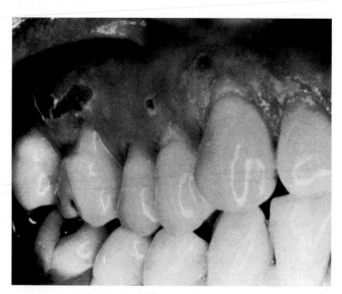

FIGURE 42–12. Toothbrush trauma.

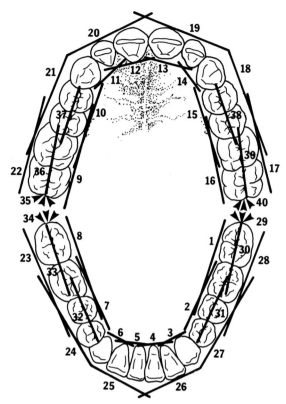

FIGURE 42–13. Bass method. Recommended sequence of brush positions.

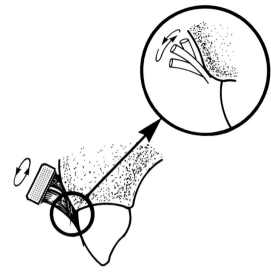

FIGURE 42–15. Charters method. The bristles are pressed sideward against the teeth and gingiva. The brush is activated with short circular or back-and-forth strokes.

such as the distal surfaces of the third molars, furcations, or gingival clefts. The methods described for manual brushing are also suitable for application with powered toothbrushes (Fig. 42–16).

back-and-forth strokes (see Fig. 42–11). The procedures are repeated systematically until all chewing surfaces are cleaned.

The Charters method is especially suitable for gentle plaque removal and gingival massage. When using a soft brush, this technique can be recommended for temporary cleaning in areas of healing wounds after periodontal surgery.

Methods of Cleaning With Powered Brushes

The various mechanical motions built into powered toothbrushes do not require special techniques of application. However, patients must be reminded to place the brush head next to the teeth at the gingival margin and to proceed systematically around the dentition. Additional hand movements can also be used to clean difficult areas,

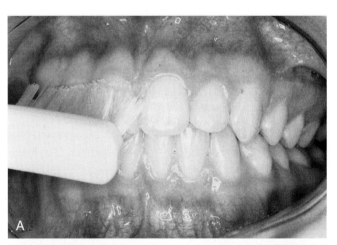

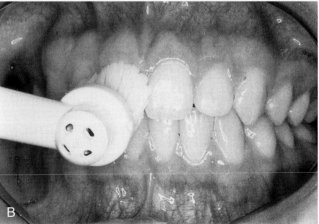

FIGURE 42–16. Powered toothbrushing using the Bass method. *A,* With a conventional toothbrush head (Waterpik). *B,* With a reciprocating round head (Braun).

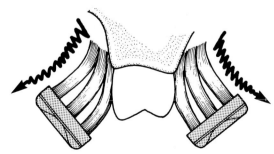

FIGURE 42–14. Modified Stillman method. The sides of the bristles are pressed against the teeth and gingiva while moving the brush with short back-and-forth strokes in a coronal direction.

INTERDENTAL CLEANING AIDS

It has been shown that a toothbrush, regardless of the brushing method used, does not completely remove interdental plaque, either in individuals with healthy periodontal conditions or in periodontally involved patients with open embrasures.[38,42,90] Because the majority of dental and periodontal disease appears to originate in interproximal areas, interdental plaque removal is crucial to augment the effects of tooth brushing.

The purpose of interdental cleaning is to remove plaque, not to dislodge fibrous threads of food wedged between two teeth. Although interdental cleaning will dislodge food fragments, chronic food impaction should be treated by correcting proximal tooth contacts and plunger cusps.

To achieve optimal plaque control, toothbrushing should be supplemented with a more effective method of interdental cleaning. The specific aids required for this procedure depend on various criteria such as the size of the interdental spaces, the presence of open furcations, tooth alignment, and the presence of orthodontic appliances or fixed prostheses.

Among the numerous aids available, dental floss and interdental cleaners such as wooden or plastic tips and interdental brushes are the most commonly recommended.

Dental Floss

Dental flossing is the most widely recommended method of removing plaque from proximal tooth surfaces.[37] Floss is available as a multifilament nylon yarn that is either twisted or nontwisted, bonded or nonbonded, waxed or unwaxed, and thick or thin. There are also monofilament flosses made of a Teflon-type material that are preferred by some individuals because they do not fray. A variety of individual factors, such as the tightness of tooth contacts, the roughness of proximal surfaces, and the patient's manual dexterity, not the superiority of any one product, determine the choice of dental floss. Clinical research so far has not been able to show any significant differences in the ability of the various types of floss to remove dental plaque.[32,49,56,57,88] In the past, waxed dental floss was thought to leave a waxy film on proximal surfaces, thus contributing to plaque accumulation and gingivitis. It has been shown, however, that wax is not deposited on tooth surfaces[84] and that improvement in gingival health is unrelated to the type of floss used.[32] Therefore, recommendations about type of floss should be based on ease of use and personal preference.

There are several ways of using dental floss. The floss must contact the proximal surface from line angle to line angle to clean effectively. Start with a piece of floss long enough to grasp securely; 12 to 18 inches is usually sufficient. It may be wrapped around the fingers, or the ends may be tied together in a loop. Stretch the floss tightly between the thumb and forefinger (Fig. 42–17), or between both forefingers, and pass it gently through each contact area with a firm back-and-forth motion. Do not snap the floss past the contact area, because this may injure the interdental gingiva. In fact, proximal grooves are created by zealous snapping of floss through contact areas. Once the

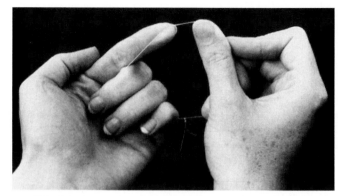

FIGURE 42–17. Dental flossing using the loop technique.

floss is under the contact area between the teeth, wrap the floss around the proximal surface of one tooth, and slip it under the marginal gingiva. Move the floss firmly along the tooth up to the contact area and gently down into the sulcus again, repeating this up-and-down stroke more than once (Fig. 42–18). Then move the floss across the interdental gingiva and repeat the procedure on the proximal surface of the adjacent tooth. Continue through the whole dentition, including the distal surface of the last tooth in each quadrant. When the working portion of the floss becomes soiled or begins to shred, move to a fresh portion of floss.

Flossing can be made easier by using a floss holder (Fig. 42–19). Although use of such devices is considerably more time consuming than finger flossing, they are helpful for patients lacking manual dexterity and for nursing personnel assisting handicapped and hospitalized patients in cleaning their teeth. A floss holder should feature (1) one or two forks that are rigid enough to keep the floss taut even when it is moved past tight contact areas and (2) an effective and simple mounting mechanism that holds the floss firmly in place yet allows quick rethreading of the floss whenever its working portion becomes soiled or begins to shred.

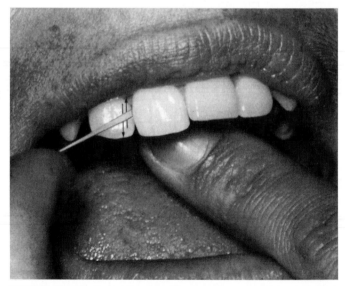

FIGURE 42–18. Dental flossing. The floss is wrapped around each proximal surface and is activated with repeated up-and-down strokes.

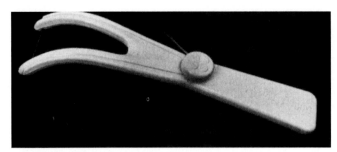

FIGURE 42-19. Floss holder. This device can simplify the manipulation of dental floss.

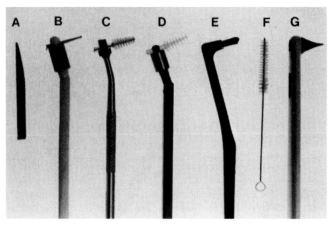

FIGURE 42-21. Interdental cleansers. Wooden tips: *A,* Stim-U-Dent; and *B,* Perio-Aid. Interdental brushes: *C,* Cone-shaped bristle brush; *D,* cone-shaped plastic brush; *E,* unitufted brush; and *F,* miniature bottle brush. *G,* Rubber tip.

Disposable, single-use floss holders with floss already threaded are available and may be useful for some patients. Short-term clinical evidence suggests that plaque reduction and improvement in gingivitis scores are similar for individuals instructed in the use of disposable flossers when compared with scores for those instructed in finger flossing.[93]

The establishment of lifelong habits of flossing the teeth is difficult to achieve. There is no information available about the establishment of long-term flossing habits comparing the various tools and finger flossing. However, the tools may help some individuals begin flossing or make flossing possible if they have limited dexterity.

Interdental Cleaning Devices

For cleaning in narrow gingival embrasures that are occupied by intact papillae and bordered by tight contact zones, dental floss is probably the most effective dental hygiene aid. Proper manipulation of the floss requires good dexterity, intensive instruction, and repeated reinforcement, so it is not suitable in every case. Concave root surfaces and furcations cannot be reached with dental floss (Fig. 42–20A). Therefore, special cleaning aids that are easy to handle and that adapt better than floss to irregular tooth surfaces and to long, exposed root surfaces (Fig. 42–20B) are recommended for proximal cleaning of teeth with large or open interdental spaces. This type of gingival

architecture is common in periodontally involved dentitions.

A wide variety of interdental cleaning devices are available for removing soft debris from tooth surfaces that are not accessible to a full-size toothbrush (Fig. 42–21). Clinical research has shown that they are effective on lingual and facial tooth surfaces, as well as on proximal surfaces.[90,99] The most common types are tapered wooden toothpicks that are round or triangular in cross section, small conical or cylindric brushes, and single tufted brushes. Many interdental devices can be attached to a handle for convenient manipulation around the teeth.

Interdental Brushes. Interdental brushes are cone-shaped brushes made of bristles mounted on a handle (see Fig. 42–21C,D), single-tufted brushes (see Fig. 42–21E),

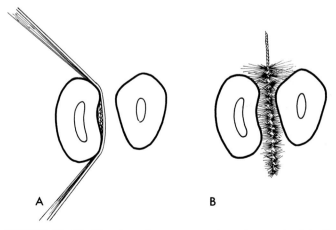

FIGURE 42-20. Cleaning of concave or irregular proximal tooth surfaces. Dental floss *(A)* is less effective than an interdental brush *(B).*

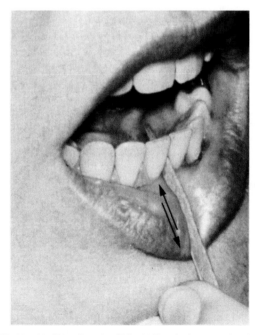

FIGURE 42-22. Wooden tip (Stim-U-Dent). Interproximal cleaning and massage with the tip inserted between the teeth and resting on the gingival papilla.

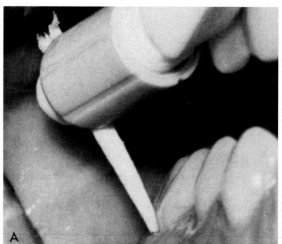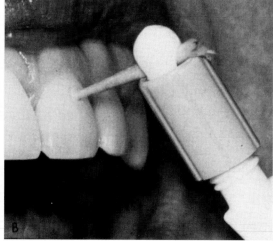

FIGURE 42–23. Wooden tip (Perio-Aid). *A,* Side of tip is used to clean along gingival margins and subgingivally. *B,* Frayed end of tip cleans large surface areas.

or small conical brushes (see Fig. 42–21*F*). Interdental brushes are particularly suitable for cleaning large, irregular, or concave tooth surfaces adjacent to wide interdental spaces. They are inserted interproximally and are activated with short back-and-forth strokes in between the teeth. For best cleaning efficiency, the diameter of the brush should be slightly larger than the gingival embrasures so that the bristles can exert pressure on the tooth surfaces, working their way into concavities on the roots. Single-tufted brushes are highly effective on the lingual surface of mandibular molars and premolars, where a regular toothbrush is often impeded by the tongue, and for isolated areas of deep recession.

Wooden Tips. Wooden tips are used either with or without a handle. Soft triangular wooden toothpicks such as a Stim-U-Dent (see Fig. 42–21*A*) are placed in the interdental space in such a way that the base of the triangle rests on the gingiva and the sides are in contact with the proximal tooth surfaces (Fig. 42–22). The Stim-U-Dent is then repeatedly moved in and out of the embrasure, removing soft deposits from the teeth and mechanically stimulating

the papillary gingiva. Its usefulness is limited to the facial surfaces in the anterior region of the mouth.

Wooden toothpicks can be attached to a handle such as the Perio-Aid (see Fig. 42–21*B*) and used on the facial or lingual surfaces throughout the mouth. Deposits are removed by using either the sides (Fig. 42–23*A*) or the tip of the toothpick (Fig. 42–23*B*). This device is particularly efficient for cleaning along the gingival margin[90] and into periodontal pockets.

Conclusion. There is a large and changing variety of interdental cleaning aids available for patients. Experience will help the clinician determine which is appropriate for any particular situation. In general, the largest brush or device that fits into a space will clean most efficiently. Figure 42–24 shows three types of embrasures and the kind of interdental cleaner most frequently recommended. However, some devices are more difficult to assemble and use than others, so a favorite tool of one individual may be impossible for another to use. It is useful to have a variety of aids available so the clinician and the patient can decide what fits best and is most convenient to use.

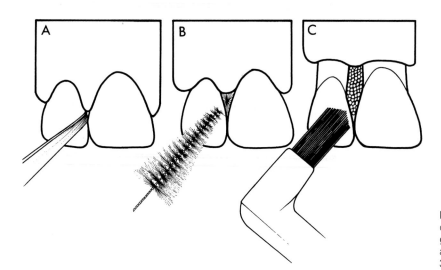

FIGURE 42–24. Interproximal embrasure types and corresponding interdental cleansers. *A,* Type 1—no gingival recession: dental floss. *B,* Type 2—moderate papillary recession: interdental brush. *C,* Type 3—complete loss of papillae: unitufted brush.

GINGIVAL MASSAGE

Massaging the gingiva with a toothbrush or interdental cleaning devices produces epithelial thickening, increased keratinization, and increased mitotic activity in the epithelium and connective tissue.[20,22,41,94] *It is questionable whether epithelial thickening, increased keratinization, and improved blood circulation provide substantial protection against microorganisms and other local irritants and are therefore beneficial or necessary for gingival health.*[40] Because keratinization occurs in the oral gingiva and not in the sulcular gingiva, which is more vulnerable to microbial attack, it appears that the improved gingival health associated with interdental stimulation results more from plaque removal than from gingival massage. In addition, studies with chemotherapeutic mouthrinses such as chlorhexidine have shown that gingival health can be maintained in the absence of mechanical oral hygiene procedures.[71] These data underscore the importance of altering or removing plaque rather than thickening the keratinized surface.

Toothbrushing methods designed to massage the gingiva and devices such as the rubber tip stimulator (see Fig. 42–21G) result in plaque removal in addition to massage. The plaque removal effect is likely far more important to periodontal health.

ORAL IRRIGATION DEVICES

Oral irrigators for daily home use by patients work by directing a high-pressure, steady or pulsating stream of water through a nozzle to the tooth surfaces. The pressure is generated by a built-in pump or a water faucet to which the device is attached (Fig. 42–25). Oral irrigators clean nonadherent bacteria and debris from the oral cavity more effectively than do toothbrushes and mouthrinses. They are particularly helpful for removing nonstructured debris from inaccessible areas around orthodontic appliances and fixed prostheses. When used as adjuncts to toothbrushing, these devices can have a beneficial effect on periodontal health by retarding the accumulation of plaque and calculus[54,69,85] and by reducing gingival inflammation and pocket depth.[21,85]

Oral irrigation has been shown to disrupt and detoxify subgingival plaque and can be useful in delivering antimicrobial agents into periodontal pockets.[79] Irrigation can be used supragingivally and subgingivally. Used supragingivally with dilute antiseptic chlorhexidine, daily use for 6 months resulted in significant reductions in bleeding and gingivitis compared with controls. Irrigation with water alone also reduced gingivitis, but not as much.[34] The common, home-use irrigator tip is a plastic nozzle with a 90-degree bend at the tip, attached to a pump providing pulsating beads of water at speeds regulated by a dial. Patients should be instructed to aim the pulsating jet across the proximal papilla, hold it there for 10 to 15 seconds, then trace along the gingival margin to the next proximal space and repeat the procedure. It can be used both buccally and lingually. This cleaning must be done while leaning across the bathroom sink, because water will drip down the pa-

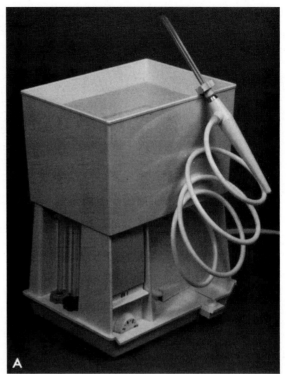

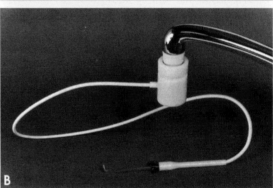

FIGURE 42–25. Oral irrigation devices. *A*, Built-in pump and reservoir. *B*, Faucet attachment.

tient's arm. Patients with gingival inflammation usually start at lower pressure and then can increase the pressure comfortably to medium as tissue health improves. Some individuals like to use the device on the highest pressure setting, with no reported harm. Patient comfort should be the guide for pressure setting.

Subgingival irrigation performed both in the dental office and by the patient at home, particularly with antimicrobial agents, has been shown to provide some site-specific therapy. Irrigation done in the dental office, also called *lavage* or *flushing* of the periodontal pocket, after scaling and root planing may be helpful in reducing bleeding and pocket depths, but data are not consistent.[45,91]

Subgingival irrigation, with antiseptic chlorhexidine diluted to one-third strength, performed regularly at home after scaling, root planing, and in-office irrigation therapy has produced significant gingival improvement compared with controls.[55] These improvements in gingival health, along with other results,[45,91] suggest that patients can and should use subgingival irrigation at least in difficult sites such as

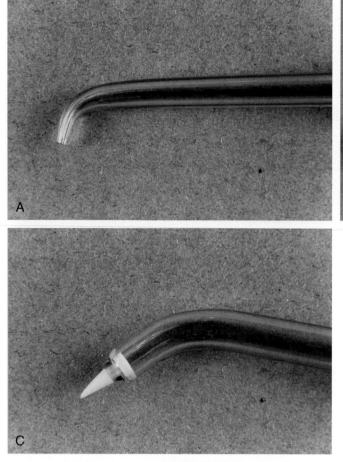

FIGURE 42–26. Irrigator tips. *A,* Conventional. *B,* Soft rubber. *C,* Cannula.

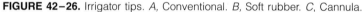

furcations and residual pockets. Currently available sub-gingival irrigation tips (Fig. 42–26) have been shown to disrupt plaque about half the depth of pockets up to 7 mm, much farther than a toothbrush or floss can reach.[28]

Currently there are two types of irrigator tips useful for subgingival irrigation (see Fig. 42–26*B,C*). One is the cannula type tip recommended for office use, and the other is a soft rubber tip for patient use at home. Both reduce the pressure and flow of the pulsating jet of water. Effective penetration of irrigant of up to 70% has been shown when using the cannula tip for deeper pockets.[53] Similar results have been reported for the soft rubber tip.[19] The soft rubber tip, designed to irrigate at low pressure and reduced flow, is recommended for patient use at home.[24]

One cautionary note must be considered. Transient bacteremia has been reported[31] after water irrigation in patients with periodontitis and in patients on periodontal maintenance.[100] However, bacteremia has also been found after toothbrushing[81] and scaling alone.[100] According to the Council on Dental Therapeutics of the ADA, bacteremia can occur in the absence of dental procedures.[25] Therefore, dentists should make every attempt to reduce gingival inflammation in susceptible patients by the use of toothbrushes, floss, and mouthwashes. Subgingival irrigation at home may not be the oral hygiene procedure of choice for patients requiring antibiotic prophylaxis prior to dental treatment, particularly if inflammation is present.

CHEMICAL PLAQUE CONTROL

Mechanical plaque removal remains the primary method used to prevent dental diseases and maintain oral health. However, an improved understanding of the infectious nature of dental diseases has dramatically revitalized interest in chemical methods of plaque control.

The ADA Council on Dental Therapeutics has adopted a program for acceptance of plaque control agents. The agents must be evaluated in placebo-controlled clinical trials of 6 months or longer and demonstrate significantly improved gingival health compared with controls. To date, two agents have been accepted by the ADA for treatment of gingivitis: two prescription solutions of chlorhexidine mouthwash (Peridex and PerioGard) and a nonprescription essential oil mouthwash (Listerine).

Chlorhexidine. The agent that has shown the most positive results to date is chlorhexidine, a diguanidohexane with pronounced antiseptic properties. The initial finding that two daily rinses with 10 ml of a 0.2% aqueous solution of chlorhexidine gluconate almost completely inhibited the development of dental plaque, calculus, and gingivitis in the human model for experimental gingivitis[71] has been confirmed by a number of other clinical investigations. Clinical studies of several months' duration have reported plaque reductions of 45% to 61% and, more importantly, gingivitis reductions of 27% to 67%.[46,63] The 0.12% chlorhexidine preparation available in the United States is the most effective agent currently available in America for reducing plaque and gingivitis.[61]

There are local, reversible side effects to chlorhexidine use, primarily brown staining of teeth, tongue, and silicate and resin restorations[61] and transient impairment of taste perception.[70] Chlorhexidine has very low systemic toxic activity in humans, has not produced any appreciable resistance of oral microorganisms, and has not been associated with any teratogenic alterations.[61]

Essential Oil Mouthwash. Essential oil or phenol mouthwashes have been evaluated in three long-term clinical studies. Plaque reductions of 20% to 35% and gingivitis reductions of 25% to 35% have been reported.[27,43,60] This type of mouthwash has a long history of use and safety dating back to the 19th century.

Other Products. Several other products on the market have shown some evidence of plaque reduction, although long-term improvement in gingival health has not been substantiated; these are stannous fluoride,[66,103] cetylpyridinium chloride (quaternary ammonia compounds),[7,8] and sanguinarine.[75,82] Evidence suggests that these and other mouthwash products do not possess the antimicrobial potential of either chlorhexidine products or essential oil preparations. However, they can be useful for patients who perceive benefits from the preparations.

One type of agent has been marketed as a prebrushing mouthrinse to improve the effectiveness of brushing. The active ingredient is sodium benzoate. Research to support its effectiveness is contradictory, but the preponderance of evidence suggests that using a prebrushing rinse is no more effective than brushing alone.[15,16]

Chemical plaque control has been shown to be effective for both plaque reduction and improved wound healing after periodontal surgery. Both chlorhexidine[4] and essential oil[104] mouthwashes have significant positive effects when prescribed for use after periodontal surgery for periods of 1 to 4 weeks.

Conclusion. Mechanical plaque control is necessary and not replaceable by chemical plaque control. Chlorhexidine rinses are very effective agents to augment plaque control for patients with recurrent problems, for ineffective plaque control for any reason, for some uncommon oral mucous membrane diseases, and for use after periodontal or oral surgery. Essential oil mouthwashes are effective to a lesser degree, but they have fewer side effects and are available without prescription. The use of other agents can be encouraged if patients perceive benefits from them, but active recommendation of their use should await confirmation by clinical research.

DISCLOSING AGENTS

Disclosing agents are solutions or wafers capable of staining bacterial deposits on the surfaces of teeth, tongue, and gingiva. They are excellent oral hygiene aids, because they can provide the patient with an educational and motivational tool to improve the efficiency of plaque control procedures[5] (Fig. 42–27).

Solutions and wafers are available commercially. Solutions are applied to the teeth as concentrates on cotton swabs or diluted in mouthwashes. They usually produce

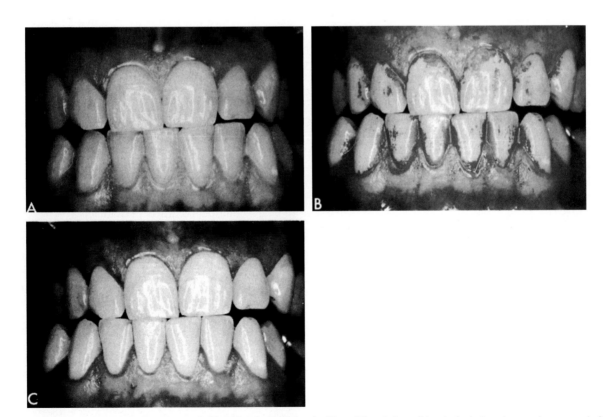

FIGURE 42–27. Effect of a disclosing agent. *A,* Unstained. *B,* Stained with a 6% solution of basic fuchsin; plaque shows as dark particulate patches. *C,* Restained with basic fuchsin after thorough tooth cleaning.

heavy staining of bacterial plaque, gingiva, tongue, lips, fingers, and sink. Wafers are crushed between the teeth and swished around the mouth for a few seconds and then spit out. Either should be used in the office for plaque control instruction and dispensed as needed for home use to aid periodontal patients.

FREQUENCY OF PLAQUE REMOVAL

In the controlled and supervised environment of clinical research, where well-trained individuals remove all visible plaque, gingival health can be maintained by one thorough cleaning exercise with brush, floss, and toothpicks every 24 to 48 hours.[62,71] Most patients, however, fall far short of this goal. The average cleaning lasts just 2 minutes every day and removes only 40% of plaque.[26] Several studies report improved periodontal health associated with increasing the frequency of brushing up to twice per day.[77,99] Cleaning three or more times per day does not appear to further improve periodontal conditions. Cleaning once a day with all necessary tools is sufficient if it is performed meticulously. If plaque control is not adequate, a second brushing will help.

Conclusion. Emphasis must be placed on the efficiency of complete plaque removal at least once per day, rather than the frequency of brushing alone. However, poor performance of plaque removal can be improved by brushing twice per day.

RECOMMENDATIONS FOR PLAQUE CONTROL INSTRUCTION

In periodontal therapy, plaque control has two important purposes: to minimize gingival inflammation and to prevent the recurrence or progression of periodontal disease. Daily mechanical removal of plaque by the patient, including the use of appropriate antimicrobials, appears to be the only practical means for improving oral hygiene on a long-term basis. The process requires motivation on the part of the patient, education and instruction, followed by encouragement and reinforcement.

Motivation

Motivation for effective plaque control is one of the most critical and difficult elements of long-term success in periodontal therapy. To be successful, the patient is required to make the following efforts:

1. *Receptiveness:* required to understand the concepts of the pathogenesis, treatment, and prevention of periodontal disease.
2. *Change the habits of a lifetime:* required to adopt a successful, self-administered daily plaque control regimen.
3. *Behavioral changes:* required to adjust the hierarchy of one's beliefs, practices, and values to accommodate the required new oral hygiene habits and return for regular periodontal maintenance visits.

The patient must understand what periodontal disease is, what its effects are, that he or she is susceptible to it, and what his or her responsibility is in achieving and maintain-

ing oral health. Manual skills must be developed and used to establish a plaque control regimen. In addition, the benefits of a clean mouth must be understood. If not, long-term failure of any individual plaque control program is inevitable and leads to frustration for both the dentist and the patient. Changes in the habits of individuals' entire lives are difficult to achieve. However, improvements in plaque control are necessary for successful periodontal therapy.

Education

Many patients believe that visits to the dental office for periodontal care will eliminate the disease process. It is incumbent on the dentist to inform and reinforce patient responsibility for long-term success of therapy and cure. *Patient-administered plaque control currently is the most important preventive and therapeutic procedure in periodontal therapy.* Our health-conscious society is an advantage with regard to patient education. Most patients know what gingivitis is because they have heard about it on television or read about in magazines. They are willing to spend time and money to try new products such as toothbrushes and mouthwashes. Each patient education experience must be individualized according to need and level of understanding.

Patients must be informed that periodic assessment and debridement of the teeth in the dental office are helpful preventive measures against periodontal disease, but only if these are combined with individualized oral hygiene procedures practiced daily at home. Therefore, time spent in the dental office teaching the patient how to perform plaque control procedures is as valuable a service as cleaning the teeth. It must be explained that dental visits two or three times a year are not nearly as effective as daily home oral care. This information gives each patient responsibility for health care and control over the disease process. Only the combination of regular office visits with conscientious home care significantly reduces gingivitis and loss of supporting periodontal tissues over the long term.[67,98]

A periodontal patient should be shown that periodontal disease has manifested itself in his or her own mouth. Stained dental plaque, the bleeding of inflamed gingiva, and a periodontal probe inserted into a pocket are impressive and convincing demonstrations of the presence of pathogens and actual disease. It is also of educational value to a patient to have his or her oral cleanliness and periodontal condition recorded periodically.[10] The patient and the dentist can use this as feedback information about the level of performance and improvement. The Plaque Control Record and the Bleeding Points Index are simple indices and are commonly used for patient reinforcement.

Plaque Control Record.[80] Disclosing solution is applied to all supragingival tooth surfaces. After the patient has rinsed, each tooth surface (except occlusal surfaces) is examined for the presence or absence of stained deposits at the dentogingival junction, four surfaces for each tooth. Plaque, if present, is recorded by coloring the appropriate box in a diagram (Fig. 42–28). After all teeth have been scored, the index is calculated by dividing the number of surfaces with plaque by the total number of surfaces scored. Multiply by 100 to get a percentage of surfaces with plaque present. A reasonable goal for patients is 10%

Plaque Control Record

Previous Index _____ _____ Present Index

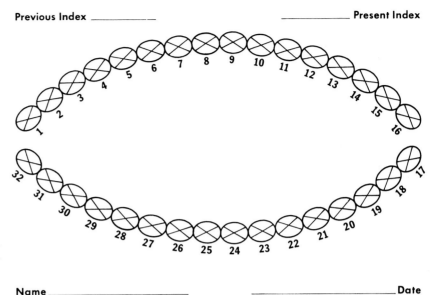

FIGURE 42–28. The plaque control record. An oral hygiene aid to patient motivation and instruction. This same chart can be used for the bleeding index. (From O'Leary TJ, Drake RB, Naylor JE. The plaque control record. J Periodontol *43*:38, 1972.)

Name _____ _____ Date

or fewer surfaces with plaque, unless plaque is always present in the same areas. If so, special instructions should be directed toward improving performance in that area. It is extremely difficult to achieve a perfect score of 0, so patients should be rewarded for approaching it.

Bleeding Points Index.[64] The Bleeding Points Index provides an evaluation of bleeding gingiva around each tooth in the patient's mouth. Retract the cheek, and place the periodontal probe 1 mm into the sulcus or pocket at the distal aspect of the most posterior tooth in the quadrant. Carry the probe lightly across the length of the sulcus to the mesial interproximal area on the facial aspect. Continue along all the teeth in the quadrant from the facial aspect. Wait 30 seconds, and record the presence of bleeding on the distal, facial, and mesial surfaces on the chart. Repeat on the lingual-palatal aspect, recording bleeding only for the direct lingual surface, not for the mesial or distal surfaces. Repeat the steps for each quadrant.

The percentage of the number of bleeding surfaces is then calculated to provide the patient's score. Divide the number of surfaces that bled by the total number of tooth surfaces (4 per tooth) and convert the number to a percentage by multiplying by 100.

This index is designed to demonstrate bleeding gingiva, rather than the presence of plaque. Again, a goal of 10% or fewer bleeding points is good, but 0 is ideal. If a few bleeding points repeatedly occur in the same areas, reinstruction in plaque control for those areas is needed.

Instruction

With repeated instruction and encouragement, patients can reduce the incidence of plaque and gingivitis far more effectively than with self-acquired oral hygiene habits.[44,98] However, instruction in how to clean teeth must be more than a cursory chairside demonstration of the use of a toothbrush and oral hygiene aids. It is a painstaking procedure that requires patient participation, careful supervision

with correction of mistakes, and reinforcement during return visits until the patient demonstrates that he or she has developed the necessary proficiency.[3,65]

At the first instruction visit, the patient should be given a new toothbrush, an interdental cleaner, and a disclosing agent. First, the patient's plaque is identified. Unstained, small amounts of bacterial deposits are difficult for the patient to see (see Fig. 42–27A); heavier accumulations of plaque and debris may be visible as gray, yellow, or white material on the teeth, along the gingival margin, and in faciolingual embrasures. Loose debris should be rinsed off. Then a disclosing solution or wafer is used to stain the invisible plaque. After a brief water rinse to remove excess dye and stained saliva, which would obscure the picture, the stained plaque and pellicle can be clearly demonstrated to the patient (see Fig. 42–27B). Polished dental restorations do not take up the stain, but the oral mucosa and the lips may retain it for up to several hours. Covering the lips lightly with petroleum jelly before using the dye is helpful.

Toothbrushing should be demonstrated in the patient's mouth while he or she observes with a hand mirror. The patient then takes over and repeats the procedures on his or her own teeth with the instructor giving assistance, correction, and positive reinforcement.

Repeat the demonstration and instruction process with dental floss and interdental cleaning aids according to the patient's needs. The teeth can be restained to evaluate the efficiency of plaque removal, but even after vigorous cleaning, some stain usually remains on proximal surfaces (see Fig. 42–27C). Teaching videos and pamphlets can be used to augment personalized instruction, but they are not a substitute; reminder pamphlets may be useful for the patient to take home.

After the instruction session, the patient should be given the hygiene aids needed to get started. He or she must be encouraged to clean the teeth at least once a day, with thorough attention to all areas. Home care procedures on a full dentition take 5 to 10 minutes; in complex periodontal maintenance cases, such procedures may require up to 30 minutes. The patient should set aside a convenient time and place in his or her daily schedule to perform the procedures reliably every day.

Subsequent instruction visits should be used to reinforce or modify previous instructions, periodically recording the state of gingival health and amount of plaque. Reinforcement and encouragement should be given often to help patients modify long-standing habits, adopt new ones, and understand that their plaque control is also important to the clinician. *Patience and reinforcement are the secrets of success in plaque control instruction.*

REFERENCES

1. Abrasivity of current dentifrices: Report of the Council of Dental Therapeutics. J Am Dent Assoc *81:*117, 1970.
2. Accepted Dental Therapeutics. 3rd ed. Chicago, American Dental Association, 1969–1970, p 225.
3. Anderson JL. Integration of plaque control into the practice of dentistry. Dent Clin North Am *16:*621, 1972.
4. Anderson L, Sanz M, Newman MG, et al. Clinical effects of a 0.12% chlorhexidine mouthrinse on periodontal surgical wounds without periodontal dressing. Abstract 1728. J Dent Res *67:*329, 1988.
5. Arnim SS. The use of disclosing agents for measuring tooth cleanliness. J Periodontol *34:*227, 1963.
6. Ash MM. A review of the problems and results of studies on manual and power toothbrushes. J Periodontol *35:*202, 1964.
7. Ashley FP, Skinner A, Jackson P, et al. The effect of a 0.1% cetylpyridinium chloride mouthrinse on plaque and gingivitis in adult subjects. Br Dent J *157:*191, 1984.
8. Ashley FP, Skinner A, Jackson PY, Wilson RF. Effect of a 0.1% cetylpyridinium chloride mouthrinse on the accumulation and biochemical composition of dental plaque in young adults. Caries Res *18:*465, 1984.
9. Axelsson P, Lindhe J. The effect of a preventive programme on dental plaque, gingivitis and caries in school-children: Results after one and two years. J Clin Periodontol *1:*126, 1974.
10. Barrikman R, Penhall O. Graphing indexes reduce plaque. J Am Dent Assoc *87:*1904, 1973.
11. Bass CC. The optimum characteristics of toothbrushes for personal oral hygiene. Dent Items Int *70:*696, 1948.
12. Bass CC. Optimum characteristics of dental floss for personal oral hygiene. Dent Items Int *70:*921, 1948.
13. Bass CC. An effective method of personal oral hygiene. Part II. J La State Med Soc *106:*100, 1954.
14. Bay I, Kardel K, Skougaard MR. Quantitative evaluation of the plaque-removing ability of different types of toothbrushes. J Periodontol *38:*526, 1967.
15. Beiswander BB, Mallott MC, Mau MS, Katz BP. The relative plaque removal effect of a prebrushing mouthrinse. J Am Dent Assoc *120:*190, 1990.
16. Binney A, Addy M, Newcombe RG. The plaque removal effects of single rinsings and brushings. J Periodontol *64:*181, 1993.
17. Bjorn H, Lindhe J. On the mechanics of toothbrushing. Odont Revy *17:*9, 1966.
18. Brandtzaeg P. The significance of oral hygiene in the prevention of dental diseases. Odont T *72:*460, 1964.
19. Braun RE, Ciancio SG. Subgingival delivery by an oral irrigation device. J Periodontol *63:*469, 1992.
20. Cantor MT, Stahl SS. The effects of various interdental stimulators upon the keratinization of the interdental col. Periodontics *3:*243, 1965.
21. Cantor MT, Stahl SS. Interdental col tissue responses to the use of a water pressure device. J Periodontol *40:*292, 1969.
22. Castenfelt T. Toothbrushing and Massage in Periodontal Disease. An Experimental *Clinical Histologic Study.* Stockholm, Nordisk Rotegravyr, 1952, p 109.
23. Charters WJ. Eliminating mouth infections with the toothbrush and other stimulating instruments. Dent Digest *38:*130, 1932.
24. Ciancio SC. Clinical benefits of powered subgingival irrigation. Biol Ther Dentist *8:*13, 1992.
25. Council on Dental Therapeutics, American Dental Association. Preventing bacterial endocarditis: A statement for the dental professional. J Am Dent Assoc *122:*87, 1991.
26. De la Rosa MR, Guerra JZ, Johnston DA, Radike AW. Plaque growth and removal with daily toothbrushing. J Periodontol *50:*661, 1979.
27. De Paola LG, Overholser CD, Meiller TF, et al. Chemotherapeutic reduction of plaque and gingivitis development, a 6 month investigation. J Dent Res *65:*274, 1986.
28. Eakle WS, Ford C, Boyd RL. Depth of penetration in periodontal pockets with oral irrigation. J Clin Periodontol *13:*39, 1985.
29. Eriksen HM, Gjermo P, Johansen JR. Results from two years' use of chlorhexidine (CH)-containing dentifrices. Helv Odontol Acta *17:*52, 1973.
30. Ervin JC, Bucher ET. Prevalence of tooth root exposure and abrasion among dental patients. Dent Items Int *66:*7601, 1944.
31. Felix JA, Rosen S, App GR. Detection of bacteremia after the use of an oral irrigation device in subjects with periodontitis. J Periodontol *42:*785, 1971.
32. Finkelstein P, Grossman E. The effectiveness of dental floss in reducing gingival inflammation. J Dent Res *58:*1034, 1979.
33. Fones AC. Mouth Hygiene. 4th ed. Philadelphia, Lea & Febiger, 1934, p 300.
34. Flemmig TF, Newman MG, Doherty FM, et al. Supragingival irrigation with 0.06% chlorhexidine in naturally occurring gingivitis 1. Six month clinical observations. J Periodontol *61:*112–117, 1990.
35. Gillette WB, Van House RL. Ill effects of improper oral hygiene procedures. J Am Dent Assoc *101:*476, 1980.
36. Gilson CM, Charbeneau GT, Hill HC. A comparison of physical properties of several soft toothbrushes. J Mich Dent Assoc *51:*347, 1969.
37. Gjermo P, Flotra L. The plaque removing effect of dental floss and toothpicks: A group comparison study. J Periodont Res *4:*170, 1969.
38. Gjermo P, Flotra L. The effect of different methods of interdental cleaning. J Periodont Res *5:*230, 1970.
39. Glass RL. A clinical study of hand and electric toothbrushing. J Periodontol *36:*322, 1965.
40. Glickman I, Petralis R, Marks R. The effect of powered toothbrushing plus interdental stimulation upon the severity of gingivitis. J Periodontol *35:*519, 1964.
41. Glickman I, Petralis R, Marks R. The effect of powered toothbrushing and interdental stimulation upon microscopic inflammation and surface keratinization of the interdental gingiva. J Periodontol *36:*108, 1965.
42. Goldman HM. The effect of single and multiple toothbrushing in the normal and periodontally involved dentition. Oral Surg *9:*203, 1956.
43. Gordon JM, Lamster IV, Seiger MC. Efficacy of Listerine antiseptic in inhibiting the development of plaque and gingivitis. J Clin Periodontol *12:*697, 1985.
44. Gravelle HR, Shackelford NF, Lovett JT. The oral hygiene of high school students as affected by three different educational programs. J Public Health Dent *27:*91, 1967.
45. Greenstein G. Effects of subgingival irrigation on periodontal status. J Periodontol *58:*829, 1987.
46. Grossman E, Reiter G, Sturzenberger OP, et al. Six-month study of the effects of a chlorhexidine mouthrinse on gingivitis in adults. J Periodont Res (Suppl) *16:*33, 1986.
47. Harrington JH, Terry IA. Automatic and hand toothbrushing abrasion studies. J Am Dent Assoc *68:*343, 1964.
48. Harris NO. Dentifrices, mouth rinses, and oral irrigators. In Harris NO, Christen AG, eds. Primary Preventive Dentistry. 3rd ed. East Norwalk, CT, Appleton & Lange, 1991, p 141.
49. Hill HC, Levi PA, Glickman I. The effects of waxed and unwaxed dental floss on interdental plaque accumulation and interdental gingival health. J Periodontol *44:*411, 1973.
50. Hine MK. Toothbrush. Int Dent J *6:*15, 1956.
51. Hiniker JJ, Forscher BK. The effect of toothbrush type on gingival health. J Periodontol *25:*40, 1954.
52. Hirschfeld I. The toothbrush, its use and abuse. Dent Items Int *3:*833, 1931.
53. Hollander BN, Boyd RL, Eakle WS. Comparison of cannula versus standard tip for oral irrigation. J Clin Periodontol *5:*340, 1992.
54. Hoover DR, Robinson HBG, Billingsley A. The comparative effectiveness of the Water-Pik in a noninstructed population. J Periodontol *39:*43, 1968.
55. Jolkovsky DL, Waki MY, Newman MN, et al. Clinical and microbiological effects of subgingival and gingival marginal irrigation with chlorhexidine gluconate. J Periodontol *61:*663, 1990.
56. Keller SE, Manson-Hing LR. Clearance studies of proximal tooth surfaces. Part II. In vivo removal of interproximal plaque. Ala J Med Sci *6:*266, 1969.
57. Keller SE, Manson-Hing LR. Clearance studies of proximal tooth surfaces. Parts III and IV. In vivo removal of interproximal plaque. Ala J Med Sci *6:*399, 1969.
58. Khocht A, Simon G, Person P, Denepitiya JL. Gingival recession in relation to history of hard toothbrush use. J Periodontol *64:*900, 1993.
59. Khocht A, Spindel L, Person P. Comparative clinical study of three toothbrushes. J Periodontol *63:*603, 1992.
60. Lamster IB, Alfano MC, Seiger MC, Gordon JM. The effect of Listerine antiseptic on reduction of existing plaque and gingivitis. J Clin Prev Dent *5:*12, 1983.
61. Lang NP, Brecx MC. Chlorhexidine digluconate—an agent for chemical plaque control and prevention of gingival inflammation. J Periodont Res (Suppl) *21:*74, 1986.
62. Lang NP, Cumming BR, Löe H. Toothbrushing frequency as it relates to plaque development and gingival health. J Periodontol *44:*396, 1973.
63. Lang NP, Hotz P, Graf H, et al. Effects of supervised chlorhexidine mouthrinses in children. A longitudinal clinical trial. J Periodont Res *17:*101, 1982.
64. Lenox JA, Kopczyk RA. A clinical system for scoring a patient's oral hygiene performance. J Am Dent Assoc *86:*849, 1973.
65. Less W. Mechanics of teaching plaque control. Dent Clin North Am *16:*647, 1972.
66. Leverett DH, McHugh WD, Jensen DE. Effect of daily rinsing with stannous fluoride on plaque and gingivitis: Final report. J Dent Res *63:*1083, 1984.

67. Lindhe J, Nyman S. The effect of plaque control and surgical pocket elimination on the establishment and maintenance of periodontal health. A longitudinal study of periodontal therapy in cases of advanced disease. J Clin Periodontol 2:67, 1975.
68. Lobene RR. The effect of an automatic toothbrush on gingival health. J Periodontol 35:137, 1964.
69. Lobene RR. The effect of a pulsed water pressure cleaning device on oral health. J Periodontol 40:667, 1969.
70. Löe H. Does chlorhexidine have a place in the prophylaxis of dental disease? J Periodont Res 8(suppl 12):93, 1973.
71. Löe H, Schiott CR. The effect of mouthrinses and topical application of chlorhexidine on the development of dental plaque and gingivitis in man. J Periodont Res 5:79, 1970.
72. Löe H, Theilade E, Jensen SB. Experimental gingivitis in man. J Periodontol 36:177, 1965.
73. Manhold JH. Gingival tissue health with hand and power brushing: A retrospective with corroborative studies. J Periodontol 38:23, 1967.
74. Manly RS, Brudevold F. Relative abrasiveness of natural and synthetic toothbrush bristles on cementum and dentin. J Am Dent Assoc 55:779, 1957.
75. Mauriello SM, Bader JD. Six-month effects of a sanguinarine dentifrice on plaque and gingivitis. J Periodontol 59:238, 1988.
76. McKendrick AJW, Barbenel LMH, McHugh WD. A two year comparison of hand and electric toothbrushes. J Periodont Res 3:224, 1968.
77. McKendrick AJW, Barbenel LMH, McHugh WD. The influence of time of examination, eating, smoking, and frequency of brushing on the oral debris index. J Periodont Res 5:205, 1970.
78. Mintzer MA. A Symposium: The Formation and Control of Dental Calculus. Procter & Gamble, Cinncinatti, Ohio, 1986.
79. Mueller-Joseph LM, Davis C, Jones B. Oral irrigation and antimicrobial plaque control. In Woodall IR, ed. Comprehensive Dental Hygiene Care. 4th ed. St Louis, CV Mosby, 1993, p 616.
80. O'Leary TJ, Drake RB, Naylor JE. The plaque control record. J Periodontol 43:38, 1972.
81. O'Leary TJ, Shafer WG, Swenson HM, Nesler DC. Possible penetration of crevicular tissue from oral hygiene procedures. II. Use of the toothbrush. J Periodontol 41:163, 1970.
82. Parsons LG, Thomas LG, Southard GL, et al. Effect of sanguinaria extract on established plaque and gingivitis when supragingivally delivered as a manual rinse or under pressure in an oral irrigator. J Clin Periodontol 14:381, 1987.
83. Pattison GA. Self-inflicted gingival injuries: Literature review and case report. J Periodontol 54:299, 1983.
84. Perry DA, Pattison G. The investigation of wax residue on tooth surfaces after the use of waxed dental floss. Dent Hygiene 60:16, 1986.
85. Robinson HBG, Hoover PR. The comparative effectiveness of a pulsating oral irrigator as an adjunct in maintaining oral health. J Periodontol 42:37, 1971.
86. Sanders WE, Robinson HBG. The effect of toothbrushing on deposition of calculus. J Periodontol 33:386, 1962.
87. Sangnes G. Traumatization of teeth and gingiva related to habitual tooth cleaning procedures. J Clin Periodontol 3:94, 1976.
88. Sangnes G, Gjermo P. Prevalence of oral soft and hard tissue lesions related to mechanical tooth cleaning procedures. Commun Dent Oral Epidemiol 4:77, 1976.
89. Saxton CA. The effects of dentifrices on the appearance of the tooth surface observed with the scanning electron microscope. J Periodont Res 11:74, 1976.
90. Schmid MO, Balmelli O, Saxer UP. The plaque removing effect of a toothbrush, dental floss and a toothpick. J Clin Periodontol 3:157, 1976.
91. Shiloah J, Hovious LA. The role of subgingival irrigations in the treatment of periodontitis. J Periodontol 64:835, 1993.
92. Silverstone LM, Featherstone MJ. A scanning electron microscope study of the end rounding of bristles in eight toothbrush types. Quint Int 19:3, 1988.
93. Spolsky VA, Perry DA, Meng Z, Kissel P. Evaluating the efficacy of a new flossing aid. J Clin Periodontol 20:490, 1993.
94. Stahl SS, Wachtel N, DeCastro C, Pelletier G. The effect of toothbrushing on the keratinization of the gingiva. J Periodontol 24:20, 1953.
95. Stillman PR. A philosophy of the treatment of periodontal disease. Dent Digest 38:314, 1932.
96. Stookey G. Are all fluoride dentifrices the same? In Wei SHY, ed. Clinical Uses of Fluorides. Philadelphia, Lea & Febiger, 1985.
97. Stookey GK, Muhler JC. Laboratory studies concerning the enamel and dentin abrasion properties of common dentifrice polishing agents. J Dent Res 47:524, 1968.
98. Suomi JD, Green JC, Vermillion JR, et al. The effect of controlled oral hygiene procedures on the progression of periodontal disease in adults: Results after two years. J Periodontol 40:416, 1969.
99. Waerhaug J. The interdental brush and its place in operative and crown and bridge dentistry. J Oral Rehabil 3:107, 1976.
100. Waki MY, Jolkovsky DL, Otomo-Corgel J, et al. Effects of subgingival irrigation on bacteremia following scaling and root planing. J Periodontol 61:405, 1990.
101. Wilson T. Compliance—a review of the literature with possible applications to periodontics. J Periodontol 58:706, 1987.
102. Wolff LF, Philstrom BL, Bakdash MD, et al. Effect on gingivitis of toothbrushing with 0.04% stannous fluoride and 0.22% sodium fluoride gel on gingivitis for 18 months. J Am Dent Assoc 119:283, 1989.
103. Yankell SL. Toothbrushing and toothbrushing techniques. In Harris NO, Christen AG, eds. Primary Preventive Dentistry. 3rd ed. East Norwalk, CT, Appleton & Lange, 1991, p 93.
104. Yukna RA, Broxson AW, Mayer ET, et al. Comparison of Listerine mouthwash and periodontal dressing following periodontal flap surgery. Clin Prev Dent 4:14, 1986.

43

Treatment of Uncomplicated Chronic Gingivitis

FERMIN A. CARRANZA, JR.

Treatment
Causes of Failure

Uncomplicated chronic gingivitis is the most common disease of the gingiva, affecting both the interdental and the marginal gingivae. It should be detected in its earliest stages and treated as soon as detected (Figs. 43–1 and 43–2). Usually painless, it is the most common cause of gingival bleeding. Failure to treat it invites destruction of the underlying periodontal tissues and premature tooth loss.

Although chronic gingivitis may never progress to bone loss, it often is the initial stage of periodontitis and should be treated before pockets develop. There is no method available at present to prognosticate whether gingivitis will remain as such or will progress to periodontitis.

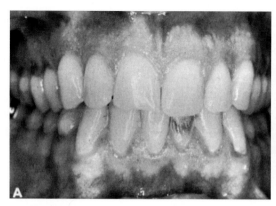
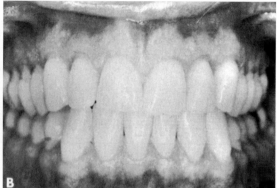

FIGURE 43–1. Uncomplicated chronic marginal gingivitis. *A*, Before treatment. *B*, After treatment.

Chronic gingivitis is always caused by plaque accumulation. The classic study on experimental gingivitis by Löe and coworkers[5,6] has shown the association of plaque accumulation and maturation with gingivitis and how plaque removal and/or interference with its maturation will result in elimination of the gingivitis.

Systemic conditions may aggravate or modify the inflammation caused by plaque and should be appropriately dealt with (see Chapter 14), but no systemic conditions by themselves cause chronic gingivitis.

TREATMENT

Treatment should be preceded by a careful examination to detect all sources of local irritation, such as dental plaque, calculus, food impaction, overhanging or improperly contoured restorations, or irritating removable prostheses. The teeth should be stained with disclosing solution to reveal plaque and should be carefully probed with a no. 17 or no. 3A explorer to locate small particles of calculus.

First Visit. The treatment of uncomplicated gingivitis is started by explaining the importance of plaque control and teaching the patient how to achieve it (see Chapter 42). This gives the patient a realistic perspective regarding the treatment of gingivitis: It includes something he or she must do, as well as something the dentist does for him or her. It also provides an opportunity to demonstrate that plaque control really benefits the tissues. After the patient is instructed in plaque control, an appointment for the next visit is made.

Second Visit. The gingival condition is examined with the patient, and improvement is pointed out. The teeth are stained with disclosing solution and plaque control is reviewed, with the patient demonstrating the various procedures used.

The teeth are scaled to remove all deposits, and all tooth surfaces are polished with a paste of fine pumice. Polishing is an important preventive measure against the recurrence of gingivitis. Plaque, the most important cause of gingivitis and the initial stage in the formation of calculus, tends to form more readily on rough surfaces.

Other sources of local irritation listed earlier should also be eliminated.

Third Visit. The gingivae are examined, and plaque control is reviewed. Special attention is given to areas of persistent inflammation; this usually entails rescaling and emphasizing patient technique for cleansing the areas. Chlorhexidine mouthwashes (Peridex or PerioGard), once or twice a day for 2 to 4 weeks or more, can be prescribed for these persistent cases; the patient should be informed that this mouthwash may stain the teeth after several weeks of use. A thorough prophylaxis should be given when the stain appears.[4,7] Daily oral irrigation by the patient with 0.06% chlorhexidine has been shown to be a most effective method for the treatment of gingivitis.[1,3]

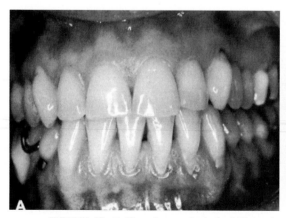
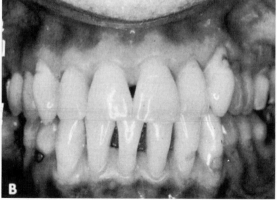

FIGURE 43–2. Chronic marginal gingivitis and recession. *A*, Before treatment. *B*, After treatment.

A recent study[2] has shown that mouthrinses are not as effective in preventing and treating interdental gingivitis as other mechanical methods of plaque removal, such as dental floss or Stim-U-Dents. This should be taken into consideration when papillary inflammation persists.

When the gingivitis disappears, the patient is placed on "recall," with a careful explanation of the reasons for periodic visits and the importance of the care given the mouth in the intervening periods.

CAUSES OF FAILURE

The treatment of chronic gingivitis should present no problems. However, if disease persists, the following are the most likely causes:

1. Failure to remove minute particles of calculus, often just beneath the cemento-enamel junction.
2. Failure to polish the tooth surfaces after deposits are removed.
3. Failure to eliminate sources of irritation other than deposits on the teeth. Subgingival margins of restorations, even if clinically adequate, may harbor bacteria that will perpetuate gingival inflammation; areas of food impaction are often overlooked as irritating factors.
4. Inadequate plaque control because of insufficient patient instruction, dismissal of the patient before he or she demonstrates competence in plaque control, or lack of patient cooperation.
5. A tendency to seek a remote systemic etiology for persistent gingivitis caused by overlooked local irritants.
6. Dependence on vitamins and hormones, antibiotics, and oxidizing agents for treatment. Except for some antibacterial agents (i.e., Peridex, Listerine) and topical anesthetics, drugs serve no significant purpose in the treatment of chronic gingivitis.

REFERENCES

1. Brownstein CN, Brigs SD, Schweitzer KL, et al. Irrigation with chlorhexidine to resolve naturally occurring gingivitis. J Clin Periodontol 17:588, 1990.
2. Caton JG, Blieden TM, Lowenguth RA, et al. Comparison between mechanical cleaning and an antimicrobial rinse for the treatment and prevention of interdental gingivitis. J Clin Periodontol 20:172, 1993.
3. Flemmig TF, Newman MG, Doherty FM, et al. Supragingival irrigation with 0.06 per cent chlorhexidine in naturally occurring gingivitis. I. Six month clinical observations. J Periodontol 61:112, 1990.
4. Lang NP, Brecx MC. Chlorhexidine digluconate: An agent for chemical control and prevention of gingival inflammation. J Periodont Res 21(suppl 16):74, 1986.
5. Löe H, Theilade E, Jensen SB. Experimental gingivitis in man. J Periodontol 36:177, 1965.
6. Löe H, Theilade E, Jensen SB, Schiott CR. Experimental gingivitis in man. III. The influence of antibiotics on gingival plaque development. J Periodont Res 2:282, 1967.
7. Siegrist BE, Gusberti FA, Brecx MC, et al. Efficacy of supervised rinsing with chlorhexidine gluconate in comparison to phenolic and plant alkaloid compounds. J Periodont Res 21(suppl 16):60, 1986.

44

Antimicrobial and Other Chemotherapeutic Agents in Periodontal Therapy

DAVID L. JOLKOVSKY and SEBASTIAN C. CIANCIO

Systemic Administration of Antibiotics
Tetracyclines
Metronidazole
Ciprofloxacin
Penicillins
Clindamycin
Erythromycin
Spiramycin

Serial and Combination Therapy
Nonsteroidal Anti-inflammatory Drugs
Local Administration of Antibiotics and Antimicrobial Agents
Vehicles for Local Delivery
Local Delivery Methods
Irrigation Agents
Conclusions

Numerous attempts have been made to use antimicrobial agents to control the microbial causes of periodontal diseases.[65,66,135] W. D. Miller was the first to investigate the relationship between periodontal diseases and bacteria.[74] In the 1880s he suggested the use of an antimicrobial mouthrinse (Listerine) to aid in fighting what was then known as pyorrhea alveolaris.[87] Currently there is a large body of information concerning the use of antimicrobial agents to control periodontal disease.

The authors are grateful to Dr. Gary Greenstein for his constructive critical analysis of this chapter.

Chemotherapeutic agent is a general term that refers to the ability of an active chemical substance to provide a therapeutic clinical benefit. *Antimicrobial agents* are chemotherapeutic agents that reduce the amount of bacteria present, either by specifically targeting certain organisms or by nonspecifically reducing all bacteria. *Antibiotics* are a form of antimicrobial agent, produced by or obtained from microorganisms, that have the capacity to kill other microorganisms or inhibit their growth. Antibiotics may be specific or cover a broad spectrum.

Chemotherapeutic agents may be administered systemically or delivered locally. Systemic antibiotic agents may reduce or eliminate bacteria that cannot be removed by scaling and root planing. This includes bacteria that have penetrated into the tissues or root surfaces.[18,20,102] It has been shown in experimental animals that systemic administration of antibiotics reduces plaque and gingivitis and slows bone loss.[63,72] By using antibiotic agents in conjunction with nonsurgical therapy, the need for periodontal surgery may be reduced or eliminated. This has been substantiated for some cases of localized juvenile periodontitis[91,92] and adult periodontitis.[76] In cases of progressive periodontal disease that may be resistant to traditional nonsurgical or surgical therapies, systemic antibiotics are also useful. These progressive forms of periodontal disease may include localized juvenile periodontitis, rapidly progressive periodontitis, or refractory periodontitis (see Chapter 45).

Other systemic chemotherapeutic agents can modify the host to promote its ability to resist bone loss or aid its ability to regenerate bone. Nonsteroidal anti-inflammatory agents can modify the host's inflammatory response to bacteria, thereby reducing bone loss. Tetracycline, aside from its antibiotic effect, has an anticollagenase effect that inhibits collagen destruction.

Many chemotherapeutic agents can be delivered locally. By delivering these agents directly to the periodontal tissues where they are needed, greater concentrations are achieved and systemic side effects are reduced. Mouthrinses provide a vehicle by which chemotherapeutic agents can be delivered locally. In addition, tetracycline has been incorporated into fibers that, when placed into the periodontal pocket, release the antibiotic slowly over time.

This chapter reviews chemotherapeutic agents used to treat periodontal disease. Other uses of chemotherapeutic agents are reviewed in other chapters. These include the following:

1. Emergency situations, including the treatment of acute periodontal abscesses, acute necrotizing ulcerative gingivitis, or postsurgical infections (see Chapters 39 and 40).
2. Premedication of patients who have medical problems requiring prophylactic systemic antibiotic coverage in association with periodontal therapy. In these cases, antibiotics are used not to treat the periodontal pocket, but to prevent systemic complications (see Chapter 34).
3. The use of chemotherapeutic mouthrinses to control gingivitis. Mouthrinses do not penetrate into the periodontal pocket; their use is reviewed elsewhere (see Chapter 42).

SYSTEMIC ADMINISTRATION OF ANTIBIOTICS

The use of antibiotics in the treatment of periodontal diseases is based on the infectious nature of these diseases.

Ideally, the causative microorganism(s) should be identified and the most effective agent selected by using antibiotic sensitivity tests. Although this appears simple, the difficulty lies primarily in identifying specific etiologic microorganism(s) rather than microorganisms simply associated with various periodontal disorders (see Chapter 9).[23]

According to Gibson, an ideal antibiotic for use in prevention and treatment of periodontal diseases should be specific for periodontal pathogens; allogenic and nontoxic; substantive; not in general use for treatment of other diseases; and inexpensive.[35] Currently there is no ideal antibiotic for treatment of periodontal diseases. Although oral bacteria are susceptible to many antibiotics, no single antibiotic at concentrations achieved in body fluids inhibits all putative periodontal pathogens.[121] Indeed, a combination of antibiotics may be necessary to eliminate all putative pathogens from some periodontal pockets.[99]

Both systemic and topical antibiotics have been evaluated as plaque-reducing agents. Systemically administered antibiotics reach therapeutic levels in the periodontium because they are excreted in the saliva and/or the gingival crevicular fluid.[5,12] Topical application has the advantage that antibiotic agents are directed to their specific target areas. Reduced drug dosages, increased drug concentrations, and reduced side effects can be benefits of topical application. Unfortunately, some antibiotics, when used topically, induce superinfections (i.e., *Candida*) or hypersensitivity reactions (see Chapter 8).

Tetracyclines

Tetracyclines are widely used in the treatment of periodontal diseases. They are frequently used in treating refractory periodontitis, including localized juvenile periodontitis. Tetracyclines have the ability to concentrate in the periodontal tissues and to destroy *Actinobacillus actinomycetemcomitans*. In addition, they exert an anticollagenase effect that can inhibit tissue destruction and may aid bone regeneration.

Pharmacology. The tetracyclines are a group of antibiotics produced naturally from certain species of *Streptomyces* or derived semisynthetically. These antibiotics are bacteriostatic and are effective against rapidly multiplying bacteria. They are generally more effective against gram-positive bacteria than gram-negative bacteria.[124] Tetracyclines are effective in treating periodontal diseases in part because their concentration in the gingival crevice is 2 to 10 times that in serum.[3,5,45] This allows a high drug concentration to be delivered into periodontal pockets. In addition, several studies have demonstrated that tetracyclines at a low gingival crevicular fluid concentration (2 to 4 μg/ml) are very effective against many periodontal pathogens.[7,8,121]

Animal Studies. Systemic administration of tetracyclines reduces plaque, gingival inflammation,[72] and bone loss in dogs[128] and rats.[123] However, a study in dogs reported that after 2 years of continuous systemic administration of tetracycline, the beneficial effect of reducing the rate of bone loss may be lost.[56] Another study showed that tetracycline therapy increases the frequency of resistant organisms.[59] These animal studies agree with long-term human clinical studies showing that tetracyclines should be used only on a short-term basis.

Clinical Use. Tetracyclines have been investigated as adjuncts in the treatment of localized juvenile periodontitis (LJP). *A. actinomycetemcomitans* is a frequent causative microorganism in LJP and is tissue invasive. Therefore, mechanical removal of calculus and plaque from root surfaces may not eliminate this bacterium from the periodontal tissues. Systemic tetracycline can eliminate tissue bacteria and, in conjunction with scaling and root planing, has been shown to arrest bone loss and suppress *A. actinomycetemcomitans* levels.[107,108] This combined form of therapy allows mechanical removal of root surface deposits and elimination of pathogenic bacteria from within the tissues. Increased post-treatment bone levels have been noted using this method.[34,107] In the treatment of adult periodontitis, the use of tetracyclines as an adjunct to scaling and root planing initially reduces inflammation[71,106] but after several weeks does not result in substantial clinical benefit.[71]

Long-term use of low doses of tetracyclines has been advocated in the past. One long-term study of patients taking low doses of tetracycline (250 mg per day for 2 to 7 years) showed persistence of deep pockets that did not bleed on probing. These sites contained high proportions of tetracycline-resistant gram-negative rods (i.e., *Fusobacterium nucleatum*). After the antibiotic was discontinued, the flora was characteristic of sites with disease.[62] Therefore, it is not advisable to engage in long-term regimens of tetracyclines because of the possible development of resistant bacterial strains. Tetracyclines should be used for 14 to 21 days around the time of active periodontal therapy.[107]

Other Chemotherapeutic Benefits. Tetracyclines in doses as low as 20 mg bid (for doxycycline) have been shown to directly inhibit the activity of collagenase and possibly other collagenolytic enzymes produced by the host tissue, resulting in a reduced rate of collagen breakdown.[38,40] Tetracycline has been shown to reduce human endogenous collagenase from polymorphonuclear leukocytes.[80] Animal studies have suggested that this anticollagenase effect may inhibit bone loss associated with experimental periodontal disease and may enhance bone regeneration.[39] Preliminary studies in humans have also suggested that this effect is present, even in low doses.[40] These nonantibiotic chemotherapeutic effects of tetracycline may be of benefit in future therapy related to new attachment procedures (e.g., guided tissue regeneration and bone grafting).

Specific Agents. Tetracycline, minocycline, and doxycycline—all semisynthetic members of the tetracycline group—have been used in periodontal therapy.

Tetracycline. Tetracycline requires administration of 250 mg qid. It is inexpensive, but compliance may be reduced by having to take four capsules per day.

Minocycline. Minocycline is effective against a broad spectrum of microorganisms. In patients with adult periodontitis, it suppresses spirochetes and motile rods as effectively as scaling and root planing, with suppression remaining evident for up to 3 months after therapy. Minocycline can be given twice a day, thus facilitating compliance when compared with tetracycline. Although it is associated with less photo- and renal toxicity than tetracycline, it may

cause reversible vertigo. Minocycline administered in a dosage of 200 mg per day for 1 week results in a reduction in total bacterial counts, complete elimination of spirochetes for periods of up to 2 months, and improvement in all clinical parameters.[21]

Doxycycline. Doxycycline has the same spectrum of activity as minocycline and may be equally as effective.[23a] Because it can be given only once daily, patients may be more compliant. Compliance is also favored because its absorption from the gastrointestinal tract is not altered by calcium, metal ions, or antacids, as is absorption of other tetracyclines. The recommended dosage is 100 mg twice daily the first day, then 100 mg once daily. To reduce stomach upset, 50 mg can be taken twice daily.

Metronidazole

Pharmacology. Metronidazole is a nitroimidazole compound developed in France to treat protozoal infections. It is bactericidal to anaerobic organisms and is believed to disrupt bacterial DNA synthesis in conditions in which a low reduction potential is present. Metronidazole is not the drug of choice for treating *A. actinomycetemcomitans* infections, but it may be effective at therapeutic levels owing to its hydroxy metabolite. However, it is effective against *A. actinomycetemcomitans* when used in combination with other antibiotics.[99,100] Metronidazole is also effective against obligate anaerobes such as *Porphyromonas gingivalis* and *Prevotella intermedia*.[48]

Clinical Use. Metronidazole has been used clinically to treat gingivitis, acute necrotizing ulcerative gingivitis, adult periodontitis, and rapidly progressive periodontitis. It has been used as monotherapy and also in combination with both root planing and surgery or with other antibiotics. Metronidazole has been used successfully for treating acute necrotizing ulcerative gingivitis.[28,77,105]

Studies in experimental animals[53] and in humans[28,69,70,76] have demonstrated the efficacy of metronidazole in the treatment of gingivitis and periodontitis. A single dose of metronidazole (250 mg orally) appears in both serum and gingival fluid in sufficient quantities to inhibit a wide range of suspected periodontal pathogens. Administered systemically (750 to 1000 mg/day for 2 weeks), this drug reduces the growth of anaerobic flora, including spirochetes, and decreases the clinical and histopathologic signs of periodontitis.[69,70] The most commonly prescribed regimen is 250 mg tid for 7 days.[48] Loesche and coworkers found that 250 mg of metronidazole given three times daily for 1 week was of benefit to patients with a diagnosed anaerobic periodontal infection. In this study, an infection was considered anaerobic when spirochetes composed 20% or more of the total microbial count. Metronidazole used as a supplement to rigorous scaling and root planing resulted in a significantly reduced need for surgery when compared with root planing alone. The bacteriologic data of this study showed that only the spirochete count was significantly reduced.[76] Currently it is not known what critical level of spirochetes is needed to diagnose an anaerobic infection, when metronidazole should be given, or what dosage or duration of therapy is ideal.[48]

As monotherapy (no concurrent root planing), metronidazole is inferior and at best only equivalent to root planing.

Therefore, if metronidazole is used, it should not be administered as monotherapy.

Metronidazole offers some benefit in the treatment of refractory periodontitis, particularly when used in combination with amoxicillin. The existence of refractory periodontitis as a diagnostic category indicates that some patients do not respond to conventional therapy, including root planing and/or surgery. Soder and coworkers showed that metronidazole was more effective than placebo in the management of sites that were not responsive to root planing.[109] Nevertheless, despite metronidazole therapy, many patients still had sites that bled on probing.

Studies have suggested that, when combined with amoxicillin or amoxicillin–clavulanate potassium (Augmentin), metronidazole may be of value in the management of patients with juvenile or refractory periodontitis (see later discussion).

Side Effects. Metronidazole has an antabuse effect when alcohol is ingested. The response is generally proportional to the amount ingested and can result in severe cramps, nausea, and vomiting. Alcohol-containing products should be avoided during therapy and for at least 1 day after therapy is discontinued. Metronidazole also inhibits warfarin metabolism. Patients undergoing anticoagulant therapy should avoid metronidazole, because it prolongs prothrombin time.[48] It should also be avoided in patients on lithium.

Ciprofloxacin

Ciprofloxacin is a quinolone active against gram-negative rods, including all facultative and some anaerobic putative periodontal pathogens. Because it demonstrates minimal effect on *Streptococcus* species, which are associated with periodontal health,[99] ciprofloxacin therapy may facilitate the establishment of a microflora associated with periodontal health. At present, ciprofloxacin is the only antibiotic in periodontal therapy to which all strains of *A. actinomycetemcomitans* are susceptible. It has also been used in combination with metronidazole.[99]

Penicillins

Penicillins are the drugs of choice for the treatment of many serious infections in humans and are the most widely used antibiotics. Penicillins are natural and semisynthetic derivatives of broth cultures of the *Penicillium* mold. They inhibit bacterial cell wall production and are therefore bactericidal. They may induce allergic reactions and bacterial resistance; up to 10% of patients may be allergic to penicillin. Penicillins other than amoxicillin and amoxicillin–clavulanate potassium (Augmentin) have not been evaluated, and their use in periodontal therapy does not appear to be justified.[125]

Amoxicillin. Amoxicillin is a semisynthetic penicillin with an extended antimicrobial spectrum that includes gram-positive and gram-negative bacteria. It demonstrates excellent absorption after oral administration. Amoxicillin is susceptible to penicillinase, a β-lactamase produced by certain bacteria that breaks the penicillin ring structure and thereby renders penicillins ineffective.[125]

Amoxicillin may be useful in the management of patients with refractory or juvenile periodontitis. Recommended dosage is 500 mg tid.

Amoxicillin–Clavulanate Potassium (Augmentin). The combination of amoxicillin with clavulanate potassium makes Augmentin not susceptible to penicillinase enzymes produced by bacteria. Augmentin may be useful in the management of patients with refractory or juvenile periodontitis.[99] Bueno and coworkers reported that Augmentin arrested alveolar bone loss in patients with periodontal disease that was refractory to treatment with other antibiotics, including tetracycline, metronidazole, and clindamycin.[17]

Clindamycin

Clindamycin is effective against anaerobic bacteria.[117] It has shown efficacy in patients with periodontitis refractory to tetracycline therapy. However, it has been associated with pseudomembranous colitis more often than other antibiotics, thereby limiting its use. When needed, however, it can be used with caution. Diarrhea or cramping that develops during the use of clindamycin may be indicative of cholitis, and clindamycin should be discontinued. If symptoms persist, the patient should be referred to an internist.

Erythromycin

Erythromycin does not concentrate in gingival crevicular fluid, and it is not effective against most putative periodontal pathogens. For these reasons, it is not recommended as an adjunct to periodontal therapy.

Spiramycin

Spiramycin is a macrolide antibiotic that is active against gram-positive organisms; it is excreted in high concentrations in saliva. It is used as an adjunct to periodontal treatment in Canada and Europe but is not available in the United States. Several studies have shown benefits—as measured by the Gingival Index, the Plaque Index, pocket depth, and crevicular fluid flow[86,113]—when spiramycin was prescribed in advanced periodontal disease. In addition, it is a safe, nontoxic drug with few and infrequent side effects and is not in general use for medical problems.[36]

SERIAL AND COMBINATION THERAPY

Rationale. Because periodontal infections may contain a wide diversity of bacteria, there may be no single antibiotic that is effective against all putative pathogens. These "mixed" infections can include a variety of aerobic, microaerophilic, and anaerobic bacteria, both gram negative and gram positive. In these instances, it may be necessary to use more than one antibiotic, either serially or in combination.[99] However, before combinations of antibiotics are used, the periodontal pathogen(s) being treated must be identified, because one drug may be adequate.

Clinical Use. Antibiotics that are *bacteriostatic* (e.g., tetracycline) generally require rapidly dividing microorganisms to be effective. They do not function well if a *bactericidal* antibiotic (e.g., amoxicillin) is given concurrently.

When both types of drugs are required, they are best given serially, not in combination.

Rams and Slots reviewed combination therapy using systemic metronidazole along with amoxicillin, Augmentin, or ciprofloxacin.[99] The metronidazole-amoxicillin and metronidazole-Augmentin combinations provided excellent elimination of many organisms in adult and juvenile periodontitis that had been treated unsuccessfully with tetracyclines and mechanical debridement. These drugs have an additive effect regarding suppression of *A. actinomycetemcomitans*. Metronidazole-ciprofloxacin is also effective against *A. actinomycetemcomitans*. Metronidazole targets obligate anaerobes, and ciprofloxacin targets facultative anaerobes. This is a powerful combination against mixed infections. Studies of this drug combination in the treatment of refractory/recurrent periodontitis have documented marked clinical improvement. This combination may provide a *therapeutic benefit* by reducing or eliminating pathogenic organisms and a *prophylactic benefit* by giving rise to a predominantly streptococcal microflora.[100]

Systemic antibiotic therapy combined with mechanical therapy appears valuable in the treatment of recalcitrant periodontal infections and localized juvenile periodontitis infections involving *A. actinomycetemcomitans*. Antibiotic treatment should be reserved for specific subsets of periodontal patients who do not respond to conventional therapy. Selection of specific agents should be guided by the results of cultures and sensitivity tests for subgingival plaque microorganisms.

NONSTEROIDAL ANTI-INFLAMMATORY DRUGS

It is only relatively recently that the role of the host's immunoinflammatory system has begun to be understood. After activation of inflammatory cells in the periodontium by bacteria, phospholipids in the plasma membranes of cells become available for actions by phospholipase. This leads to free arachidonic acid in the area.[101] Arachidonic acid can then be metabolized into prostaglandins, thromboxanes, and prostacycline by the enzyme cyclooxygenase. The lipoxygenase pathway can produce leukotrienes and hydroxyeicosatetraenoic acids from arachidonic acid. Strong evidence suggests that cyclooxygenase pathway products (e.g., prostaglandins) may be important mediators of some of the pathologic events occurring in periodontal disease.[101] Therefore, modulation of the host's inflammatory response to bacteria may alter the incidence and severity of periodontal disease. Nonsteroidal anti-inflammatory drugs (NSAIDs) may be of therapeutic value in treating periodontal disease because of their ability to interfere with arachidonic acid metabolism and thereby inhibit the inflammatory process. This expectation has been validated in studies in both animals and humans.[32,93,120,130,133] Some NSAIDs have been shown to affect the response of polymorphonuclear neutrophils (PMNs) to inflammation not related to prostaglandin inhibition.[30,58] Beneficial effects of NSAIDs have also been found after topical application.[52,119,129] Drugs studied have included flurbiprofen, ibuprofen, mefenamic acid, and naproxen.

Flurbiprofen appears to be an NSAID worthy of further investigation. It inhibits PMN migration, reduces vascular permeability, and inhibits platelet aggregation by inhibiting cyclooxygenase.[52] In a 3-year study, Williams and coworkers reported that flurbiprofen significantly inhibited radiographic alveolar bone loss when compared with placebo. Unfortunately, by 24 months, the difference in the rate of bone loss had disappeared.[131] This group also reported a return to baseline in the rate of bone loss after treatment with flurbiprofen was discontinued.[132]

Modulation of the host immune response has the potential to become a powerful tool in the treatment of periodontal disease. Owing to their apparent ability to strengthen the host's periodontium by making alveolar bone more resistant to destruction associated with periodontitis, systemic NSAIDs may become valuable adjuncts in periodontal therapy. However, clinical trials are needed to show the efficacy of these agents in humans.

LOCAL ADMINISTRATION OF ANTIBIOTICS AND ANTIMICROBIAL AGENTS

The administration of antibiotics and use of antimicrobial agents in periodontal pockets may be effective adjuncts to conventional periodontal therapy. However, these methods of delivery do not replace professional dental treatment or home oral hygiene procedures. Vehicles for local delivery of chemotherapeutic agents include dentifrices, mouthrinses, chewing gum, and slow-release devices. Methods of delivery of chemotherapeutic agents include direct professional application to the root surface during surgery (root biomodification), the Keyes technique, and both home and professional irrigation. The potential for these vehicles and methods to increase periodontal health lies in their ability to deliver the chemotherapeutic agent directly into the periodontal pocket or onto the diseased root surface. Thus, the area where disease activity occurs is directly accessed. Site-specific therapy has three potential advantages: decreased drug dosages, increased drug concentrations, and reduced systemic side effects such as gastrointestinal distress.

Vehicles for Local Delivery

Dentifrices, Mouthrinses, and Chewing Gum

These are inefficient delivery systems in periodontitis, because they fail to direct drugs into the periodontal pocket. Dentifrices with many chemotherapeutic agents, including chlorhexidine gluconate and flurbiprofen, provide limited benefit in the treatment of periodontitis. The use of a dentifrice containing flurbiprofen during a 12-month controlled study showed only a small positive effect on bone metabolism.[52] Similarly, mouthrinses can be useful in reducing inflammation associated with gingivitis,[73] but they do not penetrate well into periodontal pockets.[15,84,94] Chewing gums that release antimicrobial agents have also proved to be ineffective at treating periodontal disease.

The daily use of chlorhexidine gluconate mouthrinses is highly recommended postsurgically (1–4 weeks) and in patients with certain diseases with oral manifestations, such as acquired immunodeficiency syndrome (AIDS) and blood dyscrasias. It is also recommended for those unable to perform adequate plaque control due to physical or mental inabilities.

Controlled-Release Local Delivery Systems

Controlled-release local delivery systems* are designed to release chemotherapeutic agents into the periodontal pocket over an extended period of time. These controlled-release local delivery devices are placed into periodontal pockets in a similar manner to placement of retraction cord. The chemotherapeutic agent released from these devices can achieve high levels of concentration at precisely the site where it is needed.

Controlled-release local delivery systems that have been tested in periodontics can be classified as reservoirs without a rate-controlling system or reservoirs with a rate-controlling system.[61] Reservoirs that lack rate control include hollow fibers, gels, and dialysis tubing.[122] These systems tend to release chemotherapeutic agents very quickly and only marginally qualify as sustained-release devices. Reservoirs with rate-controlling systems include erodible polymeric matrices, polymer membranes, monolithic matrices, and coated particles.

The use of slow-release devices placed in periodontal defects, in conjunction with scaling and root planing, may offer promise in the management of such defects. These methods appear to be safe for periodontal tissues and are well tolerated by patients. Research is currently under way to determine the efficacy of resorbable subgingival delivery devices. If successful, these methods will offer the advantage of not requiring that the patient be scheduled for a separate visit for device removal.

Ethylene Vinyl Acetate (EVA). The EVA system is based on polymer technology, with tetracycline being dispersed within a solid (monolithic) polymer of EVA. EVA fibers have been found to be flexible and to sustain delivery of tetracycline for up to 9 days.[41,61] A formulation of 25% tetracycline in EVA (Actisite) has been developed as a 0.5-mm nonbiodegradable fiber (0.55 mg/cm) and has been approved by the U.S. Food and Drug Administration (FDA). This fiber is placed into a periodontal pocket and maintained there for 10 days by superficial application of a cyanoacrylate adhesive. Multicenter 6-month trials have shown that use of these fibers alone resulted in a reduction in probing depths of approximately 1 mm, compared with an approximate reduction of 0.5 mm in pockets scaled and root planed.[42,43] It should be noted that the 0.5-mm reduction in probing depth after root planing in these multicenter studies was less than that obtained in other studies of root planing efficacy, which indicates the possibility of poor root planing in the studies evaluating fibers. The discrepancy may also be accounted for by the design of the multicenter trials, in which gingival inflammation was reduced by prophylaxis prior to initiation of the study.

Newman and colleagues found that adjunctive placement of tetracycline fibers into periodontal pockets after scaling and root planing improved clinical parameters in maintenance patients when compared with scaling and root plan-

ing alone. These patients had finished an active phase of periodontal therapy and had pockets 5 to 8 mm deep. The tetracycline fiber group had significant reductions in probing depth and bleeding on probing compared with patients who underwent scaling and root planing only at 1-, 3-, and 6-month evaluations.[89] Notably, patients selected for treatment had sites that had not responded to conventional therapy.

Current drawbacks of tetracycline fiber therapy include the need for removal of the fibers, the amount of clinical time needed to place the fibers, and the need for cyanoacrylate or some other material to hold them in place. Also, tetracycline is not the only accepted drug of choice for the treatment of periodontal disease. Amoxicillin–clavulanate potassium (Augmentin), metronidazole, and ciprofloxacin have been successfully used in patients who did not respond to conventional therapy. In addition, study results have not shown significant clinical improvement with tetracycline when compared with root planing. Reductions in pocket probing depth have averaged 0.5 mm. Therefore, the clinician must decide whether such a reduction will benefit the patient. Because conventional periodontal therapy works well in the majority of patients, tetracycline fiber therapy should be used only in localized refractory sites or in the treatment of medically compromised patients who cannot receive the full complement of conventional therapy.

Acrylic and Ethylcellulose Strips. Some investigators have incorporated chemical agents into acrylic strips.[2] In most cases the drug was released in 1 day by this method, giving it short-lived antimicrobial value. Metronidazole and chlorhexidine have been studied using this methodology.[2,25] Golomb and associates reported the use of ethylcellulose strips containing either chlorhexidine or metronidazole; effective drug levels were found for up to 6 days.[37] They also found that the rate at which all formulations released minocycline decreased with time, although the rate varied for different formulations.[31]

Gels. Gels containing 2% minocycline are marketed in Europe (Dentomycin) and Japan (Periocline), and 25% metronidazole is marketed in Europe (Elyzol). These gels allow antibiotics to be syringed into the peridontal pocket.[44a]

Biodegradable Controlled-Release Devices. In vitro experiments have been performed to evaluate biodegradable devices. These devices offer the advantage of not needing to be removed.[112] However, another visit is needed to check healing.

Local Delivery Methods

Keyes Technique

The Keyes technique involves the application by toothbrushing of a slurry of sodium bicarbonate and hydrogen peroxide for the control of plaque microorganisms.[59,98] Many studies have been conducted to evaluate this treatment modality, but the results have shown that it is no more effective than conventional oral hygiene.[4,46,49,134] Greenstein reviewed 15 studies comparing the effect of a subgingival sodium bicarbonate–hydrogen peroxide mixture to conventional hygiene techniques. Only one of these studies showed any significant difference between the two techniques; the other 14 studies concluded that improve-

---

* For a review, see Kornman.[61]

ment in periodontal status was primarily due to root planing.[46] In addition, as noted earlier, toothbrushing has proved to be an ineffective means of delivering medicaments into the periodontal pocket. Therefore, minimal clinical benefit can be expected from this technique.

Root Biomodification

Application of various medicaments to root surfaces during surgical therapy has been evaluated; these agents include tetracycline, doxycycline, citric acid, and fibronectin.[11,114,115] Some authors have suggested that application of a tetracycline solution to diseased root surfaces during surgery may enhance connective tissue attachment to the roots, although data are not conclusive.[3,9,11,114] Doxycycline applied to root surfaces in a concentration of 100 mg/ml produces an antibacterial effect that lasts for 14 days.[27] At present, however, there are no clinical trials supporting the efficacy of tetracycline application to root surfaces.

Local application of citric acid to root surfaces has not been shown to effectively promote new connective attachment in humans.[83] Fibronectin application during surgical therapy suppresses epithelial cell attachment and growth and therefore may be beneficial in promoting new attachment.[3,97,115]

Home Irrigation Devices

Home irrigation devices allow the patient to deliver medicaments into the periodontal pocket at home on a more frequent basis than is practical with professional subgingival irrigation. The ability of the device to access the depth of the periodontal pocket and the manual dexterity of the patient are limiting factors. As the pocket depth increases, the difficulty in accessing the apical extent of the pocket, where the most pathogenic plaque and bacteria reside, also increases. The traditional jet tip design of oral irrigators has been augmented by irrigation tips designed to go further subgingivally, and many of the newer oral ir-

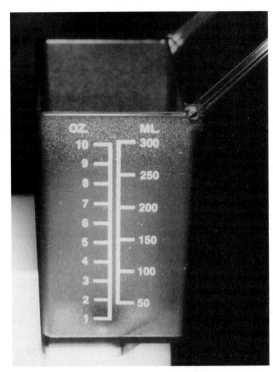

FIGURE 44–2. Graduated reservoir for accurate preparation of irrigation solutions.

rigators have graduated reservoirs so that accurate dilutions of oral mouthrinses may be prepared by the patient for delivery by irrigation (Figs. 44–1 and 44–2).

Supragingival Home Irrigation Devices. Oral irrigation devices with traditional jet tips result in greater access of medicaments to periodontal pockets when compared with rinsing alone. A 90-degree angle of application to the tooth surface provides a 71% penetration of shallow pockets (1 to 3 mm deep), a 44% penetration of moderate pockets (4 to 6 mm deep), and a 68% penetration of deep pockets (7 mm or greater depth), with a maximum pocket penetration of 4 to 5 mm. In general, a supragingival home irrigator will deliver medicaments to about one half the depth of a deeper periodontal pocket. A 45-degree angle of application does not increase penetration.[29] Therefore, although these devices may be useful in delivering medicaments in cases of gingivitis with shallow pocket depths, they are less useful in delivering medicaments in periodontitis patients with deeper pockets.

Subgingival Home Irrigation Devices. These devices generally include a blunt-end metal cannula that the patient inserts into the periodontal pocket (Fig. 44–3). This increases the depth of penetration of fluid but has the potential for injury owing to the metal tip and depending on the manual dexterity of the patient. Home subgingival irrigation may allow enhancement of periodontal health at problematic sites where access was previously limited.[47] However, the patient's manual dexterity is a limiting factor.

Marginal Home Irrigation Devices. Marginal home irrigation is a hybrid of both supragingival and subgingival irrigation. This technique uses devices that have a traditional jet tip attachment that has been modified so that it can deliver fluids subgingivally. Marginal irrigation can be performed with one of the commercially produced modified

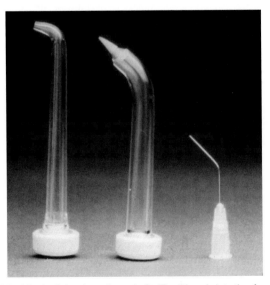

FIGURE 44–1. Irrigation tips. *Left,* Traditional jet tip for home supragingival irrigation. *Middle,* Marginal irrigation tip for home irrigation. *Right,* Blunt-end metal cannula for professional irrigation.

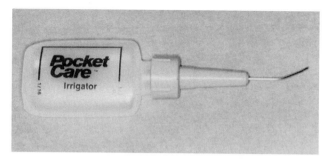

FIGURE 44-3. Home subgingival irrigator for delivery of medicaments into periodontal pockets by the patient.

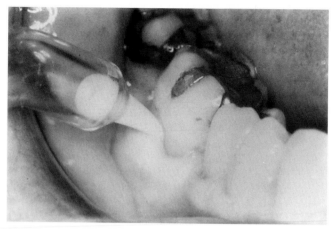

FIGURE 44-4. Marginal irrigation of medicaments into a lower molar furcation.

irrigation tips designed to deliver fluids subgingivally (Figs. 44-4 and 44-5). Home marginal irrigation allows penetration of fluid to 90% of the depth of pockets 6 mm deep or less and to 64% of the depth of pockets 7 mm deep or more.[15]

Supragingival irrigation with water is more effective at reducing gingivitis if it is a pulsating, rather than constant, flow.[10] The flushing action of water disrupts the pathogenic layer of unattached plaque, thereby improving gingival health.[57] Subgingival irrigation of saline solution with a cannula is also more effective if it is pulsed rather than constant.[55] It is not known whether the delivery of medicaments is more effective if delivered in a pulsed rather than continuous manner.

Professional Subgingival Irrigation

Professional subgingival irrigation devices include a wide array of powered and manually operated irrigators. Irrigation using a syringe with a blunt-end needle has been tried by many investigators.[19,110] Solutions reach the apical portion of the pocket by way of a syringe with a blunt-end needle, if the needle is placed 3 mm into the pocket.[51] Pocket irrigation with a blunt-end cannula (Fig. 44-6) attached to an oral irrigator can penetrate to 71.5% of the pocket depth in pockets 3.5 to 6 mm deep.[54] Professional irrigation has been performed using chlorhexidine gluconate,[14,51,57,126] stannous fluoride,[85,104] tetracycline,[78] metronidazole,[60,79] and hydrogen peroxide.[6] Irrigation with

medicaments performed in conjunction with root planing provides little, if any, additional benefit over root planing alone.[46] The effect of a one-time subgingival irrigation at a maintenance visit has a time-limited effect that precludes significant clinical improvement.[46,47,110]

Irrigation Agents*

Oral irrigation decreases gingivitis scores, even when water alone is used as the irrigant.[16,22,33,57,88,127]* The clinical improvement results from a decrease in the subgingival microflora. When antimicrobial agents are used as the irrigant, an additive beneficial effect over irrigation with water alone is possible.[22,33,57,88] Many irrigation agents have been evaluated, including many popular mouthrinses. The discussion that follows is limited to chemotherapeutic agents with proven clinical antibacterial properties.

Chlorhexidine Gluconate. This is the only prescription antimicrobial mouthrinse that is approved by both the FDA and the American Dental Association for reduction of gingival inflammation. It is marketed in the United States as a 0.12% solution (Peridex, PerioGard) and is the most stud-

---

* For a review, see Greenstein.[47]

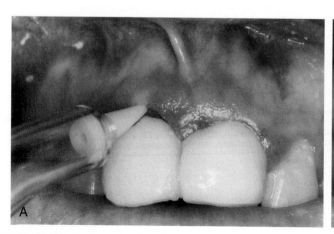
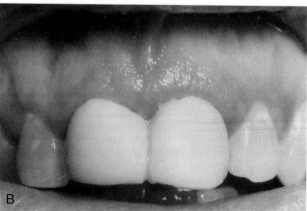

FIGURE 44-5. Marginal irrigation of temporary crowns with chlorhexidine gluconate. *A,* Gingival tissue is red and swollen after preparation of temporary crowns. *B,* After 1 week of marginal irrigation, tissue is firm and healthy.

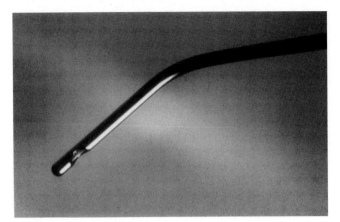

FIGURE 44–6. Blunt-end metal cannula with a side port for professional subgingival delivery of medicaments.

ied antibacterial mouthrinse.[67] Reference is made here to its use as an irrigant, not as a mouthrinse. The use of chlorhexidine gluconate as a mouthrinse for the prevention and treatment of gingivitis is discussed in Chapter 42.

Many studies have shown the effectiveness of delivering chlorhexidine gluconate into the periodontal pocket by means of an oral irrigator. Lang and Ramseier-Grossman have shown that 400 ml of a 0.02% solution of chlorhexidine gluconate (80 mg total dose) applied once daily with a supragingival oral irrigator will result in complete plaque inhibition.[68] Daily application of 200 ml of a 0.06% solution of chlorhexidine gluconate (120 mg total dose) with a supragingival oral irrigator is very effective in reducing naturally occurring gingivitis.[33] In this 6-month study, gingivitis was reduced 42.5% by irrigating once daily with chlorhexidine gluconate, 24.1% by rinsing with chlorhexidine gluconate, and 23.1% by irrigating with water. In addition, a positive microbiologic effect of irrigation was reported in patients who irrigated with chlorhexidine gluconate for 6 months.[88]

Daily patient-applied home irrigation with 180 ml of 0.04% chlorhexidine gluconate (72-mg total dose) using a marginal irrigation tip significantly reduced gingival inflammation in periodontal maintenance patients.[57] In this study there was a 33.1% reduction in gingivitis scores over baseline in patients who irrigated with chlorhexidine gluconate over a 3-month period. Daily home irrigation with chlorhexidine gluconate will improve gingival health when it is used adjunctively with routine professional dental care (supportive periodontal treatment) and routine home oral hygiene procedures.

The minimal daily dose of chlorhexidine gluconate required to be effective as a rinse in reducing gingivitis may be as low as 50 mg (50 ml of a 0.1% solution).[26] In vitro studies have indicated that chlorhexidine gluconate is bactericidal for tested organisms at concentrations of 18 to 33 $\mu g/ml$.[103] When irrigating subgingivally in vivo, blood and other materials that can interfere with chlorhexidine gluconate may be present. Therefore, the concentration may have to be as high as 125 $\mu g/ml$.[113] Investigators have used a 0.02% to 0.06% concentration of chlorhexidine gluconate as an irrigant[47] (Table 44–1). Total dosages in one irriga-

Table 44–1. PREPARATION OF IRRIGATION SOLUTIONS

	Strength	Dilution (Water:Product)	Preparation
Peridex irrigation (0.12% chlorhexidine gluconate)			
Supragingival	0.02%*	5:1	$\dfrac{300 \text{ ml}}{60 \text{ ml}} = \dfrac{1\frac{1}{4} \text{ glass water}^a}{4 \text{ capfuls Peridex}^b}$
	0.06%†	1:1	$\dfrac{100 \text{ ml water}}{100 \text{ ml Peridex}}$
Subgingival	0.12%‡	Full strength	About 1 ml per pocket
Marginal gingival	0.04%§	2:1	$\dfrac{60 \text{ ml}}{30 \text{ ml}} = \dfrac{1/4 \text{ glass water}}{2 \text{ capfuls Peridex}}$
Listerine irrigation (phenolic compound)¶			
Supragingival	11%¶	8:1	$\dfrac{360 \text{ ml}}{45 \text{ ml}} = \dfrac{1\frac{1}{2} \text{ glass water}}{3 \text{ tbsp Listerine}^c}$
Subgingival	100%¶	Full strength	About 1 ml per pocket
Marginal gingival	20%¶,#	4:1	$\dfrac{120 \text{ ml}}{30 \text{ ml}} = \dfrac{1/2 \text{ glass water}}{2 \text{ tbsp Listerine}}$

* Based on Lang and Ramsier-Grossman[68] (10-day study).
† Based on Flemmig et al.[33]
‡ No long-term clinical trials performed.
§ Based on Jolkovsky et al.[57] (Pik Pocket).
¶ Four essential oils: thymol, 0.06%; eucalyptol, 0.09%; methyl salicyate, 0.06%; menthol, 0.04%.
# Dilutions for Pik Pocket and Via-Jet are based on the fact that these tips will deliver around 80 ml/min when used at low pressure. There are no trials to support this dilution.
^a One glass equals 240 ml.
^b One capful from Peridex bottle equals 15 ml.
^c One tablespoon equals 15 ml.
Modified from Greenstein G. Supragingival and subgingival irrigation: Practical application in the treatment of periodontal diseases. Compend Contin Educ Dent 13:1098, 1992.

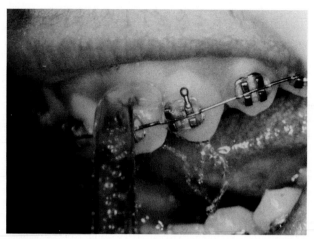

FIGURE 44–7. Oral irrigation with diluted Listerine during orthodontic therapy.

tion study ranged up to 120 mg/day.[33] In contrast, the total
dosage of chlorhexidine gluconate as a mouthrinse is 36
mg/day (30 ml of a 0.12% solution). Therefore, irrigation
with chlorhexidine gluconate generally requires a larger total dosage than does rinsing.

Phenolic Compounds. These compounds have long been
used as antiseptics and disinfectants. This group includes a
mouthrinse, Listerine, that has received American Dental
Association (ADA) approval for reduction of gingivitis
when used twice daily (Fig. 44–7).[24,101a] Generic formulations of Listerine carrying the ADA acceptance seal for
plaque and gingivitis reduction are available under a variety
of trade names.[95] One study has shown that phenolic compounds may also be effective as irrigating agents. In a 6-
week, double-blind controlled study, irrigation with Listerine provided benefits beyond those provided by a 5%
alcohol solution[22] (see Table 44–1). Benefits of irrigating
with ADA-approved phenolic compounds instead of
chlorhexidine gluconate include decreased side effects (e.g.,
staining) and decreased cost. Direct comparisons of these
two irrigants, however, indicate that chlorhexidine gluconate is more effective at reducing gingival inflammation
and plaque accumulation.

Stannous Fluoride Preparations. Stannous fluoride
preparations have antibacterial properties.[96] Direct pocket
lavage with 1.64% stannous fluoride in advanced periodontitis was found to be effective in reducing Bleeding Index
scores and in delaying repopulation of the pocket by spirochetes and motile bacteria.[85] These results, however, have
not been confirmed by other authors.[104] However, two 6-
month studies, one in abutment teeth of 61 patients and the
other in 74 orthodontic patients, in which stannous fluoride
was applied as a 0.4% gel showed a significant reduction in
plaque and gingivitis.[13,116] These two studies suggest that
there is potential value in stannous fluoride as a preventive
agent, possibly with formula modifications.

CONCLUSIONS

At the present time, the following recommendations can
be made:

1. Antibiotics may be recommended as adjuncts to conventional forms of therapy (i.e., root planing or surgery), not as
monotherapy.
2. Tetracyclines, including minocycline and doxycycline, are
effective adjuncts in the treatment of juvenile periodontitis,
rapidly progressive periodontitis, and refractory periodontitis. Also effective is metronidazole, either alone or in combination with Augmentin, amoxicillin, or ciprofloxacin.
3. When antibiotics are to be used, bacterial culturing for identification of putative pathogens and antibiotic sensitivity testing is recommended.
4. Tetracycline-impregnated EVA fibers can be used to treat localized recurrent sites that have not responded well to traditional periodontal therapy.
5. Routine home irrigation with or without medicaments reduces gingivitis scores. Such irrigation, particularly with
chlorhexidine gluconate or phenolic compounds, is beneficial in patients with gingivitis and in patients undergoing
periodontal maintenance. Marginal irrigation tips are more
effective at accessing periodontal pockets than are traditional
jet tips.
6. Professional subgingival irrigation of medicaments after root
planing provides negligible additional benefit over root planing alone.
7. The value of systemic antibiotics in enhancing the success
of new attachment and bone regeneration procedures and in
the modulation of host inflammatory responses is still uncertain at this time.

REFERENCES

1. Adams S, Burrows C, Skeldon N. Inhibition of prostaglandin synthesis and leukocyte migration by flurbiprophen. Curr Med Res Opin 5:11, 1977.
2. Addy M, Rowle L, Handley R, et al. The development and in vitro evaluation of acrylic strips and dialysis tubing for local drug delivery. J Periodontol 53:693, 1982.
3. Alger FA, Solt CW, Vuddhankanok S, Miles K. The histologic evaluation of new attachment in periodontally diseased human roots treated with tetracycline-hydrochloride and fibronectin. J Periodontol 61:447, 1990.
4. Amigone NA, Johnson GK, Kalkwarf KL. The use of sodium bicarbonate and hydrogen peroxide in periodontal therapy: A review. J Am Dent Assoc 114:217, 1987.
5. Bader HI, Goldhaber P. The passage of intravenously administered tetracycline into the gingival sulcus of dogs. J Oral Ther Pharmacol 2:324, 1968.
6. Baer PN, Limbardi RJ, Cox DS. The effects of H_2O_2 solution delivered to the base of periodontal pockets on pigmented Bacteroides. Abstract 1110. J Dent Res 65:182, 1986.
7. Baker PJ, Evans RT, Slots J, Genco RJ. Antibiotic susceptibility of anaerobic bacteria from the oral cavity. J Dent Res 65:1233, 1985.
8. Baker PJ, Evans RT, Slots J, Genco RJ. Susceptibility of human oral anaerobic bacteria to antibiotics suitable for topical use. J Clin Periodontol 12:201, 1985.
9. Baker PJ, Slots J, Genco RJ, Evans RT. Minimal inhibitory concentrations of various antimicrobial agents for human oral anaerobic bacteria. Antimicrob Agents Chemother 24:420, 1983.
10. Bhaskar SN, Cutright DE, Gross A, et al. Water jet devices in dental practice. J Periodontol 42:658, 1971.
11. Bjorvatn K, Skaug N, Selvig KA. Tetracycline-impregnated enamel and dentin: Duration of antimicrobial capacity. Scand J Dent Res 93:192, 1985.
12. Borzelleca J, Cherrick HM. Excretion of drugs in saliva. J Oral Ther Pharmacol 2:180, 1965.
13. Boyd R, Leggott P, Robertson P. Effects on gingivitis of two different 0.4% SnF₂ gels. J Dent Res 67:503, 1988.
14. Braatz L, Garrett S, Claffey N, Egelberg J. Antimicrobial irrigation of deep pockets to supplement non-surgical periodontal therapy. II. Daily irrigation. J Clin Periodontol 12:630, 1985.
15. Braun RE, Ciancio SG. Subgingival delivery by an oral irrigation device. J Periodontol 63:469, 1992.
16. Brownstein C, Briggs S, Schweitqer K, Kornman K. Gingival irrigation with chlorhexidine resolves naturally occurring gingivitis. Presented at the annual meeting of the American Academy of Periodontology, Denver, CO, 1987.
17. Bueno L, Walker C, Van Ness W, et al. Effect of augmentin on microbiota associated with refractory periodontitis. Abstract 1064. J Dent Res 67:246, 1988.
18. Carranza FA Jr, Saglie R, Newman MG, Valentin P. Scanning and transmission electron microscopic study of tissue-invading microorganisms in localized juvenile periodontitis. J Periodontol 54:598, 1983.
19. Carranza FA Sr. Experiencias clinicas sobre reinsercion. Ensayos con penicilina. Rev Asoc Odontol Argent 39:55, 1951.
20. Christersson LA, Slots J, Rosling BG, Genco RJ. Microbiological and clinical

effects of surgical treatment of localized juvenile periodontitis. J Clin Periodontol *12:*465, 1985.

21. Ciancio SG, Slots J, Reynolds HS, et al. The effect of short-term administration of minocycline HCl administration on gingival inflammation and subgingival microflora. J Periodontol *53:*557, 1982.

22. Ciancio SG, Mather ML, Zambon JJ, Reyneold HS. Effect of a chemotherapeutic agent delivered by an oral irrigation device on plaque, gingivitis, and subgingival microflora. J Periodontol *60:*310, 1989.

23. Ciancio SG. Use of antibiotics in periodontal therapy. In Newman MG, Goodman A, eds. Antibiotics in Dentistry. Chicago, Quintessence, 1983.

23a. Ciancio SG. Antibiotics in periodontal therapy. In Newman MG, Kornman K, eds. Antibiotic/Antimicrobial Use in Dental Practice. Chicago, Quintessence Publishing, 1990.

24. Council on Dental Therapeutics of the American Dental Association. Guidelines for acceptance of chemotherapeutic products for the control of supragingival plaque and gingivitis. J Am Dent Assoc *112:*529, 1986.

25. Coventry J, Newman HN. Experimental use of a slow release device employing chlorhexidine gluconate in areas of acute periodontal inflammation. J Clin Periodontol *9:*129, 1982.

26. Cummings B, Löe H. Optimal dosage and method of delivering chlorhexidine solutions for the inhibition of dental plaque. J Periodont Res *8:*57, 1973.

27. Demirel K, Baer PN, McNamara TF. Topical application of doxycycline on periodontally involved root surfaces in vitro: Comparative analysis of substantivity on cementum and dentin. J Periodontol *62:*312, 1991.

28. Duckworth R, Waterhouse JP, Britton DE, et al. Acute ulcerative gingivitis. A double-blind controlled clinical trial of metronidazole. Br Dent J *120:*599, 1966.

29. Eakle WS, Ford C, Boyle RL. Depth of penetration in periodontal pockets with oral irrigation. J Clin Periodontol *13:*39, 1986.

30. Edelson H, Kaplan H, Korchak H. Differing effects of non-steroidal anti-inflammatory agents on neutrophil functions. Clin Res *30:*469A, 1982.

31. Elkayam R, Friedman M, Stabholz A, et al. Sustained release device containing minocycline for local treatment of periodontal disease. J Controlled Release *7:*231, 1988.

32. Feldman R, Szeto B, Chauncey H, et al. Non-steroidal anti-inflammatory drugs in the reduction of human alveolar bone loss. J Clin Periodontol *10:*131, 1983.

33. Flemmig TF, Newman MG, Doherty FM, et al. Supragingival irrigation with 0.06% chlorhexidine in naturally occurring gingivitis. I. 6 month clinical observations. J Periodontol *61:*112, 1990.

34. Genco RJ, Cianciola JJ, Rosling H. Treatment of localized juvenile periodontitis. Abstract 872. J Dent Res *60:*527, 1981.

35. Gibson W. Antibiotics and periodontal disease: A selective review of the literature. J Am Dent Assoc *104:*213, 1982.

36. Gold SI. Combined therapy in the treatment of periodontosis: Case report. Periodont Case Rep *1:*12, 1979.

37. Golomb G, Freidman M, Soskolne A, et al. Sustained release device containing metronidazole for periodontal use. J Dent Res *63:*1149, 1984.

38. Golub LM, Goodson JM, Lee HM, et al. Tetracyclines inhibit tissue collagenases. Effects of ingested low-dose and local delivery systems. J Periodontol Special Issue, p. 93, 1985.

39. Golub LM, Ramamurthy NS, Kaneko H, et al. Tetracycline administration prevents diabetes-induced osteopenia in the rat: Initial observations. Res Commun Chem Pathol Pharmacol *68:*27, 1990.

40. Golub LM, Wolff M, Lee HM, et al. Further evidence that tetracyclines inhibit collagenase activity in human crevicular fluid and from other mammalian sources. J Periodont Res *20:*12, 1985.

41. Goodson JM, Offenbacher S, Farr DH, Hogan PE. Periodontal disease treatment by local delivery. J Periodontol *56:*265, 1985.

42. Goodson JM, Cugini M, Kent R, et al. Multi-center evaluation of tetracycline fiber therapy. I. Experimental design. J Periodont Res *26:*361, 1991.

43. Goodson JM, Cugini M, Kent R, et al. Multi-center evaluation of tetracycline fiber therapy. II. Clinical response. J Periodont Res *26:*371, 1991.

44. Goodson JM, Haffajee A, Socransky SS. Periodontal therapy by local delivery of tetracycline. J Clin Periodontol *6:*83, 1979.

44a. Goodson JM. Antimicrobial strategies for treatment of periodontal diseases. Periodontol 2000 *5:*142, 1994.

45. Gordon JM, Walker CB, Murphy JC. Concentration of tetracycline in human gingival fluid after single doses. J Clin Periodontol *8:*117, 1981.

46. Greenstein G. Effects of subgingival irrigation on periodontal status. J Periodontol *58:*827, 1987.

47. Greenstein G. Supragingival and subgingival irrigation: Practical application in the treatment of periodontal diseases. Compend Contin Educ Dent *13:*1098, 1992.

48. Greenstein G. The role of metronidazole in the treatment of periodontal diseases. J Periodontol *1:*1, 1993.

49. Greenwell H, Baker A, Bissada N, Debanne S. Clinical and microbiological effectiveness of Keyes' method of oral hygiene on human periodontitis with and without surgery. J Am Dent Assoc *106:*457, 1983.

50. Hardy JH, Newman HN, Strahan JD. Direct irrigation and subgingival plaque. J Clin Periodontol *9:*57, 1982.

51. Haskel E, Esquenasi J, Yussim L. Effects of subgingival chlorhexidine irrigation in chronic moderate periodontitis. J Periodontol *57:*305, 1986.

52. Heasam PA, Benn DK, Kelly PJ, et al. The use of topical flurbiprofen as an adjunct to non-surgical management of periodontal disease. J Clin Periodontol *20:*457, 1993.

53. Heijl H, Lindhe J. The effect of metronidazole on the development of plaque and gingivitis in the beagle dog. J Clin Periodontol *6:*197, 1979.

54. Hollander B, Boyd R, Eakle W. Comparison of cannula versus standard tip for oral irrigation. Abstract 1829. J Dent Res *68:*410, 1989.

55. Itic J, Serfaty R. Clinical effectiveness of subgingival irrigation with a pulsated jet irrigator versus syringe. J Periodontol *63:*174, 1992.

56. Jeffcoat MK, Williams RC, Goldhaber P. Effect of tetracycline on gingival inflammation and alveolar bone resorption in beagles: An individual tooth by tooth analysis. J Clin Periodontol *9:*489, 1982.

57. Jolkovsky DL, Waki MY, Newman MG, et al. Clinical and microbiological effects of subgingival and marginal irrigation with chlorhexidine gluconate. J Periodontol *61:*663, 1990.

58. Kaplan H, Edelson H, Korchak H, et al. Effects of non-steroidal anti-inflammatory agents on neutrophil functions in vitro and in vivo. Biochem Pharmacol *33:*371, 1984.

59. Keyes PH, Rowberry SA, Englander HA, Fitzgerald RJ. Bioassays of medicaments for the control of dentobacterial plaque, dental caries and periodontal lesions in the Syrian hamster. J Oral Ther Pharmacol *3:*157, 1966.

60. Khoo JL, Newman HN. Subgingival plaque control by a simplified oral hygiene regime plus local chlorhexidine or metronidazole. J Periodont Res *18:*607, 1983.

61. Kornman KS. Controlled-release local delivery antimicrobials in periodontics: Prospects for the future. J Periodontol *64:*783, 1993.

62. Kornman KS, Karl EH. The effect of long-term low-dose tetracycline therapy on the subgingival microflora in refractory adult periodontitis. J Periodontol *53:*604, 1982.

63. Kornman KS, Caffesse RG, Nasjleti CE. The effects of intensive antibacterial therapy on the sulcular environment in monkeys. Changes in the bacteriology of the gingival sulcus. J Periodontol *51:*34, 1980.

64. Kornman KS, Robertson PB. Clinical and microbiological evaluation of therapy for juvenile periodontitis. J Periodontol *56:*443, 1985.

65. Kritchevsky B, Seguin P. The pathogenesis and treatment of pyorrhea alveolaris. Dent Cosmos *60:*781, 1918. Translated from La Presse Medicale, Paris, May 13, 1918.

66. Krogh HW. Reduction of the gingival flora preceding operation. J Am Dent Assoc *19:*659, 1932.

67. Lang NP, Brecx MC. Chlorhexidine digluconate—an agent for chemical plaque control and prevention of gingival inflammation. J Periodont Res *21*(suppl 16):74, 1986.

68. Lang NP, Ramseier-Grossman K. Optimal dosage of chlorhexidine digluconate in clinical plaque control when applied by the oral irrigator. J Clin Periodontol *8:*189, 1981.

69. Lekovic V, Kenney EB, Carranza FA Jr, Endres B. Effect of metronidazole on human periodontal disease. A clinical and microbiologic study. J Periodontol *54:*476, 1983.

70. Lindhe J, Liljenberg B, Adielson B, Borjesson I. Use of metronidazole as a probe in the study of human periodontal disease. J Clin Periodontol *10:*100, 1983.

71. Listgarten MA, Lindhe J, Hellden L. Effect of tetracycline and/or scaling on human periodontal disease. J Clin Periodontol *5:*246, 1978.

72. Listgarten MA, Lindhe J, Parodi R. The effect of systemic antimicrobial therapy on plaque and gingivitis in dogs. J Periodont Res *14:*65, 1979.

73. Löe H. Chlorhexidine in the prevention and treatment of gingivitis. J Periodont Res *21*(suppl 16), 1986.

74. Löe H: Periodontal diseases: a brief historical perspective. Periodontology 2000 *2:*7, 1993.

75. Loesche WJ. The treatment of periodontal patients according to the specific plaque hypothesis. In Carranza FA Jr, Kenney EB, eds. Prevention of Periodontal Disease. Chicago, Quintessence, 1981.

76. Loesche WJ, Giordano JR, Hujoel P, et al. Metronidazole in periodontitis: Reduced need for surgery. J Clin Periodontol *19:*103, 1992.

77. Lozdan J, Sheiham A, Pearlman BA, et al. The use of nitrimidazine in the treatment of acute ulcerative gingivitis. A double-blind controlled trial. Br Dent J *130:*294, 1971.

78. MacAlpine R, Magnusson I, Kiger R, et al. Antimicrobial irrigation of deep pockets to supplement oral hygiene instructions and root debridement. I. Bi-weekly irrigation. J Clin Periodontol *12:*568, 1985.

79. Macaulay WJ, Newman HN. The effect on composition of subgingival plaque of a simplified oral hygiene system includine pulsating jet subgingival irrigation. J Periodontol Res *21:*375, 1986.

80. Maehara R, Hinode D, Terai H, et al. Inhibition of bacterial and mammalian collagenolytic activities by tetracyclines. J Jpn Assoc Periodontol *30:*182, 1988.

81. Mandell RL, Socransky SS. Microbiological and clinical effects of surgery plus doxycycline on juvenile periodontitis. J Periodontol *59:*373, 1988.

82. Mandell RL, Tripodi LS, Savitt E, et al. The effect of treatment on *Actinobacillus actinomycetemcomitans* in localized juvenile periodontitis. J Periodontol *57:*94, 1986.

83. Marks SC, Mehta NR. Lack of effect of citric acid treatment of root surfaces on the formation of new connective tissue attachment. J Clin Periodontol *13:*109, 1986.

84. Mashimoto PA, Umemoto T, Slots J. Pathogenicity testing of *Macaca arctoides* subgingival plaque following chlorhexidine treatment. J Periodontol *51:*190, 1980.

85. Mazza JE, Newman MG, Sims TN. Clinical and antimicrobial effect of stannous fluoride on periodontitis. J Clin Periodontol *8:*203, 1981.

86. Mills WH, Thompson GW, Beagrie GS. Clinical evaluation of spiramycin and erythromycin in control of periodontal disease. J Clin Periodontol 6:308, 1979.

87. Miller WD. Die Mikroorganismen der Mundhöhle. Leipzig, Thieme, 1889.

88. Newman MG, Flemmig TF, Nachnani S, et al. Irrigation with 0.06% chlorhexidine in naturally occuring gingivitis. II. 6 month microbiological observations. J Periodontol 61:427, 1990.

89. Newman MG, Kornman KS, Doherty FM. A 6-month multi-center evaluation of adjunctive tetracycline fiber therapy used in conjunction with scaling and root planing in maintenance patients: Clinical results. J Periodontol 65:685, 1994.

90. Reference deleted.

91. Novak JM, Polson A, Adair S. Tetracycline therapy in patients with early juvenile periodontitis. J Periodontol 59:366, 1989.

92. Novak JM, Stamatelakys C, Adair S. Resolution of early lesions of juvenile periodontitis with tetracycline therapy alone: Long-term observations of 4 cases. J Periodontol 62:628, 1991.

93. Offenbacher S, Braswell L, Loos A, et al. Effects of flurbiprophen on the progression of periodontitis in *Macaca mulatta*. J Periodont Res 22:473, 1987.

94. Oliver RE, Egelberg J, Crigger M, Rathbun E. The effect of chlorhexidine on subgingival microbial colonization. Abstract 595. J Dent Res 52:593, 1973.

95. Otomo-Corgel J. Over-the-counter and prescription mouthwashes—an update for the 1990s. Compend Contin Educ Dent 13:1086, 1992.

96. Perry DA. Fluorides and periodontal disease: A review of the literature. J West Soc Periodontol 30:92, 1982.

97. Pitaru S, Hekmati M, Geiger S, Savion N. The effects of partial demineralization and fibronectin on migration and growth of gingival epithelial cells on cementum in vitro. J Dent Res 67:1386, 1988.

98. Rams TE, Wright WE, Keyes PH, Howard SA. Long-term effects of microbiologically modulated therapy of advanced adult periodontitis. J Am Dent Assoc 111:429, 1985.

99. Rams TE, Slots J. Antibiotics in periodontal therapy: An update. Compend Contin Educ Dent 13:1130, 1992.

100. Rams TE, Feik D, Slots J. Ciprofloxacin/metronidazole treatment of recurrent adult periodontitis. Abstract. J Dent Res 71:319, 1992.

101. Research, Science and Therapy Committee. Pharmacologic blocking of host responses as an adjunct in the management of periodontal diseases: A research update. Chicago, The American Academy of Periodontology, 1992.

101a. Ross N, Charles H, Dills SS. Long-term effects of Listerine antiseptic on dental plaque and gingivitis. J Clin Dent 1:92, 1989.

102. Saglie FR, Carranza FA Jr, Newman MG, et al. Identification of tissue invading bacteria in human periodontal disease. J Periodont Res 17:452, 1982.

103. Schiott CR, Löe H. The sensitivity of oral streptococci to chlorhexidine. J Periodont Res 7:192, 1972.

104. Schmid E, Kornman KS, Tinanoff N. Changes of subgingival total colony forming units and black pigmented *Bacteroides* after a single irrigation of periodontal pockets with 1.64% SnF$_2$. J Periodontol 56:330, 1985.

105. Shinn DH. Metronidazole in acute ulcerative gingivitis. Lancet 1:1191, 1962.

105a. Siegrist BE, Gusberti FA, Brecx MC, et al. Efficacy of supervised rinsing with chlorhexidine digluconate in comparison to phenolic and plant alkaloid compounds. J Period Res 21(suppl):60, 1986.

106. Slots J, Mashimo P, Levine MJ, Genco RJ. Periodontal therapy in humans. I. Microbiological and clinical effects of a single course of periodontal scaling and root planing, and of adjunctive tetracycline therapy. J Periodontol 50:495, 1979.

107. Slots J, Rams TE. Antibiotics and periodontal therapy: Advantages and disadvantages. J Clin Periodontol 17:479, 1990.

108. Slots J, Rosling BG. Suppression of periodontopathic microflora in localized juvenile periodontitis by systemic tetracycline. J Clin Periodontol 10:465, 1983.

109. Soder P, Frithiof L, Wikner S, et al. The effects of systemic metronidazole after non-surgical treatment in moderate and advanced periodontitis in young adults. J Periodontol 61:281, 1990.

110. Soh LL, Newman HN, Strahan JD. Effects of subgingival chlorhexidine irrigation on periodontal inflammation. J Clin Periodontol 9:66, 1982.

111. Stanley A, Wilson M, Newman HN. The in vitro effects of chlorhexidine on subgingival plaque bacteria. J Clin Periodontol 16:259, 1989.

112. Steinberg D, Friedman M, Soskolne A, Sela MN. A new biodegradable controlled-release device for treatment of periodontal disease: In vitro release study. J Periodontol 61:393, 1990.

113. Sznajder N, Piovano S, Bernat MI, et al. Effect of spiramycin therapy on human periodontal disease. J Clin Periodontol 22:255, 1987.

114. Terranova VP, Franzetti LC, Hic S, et al. A biologic approach to periodontal regeneration—tetracycline treatment of dentin promotes fibroblast adhesion and growth. J Periodont Res 21:330, 1986.

115. Terranova VP, Hic S, Frenzetti L, et al. A biochemical approach to periodontal regeneration. J Periodontol 58:247, 1987.

116. Tinanoff N, Manwell M, Zameck R, Grasso J. Clinical and microbiological effects of daily brushing with either NaF or SnF$_2$ in subjects with fixed or removable dental prostheses. J Clin Periodontol 16:284, 1989.

117. Tyler K, Walker C, Gordon J, et al. Evaluation of clindamycin in adult refractory periodontitis: Antimicrobial susceptibilities. Abstract 1667. J Dent Res 64 (special issue):360, 1985.

118. van der Ouderaa F, Cummins D. Delivery systems for agents in supra and subgingival plaque control. J Dent Res 68(special issue):1617, 1989.

119. Vogel R, Schneider L, Goteinter D. The effects of a topical nonsteroidal anti-inflammatory drug on ligature induced periodontal disease in the squirrel monkey. J Clin Periodontol 12:139, 1986.

120. Waite I, Saxon C, Young A, et al. The periodontal status of subjects receiving non-steroidal anti-inflammatory drugs. J Periodont Res 16:100, 1981.

121. Walker CB, Gordon JM, Socransky SS. Antibiotic susceptibility testing of subgingival plaque samples. J Clin Periodontol 10:422, 1983.

122. Wan Yusof WZA, Newman HN, Strahan HD, Coventry JF. Subgingival metronidazole in dialysis tubing and subgingival chlorhexidine irrigation in the control of chronic inflammatory periodontal disease. J Clin Periodontol 11:166, 1984.

123. Weiner GS, DeMarco TJ, Bissada NF. Long term effects of systemic tetracycline administration on the severity of induced periodontitis in the rat. J Periodontol 50:619, 1979.

124. Weinstein L. Antimicrobial agents: Tetracyclines and chloramphenicol. In Goodman LS, Gilman A, eds. The Pharmachological Basis of Therapeutics. New York, Macmillan, 1975.

125. Weinstein L. Antimicrobial agents: Penicillins and cephalosporins. In Goodman LS, Gilman A, eds. The Pharmachological Basis of Therapeutics. New York, Macmillan, 1975.

126. Westling M, Tylenius-Bratthal G. Microbial short-term effects of repeated intracrevicular chlorhexidine rinsings. J Periodont Res 19:202, 1984.

127. White CL, Drisko CL, Mayberry WE, et al. The effect of supervised water irrigation on subgingival microflora in untreated gingivitis and periodontitis. Abstract 2298. J Dent Res 67(special issue):400, 1989.

128. Williams RC, Leone CW, Jeffcoat MK, et al. Tetracycline treatment of periodontal disease in the beagle dog. I. Clinical and radiographic course over 12 months—maximal effect on rate of alveolar bone loss. J Periodont Res 16:659, 1981.

129. Williams RC, Jeffcoat MK, Howell T, et al. Ibuprofen: An inhibitor of alveolar bone resorption in beagles. J Periodont Res 23:225, 1988.

130. Williams RC, Jeffcoat MK, Howell T, et al. Indomethacin or flurbiprofen treatment of periodontitis in beagles: Comparison of effect on bone loss. J Periodont Res 22:403, 1987.

131. Williams RC, Jeffcoat MK, Howell T, et al. Altering the progression of human alveolar bone loss with the non-steroidal anti-inflammatory drug flurbiprofen. J Periodontol 60:485, 1989.

132. Williams RC, Jeffcoat MK, Howell T, et al. Three year trial of flurbiprofen treatment in humans: Post-treatment period. Abstract #1617. J Dent Res 70:448, 1991.

133. Williams RC, Jeffcoat MK, Wechter WJ, et al. Flurbiprofen: A potent inhibitor of alveolar bone resorption in beagles. Science 227:640, 1985.

134. Wolff LR, Bandt C, Pihlstrom B, Brayer H. Phase contrast microscopic evaluation of subgingival plaque in combination with either conventional or antimicrobial home treatment of patients with periodontal inflammation. J Periodont Res 17:537, 1982.

135. Wright BL. The treatment of pyorrhea alveolaris and its secondary systemic infections by deep muscular injections of mercury. Dent Cosmos 57:1003 1915.

45

Treatment of Aggressive Forms of Periodontitis: Refractory, Rapidly Progressive, Necrotizing Ulcerative, and Juvenile

MICHAEL G. NEWMAN, DONALD F. ADAMS,
VANESSA MARINHO, and FERMIN A. CARRANZA, JR.

The majority of patients with the commonly encountered forms of chronic adult periodontitis usually respond well to conventional therapies. Typically these include nonsurgical debridement and surgery, followed by adequate long-term maintenance. However, some patients (as many as 17%) with atypical and less frequently encountered types of periodontitis do not respond to these conventional treatment approaches. The major classifications of these atypical forms of periodontitis are refractory, rapidly progressive, necrotizing ulcerative, and juvenile periodontitis.[14,22]

The treatment of all of these types of periodontitis is complex and often requires the use of the most intensive and comprehensive therapeutic modalities. Because these patients do not respond "normally" to conventional methods, the logical question is whether there are problems associated with their host response systems. Although there have been many attempts to clarify the immunologic profile of these patients, there have been no major or definitive breakthroughs important for improving the outcomes of therapy. The best treatment for these patients appears to be the combination of antimicrobial therapy with scaling and root planing. Bacterial identification appears to be of value for treatment in these patients, because the information can be used to determine the antibiotic susceptibility of suspected pathogens. Similarly, other bacterial tests have been used to monitor the microflora that recolonize after treatment.

DIAGNOSIS OF REFRACTORY PERIODONTITIS

A diagnosis of refractory periodontitis requires the gathering of baseline data and a subsequent evaluation. This is the major way in which the clinician can determine the normality of the patient's response to treatment (see Chapter 26). A few individuals may appear for the first time with unusually severe forms of periodontal destruction for their age. In these cases the initial diagnosis is not refractory periodontitis, but one of the other rapidly progressive diseases discussed later.

A patient with refractory periodontitis often does not have any distinguishing clinical characteristics on initial examination. After treatment, the differential diagnosis of refractory periodontitis should exclude the following:

1. *Improperly treated periodontitis.* Most forms of periodontitis can be treated effectively with currently available modalities if such modalities are performed properly. If, during a post-treatment examination, it is determined that the patient has not adequately responded to treatment, it must be determined whether the therapy was correctly implemented. The only way to rule out inadequately treated periodontitis is to perform the most thorough treatment available. Treatment of all etiologic factors and utilization of the most advanced techniques are essential.

2. *Periodontitis associated with poor plaque control.* Because plaque control is a prerequisite for the success of periodontal treatments,[26,33,34] special attention should be paid to the careful evaluation of plaque control before deciding on classifying a case as refractory periodontitis. Truly refractory periodontitis presupposes a type of periodontal disease that is far more nonresponsive or tenacious than the usual cases. A patient who does not comply with adequate oral hygiene procedures might also be seen by many clinicians as a failure of the dental professional to adequately motivate, educate, and control the patient. If considered from this perspective, these cases should be included in the "maltreated periodontitis" category.

3. *Endodontic lesions.* The presence of endodontic involvement

should be suspected and ruled out before a diagnosis of refractory periodontitis is made. The clinician should suspect an endodontic etiology especially in those patients with localized recurrent disease.

A true case of refractory periodontitis can be diagnosed if loss of attachment has occurred after adequate treatment has been performed and all etiologic agents have been controlled.

TREATMENT MODALITIES

Refractory Periodontitis

Estimates of prognosis and treatment predictability must be based on the evidence available from the literature and the clinician's own experience.[24] The first step in the treatment of refractory periodontitis with antimicrobial therapy must be microbial diagnostic and susceptibility tests. The results of these tests provide information about the presence and relative percentages of suspected periodontal pathogens and, more importantly, determine the organism's sensitivity to specific antimicrobials. This information enables the clinician to make the most informed and appropriate decision about antibiotic selection.

A combination of debridement and systemic antibiotic treatment can reduce bleeding on probing, suppuration, pocket depth, and incidence of active lesions and can suppress or eliminate periodontal pathogens in patients who present with refractory periodontitis. Mechanical debridement with scaling and root planing results in a dramatic reduction in the recoverable counts of most periodontopathogenic bacteria. However, local mechanical therapy often fails to completely eliminate, for example, *Actinobacillus actinomycetemcomitans* from early-onset periodontitis cases. Surgical treatment may also eliminate the marginal tissues that might be invaded by bacteria.[35] In addition, the morphology of the gingival tissues should be modified to facilitate daily plaque removal by the patient.

Antibiotic therapy in the treatment of refractory periodontitis is based on the results obtained from the microbial diagnostic tests. Many antibiotics have been used according to the target microflora (Table 45–1), with various degrees of success. For refractory periodontitis patients

Table 45–1. ANTIBIOTIC THERAPY IN THE TREATMENT OF REFRACTORY OR RAPIDLY PROGRESSIVE PERIODONTITIS

Associated Microflora	Antibiotic of Choice
Gram-positive organisms	Amoxicillin–clavulanate potassium (Augmentin)[8,51]
Gram-negative organisms	Clindamycin[12,13,50,51]
Nonoral gram-negative facultative rods	Ciprofloxacin[37]
Black-pigmented bacteria and spirochetes	Metronidazole[12,42]
Prevotella intermedia, Porphyromonas gingivalis, Actinobacillus actinomycetemcomitans	Tetracycline[19,28]
A. actinomycetemcomitans	Metronidazole/amoxicillin[12,42] Tetracycline[19,27]
P. gingivalis	Azithromycin[29]

who fail to respond to initial antibiotic therapy, subsequent treatment should include antimicrobial susceptibility testing of the remaining flora.

Patients diagnosed as having refractory periodontitis often present with a history of tetracycline therapy and microflora that is relatively resistant to this drug owing to the frequent use of this antibiotic.[15,23,48,49,51,52] Tetracycline-resistant bacteria containing the Tet M gene for resistance have been isolated from patients with refractory periodontitis.[27] However, some patients with refractory periodontitis may still benefit from the use of tetracycline.

Cases of refractory periodontitis in which the associated microflora consists primarily of gram-positive microorganisms have been successfully treated with amoxicillin–clavulanate potassium. Many efforts have been made to establish the most appropriate regimen of antibiotic therapy for these patients. Similar antimicrobials consisting of 250 mg amoxicillin and 125 mg potassium clavulanate have been administered three times a day for 14 days along with scaling and root planing and produced a reduction in attachment loss for at least 12 months. A regimen of one capsule containing the same amount of drug every 6 hours for 2 weeks, plus intrasulcular full-mouth lavage with a 10% povidone-iodine solution and chlorhexidine mouthwash rinses twice daily, showed a reduction in attachment loss that persisted at approximately 34 months.[8]

Clindamycin is a potent antibiotic that penetrates well into gingival fluid, although it is not usually effective against *A. actinomycetemcomitans* and *Eikenella corrodens*.[47] However, it has been demonstrated to be effective in controlling the extent and rate of disease progression in refractory cases in patients who have a microflora susceptible to this antibiotic.[12,37] A regimen of clindamycin hydrochloride 150 mg qid for 7 days combined with scaling and root planing produced a decrease in the incidence of disease activity from an annual rate of 8% to 0.5% of sites per patient.[12] Azithromycin may be effective in refractory periodontitis in patients infected with *P. gingivalis*.[29]

Combinations of antibiotic therapy may offer greater promise as adjunctive treatment for the management of refractory periodontitis.[1,16,23,41] The rationale is based on the diversity of putative pathogens[10,20,42] and the fact that no single antibiotic is bactericidal for all known pathogens.

Many combinations of antibiotics (e.g., metronidazole/Augmentin®[16,41] for the treatment of *A. actinomycetemcomitans*–associated periodontitis, doxycycline/metronidazole[1] for the prevention of recurrent periodontitis, metronidazole/ciprofloxacin[32] for the treatment of recurrent cases containing a microflora associated with enteric rods and pseudomonads, and amoxicillin/doxycycline[23] in the treatment of *A. actinomycetemcomitans*– and/or *Porphyromonas gingivalis*–associated periodontitis) have demonstrated significant improvement in the clinical aspects of the disease.[23]

Some cases of refractory periodontitis may not respond to a given antibiotic regimen. When this occurs, the clinician should consider a different antimicrobial therapy based on microbial susceptibility. At this point in the therapy strong consideration should be given to consulting with the patient's physician for an evaluation of a possible host immune system deficiency or a metabolic problem such as diabetes.

Although there have been no studies of the treatment of refractory periodontitis with local delivery systems, it is possible that this method could be used in localized forms of this disease, particularly localized aggressive periodontal diseases. The advantage of local therapy is that smaller dosages of topical chemotherapy can be delivered inside the pocket, avoiding the side effects of systemic antibacterial agents.[11]

The approach to restorative treatment for these patients should be made based on one single premise: "Plan for future tooth loss." The teeth with the best prognosis should be identified and considered when planning the restorative work. However, the predictive value of the traditional prognosis categorization can be as low as 43% in patients with refractory periodontitis.[14] The lower cuspids and first premolars are generally more resistant to loss. As a rule, an extensive fixed prosthesis should be avoided, and removable partial dentures should be planned in such a way as to allow for the addition of teeth. The use of dental implants should be considered with great caution, especially in partially edentulous patients.

Although a cause-and-effect relationship has not yet been established between periodontitis and peri-implantitis, a relationship between the microflora associated with periodontal and peri-implant pockets has been described.[19,30,31] Although the combination of implants and periodontally diseased teeth might be possible, the risks involved should be clearly explained to the patient and avoided until the patient's disease is stabilized.

Rapidly Progressive Periodontitis

In general the treatment of patients with rapidly progressive forms of periodontitis should be very similar to that of patients with refractory forms of the disease. To date there are no available data that suggest any alterations in the approach used for refractory forms of the disease.

The rate of disease progression may be faster in these younger individuals, and therefore, the clinician should monitor such patients more frequently. Close collaboration between members of the treatment team, which includes the periodontist, the general dentist, the dental hygienist, and the patient's physician, is required.

It is important to monitor and observe the patient's overall physical status, as weight loss, mental depression, and malaise have been reported in patients with rapidly progressive periodontitis. Similarly, flare-ups of proliferative gingival inflammation can be observed early when the patient is on a frequent monitoring cycle. Currently monitoring every 3 weeks or less is suggested while the disease is in an active phase.

Necrotizing Ulcerative Periodontitis

Patients with necrotizing ulcerative periodontits (NUP) are unusual and should be treated in consultation with the physician. As indicated in Chapter 26, these patients often have an underlying predisposing systemic factor that renders the patient susceptible to necrosis of the periodontal structures. It is mandatory that these patients be treated aggressively. This includes a medical evaluation and local, topical, and systemic antimicrobials based on the results of laboratory tests.

These patients often harbor bacteria, fungi, viruses, and other nonoral microorganisms, making the selection of treatment complicated. Oral hygiene for these patients is complicated by the sometimes painful tissues. In such cases, irrigation with diluted cleansing and antibacterial agents can be of some benefit.

The treatment of AIDS-associated NUP is presented in Chapter 46.

Juvenile Periodontitis

The prognosis for patients with juvenile periodontitis depends on whether the disease is generalized or localized and on the degree of destruction present at the time of examination. The generalized forms, which are usually associated with some systemic disease (see Chapter 27), have a worse prognosis than the localized forms. Juvenile periodontitis rarely undergoes spontaneous remission. It is important to obtain earlier radiographs to assess the stage of the disease.

The following treatments for localized juvenile periodontitis have been attempted in the past, with various degrees of success:

1. *Extraction.* After the involved teeth, usually the first molars, have been extracted, uneventful healing ensues. The enlargement of the maxillary sinus has been mentioned as an unfavorable sequela that would make future treatment of neighboring teeth difficult.[2,3] Transplantation of developing third molars to the sockets of previously extracted first molars has also been attempted.

2. *Standard periodontal therapy.* Such therapy has included scaling and root planing, curettage, flap surgery with and without bone grafts, root amputations, hemisections, occlusal adjustment, and strict plaque control.[2,5,40] However, response has been unpredictable. Frequent maintenance visits appear to be most important.[18,45,46]

3. *Antibiotic therapy.* In the late 1970s and early 1980s, the identification of *A. actinomycetemcomitans* as a major culprit and the discovery that this organism penetrates the tissues clarified the pathogenesis and provided a more solid basis for therapy. Several authors have reported success using antibiotics as adjuncts to standard therapy. Genco and coworkers[10] reported the treatment of localized juvenile periodontitis with scaling and root planing plus tetracycline (250 mg qid for 14 days every 8 weeks). Measurements of vertical defects were made at intervals of up to 18 months after the initiation of therapy. Bone loss had stopped, and one third of the defects demonstrated an increase in bone level, whereas in the control group, bone loss continued.

Liljenberg and Lindhe[17] treated patients with localized juvenile periodontitis with tetracycline (250 mg qid for 2 weeks), modified Widman flaps, and periodic recall visits (one visit every month for 6 months, then one visit every 3 months). The lesions healed more rapidly and more completely than similar lesions in patients with adult periodontitis. These investigators re-evaluated their results after 5 years and found that the treatment had resulted in resolution of gingival inflammation, gain of clinical attachment, and refill of bone in angular defects.[18]

Several investigators have noted excellent bone fill in cases of localized juvenile periodontitis treated with tetracycline plus flap surgery and placement of grafts.[21,53] Fig-

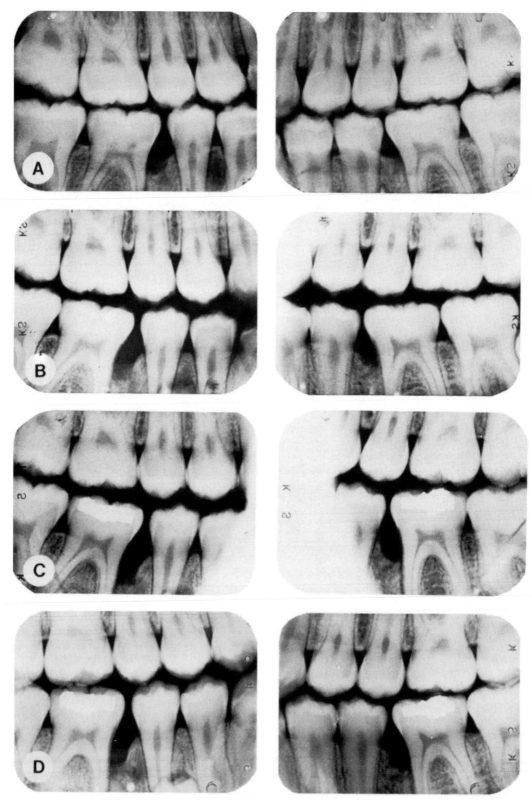

FIGURE 45–1. Radiographs depicting progression of the osseous lesion in a case of localized juvenile periodontitis. *A*, January 29, 1979: *B*, August 16, 1979; *C*, February 22, 1980; *D*. May 15, 1981. Note the progressive deterioration of the osseous level. (From Barnett ML, Baker RL. The formation and healing of osseous lesions in a patient with localized juvenile periodontitis. Case report. J Periodontol *54*:148, 1983.)

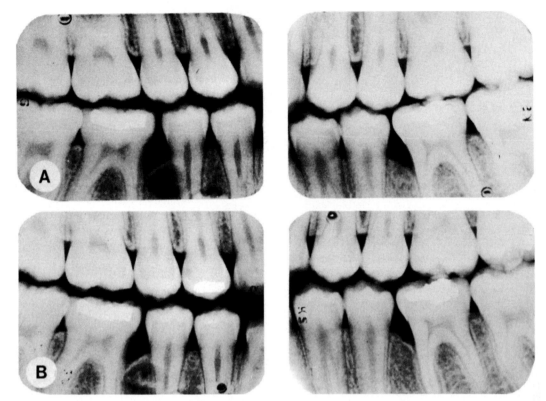

FIGURE 45–2. Postoperative radiographs of the patient shown in Figure 45–1. *A*, November 6, 1981; *B*, March 3, 1982. Treatment consisted of oral hygiene instruction; scaling and root planing concurrently with 1 gram of tetracycline per day for 2 weeks; and, finally, modified Widman flaps. (From Barnett ML, Baker RL. The formation and healing of osseous lesions in a patient with localized juvenile periodontitis. Case report. J Periodontol *54*:148, 1983.)

ures 45–1 and 45–2 show pretreatment destruction and bone repair in a patient treated by Barnett and Baker.[6]

The lack of response of juvenile periodontitis to local therapy alone has been interpreted as the result of the presence of *A. actinomycetemcomitans* in the tissues,[7,36] where it remains after therapy to reinfect the pocket. The systemic use of antibiotics is needed to eliminate bacteria from the tissues.[37]

Current Approach to Therapy. Patients who are diagnosed as having an early form of juvenile periodontitis may respond to standard periodontal therapy. In general, the earlier the disease is diagnosed (as determined by less destruction), the more conservative the therapy may be and the more predictable the outcome.

In almost all cases, systemic tetracycline (250 mg of tetracycline hydrochloride qid for at least 1 week) should be given in conjunction with local mechanical therapy. If surgery is indicated, systemic tetracycline should be prescribed, with the patient instructed to begin taking the antibiotic approximately 1 hour before surgery. Doxycycline 100 mg/day may also be used.

Chlorhexidine rinses should also be prescribed and continued for several weeks to aid healing and augment plaque control.

In refractory localized juvenile periodontitis cases, tetracycline-resistant *Actinobacillus* species have been suspected. After performing antibiotic susceptibility tests, the clinician may consider a combination of amoxicillin and metronidazole, similar to the regimen suggested for refractory periodontitis patients.[41,42]

TREATMENT ALGORITHM

Individualizing treatment based on information about the patient's bacteria can be difficult because (1) patients with the same clinical presentation can have great differences in their periodontal microflora and (2) patients with the same microflora can have great variations in their clinical presentations.[24]

Figure 45–3 shows a decision pathway, or algorithm, for a patient with refractory periodontitis. This algorithm can also be used as a general guide for many types of patients with aggressive forms of disease considered in this chapter.[25] It begins with the identification of patient's disease (A) or nondisease (B) status. The presence of periodontal disease (A) guides the clinician to perform a series of treatments (C) that usually begins with scaling and root planing and often continues to periodontal surgery.[25]

After treatment, re-evaluation of the patient (D) is done to determine whether the patient is stable (E) or not stable (F). At this stage, the patient will present with a combination of clinical signs that are a result of an etiologic agent interacting with a predisposing factor to produce the patient's observed clinical status. As an example, we will use the presence of periodontal pathogens as the target etiologic factor. There are four possible conditions that describe the patient's status (boxes 1, 2, 3, and 4 in Fig. 45–4).

Box 1 in Figure 45–4 represents a situation in which both clinical signs of disease and periodontal pathogens are present. Clinical therapy is strongly recommended, because the tooth is clearly at risk for progression of disease.

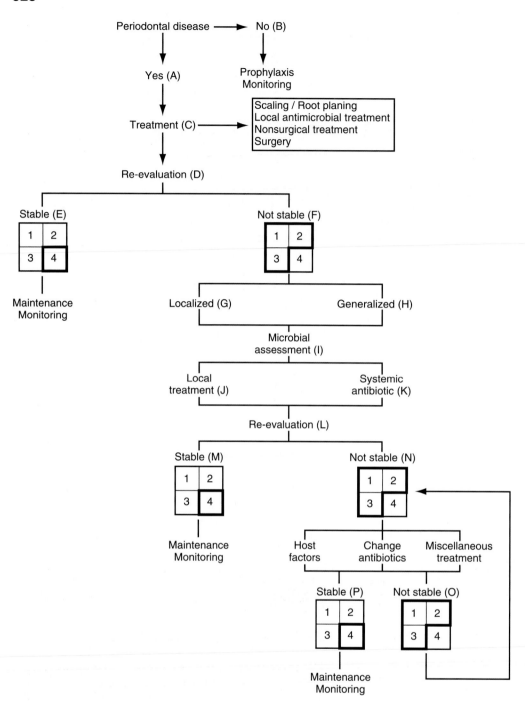

FIGURE 45-3. Decision pathway.

Box 2 in Figure 45–4 indicates a situation in which clinical signs of disease are present in the absence of periodontal pathogens as detected by the particular test used for the patient. In this case treatment should be performed. The rationale for this decision is based on the presence of disease and the fact the particular test used in this case may have "missed" some pathologic organisms because it was not designed to detect them. Similarly, in this group of patients, unusual microorganisms may be encountered, and initial testing may not be sufficient. Thus, the clinical status dictates the course of treatment.

Box 3 in Figure 45–4 represents the inverse of box 2. In this case periodontal pathogens are present in the absence of clinical signs. The presence of pathogens puts the site,

and therefore the tooth, at risk and suggests a worse prognosis. Treatment may vary considerably among patients but is aimed at the elimination of pathogens. This situation may be encountered after initial treatment is rendered and follow-up monitoring is used to determine the status of the previously diseased site.

At periodic re-evaluation (see Fig. 45–3), patients can also be "completely" stable (E), a situation in which no pathogens or clinical signs of disease (i.e., bleeding on probing, loss of attachment, or loss of bone) are found (box 4 in Fig. 45–4). Therefore, normal maintenance and monitoring are indicated.

In the three unstable situations (boxes 1, 2, and 3 in Fig. 45–4), it is important to assess whether the manifestations

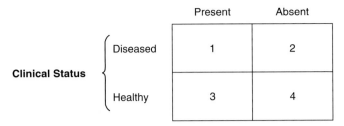

	Present	Absent
Diseased	1	2
Healthy	3	4

Clinical Status

FIGURE 45–4. Four possible combinations of the patient's microbial and clinical status. 1, Clinical signs of disease present/pathogens present. 2, Clinical signs of disease present/pathogens absent. 3, Clinical signs of disease absent (Healthy)/pathogens present. 4, Clinical signs of disease absent (Healthy)/pathogens absent. (Adapted from Newman MG, Kornman KS, Holtzman S: Association of clinical risk factors with treatment outcomes. J Periodontol 65:489, 1994.)

of the disease are localized (G) or generalized (H). As stated previously, microbial assessment (I) is recommended.

Local treatment (J) can consist of a variety of procedures, including topical chlorhexidine and local drug delivery. In cases of generalized manifestations, a systemic antibiotic (K) can be suggested based on the results of microbial testing. Topical chlorhexidine should also be prescribed during systemic antibiotic therapy.

Once again, the clinician should re-evaluate (L) to judge whether the patient is stable (M), and therefore ready for maintenance (supportive periodontal treatment [SPT]), or whether disease is still present (N). The clinician should evaluate a possible deficiency of the host immune system by consulting the patient's physician, and a different antibiotic regimen may be considered. If disease persists (O), the clinician must try to block the triggers of the disease process by employing trial-and-error approaches to treatment, which can be frustrating and often unsuccessful. When such treatment is unsuccessful, the disease is labeled *refractory* or *treatment resistant.*

If the patient responds to treatment (P), maintenance and monitoring are preferred on a regular basis.

MAINTENANCE

A supportive periodontal therapy program aimed at early detection and treatment of sites that begin to lose attachment should be established. The duration between these recall visits is usually short during the first period after the patient's evaluation, generally no longer than 3 months.

Patients with refractory periodontitis, when transferred to maintenance care, must have a stable periodontal status, similar to the situation presented in box 4 of Figure 45–4. The maintenance visit should consist of examination and evaluation of the patient's current oral health; scaling and root planing, followed by prophylaxis; and a review of oral hygiene instructions. When signs of disease recur, monitoring with bacterial testing is recommended.

REFERENCES

1. Atiken S, Birek P, Kulkarni GV, et al. Serial doxycycline and metronidazole in prevention of recurrent periodontitis in high-risk patients. J Periodontol 63:87, 1993.
2. Baer PN, Benjamin SD. Periodontal Disease in Children and Adolescents. Philadelphia, JB Lippincott, 1974.
3. Baer PN, Everett FG. The maxillary sinus as a problem in the therapy of periodontosis. J Periodontol 41:476, 1970.
4. Baer PN, Gamble JW. Autogenous dental transplants as a method of treating the osseous defect in periodontosis. Oral Surg 22:405, 1966.
5. Baer PN, Socransky SS. Periodontosis: Case report with long-term follow-up. Periodont Case Rep 1:1, 1979.
6. Barnett ML, Baker RL. The formation and healing of osseous lesions in a patient with localized juvenile periodontitis. Case report. J Periodontol 54:148, 1983.
7. Carranza FA Jr, Saglie FR, Newman MG, Valentin P. Scanning and transmission electron microscopic study of tissue-invading micro-organisms in localized juvenile periodontitis. J Periodontol 54:598, 1983.
8. Collins JG, Offenbacher S, Arnold RR. Effects of a combination of therapy to eliminate *Porphyromonas gingivalis* in refractory periodontitis. J Periodontol 64:98, 1993.
9. Christersson LA, Slots J, Rosling B, Genco RJ. Microbiological and clinical effects of surgical treatment of localized juvenile periodontitis. J Clin Periodontol 12:465, 1985.
10. Genco RJ, Ciancio SC, Rosling B. Treatment of localized juvenile periodontitis. Abstract. J Dent Res 60:527, 1981.
11. Goodson JM. Drug delivery. In: The American Academy of Periodontology. Perspectives on Oral Antimicrobial Therapeutics. Littleton MA, PSG Publishing Co., 1987, p. 61.
12. Gordon J, Walker C, Hovliaras C, Socransky S. Efficacy of clindamycin hydrochloride in refractory periodontitis: 24-month results. J Periodontol 61:689, 1990.
13. Gordon JM, Walker CB. Current status of systemic antibiotic usage in destructive periodontal disease. J Periodontol 64(8 suppl):760, 1993.
14. Hirschfeld L, Wasserman B. A long-term survey of tooth loss in 600 treated periodontal patients. J Periodontol 49:225, 1978.
15. Kornman KS, Karl EH. The effect of long-term, low-dose tetracycline therapy on the subgingival microflora in refractory adult periodontitis. J Periodontol 53:604, 1982.
16. Kornman KS, Newman MG, Flemmig T, et al. Treatment of refractory periodontitis with metronidazole plus amoxicillin or Augmentin. Abstract 403. J Dent Res 68(special issue):917, 1989.
17. Liljenberg B, Lindhe J. Juvenile periodontitis. Some microbiological, histopathological and clinical characteristics. J Clin Periodontol 7:48, 1980.
18. Lindhe J, Liljenberg B. Treatment of localized juvenile periodontitis. Results after 5 years. J Clin Periodontol 11:399, 1984.
19. Listgarten MA, Lai CH, Young V. Microbial composition and pattern of antibiotic resistance in subgingival microbial samples from patients with refractory periodontitis. J Periodontol 64:155, 1993.
20. Loesche WJ, Syed SA, Laughon B, Stoll J. The bacteriology of acute necrotizing ulcerative gingivitis. J Periodontol 53:223, 1982.
21. Mabry T, Yukna R, Sepe W. Freeze-dried bone allografts with tetracycline in the treatment of juvenile periodontitis. J Periodontol 56:74, 1985.
22. McFall WT. Tooth loss in 100 treated patients with periodontal disease in a long-term study. J Clin Periodontol 53:539, 1982.
23. Matisko MW, Bissada NF. Short-term sequential administration of amoxicillin/clavulanate potassium and doxycycline in the treatment of recurrent/progressive periodontitis. J Periodontol 64:553, 1993.
24. Newman MG, Kornman KS, Holtzman S. Association of clinical risk factors with treatment outcomes. J Periodontol 65:489, 1994.
25. Newman MG, Marinho VC. Assessing bacterial risk factors for periodontitis and peri-implantitis: Using evidence to enhance outcomes. Compend Contin Educ Dent 15(8):958, 1994.
26. Nyman S, Lindhe J, Rosling B. Periodontal surgery in plaque-infected dentitions. J Clin Periodontol 4:240, 1977.
27. Olsvik B, Teniver FC. Tetracycline resistance in periodontal pathogens. Clin Infect Dis 16(suppl 4):S310, 1993.
28. Olsvik B, Olsen I, Tenover FC. The Tet (Q) gene in bacteria isolated from patients with refractory periodontal disease. Oral Microbiol Immunol 9:251, 1994.
29. Pajukanta R. In vitro antimicrobial susceptibility of *Porphyromonas gingivalis* to azythromycin, a novel macrolide. Oral Microbiol Immunol 8:325, 1993.
30. Quiryen M, Listgarten MA. The distribution of bacterial morphotypes around natural teeth and titanium implants ad modum Brånemark. Clin Oral Impl Res 1:8, 1990.
31. Rams TE, Link CC Jr. Microbiology of failing dental implants in humans: Electron microscopy observations. J Oral Implantol 11:93, 1993.
32. Rams TE, Feik D, Slots J. Ciprofloxacin/metronidazole treatment of recurrent adult periodontitis. Abstract 1708. J Dent Res 71(special issue):319, 1992.
33. Rosling B, Nyman S, Lindhe J, Jorn B. The healing potential of the periodontal tissues following different techniques of periodontal surgery in plaque-free dentitions: A 2-year study. J Clin Periodontol 3:233, 1976.
34. Rosling B, Nyman S, Lindhe J. The effect of systemic plaque control on bone regeneration in infrabony pockets. J Clin Periodontol 3:38, 1976.
35. Saglie R, Newman MG, Carranza FA Jr, Pattison GL. Bacterial invasion of gingiva in infrabony pockets. J Clin Periodontol 53:217, 1982.
36. Saglie FR, Carranza FA Jr, Newman MG, et al. Identification of tissue invading bacteria in human periodontal disease. J Periodont Res 17:452, 1982.
37. Slots J, Feik D, Rams T. Prevalence of antimicrobial susceptibility of *Enterobacteriaceae, Pseudomonads* and *Acinetobacter* in human periodontitis. Oral Microbiol Immunol 5:149, 1990.
38. Slots J, Masimo P, Levine MJ, Genco RJ. Periodontal therapy in humans. I. Microbiological and clinical effects of a single course of periodontal scaling and

root planing and of adjunctive tetracycline therapy. J Periodontol *50:*495, 1979.

39. Sugarman MM, Sugarman EF. Precocious periodontitis: A clinical entity and a treatment responsibility. J Periodontol *48:*397, 1977.
40. Tanner ACR, Socransky SS, Goodson M. Microbiota of periodontal pockets losing crestal alveolar bone. J Periodontol Res *19:*279, 1984.
41. van Winklehoff AJ, Rodenberg JP, Goene RJ, et al. Metronidazole plus amoxicillin in the treatment of *Actinobacillus actinomycetemcomitans*–associated periodontitis. J Clin Periodontol *16:*128, 1989.
42. van Winklehoff AJ, Tijhof CJ, de Graaff. Microbial and clinical results of metronidazole plus amoxicillin therapy in *Actinobacillus actinomycetemcomitans*–associated periodontitis. J Periodontol *63:*52, 1992.
43. Vitaya CT. Antimicrobial approaches to periodontal therapy. J Dent Assoc Thai *40:*83, 1990.
44. Waerhaug J. Plaque control in the treatment of juvenile periodontitis. J Clin Periodontol *4:*29, 1977.
45. Waerhaug J. Subgingival plaque and loss of attachment in periodontosis as evaluated on extracted teeth. J Periodontol *48:*125, 1977.
46. Walker CB, Gordon JM, Cornwall HA, et al. Gingival crevicular fluid levels of clindamycin compared with its minimal inhibitory concentrations for periodontal bacteria. Antimicrob Agents Chemother *25:*867, 1981.
47. Walker CB, Gordon JM, Socransky SS. Antibiotic susceptibility testing on subgingival plaque samples. J Clin Periodontol *10:*422, 1983.
48. Walker CB, Pappas JD, Tyler KZ, Cohen JM. Antibiotic susceptibilities to eight antimicrobial agents. J Periodontol *56*(suppl):67, 1985.
49. Walker CB, Clark W, Magnusson I. Antimicrobial susceptibilities of subgingival plaque samples from patients with refractory periodontitis. Abstract. J Dent Res *66*(special issue):355, 1987.
50. Walker C, Gordon J. The effect of clindamycin on the microbiota associated with refractory periodontitis. J Periodontol *61:*692, 1990.
51. Walker CB, Gordon JM, Magnusson I, Clark WB. A role for antibiotics in the treatment of refractory periodontitis. J Periodontol *64:*772, 1993.
52. Williams BL, Osterberg KA, Jorgensen J. Subgingival microflora of periodontal patients on tetracycline therapy. J Clin Periodontol *6:*210, 1979.
53. Yukna R, Sepe W. Clinical evaluation of localized periodontosis defects with freeze-dried bone allografts combined with local and systemic tetracyclines. Internat. J Periodont Restor Dent *5:*9, 1982.

46

Periodontal Management of HIV-Infected Patients

TERRY D. REES and EDMUND CATALDO

Periodontal Treatment Protocol
Oral Candidiasis
Oral Hairy Leukoplakia
Kaposi's Sarcoma

Bacillary (Epithelioid) Angiomatosis
Nonspecific Oral Ulcerations and Recurrent Aphthae
Periodontal Disease in HIV-Positive Individuals

Acquired immunodeficiency syndrome (AIDS) is a universal epidemic that significantly affects dental practice, regardless of geographic location. The oral cavity is a frequent site for clinical manifestations of the disease. The ability to recognize and manage the oral manifestations of this disease is an important part of dental practice. The dentist should be prepared to assist human immunodeficiency virus (HIV)–infected patients in maintenance of oral health throughout the course of their disease.

The detection and diagnosis of oral lesions in HIV–positive patients has been described in Chapter 15. The clinical management of these conditions, with particular emphasis on periodontal conditions, will be presented in this chapter.

PERIODONTAL TREATMENT PROTOCOL

To safely and effectively provide periodontal therapy to HIV-infected individuals, several treatment considerations are important.

Health Status. The patient's health status should be determined from the health history, physical evaluation, and consultation with his or her physician. Treatment decisions will vary depending on the patient's state of health. For example, delayed wound healing and increased risk of postoperative infection are possible complicating factors in AIDS patients, but neither concern should significantly alter treatment planning in an otherwise healthy asymptomatic HIV-infected patient with a normal or near-normal CD4 count.[22] It is important to obtain information regarding the patient's immune status. What is the CD4$^+$ T4 lymphocyte level? How long ago was the HIV infection identified? Is it possible to identify the approximate date of original exposure? Is there a history of drug abuse, sexually transmitted diseases, multiple infections, or other factors that might alter immune response? For example, does the patient have a history of chronic hepatitis B, thrombocytopenia, nutritional deficiency, or adrenocorticoid insufficiency? What medications is the patient taking?

Infection Control Measures. Clinical management of HIV-infected periodontal patients requires strict adherence to established methods of infection control, based on guidance from the American Dental Association (ADA) and the Centers for Disease Control and Prevention (CDC).[3] Compliance, especially with universal precautions, will eliminate or minimize risks to patients and the dental staff.[17,20,31]

Immunocompromised patients are potentially at risk for acquiring as well as transmitting infections in the dental office.[18]

Goals of Therapy. Thorough oral examination will determine the patient's dental treatment needs. The primary goals of dental therapy should be the restoration and maintenance of oral health, comfort, and function. As a minimum, periodontal treatment goals should be directed toward control of HIV-associated mucosal diseases such as chronic candidiasis and recurrent oral ulcerations. Acute periodontal and dental infections should be managed, and the patient should receive detailed instructions in performance of effective oral hygiene procedures. Conservative, nonsurgical periodontal therapy should be the treatment option for virtually all HIV-positive patients, but successful performance of elective surgical periodontal procedures has been reported.[10] Necrotizing ulcerative periodontitis (NUP) or necrotizing ulcerative stomatitis (NUS) can be severely destructive to periodontal structures, but a history of these conditions does not automatically dictate extraction of involved teeth unless the patient is unable to maintain effective oral hygiene in affected areas. Decisions regarding elective periodontal procedures should be made with the informed consent of the patient and after medical consultation, when possible.

Supportive Periodontal Therapy. It is imperative that the patient maintain meticulous personal oral hygiene. In addition, periodontal maintenance recall visits should be conducted at short intervals (2 to 3 months) and any progressive periodontal disease treated vigorously. As mentioned earlier, however, systemic antibiotic therapy should be administered with caution. Blood and other medical laboratory tests may be required to monitor the patient's overall health status, and close consultation and coordination with the patient's physician are necessary.

Psychological Factors. HIV infection of neuronal cells may affect brain function and lead to outright dementia. This may profoundly influence the responsiveness of affected patients to dental treatment. However, psychological factors are numerous in virtually all HIV-infected patients, even in the absence of neuronal lesions. Patients may be greatly concerned over maintenance of medical confidentiality, and such confidentiality must be upheld. Coping with a life-threatening disease may elicit depression, anxiety, and anger in such patients, and this anger may be directed toward the dentist and the staff.[1] It is important to display concern and understanding for the patient's situation. Treatment should be provided in a calm, relaxed atmosphere, and stress to the patient must be minimized.

The dentist should be prepared to advise and counsel patients on their oral health status. Dentists often encounter HIV-infected patients who are unaware of their disease status. Early diagnosis and treatment of HIV infection can have a profound effect on the patient's life expectancy and quality of life, and the dentist should be prepared to assist the patient in being tested.[25] Patients with oral lesions suggestive of HIV infection should be informed of the findings and, if appropriate, questioned regarding any previous exposure to HIV. If HIV testing is requested, it must be accompanied by patient counseling For this reason, such tests might best be obtained through medical referral. However, if the dentist elects to request testing for HIV antibody, the patient must be thus informed. In most circumstances, written informed consent is desirable prior to testing.

ORAL CANDIDIASIS

Early oral lesions of HIV-related candidiasis are usually responsive to topical antifungal therapy (Fig. 46–1). More

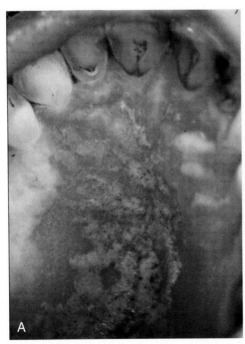
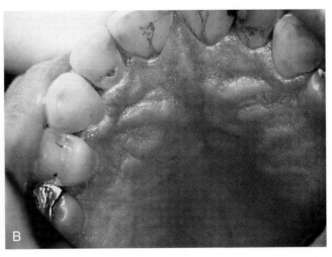

FIGURE 46–1. Erythematous and pseudomembranous candidiasis. *A,* Before treatment. *B,* Resolution after 1 week of topical clotrimazole therapy.

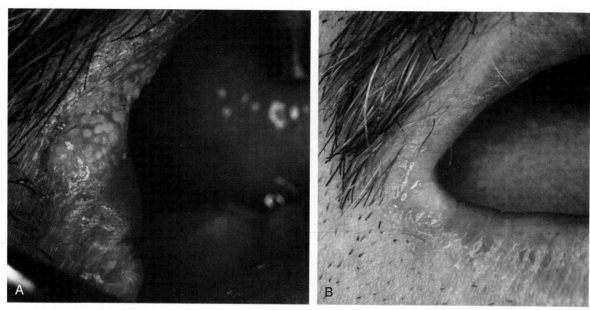

FIGURE 46-2. Marked hyperplastic candidiasis in corner of mouth. *A*, Before treatment. *B*, After 2 weeks of systemic fluconazole therapy.

advanced lesions, including hyperplastic candidiasis, may require systemic antifungal drugs; systemic therapy is mandatory for esophageal candidiasis (Fig. 46-2).

With any therapy, lesions tend to recur after the drug is discontinued, and resistant strains of candidal organisms have been described, especially with the use of systemic agents.[30] Table 46-1 identifies therapeutic agents commonly prescribed for treatment of candidal infections. Most oral topical antifungal agents contain large quantities of su-

crose, which may be cariogenic after long-term use. For this reason, some authorities recommend oral use of nystatin vaginal suppositories, as these do not contain sucrose. Chlorhexidine oral rinses may also be of some prophylactic value against oral candidal infection.[5]

Systemic antifungal agents such as ketoconazole or fluconazole are effective in treatment of oral candidiasis (see Table 46-1). As mentioned before, however, resistant strains of candidal organisms may develop with prolonged use, potentially rendering the drugs ineffective against life-threatening candidal infections in the later stages of immune suppression. In addition, long-term use of ketoconazole may induce liver damage in individuals with pre-existent liver disease. The frequency of chronic hepatitis B infection in HIV-infected individuals may put some patients at risk for ketoconazole-induced liver damage. Ketoconazole absorption may also be hampered by the gastropathy experienced by many HIV-infected individuals.[15]

Table 46-1. ANTIFUNGAL THERAPEUTIC AGENTS

Topical Drugs
1. Clotrimazole (Mycelex), 10-mg tablets: 3-5 tablets daily for 7-14 days
2. Nystatin (Mycostatin, Nilstat)
   (a) Oral suspension
     • 100,000 U/ml: Disp 240 ml
     • Rinse with 1 tsp qid
   (b) Oral suspension (extemporaneous)
     • Disp 2-4 billion U
     • Mix ⅛ tsp (500,000 U) in 4 oz water (½ cup)
     • Rinse 4 times daily
     • *Note:* Extemporaneous nystatin is sucrose free.
   (c) Tablets (500,000 U): Dissolve 1 tablet in mouth, 4-5 times daily
   (d) Pastilles (200,000 U): Dissolve 1-2 pastilles in mouth, 4-5 times daily
   (e) Vaginal troches (100,000 U): Dissolve 1 troche in mouth tid
     • *Note:* Vaginal troches are sucrose free.
   (f) Ointment (for angular cheilitis), 15-gm tube: Apply to affected area 3-4 times daily
3. Clotrimazole ointment, 15-gm tube: Apply to affected area qid
4. Miconazole 2% ointment, 15-gm tube: Apply to affected area qid

Systemic Drugs
1. Ketoconazole (Nyzoral), 200-mg tablets: Take 2 tablets immediately, then 1-2 tablets daily with food for 14 days
2. Fluconazole (Diflucan), 100-mg tablets: Take 2 tablets immediately, then 1 tablet daily for 7-14 days

ORAL HAIRY LEUKOPLAKIA

At present there appears to be little advantage in treating oral hairy leukoplakia (OHL) in most patients. Lesions can be successfully removed, however, with laser or conventional surgery. Resolution has been reported after therapy with zidovudine (Fig. 46-3) or topical vitamin A, but the systemic antiviral agent acyclovir may elicit remission more predictably (Fig. 46-4), although lesions reappear when antiviral therapy is discontinued.[2,23]

KAPOSI'S SARCOMA

Treatment of oral Kaposi's sarcoma (KS) may include laser excision, radiation therapy, or intralesional injection with vinblastine (Fig. 46-5), interferon α, or other chemotherapeutic drugs.[6,7,9,27,28] Nichols et al.[19] described

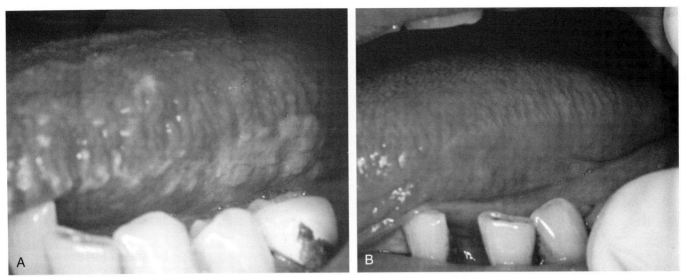

FIGURE 46–3. Oral hairy leukoplakia of 2 years' duration. *A,* Before treatment. *B,* Unexpected remission after initiation of zidovudine therapy.

the successful use of intralesional injections of vinblastine at a dosage of 0.1 mg/cm^2 using a 0.2 mg/ml solution of vinblastine sulfate in saline. In responsive patients, treatment was repeated at 2-week intervals until resolution or stabilization of the lesions. Side effects included some post-treatment pain and occasional ulceration of the lesions, but in general, the therapy was well tolerated. Total resolution was achieved in 70% of 82 intraoral KS lesions with one to six treatments. Lesions tended to recur, however, thus indicating that treatment should probably be reserved for oral KS lesions that are easily traumatized or that interfere with chewing or swallowing. On some occasions, treatment may be indicated when KS lesions create an unsightly appearance on the lips or in the anterior oral cavity.

Destructive periodontitis has also been reported in conjunction with gingival KS. In such instances, scaling and root planing and other periodontal therapy may be indicated in addition to intralesional or systemic chemotherapy.[27]

BACILLARY (EPITHELIOID) ANGIOMATOSIS

Treatment of bacillary angiomatosis consists of broad-spectrum antibiotics, such as erythromycin or doxycycline, in conjunction with conservative periodontal therapy and possibly excision of the lesion.[11]

NONSPECIFIC ORAL ULCERATIONS AND RECURRENT APHTHAE

Oral viral infections are usually treated with acyclovir (800 mg qid for at least 2 weeks). Subsequent daily main-

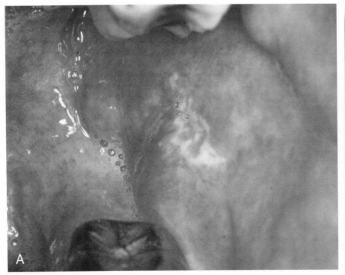
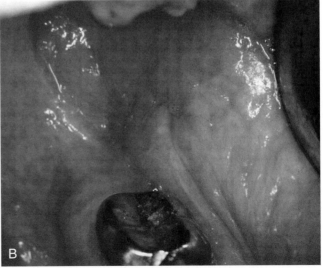

FIGURE 46–4. Oral hairy leukoplakia of left buccal mucosa. *A,* Before treatment. *B,* Remission after initiation of systemic acyclovir therapy.

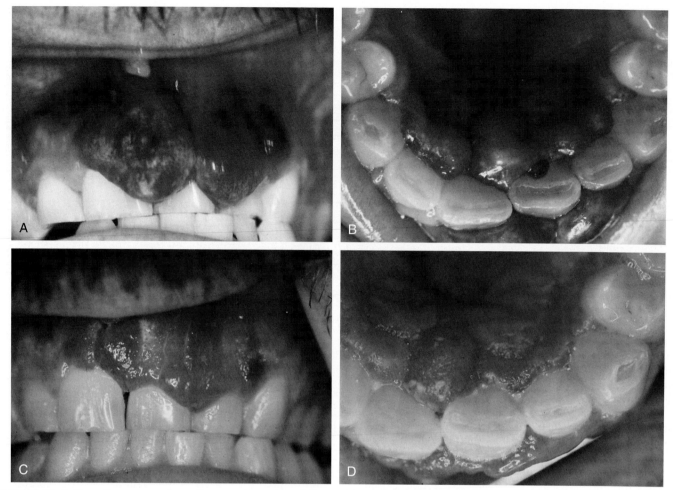

FIGURE 46–5. Kaposi's sarcoma of maxillary anterior region. *A,* Anterior facial gingiva before treatment. *B,* Palate before treatment. *C,* Partial resolution of facial gingival lesion after two vinblastine injections. *D,* Partial resolution of palatal lesion. Patient was satisfied with results and declined additional therapy.

tenance therapy (200 mg two to five times daily) may be required to prevent recurrence. Resistant viral strains are treated with foscarnet or ganciclovir.

Topical corticosteroid therapy (fluocinonide gel applied three to six times daily) is safe and efficacious for treatment of recurrent aphthous ulcer or other mucosal lesions[12,21] (Fig. 46–6). However, topical corticosteroids may predispose immunocompromised individuals to candidiasis. Consequently, prophylactic antifungal medications should be prescribed.

On occasion, large aphthae in HIV-positive individuals may prove resistant to conventional topical therapy. In this event, systemic corticosteroids (prednisone 40 to 60 mg daily) (Fig. 46–7) or alternative therapy (thalidomide, levamisole, or other) must be considered.[12,13,29]

PERIODONTAL DISEASE IN HIV-POSITIVE INDIVIDUALS

As described in Chapter 15, gingival and periodontal manifestations may be found in HIV-positive individuals. The former include linear gingival erythema and necrotizing ulcerative gingivitis (NUG), both of which may develop into rapidly progressive NUS or NUP. Management

of these conditions should be preceded by a thorough medical evaluation, including determination of the CD4 status, in consultation with the treating physician.

Linear Gingival Erythema. Linear gingival erythema is often refractory to treatment, but lesions may undergo spontaneous remission. The recommended management of this condition is as follows:

Step 1: Instruct the patient in performance of meticulous oral hygiene.
Step 2: Scale and polish affected areas and perform subgingival irrigation with chlorhexidine.
Step 3: Prescribe chlorhexidine gluconate mouthrinse.
Step 4: Re-evaluate the patient in 2 to 3 weeks. If lesions persist, evaluate for possible candidiasis.
Step 5: Re-treat if necessary.
Step 6: Place the patient on 2- to 3-month recall.

Necrotizing Ulcerative Gingivitis. There is no consensus on whether the incidence of NUG increases in HIV-positive patients. The treatment of this condition in these individuals does not differ from that in HIV-negative patients (see Chapter 39). Basic treatment consists of cleaning and debridement of affected areas with a cotton pellet soaked in peroxide after application of a topical anesthetic. Escharotic drugs should never be used for any patient and are especially contraindicated in all immunocompromised patients. The patient is to be seen daily or every other day

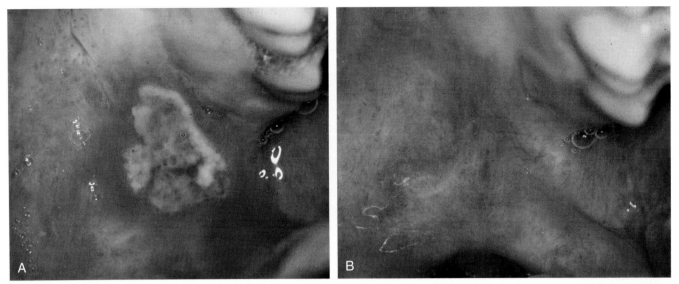

FIGURE 46–6. Major aphthae of soft palate in a 28-year-old HIV-positive man. *A,* Before treatment. *B,* Remission of lesion 1 week after prescribing topical corticosteroids.

for the first week; at each visit debridement of affected areas is repeated, and plaque control methods are gradually introduced. A meticulous plaque control program should be taught and started as soon as the sensitivity of the area allows it.

The patient should avoid tobacco, alcohol, and condiments. An antimicrobial mouthrinse, such as chlorhexidine gluconate 0.12%, is prescribed.

Systemic antibiotics such as metronidazole or amoxicillin should be prescribed for patients with moderate to severe tissue destruction and/or localized lymphadenopathy or systemic symptoms. The use of prophylactic antifungal medication should be considered if antibiotics are prescribed.

The mouth is re-evaluated 1 month after resolution of acute symptoms to assess the results of treatment and determine the need for further therapy.

Necrotizing Ulcerative Stomatitis. A severely destructive, acutely painful NUS has occasionally been reported in HIV-positive patients. This is characterized by necrosis of significant areas of oral soft tissue and underlying bone. It may occur separately or as an extension of NUP[4,8] and is commonly associated with severe depression of CD4+ immune cells.

Treatment may include prescription of an antibiotic such as metronidazole and use of an antimicrobial mouthrinse such as chlorhexidine gluconate. If osseous necrosis is present, it may be necessary to remove the affected bone to promote wound healing.[33]

Necrotizing Ulcerative Periodontitis. Therapy for NUP includes local debridement, scaling and root planing, in-office irrigation with an effective antimicrobial agent such as chlorhexidine or povidone-iodine (Betadine), and establishment of meticulous oral hygiene, including home use of an-

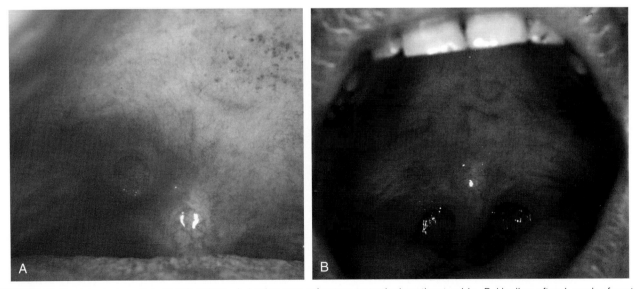

FIGURE 46–7. Persistent ulceration of soft palate. *A,* Lesion was refractory to topical corticosteroids. *B,* Healing after 1 week of systemic corticosteroid therapy (40 mg prednisone daily).

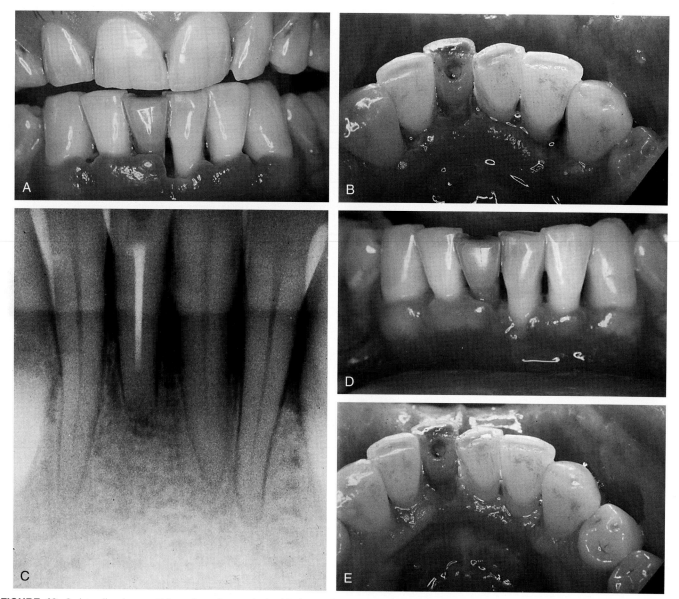

FIGURE 46–8. Localized necrotizing ulcerative periodontitis in a 43-year-old HIV-positive male. *A,* Facial view. *B,* Lingual view. *C,* Radiographic view of the mandibular anterior. *D,* Resolution 48 hours after initiation of periodontal therapy. Facial view. *E,* Resolution. Lingual view.

timicrobial rinses or irrigation[14,16,24,32] (Plate XV and Fig. 46–8).

This therapeutic approach is based on reports involving only a small number of patients.[24] In severe NUP, antibiotic therapy may be necessary but should be used with caution in HIV-infected patients to avoid an opportunistic and potentially serious localized candidiasis or even candidal septicemia. If an antibiotic is necessary, metronidazole (250 mg, with two tablets taken immediately and then one tablet qid for 5 to 7 days) is the drug of choice. Prophylactic prescription of a topical or systemic antifungal agent is prudent if an antibiotic is used.

REFERENCES

1. Asher RS, McDowell JD, Winquist H. HIV-related neuropsychiatric changes: Concerns for dental professionals. J Am Dent Assoc *124*:80–84, 1993.
2. Brockmeyer NH, Kreugfelder E, Martins L, et al. Zidovudine therapy of asymptomatic HIV-1-infected patients and combined Zidovudine-acyclovir therapy of HIV-1-infected patients with oral hairy leukoplakia. J Infect Dermatol *92*:647, 1989.
3. Centers for Disease Control. Recommended infection-control practices for dentistry, 1993. MMWR *42*(RR-8):1–12, 1993.
4. European Community Clearinghouse on Oral Problems Related to HIV Infection and WHO Collaborating Centre on Oral Manifestations of the Immunodeficiency Virus: Classification and diagnostic criteria for oral lesions in HIV infection. J Oral Pathol Med *22*:289–291, 1993.
5. Epstein JB. Antifungal therapy in oropharyngeal mycotic infections. Oral Surg Oral Med Oral Pathol *69*:32–41, 1990.
6. Epstein JB, Lozada-Nur F, McLeod A, Spindli J. Oral Kaposi's sarcoma in acquired immunodeficiency syndrome: Review of management and report of the efficacy of intralesional vinblastine. Cancer *64*:2424–2430, 1989.
7. Epstein JB, Scully C. HIV infection: Clinical features and treatment of 33 homosexual men with Kaposi's sarcoma. Oral Med Oral Surg Oral Pathol *71*:38–41, 1991.
9. Ficarra G, Berson AM, Silverman S Jr, et al. Kaposi's sarcoma of the oral cavity: A study of 134 patients with a review of the pathogenesis, epidemiology, clinical aspects and treatment. Oral Surg Oral Med Oral Pathol *66*:543–550, 1988.
10. Glick M. Clinical protocol for treating patients with HIV disease. Gen Dent *38*:418–425, 1990.
11. Glick M, Cleveland DB. Oral mucosal bacillary epitheloid angiomatosis in a pa-

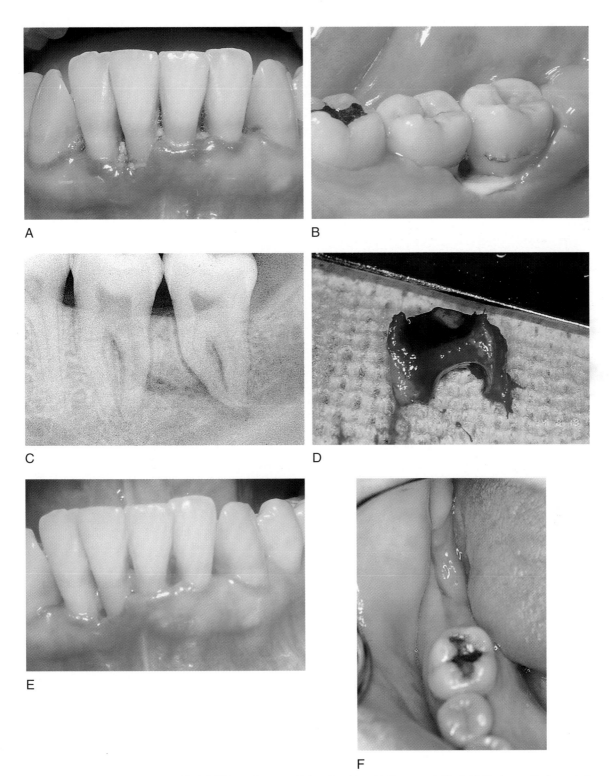

PLATE XV. Necrotizing ulcerative periodontitis (NUP) in a 28-year-old female with a CD4 count of 48. *A,* NUP of mandibular anterior region. *B,* Necrotizing stomatitis in mandibular left molar area. *C,* Radiograph of sequestra in mandibular left molar area. *D,* Sequestrae removed in conjunction with extraction of teeth #17 and 18. *E,* Mandibular anterior area 1 week post treatment. *F,* Mandibular left molar region 2 months postoperatively. Note uneventful healing.

tient with AIDS associated with rapid alveolar bone loss: A case report. J Oral Pathol Med 22:235–239, 1993.
12. Glick M, Muzyka BC. Alternative therapies for major aphthous ulcers in AIDS patients. J Am Dent Assoc 123:61–65, 1992.
13. Gorin I, Vilette B, Gehanno P, Escande P. Thalidomide in hyperalgic pharyngeal ulceration of AIDS. Lancet 335:1343, 1990.
14. Grassi M, Williams CA, Winkler JR, Murray PA. Management of HIV-associated periodontal diseases. In Robertson PB, Greenspan JS, eds. Oral Manifestations of AIDS. Littleton, MA, PSG, 1988, pp 119–130.
15. Lake-Bakaar G, Tom W, Lake-Bakaar D, et al. Gastropathy and ketoconazole malabsorption in the acquired immunodeficiency syndrome (AIDS). Ann Intern Med 109:471–473, 1988.
16. Levine RA, Glick M. Rapidly progressive periodontitis as an important clinical marker for HIV disease. Compend Contin Educ Dent XII(7):478–488, 1991.
17. Mandel ID. Occupational risks in dentistry: Comforts and concerns. J Am Dent Assoc 124:41–49, 1993.
18. Molinari JA. HIV, health care workers and patients: How to ensure safety in the dental office. J Am Dent Assoc 124:51–56, 1993.
19. Nichols CM, Flaitz CM, Hicks MJ. Treating Kaposi's lesions in the HIV-infected patient. J Am Dent Assoc 124:78–84, 1993.
20. Olsen RJ, Lynch P, Coyle MB, et al. Examination gloves as barriers to hand contamination in clinical practice. JAMA 270(3):350–353, 1993.
21. Plemons JM, Rees TD, Zachariah NY. Absorption of a topical steroid and evaluation of adrenal suppression in patients with erosive lichen planus. Oral Surg Oral Med Oral Pathol 73:138–141, 1990.
22. Porter SR, Scully C, Luker J. Complications of dental surgery in persons with HIV disease. Oral Surg Oral Med Oral Pathol 75:165–167, 1993.
23. Reichart PA, Langford A, Gelderblom HR, et al. Oral hairy leukoplakia: Observations in 95 cases and review of the literature. J Oral Pathol Med 18:410–415, 1989.
24. Robinson P. Periodontal diseases and HIV infection. J Clin Periodontol 19:609–614, 1992.
25. Schulman DJ. The dentist, HIV and the law. CDA J 21(9):45–50, 1993.
26. Schulten EAJM, ten Kate RW, van der Waal I. Oral manifestations of HIV infection in 75 Dutch patients. J Oral Pathol Med 18:42–46, 1989.
27. Shibosky CH, Winkler JR. Gingival Kaposi's sarcoma and periodontitis. Oral Med Oral Surg Oral Pathol 76:38–41, 1991.
28. Shibosky CH, Winkler JR. Gingival Kaposi's sarcoma and periodontitis. Oral Surg Oral Med Oral Pathol 76:49–53, 1993.
29. Silverman S. Color Atlas of Oral Manifestations of AIDS. Toronto, Decker, 1989.
30. Tavitian A, Raufman JP, Rosenthal LE, et al. Ketoconazole-resistant candida esophagitis in patients with acquired immune deficiency syndrome. Gastroenterology 90:443–445, 1986.
31. Verrusio AC. Risk of transmission of the human immunodeficiency virus to health care workers exposed to HIV-infected patients: A review. J Am Dent Assoc 118:339–342, 1989.
32. Winkler JR, Murray PA, Grassi M, Hammerle C. Diagnosis and management of HIV-associated periodontal lesions. J Am Dent Assoc 120(suppl):S25–S34, 1989.
33. Winkler JR, Murray PA, Hammerle C. Gangrenous stomatitis in AIDS. Lancet 2(8454):108, 1989.

47

Coronoplasty in Periodontal Therapy

WILLIAM K. SOLBERG and DONALD A. SELIGMAN

Stability of Occlusion
Forces of Occlusion
Local Environment of the Periodontium and Periodontal Health
Guidelines for Therapeutic Occlusion
Indications for Coronoplasty in Periodontal Therapy
Treatment Planning and Technique

Methods
Determining the End Point of Coronoplasty
Selecting an Occlusal Guidance Scheme
Occlusal Adjustment
Criteria for Judging the Outcome of Coronoplasty
Treatment of Bruxism and Appliance Therapy

Occlusal adjustment is the establishment of functional relationships favorable to the periodontium by one or more of the following procedures: reshaping of the teeth by grinding, dental restoration, tooth movement, tooth removal, or orthognathic surgery. *Coronoplasty* is the selective reduction of occlusal areas with the primary purpose of influencing the mechanical contact conditions and the neural pattern of sensory input.[42] It is a direct and irreversible change of the occlusal scheme.[42] There is a tendency to think of occlusal adjustment solely as eliminating injurious occlusal forces, but an equally important purpose is to provide the functional stimulation necessary for the preservation of periodontal health.

STABILITY OF OCCLUSION

Forces of Occlusion

The forces of occlusion are created by the musculature in chewing, swallowing, and speech and are transmitted through the teeth to the periodontium. Tooth position and arch form are not static; they are maintained by the balance among the forces of occlusion and oral musculature. The forces of occlusion guide the alignment of the teeth as they erupt and maintain the position of the teeth in synchronized balance. Disturbance of this balance may lead to altered tooth positions and changes in the functional environment that may be deleterious to the periodontium.

The following factors are involved in the creation and distribution of the forces of occlusion:

1. *The forces of the muscles of mastication and the counteracting oral musculature.*[81] Retrusive occlusal forces enlist the deep masseter and temporalis muscles, while protrusive forces enlist the superficial masseter muscle and medial pterygoid.[6,45] Posterior lateral forces mainly involve the temporalis muscle.[7]

2. *The anterior component of occlusal forces.* This component tends to move the teeth mesially in their sockets (Fig. 47–1). When the force is released, the teeth move back to their previous position because of the resilience of the periodontal ligament. With time, areas of proximal contact are flattened by wear, permitting mesial movement of the teeth, referred to as *adaptive mesial migration.*

3. *Proximal contacts.* The anterior component of force is transmitted through intact proximal contacts. Missing proximal contacts or deflected forces of occlusion through malpositioned contacts may cause displacement of the teeth (Fig. 47–2) and create abnormal forces on the periodontium and increased lateral loads on the contralateral condyle.[41] Unilateral contacts will reduce the occlusal forces.[45]

4. *Morphologic alignment and inclination of the teeth.* Most of the occlusal force is transferred to the teeth,[17] and the morphologic alignment and inclination of the teeth affect the transmission of occlusal forces. For example, the maxillary central incisors are shaped so that they are inclined anteromesially to provide maximal efficiency of their cutting edge and to buttress one another during function. The root of the maxillary incisors is shaped so that there is a greater area of attachment of periodontal fibers on the palatal and distal sides, which counteracts the tendency toward facial and mesial displacement during function. The molars are inclined mesially so as to transmit the mesial component of occlusal forces to the premolars and canines. The magnitude

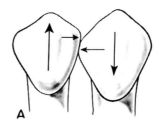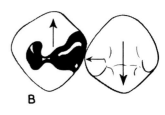

FIGURE 47–2. *A,* Improper proximal contact relationship (*horizontal arrows*). This relationship is a potential source of excessive force in the directions indicated by the vertical arrows. *B,* Improper contact relationship in the faciolingual plane (*horizontal arrow*). This relationship is a potential cause of displacement of the teeth facially and lingually, as indicated by the vertical arrows. (After R. A. Jentsch.)

of the force is also related to cusp inclines, with steepness associated with less force.[16,17]

5. *Direction of occlusal contacts.* The direction of the occlusal contacts affects the force,[80,81] with the greatest forces occurring perpendicular to the occlusal table.[45]

6. *Location of tooth contact.* The location of tooth contact affects the force,[16] with posterior teeth accepting higher force levels than anterior teeth.[80] This is not dependent on the angle of the force relative to the occlusal plane[80] but is probably due to a shorter moment arm length of the force vectors in the posterior teeth.[17,81]

7. *Atmospheric equilibrium during breathing and swallowing.* Atmospheric equilibrium during breathing and swallowing contributes to occlusal forces.

Local Environment of the Periodontium and Periodontal Health

The local environment of the periodontium is affected by two principal factors: the saliva, with its microbial population, and the occlusion of the teeth. Two environmental pollutants have an adverse impact on the periodontium: (1) dental plaque formed by oral bacteria, which leads to destructive periodontal inflammation, and (2) occlusal forces when they alter the supporting periodontal tissues in a deleterious way.

The establishment of a satisfactory local environment is essential in the treatment of periodontal disease and in the preservation of periodontal health. The urgency of controlling plaque is well recognized; coronoplasty to eliminate undesirable forces and to produce forces favorable to the periodontium is also important.

GUIDELINES FOR THERAPEUTIC OCCLUSION

Therapeutic occlusal changes are made to counteract problems related to untoward occlusal forces. Therapeutic occlusion is an occlusal treatment model used in restoring or replacing teeth so that the adaptation required of the patient and the need for compensatory tissue change are minimized.

The optimal design goal of a therapeutic occlusion is the elimination of undesirable occlusal supracontacts and the creation of a stable mandibular position. This ensures that jaw closure occurs at one functional end point wherein the temporomandibular joints (TMJs) and teeth receive stresses

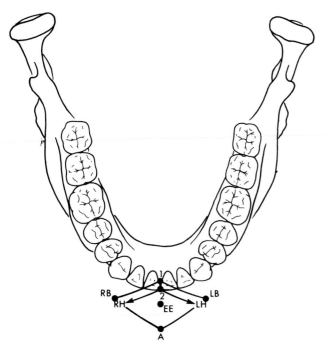

FIGURE 47–1. Anterior component of force (*arrows*) is developed as a result of contact along the occlusal plane. The forces are anteriorly directed because of the orientation and placement of the occlusal plane below the level of the axis of rotation. EE, Edge-to-edge position. RH and LH, right and left habitual movement positions. RB and LB, right and left border positions.

Table 47–1. GUIDELINES FOR OCCLUSION IN DENTAL TREATMENT*

Occlusal Stability in the ICP

1. Jaw closes to a repeatable, single end point.
2. Simultaneous masseter muscle contraction after forceful clenching in the intercuspal position.
3. Simultaneous, widely distributed posterior tooth contacts.
4. Posterior contacts are heavier than anterior contacts (patient sitting upright).
5. Forces of tooth contact directed along the long axis of the teeth.

Maxillomandibular Relationships and Tooth Contact Movement

6. Minimal mandibular shift from MCP to ICP.
7. Contact movement from RCP to ICP (mandibular shift) is sagittal in direction and less than 1 mm (no shift is acceptable).
8. Laterotrusive side guidance primarily on the ipsilateral canine-premolar teeth.
9. Protrusive guidance is symmetric and primarily on anterior teeth.

Subjective Response to Occlusion

10. Lack of unpleasantness or untoward awareness concerning the dental occlusion.
11. Acceptable free way space.
12. Acceptable speech articulation.
13. Acceptable chewing ability.
14. Acceptable mandibular position.

* These guidelines are for (1) pretreatment evaluation of dental occlusion, (2) planning occlusal changes or fabricating dental occlusion in treatment, and (3) post-treatment evaluation of the dental occlusion. The complete denture occlusion will vary from these guidelines, as taught in removable prosthodontics.

ICP, Intercuspal position; MCP, muscular contact position (mandibular position reached when the jaw is gently lifted from rest position to first point of tooth contact); RCP, retruded contact position.

with only a slight mesial component.[65] The basic guidelines for a therapeutic occlusion are generally agreed on (Table 47–1).

Comprehensive therapeutic occlusal alterations usually include stabilization of the retruded contact position (RCP) and smooth coordination of contacts between the RCP and the intercuspal position (ICP). In addition, smooth, interference-free lateral and protrusive excursions from the ICP are achieved. Disturbing retrusive supracontacts along lateral border paths are usually lessened or removed.

INDICATIONS FOR CORONOPLASTY IN PERIODONTAL THERAPY

Coronoplasty is based on the premise that tissue damage and excessive tooth mobility[53,83] caused by occlusal forces are resolved when undesirable occlusal forces are corrected.[40] A second premise is that realigning occlusal forces by creating unobstructed functional contacts provides trophic stimulation beneficial to the periodontium, the muscles, and the TMJ. In general, coronoplasty is not often indicated in periodontal therapy, except when a patient has an occlusion weakened by bone loss.[66]

Trauma From Occlusion. Occlusion is adjusted for patients who demonstrate periodontal changes manifested in the form of excessive tooth mobility,[58,89] angular thickening

of the periodontal ligament,[58] true instances of angular (vertical) bone destruction,[58] furcation involvement, and migration of teeth.[19,58]

Most people have modest retrusive supracontacts in the permanent dentition.[2,35,76] In addition, supracontacts in the lateral positions are not uncommon. However, most patients with occlusal supracontacts do not experience occlusal trauma. Trauma from occlusion may result from repetitive clamping and clenching habits (bruxism) and, less commonly, from chewing and swallowing movements. Coronoplasty may be considered in those patients with evidence of trauma from occlusion.

The absence of signs of trauma from occlusion determines that the patient's occlusal relationships merit perpetuation in periodontal restorative therapy. If the trauma is limited to a single tooth or a few teeth, localized coronoplasty of supracontacts may suffice, and no change in the mandibular position need be made. However, if there is generalized trauma from occlusion, faulty maxillomandibular relationships may be involved in the production of the trauma.[69] Normalization of these relationships may require major changes in the mandibular occlusal position in accordance with the guidelines for therapeutic occlusion (see Table 47–1) to minimize the repetitive and excessive occlusal forces. However, periodontal changes such as an elevated periodontal/gingival index or increased pocket depth have not been associated with occlusal factors[30,86] or even tooth mobility.[90]

Preventive Occlusal Adjustment. Preventive coronoplasty—the correction of what appear to be abnormal occlusal relationships in patients without signs of trauma from occlusion, for the purpose of preventing future damage—*is not recommended.* Any change in the occlusion in anticipation of future injury, without any indication that it will occur, may disrupt the established balance between the occlusion and the periodontal tissues. The occlusion should be compatible with the needs of the periodontium, the musculature, and the TMJs, not the desires of the therapist.

Planned Occlusal Reconstruction. Coordinated periodontal and restorative therapy sometimes involves major reconstruction of the disorganized or unstable occlusion. The attempt to preserve an acquired, eccentric occlusal position dictated by a few remaining teeth is unwarranted. A "therapeutic" mandibular position is more practical. That is, the occlusion and mandibular position may be changed to conform with the guidelines for therapeutic occlusion (see Table 47–1). The initial phase of oral reconstruction often begins with occlusal adjustment during periodontal therapy.

To summarize, *existing occlusion and maxillomandibular relationship is altered when it is anticipated that the resulting changes will (1) normalize the trauma from occlusion and (2) result in occlusal stabilization for future restorative or prosthetic procedures.* If a decision is made to maintain the existing ICP, then all occlusal treatments are aimed at preserving relationships while removing only traumatic contacts in localized areas. The change in the mandibular position need not be permanent; it may be reversible, as in the case of removable bite guards and splints or provisional restorations. Three categories of patients can be identified with respect to the planning of occlusal positions and maxillomandibular relationships; these are noted in Table 47–2.

Table 47–2. OCCLUSAL TREATMENT PLANNING: PATIENT CATEGORIES

Patient in Orthofunction (Normal Function)

Treatments are aimed at preserving the existing occlusion and mandibular position. An effort is made, therefore, to *avoid introducing new occlusal interferences.*

Patient in Dysfunction

Specific procedures are instituted to remove pathosis related to occlusal interferences. Partial or total alteration of the occlusion is generally indicated by either reversible or permanent means. Large-scale alterations lead to a therapeutic mandibular position and occlusion.

Patient Requiring Extensive Occlusal Reconstruction for Reasons Other Than Traumatic Occlusion

Create new intercuspal position to therapeutic occlusal standards, so that both joints and teeth receive stress with only a slight mesial component.

TREATMENT PLANNING AND TECHNIQUE

Objectives of Coronoplasty. The objective of coronoplasty is the mechanical elimination of occlusal supracontacts involved in function and parafunction. Positive results of occlusal adjustment include the following:[42]

1. Change in the pattern and degree of afferent impulses
2. Lessening of excessive tooth mobility
3. Multiple simultaneous contact spread over the occlusal scheme to effect occlusal stabilization (i.e., decrease need for muscular stabilization)
4. Beneficial change in the pattern of chewing or swallowing function
5. Multidirectional mandibular movement patterns
6. Verticalization of occlusal forces on implants

Sequencing Coronoplasty in Treatment Planning. The occlusion is usually adjusted after gingival inflammation and periodontal pockets have been eliminated, for the following reasons:

1. Evidence related to the pathogenesis and healing aspects of trauma from occlusion[60,61] suggests that the benefits of coronoplasty are not complete if inflammation is not eliminated first. Pocket depth and tooth mobility will not be improved with coronoplasty, and some enhancement in the

clinical periodontal attachment may result if inflammation is first eliminated.[9]
2. Teeth with periodontal disease often migrate. After the inflammation is eliminated, the teeth shift again, often in the direction of their original position (Fig. 47–3). If the occlusion is adjusted before the inflammation is alleviated, it may have to be readjusted after gingival health is restored.

This sequence of treatment is modified under the following conditions:

1. In infrabony pockets. In cases of infrabony pockets, excessive occlusal forces are important in determining the pattern of the osseous defects; to provide optimal conditions for repair of the bony defect, the occlusion is adjusted before or at the same time as the pocket elimination procedures.[72]
2. In mucogingival surgery, because occlusal forces affect the post-treatment contour of the facial bony plate.[23]
3. In cases of excessive tooth mobility, in which trauma from occlusion is a major causative factor (the occlusion is adjusted before or with treatment of the inflammation).
4. If a cracked tooth is suspected.[1]

Occlusal Analysis. Prior to extensive coronoplasty, casts from dental impressions should be made. These records are useful for reference during the procedure and at follow-up visits and for determining a reasonable prediction of the biomechanical result, which is a necessity. Mounting the casts on an articulator using a facebow transfer and a retruded position intermaxillary record assists in attaining this objective.[13] Trial carving of the casts allows rehearsal of the planned adjustment with greater confidence and efficiency.

Suggested Materials. To identify and mark tooth contacts, it is best to use multiple products; selected products are listed in Table 47–3, with recommendations for specific application in the coronoplasty process. Marking ribbon and marking paper work best on a dry tooth surface and therefore should be used in combination with adequate isolation. Blotting paper and cotton rolls are useful for this purpose.

Informed Consent. Patients are often concerned about whether coronoplasty will change their appearance, cause tooth decay, or increase tooth sensitivity. The clinician should explain that the teeth are not going to be ground down, but reshaped so that they will function better. The reshaping is done in areas where tooth decay rarely occurs. The patient should understand that the teeth and the occlusion change with time and that minor adjustments will be made on subsequent recall, if necessary.

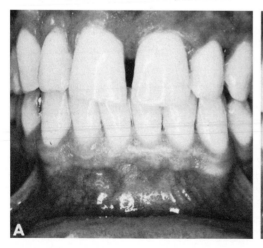 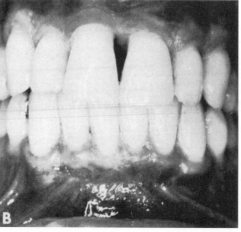

FIGURE 47–3. Change in tooth position after periodontal treatment. *A,* Before treatment. Note the diastema between the maxillary central incisors. *B,* In the course of treatment, the teeth return to their normal position after resolution of inflammation.

Products

Occlusal registration strips (Artus Corp, Englewood, NJ)
Occlusal indicator wax (Kerr Corp, Romulus, MI)
Marking ribbon, red, green (Columbia Ribbon, Cucamonga, CA);
  blue Mylar ribbon (Parkel, Farmingdale, NJ)
Articulating paper, blue (Holg Mark-Rite Interstate Dental Co,
  New Hyde Park, NY)

Suggested Applications of Products

ICP contact
RCP contact
Protusive and lateral contact
Intensity/area of contact

ICP, Intercuspal position; retruded contact position.

METHODS

Determining the End Point of Coronoplasty

Clinicians have placed an enormous emphasis on the significance of the relationship between RCP and ICP in planning coronoplasty. Selection of an intraborder position as the end point in coronoplasty is logical, as there is little doubt that the ICP is the functional end point of the occlusion.[22] Retruded contact position adjustment is practical in more complex cases, because the RCP adjustment provides an objective method by which to align the mandible. In the end, stability of the occlusion is more important than whether RCP, ICP, or the habitual closure position is selected for the occlusal end point.[39]

This controversial topic has been reviewed by Møller[52] and by Gibbs and Lundeen.[21] Møller[52] has characterized ICP as a working position because of its importance as an entry and exit position in chewing and because it represents a position selected by the central nervous system primarily to withstand the exertion of strong force. A wide range of ICPs are tolerated by the system, and regardless of where ICP is located with respect to RCP, adequate occlusal force can be supplied as long as there are stable contact relationships at ICP.[39] Instability at ICP causes reflex inhibition of the elevators and promotes increased neuromuscular control over mandibular positioning.[3] The positioning of the jaws at ICP can therefore be thought of as a morphofunctional reflex adaptation. Whether this adaptation is successful depends on the positional tolerances of the masticatory muscles and the ability of the TMJs to resist destabilizing forces.[52]

These concepts are supported by the studies of Gibbs and Lundeen,[21] who showed that the neuromuscular system exerts fine control during chewing to avoid particular supracontacts. In subjects with good occlusions, such fine control does not appear to be necessary. This concept also applies to the anterior teeth if they encroach on chewing and speaking motion. Therefore, occlusal form should be harmonious with the envelope of jaw movement during chewing.[21]

On the basis of jaw tracking and electromyography (EMG) studies, it seems reasonable to suggest that RCP, although rarely approached during function[50] and seen only as a postural end point of occlusion in a minority of subjects,[31,63] is nevertheless a useful reference position from which to judge the alignment and positional requirements for an optimal therapeutic position during coronoplasty. The alignment is most physiologic if the articular disc and the condyle are stable in their relationship to each other against the temporal surface. From a practical standpoint, this would involve establishing a compatible relationship between RCP and ICP, with bilateral posterior contact in both positions.[67] The presence of a symmetric occlusal glide from RCP to ICP, as experienced by 70% to 90% of healthy populations,[2,76] is compatible with a favorable RCP–ICP relationship. Because RCP induces more positioning muscle activity than ICP,[39] its choice as the sole occlusal end point for coronoplasty is rarely indicated. However, discrepancies between RCP and ICP of more than 2 mm in magnitude should be carefully evaluated for coronoplasty, because they induce earlier onset of heightened muscle activity[37] and are not characteristic of healthy populations.[64] After the entire dentition is reconstructed so that RCP is stable and on the same horizontal plane as ICP, a patient may persist in using ICP.[24]

The concept of using RCP analysis does not necessarily apply to unstable or painful joints; for example, TMJ derangements involving chronic clicking near the closed position and arrested jaw motion as a result of locking of the articular disc require special evaluation and treatment.

Selecting an Occlusal Guidance Scheme

Balanced Occlusion. The term *balanced occlusion* refers to simultaneous contact between the right and left posterior segments of the arch in lateral excursion of the mandible and between the posterior and anterior segments of the arch in protrusive excursion. Although balanced occlusion was at one time hypothesized to be the "ideal" excursive contact pattern, its occurrence in modern dentitions is rare.[36] The putative benefits of attempting to create bilateral balance by occlusal adjustment or prosthetic restorations include decreased dental loading forces with bilaterally similar cuspal inclines.[17] Nonetheless, the creation of mediotrusive contacts may introduce the risk of damage to the periodontium,[73,77] especially if such contacts are not carefully balanced with the contralateral working contacts. In patients with periodontal disease, molars with unilateral non–working side contact showed significantly greater loading forces,[17] and greater mobility, bone loss, and pocket depth have been reported in such teeth compared with teeth that do not contact on the nonworking side.[89] Furthermore, the highest compressive condyle forces occur with balanced occlusions.[41]

Canine-Protected Occlusion. According to the concept of canine-protected occlusion,[14] the maxillary canines act to guide the mandible so that the posterior teeth come into closure with minimal horizontal forces (Fig. 47–4A). In lateral and protrusive excursions, the mandibular canines and first premolars engage the lingual surface of the maxillary canines so as to disclude the incisors, premolars, and

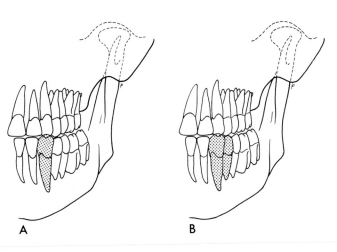

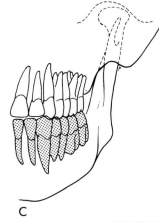

FIGURE 47–4. Types of occlusion. *A,* Canine-protected occlusion. The canine teeth act as the discluders of the other teeth. *B,* Canine–premolar disclusion as found in normal young adults. *C,* Group function occlusion.

molars and protect them from undesirable horizontal forces. The hypothesis that the maxillary canines are especially equipped to absorb lateral forces because of the size of the root and radicular bone and because of an especially sensitive proprioceptive mechanism that reflexly reduces muscle forces when the canines make occlusal contact has not been shown to be valid.[25] Results from a study combining EMG and kinesiography suggest that canine-protected occlusions do not significantly reduce muscle activity during parafunctional clenching.[5] Other studies have verified that canine-protected occlusions exhibit reduced masticatory muscle activity when compared with occlusions with group function,[5,8,49,74,76] but this phenomenon seems related more to the number of contacts during laterotrusion than to any specific property of the canines themselves.[25] In support of canine-protected occlusal schemes, however, the teeth of individuals having canine-protected occlusions in one study had significantly lower mean Periodontal Disease Index scores than did those of individuals having progressive disclusion (Fig. 47–4*B*) or group function (Fig. 47–4*C*).

Group Function. Group function, or the simultaneous gliding contact of teeth on the laterotrusive side during laterotrusion (see Fig. 47–4*C*), is much more common than canine-protected guidance and is highly variable.[88] In group function, both functional and parafunctional occlusal forces exceed those in canine function,[11,41] so it is not indicated for periodontally compromised dentitions. Nonetheless, the tendency to progress from canine guidance to group function over time should be respected in older patients,[87] and if group function is chosen as an occlusal guidance scheme, tooth loads can be minimized by steepening the guidance pattern.[17] Although group function is physiologically acceptable as a disclusion system, it is not a requirement in restorative therapy.

None of the preceding concepts fulfills the needs of the clinician, who must evaluate cuspal guidance in individual patients presenting with a variety of dental and skeletal malocclusions. Individualization of the disclusion pattern is ultimately necessary.

Occlusion, like other physiologic body processes, is variable and changes with age. The dentist should consider the needs of the individual occlusion rather than attempt a standard occlusion for all patients.

Occlusal Adjustment

Clinical Goals. The clinical goals of ICP and RCP adjustment are to reduce the supracontacts so as to create unobstructed closure of cusps into fossae and marginal ridges, while at the same time conserving original crown structure. Rough grinding down of supracontacts is to be avoided, because it creates flattened planes that further disrupt the occlusion.

The correction of occlusal supracontacts consists of grooving, spheroiding, and pointing. *Grooving* entails restoring the depth of developmental grooves; it is done with a tapered cutting tool until the desired depth is attained (Fig. 47–5).

Spheroiding consists of reducing the supracontact while restoring the original tooth contour. Starting 2 or 3 mm

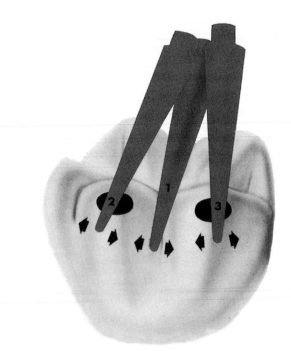

FIGURE 47–5. Grooving to restore the depth of developmental grooves on worn tooth surfaces. A tapered diamond stone (1) is rotated slowly in the groove as indicated. After the desired depth is attained, the stone is moved (2) and (3) to spheroid the adjacent tooth surface.

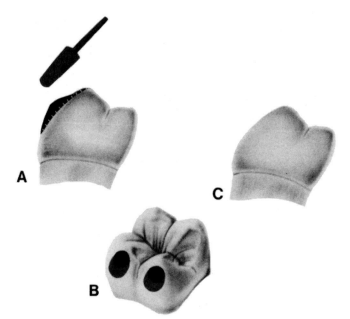

FIGURE 47–6. Spheroiding to restore the original tooth contour. *A,* Recontouring prematurity. *B,* Recontouring extends several millimeters below the black marking. *C,* Corrected contour.

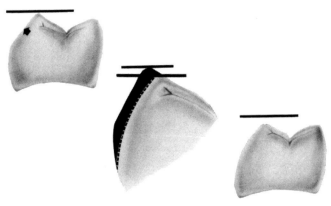

FIGURE 47–8. Incorrect method of spheroiding (*broken line*) results in excessive reduction in buccal cusp height (*horizontal lines*). The *arrow* points to the prematurity.

mesial or distal to the prematurity, the tooth is recontoured from the occlusal margin to a distance 2 or 3 mm apical to the marking (see Fig. 47–5; Fig. 47–6). This is done with a light "paintbrush" stroke, gradually blending the area of the prematurity with the adjacent tooth surface. Effort is made to preserve the occlusal height of the cusps (Figs. 47–7 and 47–8).

When teeth are flattened by wear or poor dental restoration, the buccolingual diameter of the occlusal surface is increased. Spheroiding restores the buccolingual width of the occlusal surface to normal dimensions (Fig. 47–9).

Pointing consists of restoring cusp point contours (Fig. 47–10); it is done by reshaping the tooth with rotating cutting tools.

Sequence for Coronoplasty (Nine Steps). Coronoplasty can be accomplished using a variety of different sequences, particularly if the area to be corrected involves only a few

teeth. However, when a comprehensive coronoplasty is to be accomplished, a step-by-step approach is required, although experienced clinicians tend to blend the steps.

The occlusion is adjusted systematically according to the schedule in Table 47–4. The series of steps is normally accomplished over two or more appointments, with each visit lasting no more than 30 minutes.

Many situations in periodontal therapy require coronoplasty of only one or two teeth, and comprehensive oc-

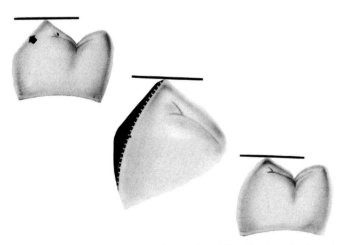

FIGURE 47–7. Correct method of spheroiding (*broken line*) and preserving the height of the buccal cusp (*horizontal lines*). The *arrow* points to the prematurity.

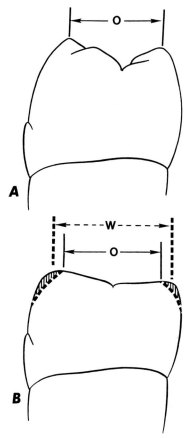

FIGURE 47–9. Flattened occlusal surface restored to unworn width. *A,* Occlusal diameter (O) of unworn mandibular molar. *B,* Widened occlusal diameter (W) of worn molar restored to diameter of unworn surface (O) by recontouring (*shaded areas*).

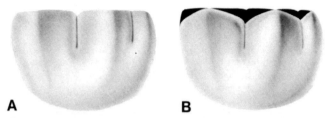

FIGURE 47-10. Pointing. *A,* Buccal margin of mandibular molar flattened by wear. *B,* Tooth recontoured to restore cusp points.

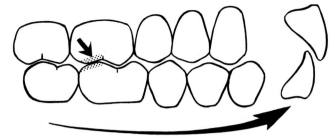

FIGURE 47-11. Shift from retruded contact position to intercuspal position. When contact is located on terminal hinge closure (retruded contact position), prematurities *(short arrow)* may cause the mandible to glide mesially into the intercuspal position *(long arrow).*

clusal adjustment is not warranted. In these cases, localized coronoplasty is often limited to intraborder reduction of supracontacts on the involved teeth (steps 2, 4, and 5 in the discussion that follows). As discussed earlier, the decision to include RCP adjustments (step 1) is usually based on the use of RCP as a reference position rather than as the occlusal end point position.

Step 1: Remove Retrusive Supracontacts and Minimize the Deflective Shift from RCP to ICP. The purpose of this step is to reduce supracontacts that interfere with posterior border closure of the mandible to a stable bilateral RCP. When contact is located on the retruded path of closure, supracontacts may cause the mandible to deflect forward and sometimes laterally into the ICP. This contact movement is termed the *shift* or *slide* from RCP to ICP (Fig. 47-11). Retrusive adjustment results in the elimination of the RCP-to-ICP shift. In general, it neutralizes or removes asymmetric shifts from RCP to ICP (Fig. 47-12). The target areas of contact at RCP or ICP are referred to as *vertical* (or *centric*) *stops.*

How to Locate the RCP. Locating the RCP is the key to controlled coronoplasty. The patient is placed in the supine position, which has been shown to reduce most completely the activity of the protruder and postural elevator muscles.[20,34,44,51] The clinician should test and rehearse hinge closure to RCP. Some patients allow their mandibles to be passively retruded quite easily; other patients resist because of reflex guarding by the protruder muscles. Arriving at the RCP is dependent on specific verbal and motor actions by the operator. Figure 47-13 shows two hand-grasp methods that have proved effective for manipulation of the mandible.[15,32,66] A common error is to grasp the chin and nervously order the patient to relax. In the supine position,

the patient's mandible will fall passively to the RCP. The operator's main function is to create an arcing retruded movement over the initial 10 mm of mouth opening. Experience has shown that some statements and/or actions are better than others in obtaining the desired result:

1. With light pressure, encourage small arcing movements and say, "Let your mouth drop open."
2. As the jaw falls downward and backward to the retruded position, exert more chin pressure backward and upward and seek out the ligamentous resistance of the TMJs. Muscular resistance (guarding) may be encountered; when this is sensed, remove the hands completely and begin the manipulation again. Talk in low tones using repetitive phrases such as, "Just let it go." At this point the jaw should be arcing. Then say, "Let your jaw come together . . . just so the teeth first touch."
3. After the initial contact is perceived, say, "Squeeze." The shift from RCP to ICP, if present, should be apparent. Remember: Locating RCP is dependent on the ability to detect the "ligamentous signal" from the patient. A stiff wrist and forearm will improve receptivity to this joint feel. Generally,

---

Table 47-4. SCHEDULE OF CORONOPLASTY

Step 1: Remove retrusive prematurities and eliminate the deflective shift from RCP to ICP. (The retrusive pathway prematurities are eliminated.)

Step 2: Adjust ICP to achieve stable, simultaneous, multipointed, widely distributed contacts.

Step 3: Test for excessive contact (fremitus) on the incisor teeth.

Step 4: Remove posterior protrusive supracontacts and establish contacts that are bilaterally distributed on the anterior teeth.

Step 5: Remove or lessen mediotrusive (balancing) interferences.

Step 6: Reduce excessive cusp steepness on the laterotrusive (working) contacts.

Step 7: Eliminate gross occlusal disharmonies.

Step 8: Recheck tooth contact relationships.

Step 9: Polish all rough tooth surfaces.

ICP, Intercuspal position; RCP, retruded contact position.

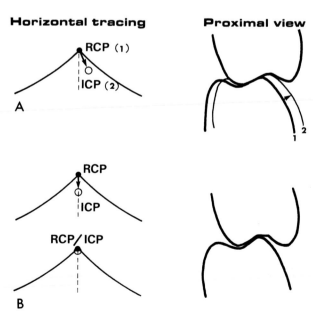

FIGURE 47-12. Shift from retruded contact position (RCP) to intercuspal position (ICP). *A,* Before occlusal adjustment. Mandibular teeth shift from point 1 to point 2 (asymmetric shift). The same movement is seen in the arrow point tracing in the horizontal plane. *B,* After occlusal adjustment. Asymmetric shift from RCP to ICP is removed, and resulting intercuspal position is nearer or identical to RCP.

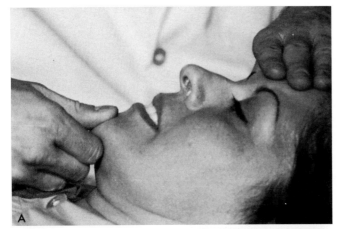

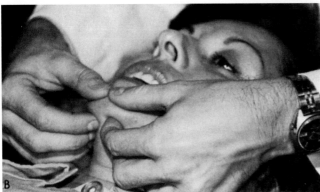

FIGURE 47–13. Methods for locating retruded contact position. *A,* Patient is supine. Forefinger and thumb are "butted" against the chin, with the other hand stabilizing the head. *B,* Dawson[15] method. All four fingers of each hand are placed on the lower border of the mandible. This creates an upward pressure on the condyle during the manipulation. The thumbs are placed in the notch over the symphysis, exerting a downward pressure. The thumbs should touch each other.

if the mandible cannot be manipulated to RCP, a coronoplasty in the retruded position should not be attempted. Instead, removable interocclusal splints are indicated for reducing the neuromuscular guarding prior to coronoplasty.

4. Retrusive prematurities can be marked with green wax or red marking tape. Red tape should be placed in a ribbon forceps and inserted between the desired teeth after they are properly dried (Fig. 47–14). Occlusal registration wax is placed on the maxillary or mandibular posterior quadrant, with the adhesive (shiny) surface pressed lightly against the teeth (Fig. 47–15). The occlusal surface of the wax is moistened with a wet finger to prevent adherence of the opposing teeth. The mandible is manipulated to strike against the wax in short, interrupted closures. Mobile teeth are stabilized with the fingers so that supracontacts will not be pushed aside. If there are no supracontacts on retruded closure of the jaw, the wax will be uniformly transparent at the contact areas. Significant supracontacts will cause perforation of the wax. The supracontacts are marked on the teeth through the wax with a pencil, and the wax strips are removed (Fig. 47–16).

5. Question the patient as to which teeth seem to "hit first" as the jaws close. The patient's confirmation in locating the areas of supracontact should be invited. Typical sites of supracontacts are the mesial inclines of the maxillary lingual cusps and their opposing tooth surfaces. The mesial inner incline of the lingual cusp of the maxillary first premolars is the most common initial supracontact at the RCP.

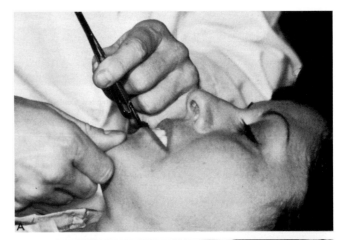

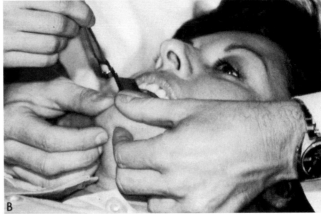

FIGURE 47–14. Techniques for marking retruded contact position contacts on the teeth. *A,* Chin grasp technique. *B,* Technique after Dawson.[15]

Principles Not To Be Violated in the Retrusive Coronoplasty

1. Remove the inclines between RCP and ICP that cause supracontacts when the mandible moves from RCP to ICP, without removing the vertical stop or supporting cusp tip (see Fig. 47–16C–E). These inclines, called *retrusive prematurities,* are usually found on mesial facing inclines of the maxillary teeth and distal facing inclines of the mandibular teeth (MUDL rule).

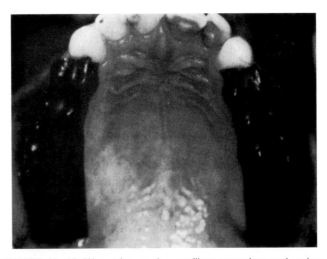

FIGURE 47–15. Wax strips on the maxillary premolars and molars. The anterior teeth are not covered.

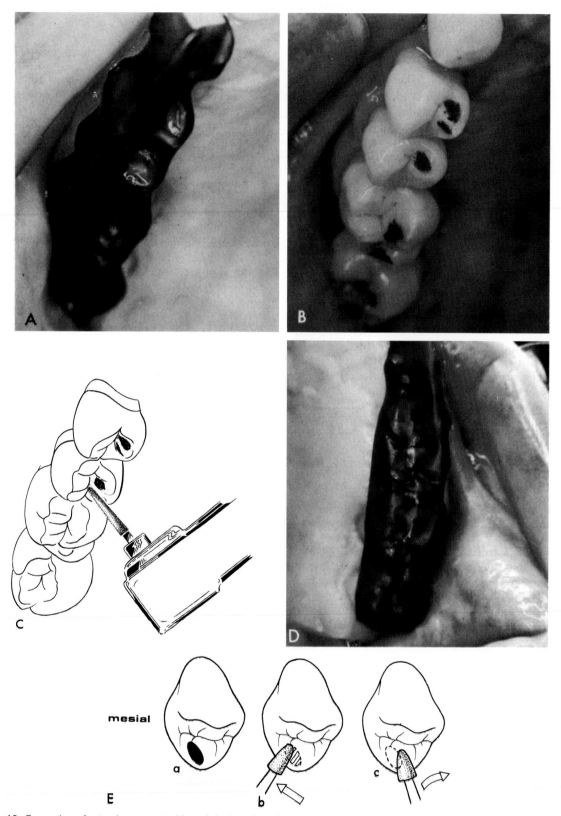

FIGURE 47–16. Correction of retrusive prematurities. *A,* Indentations in wax show retrusive prematurities on the mesial inner inclines of the maxillary lingual cusps. *B,* Retrusive prematurities marked on the teeth. *C,* Prematurities corrected with a diamond point. *D,* After correction, wax shows evenly distributed contact on cusp tips and fossae. *E,* Correction of retrusive interferences involves flat reduction (a and b) but should be followed by spheroiding (c).

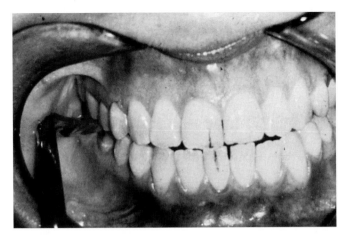
FIGURE 47–17. Mylar occlusal strips are used in confirming areas of contact.

2. Strive to achieve vertical stops at RCP on each tooth. Avoid losing them when grinding excursive supracontacts. If the vertical cusps are not aligned within the desired opposing fossa, corrections are made on the opposing cusp slope or incline to place the cusp more nearly within the fossa. If the cusp and fossa are in alignment, either the fossa is deepened or the cusp is shortened, depending on which element is more out of harmony with the other like elements in the arch.[68]

3. Reshape, if possible, at the expense of the fossae, ridges, or cusp inclines. Preserve the marginal ridges; adjust the cusp tip as a last resort. Adjust worn facets to achieve point-to-surface rather than surface-to-surface contact.

4. Mobile teeth are stabilized with the fingers so that prematurities are accurately registered and not pushed aside. To avoid excessive grinding of one dental arch, do part of the correction on the other arch.

5. Remove the lateral thrust in the RCP-to-ICP shift. In lateral shifts, the significant retrusive markings on the maxillary teeth face in the direction in which the mandible shifts from RCP to ICP. Adjustment of these prematurities eliminates the lateral component of the shift. This simple observation can be of great help in rapidly achieving the end point in retrusive range adjustment.

6. Continue to adjust the RCP vertical stops so that they approach the same vertical level as the previous ICP. If the RCP stops appear stable but still require reduction to approach the same level as ICP, use the following guidelines: (1) reduce the cusp tip when supracontacts in excursions are associated with the movement of that cusp; (2) otherwise, reduce the fossa, especially if it appears too shallow. Both the cusps and the fossae may eventually require adjustment to obtain RCP and ICP at the same level. After this relationship is obtained, both the cranial and the lateral components of the RCP-to-ICP shift are removed. The therapeutic result is to allow sagittal movement between RCP and ICP at the same level; alternatively, RCP may be made slightly cranial to the preoperative ICP, in which case RCP and ICP may be nearly identical after coronoplasty.

7. The retrusive range adjustment is complete when the following conditions are achieved: (1) the contact pattern is bilateral with multi-pointed contacts; (2) the deflective shift from RCP to ICP has been eliminated; (3) both RCP and ICP approach the same vertical dimension of occlusion; (4) the pathway from RCP to ICP, if present, is smooth and gliding; and (5) repeated closure of the teeth together in the hinge position produces a sharp, resonant sound.

Step 2: Adjustment of the ICP. A task common to many dental procedures is the localized adjustment of ICP contacts on one or more teeth. The adjustment of ICP is also a major step in comprehensive coronoplasty. The purpose of this step is to achieve a stable ICP and to refine occlusal anatomic relationships. The main feature of this step is that the supracontacts are identified without guidance by the operator's hand. The reshaping is accomplished by progressive adjustment of supracontacts or undesirable contacts during one or more visits. The posterior teeth are adjusted first, followed by conservative adjustment of the anterior teeth, if necessary.

How to Locate Supracontacts in ICP. Instruct the patient, "Tap your back teeth together, both sides at the same time, slow and hard." Ask the patient to repeat this process once or twice. The teeth normally will meet in the same position. This is the ICP, or habitual occlusion. Because relatively heavy muscular force is used, the choice of marking medium is less critical. The combined use of more than one medium for cross comparison is advantageous. Occlusal indicator wax, blue marking paper, and marking tape work well. Physical ICP contact can be assessed by using Mylar occlusal indicator strips inserted between clenched teeth and tested with a "tugging" motion (Fig. 47–17). The strips should be less than 2 μm thick and possess plastic deformation properties.[28] If wax is used, it is placed on the

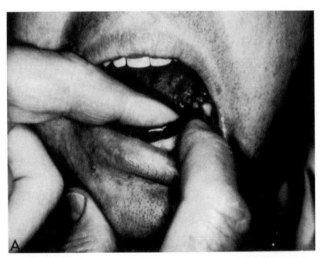

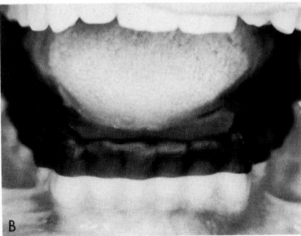
FIGURE 47–18. Correcting prematurities in the intercuspal position. *A,* Placing the wax on the mandibular teeth. *B,* Wax in position.

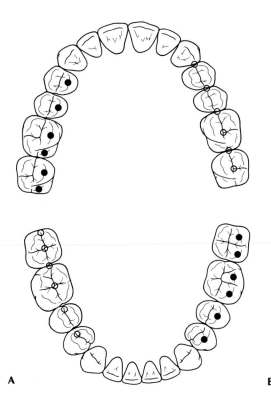

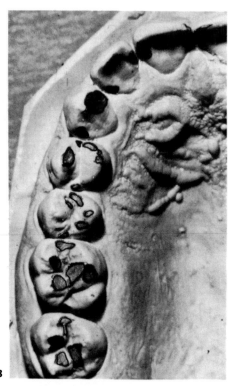

FIGURE 47–19. Normal zones of contact in the intercuspal position. *A,* Open circles denote vertical (centric) stops; solid circles denote centric cusps. *B,* Zones of contact in a natural dentition.

occlusal and incisal surfaces of the mandibular teeth (Fig. 47–18). The patient is then asked to open and close again, as before. The translucent areas are marked on the mandibular teeth with a pencil, and the wax is removed.

The goal of ICP adjustment is to achieve occlusal stability between tooth pairs. Correction of ICP contacts should be made, keeping in mind those occlusal schemes found in individuals with normally aligned teeth (Fig. 47–19). Two major conditions must be met to fulfill these objectives of ICP adjustment: (1) if the contact is at an unfavorable location on the tooth, the correction is made to favor a more

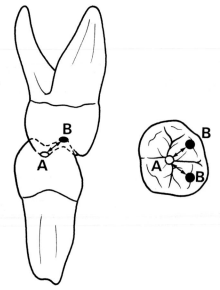

FIGURE 47–20. The establishment or preservation of cross-tooth contacts is a goal in occlusal adjustment. Cross-tooth contacts (A–B) are shown in proximal *(left)* and occlusal *(right)* views.

ideal contact position; and (2) if the contact is too high (true supracontact), one should either create fossa depth or remove cuspal height, depending on the individual cusp-to-fossa relationship. Take care not to induce unwanted heavy incisal pressure by decreasing the vertical dimension of occlusion on the posterior teeth. The rule is to be judicious in the reduction of true supracontacts. It is desirable to achieve cross-tooth vertical stops in ICP wherever possible (Fig. 47–20), but it is not necessary to achieve the maximum number of contacts in the posterior teeth to reach maximum muscle activity levels.[40] Among the alterations that commonly are made in conjunction with this step are reduction of cuspal size, alteration of occlusal table width, and lessening of plunger cusp height. Figures 47–21 and 47–22 illustrate typical problems encountered in ICP adjustment.

Step 3: Test for Excessive Contact on the Incisor Teeth in ICP. The incisor teeth should be slightly out of contact or in light contact over the maximum number of teeth.[45] The firmness of contact can be detected by using Mylar occlusal strips held with a hemostat. The Mylar strip should just slip through the incisor teeth when the patient clenches firmly in ICP. In addition, closing contacts should be tested for fremitus, a vibration or displacement perceptible on palpation of the facial tooth surface with a moistened forefinger during repeated firm closure to ICP. If a supracontact is present, it may be marked with wax or marking ribbon and reduced (Fig. 47–22). No fremitus should be detectable on firm intercuspal closure of the teeth.

The ICP adjustment is complete when the following conditions are achieved:

1. The contact pattern is bilateral, stable, and many-pointed (see Fig. 47–19A,B).
2. Each posterior vertical step holds a Mylar occlusal strip with equal resistance.

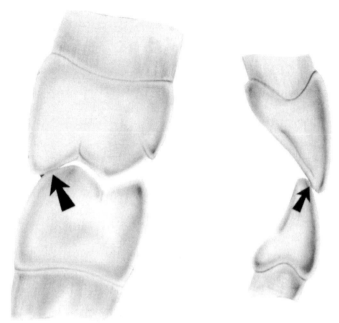

FIGURE 47–21. Class I prematurities in the intercuspal position. Class I prematurities on the facial surface of the mandibular anterior and posterior teeth are indicated by *arrows*.

3. Sharp, resonant sounds are heard when the patient taps his or her teeth together in ICP (with a stethoscope placed over the infraorbital skin area[85]) (Fig. 47–23).
4. The patient responds negatively to the following question: "Tap on your back teeth, slow and hard—do you feel any difference between the two sides?"
5. No fremitus is detected in the anterior teeth.

Step 4: Remove Posterior Protrusive Supracontacts; Obtain Bilateral Protrusive Contact Movement on the Anterior Teeth. *Protrusive excursion* refers to the path of the mandible as it moves anteriorly between the ICP and the edge-to-edge relationship of the anterior teeth. The latter is called the *incisal position*. Any position away from the ICP on this path is a *protrusive position*. The protrusive path and excursion are altered separately. Figure 47–24 illustrates and defines these supracontacts in term of jaw movement.

Correction of Protrusive Position. The objective of this step is to attain bilateral, well-distributed contact on the incisal edges of the maxillary and mandibular incisor teeth. This is completed as follows: From ICP contact, instruct the patient to protrude the mandible slowly. There should be bilateral contact in this segment, with little or no deviation of the mandible. Deviation usually is caused by a molar interference or an asymmetric incisal plane. Use finger pressure to help guide the patient's jaw along a precise, symmetric excursion (Fig. 47–25A). The patient is instructed to open and close in this position with marking ribbon or wax strips between the teeth. Progressive adjustment of the marked areas permits the unmarked incisal edges to come into contact (Fig. 47–25B–E). Wherever possible, adjustment is confined to the maxillary teeth to protect mandibular functional cusp height. If such contact is not maintained, the mandibular teeth tend to extrude and re-create prematurities. The mandibular teeth are ground (1) when, because of pain, proximity to the pulp, or aesthetic reasons, the limit of grinding of the maxillary teeth has been reached; or (2) when individual mandibular teeth protrude either incisally or facially.

FIGURE 47–22. Correction of class I prematurities in the intercuspal position. *A,* Prematurities are marked through the wax onto the teeth. *B,* Prematurities marked on the teeth. *C,* Grooving the buccal surface with a tapered diamond. *D,* After correction, contact is shown on the cusp tips.

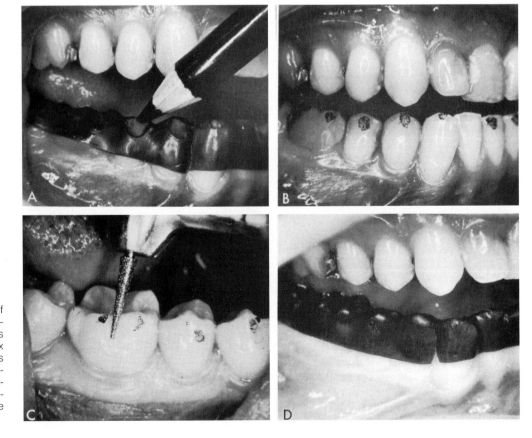

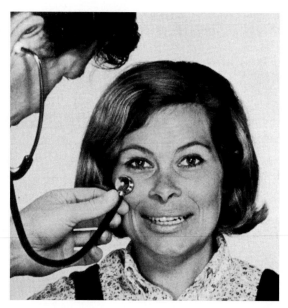

FIGURE 47–23. Occlusal sounds are tested by instructing the patient to tap *slowly* and *firmly* in the intercuspal position. Ideally, the sounds should be sharp. Dull or mixed sounds are the result of discrepancy between the muscular contact position and the intercuspal position.[85] Muscular contact position–intercuspal position discrepancies can be caused by occlusal prematurities, muscle imbalance, or both.

The production of flat, broad incisal surfaces by grinding should be avoided. After a maximum number of anterior teeth are in contact, the width of the incisal edges is reduced by grinding the facial margin of the maxillary teeth and the lingual margin of the mandibular teeth. Caution should be exercised in reshaping the anterior teeth merely to improve aesthetics. The ideal result of correction of the protrusive path is several contact points equally distributed between the right and left anterior teeth.[45] This may not be fully attainable in cases of tooth irregularity.

Correction of Protrusive Excursion. If any posterior teeth interfere or contact in the protrusive excursion, tooth structure is removed from the offending cusps until all articulating contacts between the posterior teeth have been eliminated. Harmonious protrusive contact that occurs during the first millimeter of jaw movement is acceptable. Protrusive interferences are on the distal facing inclines of the maxillary teeth and the mesial facing inclines of the mandibular teeth. A practical method for marking excursive contact is the two-color method. The protrusive contacts are first marked by drying and isolating the teeth, inserting red marking tape, and directing the patient to produce multiple protrusive glides. The vertical stops are then marked with blue marking paper by directing the patient to tap the teeth together in ICP. As a result, the target protrusive supracontacts (red) are clearly distinguished from the vertical stops (blue), which are to be preserved. It is important not to disturb the cusp tips and vertical stops required for maintenance of the ICP. Mobile teeth should be stabilized by the operator's fingers to prevent them from moving away from the forces of contact. The absence of posterior protrusive interferences is confirmed by the use of Mylar strips.

The lingual surfaces of the anterior maxillary teeth are

also marked using the two-color method (protrusive gliding contacts in red; ICP stops, if present, in blue). The protrusive contacts are reduced to provide a bilateral, smooth contact glide along the path approaching the previously established protrusive position. Attempts should be made to limit the protrusive glide adjustment to the lingual surfaces of the anterior maxillary teeth in most cases. There are several types of problems that require the use of clinical judgment in the protrusive excursion adjustment. Occasionally, an open bite situation does not permit edge-to-edge contact of the anterior teeth. The posterior teeth must then be recruited to play a role in the protrusive guidance (i.e., the preservation of smooth protrusive posterior contact).

Similarly, the anterior teeth may not be suitable for use as sole discluders of the teeth on protrusive excursion because of loss of bony support. In such instances, the anterior and posterior teeth should be brought into contact during the protrusive glide (especially the first 2 mm of contact movement). Attempts should also be made to evaluate habitual incisal "lock-and-key" bruxism facets. Any sig-

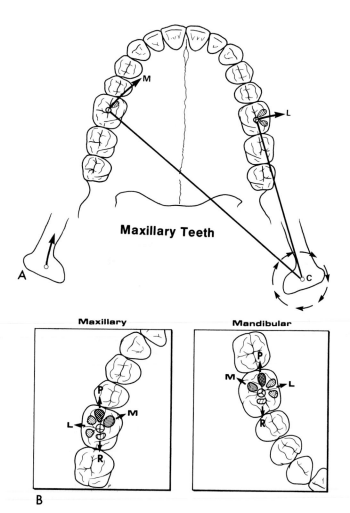

FIGURE 47–24. Excursive interferences. These are named after the mandibular movement that caused the contact to occur. *A,* Note that the potential for interferences occurs over pathways determined by the rotating (working) condyle (C). L, Laterotrusive interference; M, mediotrusive interference. *B,* The four main occlusal interferences. L, Laterotrusive; M, mediotrusive; P, protrusive; R, retrusive. Open circle denotes the intercuspal position contact area.

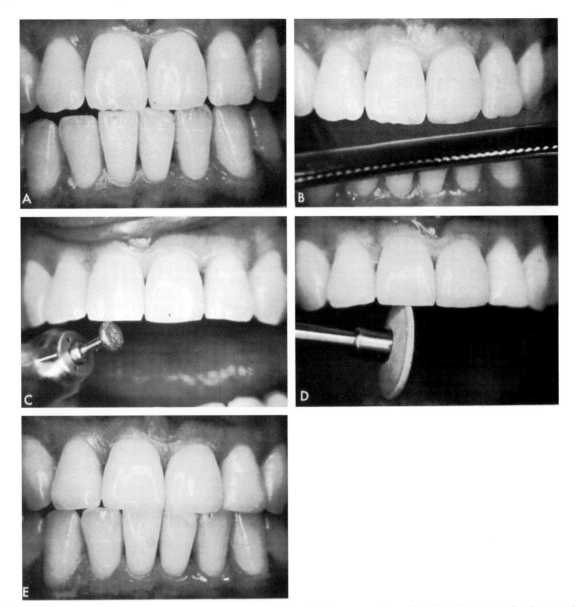

FIGURE 47–25. Correction of the anterior teeth in protrusive position. *A,* Before correction. *B,* Articulating paper in place to detect areas of contact. *C,* Marked areas on maxillary teeth reduced. *D,* Smoothing the ground surfaces with rubber wheel. *E,* Multipointed, bilateral contact of anterior teeth in protrusive position.

nificant facets on teeth in the anterior segment should be rounded over without shortening the clinical crowns.

Step 5: Remove or Lessen Mediotrusive (Balancing) Supracontacts. Mediotrusive (balancing) supracontacts complicate correction of the laterotrusive (working) guidance. They may even prevent laterotrusive side guidance. Mediotrusive supracontacts are routinely observed as oblique facets on the first and second molar teeth (the inner inclines of the mandibular buccal cusps and the inner inclines of the maxillary lingual cusps) (Fig. 47–26). Mediotrusive supracontacts should be lessened or removed to facilitate a dominant disclusion on the laterotrusive side. It is recommended that both habitual excursion and passive (border) manipulation of the mandible be employed to identify mediotrusive interferences originating from both ICP and RCP. To record these supracontacts, the mediotrusive contact should be marked with red marking ribbon and the ICP stops located with blue marking paper (two-color

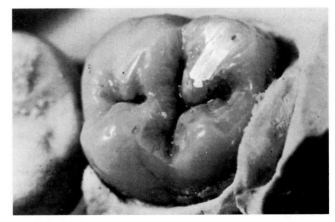

FIGURE 47–26. Mediotrusive (balancing) interferences appear as oblique facets on the molar teeth. Example shows extracted mandibular tooth set in dental cast.

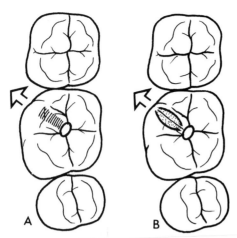

FIGURE 47–27. *A* and *B*, Adjustment of mediotrusive (balancing) interference often involves grooving to allow freedom for the opposing cusp movement.

method). Often reduction is achieved by grinding new grooves or shallow depressions for the opposing cusp pathway (Fig. 47–27).

The integrity of the vertical stops can be checked intermittently by the use of Mylar occlusal strips. Care should be taken, because complete removal of mediotrusive supracontacts may disrupt ICP contact. Therefore, the advantages of complete removal of all mediotrusive interferences must be weighed in relation to the effect of such removal on mandibular stability in the ICP. It should be stressed that mediotrusive contact is necessarily pathologic per se. It hardly could be, because the probability of observing a mediotrusive contact on at least one side in healthy young adults is at least 84%.[32] It is probable that the traumatic potential of mediotrusive interferences is related to the intensity of the contact combined with the lack of adequate cross-arch canine guidance. Thus, correct adjustment of mediotrusive supracontacts may involve reducing them so that they are compatible with good contact movement. A functional chewing test is helpful in making this assessment. The test is conducted as follows: Place a strip of adhesive occlusal registration wax over the mandibular quadrant in question. Give another strip of folded occlusal registration wax to the patient, and instruct the patient to chew the wax bolus on the opposite side up to five times. If there are significant mediotrusive supracontacts, oblique perforations of the applied wax strip will be observed. Repeat the test after adjustment for comparison and evaluation.

When the mediotrusive supracontacts have been dealt with on one side, the laterotrusive interferences are adjusted on the opposite side (step 6). Thus, the lateral excursion of one laterotrusive (working) side and its corresponding mediotrusive (balancing) side is completely corrected before the other lateral excursion is treated. Repeated checking of both sides is appropriate for lateral excursion.

Step 6: Reduce Supracontacts on the Laterotrusive (Working) Side. Lateral guidance is dominated by the canine and first premolar teeth in healthy young adults. The canine tooth is most frequently involved in disclusion.[68,71] The disclusion scheme is likely to include more posterior teeth with advancing age and in individuals with acceler-

ated wear. The lack of adequate guidance in the canine area increases the risk for single-tooth molar supracontacts that may result in trauma from functional and parafunctional movement. The first 2 mm of excursive guidance from ICP and RCP are especially important, because maximum force can be applied near the closed position.

The disclusing guidances and the periodontal status of all potential disclusing teeth should be systematically assessed. Laterotrusive disclusing contact should be on the ipsilateral canine and frequently on the first premolar, unless these teeth are weakened periodontally. In the case of mobile canines, all the teeth on the laterotrusive side, except the second molar, should assist in lateral guidance. An attempt should be made to remove or neutralize single-tooth supracontacts on the molar teeth. Contact area may be reduced on the canine and premolars if extensive surface-to-surface faceting predominates. Existing lock-and-key facets on laterotrusive cusps should be rounded over without shortening the clinical crown.

In lateral function, whether limited to the canine or involving multiple teeth, the disclusing angle should be acute enough to prevent mediotrusive contact on the contralateral side and allow for a definite separation of the ipsilateral molar teeth (Fig. 47–28). Normally, little reduction is attempted on the canine and premolar teeth, as these supracontacts are considered important for disclusion of the molar teeth in lateral movement. Unrestricted smooth contact movement in laterotrusion is more important than the number or location of contacts that are brought into lateral function.

Laterotrusive contacts can be marked with the two-color

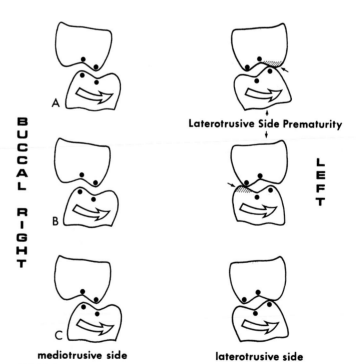

FIGURE 47–28. Correction of laterotrusive interferences (*hatched areas*) on posterior teeth to gain smooth contact movement patterns; mandibular movement indicated by *arrows*. *A,* Laterotrusive interference on buccal cusps. *B,* Laterotrusive interference on lingual cusps. *C,* Unrestricted glide after correction of laterotrusive interferences. Note absence of contact on the mediotrusive side.

method described in preceding discussions. If possible, reshape the inner inclines of the maxillary facial cusps, because grinding of the mandibular buccal cusps jeopardizes the functional ICP cusps. Always avoid grinding the vertical stop. Adjustment of the facial inclines often can be achieved through the process of grooving. All reductions should result in spherical or grooved surfaces. Avoid creating flat planes. Check your adjustment using Mylar strips.

Step 7: Eliminate Undesirable Gross Occlusal Features. At this point in the complete coronoplasty, all targeted supracontacts have been removed or lessened. However, gross undesirable occlusal features harmful to the periodontal structures may remain, and these should be modified. Care should be taken to avoid changing or removing previously attained occlusal contact relationships. Elimination of gross occlusal disharmonies at the beginning of the coronoplasty may be tempting and is permissible. Early gross adjustment should be done only to the extent that tooth contacts important to the future stability of the occlusion are not destroyed in the process. Some examples of undesirable gross occlusal features are described in the following sections.

Extruded Teeth. Extruded teeth are reduced to the level of the occlusal plane by grinding and reshaping within the limits permitted by proximity to the pulp (Fig. 47–29). If large areas are exposed by grinding, a dental restoration in conformity with the corrected occlusal relationship is indicated. Extruded unopposed molars may irritate the mucosa of the opposing jaw, interfere with closure to the ICP, and deflect the mandible on its way to a secure functional end point. Food impaction is also common between extruded third molars and the second molar.

When an unopposed maxillary third molar is removed, the interdental space between the adjacent first and second

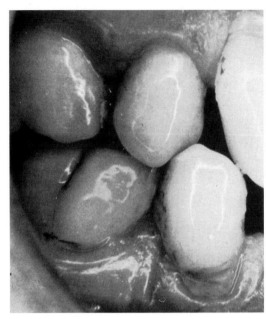

FIGURE 47–30. Plunger cusp on the maxilla. The premolar forces food between the mandibular teeth, causing gingival inflammatiion.

molars should be watched for evidence of food impaction. Distal thrusts produced on occlusal contact may momentarily break the contact between the maxillary first and second molars and permit impaction of food (Fig. 47–30). At the first sign of such impaction, ICP contacts should be evaluated and adjusted if their incline contact relationships promote distal movement of the second molar. If subsequent adjustment fails to result in closure of the contact, it may be necessary to splint the first and second molars together.

Plunger Cusps. Plunger cusps are cusp tips that wedge into the interproximal spaces between opposing teeth and cause food impaction (see Fig. 47–30). Distolingual cusps of maxillary molars often are plunger cusps. The cusp points should be rounded and shortened or reduced entirely. This can be done without great consequence to the stability of the occlusion.

Uneven Adjacent Marginal Ridges. Differences in the height of adjacent marginal ridges may cause food impaction and should be corrected by either reducing the height of the comparatively high marginal ridge or increasing the height of the lower one with a restoration (Fig. 47–31). Extreme differences are overcome by using both procedures. In grinding the marginal ridges the natural tooth contour should be preserved. The marginal ridge should not be reduced if this entails sacrifice of occlusal contact or threat of food impaction.

Rotated, Malposed, and Tilted Teeth. Teeth that are rotated or tilted facially or lingually may interfere with functional movement of the mandible and cause food accumulation and impaction. Depending on the extent of malposition, such conditions can be corrected by coronoplasty or orthodontic procedures (see Chapter 48) or by restorations that conform to the corrected occlusal and proximal relationship of the dentition (Fig. 47–32).

Facets and Flat Occlusal Wear. *Facets* are flattened planes produced by tooth-to-tooth wear on a convex tooth surface.[79] Facets vary in size and outline (Fig. 47–33).

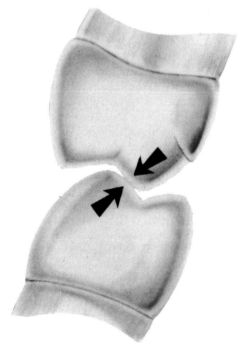

FIGURE 47–29. Class III prematurity in the intercuspal position. The buccal surface of the lingual cusp of the maxillary molars and premolars, with the lingual aspect of the buccal cusps of the mandibular teeth (*arrows*).

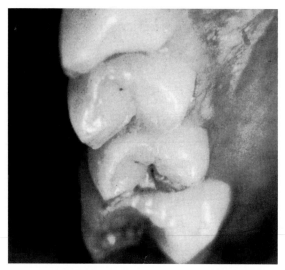

FIGURE 47–31. Uneven marginal ridges.

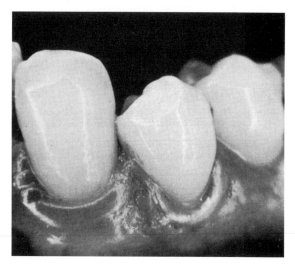

FIGURE 47–33. Prominent facets on the premolars.

They are detected by mirror examination after the teeth have been dried. Study casts are also helpful for locating facets not easily seen directly in the mouth owing to their location. Occlusal contact at the periphery of broad facets may create lateral or tipping forces potentially deleterious to the periodontium and should be adjusted so that only a small area remains in occlusal contact (Fig. 47–34).

Flat Occlusal Wear. When excessive occlusal wear produces broad, flat, or cupped-out occlusal surfaces, forces applied at the periphery are directed outside the confines of the root and may create tipping forces injurious to the periodontium. The occlusal surface is modified by grinding to restore the normal faciolingual and mesiodistal occlusal table and occlusal anatomy (Fig. 47–35). Incisal edges flattened by excessive occlusal wear can be reshaped by grinding (Fig. 47–36). In dentitions with advanced wear, it is unnecessary and usually undesirable to restore the occlusion to an idealized steep cusp–fossa scheme.

Step 8: Recheck Tooth Contact Relationships. Tooth contact relationships in all positions and movements are rechecked to verify that the seven criteria listed below are met. These criteria also can serve as guidelines to help determine the feasibility of achieving a satisfactory result by means of occlusal adjustment. There are many instances when restorative or prosthetic treatments are necessary, sometimes in combination with orthodontic and surgical intervention. In questionable cases, a trial carving of articulated casts is the best means by which to judge the anticipated fulfillment of the foregoing criteria. (Refer to Fig.

47–37 for recommended instruments for completing the above steps.)

Step 9: Finishing Techniques and Patient Instruction. The occlusal surfaces are smoothed and polished so that they feel "comfortable" to the patient.

Results. There is evidence that the method of coronoplasty recommended in this chapter provides stability for the short term. Teeth and dental restorations wear over time. As a result, the occlusion changes over longer periods. No method of occlusal adjustment creates a permanent occlusal relationship. The occlusion must be checked periodically, after which minor adjustments can be made. The patient should be advised accordingly.

CRITERIA FOR JUDGING THE OUTCOME OF CORONOPLASTY

1. There is no asymmetric shift from RCP to ICP. If a shift is present, it is smooth, symmetric, and less than 1 mm in magnitude.
2. The completed adjustments have light contact or no contact between the incisor teeth and firm contact between as many posterior teeth as possible.
3. The patient perceives "even" (bilateral) contact when closing the teeth to ICP.
4. Sharp occlusal sounds are produced when the patient taps slowly and firmly into ICP.
5. Molar excursive supracontacts are neutralized or significantly reduced so that unrestricted glide paths are available for the posterior cusps.

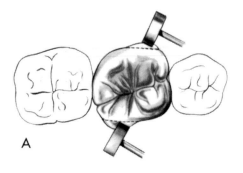

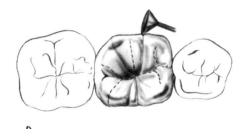

A   B

FIGURE 47–32. Reshaping slightly rotated tooth by grinding. *A,* Slightly rotated molar. Areas to be removed by grinding are indicated by dashed lines. *B,* Occlusal surface recontoured (*dashed lines*) and buccal grooves relocated.

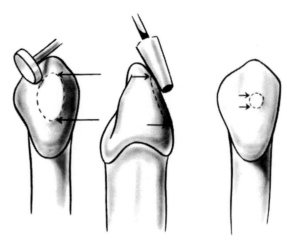

FIGURE 47–34. Reduction of facet by grinding. The dimensions of the facet before and after reduction are indicated by *arrows* and *dashes.*

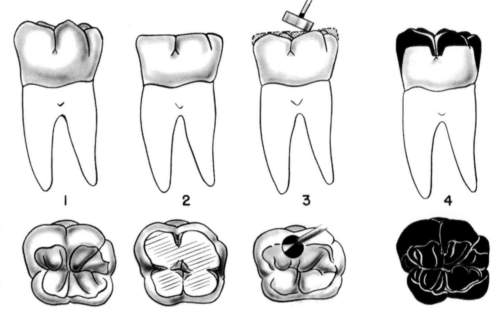

FIGURE 47–35. Reshaping the occlusal surface of a mandibular molar altered by functional wear. 1, The unworn molar crown. 2, The molar crown altered by wear. 3, Reshaping the molar crown to reduce the area of the occlusal surface and to restore cuspal inclines and marginal ridges. (The outlined stippled area is the portion of the tooth surface removed.) 4, The use of restoration to reshape a worn molar crown when correction by grinding is not feasible.

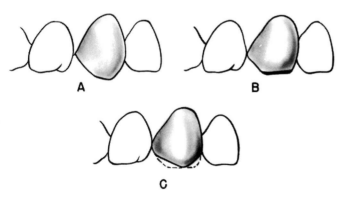

FIGURE 47–36. Recontouring a canine tooth altered by incisal wear. *A,* Contour of unworn maxillary canine. *B,* Facet frequently seen at incisal edge of canine. *C,* Correction of facet. Areas of tooth removed are indicated by the dashed line.

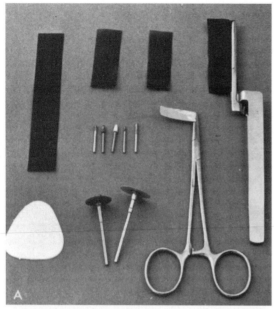

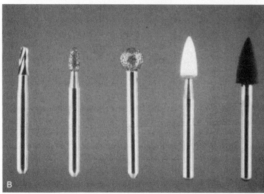

FIGURE 47–37. Instruments and materials used in performing coronoplasty. *A,* Clockwise from lower right: Mylar strip in hemostat, abrasive disc and wheel, blotting paper to reduce salivary flow, inked marking ribbons and ribbon holder; *center:* Friction grip burs and stones. *B,* Cutting and abrasive burs used in performing coronoplasty. Left to right: Rounded, tapered fissure; football diamond; round diamond; Arkansas stone; and rubber polishing cone.

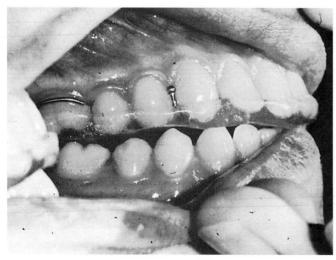

FIGURE 47–38. Removable full-arch stabilization appliance used for bruxism patients and patients with temporomandibular joint disorders. The appliance may be constructed for either the maxillary or the mandibular arch.

6. Tooth guidance under lateral and protrusive excursions is smooth and without effort.
7. The displacement of mobile teeth is minimized under closure and gliding movements.

TREATMENT OF BRUXISM AND APPLIANCE THERAPY

There are several short-term modalities by which the patient with bruxism can be treated. The *behavioral modality* is initiated by the dentist through explanation and arousal of the patient's awareness of the habit. Specific behavioral therapies such as EMG biofeedback may be prescribed.[57,70] If musculoskeletal pain and stiffness are associated with bruxism, a brief course of physical therapy is appropriate. Medications prescribed for a few days aimed at altering sleep arousal or anxiety level, such as diazepam, may be helpful. Ware and associates[84] have proposed the use of low doses of tricyclic antidepressants as a means of inhibiting the amount of REM sleep, during which bruxism may occur. Although antidepressants at this dose fail to have an antidepressant effect, their effect on sleep improvement is rapid.[56]

The *maxillary stabilization appliance* remains the most universal and effective long-term means of interfering with the effects of bruxism (Figs. 47–38 and 47–39). The aim of this appliance is to protect the tooth surface and to dissipate forces built up in the musculoskeletal system through bruxism.[18,62] There is evidence that these appliances effect a significant decrease in the bruxism habit of some individuals,[59,75] but these results are not uniform.[43] In application, the stabilization appliance is more practical for treating nocturnal bruxism than for correcting daytime clenching habits.

The stabilization appliance results in an immediate reduction in masseter[48] and temporalis[82] muscle activity lev-

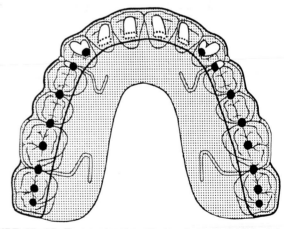

FIGURE 47–39. The occlusal contact scheme established for the maxillary full-arch stabilization appliance. Large black dots denote posterior vertical stops of positive contact in the intercuspal position. Dotted lines denote light incisal contact. Clear areas are the pathways of protrusive and lateral guidance. Note that there is freedom from lateral or protrusive posterior contact. If heavy lateral and protrusive facets are observed at the follow-up visit, these areas should be reduced. Wrought-wire ball clasps (between canines and premolars) and retentive arms (molars) are used to aid in retention.

Table 47–5. CRITERIA FOR MAXILLARY STABILIZATION APPLIANCE

Occlusal Criteria

1. *Appliance:* Stable
2. *RCP, ICP:* Stable, multipointed, widely distributed contacts.
3. *ICP:* Posterior vertical stops in firm contact; incisor teeth in slight infracontact.
4. *RCP–ICP relationship:* RCP and ICP in same sagittal plane; ICP and RCP are nearly identical.
5. Smooth gliding contact in all excursions (incisal and/or canine disclusion optional).
6. *MCP:* Stable, repeatable.

Technique for Verification of Criteria

1. *Criterion 1 (appliance stability):* No hint of movement to tipping forces.
2. *Criterion 2 (RCP):* Red-inked ribbon on dry surface.
3. *Criterion 3 (vertical stops):* Mylar strips held firmly by telling subject, "Close your back teeth, both sides at the same time."
4. *Criterion 4 (RCP–ICP):* No slide from RCP to ICP.
5. *Criterion 5 (guidance):* Use full arch red-blue paper. Mark excursion in red, then vertical stops in blue.
6. *Criterion 6 (MCP):* Solid MCP tapping by patient in upright position; patient verifies even contact.

ICP, Intercuspal position; MCP, muscular contact position; RCP, retruded contact position.

els, and these effects persist throughout the treatment period.[10,29,75] Appliances to control bruxing in TMD patients are more effective if the symptoms are not severe,[12] and hard appliances are more effective than soft appliances.[55]

The purpose of the stabilization appliance is to redistribute the forces created by bruxism that alter mandibular behavior.[54] The occlusal criteria for adjusting the occluding surface of the appliance are summarized in Table 47–5. The recommended contact scheme is shown in Figure 47–39.

The stabilization appliance is delivered and carefully adjusted to conform to the criteria listed in Table 47–5. The patient is instructed to wear the appliance during sleep and perhaps at other times when bruxist activity has been identified. The appliance should be readjusted in 2 to 4 weeks and thereafter over longer intervals. At follow-up visits, the occlusal surface of the appliance should be observed for bruxofacets in the hard acrylic resin. Bruxofacets on the appliance surface should be burnished away with a smooth, pumice-impregnated rubber wheel. Careful balancing of the occlusion on the nightguard should be completed before patient dismissal. The dentist must determine whether the appliance should be used indefinitely at night or whether the appliance therapy should be discontinued with no further use, with reintroduction of appliance use during periods when symptoms return.

REFERENCES

1. Agar JR, Weller RN. Occlusal adjustment for initial treatment and prevention of the cracked tooth syndrome. J Prosthet Dent 60:145–147, 1988.
2. Agerberg G, Sandström R. Frequency of occlusal interferences: A clinical study in teenagers and young adults. J Prosthet Dent 59:212, 1988.
3. Bakke M, Møller E. Distortion of maximal elevator activity by unilateral premature contact. Scand J Dent Res 88:67, 1980.
4. Balthazar Y, Ziebert G, Donegan S. Limited mandibular mobility and potential jaw dysfunction. J Oral Rehabil 14:569–574, 1987.
5. Belser UC, Hannam AG. The influence of altered working-side occlusal guidance on masticatory muscles and related jaw movements. J Prosthet Dent 53:406–413, 1985.
6. Belser UC, Hannam AG. The contribution of the deep fibers of the masseter muscle to selected tooth-clenching and chewing tasks. J Prosthet Dent 56:629–635, 1986.
7. Blanksma NG, Van Eijden TMGJ. Electromyographic heterogeneity in the human temporalis muscle. J Dent Res 69:1686–1690, 1990.
8. Brose M, Tanquist RA. The influence of anterior coupling on mandibular movement. J Prosthet Dent 57:345–353, 1987.
9. Burgett FG, Charbeneau TD, Nissle RR, et al. A randomized occlusal adjustment in periodontitis patients. Abstract 93. J Dent Res 67(special issue):124, 1988.
10. Carr AB, Christiansen LV, Donegan SJ, Ziebert GJ. Postural contractile activities of human jaw muscles following use of an occlusal splint. J Oral Rehabil 18:185–191, 1991.
11. Christensen LV, Hutchins MO. Methodological observations on positive and negative work (teeth grinding) by human jaw muscles. J Oral Rehabil 19:399–411, 1992.
12. Clark GT, Beemsterboer PL, Solberg WK, Rugh JD. Nocturnal electromyographic evaluation of myofascial pain-dysfunction in patients undergoing occlusal splint therapy. J Am Dent Assoc 99:607, 1979.
13. Clayton JA, Kotowicz WE, Zahler JM. Pantographic tracings of mandibular movements and occlusion. J Prosthet Dent 25:389, 1971.
14. D'Amico A. The canine teeth: Normal functional relation of the natural teeth of man. J South Calif Dent Assoc 26:6, 49, 127, 175, 194, 239, 1958.
15. Dawson PE. Evaluation, Diagnosis, and Treatment of Occlusal Problems. St Louis, CV Mosby, 1975, p 56.
16. dos Santos J Jr, Ash MM Jr, Warshawsky P. Learning to reproduce a consistent functional jaw movement. J Prosthet Dent 65:294–302, 1991.
17. dos Santos J Jr, Blackman RB, Nelson SJ. Vectoral analysis of the static equilibrium of forces generated in the mandible in centric occlusion, group function, and balanced occlusal relationships. J Prosthet Dent 65:557–567, 1991.
18. dos Santos J Jr, Suzuki H, Ash MM Jr. Mechanical analysis of the equilibrium of occlusal splints. J Prosthet Dent 59:346–352, 1988.
19. Ehrlich J, Hochman N, Yaffe A. The masticatory pattern as an adjunct for diagnosis and treatment. J Oral Rehabil 19:393–398, 1992.
20. Federick DR, Pameijer CH, Stallard RE. A correlation between force and distalization of the mandible in obtaining centric relation. J Periodontol 45:70, 1974.
21. Gibbs CH, Lundeen HC. Jaw movements and forces during chewing and swallowing and their clinical significance. In Lundeen HC, Gibbs CH, eds. Advances in Occlusion. Postgraduate Dental Handbook Series. Vol 14. Bristol, John Wright & Sons, 1982, pp 7, 22.
22. Glickman I, Pameijer JH, Roeber FW, Brion MAM. Functional occlusion as revealed by miniaturized radio transmitters. Dent Clin North Am 13:666, 1969.
23. Glickman I, Smulow JB, Vogel G, Passamonti G. The effect of occlusal forces on healing following mucogingival surgery. J Periodontol 37:319, 1966.
24. Glickman I, Haddad AW, Martignoni M, et al. Telemetric comparison of centric relation and centric occlusion reconstructions. J Prosthet Dent 31:527, 1974.
25. Graham GS, Rugh JD. Maxillary splint occlusal guidance patterns and electromyographic activity of the jaw-closing muscles. J Prosthet Dent 59:73–77, 1988.
26. Greene CS. A survey of current professional concepts and opinions about the myofascial pain dysfunction (MPD) syndrome. J Am Dent Assoc 86:128–135, 1973.
27. Haddad AW. The functioning dentition. In Kawamura J, ed. Frontiers of Oral Physiology: Physiology of Oral Tissues. Basel, S Karger, 1976.
28. Halperin GC, Halperin AR, Norling BK. Thickness, strength, and plastic deformation of occlusal registration strips. J Prosthet Dent 48:575–578, 1982.
29. Hamada T, Kotani H, Kawazoe Y, Yamada S. Effects of occlusal splints on the EMG activity of masseter and temporalis muscles in bruxism with clinical symptoms. J Oral Rehabil 9:119–123, 1982.
30. Hanson ML, Andrianopoulos MV. Tongue thrust, occlusion, and dental health in middle-aged subjects: A pilot study. Int J Orofacial Myol 13:3–9, 1987.
31. Helkimo M. Studies on function and dysfunction of the masticatory system. Swed Dent J 67:1–18, 1974.
32. Hellsing G, Isberg-Holm A, McWilliam J. A comparative study of two techniques for recording centric relation. Dentomaxillofac Radiol 12:5–12, 1983.
33. Hellsing G. Occlusal adjustment and occlusal stability. J Prosthet Dent 59:696–702, 1988.
34. Holmgren K, Sheiksholeslam A, Riise C. An electromyographic study of the immediate effect of an occlusal splint on the postural activity of the anterior temporalis and masseter muscles in different body positions with and without visual input. J Oral Rehabil 12:483–490, 1985.
35. Ingervall B. Retruded contact position of mandible. A comparison between children and adults. Odontol Rev 15:150, 1964.
36. Ingervall B. Tooth contacts on the functional and nonfunctional side in children and young adults. Arch Oral Biol 17:191, 1972.
37. Ingervall B, Egermark-Eriksson I. Function of temporal and masseter muscles in individuals with dual bite. Angle Orthodont 49:131–140, 1979.
38. Jankelson B. Physiology of human dental occlusion. J Am Dent Assoc 50:664, 1955.

39. Jiminez ID. Electromyography of the masticatory muscles in three jaw registration positions. Am J Orthodont Dentofac Orthop *95:*282–288, 1989.

40. Karlsen K. Traumatic occlusion as a factor in the propagation of periodontal disease. Int Dent J *22:*387, 1972.

41. Korioth TWP, Hannam AG. Effect of bilateral asymmetric tooth clenching on load distribution at the mandibular condyle. J Prosthet Dent *64:*62–73, 1990.

42. Krogh-Poulsen WG, Olsson A. Management of the occlusion of the teeth. In Schwartz LS, Chayes CM, eds. Facial Pain and Mandibular Dysfunction. Philadelphia, WB Saunders, 1968.

43. Kydd WL, Daley C. Duration of nocturnal contacts during bruxing. J Prosthet Dent *53:*717–721, 1985.

44. Lund P, Nishiyama T, Møller E. Postural activity in the muscles of mastication with the subject upright, inclined, and supine. Scand J Dent Res *78:*417, 1970.

45. MacDonald JWC, Hannam AG. Relationship between occlusal contacts and jaw closing muscle activity during tooth clenching: Part I. J Prosthet Dent *52:*718–729, 1984.

46. Magnussen T, Carlsson GE. Treatment of patients with functional disturbances in the masticatory system: A survey of 80 consecutive patients. Swed Dent J *4:*145–153, 1980.

47. Manns A, Chan C, Turalles R. Influence of group function and canine guidance on electromyographic activity of elevator muscles. J Prosthet Dent *57:*494–501, 1987.

48. Manns A, Miralles R, Cumsille F. Influence of vertical dimension on masseter muscle electromyographic activity in patients with mandibular dysfunction. J Prosthet Dent *53:*243–246, 1985.

49. Miralles R, Bull R, Manns A, Roman E. Influence of balanced occlusion and canine guidance on electromyographic activity of elevator muscles in complete denture wearers. J Prosthet Dent *61:*494–498, 1989.

50. Mohamed SE, Christensen LV. Mandibular reference positions. J Oral Rehabil *12:*355–367, 1985.

51. Møller E, Sheikholeslam A, Lous L. Deliberate relaxation of the temporal and masseter muscles in subjects with functional disorders of the chewing apparatus. Scand J Dent Res *78:*478, 1971.

52. Møller E. The myogenic factor in headache and facial pain. In Kawamura Y, Dubner R, eds. Oral-Facial Sensory and Motor Functions. Tokyo, Quintessence Publishing, 1981, pp 225–239.

53. Muhlemann HR, Herzog H, Rateitschak KH. Quantitative evaluation of the therapeutic effect of selective grinding. J Periodontol *28:*11, 1957.

54. Naeije M, Hansson T. Short term effect of the stabilization appliance on masticatory muscle activity in myogenous craniomandibular disorder patients. J Craniomandib Dis Fac Oral Pain *5:*245–250, 1991.

55. Okeson JP. The effects of hard and soft occlusal splints on nocturnal bruxism. J Am Dent Assoc *114:*788, 1987.

56. Olkinuora M. Bruxism as a psychosomatic phenomenon. Academic dissertation. Helsinki, Forssan Kirjapaino Oy-Forssa, 1972.

57. Pertes R, Vella M, Milone A. Vertical skeletal facial types and condylar position in TMJ patients. Abstract 109. J Dent Res (special issue) *68:*195, 1989.

58. Philstrom B, Anderson K, Aeppli D, Schaffer E. Association between signs of trauma from occlusion to periodontitis. J Periodontol *57:*1, 1986.

59. Pierce CJ, Gale EN. A comparison of different treatments for nocturnal bruxism. J Dent Res *67:*597–601, 1988.

60. Polson AM, Meitner SW, Zander HA. Trauma and progression of marginal periodontitis in squirrel monkeys. III. Adaptation of interproximal alveolar bone to repetitive injury. J Periodont Res *11:*279, 1976.

61. Polson AM, Meitner SW, Zander HA. Trauma and progression of marginal periodontitis in squirrel monkeys. IV. Reversibility of bone loss due to trauma alone and trauma superimposed upon periodontitis. J Periodont Res *11:*290, 1976.

62. Posselt V, Wolff IB. Treatment of bruxism by bite guards and bite plates. J Can Dent Assoc *29:*773, 1963.

63. Pullinger AG, Seligman DA. The degree to which attrition characterizes diagnostic groups of temporomandibular disorders. J Craniomandib Disord Facial Oral Pain. J Orofacial Pain *7:*196, 1993.

64. Pullinger AG, Seligman DA, Gornbein JA. A multiple regression analysis of the risk and relative odds of temporomandibular disorders as a function of common occlusal factors. J Dent Res *72:*968, 1993.

65. Ramfjord SP. Occlusion. Indent *1:*20, 1973.

66. Ramfjord SP, Ash MM. Occlusion. 2nd ed. Philadelphia, WB Saunders, 1971, p 206.

67. Ramfjord SP, Ash MM. Occlusion. 3rd ed. Philadelphia, WB Saunders, 1983.

68. Reynolds JM. Occlusal adjustment. Personal communication. Augusta, GA, 1975.

69. Richardson E, Seibert W, Semenya K, Lemeh D. Effects of malaligned teeth on periodontal disease. Abstract 1026. J Dent Res *65*(special issue)*:*283, 1986.

70. Rugh JD, Solberg WK. Electromyographic evaluation of bruxist behavior before and after treatment. Can Dent Assoc J *3:*56, 1975.

71. Scaife RR Jr, Holt JE. Natural occurrence of cuspid guidance. J Prosthet Dent *22:*225, 1969.

72. Scharer P, Butler J, Zander H. Die heilung parodon-taler Knochentaschen bei okklusalar Dysfunktion. Schweiz Monatsschr Zahnheilkd *79:*244, 1969.

73. Schuyler CH. Factors contributing to traumatic occlusion. J Prosthet Dent *11:*708, 1961.

74. Shupe RJ, Mohamed SE, Christensen LV, et al. Effects of occlusal guidance on jaw muscle activity. J Prosthet Dent *51:*811–818, 1984.

75. Solberg WK, Clark GT, Rugh JD. Nocturnal electromyographic evaluation of bruxism patients undergoing short term splint therapy. J Oral Rehabil *2:*215, 1975.

76. Solberg WK, Woo MW, Houston JB. Prevalence of mandibular dysfunction in young adults. J Am Dent Assoc *98:*25, 1979.

77. Stallard H, Stuart CE. Eliminating tooth guidance in natural dentitions. J Prosthet Dent *11:*47, 1961.

78. Tallgren A, Melsen B, Hansen MA. An electromyographic and roentgen cephalometric study of occlusal morphofunctional disharmony in children. Am J Orthod *76:*394–409, 1979.

79. Thomas BOA, Gallagher JW. Practical management of occlusal dysfunctions in periodontal therapy. J Am Dent Assoc *46:*18, 1953.

80. Van Eijden TMG. Three dimensional analysis of human bite-force magnitude and moment. Arch Oral Biol *36:*535–539, 1991.

81. Van Spronsen PH, Weijs WA, Valk J, et al. A comparison of jaw muscle cross-section of long-face and normal adults. J Dent Res *71:*1279–1285, 1992.

82. Vissar A, McCarroll RS, Naeije M. Masticatory muscle activity in different jaw relations during submaximal clenching efforts. J Dent Res *71:*372–379, 1992.

83. Vollmer WH, Rateitschak KH. Influence of occlusal adjustment by grinding on gingivitis and mobility of traumatized teeth. J Clin Periodontol *2:*113, 1975.

84. Ware JC, Rugh JD, Brown FW, et al. Sleep related bruxism: Differences in patients with dental sleep complaints. Sleep Res *11:*182, 1982.

85. Watt D. A study of the average duration of occlusal sounds in different age groups. Br Dent J *138:*385, 1975.

86. Wise MD. Occlusion and restorative dentistry for the general practitioner. Part I: Preliminary considerations and examination procedure. Br Dent J *152:*117–122, 1982.

87. Woda A, Gourdon AM, Faraj M. Occlusal contact and tooth wear. J Prosthet Dent *57:*85–93, 1987.

88. Yaffe A, Ehrlich J. The functional range of tooth contact in lateral grinding movements. J Prosthet Dent *57:*730–733, 1987.

89. Yuodelis RA, Mann WV Jr. The prevalence and possible role of nonworking contacts in periodontal disease. Periodontics *3:*219, 1965.

90. Zahn M, Burgett F, Dennison J, Krostoffersen T. Three clinical factors used as predictors of future attachment loss. Abstract 2555. J Dent Res *70*(special issue)*:*585, 1991.

48

Orthodontic Considerations in Periodontal Therapy

FERMIN A. CARRANZA, JR. and NEAL C. MURPHY

RATIONALE FOR ORTHODONTIC MOVEMENT IN PERIODONTAL THERAPY

Orthodontic procedures are sometimes required in periodontal therapy to change the position of the teeth. The advisability of undertaking orthodontic correction depends on (1) the severity of the periodontal problem and the possibility of improving it by orthodontics, (2) the level of the remaining bone, and (3) the possibility that the periodontal condition would worsen without orthodontic correction. *Although there is no consistent relationship between malocclusion and periodontal disease, certain characteristics of malocclusions can promote a pathologic environment and hinder periodontal therapy.*

Orthodontic movement can be justified as a part of periodontal therapy if it is used to reduce plaque retention, improve gingival and osseous form, facilitate prosthetic replacements, and improve aesthetics.

Reducing Plaque Retention. Crowded teeth (arch length deficiency) are frequently difficult to clean, making the introduction of dental floss and other cleaning devices practically impossible. This occurs most frequently in lower anterior areas of the mouth. Mesially tipped teeth, usually in an edentulous area, create plaque accumulation sites that are difficult to clean. In addition, they open the distal contact, creating an area of food impaction.[2,10,17] Arch length deficiencies also create abnormal occlusal relationships that may favor trauma from occlusion. This creation of abnormal contacts with the opposing jaw may trigger the development of bruxing habits. Crowding also creates enlarged contact surfaces and altered embrasure spaces, the latter housing smaller papillae and a soft tissue facial ridge. Most importantly, as the contact point is distorted by arch length deficiency, the gingival embrasure, an area of abundant plaque accumulation, is displaced apically, thereby becoming less accessible to floss and other plaque-removing devices.

Improving Gingival and Osseous Form. There is an interrelationship between the position of a tooth and the shape of the gingiva and bone that surround it. A typical example is a lower first or second molar tilted into an edentulous mesial space. This tooth has a narrow space between its crown and the bone that easily becomes inflamed and in which a pocket may develop. Osseous contouring may correct the bony defect but will also create a topography inconsistent with a healthy gingival sulcus. Orthodontic therapy may improve the shape of the periodontium and reduce the indications for bone surgery.

Facilitating Prosthetic Replacements. The uprighting of tilted abutment teeth may be important in restorative dentistry. Parallel abutment teeth less frequently require hemisection or removal, are less likely to sustain pulpal damage, and can accommodate better contoured crowns, all of which will benefit the periodontal condition.

Improving Aesthetics. Migration and diastemata between anterior teeth are relatively frequent features of moderate and advanced periodontal disease. These changes may be due in part to tongue thrusting or other habits. Posterior tooth prematurities are usually combined with loss of periodontal support.

Indications

The most common problems that can be solved by minor orthodontic therapy include crowded teeth, closure of anterior diastemata, mesial tilting of molars, and open contacts. These problems involve treatment within one dental arch and rarely involve intermaxillary mechanotherapy.

In most cases, consultation with an orthodontist or patient referral for this particular phase of therapy is in the best interest of the patient. In all phases of combined orthodontic and periodontal therapy, a close collaboration between the orthodontist and the periodontist is highly desirable.

Contraindications

The only contraindication to orthodontic treatment in patients with periodontal disease is the persistence of active disease in spite of adequate Phase I therapy procedures. The superimposition of tooth movement on inflamed gingiva may exacerbate the periodontal problem. This can occur by shifting the position of plaque subgingivally, increasing the rate of periodontal attachment loss and altering the morphology of the bone. A buccolingual movement can cause gingival and bony dehiscence, especially if the buccal gingiva is thin.[20] Even though the primary etiologic factor may be plaque, prophylactic gingival augmentation may be prudent in the periodontally vulnerable orthodontic patient.

Where vertical defects are present, the movement of teeth, whether tipping or bodily movement, may produce additional loss of connective tissue.[20] The potential destructive effects are so significant that periodontal evaluation before the initiation of orthodontic tooth movement and frequent periodontal care during orthodontic treatment are recommended for all orthodontic patients, regardless of disease activity at the initial examination.[20]

Age is not a contraindication to orthodontic treatment, although it is generally assumed that bone remodeling processes occur more slowly in older patients. Sometimes, limited therapeutic goals or termination of therapy before ideal results are achieved may be justified to minimize the risk of attachment loss in patients who are periodontally vulnerable.

TIMING OF ORTHODONTIC PROCEDURES IN PERIODONTAL TREATMENT

Orthodontic treatment should not be started until inflammation of the gingiva has been reduced to a minimum through adequate scaling, root planing, and correction of other irritational factors. Furthermore, the patient should be aware of and willing to perform the most fastidious home care technique.

Periodically during orthodontic treatment, the periodontist should check the condition of the tissues, remove all irritants, and reinforce the patient's oral hygiene as needed; these examinations are usually conducted every 8 to 12 weeks. The reason for these controls is twofold: (1) the reduction of inflammation diminishes the chances for increased forces on the teeth to become detrimental to the tissues; and (2) if the patient experiences an exacerbation of the periodontal disease, the orthodontist may wish to modify the treatment objectives based on the periodontist's consultation.

After elimination of inflammation, tooth position may change. Major occlusal adjustment and surgical procedures are better performed after the completion of orthodontic therapy. In any case, after orthodontic treatment, a final coronoplasty should be performed.

The necessary surgical procedures are therefore done *after* orthodontic treatment because orthodontics may change the shape of the periodontium, reducing the need for or the extent of surgery; in addition, the removal of supracrestal periodontal fibers during surgery may facilitate retention, because new, reoriented fibers form. On the other hand, performing periodontal surgery *before* orthodontic therapy can open embrasures, ensure more complete elimination of irritants and inflammatory changes, and allow the patient better access during orthodontic therapy.

Clearly, there are cogent arguments for periodontal surgery at different stages of orthodontic treatment. Therefore, the sequence of periodontal and orthodontic procedures should be determined by close consultation between the orthodontist and the periodontist.

ORTHODONTIC TREATMENT MODALITIES

Methods for tooth movement fall into two basic categories: fixed appliances and removable appliances. Some of the simpler methods of tooth movement are described here as examples of what can be done; the reader is urged to study some of the textbooks on adult orthodontics and to consult an orthodontist for evaluation and/or performance of the methods.

Correction of Pathologic Migration

The following factors should be considered when orthodontic correction of migrated teeth is contemplated:

1. The availability of space for the teeth to be repositioned or the possibility of creating space by extraction or interproximal enamel reduction (stripping).
2. The absence of interference from teeth in the opposing arch and the threat of occlusal trauma during tooth movement.
3. The extent to which loss of posterior tooth support, reduced vertical dimension, and accentuated anterior overbite complicate orthodontic movement.
4. The availability of sufficient anchorage from which forces can be applied.
5. Aesthetic demands and limits on patient compliance.
6. Habits that may interfere with the desired tooth movement.

Removable Appliances. Three basic appliances that can be used for intra-arch tipping movements are the Hawley appliance, the Crozat appliance, and the spring retainer.

The *Hawley appliance* is a removable tissue-borne appliance with an anterior wire frame extension or "labial bow," posterior tooth clasps, and an acrylic body (Figs. 48–1 and 48–2). It may be modified in a variety of ways for moving individual teeth and has the advantage of incorporating a maxillary bite plane to disarticulate posterior teeth. The tissue-borne acrylic portion covers the palate or the lingual gingiva. The margin of the appliance is cut away when necessary to create space for the desired tooth movement. The principal disadvantage of this appliance is that the acrylic accumulates plaque where it is in contact with the gingival tissue.

The *Crozat appliance* is more hygienic than the Hawley appliance and can therefore be used for patients with less than ideal plaque control (Fig. 48–3). The appliance is made of stainless steel or gold wire and is essentially tooth borne, giving the patient free access to the gingival margin for plaque removal.

The *spring retainer* is a wire and acrylic appliance that uses buccal and lingual panels of acrylic to align mandibu-

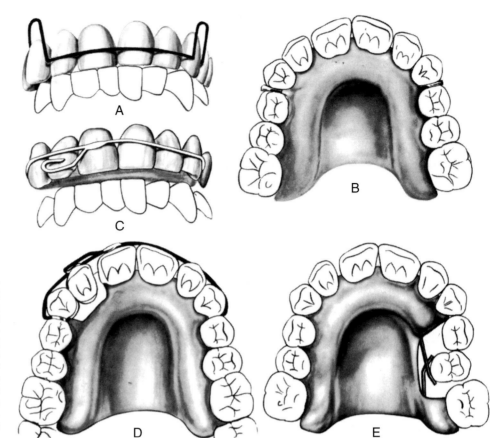

FIGURE 48–1. The Hawley appliance. *A*, Hawley appliance with labial bow. *B*, Acrylic tissue–borne portion covers approximately one third of the length of the crowns. *C*, Wire soldered to labial bow to move lateral incisor. The palatal acrylic is used as an anterior bite plate. *D*, Palatal view showing acrylic cut away to provide space for the lateral incisor. *E*, Wire spring embedded in acrylic to move the second premolar buccally. If necessary, the proximal tooth surfaces are stripped to provide space.

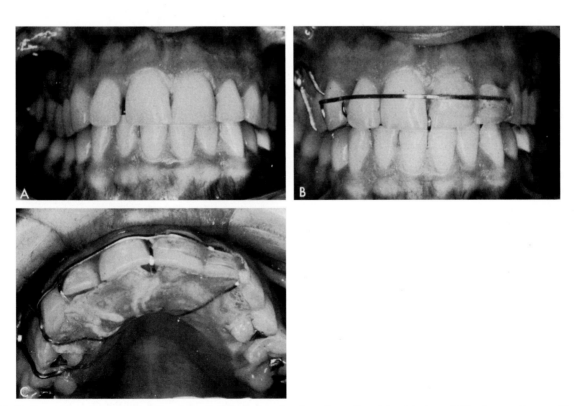

FIGURE 48–2. Correction of pathologic migration. *A*, Pathologic migration of maxillary lateral incisor. *B*, Hawley appliance with wire spring on distal surface of lateral incisor accomplishes desired movement. *C*, Lingual view of labial bow with wire spring to lateral incisor.

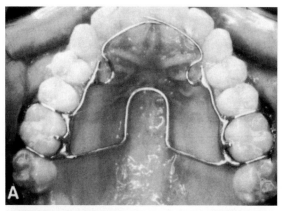
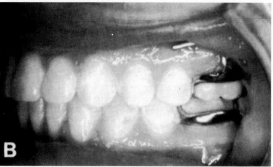

FIGURE 48–3. The Crozat appliance. *A,* Occlusal view. *B,* Lateral view.

lar anterior teeth. It is particularly effective when the malposition of the lower incisors necessitates simple buccolingual movement and crowding is mild to moderate (Fig. 48–4). The appliance is activated by constricting the labial bow adjacent to the acrylic panels. The spring retainer can be incorporated in the larger framework of the Hawley or the Crozat appliance.

Fixed Appliances. The fixed appliances consist essentially of brackets and an arch wire. The brackets may be attached to each tooth with a stainless steel band or directly bonded to the tooth surface. Bands often produce overhangs that irritate the gingiva and should be festooned interproximally (Fig. 48–5). The directly bonded brackets are preferred for the periodontally vulnerable patient, because they are less irritating to the gingiva and provide access for interproximal plaque removal. The arch wire should produce a low profile with minimal loops, and brackets should be as small as possible to facilitate plaque removal from the gingival margin. Excess bonding material should be removed from the bracket margin during placement.

Correction of Mesially Tipped Teeth

A number of methods have been proposed for uprighting molar teeth that have tilted into an edentulous mesial space.[9,16,18,19] Figure 48–6 shows the bone response to uprighting of a tipped molar with a spring formed by rectangular wire engaged into a horizontal tube on the molars to be uprighted. This so-called uprighting spring can be used in conjunction with a coiled spring or nickel titanium wire.

Pockets mesial to uprighted molars are shallower than pockets mesial to control teeth that have not been uprighted. This is due to a reduction in soft tissue height while the bone height remains unchanged. Gingival inflammation does not differ from that around control teeth.[3,12]

The presence of other discrepancies, such as lingual inclination, necessitates treatment by an orthodontist.

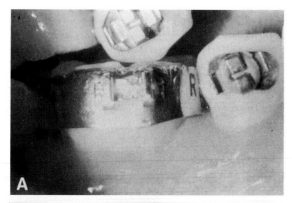
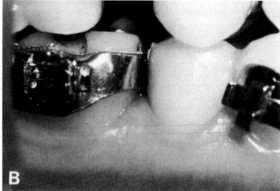

FIGURE 48–5. Festooned band. *A,* Inadequately festooned band will promote plaque accumulation. *B,* Festooning the band away from the gingival margin will reduce the chances of plaque accumulation and gingivitis.

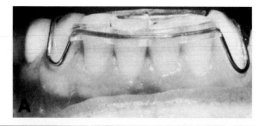
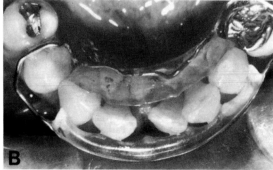

FIGURE 48–4. Spring retainer. *A,* Facial view. *B,* Occlusal view.

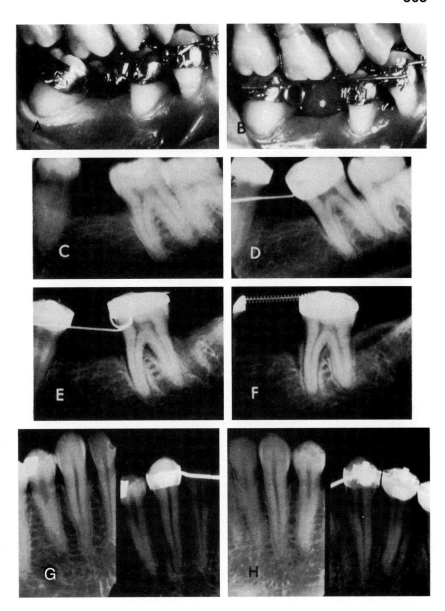

FIGURE 48–6. Molar uprighting: reciprocal spring. A variety of mechanisms have been devised to upright tipped molars. *A* and *B*, Reciprocal spring formed from a rectangular wire engaged into a horizontal tube on the molars to be uprighted. *C* and *D*, Typical radiographic changes noted as a molar is uprighted. *E*, As the molar begins to move, bone forms on the mesial aspect. *F*, Final tooth position. *G*, Even with proper anchorage, some undesired movement can occur. A shift in root position is observed on the contralateral side of a molar uprighting, and external tooth resorption and change in the position of the root are noted on the ipsilateral side *(H)*. (From Swanson JC, Rosenberg F. Orthodontic movement in periodontal therapy. Dent Clin North Am *24*:231, 1980.)

Correction of Crowded and Malposed Teeth

Although grassline ligatures and rubber dam elastics[9] have proved effective for the correction of malposed individual teeth, the potential for iatrogenic damage to the periodontium[15] and accumulation of plaque renders these methods less desirable than modern orthodontic methods.

Correction of Crowded Mandibular Anterior Teeth. Crowded and malposed lower incisors frequently present both periodontal and orthodontic problems. The gingiva around teeth in labial version is often attached apical to the level of gingiva around the adjacent teeth; gingival and bony dehiscences are often common on these teeth.[7] On teeth in lingual version, the labial gingiva is often enlarged and attracts irritating plaque and debris. Orthodontic correction of malposed teeth creates gingival contours that are more conducive to periodontal health.

A lower incisor may be extracted to correct crowding (Fig. 48–7), provided the extraction creates sufficient space for proper alignment of the remaining teeth and ade-

anterior guidance can be established in excursive movements. Injudicious extraction of mandibular incisors, although it corrects localized crowding, may result in an increase in the overjet and create undesirable periodontal and aesthetic sequelae. Consultation with an orthodontist is recommended before a lower incisor is extracted to eliminate crowding.

When possible, it is preferable to "strip" or reduce interproximal enamel surfaces to create space for the crowded teeth. However, when excessive interproximal reduction is performed, close root proximity and lack of adequate embrasure space may result. Enough interradicular space should be maintained to allow efficient root instrumentation.

Retention

Some type of permanent retention is usually necessary after the desired tooth movement has been completed. Although many patients tolerate an extracoronal retainer at night or even 24 hours a day, extracoronal splinting or ex-

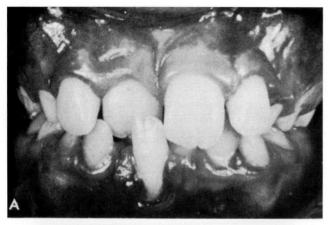

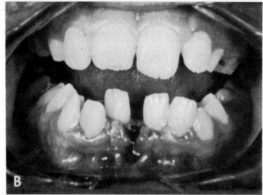

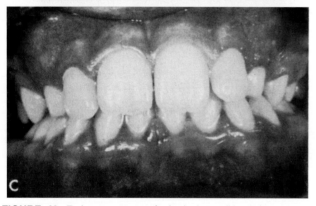

FIGURE 48–7. Improvement of gingival condition after correction of crowding in the mandibular anterior region. *A,* Marked gingival disease associated with malocclusion. *B,* Central incisor removed. *C,* Improved condition of the gingiva associated with improvement in the tooth relationship after orthodontic treatment.

tracoronal wire and composite splinting provide a reasonable alternative to indefinite removable appliance wear.

PERIODONTAL MAINTENANCE IN THE ORTHODONTIC PATIENT

Close cooperation between the periodontist and the orthodontist is necessary in all orthodontic cases to establish an effective periodontal maintenance program and ensure

minimal tissue damage during orthodontic therapy. Proper periodontal management of patients in orthodontic therapy concerns principally the management of attached gingiva, plaque control, and control of occlusion.

Management of Attached Gingiva. Although minimal attached gingiva can be maintained in a state of health, a wider band may be necessary during orthodontic treatment. This is particularly true in the mandibular incisor area, because an anterior movement of these teeth often accompanies orthodontic treatment. A free gingival graft should be considered in these cases.

Plaque Control. The presence of fixed orthodontic appliances may make plaque control measures, particularly flossing, difficult but not impossible. The orthodontist should reinforce at each visit the oral hygiene techniques taught as part of periodontal therapy.[9]

Control of Occlusion. Some studies suggest that when trauma from occlusion is superimposed on existing periodontal infection, the pattern of bone loss may be altered and its rate accelerated.[11,14] The orthodontic movement per se does not induce pathologic changes; however, when tooth movement is countered by heavy bruxing forces, traumatic lesions may result.

REFERENCES

1. Artun J, Osterberg S. Periodontal status of teeth facing extraction sites long after orthodontic treatment. J Periodontol *58:*24, 1987.
2. Behfelt K, Ericsson L, Jacobson L, Linder-Aronson S. The occurrence of plaque and gingivitis and its relationship to tooth alignment within the dental arches. J Clin Periodontol *8:*329, 1981.
3. Brown JS. The effect of orthodontic therapy on certain types of periodontal defects. I. Clinical findings. J Periodontol *44:*742, 1973.
4. Cooper ME. Minor tooth movement in the management of the periodontal patient. In Prichard J, ed. The Diagnosis and Treatment of Periodontal Disease. Philadelphia, WB Saunders, 1979.
5. Ewen SJ, Pasternak R. Periodontal surgery, an adjunct to orthodontic therapy Periodontics *2:*162, 1964.
6. Feliu J. Long-term benefits on orthodontic treatment of oral hygiene. Am J Orthod *82:*473, 1982.
7. Hall WB. Pure Mucogingival Problems. Chicago, Quintessence Publishing, 1984.
8. Hirschfeld L. Minor tooth movement in periodontal therapy. In Schluger S, Youdelis R, Page RC, eds. Periodontal Disease. Philadelphia, Lea & Febiger, 1977.
9. Hirschfeld L, Geiger A. Minor Tooth Movement in General Practice. St Louis, CV Mosby, 1966.
10. Hug HU. Periodontal status and its relationship to variations in tooth position. An analysis of the findings reported in the literature. Helv Odontol Acta *26:*11, 1982.
11. Kaufman H, Carranza FA Jr, Endres B, et al. The influence of trauma from occlusion on the bacterial repopulation of periodontal pockets in dogs. J Periodontol *55:*86, 1984.
12. Kraal JH, Digiancinto JJ, Dayl RA, et al. Periodontal conditions in patients after molar uprighting. J Prosthet Dent *43:*156, 1980.
13. Lang N, Löe H. The relationship between the width of the attached gingiva and gingival health. J Periodontol *43:*623, 1972.
14. Lindhe J, Svanberg G. Influence of trauma from occlusion on progression of experimental periodontitis in the beagle dog. J Clin Periodontol *1:*3, 1974.
15. Marino VA, Fry HR, Behrents RG. Severe localized destruction of the periodontium secondary to subgingival displacement of an elastic band. Report of a case. J Periodontol *59:*472, 1988.
16. Proffit W. Contemporary Orthodontics. St Louis, CV Mosby, 1987.
17. Stoner JE, Mazdyasna S. Gingival recession in the lower incisor region of 15 year old subjects. J Periodontol *51:*74, 1980.
18. Swanson JC, Rosenberg F. Orthodontic movement in periodontal therapy. Dent Clin North Am *24:*231, 1980.
19. Wagenberg BD, Eskow RN, Langer B. Orthodontic procedures that improve periodontal prognosis. J Am Dent Assoc *100:*370, 1980.
20. Wennstrom J, Stockland BL, Nyman S, Thilander B. Periodontal tissue response to orthodontic movement of teeth with infrabony pockets. Am J Orthod Dentofac Orthop *103:*313, 1993.

49

The Surgical Phase of Therapy

FERMIN A. CARRANZA, JR.

Objectives of the Surgical Phase
Surgical Pocket Therapy
Results of Pocket Therapy
Pocket Elimination Versus Pocket Maintenance

Re-evaluation After Phase I Therapy
Indications for Periodontal Surgery
Methods of Pocket Elimination
Criteria for Method Selection

Although in a strict sense all instrumental therapy can be considered surgical, this chapter refers only to those techniques that include the intentional severing or incising of gingival tissue with the purpose of controlling or eliminating periodontal disease. Therefore, scaling and root planing is not included, because this procedure does not intentionally act on the gingival tissue.

OBJECTIVES OF THE SURGICAL PHASE

The surgical phase of periodontal therapy seeks to (1) improve the prognosis of teeth and (2) improve aesthetics. It consists of techniques performed for pocket therapy and for the correction of related morphologic problems (i.e., mucogingival defects). In many cases procedures are combined so that one surgical intervention fulfills both objectives.

The purpose of surgical pocket therapy is to eliminate the pathologic changes in the pocket walls; to create a stable, easily maintainable state; and, if possible, to promote periodontal regeneration. To fulfill these objectives, surgical techniques (1) increase accessibility to the root surface, making it possible to remove all irritants; (2) reduce or eliminate pocket depth, making it possible for the patient to maintain the root surfaces free of plaque; and (3) reshape soft and hard tissues to attain a harmonious topography.

The other objective of the surgical phase of periodontal therapy is the correction of morphologic defects that may favor plaque accumulation and pocket recurrence. This involves mucogingival techniques used to create attached gingiva or to cover denuded roots; these are dealt with in Chapter 59.

In addition, there are surgical techniques aimed at surgical preprosthetic preparation of the mouth, including the placement of dental implants. These are covered in Chapter 64. This chapter deals only with surgical pocket therapy.

Surgical Pocket Therapy

Surgical pocket therapy can be directed toward (1) opening up the pocket area to ensure the removal of irritants from the tooth surface or (2) eliminating or reducing the depth of the periodontal pocket.

The effectiveness of periodontal therapy is based on total elimination of plaque, calculus, and diseased cementum from the tooth surface. Numerous investigations have shown that the difficulty of this task increases as the pocket becomes deeper.[2,5] There are many irregularities on the root surface that increase the difficulty of the procedure. As the pocket gets deeper, the surface to be scaled increases, more irregularities appear on the root surface, and accessibility is impaired.[11,17] The presence of furcation involvements sometimes creates insurmountable problems (see Chapter 31).

All of these problems can be reduced by resecting or displacing the soft tissue wall of the pocket, thereby increasing the visibility and accessibility of the root surface.[3] The flap approach and the gingivectomy technique attain this result.

The need to eliminate or reduce the depth of the pocket is another important consideration. Pocket elimination consists of reducing the depth of periodontal pockets to that of a physiologic sulcus to enable cleansing by the patient. The presence of a pocket produces areas that are impossible for the patient to keep clean, and therefore the vicious cycle depicted in Figure 49–1 is established.

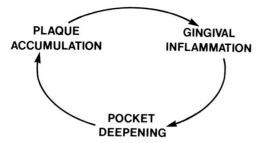

FIGURE 49–1. Accumulation of plaque leads to gingival inflammation and pocket deepening, which in turn increases plaque accumulation.

Results of Pocket Therapy

A periodontal pocket can be in an active state or in a period of inactivity or quiescence. An active pocket is one under which bone is being lost (Fig. 49–2, *top left*) and may be suspected clinically by the presence of bleeding and secretion, either spontaneously or on probing. After Phase I therapy, the inflammatory changes in the pocket wall subside, rendering the pocket inactive and reducing its depth (Fig. 49–2, *top center*). The extent of this reduction depends on the depth before treatment and on the degree to which the depth is due to the edematous and inflammatory component of the pocket wall.

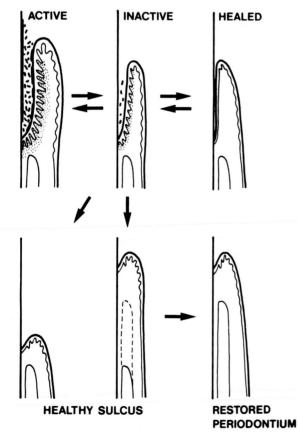

FIGURE 49–2. Possible results of pocket therapy. An active pocket can become inactive and heal by means of a long junctional epithelium. Surgical pocket therapy can result in a healthy sulcus, with or without gain of attachment. Improved gingival attachment promotes restoration of bone height, with re-formation of periodontal ligament fibers and layers of cementum.

Whether the pocket remains inactive depends on the characteristics of the plaque components and the host response. Recurrence of the initial activity is likely.

Inactive pockets can sometimes heal with a long junctional epithelium (Fig. 49–2, *top right*). However, this condition may be unstable, and the chance of recurrence and reformation of the original pocket is always present because the epithelial union to the tooth is a weak one. However, one study in monkeys has shown that the long junctional epithelial union may be as resistant to plaque infection as a normal connective tissue attachment.[9]

Studies have shown that inactive pockets can be maintained for long periods with little loss of attachment by means of frequent scaling and root planing procedures.[6,10,12] A more reliable and stable result is obtained, however, by transforming the pocket into a healthy sulcus. The bottom of the healthy sulcus can be located either where the bottom of the pocket was localized or coronal to it. In the first case there is no gain of attachment (Fig. 49–2, *bottom left*), and the area of the root that was previously the tooth wall of the pocket becomes exposed. This does not mean that the periodontal treatment has caused recession, but rather that it has uncovered the recession previously induced by the disease.

The healthy sulcus can also be located coronal to the bottom of the pre-existent pocket (Fig. 49–2, *bottom center and right*). This is conducive to a restored marginal periodontium; the result is a sulcus of normal depth with gain of attachment. The creation of a healthy sulcus and a restored periodontium is termed *new attachment* and entails a total restoration of the status that existed before periodontal disease began. This is, of course, the ideal result of treatment.

POCKET ELIMINATION VERSUS POCKET MAINTENANCE

Total pocket elimination has traditionally been considered one of the main goals of periodontal therapy. Elimination was considered vital because of the need to improve the accessibility of the root surfaces for the therapist during treatment and for the patient after healing.

Another viewpoint has emerged and is supported by clinical longitudinal studies.[18] It has been shown that after surgical therapy, pockets of 4 and even 5 mm can be maintained in a healthy state and without radiographic evidence of advancing bone loss. This was accomplished after pocket therapy, by maintenance visits consisting of scaling and root planing, with oral hygiene reinforcement performed at regular intervals of not more than 3 months. In these cases the residual defect can be penetrated with a thin periodontal probe, but no pain, exudate, or bleeding results; this appears to indicate that no plaque has formed on the subgingival root surfaces.

These findings do not alter the indications for periodontal surgery, because the results obtained are based on surgical exposure of the root surfaces for a thorough and complete elimination of irritants. They do, however, emphasize the importance of the maintenance phase and of the close monitoring of both level of attachment and pocket depth, together with the other clinical variables (i.e., bleeding, exdation, and tooth mobility). *The transformation of the initial deep, active lesion into a shallower, inactive, maintainable one requires some form of definitive pocket therapy and constant supervision thereafter.*

Pocket depth is an extremely useful and widely employed clinical parameter, but it must be evaluated together with level of attachment and the presence of bleeding, exudation, and pain. The most important variable for evaluating whether a pocket (or deep sulcus) is progressive is the level of attachment, which is measured in millimeters from the cemento-enamel junction; it is the apical displacement of the level of attachment that places the tooth in jeopardy, not the increase in pocket depth, which may be due to coronal displacement of the gingival margin.

Pocket depth remains an important clinical variable on which decisions about treatment can be partially based. Lindhe and colleagues compared the effect of root planing alone and in conjunction with a modified Widman flap on the resultant level of attachment and in relation to initial pocket depth.[7] They reported that scaling and root planing procedures induce loss of attachment if performed in pockets shallower than 2.9 mm, whereas in deeper pockets, gain of attachment occurs. The modified Widman flap induces loss of attachment if done in pockets shallower than 4.2 mm but results in a greater gain of attachment than does root planing in pockets deeper than 4.2 mm. The loss is a true loss of connective tissue attachment, whereas the gain can be considered a false gain owing to reduced penetrability of connective tissues apical to the bottom of the pocket after treatment.[8,19]

Furthermore, probing depths established after active therapy and healing (approximately 6 months after treatment) can be maintained unchanged or reduced even further during a maintenance care program involving careful prophylaxis once every 3 months.[7]

Ramfjord and associates[12] and Rosling and colleagues[13] showed that regardless of the surgical technique used for pocket therapy, a certain pocket depth recurs. *Therefore, maintenance of this depth without any further loss of attachment becomes the goal.*

RE-EVALUATION AFTER PHASE I THERAPY

Several longitudinal studies carried out since the 1970s have noted that all patients should be treated initially with scaling and root planing and that a final decision on the need for periodontal surgery should be made only after a thorough evaluation of the effects of Phase I therapy. The assessment is generally made 1 to 3 months after completion of Phase I therapy, although sometimes periods as long as 9 months have been recommended.[1] This re-evaluation of the periodontal condition should include reprobing the entire mouth, rechecking for the presence of calculus, root caries, defective restorations, and all signs of persistent inflammation.

There are several different surgical techniques for pocket therapy. The criteria for their selection are based on clinical findings in the soft tissue pocket wall, in the tooth surface, in the underlying bone, and in the attached gingiva.

Zone 1: The Soft Tissue Wall. The morphologic features, thickness, and topography of the soft tissue pocket wall and the persistence of inflammatory changes in it should be determined.

Zone 2: The Tooth Surface. The presence of deposits and alterations on the cementum surface and the accessibility of the root surface to instrumentation should be identified. Phase I therapy should have solved many if not all of the problems on the tooth surface. Evaluation of the results of Phase I therapy should determine the need for further therapy and the method to be used.

Zone 3: The Bone. The shape and height of the alveolar bone next to the pocket wall should be established by careful probing and clinical and radiographic examination. Bony craters, angular bone losses, and other bone deformities are important criteria for the selection of the pocket therapy technique.

Zone 4: The Attached Gingiva. The presence or absence of an adequate band of attached gingiva is a factor to be considered when selecting the pocket eradication method. Diagnostic techniques for mucogingival problems are described in Chapter 59. An inadequate attached gingiva may be due to a high frenum attachment, marked gingival recession, or a deep pocket that reaches the level of the mucogingival junction. All of these possible conditions should be explored and their influence on pocket elimination determined.

INDICATIONS FOR PERIODONTAL SURGERY

The following findings may indicate the need for surgical therapy:

1. Areas with irregular bony contours or deep craters.
2. Pockets on teeth in which a complete removal of root irritants is not considered clinically possible. This occurs frequently in molar and premolar areas.
3. In cases of grade II or III furcation involvement, a surgical approach ensures the removal of irritants; any necessary root resection or hemisection also requires surgical intervention.
4. Infrabony pockets in distal areas of last molars, which are frequently complicated by mucogingival problems, are usually unresponsive to nonsurgical methods.
5. Persistent inflammation in areas with moderate to deep pockets may require a surgical approach. In areas with shallow pockets or normal sulci, persistent inflammation may point to the presence of a mucogingival problem that requires a surgical solution.

METHODS OF POCKET ELIMINATION

The methods of pocket elimination are classified as follows:

1. *New attachment techniques* offer the ideal result, because they eliminate pocket depth by reuniting the gingiva to the tooth at a position coronal to the bottom of the pre-existing pocket. New attachment is usually associated with filling in of bone and regeneration of periodontal ligament and cementum.
2. *Removal of the pocket wall* is the most common method. The wall of the pocket consists of soft tissue and may also include bone in the case of infrabony pockets. It can be removed by (a) retraction or shrinkage, in which scaling and

root planing procedures resolve the inflammatory process and the gingiva shrinks, thereby reducing the pocket depth; (b) surgical removal performed by the gingivectomy technique or by means of an undisplaced flap (internal gingivectomy); and (c) apical displacement with an apically displaced flap.

3. *Removal of the tooth side of the pocket,* which is accomplished by tooth extraction or by partial tooth extraction (hemisection or root resection).

These techniques, their results, and the factors governing their selection are presented in Chapters 53 to 60.

Criteria for Method Selection

Scientific criteria to establish the indications for each technique are difficult to determine. Longitudinal studies that follow a significant number of cases over a number of years, standardizing multiple factors and different variables, are needed. Clinical experience, however, has suggested the criteria for selecting the method to be used to eliminate the pocket in individual cases. The selection of a technique for treatment of a particular periodontal lesion is based on a number of considerations:

1. Characteristics of the pocket: depth, relation to bone, and configuration.
2. Accessibility to instrumentation, including presence of furcation involvements.
3. Existence of mucogingival problems.
4. Response to Phase I therapy.
5. Patient cooperation and ability to perform effective oral hygiene.
6. Age and general health of the patient.
7. Overall diagnosis of the case: various types of gingival enlargement and types of periodontitis (slowly or rapidly progressing periodontitis, juvenile periodontitis, and so forth).
8. Aesthetic considerations.
9. Previous periodontal treatments.

Each of these variables is analyzed in relation to the pocket therapy techniques available, and a specific technique is selected. Of the many techniques available, the one that will most successfully solve the problems with the fewest undesirable effects should be chosen. *Clinicians who adhere to one technique to solve all problems do not use the wide repertoire of techniques available to the advantage of the patient.*

Therapy for Gingival Pockets. Two factors are taken into consideration: the character of the pocket wall and pocket accessibility. The pocket wall may be edematous or fibrotic. Edematous tissue shrinks after the elimination of local factors, thereby reducing or totally eliminating pocket depth. Therefore, scaling and root planing is the technique of choice in these cases.

Pockets with a fibrotic wall are not appreciably reduced in depth after scaling and root planing and therefore are eliminated surgically. Until relatively recently gingivectomy was the only technique available; it solves the problem successfully, but in cases of marked gingival enlargement (e.g., severe phenytoin enlargement), it may leave a large wound that goes through a painful and prolonged healing process. In these cases a modified flap technique can adequately solve the problem with fewer postoperative problems[15] (see Chapter 60).

Therapy for Mild Periodontitis. In mild or incipient periodontitis, bone loss has occurred to a small degree and

pockets are shallow to moderate. In these cases a conservative approach and adequate oral hygiene are generally sufficient to control the disease. Incipient periodontitis occurring as recurrence in previously treated sites may require a thorough analysis of the causes for the recurrence and, infrequently, a surgical approach to correct them.

Therapy for Moderate to Severe Periodontitis in the Anterior Sector. The anterior teeth are important aesthetically; therefore, the techniques that induce the least amount of visual root exposure should be considered first. However, the importance of aesthetics may be different for different patients, and nonelimination of the pocket may place the tooth in jeopardy. The final decision may entail a compromise between health and aesthetics, with ideal results not attained in either respect.

Anterior teeth offer some advantages to a conservative approach. First, they are all single rooted and easily accessible; second, patient compliance and thoroughness in plaque control are easier to attain. *Therefore, scaling and root planing is the technique of choice for the anterior teeth.*

Sometimes, however, a surgical technique may be necessary owing to the need for improved accessibility for root planing or reconstructive surgery of osseous defects. The *papilla preservation flap* can be used for both purposes and also offers a better postoperative result with less recession and reduced soft tissue crater formation interproximally.[16] It is the first choice when a surgical approach is needed.

When the teeth are too close interproximally, the papilla preservation technique may not be feasible, and a technique that splits the papilla must be used. The *sulcular incision flap* offers good aesthetic results and is the next choice.

When aesthetics are not the primary consideration, the so called *modified Widman flap* can be chosen. This technique uses an internal bevel incision about 1 to 2 mm from the gingival margin and therefore results in some degree of recession.

In some infrequent cases, bone contouring may be needed in spite of the resultant root exposure. The technique of choice is the *apically displaced flap with bone contouring.*

Therapy for Moderate to Severe Periodontitis in the Posterior Area. Treatment for premolars and molars usually poses no aesthetic problem and frequently involves difficult accessibility. Bone defects are more frequent than in the anterior sector, and root morphologic features, particularly in relation to furcations, may offer insurmountable problems for instrumentation in a close field. Therefore, surgery is frequently indicated in this region.

The purpose of surgery in the posterior area is either enhanced accessibility or need for osseous surgery. Accessibility can be obtained by a modified Widman flap. However, if pocket reduction is also desired, then an apically displaced flap is the technique of choice.

Most cases of moderate to severe periodontitis have developed osseous defects that require some degree of osseous remodeling or reconstructive procedures. When osseous defects amenable to reconstruction are present, the papilla preservation flap is the technique of choice, because it better protects the interproximal areas where defects are frequently present. Second and third choices are the sulcular flap and the modified Widman flap, respectively. These techniques allow adequate exposure of the area but do not offer adequate protection of the interproximal grafted area. They are resorted to when the papilla preservation flap is not possible owing to anatomic factors.

When osseous defects with no possibility of reconstruction, such as interdental craters, are present, the technique of choice is the apically displaced flap with osseous contouring.

REFERENCES

1. Badersten A, Nilveus R, Egelberg J. Effect of nonsurgical periodontal therapy. II. Severely advanced periodontitis. J Clin Periodontol *11:*63, 1984.
2. Bower RC. Furcation morphology relative to periodontal treatment. Furcation root surface anatomy. J Periodontol *50:*366, 1979.
3. Caffesse RG, Sweeney PL, Smith BA. Scaling and root planing with and without periodontal flap surgery. J Clin Periodontol *13:*205, 1986.
4. Davies WIR. Open curettage and pocket elimination. In Shanley D, ed. Efficacy of Treatment Procedures in Periodontics. Chicago, Quintessence Publishing, 1980.
5. Gher ME, Vernino AR. Root morphology—clinical significance in pathogenesis and treatment of periodontal disease. J Am Dent Assoc *101:*627, 1980.
6. Hill RW, Ramfjord SP, Morrison GC, et al. Four types of periodontal treatment compared over two years. J Periodontol *52:*655, 1981.
7. Lindhe J, Socransky S, Nyman S, et al. Critical probing depths in periodontal therapy. J Clin Periodontol *9:*323, 1982.
8. Lindhe J, Socransky SS, Nyman S. Dimensional alteration of the periodontal tissues following therapy. Int J Periodont Restor Dent *7:*8, 1987.
9. Magnusson I, Runstad L, Nyman S, Lindhe J. A long junctional epithelium—a locus minoris resistentiae in plaque infection. J Clin Periodontol *10:*333, 1983.
10. Pihlstrom BL, Ortiz Campos C, McHugh RB. A randomized four year study of periodontal therapy. J Periodontol *52:*227, 1981.
11. Rabbani GM, Ash MM, Caffesse RG. The effectiveness of subgingival scaling and root planing in calculus removal. J Periodontol *52:*119, 1981.
12. Ramfjord SP, Knowles JW, Nissle RR, et al. Results following three modalities of periodontal therapy. J Periodontol *46:*522, 1975.
13. Rosling B, Nyman S, Lindhe J, et al. The healing potential of the periodontal tissues following different techniques of periodontal surgery in plaque-free dentitions. A 2 year clinical study. J Clin Periodontol *3:*233, 1976.
14. Socransky SS, Haffajee AD. Problems in the evaluation of therapeutic procedures in view of periodontal research findings. Int J Periodont Restor Dent *5:*69, 1985.
15. Takei HH. A modified flap technique for the removal of gingival enlargements. Unpublished manuscript. UCLA, 1985.
16. Takei HH, Han TJ, Carranza FA Jr, et al. Flap technique for periodontal bone implants—the papilla preservation technique. J Periodontol *56:*204, 1985.
17. Waerhaug J. Healing of the dento-epithelial junction following subgingival plaque control. II. As observed on extracted teeth. J Periodontol *49:*119, 1978.
18. Weeks PR. Pros and cons of periodontal pocket elimination procedures. J West Soc Periodontol *28:*4, 1980.
19. Westfelt E, Bragd L, Socransky SS, et al. Improved periodontal conditions following therapy. J Clin Periodontol *12:*283, 1985.
20. Zamet JS. A comparative clinical study of three periodontal surgical techniques. J Clin Periodontol *2:*87, 1975.

50

General Principles of Periodontal Surgery

FERMIN A. CARRANZA, JR.

Outpatient Surgery
Preparation of the Patient
Emergency Equipment
Measures to Prevent Transmission of Infection
Sedation and Anesthesia
Tissue Management
Scaling and Root Planing
Hemostasis
Periodontal Dressings (Periodontal Packs)
Instructions for the Patient After Surgery
The First Postoperative Week
Removal of the Periodontal Pack and Return Visit Care

Care of the Mouth Between Periodontal Surgery Procedures
Hospital Periodontal Surgery
Indications
Hospital Admission and Presurgical Medical Examination
Premedication and Anesthesia
The Operation
Postoperative Instructions at the Hospital
First Postoperative Office Visit

All surgical procedures should be very carefully planned. The patient should be adequately prepared medically, psychologically, and practically for all aspects of the intervention. This chapter covers the preparation of the patient and the general considerations that are common to all periodontal surgical techniques. Complications that may occur during or after surgery are also discussed.

Surgical periodontal procedures are usually performed in the dental office. The indications for performing periodontal surgery in the hospital will be discussed.

OUTPATIENT SURGERY

Preparation of the Patient

Re-evaluation After Phase I Therapy. Almost every patient undergoes the initial or preparatory phase of therapy, which basically consists of thorough scaling and root planing and removal of all irritants responsible for the periodontal inflammation. These procedures will (1) eliminate some lesions entirely; (2) render the tissues more firm and consistent, thus permitting more accurate and delicate surgery; and (3) acquaint the patient with the office and with the operator and assistants, thereby reducing the patient's apprehension and fear.

The re-evaluation phase consists of reprobing and re-examining all the pertinent findings that previously indicated the need for the surgical procedure. Persistence of these findings will confirm the indication for surgery. The number of surgical procedures to be performed, the dates for all the procedures, the expected outcome, and the postoperative care that is needed are all decided beforehand. These are discussed with the patient, and a final decision is made, incorporating any necessary adjustments to the original plan.

Premedication. For patients who are not medically compromised,* the value of administering antibiotics routinely for periodontal surgery has not been clearly demonstrated,[40] although some studies have shown reduced postoperative complications, including reduced pain and swelling, when antibiotics are administered starting prior to periodontal surgery and continuing for 4 to 7 days after surgery.[4,14,29,46]

The prophylactic use of antibiotics has been advocated for bone-grafting procedures in periodontal patients who are otherwise healthy and has been claimed to enhance the chances of new attachment. Although the rationale for such use appears logical, there is no research evidence to support it. In any case, the risks inherent in the administration of antibiotics should be evaluated together with the potential benefits.

Other presurgical medications include the administration of one 800-mg tablet of ibuprofen (Motrin) 1 hour before the procedure[15] and one oral rinse with 0.12% chlorhexidine gluconate (Peridex or PerioGard).

Informed Consent. The patient should be informed at the time of the initial visit about the diagnosis, the prognosis, the different possible treatments and their expected results, and the advantages and disadvantages of each approach. At the time of surgery, the patient should again be informed, both verbally and in writing, of the procedure to be performed, and he or she should indicate agreement by signing the consent form.

Emergency Equipment

The operator, all assistants, and office personnel should be trained to handle all possible emergencies that may arise. Drugs and equipment for emergency use should be readily available at all times.

The most common emergency is *syncope,* or a transient loss of consciousness owing to a reduction in cerebral blood flow. The most common cause is fear and anxiety. Syncope is usually preceded by a feeling of weakness, which is followed by pallor, sweating, coldness of the extremities, dizziness, and slowing of the pulse. The patient should be placed in a supine position with the legs elevated; tight clothes should be loosened and an open airway ensured; administration of oxygen is also useful. Unconsciousness persists for a few minutes. A history of previous

syncopal attacks during dental appointments should be explored before treatment is begun, and if such attacks are reported, extra efforts should be made to relieve the patient's fear and anxiety. The reader is referred to other texts[3] for a complete analysis of this important topic.

Measures to Prevent Transmission of Infection

The danger of transmitting infections to the dental team or to other patients has become apparent, particularly with the threat of acquired immunodeficiency syndrome (AIDS) and hepatitis B. Protective attire and barrier techniques are strongly recommended. These include the use of disposable sterile gloves, surgical masks, and protective eye wear. All surfaces that may be contaminated with blood or saliva and cannot be sterilized (e.g., light handles and unit syringes) must be covered with aluminum foil or plastic wrap. Aerosol-producing devices (e.g., the Cavitron) should not be used in patients with suspected infections, and their use should be kept to a minimum in all other patients. Special care should be taken when using and disposing of sharp items such as needles and scalpel blades.

Sedation and Anesthesia

Periodontal surgery should be painless. The patient should be assured of this at the outset and thoroughly anesthetized by means of local block and infiltration injections. Injections directly into the interdental papillae may be helpful.

Apprehensive and neurotic patients require special management. The history, physical condition, and personality of the patient should be taken into consideration to determine the medications required, if any. Diazepam (Valium), 10 mg orally before surgery, can be used in apprehensive patients.

Intravenous sedation with diazepam or inhalation analgesia with nitrous oxide–oxygen is also helpful in some cases. The operator should receive training in the techniques for administering these agents and should understand their indications, contraindications, and risks before attempting to use them in patients.[3] Many of these drugs require that the patient come to the dental office accompanied by a responsible adult who can drive him or her home if necessary.

Tissue Management

1. *Operate gently and carefully.* In addition to being most considerate to the patient, this is also the most effective way to operate. Tissue manipulation should be gentle. Thoroughness is essential, but roughness must be avoided, because it produces excessive tissue injury, causes postoperative discomfort, and delays healing.
2. *Observe the patient at all times.* It is essential to pay careful attention to the patient's reactions. The facial expression indicates whether the patient is in pain; pallor and perspiration are warning signs of patient anxiety.
3. *Be certain the instruments are sharp.* Instruments must be sharp to be effective; successful treatment is not possible without sharp instruments. Dull instruments inflict unnecessary trauma because of the excess force usually applied to

---

* Precautions to be taken with medically compromised patients can be found in Chapter 34.

compensate for their ineffectiveness. A sterile sharpening stone should be available on the operating table at all times (see Chapter 36).

Scaling and Root Planing

Although scaling and root planing have been performed previously as part of Phase I therapy, all exposed root surfaces should be carefully explored and planed as needed as part of the surgical procedure. In particular, areas of difficult access, such as furcations or deep pockets, often are still rough or even have calculus that was undetected during the preparatory sessions. The assistant who is separating the tissues and using the aspirator should also, from a different angle, check for the presence of calculus and the smoothness of each surface.

Hemostasis

An aspirator is indispensable for performing periodontal surgery. It provides the operator with a clear view of each root surface, which is necessary for thorough removal of deposits and planing. Furthermore, it permits an accurate appraisal of the extent and pattern of soft tissue and bone involvement and prevents seepage of blood into the floor of the mouth and oropharynx.

Periodontal surgery produces profuse bleeding in its initial incisional steps. However, after granulation tissue has been removed, bleeding disappears or is considerably reduced. Packing with gauze squares and the use of an aspirator are necessary to keep a dry field.

Excessive hemorrhaging after these initial steps may be due to lacerated capillaries and arterioles or to damage to larger vessels as a result of surgical invasion of anatomic areas (e.g., the palate halfway from the teeth to the midpalate, where the palatine arteries run). Bleeding from vessels emerging from the retroincisal foramina or from the inferior alveolar artery is rare. Proper design of the flaps, taking into consideration these anatomic structures, prevents accidents (see Chapter 51).

Minor areas of persistent bleeding can be stopped by applying pressure with gauze for a few minutes. A cotton pellet dipped in ferric subsulfate powder may sometimes be needed.

Thrombin is a drug capable of hastening the process of blood clotting. It is intended for topical use only and is applied as a liquid or a powder. Oxidized cellulose (Novocell, Oxycel) and absorbable gelatin sponges (Gelfoam) are useful hemostatics in deep wounds. Patients with bleeding disorders should be carefully prepared for surgery, frequently by a hematologist (see Chapter 34).

Periodontal Dressings (Periodontal Packs)

In most cases, after the surgical periodontal procedures are completed, the area is covered with a surgical pack. In general, dressings have no curative properties; they assist healing by protecting the tissue rather than by providing "healing factors." The pack minimizes the likelihood of postoperative infection and hemorrhage, facilitates healing by preventing surface trauma during mastication, and protects against pain induced by contact of the wound with food or with the tongue during mastication. For a complete literature review on this subject, the reader is referred to the work of Sachs et al.[50]

Types of Dressings

Zinc Oxide–Eugenol Packs. Packs based on the reaction of zinc oxide and eugenol include the Wondr-Pak developed by Ward[57] in 1923 and several others that modified Ward's original formula. The addition of accelerators, such as zinc acetate, gives the dressing a better working time. Other substances that have been added include asbestos, used as a binder and a filler, and tannic acid. However, asbestos can induce lung diseases, and tannic acid may lead to liver damage; therefore, both substances have been eliminated.

Zinc oxide–eugenol dressings are supplied as a liquid and a powder that are mixed prior to use. Eugenol may induce an allergic reaction that produces reddening of the area and burning pain in some patients.

Noneugenol Packs. The reaction between a metallic oxide and fatty acids is the basis for Coe-Pak, the most widely used type of dressing in the United States. This is supplied in two tubes, the contents of which are mixed immediately before use until a uniform color is obtained. One of the tubes contains zinc oxide, an oil (for plasticity), a gum (for cohesiveness), and bithionol (Lorothidol) (a fungicide); the other tube contains liquid coconut fatty acids, thickened with colophony resin (or rosin) and chlorothymol (a bacteriostatic agent).[50,52] This dressing does not contain asbestos or eugenol and thereby avoids the problems associated with these substances.

Other noneugenol packs include cyanoacrylates[6,27,32] and tissue conditioners (methacrylic gels).[1] However, these are not commonly used.

Retention of Packs. Periodontal dressings are usually kept in place mechanically by interlocking in interdental spaces and by joining the lingual and facial portions of the pack.

In isolated teeth or when there are several missing teeth in an arch, retention of the pack may be difficult. Numerous reinforcements and splints and stents for this purpose have been described.[23,24,59] Placement of dental floss tied loosely around the teeth enhances retention of the pack.

Antibacterial Properties of Packs. Improved healing and patient comfort with less odor and taste[6] have been reported by incorporating antibiotics in the pack. Bacitracin,[5] oxytetracycline (Terramycin),[17] neomycin, and nitrofurazone have been tried, but all may produce hypersensitivity reactions.[38] The emergence of resistant organisms and opportunistic infection have been reported.[48]

Incorporation of tetracycline powder into the Coe-Pak is generally recommended, particularly when long and traumatic surgeries are performed.

Allergy. Contact allergy to eugenol and to rosin has been reported.[47]

Preparation and Application of the Periodontal Dressing. Zinc oxide packs are mixed with eugenol or noneugenol liquids on a wax paper pad with a wooden tongue depressor. The powder is gradually incorporated with the liquid until a thick paste is formed.

Coe-Pak is prepared by mixing equal lengths of paste from the tubes containing the accelerator and the base until

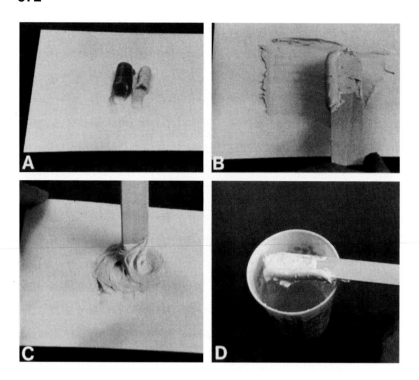

FIGURE 50–1. Preparing the surgical pack (Coe-Pak). *A,* Equal lengths of the two pastes are placed on the paper pad. *B,* The pastes are mixed with a wooden tongue depressor for 2 or 3 minutes until the paste loses its tackiness *(C). D,* Paste is placed in a paper cup of water at room temperature. It is then rolled into cylinders with lubricated fingers and placed on the surgical wound.

the resulting paste is a uniform color. A capsule of tetracycline powder can be added at this time. The pack is then placed in a cup of water at room temperature. In 2 to 3 minutes the paste loses its tackiness (Fig. 50–1), and 3 to 5 minutes after mixing, it can be handled and molded; it remains workable for 15 to 20 minutes. Working time can be shortened by adding a small amount of zinc oxide to the accelerator (pink paste) before spatulating.

The pack is then rolled into two strips approximately the length of the treated area. The end of one strip is bent into a hook shape and fitted around the distal surface of the last tooth, approaching it from the distal surface (Fig. 50–2A). The remainder of the strip is brought forward along the facial surface to the midline and gently pressed into place along the gingival margin and interproximally. The second strip is applied from the lingual surface. It is joined to the pack at the distal surface of the last tooth and then brought forward along the gingival margin to the midline (Fig. 50–2B). The strips are joined interproximally by applying gentle pressure on the facial and lingual surfaces of the pack (Fig. 50–2C). For isolated teeth separated by edentulous spaces, the pack should extend continuously from tooth to tooth, covering the edentulous areas (Fig. 50–3).

When split flaps have been performed, the area should be covered with tin foil to protect the sutures before placing the pack (see Chapter 59).

The pack should cover the gingiva, but overextensions onto uninvolved mucosa should be avoided. *Excess pack irritates the mucobuccal fold and floor of the mouth and interferes with the tongue.* Overextension also jeopardizes the remainder of the pack, because the excess tends to break off, taking pack from the operated area with it. *Pack that interferes with the occlusion should be trimmed away before the patient is dismissed* (Fig. 50–4). Failure to do so causes discomfort and jeopardizes retention of the pack.

The operator should have the patient move the tongue forcibly out and to each side, and the cheek and lips should

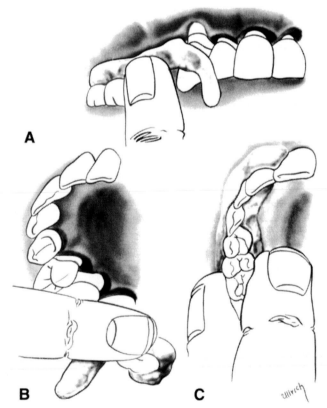

FIGURE 50–2. Inserting the periodontal pack. *A,* A strip of the pack is hooked around the last molar and pressed into place anteriorly. *B,* The lingual pack is joined to the facial strip at the distal surface of the last molar and is fitted into place anteriorly. *C,* Gentle pressure on the facial and lingual surfaces joins the pack interproximally.

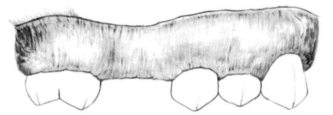

FIGURE 50–3. Continuous pack covers edentulous space.

be displaced in all directions to mold the pack while it is still soft. After the pack has set, it should be trimmed to eliminate all excess.

As a general rule, the pack is kept on for 1 week after surgery. This guideline is based on the usual timetable of healing and clinical experience. It is not a rigid requirement; the period may be extended, or the area may be repacked for an additional week.

Fragments of the surface of the pack may come off during the week, but this presents no problem. If a portion of the pack is lost from the operated area and the patient is uncomfortable, it is usually best to repack the area. The clinician should remove the remaining pack, wash the area with warm water, and apply a topical anesthetic before replacing the pack, which is then retained for 1 week. Again, patients may develop pain from an overextended margin that irritates the vestibule, the floor of the mouth, or the tongue. The excess pack should be trimmed away, making sure that the new margin is not rough, before the patient is dismissed.

Instructions for the Patient After Surgery

After the pack is placed, the following printed instructions are given to the patient to be read before he or she leaves the chair:

INSTRUCTIONS FOR (Patient's Name)

The following information on your gum operation has been prepared to answer questions you may have about how to take care of your mouth. Please read the instructions carefully; our patients have found them very helpful.

Although there will be little or no discomfort when the anesthesia wears off, you should *take two acetaminophen (Tylenol) tablets every 6 hours for the first 24 hours.* After that, take the same medication if you have some discomfort. Do not take aspirin, as this may increase bleeding.

We have placed a periodontal pack over your gums to protect them from irritation. The pack prevents pain, aids healing, and enables you to carry on most of your usual activities. The pack will harden in a few hours, after which it can withstand most of the forces of chewing without breaking off. It may take a little while to become accustomed to it.

The pack should remain in place until it is removed in the office at your next appointment. If particles of the pack chip off during the week, do not be concerned as long as you do not have pain. If a piece of the pack breaks off and you are in pain, or if a rough edge irritates your tongue or cheek, please call the office. The problem can be easily remedied by replacing the pack.

For the first 3 hours after the operation, avoid hot foods to permit the pack to harden. It is also convenient to avoid hot liquids for the first 24 hours. You can eat anything you can manage, but

try to chew on the nonoperated side of your mouth. Semisolid or finely minced foods are suggested. Avoid citrus fruits or fruit juices, highly spiced foods, and alcoholic beverages; these will cause pain. Food supplements and/or vitamins are generally not necessary. We will prescribe them if needed.

Do not smoke. The heat and smoke will irritate your gums and delay healing. If at all possible, use this opportunity to give up smoking. In addition to all other well-known health risks, smokers have more gum disease than nonsmokers.

Do not brush over the pack. Brush and floss normally the areas of the mouth not covered by the pack. Use chlorhexidine (Peridex) mouthrinses after brushing. (The prescription for this mouthrinse has been given to you.)

During the first day, apply ice intermittently on the face over the operated area.

You may experience a slight feeling of weakness or chills during the first 24 hours. This is not a cause for alarm but should be reported at the next visit. *Follow your regular daily activities, but avoid excessive exertion of any type.* Golf, tennis, skiing, bowling, swimming, or sunbathing should be postponed for a few days after the operation.

Swelling is not unusual, particularly in areas that required extensive surgical procedures. The swelling generally begins 1 to 2 days after the operation and subsides gradually in 3 or 4 days. If this occurs, apply moist heat over the operated area. If the swelling is painful or appears to become worse, please call the office.

There may be occasional blood stains in the saliva for the first 4 or 5 hours after the operation. This is not unusual and will correct itself. If there is considerable bleeding beyond this, take a piece of gauze, form it into the shape of a U, hold it in the thumb and index finger, and apply it to both sides of the pack; hold it there under pressure for 20 minutes. Do not remove it during this period to examine it. If the bleeding does not stop at the end of 20 minutes, please contact the office. *Do not try to stop bleeding by rinsing.*

After the pack is removed, the gums will most likely bleed more than they did before the operation. This is perfectly normal in the early stages of healing and will gradually subside. Do not stop cleaning because of it.

If any other problems arise, please call the office.

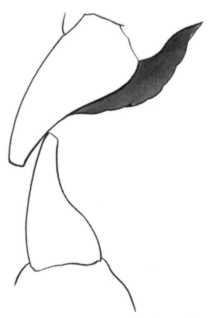

FIGURE 50–4. The pack should not interfere with occlusion.

The First Postoperative Week

Properly performed, periodontal surgery presents no serious postoperative problems. Patients should be told to rinse with 0.12% chlorhexidine gluconate (Peridex, PerioGard) immediately after the surgical procedure and twice daily thereafter until normal plaque control technique can be resumed.[39,51,56] The following complications may arise in the first postoperative week, although they are the exception rather than the rule:

1. *Persistent bleeding after surgery.* The pack is removed; the bleeding points are located; and the bleeding is stopped with pressure, sutures, electrosurgery, or electrocautery. After the bleeding is stopped, the pack is replaced.

2. *Sensitivity to percussion.* Sensitivity to percussion may be caused by the extension of inflammation into the periodontal ligament. The patient should be questioned regarding the progress of the symptoms. Gradual diminution of severity is a favorable sign. The pack should be removed and the gingiva checked for localized areas of infection or irritation; these should be cleaned or incised to provide drainage. Particles of calculus that may have been overlooked should be removed. Relieving the occlusion is usually helpful. Sensitivity to percussion may also be caused by excess pack, which interferes with the occlusion. Removal of the excess usually corrects the condition.

3. *Swelling.* Sometimes within the first 2 postoperative days patients report a soft, painless swelling of the cheek in the area of operation. There may be lymph node enlargement, and the temperature may be slightly elevated. The area of operation itself is usually symptom free. This type of involvement results from a localized inflammatory reaction to the operative procedure and generally subsides by the fourth postoperative day, without necessitating removal of the pack. Amoxicillin 500 mg should be taken every 8 hours for 1 week, and the patient should be instructed to apply moist heat intermittently over the area. The antibiotic should also be used as a prophylactic measure for the next operation, starting before the surgical appointment.

4. *Feeling of weakness.* Occasionally patients report experiencing a "washed-out," weakened feeling for about 24 hours after the operation. This represents a systemic reaction to a transient bacteremia induced by the operative procedure. It is prevented by premedication with amoxicillin, 500 mg every 8 hours, beginning 24 hours before the next operation and continuing for a 5-day postoperative period.

Removal of the Periodontal Pack and Return Visit Care

When the patient returns after 1 week, the pack is taken off by inserting a surgical curette along the margin and exerting gentle lateral pressure (Fig. 50–5). Pieces of pack retained interproximally and particles that adhere to the tooth surfaces and to ceramic and gold crowns are removed with scalers. Particles may be enmeshed in the cut surface and should be carefully picked off with fine cotton pliers. The entire area is swabbed with peroxide to remove superficial debris.

Findings at Pack Removal. The following are usual when the pack is removed:

If a gingivectomy has been performed, the cut surface is covered with a friable meshwork of new epithelium, which should not be disturbed. If calculus has not been completely removed, red, bead-like protuberances of granulation tissue will persist. This granulation tissue must be

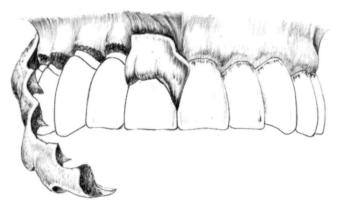

FIGURE 50–5. Removal of the periodontal pack.

removed with a curette, exposing the calculus so that it can be removed and the root can be planed. Removal of the granulation tissue without removal of calculus will be followed by recurrence.

After a flap operation, the areas corresponding to the incisions are epithelialized but may bleed readily when touched; they should not be disturbed. Pockets should not be probed.

The facial and lingual mucosa may be covered with a grayish yellow or white granular layer of food debris that has seeped under the pack. This is easily removed with a moist cotton pellet. The root surfaces may be sensitive to a probe or to thermal changes, and the teeth may be stained.

Fragments of calculus delay healing. Each root surface should be rechecked visually to be certain no calculus is present. Sometimes the color of the calculus is similar to that of the root. The grooves on proximal root surfaces and the furcations are areas in which calculus is likely to be overlooked.

Repacking. After the pack is removed, it is usually not necessary to replace it. However, it is advisable to repack for an additional week for patients with (1) a low pain threshold who are particularly uncomfortable when the pack is removed, (2) unusually extensive periodontal involvement, or (3) slow healing. Clinical judgment helps in deciding whether to repack the area or leave the initial pack on longer than 1 week.

Tooth Mobility. Tooth mobility is increased immediately after surgery[10] but by the fourth week diminishes below the pretreatment level.[33]

Final Check on Smoothness of the Root Surfaces. One week after the pack is removed from the final quadrant, all root surfaces are checked to see that they are smooth and firm. A rubber cup with fine pumice and polishing strips are used for the final smoothing of the root at this time.

Care of the Mouth Between Periodontal Surgery Procedures

Care of the mouth by the patient between treatment of the first and treatment of the final areas, as well as after surgery is completed, is extremely important.[60] These measures should begin after the pack is removed from the first operation. Even though the patient has been through a presurgical period of instruction in plaque control, he or she should be reinstructed at this time.

Vigorous brushing is not feasible during the first week after the pack is removed. However, the patient is informed that plaque and food accumulation retard healing and is advised to try to keep the area as clean as possible by the gentle use of soft toothbrushes and light water irrigation. Rinsing with chlorhexidine (Peridex, PerioGard) mouthwash or topical application with cotton-tipped applicators (Q-tips) is indicated for the first few postoperative weeks, particularly in advanced cases. Brushing is introduced when healing of the tissues permits it; the vigor of the overall hygiene regimen is increased as healing progresses. Patients should be told that there will most likely be more gingival bleeding than before the operation, that this is perfectly normal and will subside as healing progresses, and that it should not deter them from following their oral hygiene regimen.

Management of Postoperative Pain. Periodontal surgery performed following the basic principles outlined here should produce only minor pain and discomfort.[53] One study of 304 consecutive periodontal surgical interventions revealed that 51.3% of the patients reported minimal or no postoperative pain, and only 4.6% reported severe pain. Only 20.1% took five or more doses of analgesic.[13] The same study showed that mucogingival procedures result in six times more discomfort and osseous surgery in 3.5 times more discomfort than plastic gingival surgery. In the few cases in which severe pain may be present, its control becomes an important part of patient management.[38]

A common source of postoperative pain is overextension of the periodontal pack onto the soft tissue beyond the mucogingival junction or onto the frena. Overextended packs cause localized areas of edema that are usually noticed 1 to 2 days after surgery. Removal of excess pack is followed by resolution in about 24 hours. Extensive and excessively prolonged exposure and dryness of bone will also induce severe pain.

All patients are given one 800-mg tablet of ibuprofen before the procedure. The written patient instructions include the indication to take one tablet of acetaminophen every 6 hours after the procedure for 1 day and as needed thereafter. If pain persists, acetaminophen plus codeine (Tylenol 3) can be prescribed.

When severe postoperative pain is present, the patient should be seen at the office on an emergency basis. The area is anesthetized either by infiltration or topically, the pack is removed, and the wound is examined. Postoperative pain related to infection is accompanied by localized lymphadenopathy and a slight elevation in temperature; it should be treated with systemic antibiotics and analgesics.

Treatment of Sensitive Roots. Root hypersensitivity is a relatively common problem in periodontal practice. It may occur spontaneously when the root becomes exposed as a result of gingival recession or pocket formation, or it may appear after scaling and root planing and surgical procedures. (For a complete review of the literature, see the July 1990 issue of *Dental Clinics of North America*, edited by F. A. Curro and entitled "Tooth Hypersensitivity.") It is manifested as pain induced by cold or hot temperature, more commonly cold; by citrus fruits or sweets; or by contact with a toothbrush or a dental instrument.

Root sensitivity occurs more frequently in the cervical area of the root, where the cementum is extremely thin. Scaling and root planing procedures may entirely remove this thin cementum, inducing the hypersensitivity.

Transmission of stimuli from the surface of the dentin to the nerve endings located in the dental pulp or in the pulpal region of the dentin may occur through the odontoblastic process or owing to a hydrodynamic mechanism (e.g., by displacement of dentinal fluid). The latter process seems more likely and would explain the importance of burnishing desensitizing agents to obturate the dentinal tubule.

An important factor for reducing or eliminating hypersensitivity is adequate plaque control. However, hypersensitivity may prevent plaque control, and therefore a vicious cycle of escalating hypersensitivity and plaque accumulation may be created.

Desensitizing Agents. A number of agents have been proposed to control root hypersensitivity. Clinical evaluation of the many agents proposed has proved problematic, in part because (1) it is difficult to measure and compare different persons' pain, (2) hypersensitivity disappears by itself after a time, and (3) desensitizing agents usually take a few weeks to act.

The patient should be informed about the possibility of root hypersensitivity before treatment is undertaken. The following information on how to cope with the problem should also be given to the patient:

1. Hypersensitivity appears as a result of exposure of dentin, which is inevitable if calculus and plaque and their products, buried in the root, are to be removed.
2. Hypersensitivity slowly disappears over a few weeks.
3. Plaque control is important for the reduction of hypersensitivity.
4. Desensitizing agents do not produce immediate relief. They must be used for several days or even weeks to produce results.

Desensitizing agents can be applied by the patient at home or by the dentist or hygienist in the dental office. The most likely mechanism of action is the reduction in the diameter of the dentinal tubules so as to limit the displacement of fluids in them. According to Trowbridge and Silver,[55] this can be attained by (1) formation of a smear layer produced by burnishing the exposed surface, (2) topical application of agents that form insoluble precipitates within the tubules, (3) impregnation of tubules with plastic resins, or (4) sealing off the tubules with plastic resins.

Agents Used by the Patient. The most common agents are dentifrices used by the patient for oral hygiene. The following dentifrices have been approved by the American Dental Association for desensitizing purposes: Sensodyne and Thermodent, which contain strontium chloride[9,11,49]; Denquel and Promise, which contain potassium nitrate[11]; and Protect, which contains sodium citrate. Fluoride rinsing solutions and gels can also be used after the usual plaque control procedures.[54]

Agents Used in the Dental Office. Table 50–1 lists various office treatments for the desensitization of hypersensitive dentin. The reader is again referred to the paper by Trowbridge and Silver[55] for a more detailed consideration of these methods.

Fluoride solutions and pastes historically have been the agents of choice. In addition to their antisensitivity properties, they have the advantage of anticaries activity, which is particularly important for patients with a tendency to develop root caries.

Table 50–1. OFFICE TREATMENTS FOR DENTINAL HYPERSENSITIVITY

Cavity varnishes
Anti-inflammatory agents
Treatments that partially obturate dentinal tubules
  Burnishing of dentin
  Silver nitrate
  Zinc chloride–potassium ferrocyanide
  Formalin
  Calcium compounds
    Calcium hydroxide
    Dibasic calcium phosphate
  Fluoride compounds
    Sodium fluoride
    Sodium silicofluoride
    Stannous fluoride
  Iontophoresis
  Strontium chloride
  Potassium oxalate
Restorative resins
Dentin bonding agents

From Trowbridge HO, Silver DR. A review of current approaches to in-office management of tooth hypersensitivity. Dent Clin North Am *34*(3): 566, 1990.

Currently potassium and ferric oxalate solutions are the preferred agents. They form insoluble calcium oxalate crystals that occlude the dentinal tubules.[41,43] Potassium oxalate is available under the name Protect and ferric oxalate under the name Sensodyne Sealant. Special applicators have been developed for their use.

HOSPITAL PERIODONTAL SURGERY

Ordinarily, periodontal surgery is an office procedure performed in quadrants or sextants, usually at biweekly intervals. Under certain circumstances, however, it is in the best interest of the patient to treat the mouth in one operation with the patient hospitalized.

Indications

Patient Protection. Some patients have systemic conditions that are not severe enough to contraindicate elective surgery but may require special precautions best provided in a hospital. These include some patients with cardiovascular disease, abnormal bleeding tendencies, or hyperthyroidism; those undergoing prolonged steroid therapy; and those with a history of rheumatic fever.

The purpose of hospitalization is to protect patients by anticipating their special needs, not to perform periodontal surgery when it is contraindicated by the patient's general condition. There are patients for whom elective surgery is contraindicated, regardless of whether it is performed in the dental office or in the hospital. When consultation with the patient's physician leads to this decision, palliative periodontal therapy in the form of scaling and curettage, if permissible, is the necessary compromise.

The Apprehensive Patient. Gentleness, understanding, and preoperative sedation are usually sufficient to calm the fears of most patients. For some patients, however, the prospect of a series of surgical procedures is sufficiently stressful to trigger disturbances that jeopardize the well-being of the patient and hamper treatment. Explaining that the treatment at the hospital will be performed painlessly and it will be preceded by a depth of sedation that is not practical for ambulatory patients in a dental office is an important step in allaying their fears. The thought of completing the necessary surgical procedures in one session rather than in repeated visits is an added comfort to the patient, because it eliminates the prospect of repeated anxiety in anticipation of each treatment.

With complete mouth surgery, there is less stress for the patient. It is performed after a night's rest in the hospital and under ample sedation rather than after coming straight from the street into the dental office (sometimes after rushing to be on time for the appointment). The patient is returned to the hospital room after surgery for a check of her or his physical condition and for a restful postoperative sleep, instead of having to leave the dental office and make the trip home.

Patient Convenience. For patients whose occupation entails considerable contact with the public, surgery performed at biweekly intervals sometimes presents a special problem. It means that for a period of several weeks, some area of the mouth will be covered by a periodontal pack. With the complete mouth technique, the pack is ordinarily retained for only 1 week. Patients find this an acceptable alternative to several weeks of pack placement. For a variety of other reasons, patients may desire to attend to their surgical needs in one session under optimal conditions.

Hospital Admission and Presurgical Medical Examination

If, after consideration of all factors, complete mouth operation is selected as the procedure of choice, a hospital appointment is made.

The length of the hospital stay is 48 hours. The patient usually is admitted early in the afternoon preceding the day of the operation to allow time for a physical examination, a hemogram and other laboratory procedures, and medical consultations as necessary. Preparations are made for special precautionary measures that may be required before, during, or after surgery. For example, diabetics who consider their disease to be "under control" sometimes require a short period of dietary supervision and regulation of insulin before surgery. The medical examination occasionally reveals a disease of which the patient is not aware, as well as conditions that the patient believed were not relevant to his or her dental problem and were omitted from the case history taken in the dentist's office.

Premedication and Anesthesia

Premedication. Patients should be given a sedative or tranquilizer the night before surgery. Barbiturates may be used, but frequently diazepam (10 mg orally) is sufficient to ensure a restful night. Another 10-mg tablet of diazepam is administered 1 hour prior to the procedure. If a higher level of sedation is necessary, intravenous diazepam (10 to 20 mg), together with 25 to 50 mg of meperidine hydrochloride to prolong the sedative effect, is the method of choice. Deeper levels of sedation may be achieved with the use of intravenous barbiturates either alone or in combination with other agents, as in the Jorgensen technique.[3] Patients undergoing complete mouth surgery as an outpatient procedure are also usually medicated before and during surgery with oral or intravenous diazepam. Patients with systemic problems (e.g., a history of rheumatic fever, cardiovascular problems, etc.) are premedicated as needed (see Chapter 34).

Anesthesia. Local or general anesthesia[34] may be used. Local anesthesia is the method of choice, except for especially apprehensive patients. It permits unhampered movement of the head, which is necessary for optimal visibility and accessibility to the various root surfaces. Local anesthesia is utilized in the same manner as for routine periodontal surgery.

When general anesthesia is indicated, it is administered by an anesthesiologist; it is important that the patient also receive local anesthesia to ensure reduced bleeding during the procedure.

The Operation

Surgery in the operating room is performed on the operating table with the patient's back elevated at an angle of approximately 30 degrees and the head at the level of the operator's elbows. The assistant responsible for the aspirator stands on the side of the table opposite the operator. When general anesthesia has been utilized, it is wise to delay placing the periodontal dressing until the patient has recovered sufficiently to have a demonstrable cough reflex. Periodontal dressings placed before the end of general anesthesia can be displaced during the recovery period, resulting in the serious risk of their being inhaled.

Postoperative Instructions at the Hospital

The patient is returned to his or her room, and the following postoperative instructions are entered in the record:
Cold, semisolid foods only.
Demerol, 50 mg every 4 hours, if necessary.

The patient is discharged from the hospital the morning after the operation, with an appointment scheduled for 1 week later at the dentist's office. Postoperative instructions and care for patients after complete mouth periodontal surgery are the same as those outlined in the preceding discussion of surgery in the office setting.

First Postoperative Office Visit

The patient is seen at the office 1 week after the operation. The pack is usually removed, and plaque control methods are reviewed. If necessary, one or more areas of the mouth may be repacked for another week.

REFERENCES

1. Addy M, Douglas WH. A chlorhexidine-containing methacrylic gel as a periodontal dressing. J Periodontol 46:465, 1975.
2. Addy M, Dowell P. Dentine hypersensitivity—a review. Clinical and in vitro evaluation of treatment agents. J Clin Periodontol 10:351, 1983.
3. Allen GD. Dental Anesthesia and Analgesia (Local and General). 2nd ed. Baltimore, Williams & Wilkins, 1979.
4. Ariaudo AA. The efficacy of antibiotics in periodontal surgery. J Periodontol 40:150, 1969.
5. Baer PN, Goldman HM, Scigliano J. Studies on a bacitracin periodontal dressing. Oral Surg 11:712, 1958.
6. Baer PN, Summer CF III, Miller G. Periodontal dressings. Dent Clin North Am 13:181, 1969.
7. Bailey BA. Informed consent in dentistry. J Am Dent Assoc 110:709, 1985.
8. Berman LH. Dentinal sensation and hypersensitivity. A review of mechanisms and treatment alternatives. J Periodontol 56:216, 1984.
9. Blitzer B. A consideration of the possible causes of dental hypersensitivity: Treatment by a strontium ion dentifrice. Periodontics 5:318, 1967.
10. Burch J, Conroy CW, Ferris RT. Tooth mobility following gingivectomy. A study of gingival support of the teeth. Periodontics 6:90, 1960.
11. Collins JF, Gingold J, Stanley H, Simring M. Reducing dentinal hypersensitivity with strontium chloride and potassium nitrate. Gen Dent 32:40, 1984.
12. Curro FA, ed. Tooth hypersensitivity. Dent Clin North Am 34(3):403–587, 1990.
13. Curtis JW Jr, McLain JB, Hutchinson RA. The incidence and severity of complications and pain following periodontal surgery. J Periodontol 56:597, 1985.
14. Dal Pra DJ, Strahan JD. A clinical evaluation of the benefits of a course of oral penicillin following periodontal surgery. Aust Dent J 17:219, 1972.
15. Dionne RA. New approaches to preventing and treating postoperative pain. J Am Dent Assoc 123:27, 1992.
16. Forrest JO. A clinical assessment of three desensitizing toothpastes containing formalin. Br Dent J 114:103, 1963.
17. Fraleigh CM. An evaluation of topical Terramycin in postgingivectomy pack. J Periodontol 27:201, 1956.
18. Frisch J, Levin MP, Bhaskar SN. The use of tissue conditioners in periodontics. J Periodontol 38:359, 1968.
19. Gangarosa L. Iontophoretic application of fluoride by tray techniques for desensitizing multiple teeth. J Am Dent Assoc 95:50, 1981.
20. Glendinning DEH. A method for retention of the periodontal pack. J Periodontol 47:236, 1976.
21. Greenhill JD, Pashley DH. The effects of desensitizing agents on the hydraulic conductance of human dentin "in vitro." J Dent Res 60:686, 1981.
22. Haugen E, Espevik S, Mjor IA. Adhesive properties of periodontal dressings—an "in vitro" study. J Periodontal Res 14:487, 1979.
23. Hirschfeld AS, Wasserman BH. Retention of periodontal packs. J Periodontol 29:199, 1958.
24. Holmes CH. Periodontal pack on single tooth retained by acrylic splint. J Am Dent Assoc 64:831, 1962.
25. Holroyd SF. Antibiotics in the practice of periodontics. J Periodontol 42:584, 1971.
26. Hoyt WH, Bibby BG. Use of sodium fluoride for desensitizing dentine. J Am Dent Assoc 30:1372, 1943.
27. Javelet J, Torabinejad M, Danforth A. Isobutyl cyanoacrylate: A clinical and histological comparison with sutures in closing mucosal incisions in monkeys. Oral Surg 59:91, 1985.
28. Kanouse MC, Ash MM Jr. The effectiveness of a sodium monofluorophosphate dentifrice on dental hypersensitivity. J Periodontol 40:38, 1969.
29. Kidd EA, Wade AB. Penicillin control of swelling and pain after periodontal osseous surgery. J Clin Periodontol 1:52, 1974.
30. Koch G, Magnusson B, Nyquist G. Contact allergy to medicaments and materials used in dentistry. II. Sensitivity to eugenol and rosin. Odontol Revy 22:375, 1971.
31. Koch G, Magnusson B, Nobreus N, et al. Contact allergy to medicaments and materials used in dentistry. IV. Sensitizing effect of eugenol/rosin in surgical dressing. Odontol Revy 24:109, 1973.
32. Levin MP, Cutright DE, Bhaskar SN. Cyanoacrylate as a periodontal dressing. J Oral Med 30:40, 1975.
33. Majewski I, Sponholz H. Ergebnisse nach parodonal therapeutischen Massnahmen unter besonderer Berucksichtigung der Zahnbeweglichkeitssung mit dem Makroperiodontometer nach Muhlemann. Zahnaerztl Rundsch 75:57, 1966.
34. Manson JD, Millar Danks S. General anesthesia for periodontal surgery. J Clin Periodontol 5:163, 1978.
35. McFall WT Jr, Morgan WC Jr. Effectiveness of a dentifrice containing formalin and sodium monofluorophosphate on dental hypersensitivity. J Periodontol 56:288, 1985.
36. Meyler A. Side Effects of Drugs. Vol 5. Amsterdam, Excerpta Medica, 1966.
37. Miller JT, Shannon KL, Kilyore WG, Bookman JE. Use of water-free stannous fluoride-containing gel in the control of dental hypersensitivity. J Periodontol 40:490, 1969.
38. Murphy NC, DeMarco TJ. Controlling pain in periodontal patients. Dent Surv 55:46, 1979.
39. Newman MG, Sanz M, Nachnani S, et al. Effect of 0.12 per cent chlorhexidine on bacterial recolonization following periodontal surgery. J Periodontol 60:577, 1989.
40. Pack PO, Haber J. The incidence of clinical infection after periodontal surgery. A retrospective study. J Periodontol 54:441, 1983.
41. Pashley DH, Galloway SE. The effects of oxalate treatment on the smear layer of ground surfaces of human dentine. Arch Oral Biol 30:731, 1985.
42. Pashley DH, Leibach JG, Horner JA. The effects of burnishing NaF/kaolin/glycerin paste on dentin permeability. J Periodontol 58:19, 1987.
43. Pashley DH, Livingston MJ, Reeder OW, Horner JA. Effects of the degree of tubule occlusion on the permeability of human dentin in vitro. Arch Oral Biol 23:1127, 1978.
44. Pattison GL, Pattison AM. Periodontal Instrumentation. Reston, VA, Reston Publishing, 1979.

45. Peden JW. Dental hypersensitivity. J West Soc Periodontol 25:75, 1977.
46. Pendrill K, Reddy J. The use of prophylactic penicillin in periodontal surgery. J Periodontol 51:44, 1980.
47. Romanow I. Allergic reactions to periodontal pack. J Periodontol 28:151, 1957.
48. Romanow I. Relationship of moniliasis to the presence of antibiotics in periodontal packs. Periodontics 2:298, 1964.
49. Ross MR. Hypersensitive teeth: Effect of strontium chloride in a compatible dentifrice. J Periodontol 32:49, 1961.
50. Sachs HA, Farnoush A, Checchi L, Joseph CE. Current status of periodontal dressings. J Periodontol 55:689, 1984.
51. Sanz M, Newman MG, Anderson L, et al. Clinical enhancement of post-periodontal surgical therapy by a 0.12 per cent chlorhexidine gluconate mouthrinse. J Periodontol 60:570, 1989.
52. Smith DC. A materialistic look at periodontal packs. Dent Pract Dent Rec 20:273, 1970.
53. Strahan JD, Glenwright HD. Pain experience in periodontal surgery. J Periodont Res 1:163, 1967.
54. Tarbet WJ, Silverman G, Stolman JW, Fratarcangelo PA. A clinical evaluation of a new treatment for dentinal hypersensitivity. J Periodontol 51:535, 1980.
55. Trowbridge HO, Silver DR. A review of current approaches to in-office management of tooth hypersensitivity. Dent Clin North Am 34:583, 1990.
56. Vaughan ME, Garnick JJ. The effect of a 0.125 per cent chlorhexidine rinse on inflammation after periodontal surgery. J Periodontol 60:704, 1989.
57. Ward AW. Inharmonious cusp relation as a factor in periodontoclasia. J Am Dent Assoc 10:471, 1923.
58. Watts TAP, Combe EC. Periodontal dressing materials. J Clin Periodontol 6:3, 1979.
59. Watts TAP, Combe EC. Adhesion of periodontal dressings to enamel "in vitro." J Clin Periodontol 7:62, 1980.
60. Westfelt E, Nyman S, Socransky SS. Significance of frequency of professional cleaning for healing following periodontal surgery. J Clin Periodontol 10:148, 1983.

51

Surgical Anatomy of the Periodontium and Related Structures

FERMIN A. CARRANZA, JR.

Mandible
Maxilla
Muscles
Anatomic Spaces

A sound knowledge of the anatomy of the periodontium and the hard and soft structures that surround it is essential to determine the scope and possibilities of surgical periodontal procedures and to minimize their risks. Bones, muscles, blood vessels and nerves, as well as the anatomic spaces located in the vicinity of the periodontal surgical field, are particularly important. Only those features of periodontal relevance will be mentioned; the reader is referred to books on oral anatomy[3,4] for a more comprehensive description of these structures.

MANDIBLE

The mandible is a horseshoe-shaped bone connected to the skull by the temporomandibular joints. It presents several landmarks of great surgical importance.

The *mandibular canal,* occupied by the inferior alveolar nerve and vessels, begins at the mandibular foramen on the medial surface of the mandibular ramus and curves downward and forward, becoming horizontal below the apices of

the molars (Fig. 51–1). The distance from the canal to the apices of the molars is shorter in the third molar area and increases as it goes forward. In the premolar area the canal divides in two: the incisive canal, which continues horizontally to the midline, and the mental canal, which turns upward and opens in the mental foramen.

The *mental foramen,* from which the mental nerve and vessels emerge, is located on the buccal surface of the mandible below the apices of the premolars, sometimes closer to the second premolar and usually halfway between the lower border of the mandible and the alveolar margin (Fig. 51–2). The opening of the mental foramen faces upward and distally, with its posterosuperior border slanting gradually to the bone surface. As it emerges, the mental nerve divides into three branches. One branch of the nerve turns forward and downward to supply the skin of the chin. The other two branches course anteriorly and upward to supply the skin and mucous membrane of the lower lip and the mucosa of the labial alveolar surface.

Surgical trauma to the mental nerve can produce paresthesia of the lip, which recovers slowly. Familiarity with the location and appearance of the mental nerve reduces the likelihood of injuring it (Fig. 51–3).

In partially or totally edentulous jaws, the disappearance

The author is grateful to Dr. Andrew D. Dixon for his constructive analysis of this chapter.

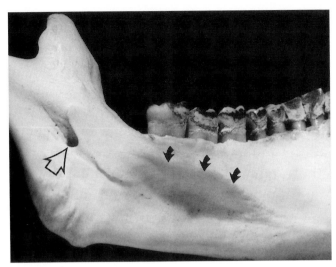

FIGURE 51–1. Mandible, lingual surface view. Note the lingual or mandibular foramen (*open arrow*) where the inferior alveolar nerve enters the mandibular canal and the mylohyoid ridge (*solid arrows*).

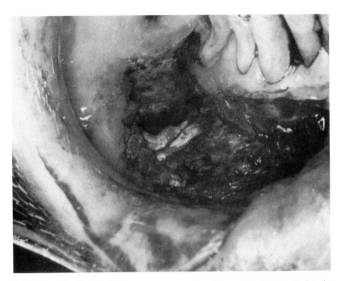

FIGURE 51–3. Mental nerve emerging from the foramen in the premolar area.

of the alveolar portion of the mandible brings the mandibular canal closer to the superior border. When these patients are evaluated for placement of implants, the distance between the canal and the superior surface of the bone must be carefully determined to avoid surgical injury to the nerve.

The *lingual nerve*, along with the inferior alveolar nerve, is a branch of the posterior division of the mandibular nerve and descends along the mandibular ramus medial to and in front of the inferior alveolar nerve. It lies close to the surface of the oral mucosa in the third molar area and goes deeper as it goes forward (Fig. 51–4; see also Fig. 51–18). It can be damaged during anesthetic injections and during oral surgery procedures such as third molar extractions.[7] Less commonly it may be injured when a periodon-

tal partial thickness flap is raised in the third molar region or releasing incisions are made.

The *alveolar process,* which provides the supporting bone to the teeth, has a narrower distal curvature than the body of the mandible (Fig. 51–5), creating a flat surface in the posterior area between the teeth and the anterior border of the ramus. This results in the formation of the *external oblique ridge,* which runs downward and forward to the region of the second or first molar (Fig. 51–6), creating a shelf-like bony area. Resective osseous therapy may be difficult or impossible in this area owing to the amount of bone that would have to be removed.

Distal to the third molar, the external oblique ridge circumscribes the *retromolar triangle* (see Fig. 51–6). This region is occupied by glandular and adipose tissue covered by unattached nonkeratinized mucosa. If sufficient space exists distal to the last molar, a band of attached gingiva

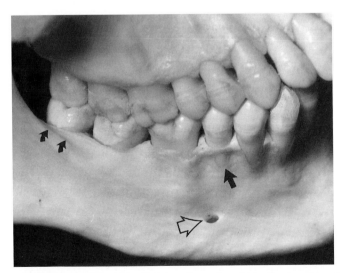

FIGURE 51–2. Mandible, facial surface view. Note the location of the mental foramen (*open arrow*), slightly distal and apical to the apex of the second premolar, and the shelf-like area in the region of the molars (*curved solid arrows*), created by the external oblique ridge. Note also the fenestration present in the second premolar (*straight solid arrow*).

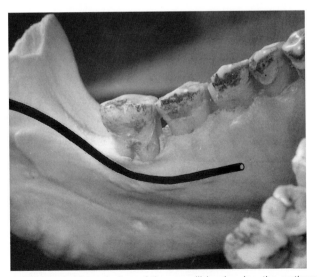

FIGURE 51–4. Lingual view of the mandible showing the pathway of the lingual nerve, which goes near the gingiva in the third molar area and then continues forward, going deeper and medially.

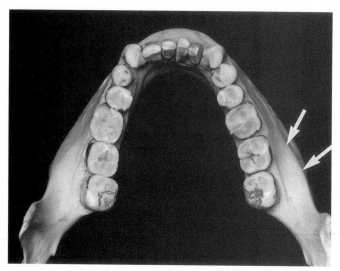

FIGURE 51–5. Occlusal view of mandible. Note the shelf created in the facial molar areas by the external oblique ridge. *Arrows* on the right show the attachment of the buccinator muscle.

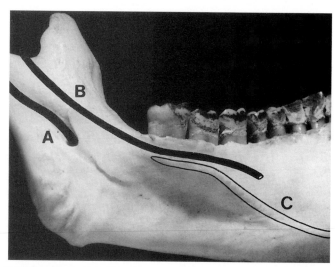

FIGURE 51–7. Mandible: lingual view showing the inferior alveolar nerve entering the mandibular canal (A), the lingual nerve traversing near the lingual surface of the third molar (B), and, inferiorly, the attachment of the mylohyoid muscle (C).

may be present; only in such a case can a distal wedge operation be performed.

The inner side of the body of the mandible is traversed obliquely by the *mylohyoid ridge*, which starts close to the alveolar margin in the third molar area and continues anteriorly, increasing its distance from the osseous margin as it goes forward (Fig. 51–7). The mylohyoid muscle, inserted at this ridge, separates the sublingual space, located more anteriorly and superiorly, from the submandibular space, located more posteriorly and inferiorly (see Fig. 51–18).

MAXILLA

The maxilla is a paired bone that is hollowed out by the maxillary sinus and has four processes: the *alveolar process*, which contains the sockets for the upper teeth; the *palatine process*, which extends horizontally to meet its counterpart from the other maxilla at the midline intermaxillary suture, and posteriorly with the horizontal plate of the palatine bone to form the hard palate; the *zygomatic process*, which extends laterally from the area of the first molar and determines the depth of the vestibular fornix; and the *frontal process*, which extends in an ascending direction and articulates with the frontal bone at the frontomaxillary suture.

In the midline anterior area of the palate opens the *incisive canal*, through which pass the terminal branches of the nasopalatine nerve and vessels (Fig. 51–8). The mucosa overlying the incisive canal presents a slight protuberance called the *incisive papilla*. Vessels emerging through the in-

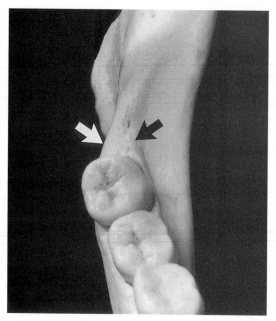

FIGURE 51–6. Mandible: occlusal view of ramus and molars. Note the retromolar triangle area distal to the third molar (*arrows*).

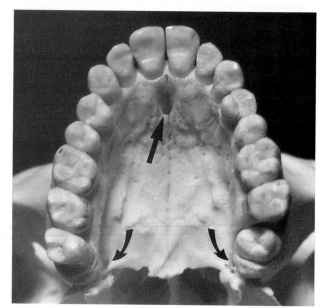

FIGURE 51–8. Occlusal view of maxilla and palatine bone. Note the opening of the incisive canal or anterior palatine foramen (*straight arrow*) and the greater palatine foramen (*curved arrows*).

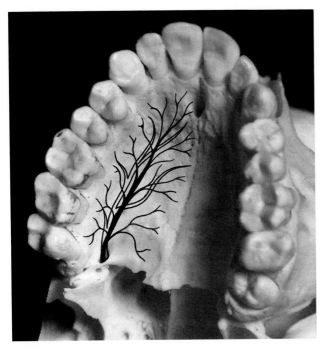

FIGURE 51–9. Occlusolateral view of palate showing nerves and vessels emerging from the greater palatine foramen and continuing anteriorly on the palate.

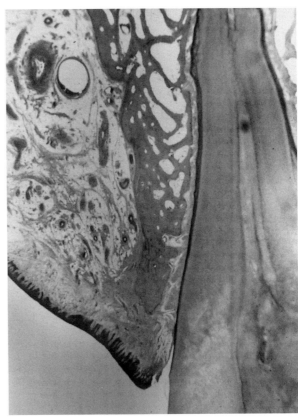

FIGURE 51–10. Histologic frontal section of human palate at the level of the first molar, showing the location of vessels and nerve, surrounded by adipose and glandular tissue.

cisive canal are of small caliber, and their surgical interference is of little consequence.

The *greater palatine foramen* opens 3 to 4 mm anterior to the posterior border of the hard palate (Fig. 51–9). The greater palatine nerve and vessels emerge through this foramen and run anteriorly in the submucosa of the palate, between the palatal and alveolar processes (Fig. 51–10). Palatal flaps and donor sites for gingival grafts should be carefully performed and selected to avoid invading these areas, as profuse hemorrhages may ensue, particularly if vessels are damaged at the palatine foramen.

The mucous membrane covering the hard palate is firmly attached to the underlying bone. The submucous layer of the palate posterior to the first molars contains the *palatal glands*, which are more compact in the soft palate and extend anteriorly, filling the gap between the mucosal connective tissue and the periosteum and protecting the underlying vessels and nerve (see Fig. 51–17).

The area distal to the last molar is called the *maxillary tuberosity* and consists of the posteroinferior angle of the infratemporal surface of the maxilla; medially it articulates with the pyramidal process of the palatine bone. It is covered by fibrous connective tissue and contains the terminal branches of the middle and posterior palatine nerves. Excision of the area for distal wedge surgery may reach medially to the tensor palati muscle, which comes from the greater wing of the sphenoid bone and ends in a tendon that forms the palatine aponeurosis, which expands, fan-like, to attach to the posterior border of the hard palate.

The body of the maxilla is occupied by the *maxillary sinus* or *antrum,* which is a hollow pyramidal area with its base toward the nose and lined by respiratory epithelium. The inferior wall of the maxillary sinus is frequently separated from the apices and roots of the maxillary posterior teeth by a thin, bony plate (Fig. 51–11). In edentulous pos-

terior areas the maxillary sinus bony wall may be only a thin plate in intimate contact with the alveolar mucosa (Fig. 51–12). Adequate determination of the extension of the maxillary sinus into the surgical site is important to avoid creating an oroantral communication, particularly in relation to the placement of implants. In edentulous jaws it is also critical to determine the amount of available bone in the anterior area, below the floor of the nasal cavity.

Both the maxilla and the mandible may have exostoses or tori, which are considered to be within the normal range

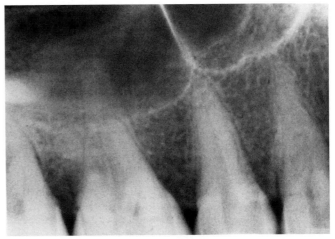

FIGURE 51–11. Radiograph of upper molars and premolars, with the maxillary sinus apparently near the apices.

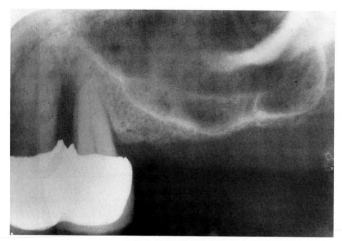

FIGURE 51–12. Radiograph of edentulous molar maxillary area with the sinus very close to the surface.

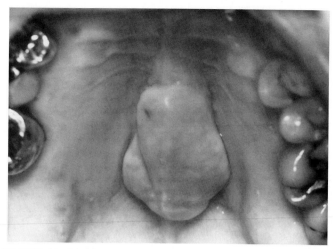

FIGURE 51–14. Clinical photograph of palatal torus, located in the midline of the palate.

of anatomic variation. Sometimes they may hinder the removal of plaque by the patient and may have to be removed to improve the prognosis of neighboring teeth. The most common location of a *mandibular torus* is in the lingual area of canine and premolars, above the mylohyoid muscle (Fig. 51–13). *Maxillary tori* are usually located in the midline of the hard palate (Fig. 51–14); smaller tori may be seen over the palatal roots of the molars (Fig. 51–15).

MUSCLES

Several muscles may be encountered when performing periodontal flaps, particularly in mucogingival surgery. These are the *mentalis, incisivus labii inferioris, depressor labii inferioris, depressor anguli oris (triangularis), incisivus labii superioris,* and *buccinator.* Their bony attachment is shown in Figure 51–16, and they provide mobility to the lips and cheeks.

ANATOMIC SPACES

Several anatomic spaces or compartments are found close to the operative field of periodontal surgery. These

spaces contain loose connective tissue but can be easily distended by inflammatory fluid and infection.

Surgical invasion of these areas may result in dangerous infections and should be carefully avoided. Some of these spaces will be briefly described. For further information, the reader is referred to references 2, 5, 6, 9, and 10.

The *canine fossa* contains varying amounts of connective tissue and fat and is bounded superiorly by the quadratus labii superioris muscle, anteriorly by the orbicularis oris, and posteriorly by the buccinator. Infection of this area results in swelling of the upper lip, obliterating the nasolabial fold, and of the upper and lower eyelids, closing the eye.

The *buccal space* is located between the buccinator and the masseter muscles. Infection of this area results in swelling of the cheek but may extend to the temporal space or the submandibular space, with which the buccal space communicates.

The *mental* or *mentalis space* is located in the region of the mental symphysis, where the mental muscle, the depressor muscle of the lower lip, and the depressor muscle of the corner of the mouth are attached. Infection of this

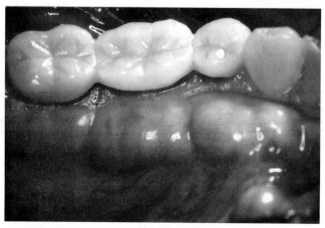

FIGURE 51–13. Clinical photograph of mandibular torus.

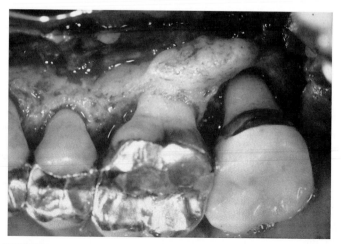

FIGURE 51–15. Clinical photograph after flap elevation, showing a palatal torus located near the osseous margin. Note also the circumferential bone loss around the second molar.

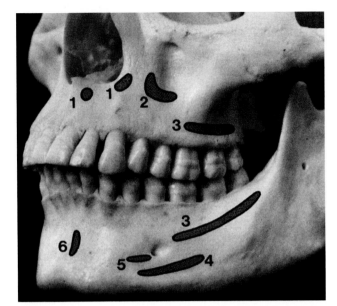

FIGURE 51–16. Muscle attachments that may be encountered in mucogingival surgery. 1, Nasalis; 2, levator anguli oris; 3, buccinator; 4, depressor anguli oris; 5, depressor labii inferioris; 6, mentalis.

area results in large swelling of the chin, extending downward.

The *masticator space* contains the masseter muscle, the pterygoid muscles, the tendon of insertion of the temporalis muscle, and the mandibular ramus and posterior part of the body of the mandible. Infection of this area

results in swelling of the face and severe trismus and pain. If the abscess occupies the deepest part of this compartment, facial swelling may not be obvious, but the patient may complain of pain and trismus. Patients may also have difficulty and discomfort when moving the tongue and swallowing.

The *sublingual space* is located below the oral mucosa in the anterior part of the floor of the mouth and contains the sublingual gland and its excretory duct, the submandibular or Wharton's duct, and is traversed by the lingual nerve and vessels and the hypoglossal nerve (Fig. 51–17). Its boundaries are the geniohyoid and genioglossus muscles medially and the lingual surface of the mandible and below the mylohyoid muscle laterally and anteriorly (Fig. 51–18). Infection of this area raises the floor of the mouth and displaces the tongue, resulting in pain and difficulty in swallowing but little facial swelling.

The *submental space* is found between the mylohyoid muscle superiorly and the platysma inferiorly. It is bounded laterally by the mandible and posteriorly by the hyoid bone and is traversed by the anterior belly of the digastric muscle. Infections of this area arise from the region of the mandibular anterior teeth and result in swelling of the submental region; they become more dangerous as they proceed posteriorly.

The *submandibular space* is found external to the sublingual space, below the mylohyoid and hyoglossus muscles (see Figs. 50–17 and 50–18). This space contains the submandibular gland, which extends partially above the mylohyoid muscle, thus communicating with the sublingual space, and numerous lymph nodes. Infections of this area

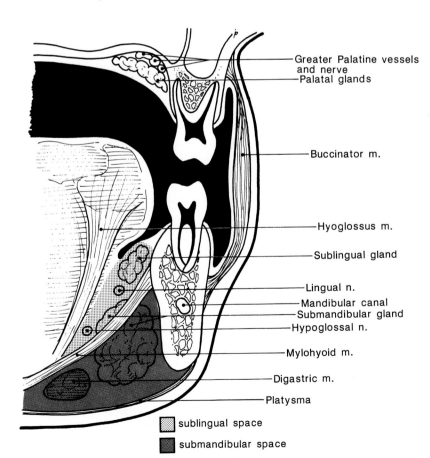

Greater Palatine vessels and nerve
Palatal glands

Buccinator m.

Hyoglossus m.

Sublingual gland

Lingual n.
Mandibular canal
Submandibular gland
Hypoglossal n.

Mylohyoid m.

Digastric m.

Platysma

sublingual space
submandibular space

FIGURE 51–17. Diagram of a frontal section of the human head at the level of the first molars, depicting the most important structures in relation to periodontal surgery. Note the location of the sublingual space, the submandibular space, and the greater palatine nerve and vessels.

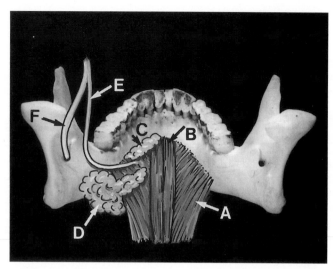

FIGURE 51–18. Posterior view of mandible, showing the attachment of the mylohyoid muscles (A); the geniohyoid muscles (B); the sublingual gland (C); the submandibular gland (D), which extends below and also to some extent above the mylohyoid muscle; and the sublingual (E) and inferior alveolar (F) nerves.

fection of this space that may extend to the sublingual and submental spaces; it results in hardening of the floor of the mouth and may lead to asphyxiation from edema of the neck and glottis. Although the bacteriology of these infections has not been completely determined, they are presumed to be mixed infections with an important anaerobic component.[1,8]

REFERENCES

1. Bartlett JG, Gorbach SL. Anaerobic infections of the head and neck. Otolaryngol Clin North Am *9:*655, 1976.
2. Clarke MA, Bueltmann KW. Anatomical considerations in periodontal surgery. J Periodontol *42:*610, 1971.
3. Dixon AD. Anatomy for Students of Dentistry. 5th ed. New York, Churchill Livingstone, 1986.
4. DuBrul EL. Sicher and DuBrul's Oral Anatomy. 8th ed. St Louis, Ishiyaku EuroAmerica, 1988.
5. Gregg JM. Surgical Anatomy. In Laskin DM. Oral and Maxillofacial Surgery. Vol 1. St Louis, CV Mosby, 1980.
6. Hollinshead WH. Anatomy for Surgeons. Vol 1: The Head and Neck. New York, Hoeber-Harper, 1954.
7. Kieselbach JE, Chamberlain JG. Clinical and anatomic observations on the relationship of the lingual nerve to the mandibular third molar region. J Oral Maxillofac Surg *42:*565, 1984.
8. Mulligan ME. Ear, nose, throat, and head and neck infections. In Finegold SM, George WL, eds. Anaerobic Infections in Humans. San Diego, Academic Press, 1989.
9. Spilka CJ. Pathways of dental infections. J Oral Surg *24:*111, 1966.
10. Topazian RG, Goldberg MH. Oral and Maxillofacial Infections. 2nd ed. Philadelphia, WB Saunders, 1987.

originate in the molar or premolar area and result in swelling that obliterates the submandibular line and pain when swallowing. Ludwig's angina is a severe form of in-

52

Gingival Curettage

FERMIN A. CARRANZA, JR.

Rationale
Indications
Procedure
Basic Technique

Other Techniques
Healing After Scaling and Curettage
Clinical Appearance After Curettage

The word *curettage* is used in periodontics to mean the scraping of the gingival wall of a periodontal pocket to remove inflamed soft tissue. *Scaling* refers to the removal of deposits from the root surface, whereas *planing* means smoothing the root to remove infected and necrotic tooth substance. Scaling and root planing may inadvertently include various degrees of curettage. However, they are different procedures, with different rationales and indications, and should be considered separate parts of periodontal treatment.

A differentiation has been made between gingival and subgingival curettage (Fig. 52–1). *Gingival curettage* con-

sists of the removal of inflamed soft tissue lateral to the pocket wall, whereas *subgingival curettage* refers to the procedure that is performed apical to the junctional epithelium, in which the connective tissue attachment is severed down to the osseous crest.

Some degree of curettage is done unintentionally when scaling and root planing is performed. This is called *inadvertent curettage*. This chapter refers to the deliberate curettage performed during the same visit as scaling and root planing or as a separate operation; the aim of curettage is to reduce pocket depth by enhancing gingival shrinkage and/or new connective tissue attachment.

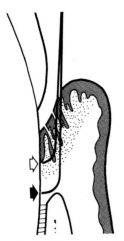

FIGURE 52–1. Extent of gingival curettage (*white arrow*) and subgingival curettage (*black arrow*).

RATIONALE

Curettage accomplishes removal of chronically inflamed granulation tissue in the lateral wall of the periodontal pocket. In addition to the usual components of granulation tissue (e.g., fibroblastic and angioblastic proliferation), this tissue contains areas of chronic inflammation and may have also pieces of dislodged calculus and bacterial colonies. The calculus and bacterial colonies may perpetuate the pathologic features of the tissue and hinder healing.

This inflamed granulation tissue is lined with epithelium, and deep strands of epithelium penetrate into the tissue. The presence of this epithelium is construed as a barrier to the attachment of new fibers in the area.

When the root is thoroughly planed, the major source of bacteria disappears and the pocket pathologic changes resolve, with no need to eliminate the inflamed granulation tissue using curettage. The existing granulation tissue is slowly resorbed; the bacteria, in the absence of replenishment of their numbers by pocket plaque, are destroyed by the defense mechanisms of the host. Therefore, *the need for curettage just to eliminate inflamed granulation tissue is questionable.** It has been shown that scaling and planing with and without additional curettage does not improve the condition of the periodontal tissues beyond the improvement caused by scaling and root planing alone.[9]

Curettage may also eliminate all or most of the epithelium that lines the pocket wall, epithelial extensions that penetrate the granulation tissue, and the underlying junctional epithelium. This purpose of curettage may still be valid, particularly when an attempt is made at new attachment, as occurs in infrabony pockets. However, opinions differ regarding whether scaling and curettage consistently

remove the pocket lining and the junctional epithelium. Some investigators report that scaling and root planing tear the epithelial lining of the pocket without removing either it or the junctional epithelium,[17] but both epithelial structures,[3,4,16] sometimes including underlying inflamed connective tissue,[18] are removed by curettage. Other investigators report that the removal of pocket lining and junctional epithelium by curettage is not complete.[26,29,30]

Curettage and Aesthetics. The awareness of aesthetics in periodontal therapy has become an integral part of care in the modern practice of periodontics. In the past, pocket elimination was the primary goal of therapy, and little regard was given to the aesthetic result. Maximal, rapid shrinkage of gingival tissue was the aim to eliminate the pocket. Currently aesthetics is a major consideration of therapy, particularly in the anterior maxilla (teeth #6–11) and *requires preservation of the interdental papilla.*

When regenerative therapy is not possible, every effort should be made to minimize shrinkage or loss of the interdental papilla. A compromise therapy that is feasible in the anterior maxilla, where access is not difficult, consists of thorough subgingival root planing, attempting not to detach the connective tissue beneath the pocket and *avoiding gingival curettage.* The granulation tissue in the lateral wall of the pocket, in an environment free of plaque and calculus, will become connective tissue, thereby minimizing shrinkage. Thus, although complete pocket elimination is not accomplished, the inflammatory changes are reduced or eliminated while the interdental papilla and the aesthetic appearance of the area are preserved.

Surgical techniques specially designed to preserve the interdental papilla, such as the papilla preservation technique (see Chapter 54), result in a better aesthetic appearance of the anterior maxilla than do aggressive scaling and curettage of the area.

INDICATIONS

Indications for curettage are very limited. It can be used after scaling and root planing for the following purposes:

1. Curettage can be performed as part of new attachment attempts in moderately deep infrabony pockets located in accessible areas where a type of "closed" surgery is deemed advisable. However, technical difficulties and inadequate accessibility frequently contraindicate such surgery.
2. Curettage can be done as a nondefinitive procedure to reduce inflammation prior to pocket elimination using other methods or in patients in whom more aggressive surgical techniques (e.g., flaps) are contraindicated owing to age, systemic problems, psychologic problems, and so forth. It should be understood that in these patients, the goal of pocket elimination is compromised, and prognosis is impaired. The clinician should resort to this approach only when the indicated surgical techniques cannot be performed, and both clinician and patient must have a clear understanding of its limitations.
3. Curettage is also frequently performed on recall visits[23] as a method of maintenance treatment for areas of recurrent inflammation and pocket deepening, particularly where pocket reduction surgery has previously been performed.

---

* This should not be confused with elimination of granulation tissue during flap surgery. The reason for the latter is to remove the bleeding tissue that obstructs the view and does not allow the necessary examination of the root surface and the bone morphology. Thus, removal of granulation tissue during surgery is done for technical rather than biologic reasons.

PROCEDURE

Basic Technique

Curettage does not eliminate the causes of inflammation (i.e., bacterial plaque and deposits). *Therefore, it should always be preceded by scaling and root planing, which is the basic periodontal therapy procedure.*

Scaling and root planing are described in detail in Chapters 37 and 41; the use of local infiltrative anesthesia for these procedures is optional. However, gingival curettage always requires some type of local anesthesia.

The curette is selected so that the cutting edge will be against the tissue; the Gracey curette no. 13–14 is used for mesial surfaces and the Gracey curette no. 11–12 for distal surfaces. Curettage can also be performed with a 4R–4L Columbia universal curette. The instrument is inserted so as to engage the inner lining of the pocket wall and is carried along the soft tissue, usually in a horizontal stroke (Fig. 52–2). The pocket wall may be supported by gentle finger pressure on the external surface. The curette is then placed under the cut edge of the junctional epithelium to undermine it.

In subgingival curettage, the tissues attached between the bottom of the pocket and the alveolar crest are removed with a scooping motion of the curette to the tooth surface (Fig. 52–3). The area is flushed to remove debris, and the tissue is partly adapted to the tooth with gentle finger pressure. Sometimes suturing of separated papillae and application of a periodontal pack may be indicated.

Other Techniques

Other techniques for gingival curettage include the excisional new attachment procedure, ultrasonic curettage, and the use of caustic drugs.

Excisional New Attachment Procedure (ENAP). This technique, developed and used by the U.S. Naval Dental Corps,[22,33,34] is a definitive subgingival curettage procedure performed with a knife. The technique is as follows:

1. After adequate anesthesia, an internal bevel incision is made with a surgical blade from the margin of the free gingiva apically to a point below the bottom of the pocket (Fig. 52–4). The incision is carried interproximally on both the

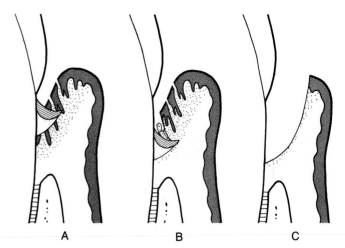

FIGURE 52–3. Subgingival curettage. *A,* Elimination of pocket lining. *B,* Elimination of junctional epithelium and granulation tissue. *C,* Procedure completed.

facial and the lingual sides, attempting to retain as much interproximal tissue as possible. The intention is to cut the inner portion of the soft tissue wall of the pocket, all around the tooth.

2. Remove the excised tissue with a curette, and carefully root plane all exposed cementum to a smooth, hard consistency. Preserve all connective tissue fibers that remain attached to the root surface.

3. Approximate the wound edges; if they do not meet passively, recontour the bone until good adaptation of the wound edges is achieved. Place sutures and a periodontal dressing.

Ultrasonic Curettage. The use of ultrasonic devices has been recommended for gingival curettage.[19] When applied to the gingiva of experimental animals, ultrasonic vibrations disrupt tissue continuity, lift off epithelium, dismember collagen bundles, and alter the morphologic features of fibroblast nuclei.[11] Thus, ultrasound is effective for debriding the epithelial lining of periodontal pockets[11]; it results in a narrow band of necrotic tissue (microcauterization), which strips off the inner lining of the pocket.

The Morse scaler and the rod-shaped ultrasonic instru-

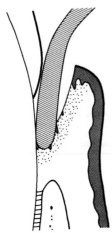

FIGURE 52–2. Gingival curettage performed with a horizontal stroke of the curette.

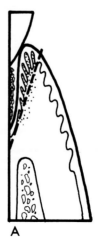 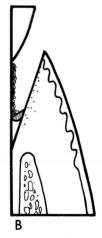

FIGURE 52–4. Excisional new attachment procedure. *A,* Internal bevel incision to a point below the bottom of the pocket. *B,* After excision of tissue, scaling and root planing are performed.

ment are used for this purpose. Some investigators found ultrasonic instruments to be as effective as manual instruments for curettage,[19,25,35] but resulting in less inflammation and less removal of underlying connective tissue than manual instruments. The gingiva can be made more rigid for ultrasonic curettage by injecting anesthetic solution directly into it.[7]

Caustic Drugs. Since early in the development of periodontal procedures,[28,32] the use of caustic drugs has been recommended to induce a chemical curettage of the lateral wall of the pocket or even the selective elimination of the epithelium. Drugs such as sodium sulfide, alkaline sodium hypochlorite solution (Antiformin),[5,12,13] and phenol[1,6] have been proposed and then discarded after studies showed their ineffectiveness.[2,10,13] The extent of tissue destruction with these drugs cannot be controlled, and they may increase rather than reduce the amount of tissue to be removed by enzymes and phagocytes.

HEALING AFTER SCALING AND CURETTAGE

Immediately after curettage, a blood clot fills the gingival sulcus, which is totally or partially devoid of epithelial lining. Hemorrhage is also present in the tissues with dilated capillaries, and abundant polymorphonuclear leukocytes appear shortly thereafter on the wound surface. This is followed by a rapid proliferation of granulation tissue, with a decrease in the number of small blood vessels as the tissue matures.

Restoration and epithelialization of the sulcus generally require from 2 to 7 days,[15,18,20,30] and restoration of the junctional epithelium occurs in animals as early as 5 days after treatment. Immature collagen fibers appear within 21 days. Healthy gingival fibers inadvertently severed from the tooth and tears in the epithelium[17,24] are repaired in the healing process. Several investigators have reported that in monkeys[8,33] and humans[31] treated by scaling and curettage procedures, healing results in the formation of a long, thin junctional epithelium with no new connective tissue attachment. Sometimes this long epithelium is interrupted by "windows" of connective tissue attachment.[8]

CLINICAL APPEARANCE AFTER CURETTAGE

Immediately after scaling and curettage, the gingiva appears hemorrhagic and bright red.

After 1 week, the gingiva appears reduced in height owing to an apical shift in the position of the gingival margin. The gingiva is also slightly redder than normal, but much less so than on previous days.

After 2 weeks, and with proper oral hygiene by the patient, normal color, consistency, surface texture, and contour of the gingiva are attained, and the gingival margin is well adapted to the tooth.

REFERENCES

1. Barkann A. A conservative technique for the eradication of a pyorrhea product. J Am Dent Assoc 26:61, 1939.
2. Beube FE. An experimental study of the use of sodium sulphide solution in treatment of periodontal pockets. J Periodontol 10:49, 1939.
3. Beube FE. Treatment methods for marginal gingivitis and periodontitis. Tex Dent J 71:427, 1953.
4. Blass JL, Lite T. Gingival healing following surgical curettage: A histopathologic study. NY Dent J 25:127, 1959.
5. Box KF. Periodontal disease and treatment. J Ontario Dent Assoc 29:194, 1952.
6. Bunting RW. The control and treatment of pyorrhea by subgingival surgery. J Am Dent Assoc 15:119, 1928.
7. Burman LR, Alderman NE, Ewen SJ. Clinical application of ultrasonic vibrations for supragingival calculus and stain removal. J Dent Med 13:156, 1958.
8. Caton JC, Zander HA. The attachment between tooth and gingival tissues after periodic root planing and soft tissue curettage. J Periodontol 50:462, 1979.
9. Echeverria JJ, Caffesse RG. Effects of subgingival curettage when performed one month after root instrumentation: A biometric evaluation. J Clin Periodontol 10:277, 1983.
10. Glickman J, Patur B. Histologic study of the effect of Antiformin on the soft tissue wall of periodontal pockets in humans. J Am Dent Assoc 51:420, 1955.
11. Goldman HM. Histologic assay of healing following ultrasonic curettage versus hand instrument curettage. Oral Surg Oral Med Oral Pathol 14:925, 1961.
12. Hunter HA. A study of tissues treated with Antiformin citric acid. J Can Dent Assoc 21:344, 1955.
13. Johnson RW, Waerhaug J. Effect of Antiformin on gingival tissue. J Periodontol 27:24, 1956.
14. Kalkwarf KL, Tussing GJ, Davis MJ. Histologic evaluation of gingival curettage facilitated by sodium hypochlorite solution. J Periodontol 53:63, 1982.
15. Kon S, Novaes AB, Ruben MP, et al. Visualization of microvascularization of the healing periodontal wound. II. Curettage. J Periodontol 40:96, 1969.
16. Morris ML. The removal of the pocket and attachment epithelium in humans: A histological study. J Periodontol 25:7, 1954.
17. Moskow BS. The response of the gingival sulcus to instrumentation: A histologic investigation. I. The scaling procedure. J Periodontol 33:282, 1962.
18. Moskow BS. The response of the gingival sulcus to instrumentation: A histologic investigation. II. Gingival curettage. J Periodontol 35:112, 1964.
19. Nadler H. Removal of crevicular epithelium by ultrasonic curettes. J Periodontol 33:220, 1962.
20. O'Bannon JY. The gingival tissues before and after scaling the teeth. J Periodontol 35:69, 1964.
21. Pattison GL, Pattison AM. Periodontal Instrumentation. 2nd ed. Norwalk, CT, Appleton & Lange, 1992.
22. Periodontics Syllabus. NAVED P5110. US Naval Dental Corps, 1975, pp 113–115.
23. Ramfjord SP, Ash MM Jr. Periodontology and Periodontics. Philadelphia, WB Saunders, 1979.
24. Ramfjord SP, Kiester G. The gingival sulcus and the periodontal pocket immediately following scaling of the teeth. J Periodontol 25:167, 1954.
25. Sanderson AD. Gingival curettage by hand and ultrasonic instruments—a histologic comparison. J Periodontol 37:279, 1966.
26. Sato M. Histopathological study of the healing process after surgical treatment for alveolar pyorrhea. Bull Tokyo Dent Coll 1:71, 1960.
27. Sorrin S, Miller SCh. The action of sodium sulphide as an epithelial solvent. Dent Cosmos 69:1113, 1927.
28. Stewart H. Partial removal of cementum and decalcification of tooth in the treatment of pyorrhea alveolaris. Dent Cosmos 41:617, 1899.
29. Stone S, Ramfjord SP, Waldron J. Scaling and gingival curettage—a radioautographic study. J Periodontol 37:415, 1966.
30. Waerhaug J. Microscopic demonstration of tissue reaction incident to removal of subgingival calculus. J Periodontol 26:26, 1955.
31. Waerhaug J. Healing of the dentoepithelial junction following subgingival plaque control. I. As observed in human biopsy material. J Periodontol 49:1, 1978.
32. Younger WJ. Some of the latest phases in implantations and other procedures. Dent Cosmos 35:102, 1893.
33. Yukna RA. A clinical and histological study of healing following the excisional new attachment procedure in rhesus monkeys. J Periodontol 47:701, 1976.
34. Yukna RA, Bowers GM, Lawrence JJ, Fedi PF Jr. A clinical study of healing in humans following the excisional new attachment procedure. J Periodontol 47:696, 1976.
35. Zach L, Cohen G. The histology of the response to ultrasonic curettage. J Dent Res 40:751, 1961.

53

The Gingivectomy Technique

FERMIN A. CARRANZA, JR.

Indications and Contraindications
Surgical Gingivectomy
Gingivoplasty
Healing After Surgical Gingivectomy

Gingivectomy by Electrosurgery
Healing After Electrosurgery
Laser Gingivectomy
Gingivectomy by Chemosurgery

The term *gingivectomy* means excision of the gingiva. By removing the diseased pocket wall that obscures the tooth surface, gingivectomy provides the visibility and accessibility necessary for complete removal of surface deposits and thorough smoothing of the roots (Fig. 53–1). By removing diseased tissue and local irritants, it also creates a favorable environment for gingival healing and the restoration of a physiologic gingival contour.

The gingivectomy technique was widely performed in the past. Improved understanding of healing mechanisms and the development of more sophisticated flap methods have relegated the gingivectomy technique to a lesser role in the current repertoire of available techniques. However, it remains an effective form of treatment when indicated (Fig. 53–2).

INDICATIONS AND CONTRAINDICATIONS

The gingivectomy technique may be performed for (1) elimination of suprabony pockets, regardless of their depth, if the pocket wall is fibrous and firm; (2) elimination of gingival enlargements; or (3) elimination of suprabony periodontal abscesses.[11] Contraindications include (1) the need for bone surgery or even for examination of the bone shape and morphologic features, (2) the bottom of the pocket located apical to the mucogingival junction, and (3) aesthetic considerations, particularly in the anterior maxilla.

The gingivectomy technique may be performed surgically by means of scalpels, electrodes, laser beams, or chemicals. All of these methods will be reviewed in this chapter, although the first one is the only one generally recommended.

SURGICAL GINGIVECTOMY

Step 1. The pockets on each surface are explored with a periodontal probe and marked with a pocket marker (Figs. 53–3 and 53–4). Each pocket is marked in several areas to outline its course on each surface.

Step 2. Periodontal knives (e.g., Kirkland knives) are used for incisions on the facial and lingual surfaces and

those distal to the terminal tooth in the arch. Orban periodontal knives are used for supplemental interdental incisions, if necessary, and Bard-Parker blades no. 11 and 12 and scissors are used as auxiliary instruments.

The incision is started apical to the points marking the course of the pockets[36,43] and is directed coronally to a point between the base of the pocket and the crest of the bone. It should be as close as possible to the bone without exposing it, to remove the soft tissue coronal to the bone. Exposure of bone is undesirable. If it occurs, healing usually presents no problem if the area is adequately covered by the periodontal pack.

Discontinuous or continuous incisions may be used. Figure 53–5 shows the design of each of these two incisions. *The incision should be beveled at approximately 45 degrees to the tooth surface and should re-create, as far as possible, the normal festooned pattern of the gingiva.* Failure to bevel leaves a broad fibrous plateau that takes more time than is ordinarily required to develop a physiologic contour. In the interim, plaque and food accumulation may lead to recurrence of pockets.

Step 3. Remove the excised pocket wall, clean the area, and closely examine the root surface. The most apical zone will consist of a band-like light zone where the tissues were attached, and coronally to it some calculus remnants, root caries, or root resorption may be found. Granulation tissue may be seen on the excised soft tissue (Fig. 53–6).

Step 4. Carefully curette out the granulation tissue and remove any remaining calculus and necrotic cementum, so as to leave a smooth and clean root surface.

Step 5. Cover the area with a surgical pack (see Chapter 50).

Gingivoplasty

Gingivoplasty is similar to gingivectomy, but its purpose is different. Gingivectomy is performed to eliminate periodontal pockets and includes reshaping as part of the technique. Gingivoplasty is a reshaping of the gingiva to create physiologic gingival contours, with the sole purpose of recontouring the gingiva in the absence of pockets.

Gingival and periodontal disease often produces deformities in the gingiva that interfere with normal food excursion, collect plaque and food debris, and prolong and ag-

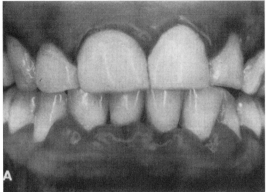
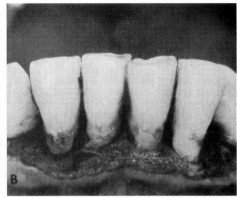

FIGURE 53-1. Visibility and accessibility of calculus. *A,* Gingival enlargement. *B,* Removal of diseased gingiva exposes calculus. Phase I therapy is sometimes omitted when the indication for a gingivectomy is obvious; it can never be omitted when a flap appears to be indicated.

gravate the disease process. Gingival clefts and craters and the shelf-like interdental papillae caused by necrotizing ulcerative gingivitis are examples of such deformities.

Gingivoplasty may be done with a periodontal knife, a scalpel, rotary coarse diamond stones,[8] or electrodes.[7] It consists of procedures that resemble those performed in festooning artificial dentures—namely, tapering the gingival margin, creating an escalloped marginal outline, thinning the attached gingiva, and creating vertical interdental grooves and shaping the interdental papillae to provide sluiceways for the passage of food.

Healing After Surgical Gingivectomy

The initial response after gingivectomy is the formation of a protective surface clot; the underlying tissue becomes acutely inflamed, with some necrosis. The clot is then replaced by granulation tissue. By 24 hours, there is an increase in new connective tissue cells, mainly angioblasts, just beneath the surface layer of inflammation and necrosis; by the third day, numerous young fibroblasts are located in the area.[35] The highly vascular granulation tissue grows coronally, creating a new free gingival margin and sulcus.[29] Capillaries derived from blood vessels of the periodontal

ligament migrate into the granulation tissue, and within 2 weeks they connect with gingival vessels.[44]

After 12 to 24 hours, epithelial cells at the margins of the wound start to migrate over the granulation tissue, separating it from the contaminated surface layer of the clot. Epithelial activity at the margins reaches a peak in 24 to 36 hours[7]; the new epithelial cells arise from the basal and deeper spinous layers of the wound edge epithelium and migrate over the wound over a fibrin layer that is later resorbed and replaced by a connective tissue bed.[17] The epithelial cells advance by a tumbling action, with the cells becoming fixed to the substrate by hemidesmosomes and a new basement lamina.[18]

Surface epithelialization is generally complete after 5 to 14 days. During the first 4 weeks after gingivectomy, keratinization is less than it was prior to surgery. Complete epithelial repair takes about 1 month.[41] Vasodilation and vascularity begin to decrease after the fourth day of healing and appear to be almost normal by the 16th day.[26] Complete repair of the connective tissue takes about 7 weeks.[41]

The flow of gingival fluid in humans is initially increased after gingivectomy and diminishes as healing progresses.[1,37] Maximal flow is reached after 1 week, coinciding with the time of maximal inflammation.

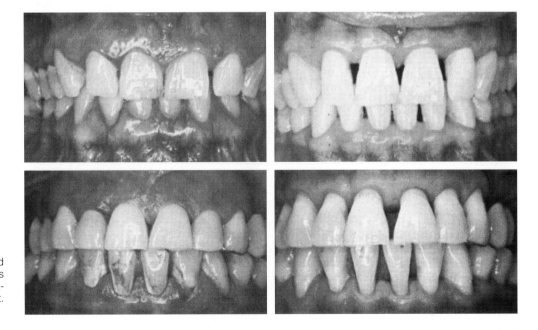

FIGURE 53-2. Results obtained by treating suprabony pockets of different depths with gingivectomy. *Left,* Before treatment. *Right,* After treatment.

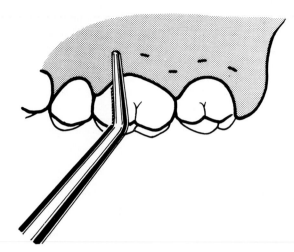

FIGURE 53–3. Pocket marker makes pinpoint perforations that indicate pocket depth.

Although the tissue changes that occur in postgingivectomy healing are the same in all individuals, the time required for complete healing varies considerably, depending on the extent of the cut surface and interference from local irritation and infection. In patients with physiologic gingival melanosis, pigmentation is diminished in the healed gingiva.

GINGIVECTOMY BY ELECTROSURGERY

Advantages. Electrosurgery permits adequate contouring of the tissue and controls hemorrhage.[9,28]

Disadvantages. Electrosurgery cannot be used in patients who have a noncompatible or a poorly shielded cardiac pacemaker. The treatment causes an unpleasant odor. If the electrosurgery point touches the bone, irreparable damage can be done[2,12,25,32]; furthermore, the heat generated by injudicious use can cause tissue damage and loss of periodontal support when the electrode is used close to bone.

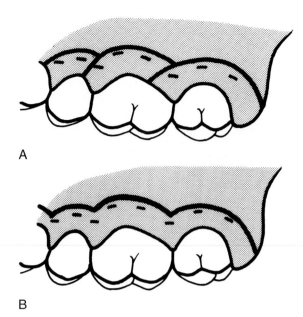

FIGURE 53–5. *A,* Discontinuous incision apical to the bottom of the pocket, indicated by pinpoint markings. *B,* Continuous incision begins on the molar and extends anteriorly without interruption.

When the electrode touches the root, areas of cementum burn are produced.[45] *Therefore, the use of electrosurgery should be limited to superficial procedures such as removal of gingival enlargements, gingivoplasty, relocation of frenum and muscle attachments, and incision of periodontal abscesses and pericoronal flaps; extreme care should be exercised to avoid contacting the tooth surface. It should not be used for procedures that involve proximity to the bone, such as flap operations or mucogingival surgery.*

Technique. The removal of gingival enlargements and gingivoplasty[28] is performed with the needle electrode, supplemented by the small ovoid loop or the diamond-shaped electrodes for festooning. A blended cutting and coagulating (fully rectified) current is used. In all reshaping procedures the electrode is activated and moved in a concise "shaving" motion.

In the treatment of acute periodontal abscesses, the incision to establish drainage can be made with the needle electrode without exerting painful pressure. The incision remains open because the edges are sealed by the current. Af-

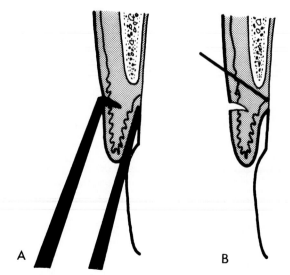

FIGURE 53–4. Marking the depth of a suprabony pocket. *A,* Pocket marker in position. *B,* Beveled incision extends apical to the perforation made by the pocket marker.

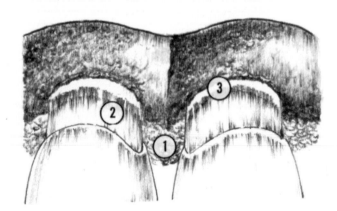

FIGURE 53–6. Field of operation immediately after removing pocket wall. 1, Granulation tissue. 2, Calculus and other root deposits. 3, Clear space where bottom of pocket was attached.

ter the acute symptoms subside, the regular procedure for the treatment of the periodontal abscess is followed (see Chapter 40).

For hemostasis, the ball electrode is used. Hemorrhage must be controlled by direct pressure (via air, compress, or hemostat) first; then the surface is lightly touched with a coagulating current. Electrosurgery is helpful for the control of isolated bleeding points. Bleeding areas located interproximally are reached with a thin, bar-shaped electrode.

Frenum and muscle attachments can be relocated to facilitate pocket elimination using a loop electrode. For this purpose, the frenum or muscle is stretched and sectioned with the loop electrode and a coagulating current. For cases of acute pericoronitis, drainage may be obtained by incising the flap with a bent needle electrode. A loop electrode is used to remove the flap after the acute symptoms subside.

Healing After Electrosurgery

Some investigators report no significant differences in gingival healing after resection by electrosurgery and resection with periodontal knives[6,23]; other researchers, however, have reported delayed healing, greater reduction in gingival height, and more bone injury after electrosurgery.[32] There appears to be little difference in the results obtained after shallow gingival resection with electrosurgery and those obtained with periodontal knives. However, *when used for deep resections close to bone, electrosurgery can produce gingival recession, bone necrosis and sequestration, loss of bone height, furcation exposure, and tooth mobility, which do not occur with the use of periodontal knives.*[2,12]

LASER GINGIVECTOMY

The lasers most commonly used in dentistry are the carbon dioxide (CO_2) and the neodymium:yttrium-aluminum-garnet (Nd:YAG) lasers, which have wavelengths of 10,600 nm and 1064 nm, respectively, both in the infrared range; they must be combined with other types of visible lasers for the beam to be seen and aimed.[14]

The CO_2 laser beam has been used for the excision of gingival overgrowths,[3,30] although healing is delayed when compared with healing after conventional scalpel gingivectomy.[14,22,31] The use of a laser beam for oral surgery requires precautionary measures to avoid reflecting the beam on instrument surfaces, which could result in injury to neighboring tissues or the eyes of the operator.

At present, the use of lasers for periodontal surgery is not supported by research and is therefore discouraged. The use of lasers for other periodontal purposes, such as subgingival curettage, is equally unsubstantiated and is also not recommended.

GINGIVECTOMY BY CHEMOSURGERY

Several techniques using chemicals (5% paraformaldehyde[27] or potassium hydroxide[21]) to remove the gingiva have been described. These methods have the following disadvantages: (1) their depth of action cannot be con-

trolled, and therefore, healthy attached tissue underlying the pocket may be injured; (2) gingival remodeling cannot be accomplished effectively; and (3) epithelialization and reformation of the junctional epithelium and re-establishment of the alveolar crest fiber system are slower in chemically treated gingival wounds than in those produced by a scalpel.[42] *Their use, therefore, is not recommended.*

REFERENCES

1. Arnold R, Lunstad G, Bissada N, Stallard R. Alterations in crevicular fluid flow during healing following gingival surgery. J Periodont Res *1:*303, 1966.
2. Azzi R, Kenney EB, Tsao TF, Carranza FA Jr. The effect of electrosurgery upon alveolar bone. J Periodontol *54:*96, 1983.
3. Barak S, Kaplan I. The CO_2 laser in the surgical excision of gingival hyperplasia caused by nifedipine. J Clin Periodontol *15:*633, 1988.
4. Bernier J, Kaplan H. The repair of gingival tissue after surgical intervention. J Am Dent Assoc *35:*697, 1947.
5. Donnenfeld OW, Glickman I. A biometric study of the effects of gingivectomy. J Periodontol *37:*447, 1966.
6. Eisenmann D, Malone WF, Kusek J. Electron microscopic evaluation of electrosurgery. Oral Surg *29:*660, 1970.
7. Engler WO, Ramfjord S, Hiniker JJ. Healing following simple gingivectomy. A tritiated thymidine radioautographic study. I. Epithelialization. J Periodontol *37:*298, 1966.
8. Fisher SE, Frame JW, Browne RM, Tranter RMD. A comparative histological study of wound healing following CO_2 laser and conventional surgical excision of the buccal mucosa. Arch Oral Biol *28:*287, 1983.
9. Flocken JE. Electrosurgical management of soft tissues and restoration dentistry. Dent Clin North Am *24:*247, 1980.
10. Fox L. Rotating abrasives in the management of periodontal soft and hard tissues. Oral Surg *8:*1134, 1955.
11. Glickman I. The results obtained with the unembellished gingivectomy technic in a clinical study in humans. J Periodontol *27:*247, 1956.
12. Glickman I, Imber LR. Comparison of gingival resection with electrosurgery and periodontal knives: A biometric and histologic study. J Periodontol *41:*142, 1970.
13. Goldman HM. The development of physiologic gingival contours by gingivoplasty. Oral Surg *3:*879, 1950.
14. Gottsegen R, Ammons WF Jr. Research in Lasers in Periodontics. Position paper. American Academy of Periodontology, Chicago, IL, May 1992.
15. Henning F. Healing of gingivectomy wounds in the rat: Reestablishment of the epithelial seal. J Periodontol *39:*265, 1968.
16. Henning F. Epithelial mitotic activity after gingivectomy. Relationship to reattachment. J Periodont Res *4:*319, 1969.
17. Innes PB. An electron microscopic study of the regeneration of gingival epithelium following gingivectomy in the dog. J Periodont Res *5:*196, 1970.
18. Krawczyk WS. A pattern of epithelial cell migration during wound healing. J Cell Biol *49:*247, 1971.
19. Reference deleted.
20. Listgarten MA. Electron microscopic features of the newly formed epithelial attachment after gingival surgery. J Periodont Res *2:*46, 1967.
21. Loe H. Chemical gingivectomy. Effect of potassium hydroxide on periodontal tissues. Acta Odontol Scand *19:*517, 1961.
22. Loumanen M. A comparative study of healing of laser and scalpel incision wounds in the rat oral mucosa. Scand J Dent Res *95:*65, 1987.
23. Malone WF, Eisenmann D, Kusck J. Interceptive periodontics with electrosurgery. J Prosthet Dent *22:*555, 1969.
24. Morris ML. Healing of human periodontal tissues following surgical detachment from vital teeth: The position of the epithelial attachment. J Periodontol *32:*108, 1961.
25. Nixon KC, Adkins KF, Keys DW. Histological evaluation of effects produced in alveolar bone following gingival incision with an electrosurgical scalpel. J Periodontol *46:*40, 1975.
26. Novaes AB, Kon S, Ruben MP, Goldman H. Visualization of the microvascularization of the healing periodontal wound. III. Gingivectomy. J Periodontol *40:*359, 1969.
27. Orban B. New methods in periodontal treatment. Bur *42:*116, 1942.
28. Oringer MJ. Electrosurgery for definitive conservative modern periodontal therapy. Dent Clin North Am *13:*53, 1969.
29. Persson PA. The healing process in the marginal periodontium after gingivectomy with special regard to the regeneration of epithelium (an experimental study on dogs). Odontol T *67:*593, 1959.
30. Pick RM, Pecaro BC, Silberman CJ. The laser gingivectomy: The use of CO_2 laser for the removal of phenytoin hyperplasia. J Periodontol *56:*492, 1985.
31. Pogrel MA, Yen CK, Hansen LS. A comparison of carbon dioxide laser, liquid nitrogen cryosurgery and scalpel wounds in healing. Oral Surg Med Pathol *69:*269, 1990.
32. Pope JW, Gargiulo AW, Staffileno H, Levy S. Effects of electrosurgery on wound healing in dogs. Periodontics *6:*30, 1968.
33. Prandi EC, Blitzer B, Carranza FA Jr. Evaluación biométrica de la técnica de gingivectomía en humanos. Rev Asoc Odontol Argent *57:*84, 1969.

34. Ramfjord S, Costich ER. Healing after simple gingivectomy. J Periodontol *34*:401, 1963.
35. Ramfjord SP, Engler WD, Hiniker JJ. A radiographic study of healing following simple gingivectomy. II. The connective tissue. J Periodontol *37*:179, 1966.
36. Ritchey B, Orban B. The periodontal pocket. J Periodontol *23*:199, 1952.
37. Sandalli P, Wade AB. Alterations in crevicular fluid flow during healing following gingivectomy and flap procedures. J Periodont Res *4*:314, 1969.
38. Stahl SS. Soft tissue healing following experimental gingival wounding in female rats of various ages. Periodontics *1*:142, 1963.
39. Stahl SS. Periodontal Surgery: Biologic Basis and Technique. Springfield, IL, Charles C Thomas, 1976.
40. Stahl SS, Witkin GJ, Cantor M, Brown R. Gingival healing. II. Clinical and histologic repair sequences following gingivectomy. J Periodontol *39*:109, 1968.

41. Stanton G, Levy M, Stahl SS. Collagen restoration in healing human gingiva. J Dent Res *48*:27, 1969.
42. Tonna E, Stahl SS. A polarized light microscopic study of rat periodontal ligament following surgical and chemical gingival trauma. Helv Odontol Acta *11*:90, 1967.
43. Waerhaug J. Depth of incision in gingivectomy. Oral Surg *8*:707, 1955.
44. Watanabe Y, Suzuki S. An experimental study in capillary vascularization in the periodontal tissue following gingivectomy or flap operation. J Dent Res *42*:758, 1963.
45. Wilhelmsen NR, Ramfjord SP, Blankenship JR. Effects of electrosurgery on the gingival attachment in Rhesus monkeys. J Periodontol *47*:160, 1976.

54

The Periodontal Flap

HENRY H. TAKEI and FERMIN A. CARRANZA, Jr.

Classification of Flaps	Incisions for the Papilla Preservation Flap
Design of the Flap	**Elevation of the Flap**
Incisions	**Suturing Techniques**
Incisions for the Conventional Flap	**Healing After Flap Surgery**

A *periodontal flap* is a section of gingiva and/or mucosa surgically elevated from the underlying tissues to provide visibility of and access to the bone and root surface. The flap also allows the gingiva to be displaced to a different location. The elevated flap has to maintain an adequate blood supply in order to avoid tissue necrosis during healing (Plates XVI and XVII).

CLASSIFICATION OF FLAPS

Periodontal flaps are classified as either full-thickness (mucoperiosteal) or partial-thickness (mucosal) flaps (Fig. 54–1).

In a *full-thickness flap,* all the soft tissue, including the periosteum, is reflected to expose the underlying bone. This complete exposure of and access to the underlying bone is needed if osseous surgery is contemplated.

The *partial-thickness flap* includes only the epithelium and a layer of the underlying connective tissue; the bone remains covered by a layer of connective tissue, including the periosteum. This type of flap is also called the *split-thickness flap.* The partial-thickness flap is indicated when the flap is to be positioned apically or when the operator does not desire to expose bone.

There are conflicting data regarding the advisability of uncovering the bone when this is not actually needed.

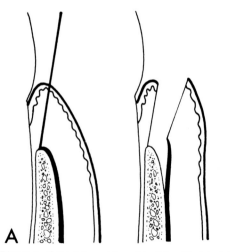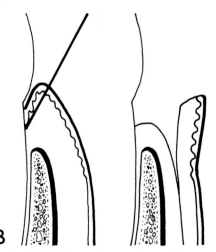

FIGURE 54–1. *A,* Diagram of the internal bevel incision (first incision) to reflect a full-thickness (mucoperiosteal) flap. Note that the incision ends on the bone to allow for reflection of the entire flap. *B,* Diagram of the internal bevel incision to reflect a partial-thickness flap. Note that the incision ends on the root surface to preserve the periosteum on the bone.

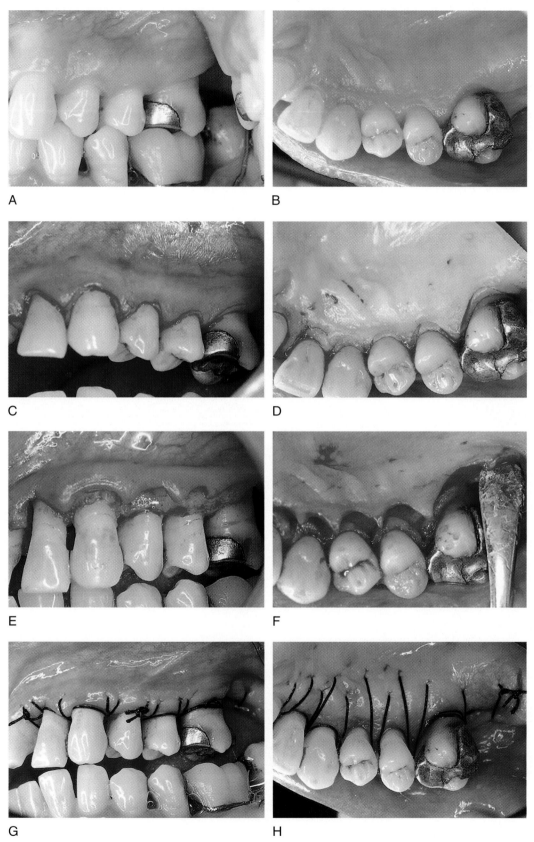

PLATE XVI. The periodontal flap technique. Facial view *(A)* and palatal view *(B)* of case preoperatively. A thorough scaling and root planing had been performed 6 weeks before. Five- to 6-mm pockets persisted in palatal areas. *C,* Facial incisions (internal bevel and crevicular) performed. *D,* Palatal incisions performed. Note the scalloping. *E* and *F,* Facial and palatal flaps elevated. A wedge of marginal tissue has not yet been removed in the palate. After thorough debridement, the root is examined for any remaining accretions, and the bone is examined to determine the need for osseous surgery. *G* and *H,* Continuous mattress suture in place.

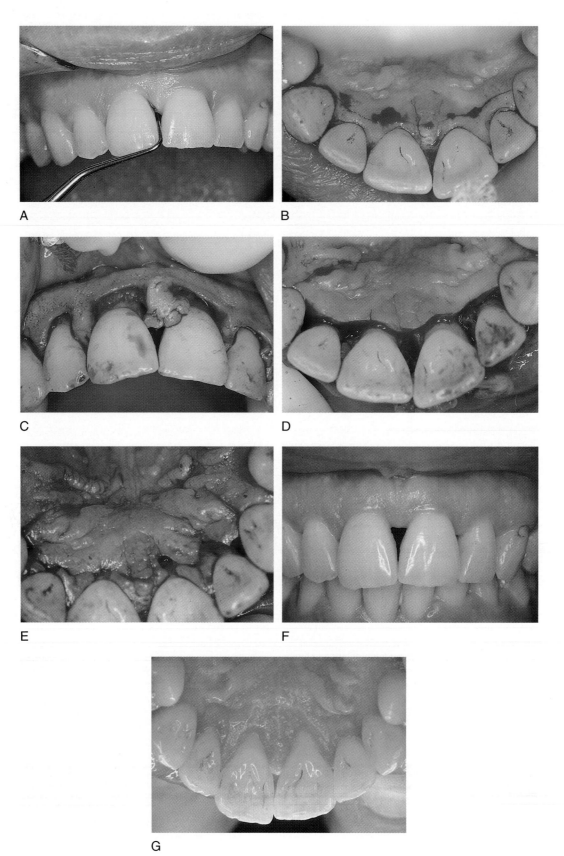

PLATE XVII. The papilla preservation flap. *A,* Facial view after sulcular incisions have been made. *B,* Straight line incision in the palatal area about 3 mm from gingival margins. This incision is then connected to the margins with vertical incisions in the mid-part of each tooth. *C,* The papillae are reflected with the facial flap. *D,* Lingual view after reflection of the flap. *E,* Lingual view after the flap is brought back to its original position; it is then sutured with independent sutures. *F,* Facial view after healing. *G,* Palatal view after healing.

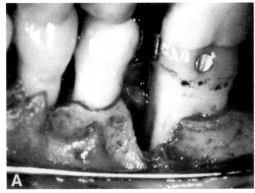
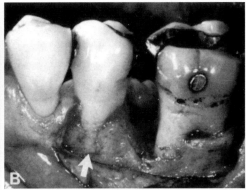

FIGURE 54–2. Loss of marginal bone as a result of uncovering the osseous crest. *A,* Mucoperiosteal flap elevated as part of a clinical study. *B,* Re-entry performed 6 months later reveals loss of marginal bone facial to second premolar *(arrow).* (Courtesy of Dr. Silvia Oreamuno.)

When bone is stripped of its periosteum, marginal bone is lost; this loss is prevented when the periosteum is left on the bone.[4] The differences, however, are usually not clinically significant,[7] although sometimes they may be (Fig. 54–2). The partial-thickness flap may be necessary in cases in which the crestal bone margin is thin and is exposed when the flap is placed apically, or when dehiscences or fenestrations are present. The periosteum left on the bone may also be used for suturing the flap when it is displaced apically.

Flaps can also be classified as (1) repositioned (positioned, displaced) flaps or (2) unrepositioned (undisplaced) flaps, depending on the placement of the flap at the conclusion of the surgical procedure. An *undisplaced flap* is located in the position it had before surgery, whereas a *displaced flap* can be located apical, coronal, or lateral to its original position. Displacement of a flap is made possible by totally separating the attached gingiva from the underlying bone, thereby enabling the unattached portion of the gingiva to be moveable. Palatal flaps cannot be displaced owing to the absence of unattached gingiva.

Apically displaced flaps have the important advantage of preserving the outer portion of the pocket wall and transforming it into attached gingiva. They therefore accomplish the double objective of eliminating the pocket and increasing the width of the attached gingiva.

This chapter presents general considerations for undisplaced and apically displaced flaps. The indications and technique for these flaps are presented in Chapter 55. Coronally and laterally positioned flaps are discussed in Chapter 59.

DESIGN OF THE FLAP

The design of the flap is dictated by the surgical judgment of the operator and may depend on the objectives of the operation. The degree of necessary access to the underlying bone and root surfaces and the final position of the flap must be considered when designing the flap. Preservation of good blood supply to the flap is an important consideration.

Two basic flap designs are used. Depending on how the interdental papilla is dealt with, flaps can either split the papilla or preserve it.

In the *conventional flap,* the incisions for the facial flap and the lingual or palatal flap reach the tip of the interdental papilla or its vicinity, thereby splitting the papilla into a facial half and a lingual or palatal half (Figs. 54–3 and 54–4). Conventional flaps include the modified Widman flap, the undisplaced flap, and the apically displaced flap;

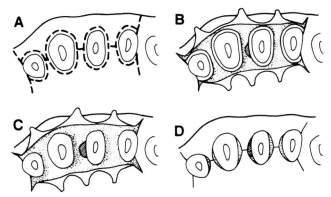

FIGURE 54–3. Flap design for the conventional or traditional flap technique. *A,* Design of the incisions. The internal bevel incision, splitting the papilla, and the vertical incisions are drawn in dashed lines. *B,* The flap has been elevated, and the wedge of tissue next to the tooth is still in place. *C,* All marginal tissue has been removed, exposing the underlying bone (see defect in one space). *D,* Tissue returned to its original position. Proximal areas are not totally covered.

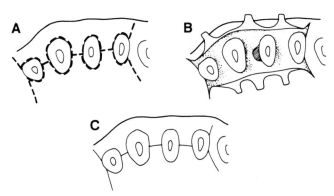

FIGURE 54–4. Flap design for a sulcular incision flap. *A,* Design of the incisions. The sulcular incisions and the vertical incisions are depicted by interrupted lines. *B,* The flap has been elevated, exposing the underlying bone (see defect in one space). *C,* Tissue returned to its original position covers the entire interdental spaces.

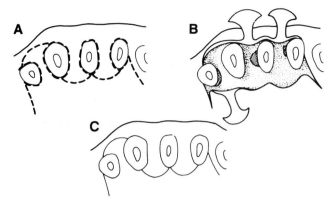

FIGURE 54–5. Flap design for a papilla preservation flap. *A,* Incisions for this type of flap are depicted by interrupted lines. The preserved papilla can be incorporated into the facial or the lingual-palatal flap. *B,* The reflected flap exposes the underlying bone. Several osseous defects are seen. *C,* The flap returned to its original position covering the entire interdental spaces.

these techniques are discussed in detail in Chapter 55. The conventional flap is used (1) when the interdental spaces are too narrow, thereby precluding the possibility of preserving the papilla, and (2) when the flap is to be displaced.

In the *papilla preservation flap,* the incisions are such that the entire papilla is incorporated into one of the flaps[14] (Fig. 54–5). This flap offers the advantage of better postsurgical aesthetics and more protection for the interdental bone, which is especially important when bone regeneration techniques are attempted.

The entire surgical procedure should be planned in every detail before the intervention is begun. This should include the type of flap, the exact location and type of incisions, the management of the underlying bone, and the final closure of the flap and sutures. Although some details may be modified during the actual performance of the procedure, detailed planning allows for a better clinical result.

INCISIONS

Incisions for the Conventional Flap

Horizontal Incisions. Periodontal flaps utilize horizontal and vertical incisions. Horizontal incisions are directed along the margin of the gingiva in a mesial or a distal direction (Fig. 54–6). Two types of horizontal incisions have been recommended: the internal bevel incision,[6] which starts at a distance from the gingival margin and is aimed at the bone crest, and the crevicular incision, which starts at the bottom of the pocket and is directed to the bone margin. A third type, the interdental incision, is performed after the flap is elevated.

The *internal bevel incision* is basic to most periodontal flap procedures. It is the incision from which the flap will be reflected to expose the underlying bone and root. The internal bevel incision accomplishes three important objectives: (1) it removes the pocket lining; (2) it conserves the relatively uninvolved outer surface of the gingiva, which, if apically positioned, becomes attached gingiva; and (3) it produces a sharp, thin flap margin for adaptation to the bone–tooth junction. This incision has also been termed the *first incision,* because it is the initial incision in the reflection of a periodontal flap, and the *reverse bevel incision,* because its bevel is in a reverse direction from that of the gingivectomy incision. The no. 15 or no. 11 surgical scalpel is used most commonly. The portion of the gingiva that is left around the tooth contains the epithelium of the pocket lining and the adjacent granulomatous tissue. It will be discarded after the crevicular (second) and interdental (third) incisions are performed (Fig. 54–6).

The internal bevel incision starts from a designated area on the gingiva and is directed to an area at or near the crest of the bone (Fig. 54–7). The starting point on the gingiva is determined by whether the flap will be apically displaced or not displaced (Fig. 54–8).

The *crevicular incision,* also termed the *second incision,* is made from the base of the pocket to the crest of the bone (Fig. 54–9). This incision, together with the initial reverse bevel incision, forms a V-shaped wedge ending at or near the crest of bone; this wedge of tissue contains most of the inflamed and granulomatous areas that constitute the lateral wall of the pocket, as well as the junctional epithelium and the connective tissue fibers that still persist between the bottom of the pocket and the crest of the bone. The incision is carried around the entire tooth. The beak-shaped no. 12B blade is usually used for this incision.

A periosteal elevator is inserted into the initial internal bevel incision, and the flap is separated from the bone. The

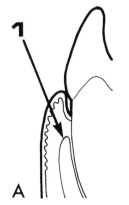
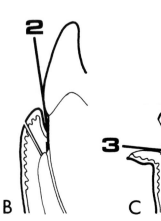

FIGURE 54–6. *A* to *C,* The first (internal bevel), second (crevicular), and third (interdental) incisions are the three incisions necessary for flap surgery.

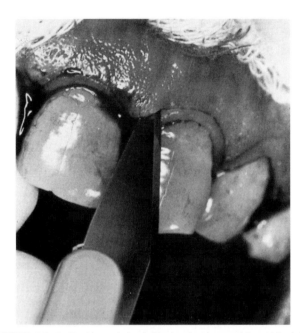

FIGURE 54–7. Position of the knife for the internal bevel incision.

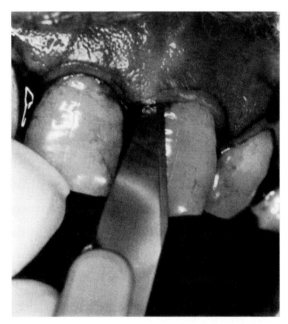

FIGURE 54–9. Position of knife for the crevicular incision.

most apical end of the internal bevel incision is more exposed and visible. With this access, the surgeon is able to make the *third* or *interdental incision* to separate the collar of gingiva that is left around the tooth. The Orban knife is usually utilized for this incision. The incision is made not only around the facial and lingual radicular area, but also interdentally, connecting the facial and lingual segments to completely free the gingiva around the tooth (see Figs. 54–6C and 54–10).

These three incisions allow the removal of the gingiva around the tooth (i.e., the pocket epithelium and the adjacent granulomatous tissue). A curette or a large scaler (U15/30) can be used for this purpose. After removal of the large pieces of tissue, the remaining connective tissue as well as the granulation tissue in the osseous lesion should be carefully curetted out so that the entire root and the bone surface adjacent to the teeth can be observed.

Flaps can be reflected using only the horizontal incision if sufficient access can be obtained by this means and if apical, lateral, or coronal displacement of the flap is not anticipated. If no vertical incisions are made, the flap is called an *envelope flap.*

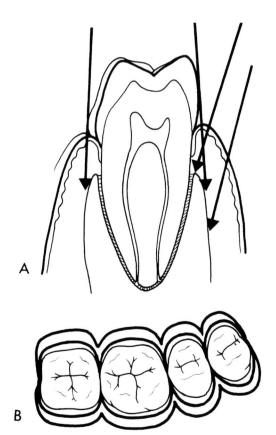

FIGURE 54–8. *A,* The internal bevel (first) incision can be made at varying locations and angles according to the different anatomic and pocket situations. *B,* An occlusal view of the different locations where the internal bevel incision can be made. Note the scalloped shape of the incisions.

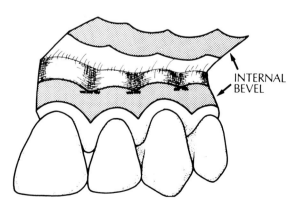

INTERNAL BEVEL

FIGURE 54–10. After the flap has been elevated, a wedge of tissue remains on the teeth, attached by the base of the papillae. An interdental incision along the horizontal lines seen in the interdental spaces will sever these connections.

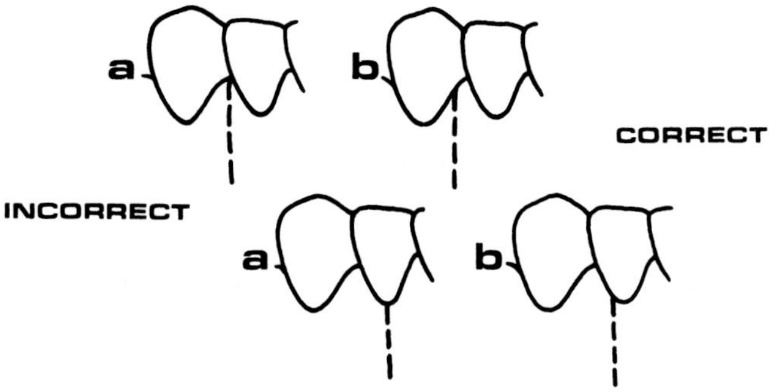

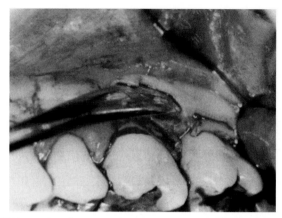

FIGURE 54–11. Correct (b) and incorrect (a) locations for a vertical incision. This incision should be made at the line angles to prevent splitting of a papilla or incision directly over a radicular surface.

Vertical Incisions. Vertical or oblique releasing incisions can be utilized on one or both ends of the horizontal incision, depending on the design and purpose of the flap. Vertical incisions at both ends are necessary if the flap is to be apically displaced. Vertical incisions must extend beyond the mucogingival line to the alveolar mucosa to allow for the release of the flap to be displaced (see Chapter 59).

In general, vertical incisions in the lingual and palatal areas are avoided. Facial vertical incisions should not be made in the center of an interdental papilla or over the radicular surface of a tooth. Incisions should be made at the line angles of a tooth either to include the papilla in the flap or to avoid it completely (Fig. 54–11). The vertical incision should also be designed so as to avoid short flaps (mesiodistally) with long, apically directed horizontal incisions, because these could jeopardize the blood supply to the flap.

Several investigators[1,2,11,12] have proposed the so-called interdental denudation procedure, which consists of horizontal, internal bevel, nonscalloped incisions to remove the gingival papillae and denude the interdental space. This technique completely eliminates the inflamed interdental areas, which heal by secondary intention, and results in excellent gingival contour. It is contraindicated when bone grafts are to be used.

Incisions for the Papilla Preservation Flap

Step 1. A crevicular incision is made around each tooth with no incisions through the interdental papilla.

Step 2. The preserved papilla can be incorporated into the facial flap or the lingual or palatal flap, although it is most commonly integrated into the facial flap. In these cases the lingual or palatal incision consists of a semilunar incision across the interdental papilla in its palatal or lingual aspect; this incision dips apically from the line angles of the tooth so that the papillary incision is at least 5 mm from the crest of the papilla.

Step 3. An Orban knife is then introduced into this incision to sever one half to two thirds of the base of the interdental papilla. The papilla is then dissected from the lingual or palatal aspect and elevated intact with the facial flap.

These incisions are illustrated in Fig. 54–5 and Plate XVII.

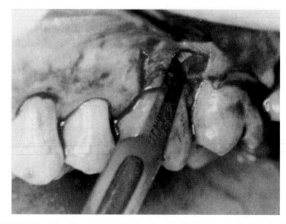

FIGURE 54–12. Elevation of the flap with a periosteal elevator to obtain a full-thickness flap.

ELEVATION OF THE FLAP

When a full-thickness flap is desired, the reflection is done by *blunt dissection.* A periosteal elevator is used to separate the mucoperiosteum from the bone by moving it mesially, distally, and apically until the desired reflection is accomplished (Fig. 54–12).

Sharp dissection is necessary to reflect a partial-thickness flap. A surgical scalpel (no. 15 or no. 11) is utilized (Fig. 54–13).

A combination of full- and partial-thickness flaps are often indicated to obtain the advantages of both. The flap is started as a full-thickness procedure, and then a partial-thickness flap is made. In this way the coronal portion of the bone, which may be subject to osseous remodeling, is exposed while the remaining bone remains protected by its periosteum.

SUTURING TECHNIQUES

After all the necessary procedures are completed, the area is re-examined and cleansed, and the flap is placed in the desired position, where it should remain *without tension.* It is convenient to keep it in place with light pressure

FIGURE 54–13. Elevation of the flap with a Bard-Parker knife to obtain a split-thickness flap.

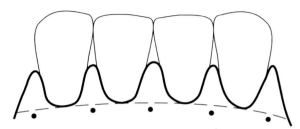

FIGURE 54–14. Placement of suture in the interdental space below the base of an imaginary triangle in the papilla.

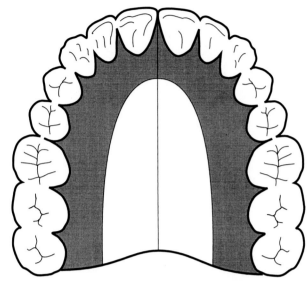

FIGURE 54–15. Placement of sutures for closing a palatal flap. For slightly or moderately elevated flaps, the sutures are placed in shaded area; for more substantial elevation of the flap, in central (unshaded) area of the palate.

through a piece of gauze, so that a small blood clot will form underneath. The purpose of suturing is to maintain the flap in the desired position until healing has progressed to the point where sutures are no longer needed.

There are many types of sutures, suture needles, and materials.[5,10] Most needs in periodontal surgery can be filled using a ³⁄₈-circle reverse-cutting eyeless needle and 3-0 black braided silk. In some cases a 5-0 resorbable (catgut) sutured is indicated.

The needle is held with the needle holder and should enter the tissues at right angles and no less than 2 to 3 mm from the incision. The needle is then carried through the tissue, following the needle's curvature. The knot should not be placed over the incision.

The periodontal flap is closed either with independent interdental sutures or with continuous, independent sling sutures. The latter method eliminates the pulling of the buccal and lingual or palatal flaps together and instead utilizes the teeth as an anchor for the flaps. There is less tendency for the flaps to buckle, and the forces on the flaps are better distributed.

Sutures of any kind placed in the interdental papillae should enter and exit the tissue at a point located below the imaginary line that forms the base of the triangle of the interdental papilla (Fig. 54–14). The location of sutures for closure of a palatal flap depend on the extent of flap elevation that has been performed. The flap is divided in four quadrants, as depicted in Figure 54–15. If the elevation of the flap is slight or moderate, the sutures can be placed in the quadrant closest to the teeth. If the flap elevation is substantial, the sutures should be placed in the central quadrants of the palate.

One may or may not utilize periodontal dressings. When the flaps are not apically displaced, there is no need to use dressings other than for patient comfort.

Interdental Ligation. Two types of interdental ligation can be used: the *direct* or *loop suture* (Fig. 54–16) or the *figure-of-eight suture* (Fig. 54–17). In the figure-of-eight suture, there is thread between the two flaps. Therefore, this suture is used when the flaps are not in close apposition because of apical flap displacement or nonscalloped incisions. It is simpler to perform than direct ligation. The direct suture permits a better closure of the interdental papilla and should be performed when bone grafts are used or when close apposition of the scalloped incision is required.

Sling Ligation. The sling ligation can be used for a flap involving two interdental spaces and where the opposite flap is not reflected (Fig. 54–18).

Horizontal Mattress Suture. This suture is often used for the interproximal areas of diastemata or for wide inter-

dental spaces to properly adapt the interproximal papilla against the bone. Two sutures are often necessary. The horizontal mattress suture can be incorporated with continuous, independent sling sutures, as shown in Figure 54–19.

The penetration of the needle is done in such a way that the mesial and distal edges of the papilla lie snugly against the bone. The needle enters the outer surface of the gingiva and crosses the undersurface of the gingiva horizontally. The mattress sutures should not be close together at the midpoint of the base of the papilla. The needle reappears on the outer surface at the other base of the papilla and continues around the tooth with the sling sutures.

Continuous, Independent Sling Suture. This is used when there are both facial and lingual flaps involving many teeth. The suture is initiated on the facial papilla closest to the midline, because this is the easiest place to position the final knot (Fig. 54–20). A continuous sling suture is laced for each papilla on the facial surface. When the last tooth is reached, the suture is anchored around it to prevent any pulling of the facial sutures when the lingual flap is sutured around the teeth in a similar fashion. The suture is again anchored around the last tooth prior to tying the final knot. This type of suture does not produce a pull on the lingual flap when the lingual flap is sutured. The two flaps are completely independent of each other owing to the anchoring around both the initial and the final tooth. The flaps are tied to the teeth and not to each other because of the sling sutures.

This type of suture is especially appropriate for the maxillary arch, because the palatal gingiva is attached and fibrous, whereas the facial tissue is thinner and mobile.

Anchor Suture. The closing of a flap mesial or distal to a tooth, as in mesial or distal wedge procedures, is best accomplished by the anchor suture. This suture closes the facial and lingual flaps and adapts them tightly against the tooth. The needle is placed at the line angle area of the facial or lingual flap adjacent to the tooth, anchored around

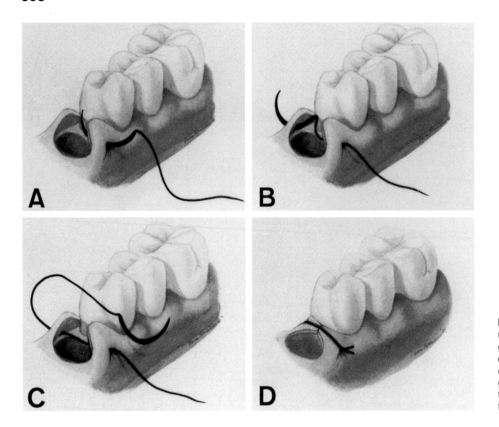

FIGURE 54–16. A simple loop suture is used to approximate the buccal and lingual flaps. *A,* The needle penetrates the outer surface of the first flap. *B,* The undersurface of the opposite flap is engaged, and the suture is brought back to the initial side *(C),* where the knot is tied *(D).*

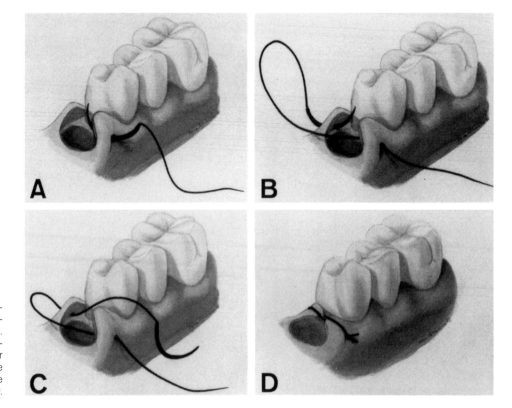

FIGURE 54–17. An interrupted figure-of-8 suture is used to approximate the buccal and lingual flaps. The needle penetrates the outer surface of the first flap *(A)* and the outer surface of the opposite flap *(B).* The suture is then brought back to the first flap *(C),* and the knot is tied *(D).*

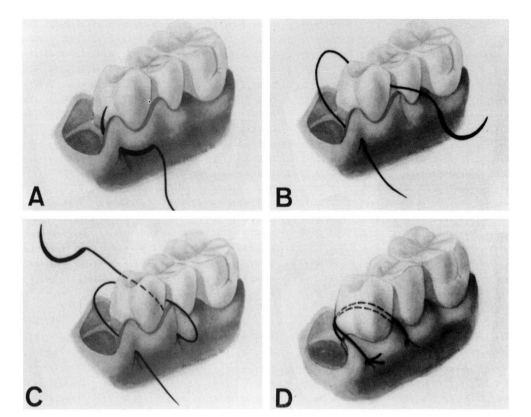

FIGURE 54–18. A single, interrupted sling suture is used to adapt the flap around the tooth. *A,* The needle engages the outer surface of the flap and encircles the tooth *(B). C,* The outer surface of the same flap of the adjacent interdental area is engaged. *D,* The suture is returned to the initial site and the knot tied.

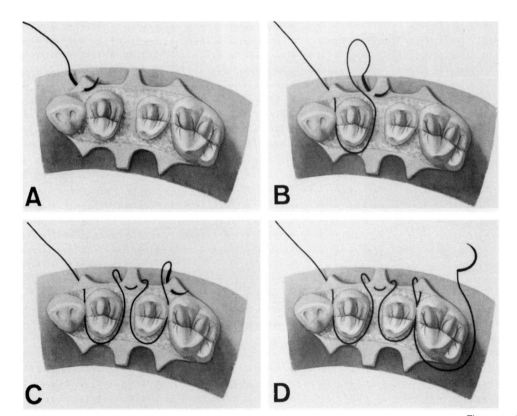

FIGURE 54–19. A continuous, independent sling suture utilizing a horizontal mattress suture around diastemata or wide interdental areas *(B* and *C).* This mattress suture is utilized on both the buccal *(D)* and the lingual *(E* and *F)* surfaces.

Figure and legend continued on the next page.

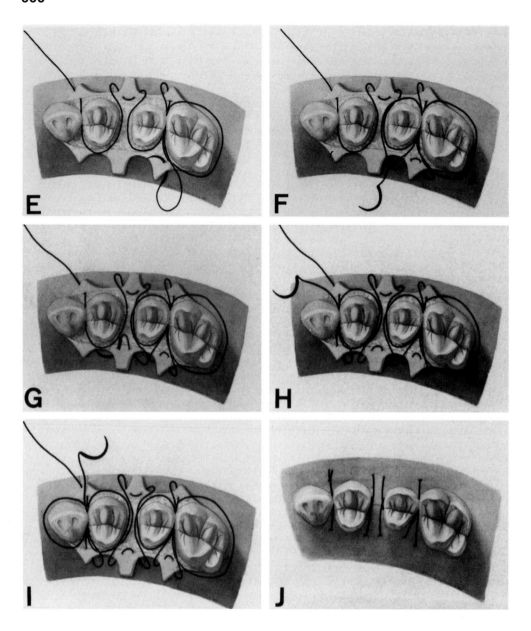

FIGURE 54–19. *Continued* Continuation of suture on lingual surfaces (*G* to *I*) and completed suture *(J).*

the tooth, passed beneath the opposite flap, and tied. The anchor suture can be repeated for each area that requires it (Fig. 54–21).

Closed Anchor Suture. Another technique for closing a flap in an edentulous area mesial or distal to a tooth consists of tying a direct suture that closes the proximal flap, carrying one of the threads around the tooth to anchor the tissue against the tooth, and then tying the two threads (Fig. 54–22).

Periosteal Suture. This type of suture is used to hold in place apically displaced partial thickness flaps. There are two types of periosteal sutures: the holding suture and the closing suture. The *holding suture* is a horizontal mattress suture placed at the base of the displaced flap to secure it in the new position. *Closing sutures* are used to secure the flap edges to the periosteum. Both types of periosteal sutures are shown in Figure 54–23.

HEALING AFTER FLAP SURGERY

Immediately after suturing (0 to 24 hours) a connection between the flap and the tooth or bone surface is established by the blood clot, which consists of a fibrin reticulum with many polymorphonuclear leukocytes, erythrocytes, debris from injured cells, and capillaries at the edge of the wound.[3] There are also bacteria and an exudate or transudate as a result of tissue injury.

One to 3 days after flap surgery the space between the flap and the tooth or bone is thinner, and epithelial cells migrate over the border of the flap, usually contacting the tooth at this time. When the flap is closely adapted to the alveolar process, there is only a minimal inflammatory response.[3]

One week after surgery an epithelial attachment to the root has been established by means of hemidesmosomes and a basal lamina. The blood clot is replaced by granulation tissue derived from the gingival connective tissue, the bone marrow, and the periodontal ligament.

Two weeks after surgery, collagen fibers begin to appear parallel to the tooth surface.[3] Union of the flap to the tooth is still weak owing to the presence of immature collagen fibers, although the clinical aspect may be almost normal.

One month after surgery a fully epithelialized gingival crevice with a well-defined epithelial attachment is present. There is a beginning functional arrangement of the supracrestal fibers.

Healing After Full-Thickness Flap Surgery. Full-thickness flaps, which denude the bone, result in a superficial bone necrosis at 1 to 3 days; osteoclastic resorption follows and reaches a peak at 4 to 6 days, declining thereafter.[13] This results in bone loss of about 1 mm[3,16]; bone loss is greater if the bone is thin.[15,16]

Healing After Osteoplasty. Osteoplasty (thinning of the buccal bone) using diamond burs, included as part of the surgical technique, results in areas of bone necrosis with reduction in bone height, which is later remodeled by new bone formation. Therefore, the final shape of the crest is

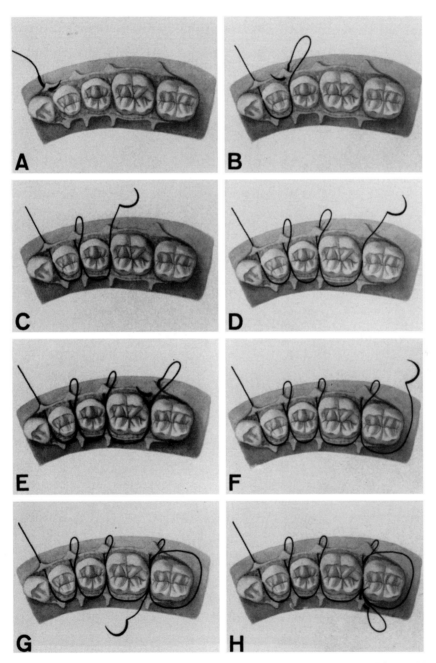

FIGURE 54–20. The continuous, independent sling suture is utilized to adapt the buccal and lingual flaps without tying the buccal flap to the lingual flap. The teeth are used to suspend each flap against the bone. It is important to anchor the suture on the two teeth at the beginning and end of the flap so that the suture will not pull the buccal flap to the lingual flap.

Figure continued on the following page.

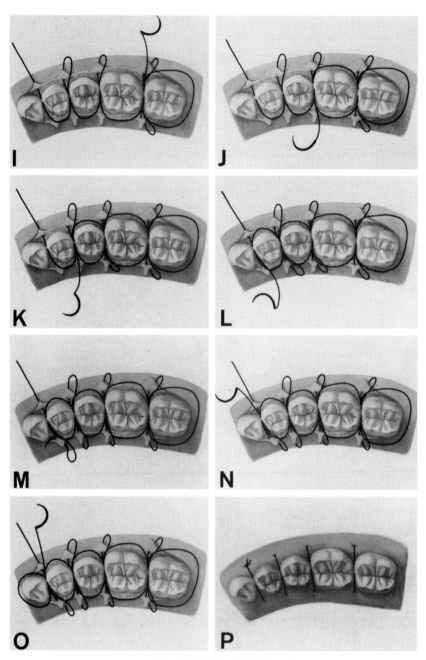

FIGURE 54–20. *Continued*

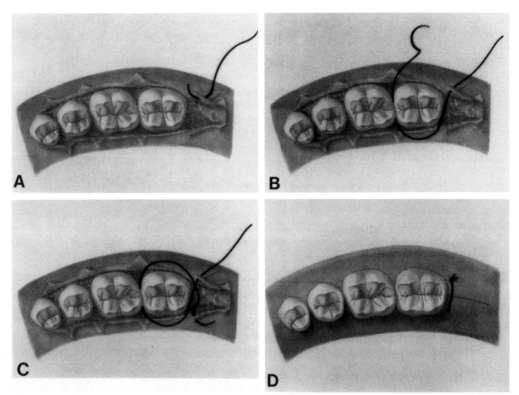

FIGURE 54–21. *A* to *D,* Distal wedge suture. This suture is also used to close flaps that are mesial or distal to a lone-standing tooth.

determined more by osseous remodeling than by surgical reshaping.[8] This may not be the case when osseous remodeling does not include excessive thinning of the radicular bone.[9] Bone repair reaches its peak at 3 to 4 weeks.[16]

Loss of bone occurs in the initial healing stages both in radicular bone and in interdental bone areas. However, in interdental areas, which have cancellous bone, the subsequent repair stage results in total restitution without any

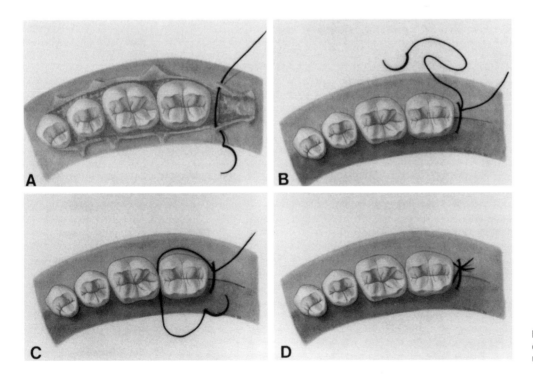

FIGURE 54–22. The closed anchor technique, another technique used to suture distal wedges.

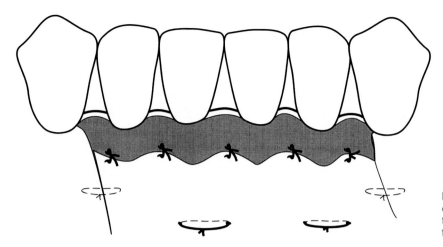

FIGURE 54–23. Periosteal sutures for an apically displaced flap. Holding sutures, shown at the bottom, are done first, followed by the closing sutures, shown at the coronal edge of the flap.

loss of bone; in radicular bone, particularly if thin and unsupported by cancellous bone, bone repair results in loss of marginal bone.[16]

REFERENCES

1. Barkann L. A conservative surgical technique for the eradication of pyorrhea pockets. J Am Dent Assoc 26:61, 1939.
2. Beube FE. Interdental tissue resection: An experimental study of a surgical technique which aids in repair of the periodontal tissues to their original contour and function. Oral Surg 33:497, 1947.
3. Caffesse RG, Ramfjord SP, Nasjleti CE. Reverse bevel periodontal flaps in monkeys. J Periodontol 39:219, 1968.
4. Carranza FA Jr, Carraro JJ. Effect of removal of periosteum on postoperative result of mucogingival surgery. J Periodontol 34:223, 1963.
5. Dahlberg WH. Incisions and suturing: Some basic considerations about each in periodontal flap surgery. Dent Clin North Am 13:149, 1969.
6. Friedman N. Mucogingival surgery: The apically repositioned flap. J Periodontol 33:328, 1962.
7. Hoag PM, Wood DL, Donnenfeld OW, Rosenfeld LD. Alveolar crest reduction following full and partial thickness flaps. J Periodontol 43:141, 1972.
8. Lobene RR, Glickman I. The response of alveolar bone to grinding with rotary stones. J Periodontol 34:105, 1963.
9. Matherson DG. An evaluation of healing following periodontal osseous surgery in monkeys. Int J Periodont Restor Dent 8:9, 1988.
10. Morris ML. Suturing techniques in periodontal surgery. Periodontics 3:84, 1965.
11. Prichard JF. Present state of the interdental denudation procedure. J Periodontol 48:566, 1977.
12. Ratcliff PA, Raust GT. Interproximal denudation: A conservative approach to osseous surgery. Dent Clin North Am 8:121, 1964.
13. Staffileno H, Wentz FE, Orban BJ. Histologic study of healing of split thickness flap surgery in dogs. J Periodontol 33:56, 1962.
14. Takei HH, Han TJ, Carranza FA Jr, et al. Flap technique for periodontal bone implants–papilla preservation technique. J Periodontol 56:204, 1985.
15. Wilderman MN. Exposure of bone in periodontal surgery. Dent Clin North Am 8:23, 1964.
16. Wilderman MN, Pennel BM, King K, Barron JM. Histogenesis of repair following osseous surgery. J Periodontol 41:551, 1970.

55

The Flap Technique for Pocket Therapy

FERMIN A. CARRANZA, JR. and HENRY H. TAKEI

The Modified Widman Flap
The Undisplaced Flap
The Palatal Flap

The Apically Displaced Flap
Distal Molar Surgery

Several techniques can be used for the treatment of periodontal pockets. The periodontal flap is one of the most frequently employed, particularly for moderate and deep pockets in posterior areas (see Chapter 49).

Techniques. Flaps can be used for pocket therapy (1) to increase accessibility to root deposits or (2) to eliminate or reduce the pocket depth. To fulfill these purposes, three flap techniques are available and in current use: the modified Widman flap; the undisplaced (unrepositioned) flap; and the apically displaced flap.

The *modified Widman flap* has been described for exposing the root surfaces for meticulous instrumentation and for

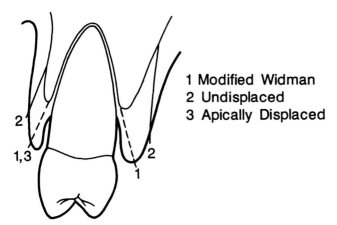

FIGURE 55–1. Locations of the internal bevel incisions for the different types of flaps.

removal of the pocket lining[7]; it is not intended to eliminate or reduce pocket depth, except for the reduction that occurs in healing by tissue shrinkage.

The *undisplaced (unrepositioned) flap,* in addition to improving accessibility for instrumentation, is created to remove the pocket wall to reduce or eliminate the pocket. This is essentially an excisional procedure of the gingiva.

The *apically displaced flap* also improves accessibility and eliminates the pocket but does the latter by apically repositioning the soft tissue wall of the pocket.[3] In so doing it preserves and/or increases the width of the attached gingiva by transforming the previously unattached keratinized pocket wall into attached tissue. This increase in width of the band of attached gingiva is supposedly based on an apical shift of the mucogingival junction, which includes apical displacement of the muscle attachments. A study made before and 18 years after apically displaced flaps failed to show a permanent relocation of the mucogingival junction.[1] All three techniques use the basic incisions described in Chapter 54: the internal bevel incision, the crevicular incision, and the interdental incision. However, there are important variations in the way in which these incisions are performed for the different types of flaps.

The modified Widman flap does not intend to remove the pocket wall but does eliminate the pocket lining. Therefore, the internal bevel incision starts close (no more than 1 to 2 mm apical) to the gingival margin and follows the normal scalloping of the gingival margin (Figs. 55–1 and 55–2).

For the apically displaced flap, the pocket wall also must be preserved to be repositioned apically while its lining is removed. The purpose of this surgical technique is to preserve the maximal amount of keratinized gingiva of the pocket wall to displace it apically and transform it into attached gingiva. For this reason, the internal bevel incision should be made as close to the tooth as possible (0.5 to 1.0 mm) (see Fig. 55–1). There is no need to determine where the bottom of the pocket is in relation to the incision, as one would for the undisplaced flap; the flap is placed approximately at the tooth–bone junction by apically displacing the flap. Its final position is not determined by the placement of the first incision.

For an undisplaced flap, the internal bevel incision is started at or near a point just coronal to the projection of the bottom of the pocket on the outer surface of the gingiva (see Fig. 55–1). This incision can be accomplished only if there is sufficient attached gingiva remaining apical to the incision. Because the pocket wall is not displaced apically, the initial incision should also eliminate the pocket wall. If the incision is made too close to the tooth, it will not eliminate the pocket wall and may result in re-creation of a soft tissue pocket. If the tissue is thick, it should also be thinned by the initial incision so that the bone can be covered properly during flap closure. Proper placement of the flap during closure is essential to prevent recurrence of pockets or bone exposure; placement is determined by where this first incision is made. The internal bevel incision should be scalloped to preserve, as much as possible, the interdental papilla (see Fig. 55–2). This allows better coverage of the bone at both the radicular and the interdental areas.

If the surgeon contemplates osseous surgery, the first incision should be placed in such a way as to compensate for the removal of bone tissue so that the flap ends at the tooth–bone junction.

THE MODIFIED WIDMAN FLAP

In 1965 Morris revived a technique described early in this century in the periodontal literature; he called it the *unrepositioned mucoperiosteal flap.*[5] Essentially the same procedure was presented in 1974 by Ramfjord and Nissle, who called it the *modified Widman flap* (Fig. 55–3).[7] This tech-

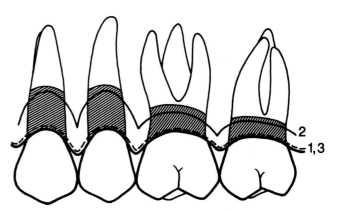

FIGURE 55–2. Scallopings required for the different types of flaps. Shaded areas on teeth denote pockets.

1 Modified Widman 2 Undisplaced 3 Apically Displaced

nique offers the possibility of establishing an intimate postoperative adaptation of healthy collagenous connective tissue to tooth surfaces[6,7] and provides access for adequate instrumentation of the root surfaces and immediate closure of the area.

Step 1. The initial incision is an internal bevel incision to the alveolar crest starting ½ to 1 mm away from the gingival margin (Fig. 55–3C). Scalloping follows the gingival margin. Care should be taken to insert the blade in such a way that the papilla is left with a thickness similar to that of the remaining facial flap. Vertical releasing incisions are usually not needed.

Step 2. The gingiva is reflected with a periosteal elevator (Fig. 55–3D).

Step 3. A crevicular incision is made from the bottom of the pocket to the bone, circumscribing the triangular wedge of tissue containing the pocket lining (Fig. 55–3E).

Step 4. After the flap is reflected, a third incision is made in the interdental spaces, coronal to the bone, with a curette or an interproximal knife, and the gingival collar is removed (Fig. 55–3F,G).

Step 5. Tissue tags and granulation tissue are removed with a curette. The root surfaces are checked and are scaled and planed if necessary (Fig. 55–3H). Residual periodontal fibers attached to the tooth surface should not be disturbed.

Step 6. Bone architecture is not corrected unless it prevents good tissue adaptation to the necks of the teeth. Every effort is made to adapt the facial and lingual interproximal tissue adjacent to each other in such a way that no interproximal bone remains exposed at the time of suturing (Fig. 55–3I). The flaps may be thinned to allow for close adaptation of the gingiva around the entire circumference of the tooth and to each other interproximally.

Step 7. Interrupted direct sutures are placed in each interdental space (Fig. 55–3J) and covered with tetracycline (Achromycin) ointment and with a periodontal surgical pack.

Ramfjord and coworkers performed an extensive longitudinal study comparing the Widman procedure, as modified by them, with the curettage technique and pocket elimination methods that included bone contouring when needed.[6] The patients were randomly assigned to one of the techniques, and results were analyzed yearly up to 7 years after therapy. The investigators reported approximately similar results with the three methods tested. Pocket depths initially were similar for all methods but were maintained at shallower levels with the Widman flap (Fig. 55–4); the attachment level remained higher with the Widman flap.

THE UNDISPLACED FLAP

Currently the undisplaced flap is probably the most frequently performed type of periodontal surgery. It differs from the modified Widman flap in that the soft tissue pocket wall is removed with the initial incision; thus, it may be considered an *internal bevel gingivectomy*. The undisplaced flap and the gingivectomy are the two techniques that surgically remove the pocket wall. To perform this technique without creating a mucogingival problem, the clinician should determine in advance that enough attached gingiva will remain after removal of the pocket wall.

Step 1. The pockets are measured with the periodontal probe, and a bleeding point is produced on the outer surface of the gingiva to mark the pocket bottom.

Step 2. The initial, internal bevel incision is made (Fig. 55–5) following the scalloping of the bleeding marks on the gingiva (Fig. 55–6). The incision is usually carried to a point apical to the alveolar crest, depending on the thickness of the tissue. The thicker the tissue is, the more apical will be the ending point of the incision (see Fig. 55–5). In addition, the flap should be thinned with the initial incision, because it is easier to accomplish at this time than later with a loose reflected flap that is difficult to manage. (Use of this technique in palatal areas is considered in the following discussion.)

Step 3. The second or crevicular incision is made from the bottom of the pocket to the bone to detach the connective tissue from the tooth.

Step 4. The flap is reflected with a periosteal elevator (blunt dissection) from the internal bevel incision. Usually there is no need for vertical incisions, because the flap is not displaced apically.

Step 5. The interdental incision is made with an interdental knife, separating the connective tissue from the bone.

Step 6. The triangular wedge of tissue created by the three incisions is removed with a curette.

Step 7. The area is debrided, removing all tissue tags and granulation tissue with sharp curettes.

Step 8. After the necessary scaling and root planing, the flap edge should rest on the root–bone junction. If this is not the case, owing to improper location of the initial incision or to the unexpected need for osseous surgery, the edge of the flap is rescalloped and trimmed to allow the flap edge to end at the root–bone junction.

Step 9. A continuous sling suture is utilized to secure the facial and the lingual or palatal flaps. This type of suture, which uses the tooth as an anchor, is advantageous to posi-

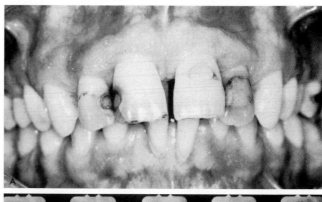
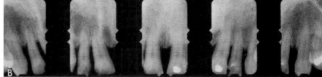

FIGURE 55–3. The modified Widman flap technique. *A*, Facial view before surgery. Probing of pockets revealed interproximal depths of 4 to 8 mm and facial and palatal depths of 2 to 5 mm. *B*, Radiographic survey of the area. Note generalized horizontal bone loss.

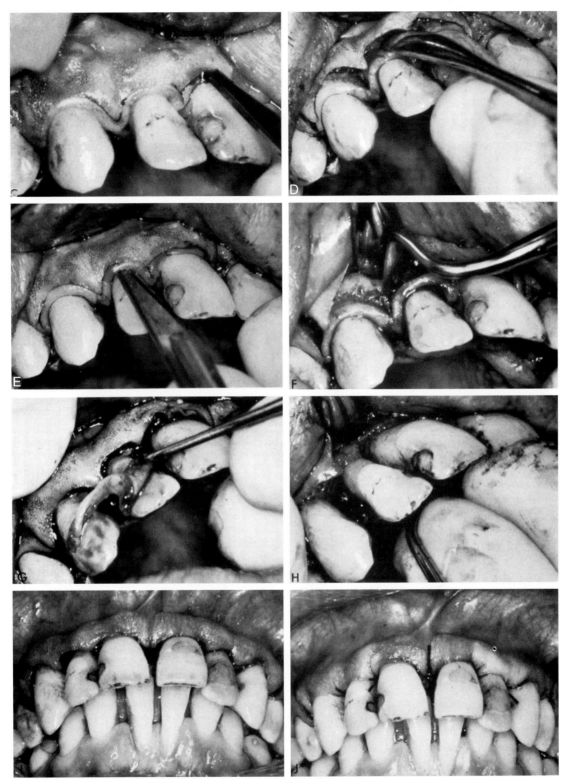

FIGURE 55–3. *Continued C,* Internal bevel incision. *D,* Elevation of the flap, leaving a wedge of tissue still attached by its base. *E,* Crevicular incision. *F,* Interdental incision sectioning the base of the papilla. *G,* Removal of tissue. *H,* Exposure of root surfaces and marginal bone; root planing and removal of remaining calculus. *I,* Replacement of the flap in its original position. *J,* Interdental sutures in place. (Courtesy of Dr. Raul G. Caffesse.)

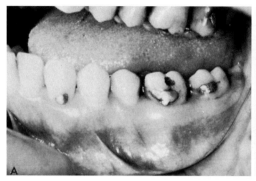
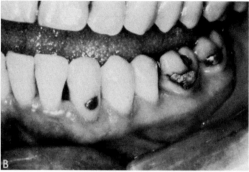

FIGURE 55–4. A patient before *(A)* and after *(B)* treatment by means of Widman flaps. Note the reduction in gingival height and concomitant pocket depth. (Courtesy of Dr. Raul G. Caffesse.)

tion and hold the flap edges at the root–bone junction. The area is covered with a periodontal pack.

The Palatal Flap

The surgical approach to the palatal area differs from that for other areas because of the character of the palatal tissue and the anatomy of the area. The palatal tissue is all attached, keratinized tissue and has none of the elastic properties associated with other gingival tissues. Therefore, the palatal tissue cannot be apically displaced, nor can a partial-thickness (split-thickness) flap be accomplished.

The initial incision for the palatal flap should be such that when the flap is sutured, it is precisely adapted at the root–bone junction. It cannot be moved apically or coronally to adapt to the root–bone junction, as can be done with flaps in other areas. *Therefore, the location of the initial incision is important for final placement of the flap.*

The palatal tissue may be thin or thick, it may or may not have osseous defects, and the palatal vault may be high or low. These anatomic variations may require changes in the location, angle, and design of the incision.

The initial incision for a flap varies with the anatomic situation. As shown in Figure 55–7, the initial incision may be the usual internal bevel incision, followed by crevicular and interdental incisions. If the tissue is thick, a horizontal gingivectomy incision may be made, followed

by an internal bevel incision that starts at the edge of this incision and ends on the lateral surface of the underlying bone. The placement of the internal bevel incision must be such that the flap fits around the tooth without exposing the bone.

Before the flap is reflected to the final position for scaling and management of the osseous lesions, its thickness must be checked. Flaps should be thinned to adapt to the underlying osseous tissue and provide a thin, knife-like gingival margin. Often flaps, particularly palatal flaps, are too thick and may have a propensity to separate from the tooth and may delay and complicate healing. It is best to thin the flaps prior to their complete reflection, because a free, mobile flap is difficult to hold for thinning (Fig. 55–8). A sharp, thin papilla positioned properly around the interdental areas at the tooth–bone junction is essential to prevent recurrence of soft tissue pockets.

The purpose of the palatal flap should be considered before the incision is made. If the intent of the surgery is debridement, the internal bevel incision is planned so that the flap adapts at the root–bone junction when sutured. If osseous resection is necessary, the incision should be planned to compensate for the lowered level of the bone when the flap is closed. Probing and sounding of the osseous level and the depth of the infrabony pocket should be used to determine the position of the incision.

The apical portion of the scalloping should be narrower than the line angle area, because the palatal root tapers apically. A rounded scallop will result in a palatal flap that does not fit snugly around the root. This procedure should be done prior to the complete reflection of the palatal flap, as a loose flap is difficult to grasp and stabilize for dissection.

It is sometimes necessary to thin the palatal flap after it has been reflected. This can be accomplished by holding the inner portion of the flap with a mosquito hemostat or Adson forceps as the inner connective tissue is carefully dissected away with a sharp no. 15 scalpel blade. Care must be taken not to perforate or overthin the flap. The edge of the flap should be thinner than the base, and therefore, the blade should be angled toward the lateral surface of the palatal bone. The dissected inner connective tissue is removed with a hemostat. As with any flap, the triangular papilla portion (Fig. 55–9) should be thin enough to fit snugly against the bone and into the interdental area.

The principles for the use of vertical releasing incisions are similar to those for using other incisions. Care must be

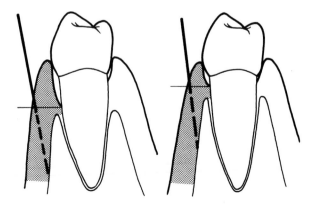

FIGURE 55–5. Diagram showing the different areas where the internal bevel incision is made in a nondisplaced flap. The incision is made at the level of the pocket to discard the tissue coronal to it if there is sufficient remaining attached gingiva.

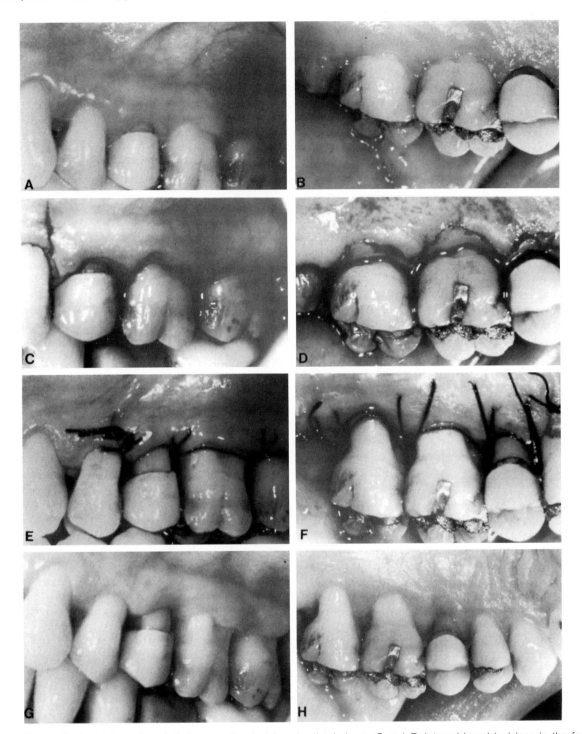

FIGURE 55–6. The undisplaced flap. *A* and *B*, Preoperative facial and palatal views. *C* and *D*, Internal bevel incisions in the facial and palatal aspects. Note the deeper scalloping palatally for the undisplaced flap. *E* and *F*, After the necessary osseous surgery, the flaps have been sutured. The facial flap is apically displaced, whereas the palatal flap is nondisplaced. *G* and *H*, Ten-week postoperative results. (Courtesy of Dr. Silvia Oreamuno.)

exercised so that the length of the incision is minimized to avoid the numerous vessels located in the palate.

THE APICALLY DISPLACED FLAP

This technique, with some variants, can be used for pocket eradication and/or preserving or widening the zone of attached gingiva. Depending on the purpose, it can be a full-thickness (mucoperiosteal) or a split-thickness (mucosal) flap. The split-thickness flap requires more precision and time but can be more accurately positioned and sutured in an apical position using a periosteal suturing technique.

Step 1. An internal bevel incision is made (Fig. 55–10). To preserve as much of the keratinized and attached gingiva as possible, the incision should be no more than about 1 mm from the crest of the gingiva and directed toward

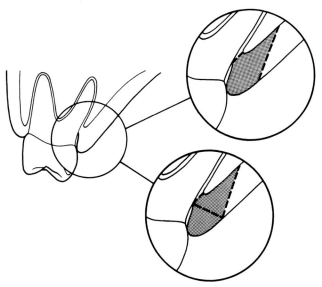

FIGURE 55–7. Examples of two methods for eliminating a palatal pocket. One incision is an internal bevel incision made at the area of the apical extent of the pocket. The other procedure uses a gingivectomy incision, which is followed by an internal bevel incision.

the crest of the bone (see Fig. 55–1). The incision is made following the existing scalloping; there is no need to mark the bottom of the pocket in the external gingival surface, because the incision is unrelated to pocket depth. It is also not necessary to accentuate the scallop interden-

tally, as the flap is displaced apically and not placed interdentally.

Step 2. Crevicular incisions are made, followed by initial elevation of the flap, and then interdental incisions are performed, and the wedge of tissue that contains the pocket wall is removed.

Step 3. Vertical incisions extending *beyond the mucogingival junction* are made, and for a full-thickness flap, the flap is elevated by blunt dissection with a periosteal elevator. If a split-thickness flap is required, it is elevated using sharp dissection with a Bard-Parker knife to split it, leaving a layer of connective tissue (including the periosteum) on the bone.

Step 4. After removal of all granulation tissue, scaling and root planing, and osseous surgery, if necessary, the flap is displaced apically to its original position. It is important that the vertical incisions and, consequently, the flap elevation reach past the mucogingival junction to provide adequate mobility to the flap for its apical displacement.

Step 5. Appropriate sutures prevent the flap from sliding to a position more apical than that desired, and the periodontal dressing avoids its movement in a coronal direction. For a full-thickness flap, a continuous, individually anchored suture is made, whereas a partial-thickness flap is sutured to the periosteum using a direct loop suture or a combination of loop and anchor sutures. A dry foil is placed over the flap prior to covering it with the dressing to prevent the introduction of pack under the flap.

After 1 week, dressings and sutures are removed. The area is usually repacked for another week, after which the patient is instructed to use chlorhexidine mouthrinse or to apply chlorhexidine topically with cotton-tipped applicators for another 2 or 3 weeks.

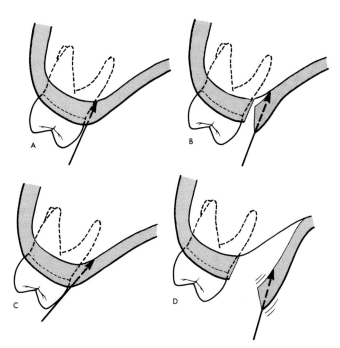

FIGURE 55–8. Diagrams illustrating the angle of the internal bevel incision in the palate and the different ways to thin the flap. *A,* The usual angle and direction of the incision. *B,* Thinning of the flap after it has been slightly reflected with a second internal incision. *C,* Beveling and thinning of the flap with the initial incision if the position and contour of the tooth allow. *D,* The problem encountered in thinning the flap once it has been reflected. The flap is too loose and free for proper positioning and incision.

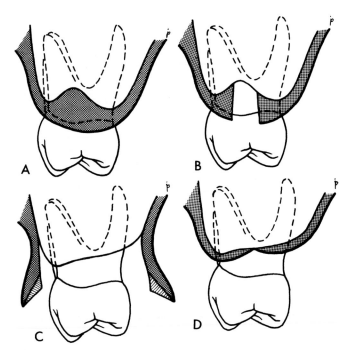

FIGURE 55–9. *A,* A distal view of incisions made to eliminate a pocket distal to the maxillary second molar. *B,* Two parallel incisions and removal of the intervening tissue. *C,* Thinning of the flap and contouring of the bone. *D,* Approximation of the buccal and palatal flaps.

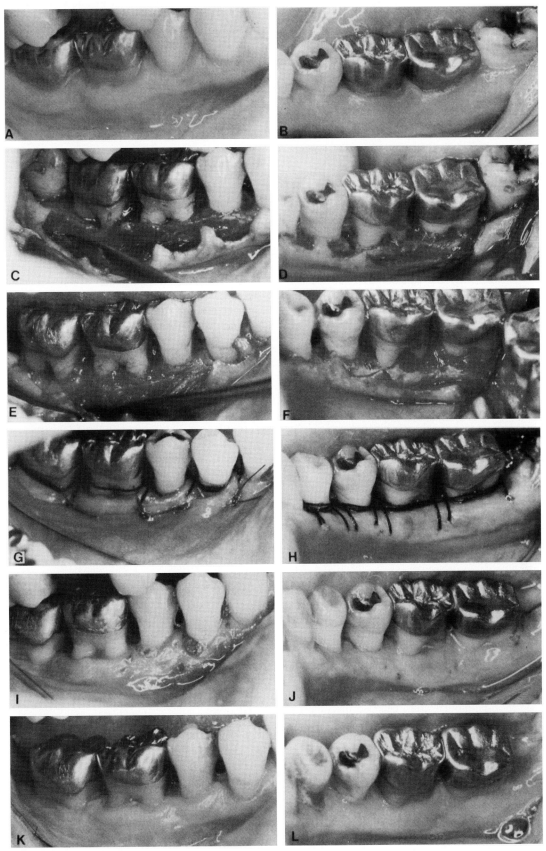

FIGURE 55–10. Apically displaced flap. *A* and *B*, Facial and lingual preoperative views. *C* and *D*, Facial and lingual flaps elevated. *E* and *F*, After debridement of the areas. *G* and *H*, Sutures in place. *I* and *J*, Healing after 1 week. *K* and *L*, Healing after 2 months. Note the preservation of attached gingiva displaced to a more apical position.

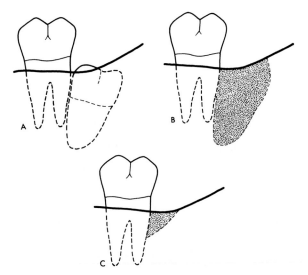

FIGURE 55–11. *A,* Impaction of a third molar distal to a second molar with little or no interdental bone between the two teeth. *B,* Removal of the third molar creates a pocket with little or no bone distal to the second molar. This often leads to a vertical osseous defect distal to the second molar *(C).*

DISTAL MOLAR SURGERY

Treatment of periodontal pockets on the distal surface of terminal molars is frequently complicated by the presence of bulbous fibrous tissue over the maxillary tuberosity or by prominent retromolar pads in the mandible. Deep vertical defects are also commonly present in conjunction with the redundant fibrous tissue. Some of these osseous lesions may result from incomplete repair after extraction of impacted third molars (Fig. 55–11).

The gingivectomy incision is the most direct approach to treating distal pockets that have adequate attached gingiva and no osseous lesions. However, the flap approach is less traumatic postsurgically, because it produces a primary closure wound rather than the open secondary wound left by a gingivectomy incision. In addition, it results in attached gingiva and provides access for examination and, if needed, correction of the osseous defect. Operations for this purpose have been described by Robinson[8] and Braden[2] and modified by several other investigators. Some representative procedures are discussed here.

Maxillary Molars. The treatment of distal pockets on the maxillary arch is usually simpler than the treatment of a similar lesion on the mandibular arch, because the tuberosity presents a greater amount of fibrous attached gingiva than does the area of the retromolar pad. In addition, the anatomy of a tuberosity extending distally and apically is more adaptable to pocket elimination than is that of the mandibular molar arch, where the tissue extends coronally. However, the lack of a broad area of attached gingiva and the abruptly ascending tuberosity sometimes complicate therapy (Fig. 55–12).

The following considerations determine the location of the incision for distal molar surgery: accessibility, the amount of attached gingiva, the pocket depth, and the available distance from the distal aspect of the tooth to the end of the tuberosity or retromolar pad.

Technique. Two parallel incisions, beginning at the distal portion of the tooth and extending to the mucogingival junction distal to the tuberosity or retromolar pad, are made (Fig. 55–13). The faciolingual distance between these two incisions depends on the depth of the pocket and the amount of fibrous tissue involved. The deeper the pocket, the greater the distance between the two parallel incisions. When the tissue between the two incisions is removed and the flaps are thinned, the two flap edges must approximate each other at a new apical position without overlapping.

When the depth of the pocket cannot be easily estimated, it is better to err on the conservative side, leaving overlapping flaps rather than flaps that are too short and result in exposure of bone. When the two flaps overlap after the surgery is completed, they should be placed one over the other, and the overlapping portion of one of them is grasped with a hemostat. Then a sharp knife or scissors is used to cut the excess.

A transversal incision is made at the distal end of the two parallel incisions so that a long, rectangular piece of tissue can be removed. These incisions are usually interconnected with the incisions for the remainder of the surgery in the involved quadrant. The parallel distal incisions should be confined to the attached gingiva, because bleeding and flap management become problems when the incision is extended into the alveolar mucosa. If access is difficult, especially if the distance from the distal aspect of the tooth to the mucogingival junction is short, a vertical incision can be made at the end of the parallel incisions.

In treating the tuberosity area, the two distal incisions are usually made at the midline of the tuberosity (Fig. 55–14). In most cases, no attempt is made to undermine the underlying tissue at this time. These incisions are made straight down into the underlying bone, where access is difficult. A no. 12B blade is generally used. It is easier to dissect out the underlying redundant tissue when the flap is partially reflected. When the distal flaps are apposed, the two flap margins should closely approximate each other.

Mandibular Molars. Incisions for the mandibular arch differ from those used for the tuberosity owing to differences in the anatomy and histologic features of the two areas. The retromolar pad area does not usually present as much keratinized attached gingiva. The keratinized gingiva,

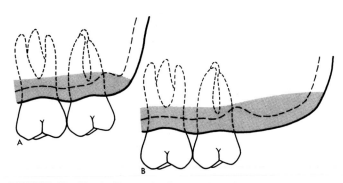

FIGURE 55–12. *A,* Removal of a pocket distal to the maxillary second molar may be difficult if there is minimal attached gingiva. If the bone ascends acutely apically, removal of this bone may make the procedure easier. *B,* A long distal tuberosity with abundant attached gingiva is an ideal anatomic situation for distal pocket eradication.

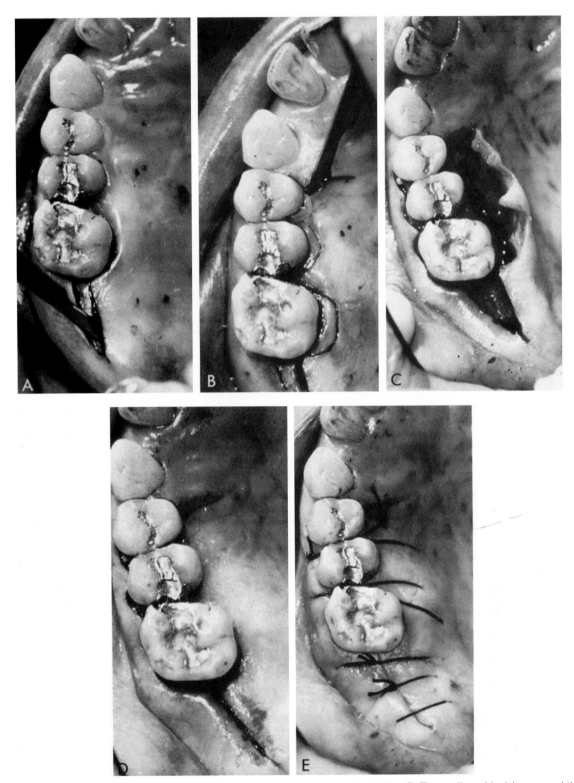

FIGURE 55–13. *A,* A distal pocket eradication procedure with the incision distal to the molar. *B,* The scalloped incision around the remaining teeth. *C,* The flap reflected and thinned around the distal incision. *D,* The flap in position prior to suturing. It should be closely approximated. *E,* The flap sutured both distally and over the remaining surgical area.

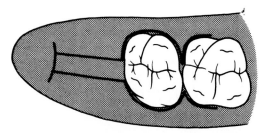

FIGURE 55–14. A typical incision design for a surgical procedure distal to the maxillary second molar.

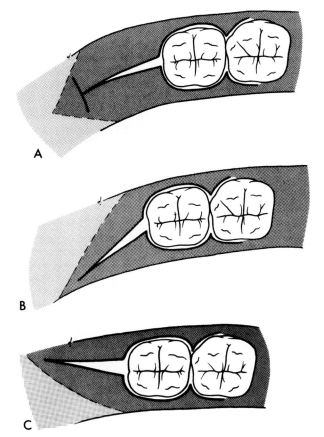

FIGURE 55–16. Incision designs for surgical procedures distal to the mandibular second molar. The incision should follow the areas of greatest attached gingiva and underlying bone.

if present, may not be found directly distal to the molar. The greatest amount may be distolingual or distofacial and may not be over the bony crest. The ascending ramus of the mandible may also create a short horizontal area distal to the terminal molar (Fig. 55–15). The shorter this area is, the more difficult it is to treat any deep distal lesion around the terminal molar.

The two incisions distal to the molar should follow the area with the greatest amount of keratinized gingiva (Fig. 55–16). Therefore, the incisions should be directed distolingually or distofacially, depending on which area has more attached gingiva. Before the flap is completely re-

flected, it is thinned with a no. 15 blade; it is easier to thin the flap before it is completely free and mobile. After reflection of the flap and removal of the redundant fibrous tissue, any necessary osseous surgery is performed. The flaps are approximated similarly to those in the maxillary tuberosity area.

REFERENCES

1. Ainamo A, Bergenholtz A, Hugoson A, Ainamo J. Location of the mucogingival junction 18 years after apically repositioned flap surgery. J Clin Periodontol *19*:49, 1992.
2. Braden BE. Deep distal pockets adjacent to terminal teeth. Dent Clin North Am *13*:161, 1969.
3. Friedman N. Mucogingival surgery: The apically repositioned flap. J Periodontol *33*:328, 1962.
4. Matelski DE, Hurt WC. The corrective phase: The modified Widman flap. In Hurt WC, ed. Periodontics in General Practice. Springfield, IL, Charles C Thomas, 1976.
5. Morris ML. The unrepositioned mucoperiosteal flap. Periodontics *3*:147, 1965.
6. Ramfjord SP. Present status of the modified Widman flap procedure. J Periodontol *48*:558, 1977.
7. Ramfjord SP, Nissle RR. The modified Widman flap. J Periodontol *45*:601, 1974.
8. Robinson RE. The distal wedge operation. Periodontics *4*:256, 1966.

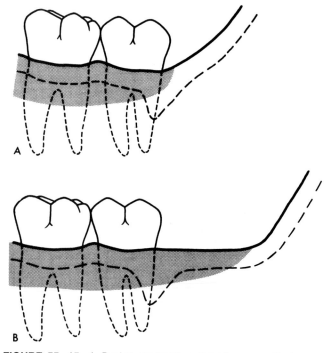

FIGURE 55–15. *A,* Pocket eradication distal to a mandibular second molar with minimal attached gingiva and a close ascending ramus is anatomically difficult. *B,* For surgical procedures distal to a mandibular second molar, abundant attached gingiva and distal space are ideal.

56

Resective Osseous Surgery

THOMAS N. SIMS and FERMIN A. CARRANZA, JR.

Selection of Treatment Technique
Rationale
Terminology

Methods of Osseous Resective Surgery
The Osseous Resection Technique
Specific Osseous Reshaping Situations

The damage resulting from periodontal disease reveals itself in variable destruction of the tooth-supporting bone. Generally, bony deformities are not uniform. They are not indicative of the alveolar housing of the tooth prior to the disease process, nor do they reflect the overlying gingival architecture. Bone loss has been classified as horizontal or vertical, but in fact, bone loss is most often a combination of horizontal and vertical loss. Horizontal bone loss generally results in a relative thickening of the marginal alveolar bone, since bone tapers as it approaches its most coronal margin.

The effect of this thickening and the development of vertical defects leave the alveolar bone with countless combinations of bony shapes. If these various topographic changes are to be altered to provide a more physiologic bone pattern, a method for osseous recontouring must be followed.

Osseous surgery may be defined as the procedure by which changes in the alveolar bone can be accomplished to rid it of deformities induced by the periodontal disease process or other related factors, such as exostosis and tooth supraeruption.

Osseous surgery can be either additive or subtractive in nature. *Additive osseous surgery* includes procedures directed at restoring the alveolar bone to its original level, whereas *subtractive osseous surgery* is designed to restore the form of pre-existing alveolar bone to the level existing at the time of surgery or slightly more apical to this level (Fig. 56–1).

Additive osseous surgery brings about the ideal result of periodontal therapy; it implies regeneration of lost bone and re-establishment of the periodontal ligament, gingival fibers, and junctional epithelium at a more coronal level. This type of osseous surgery is discussed in Chapter 57.

Subtractive osseous surgical procedures provide an alternative to additive methods and should be resorted to when the latter are not feasible. They are discussed in this chapter.

SELECTION OF TREATMENT TECHNIQUE

The morphology of the osseous defect will largely determine the treatment technique to be used. One-wall angular

defects usually have to be recontoured surgically. Three-wall defects, particularly if they are narrow and deep, can be successfully treated with techniques that aim at new attachment and bone regeneration. Two-wall angular defects can be treated with either method, depending on their depth, width, and general configuration. Therefore, except for one-wall defects, wide and shallow two-wall defects, and interdental craters, pockets are treated with the objective of obtaining optimal repair by natural healing processes.

RATIONALE

Osseous resective surgery is the most predictable pocket reduction technique. However, more than any other surgical technique, osseous resective surgery is performed at the expense of bony tissue and attachment level.[1,2,9] Thus, its value as a surgical approach is limited by the presence, quantity, and shape of the bony tissues and by the amount of attachment loss that is acceptable.

The major rationale for osseous resective surgery is centered on the tenet that discrepancies in levels and shapes of the bone and gingiva predispose patients to the recurrence of pocket depth postsurgically.[6] Although this concept is not universally accepted[3,5] and despite the fact that the procedure induces loss of radicular bone in the healing phases, there are cases in which recontouring of bone is the only logical treatment choice. The goal of osseous resective therapy is reshaping the marginal bone to resemble the alveolar process undamaged by periodontal disease. The technique is performed in combination with apically displaced flaps, and the procedure eliminates periodontal pocket depth and improves tissue contour to provide a more easily maintainable environment. The relative merits of pocket reduction procedures are discussed in Chapters 33 and 49; this chapter discusses the osseous resective technique and how and where it may be accomplished.

TERMINOLOGY

Numerous terms have been developed to describe the topography of the alveolar housing, the procedures for its

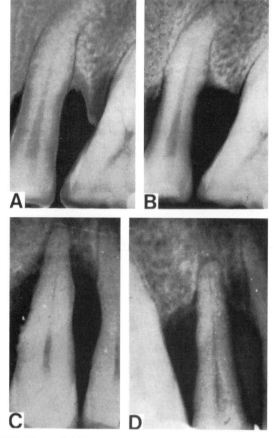

FIGURE 56–1. Additive and subtractive osseous surgery. Before *(A)* and immediately after *(B)* subtractive osseous surgery; the osseous wall of the two adjoining infrabony pockets has been removed. Before *(C)* and 1 year after *(D)* additive osseous surgery; the area has been flapped and thoroughly instrumented, resulting in regeneration of the interdental and periapical bone. (Courtesy of Dr. E. A. Albano and Dr. B. O. Barletta.)

removal, and the resulting correction. These terms should be clearly defined.

Procedures used to correct osseous defects have been classified in two groups: osteoplasty and ostectomy.[2] *Osteoplasty* refers to reshaping the bone without removing tooth-supporting bone. *Ostectomy* (or *osteoectomy*) includes the removal of tooth-supporting bone. Either or both of these procedures may be necessary to produce the desired result.

Terms that describe the bone form after reshaping can refer to morphologic features or to the thoroughness of the reshaping performed. Examples of morphologically descriptive terms include *negative, positive, flat,* and *ideal.* These terms all relate to a preconceived standard of ideal osseous form.

The terms *positive architecture* and *negative architecture* refer to the relative position of interdental bone to radicular bone. The architecture is said to be positive if the radicular bone is apical to the interdental bone. The bone is said to have negative architecture if the interdental bone is more apical than the radicular bone. *Flat architecture* is the reduction of the interdental bone to the same height as the radicular bone.

Osseous form is considered to be *ideal* when the bone is consistently more coronal on the interproximal surfaces

than on the facial and lingual surfaces. The ideal form of the marginal bone has similar interdental height, with gradual, curved slopes between interdental peaks (Fig. 56–2).

Terms that relate to the thoroughness of the osseous reshaping techniques include *definitive* and *compromise. Definitive osseous reshaping* implies that further osseous reshaping would not improve the overall result. *Compromise osseous reshaping* indicates a bone pattern that cannot be improved without significant osseous removal that would be detrimental to the overall result. References to compromise and definitive osseous architecture can be useful to the clinician, not as descriptions of morphologic features, but as terms that express the expected therapeutic result.

METHODS OF OSSEOUS RESECTIVE SURGERY

The reshaping process is fundamentally an attempt to gradualize the bone sufficiently to allow soft tissue structure to follow the contour of the bone. The soft tissue will predictably attach to the bone within certain specific dimensions. The length and quality of connective tissue and junctional epithelium that will reform in the surgical site are dependent on numerous factors, including the health of the tissue, the condition of the root surface, and the topography, as well as the proximity of the bone surrounding the tooth. Each of these factors must be controlled to the best of the clinician's ability to obtain the optimal result, making osseous resective surgery an extremely precise technique.

It is assumed in this chapter that the gingival tissue has been reflected by the apically displaced flap, described in Chapter 55. Reshaping of the bone may necessitate selective changes in gingival height. These changes must be calculated and accounted for in the initial flap design. For this reason, it is important for the clinician to have a knowledge of the underlying bone tissue prior to flap reflection. The

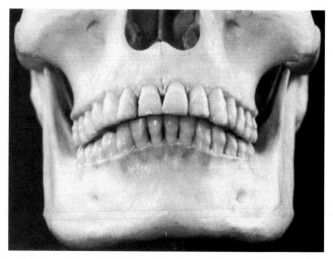

FIGURE 56–2. Skull photograph of a healthy periodontium. Note the shape of the alveolar bone housing. This bone is considered to have ideal form. It is more coronal in the interproximal areas, with a gradual slope around and away from the tooth.

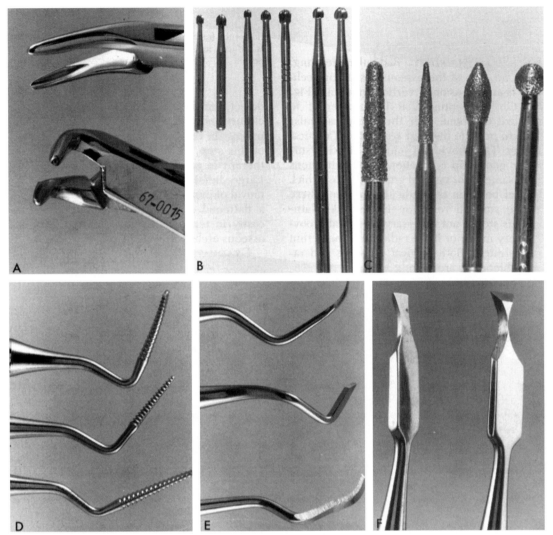

FIGURE 56–3. Instruments often used in osseous surgery. *A,* Rongeurs: Friedman *(top)* and 90-degree Blumenthal *(bottom). B,* Carbide round burs *(left to right):* friction grip, surgical-length friction grip, and slow-speed handpiece. *C,* Diamond burs. *D,* Interproximal files: Schluger and Sugarman. *E,* Back-action chisels. *F,* Ochsenbein chisels.

clinician must gain as much indirect knowledge as possible from soft tissue palpation, radiographic assessment, and transgingival probing (called *sounding*).

Radiographic examination can reveal the existence of angular bone losses in the interdental spaces; these usually coincide with infrabony pockets. The radiograph will not show the number of bony walls of the defect, nor will it determine with any accuracy the presence of angular bone defects on facial or lingual surfaces. Clinical examination and probing will determine the presence and depth of periodontal pockets on any surface of any tooth and can also give a general sense of the bony topography, but infrabony pockets can go undetected by probing. Both clinical and radiographic examinations can indicate the presence of infrabony pockets when (1) angular bone losses, (2) irregular bone losses, or (3) pockets of irregular depth in adjacent areas of the same tooth or adjacent teeth are found.

The experienced clinician can use *transgingival probing* to predict many features of the underlying bony topography. The information thus obtained can change the treat-

ment plan. For example, an area that had been selected for osseous resective surgery may be found to have a narrow defect that was unnoticed in the initial probing and radiographic assessment and is ideal for augmentation procedures. Such findings can and do change the flap design, the osseous procedure, and the result expected from the surgical intervention. Transgingival probing is extremely useful just prior to flap reflection. It is necessary to anesthetize the tissue locally prior to inserting the probe. The probe should be "walked" along the tissue–tooth interface so that the operator can feel the bony topography. The probe may also be passed horizontally through the tissue to provide more three-dimensional information regarding bony contours (i.e., the thickness, height, and shape of the underlying base). It must be remembered, however, that this information is still "blind," and although it is undoubtedly better than probing alone, it has significant limitations. Nevertheless, this step is recommended immediately prior to the surgical intervention.

The situations that can be encountered after periodontal flap reflection vary greatly. When all soft tissue is removed around the teeth, there may be large exostoses, ledges, troughs, craters, vertical defects, or combinations of any of these. For this reason, each osseous situation presents uniquely challenging problems, especially if reshaping to the optimal level is contemplated.

THE OSSEOUS RESECTION TECHNIQUE

Instruments Used. A number of hand and rotary instruments have been used for osseous resective surgery. Some excellent clinicians use only hand instruments and rongeurs, whereas others prefer a combination of hand and rotary instruments. Rotary instruments are useful for the osteoplastic steps outlined previously, whereas hand instruments provide the most precise and safe results with ostectomy procedures. Nevertheless, care and precision are required each step of the way to prevent excessive bone removal or root damage, both of which are irreversible. Figure 56–3 illustrates some of the instruments commonly used for osseous resective techniques.

Technique. In order to handle the multitude of clinical situations, the following sequential steps are suggested (Fig. 56–4A to D):

1. Vertical grooving
2. Radicular blending
3. Flattening interproximal bone
4. Gradualizing marginal bone

Not all steps are necessary in every case, but the sequencing of the steps in the order given is necessary to expedite the reshaping procedure, as well as to minimize the removal of bone.

Vertical Grooving. Vertical grooving is designed to reduce the thickness of the alveolar housing and to provide relative prominence to the radicular aspects of the teeth (see Fig. 56–4B, Fig. 56–11B, and Plate XVIII). It also provides continuity from the interproximal surface onto the radicular surface. It is the first step of the resective process, because it can define the general thickness and subsequent form of the alveolar housing. This step is usually performed with rotary instruments such as round carbide burs or diamonds. The advantages of vertical grooving are most apparent with thick, bony margins; shallow crater formations; or other areas that require maximal osteoplasty and minimal ostectomy. Vertical grooving is contraindicated in areas with close root proximity or thin alveolar housing.

Radicular Blending. Radicular blending, the second step of the osseous reshaping technique, is an extension of verti-

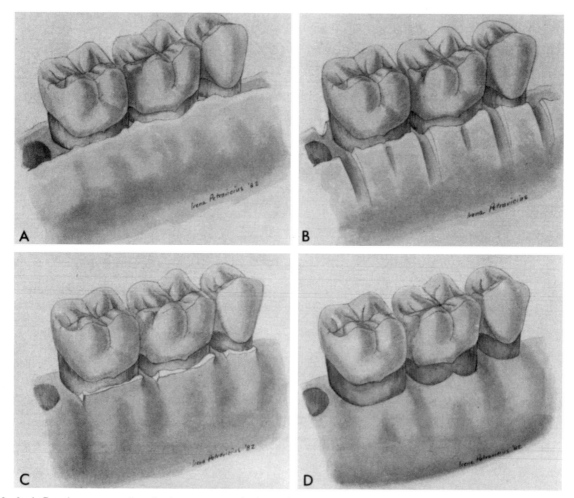

FIGURE 56–4. *A,* Drawing representing the bony topography in moderate periodontitis, with interdental craters. *B,* Vertical grooving, the first step in correction by osseous reshaping. *C,* Radicular blending and flattening of interproximal bone. *D,* Gradualizing the marginal bone. Note the area of the furcation on the first molar where the bone is preserved.

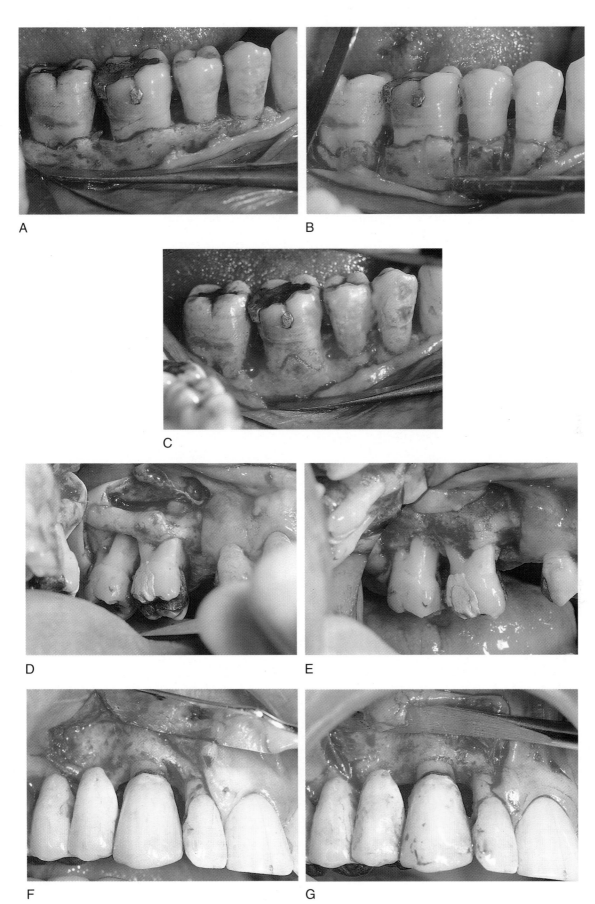

PLATE XVIII. Bone contouring in flap surgery. *A–C,* Bone contouring in interdental craters. *D* and *E,* Bone contouring in exostoses. *F* and *G,* Bone contouring in one-wall vertical defect.

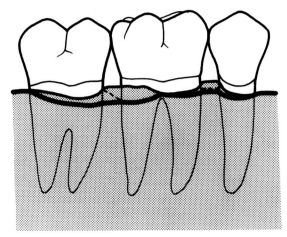

FIGURE 56–5. Diagrammatic representation of bone irregularities in periodontal disease. The thick line is the proposed correction of the defect. Note the flattening of the interproximal bone between the molars and the protection of the furcal bone on the first molar. Facial crest height is reduced in both interproximal areas to the depth of the defect.

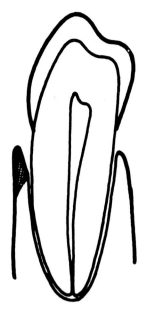

FIGURE 56–7. A one-wall defect located on the facial surface is reduced by osteoplasty. A one-wall defect located on an interproximal surface requires ostectomy for reduction.

cal grooving (see Fig. 56–4C). Conceptually, it is an attempt to gradualize the bone over the entire radicular surface to provide the best results from vertical grooving. This provides a smooth, blended surface for good flap adaptation. The indications are the same as for vertical grooving (i.e., thick ledges of bone on the radicular surface where selective surgical resection is desired). Naturally, this step is not necessary if vertical grooving is very minor or if the radicular bone is thin or fenestrated. Both vertical grooving and radicular blending are purely osteoplastic techniques that do not remove supporting bone. In most situations, they compose the bulk of osseous resective surgery. Classically, shallow crater formations, thick osseous ledges of bone on the radicular surface, and class I and early class II furcation involvements are treated almost totally with these two steps.

Flattening Interproximal Bone. Flattening of the inter-

dental bone requires the removal of very small amounts of supporting bone (Fig. 56–5). It is indicated when interproximal bone levels vary horizontally. By definition, most of the indications for this step will be one-wall interproximal defects or so-called hemiseptal defects. The omission

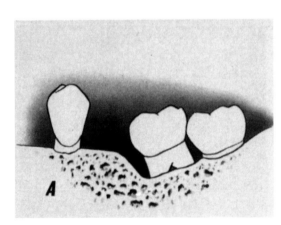

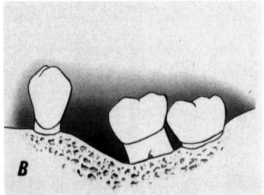

FIGURE 56–8. Reduction of a one-wall angular defect. *A,* Angular bone defect mesial to the tilted molar. *B,* Defect reduced by "ramping" angular bone.

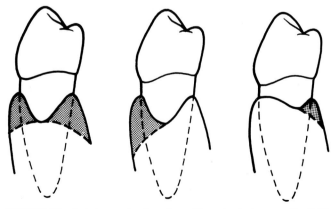

FIGURE 56–6. Interproximal craters. The shaded areas illustrate different techniques for the management of such defects. The technique that reduces the least amount of supporting bone is preferable.

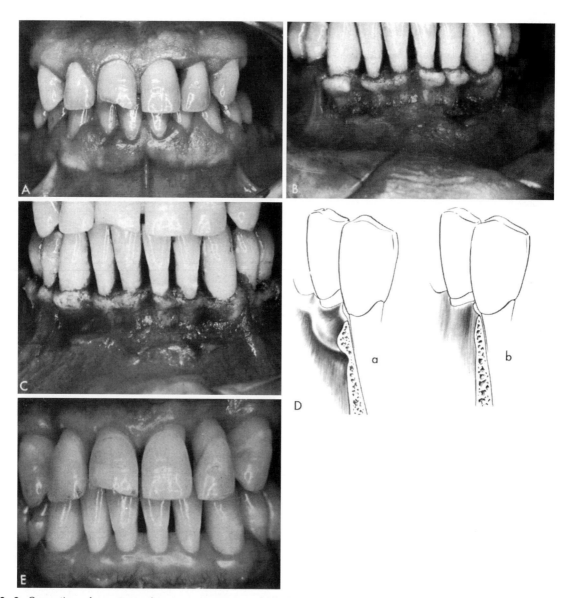

FIGURE 56–9. Correction of exostoses by osseous surgery. *A,* Periodontal disease in a patient with bulbous gingival contour in the mandible. *B,* Reflected flap reveals exostoses. *C,* Exostoses reduced, interdental grooves established, and interdental bone tapered inward and toward the crest. *D,* (a) Lateral view, showing exostosis. (b) Exostosis reduced and bone recontoured to provide interdental grooves. *E,* After 10 weeks, pockets are eliminated, and physiologic gingival contour is restored. Compare with *A.* (Courtesy of Dr. Charles A. Palioca.)

of flattening in such cases results in increased pocket depth on the most apical side of the bone loss. This step is typically not necessary in classic crater formations or in flat interproximal defects. It is best utilized in defects that have a coronally placed one-wall edge over a three-wall angular defect, and it can be helpful in obtaining good closure and, subsequently, improved healing in the three-wall defect. The limitation of this step, as with osseous resective surgical therapy in general, is in the treatment of advanced lesions. Large hemiseptal defects would require removal of inordinate amounts of bone to provide a flattened architecture, and the operation would be too costly in terms of bony support. Compromise osseous architecture is the only logical solution.

Gradualizing Marginal Bone. This final step in the osseous resective technique is also an ostectomy process.

Bone removal is minimal but necessary to provide a sound, regular base for the gingival tissue to follow. Failure to remove small bony discrepancies on the gingival line angles (often called "widow's peaks") allows the tissue to rise to a higher level than the base of the bone loss in the interdental area (see Fig. 56–4C,D). This may make the process of selective recession and subsequent pocket reduction incomplete. This step of the procedure also requires gradualization and blending of the radicular surfaces (see Fig. 56–5 and Plate XVIIIC). The two ostectomy steps should be performed with great care so as not to produce niches or grooves on the roots. When the radicular bone is thin, it is extremely easy to overdo this step, to the detriment of the entire surgical effort. For this reason, various hand instruments, such as chisels and curettes, are preferable to rotary instruments for gradualizing marginal bone.

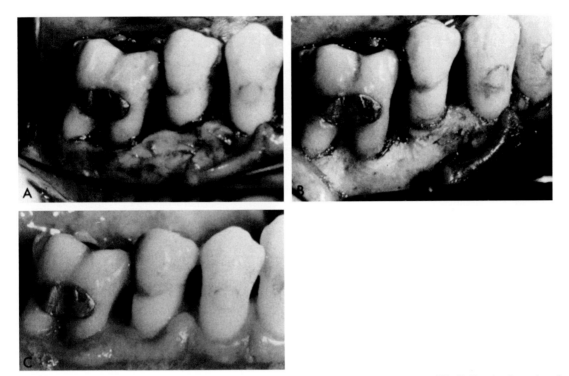

FIGURE 56–10. Photographs taken before osseous surgery *(A)* and after osseous management *(B). C,* Results 3 weeks after surgery.

SPECIFIC OSSEOUS RESHAPING SITUATIONS

The osseous corrective procedure that has been described is classically applied to shallow craters with heavy faciolingual ledges (Fig. 56–6). The correction of other osseous defects is also possible; however, careful case selection for definitive osseous surgery is very important.

Correction of one-wall hemiseptal defects requires that the bone be reduced to the level of the most apical portion of the defect. Therefore, great care should be taken to select defects that will not require unmanageable ostectomy on the well-supported tooth (Fig. 56–7). If one-wall defects occur next to an edentulous space, the edentulous ridge is reduced to the level of the osseous defect (Fig. 56–8).

Other situations that complicate osseous correction are exostoses (Fig. 56–9; see also Plate XVIII*D,E*), malpositioned teeth, and supraerupted teeth. Each of these situations is best controlled by following the four steps previously outlined. In most situations, the unique features of the bony profile will be well managed by prudently apply-

ing the same principles (Fig. 56–10; see also Plate XVIII). There are, however, situations that require deviation from the definitive osseous reshaping technique; examples include dilacerated roots, root proximity, and furcations that would be compromised by osseous surgery.

REFERENCES

1. Carranza FA Sr, Carranza FA Jr. The management of the alveolar bone in the treatment of the periodontal pocket. J Periodontol 27:29, 1956.
2. Friedman N. Periodontal osseous surgery: Osteoplasty and osteoectomy. J Periodontol 26:257, 1955.
3. Glickman I, Smulow JB, O'Brien T, Tannen R. Healing of the periodontium following mucogingival surgery. Oral Surg 16:530, 1963.
4. Knowles JN, Burgett FG, Morrison EC, et al. Comparison of results following three modalities of periodontal surgery related to tooth type and initial pocket depth. J Clin Periodontol 7:32, 1980.
5. Matherson DG. An evaluation of healing following periodontal osseous surgery in monkeys. Int J Periodont Restor Dent 8:9, 1988.
6. Ochsenbein C. Current status of osseous surgery. J Periodontol 48:577, 1977.
7. Ochsenbein C. A primer for osseous surgery. Int J Periodont Restor Dent 4:8, 1986.
8. Smith DH, Ammons WF Jr, Von Belle G. A longitudinal study of periodontal status comparing osseous recontouring with flap curettage. I. Results after six months. J Periodontol 51:367, 1980.
9. Zamet JS. A comparative clinical study of three periodontal surgical techniques. J Clin Periodontol 2:87, 1975.

57

Reconstructive Osseous Surgery

FERMIN A. CARRANZA, JR.

Evaluation of New Attachment and Bone Regeneration
Reconstructive Surgical Techniques

Non–Graft-Associated New Attachment
Graft Materials and Procedures
Summary

New attachment with bone regeneration is the ideal outcome of therapy, as it will result in obliteration of the pocket and reconstitution of the marginal periodontium (Plate XIX; Fig. 57–1). However, the techniques available are not totally dependable and the following other results of therapy may be seen (Fig. 57–2):

1. Healing with a long junctional epithelium, which can occur even if filling in of bone has occurred
2. Ankylosis of bone and tooth with resultant root resorption
3. Recurrence of the pocket
4. Any combination of the above

EVALUATION OF NEW ATTACHMENT AND BONE REGENERATION

It is sometimes difficult to determine whether new attachment has occurred and the extent to which it has occurred in clinical and experimental situations. Evidences of reconstruction of the marginal periodontium can be obtained by clinical, radiographic, surgical re-entry, or histologic procedures. All of these methods have advantages and shortcomings that should be well understood and considered in individual cases, as well as when critically evaluating the literature.

Clinical Methods. Clinical methods consist of comparison of pre- and post-treatment pocket probings, as well as determinations of clinical gingival indices. The probe can be used to determine pocket depth, attachment level, and bone level (see Chapter 28) (Fig. 57–3). Clinical determinations of attachment level are more useful than strict pocket depths, because the latter may change as a result of displacement of the gingival margin. Several studies have determined that the depth of penetration of a probe in a periodontal pocket varies according to the degree of inflammatory involvement of the tissues immediately beneath the bottom of the pocket (Fig. 57–4). Therefore, even though the forces used may be standardized with pressure-sensitive probes, there is an inherent margin of error in this method that is difficult to overcome. Fowler and colleagues[53] have calculated this error to be 1.2 mm, but it is even greater when furcations are probed.[113]

Bone probing performed under anesthesia is not subject to this error and has been found to be as accurate as bone height measurements made on surgical re-entry.[69,143,191]

Measurements of the defect should be made before and after treatment from the same exact point within the defect[134] and with the same angulation of the probe. This reproducibility of probe placement is difficult and may be facilitated in part by using a grooved stent to guide the introduction of the probe (Fig. 57–5). Preoperative and postoperative comparability of probing measurements that do not use this standardized method may be open to question.

Radiographic Methods. Radiographic evaluation of bone regeneration also requires carefully standardized techniques for reproducible positioning of the film and the tube.[128,149] Even with standardized techniques (see Chapter 30), the radiograph will not show the entire topography of the area before or after treatment. Furthermore, thin bone trabeculae may exist before treatment and go undetected radiographically because a certain minimal amount of mineralized tissue must be present to register on the radiograph. Several studies have demonstrated that radiographs, even those taken with standardized methods, are less reliable than clinical probing techniques.[88,184] Future studies with subtraction radiography will enhance the usefulness of radiographic evaluation.[191]

Surgical Re-entry. The surgical re-entry of a case after a period of healing can give a good view of the state of the bone crest that can be compared with the view taken during the initial surgical intervention and can also be subject to measurements (Fig. 57–6). Models from impressions taken of the bone at the time of the initial surgery and later at re-entry can be used to assess the results of therapy. This method is very useful but has two shortcomings: it requires a frequently unnecessary second operation, and it does not show the type of attachment that exists (i.e., new attachment or long junctional epithelium; Fig. 57–7).[29]

Histologic Methods. The type of attachment can be determined only by histologic analysis of tissue blocks obtained from the healed area. Although this method can offer clear evidence of regeneration of the attachment apparatus, it is not without problems. The need to remove a tooth with its periodontium after successful treatment limits this method to volunteers who need the extraction for prosthetic or other reasons and agree to the procedure.

Animal studies can be used to clarify some aspects of the tissue response to different materials. However, species differences should always be remembered when extrapola-

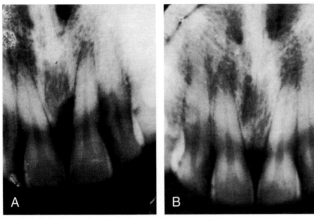

FIGURE 57–1. Bone regeneration after closed scaling, root planing, and curettage. Before *(A)* and after *(B)* radiographs are shown. (From Carranza FA Sr. J Periodontol *25*:272, 1954.)

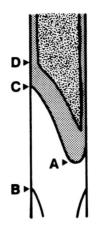

A–C: Pocket Depth
B–C: Level of Attachment
B–D: Bone Level

FIGURE 57–3. Different types of probings in an interdental space.

tions to humans are attempted. The compatibility of a material with the tissues can be shown by implanting the substance into the long bones or calvaria of rats or other rodents. This does not prove the regeneration of periodontal attachment.

Studies on the reconstruction of periodontal structures have been performed in dogs, monkeys, and pigs. Because it is difficult to find naturally occurring periodontal osseous defects that would be adequate for a study, experimentally induced bone defects must be used. Surgically produced bone defects can simulate the shape of osseous periodontal lesions but lack their chronicity and self-sustaining features. They are not exactly similar to naturally occurring disease. They can be allowed to become chronically infected, and then their similarity to chronic natural lesions is better, but it is never identical.[195] All these types of lesions have different healing sequences and provide different types of information.

In addition, the exact location of the bottom of the pocket must be determined prior to the procedure, because the surgical technique will open tissues beyond the bottom of the pocket, and healing below this point does not constitute new attachment. Notches on the root surface must be used to indicate this important point. Because the exact coronal point of the junctional epithelium is lost on surgically opening the area, a decision must be made as to whether to place the notch at the bottom of the calculus or on the crest of the alveolar bone (Fig. 57–8). The former is slightly coronal and the latter slightly apical to the real bottom of the pocket. The bottom of the calculus is a better landmark, but obviously the presence of calculus is required.

Numerous pitfalls are therefore inherent in histologic studies, and their accuracy and reliability should always be very carefully considered.

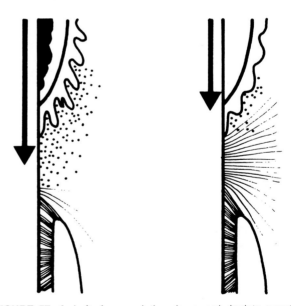

FIGURE 57–4. *Left, Arrow* pointing downward depicts penetration of a probe in an untreated periodontal pocket. The probe tip goes past the junctional epithelium and the inflamed tissue and is stopped by the first intact, attached collagen fibers. *Right,* After thorough scaling and root planing, the location of the bottom of the pocket has not changed, but the probe penetrates to only about one third the length of the junctional epithelium (see Chapter 28). *The reduction in probing depth may not reflect a change in attachment level.*

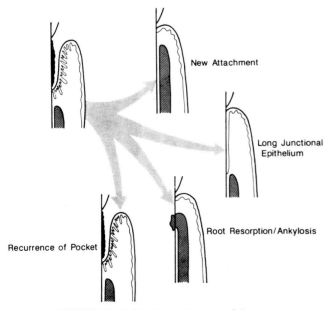

New Attachment

Long Junctional Epithelium

Recurrence of Pocket

Root Resorption/Ankylosis

FIGURE 57–2. Possible outcomes of therapy.

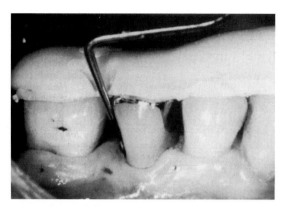

FIGURE 57–5. Grooved acrylic stent used in clinical research to standardize direction of introduction of the probe.

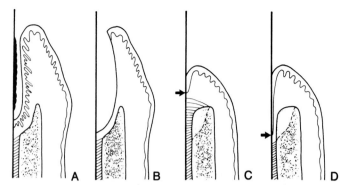

FIGURE 57–7. *A,* Periodontal pocket preoperatively. *B,* Periodontal pocket immediately after scaling, root planing, and curettage. *C,* New attachment. The arrow indicates the most apical part of the junctional epithelium. Note regeneration of bone and periodontal ligament. *D,* Healing by long junctional epithelium. Again, the *arrow* indicates the most apical part of the junctional epithelium. Note new bone but not new periodontal ligament.

RECONSTRUCTIVE SURGICAL TECHNIQUES

Reconstructive periodontics can be subdivided into two major areas: non–graft-associated new attachment and graft-associated new attachment. Many techniques, however, combine both approaches.

Non–Graft-Associated New Attachment

Periodontal reconstruction can be attained without the use of grafts in meticulously treated three-wall defects (intrabony defects)[24,64,137] and in periodontal and endodontal abscesses.[77,120] New attachment is more likely to occur when the destructive process has occurred very rapidly[120] (e.g., after treatment of pockets complicated by the formation of acute periodontal abscesses and after treatment of acute necrotizing ulcerative gingivitis).

Recommended techniques consist of careful and complete removal of all irritants, which may be done with or without exposure of the area with a flap. Trauma from occlusion may impair post-treatment healing of the supporting periodontal tissues, reducing the likelihood of new attachment. Occlusal adjustment, if needed, is therefore indicated.

This section will cover the rationale and technique for the removal of the junctional and pocket epithelium and the prevention of their migration into the healing area after therapy. It will also cover attempts at conditioning the root surface and the use of growth factors to enhance or direct healing.

Removal of Junctional and Pocket Epithelium

Since the earliest attempts at periodontal new attachment,[197] the presence of junctional and/or pocket epithelium has been perceived as a barrier to successful therapy. This perception is predicated on the fact that the presence of epithelium will interfere with the direct apposition of connective tissue and cementum and therefore will limit the height to which periodontal fibers can become inserted to the cementum.[114,140] Several methods have been recommended to remove junctional and pocket epithelia. These include curettage, chemical agents, ultrasonic methods, and surgical techniques.

Curettage. The removal of the epithelium by means of curettage has been studied histologically by several authors, and the results vary from complete removal to persistence of as much as 50% of junctional and pocket epithelia (for a complete review, see Smith and Echeverri[169]).

Chemical Agents. Chemical agents have also been used to remove pocket epithelium, in most cases in conjunction with curettage. The most commonly used drugs have been sodium sulfide, phenol camphor, antiformin, and sodium hypochlorite. However, the effect of these agents is not limited to the epithelium, and their depth of action cannot be controlled.

Ultrasonic Methods. Ultrasonics and abrasive stones have also been used, but their effects cannot be controlled

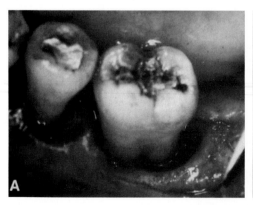

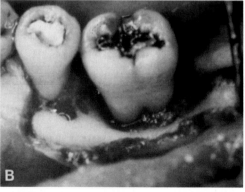

FIGURE 57–6. *A,* Osseous lesion around tooth #19 exposed by flap. *B,* Nine months later, the area is again exposed by a flap, and changes in the osseous lesion can be observed and measured. The nature of the new material, if any, present in the lesion and its connection to the tooth cannot be determined.

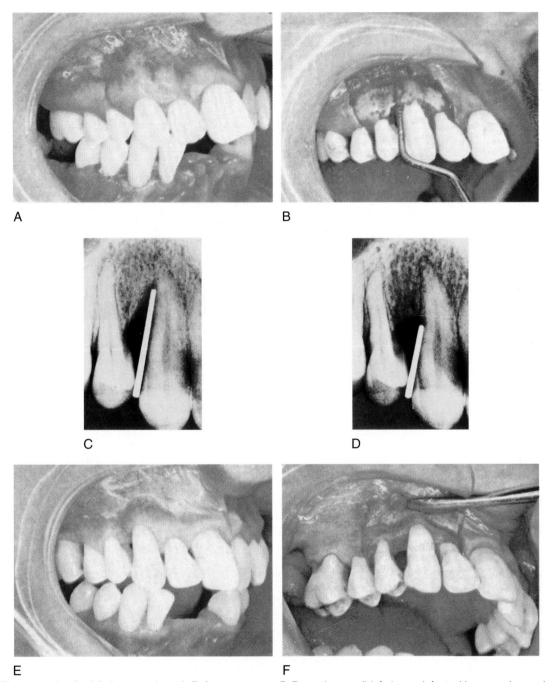

PLATE XIX. Flap operation for infrabony pocket. *A,* Before treatment. *B,* Deep three-wall infrabony defect with measuring probe inserted. *C,* Radiograph before treatment indicates angular osseous defect; gutta-percha point extends to base of pocket. *D,* Nine months after treatment. Radiograph indicates repair of osseous defect; gutta-percha point shows new level of sulcus. *E,* Nine months after treatment, the gingiva is healed with physiologic contour. *F,* Elevation of flap confirms radiographic appearance of repaired bone defect and new attachment of periodontium to tooth.

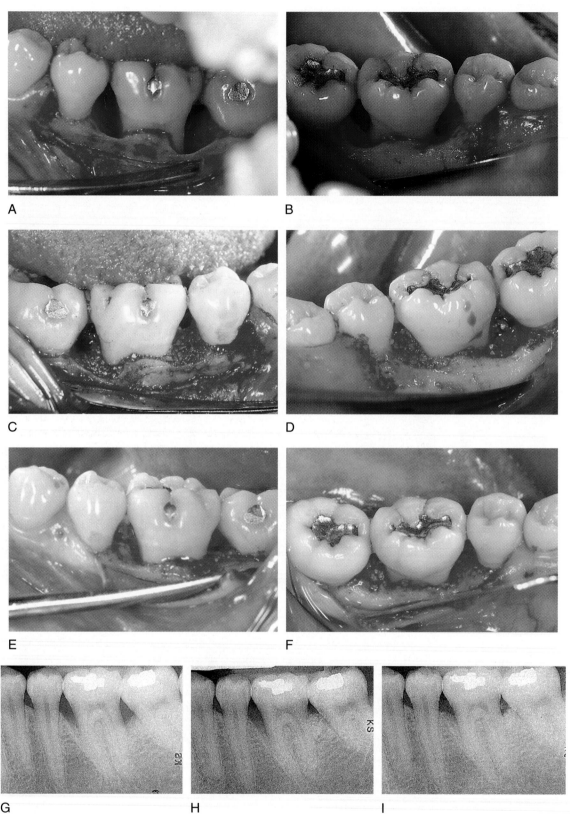

PLATE XX. Reconstructive periodontics: use of decalcified freeze-dried bone allografts (DFDBA) and porous hydroxyapatite. Facial view *(A)* and lingual view *(B)* of deep vertical lesions mesial and distal to lower first molar, exposed by a flap and debridement. Furcation is not involved. *C* and *D,* Facial and lingual views, respectively, of lesions filled with DFDBA (mesial defect) and porous hydroxyapatite (distal defect). This case was part of a study comparing both types of bone grafts. *E* and *F,* Facial and lingual views, respectively, of re-entry at 6 months postoperatively showing total fill of distal defect and partial fill of mesial defect. *G,* Preoperative radiograph. *H,* Radiograph immediately after placement of grafts. *I,* Radiograph 6 months later. (From Oreamuno S, Lekovic V, Kenney EB, et al. Comparative clinical study of porous hydroxyapatite and decalcified freeze-dried bone in human periodontal defects. J Periodontol *61:*399, 1990.)

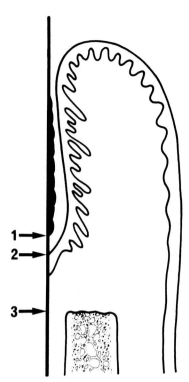

FIGURE 57–8. For future histologic reference, notches can be placed clinically at the most apical part of the calculus (1) or at the level of the osseous crest (3). However, the real landmark that will determine whether new attachment has taken place is the base of the pocket (2).

because of the clinician's lack of tactile sense when using these methods.

Surgical Techniques. Surgical techniques have been recommended to eliminate the pocket and junctional epithelia. The *excisional new attachment procedure*[198] consists of an internal bevel incision performed with a surgical knife, followed by removal of the excised tissue. No attempt is made to elevate a flap. After careful scaling and root planing, interproximal sutures are used to close the wound (see Chapter 50).

Glickman[63] and Prichard[137] have advocated performing a *gingivectomy* to the crest of the alveolar bone and then debriding the defect and removing all irritants. Excellent results have been obtained with this technique in uncontrolled human studies.[5,137]

The *modified Widman flap,* as described by Ramfjord and Nissle,[141] is similar to the excisional new attachment procedure but is followed by elevation of a flap for better exposure of the area. It eliminates the pocket epithelium with the internal bevel incision (see Chapter 55).

Another approach to delaying epithelial migration into the healing pocket area has been the use of *coronal displacement of the flap,* which increases the distance between the epithelium and the healing area. This technique is particularly suitable for the treatment of lower molar furcations and has been used mostly in conjunction with citric acid treatment of the roots.[60,101]

The technique is performed as follows (Fig. 57–9):

1. Fasten an orthodontic tube to the coronal tooth surface by means of an enamel bonding composite resin.
2. Raise a mucoperiosteal flap using intrasulcular incisions and

a vertical incision to include the mesial and distal papillae of the tooth being treated.
3. Perform meticulous scaling and root planing, and apply citric acid.
4. Make an incision fenestrating the periosteum at the base of the surgical flap to permit its elongation.
5. Displace the flap coronally and suture it to the tube with a 4-0 silk suture as follows: pass the suture through the tube, starting in its mesial opening; continue in a horizontal mattress fashion in the distal corner of the flap; pass it interdentally and around the tooth; pass it interdentally in the mesial aspects; then perform a horizontal mesial mattress suture and tie it.

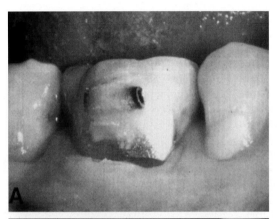

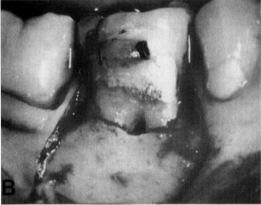

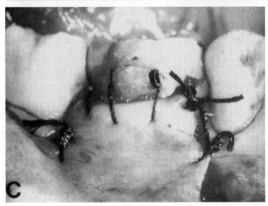

FIGURE 57–9. Coronal placement of flap. *A,* A tube attached to the crown and reinforced with bonding material. Note the relationship of the gingival margin to class V gold foil. *B,* The flap reflected, and grade II furcation debrided. *C,* The flap is coronally elevated and sutured through the tube. Note the gingival margin's relationship to gold foil. (Courtesy of Dr. Steven Garrett, Loma Linda University.)

6. Use interrupted sutures for the vertical incisions.

Periodontal regeneration after the use of this technique has been demonstrated histologically in humans.[176]

Prevention of Epithelial Migration

Elimination of junctional and pocket epithelia may not be sufficient, because the epithelium from the excised margin may rapidly proliferate apically to become interposed between the healing connective tissue and the cementum.

Several investigators have analyzed in animals[9] and in humans[10,14] the effect of excluding the epithelium by amputating the crown of the tooth and covering the root with the flap (root submergence). This experimental technique not only excludes the epithelium, but also prevents microbial contamination of the wound during the reparative stages. Successful repair of osseous lesions in the submerged environment was reported.

The following clinical methods have been proposed to prevent or retard the migration of the epithelium. Ellegaard and colleagues[42] developed a technique to be used in conjunction with bone grafts, but its purpose was the prevention of epithelial migration. It consists of total removal of the interdental papilla covering the defect to be treated and replacement of the papilla with a free autogenous graft obtained from the palate (Fig. 57–10). During healing, the epithelium necroses, and its migration is retarded.

Guided Tissue Regeneration. Another approach to the prevention of epithelial migration along the cemental wall of the pocket consists of placing barriers of different types to cover the bone and periodontal ligament.[67,68,124] This method is called *guided tissue regeneration* and is based on the assumption that only the periodontal ligament cells have the potential for regeneration of the attachment apparatus of the tooth (see Chapter 33). Excluding the epithelium and the gingival connective tissue from the root surface during the postsurgical healing phase favors repopulation of the area by periodontal ligament and bone cells.

Two types of membranes have been used: degradable and nondegradable membranes. The latter must be removed after the initial healing stages, usually 3 to 6 weeks, while the former are resorbed and therefore do not require a second intervention. Animal experiments using nondegradable membranes (e.g., Millipore filters and Teflon membranes), resulted in regeneration of cementum and alveolar bone and a functional periodontal ligament.[27,28,31,112]

Clinical case reports have shown that guided tissue regeneration results in a gain in attachment level, but this is not necessarily associated with a buildup of alveolar bone.[6,7] Histologic studies in humans have provided evidence of periodontal regeneration in most instances,[68,179] even in cases of horizontal bone losses.[174]

The use of polytetrafluoroethylene membranes (Gore-Tex periodontal material, Flagstaff, AZ) has been tested in controlled clinical studies in lower molar furcations[91,136] and has shown statistically significant decreases in pocket depths and improvement in attachment levels after 6 months; bone level measurements have been inconclusive. A study on upper molar furcations did not result in significant gain in attachment or bone levels.[111]

The recommended technique uses the Gore-Tex membrane, which can be obtained in different shapes and sizes to suit proximal spaces and facial/lingual surfaces of furcations (Fig. 57–11). The technique is as follows (Figs. 57–12 and 57–13):

Step 1: Raise a mucoperiosteal flap with vertical incisions, extending a minimum of two teeth anteriorly and one tooth distally to the tooth being treated.

Step 2: Debride the osseous defect and thoroughly plane the roots.

Step 3: Trim the membrane with sharp scissors to the approximate size of the area being treated. The apical border of the material should extend 3 to 4 mm apical to the margin of the defect and laterally 2 to 3 mm beyond the

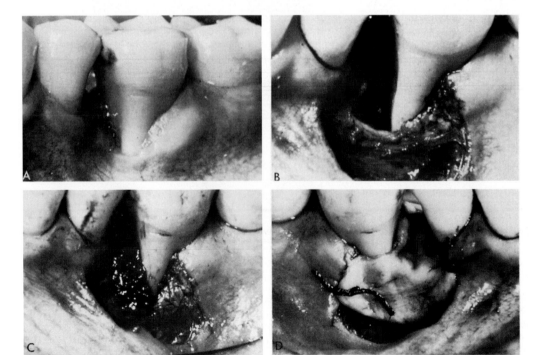

FIGURE 57–10. Ellegaard technique for preventing epithelial migration. *A,* Preoperative photograph illustrates the bone defect on the mesial aspect of the molar. *B,* The area is debrided of connective tissue. *C,* Osseous material is placed in the defect. *D,* A free gingival graft is placed over the osseous material and secured with interrupted sutures.

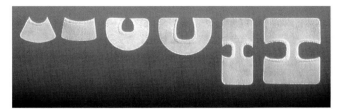

FIGURE 57–11. Different shapes and sizes of expanded polytetrafluoroethylene membranes marketed by Gore-Tex.

defect; the occlusal border of the membrane should be placed 2 mm apical to the cemento-enamel junction.[7]

Step 4: The membrane is tightly sutured around the tooth with a sling suture.

Step 5: The flap is then sutured in its original position or slightly coronal to it, using independent sutures interdentally and in the vertical sutures. The flap should cover the membrane completely.

Step 6: The use of periodontal dressings is optional, and the patient is placed on antibiotic therapy for 1 week.

After 4 to 6 weeks, the margin of the membrane becomes exposed. The membrane is removed with a gentle tug 5 weeks after the operation. If it cannot be removed easily, the tissues are anesthetized and the material is surgically removed.

The results obtained with the guided tissue regeneration technique are enhanced when the technique is combined with grafts placed in the defects.[3,13,89,102]

The Use of Biodegradable Membranes. The search for membranes that can be resorbed by the organism after a few weeks has been intense in the last decade. The materials tested include rat collagen,[130–132] bovine collagen,[11,12,30,100] Cargile membrane derived from the cecum of an ox,[23] polylactic acid,[99,195] Vycril (polyglactin 910),[52,59] synthetic skin (Biobrane),[51] and freeze-dried dura mater.[200] Of these, only a mixture of copolymers derived from polylactic acid and acetyl tributylcitrate (Guidor) has been marketed, but controlled clinical and laboratory research is needed to verify its effectiveness.[66]

The potential of autogenous periosteum to stimulate periodontal regeneration has also been explored in a controlled clinical study of grade II furcation involvements in lower molars.[90] The periosteum was obtained from patients' palates by means of a window flap. Six months after surgery, the experimental teeth showed, in comparison with the controls, significant reduction in pocket depth and gain in attachment level, as well as in vertical and horizontal measurements of the inter-radicular bone. The latter measurements were performed at re-entry surgery.

Clot Stabilization, Wound Protection, and Space Creation

Some investigators have attributed the successful results reported with graft materials, barrier membranes, and coronally displaced flaps to the fact that all of these protect the

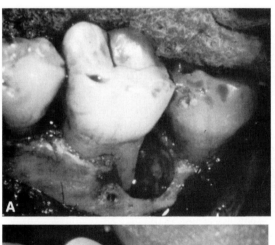

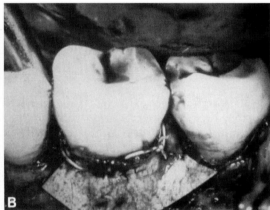

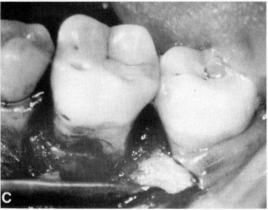

FIGURE 57–12. Patient treated according to the principles of guided tissue regeneration. *A,* Deep osseous defect on the distal root of a lower molar. *B,* After thorough instrumentation, the Gore-Tex membrane is placed. *C,* Re-entry after 9 months, showing the defect fill. (Courtesy of Dr. Burton Becker and Dr. William Becker.)

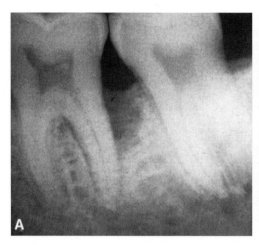
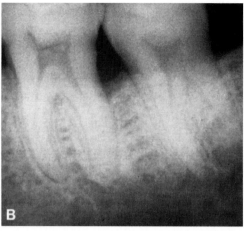

FIGURE 57–13. Before *(A)* and after *(B)* radiographs of patient shown in Fig. 57–12. (Courtesy of Dr. Burton Becker and Dr. William Becker.)

wound and create a space for undisturbed and stable maturation of the clot.[61] This hypothesis suggests that preservation of the root surface–fibrin clot interface prevents apical migration of the gingival epithelium and allows for connective tissue attachment during the early wound healing period.[61,196] However, this technique would require meticulous postoperative care to avoid any trauma to the wound, including use of resorbable sutures, carefully applied periodontal dressing, only chemotherapeutic plaque control (chlorhexidine gluconate) for 6 weeks, and very gentle professional debridement every other week for 2 months. It would also increase the need for agents to enhance the root surface's biological acceptance of fibrin clot and connective tissue attachment[61] (see later discussion).

Preparation of the Root Surface

Changes in the tooth surface wall of periodontal pockets (e.g., degeneration of remnants of Sharpey's fibers, accumulation of bacteria and their products, and disintegration of the cementum and dentin) interfere with new attachment. However, these obstacles to new attachment can be eliminated by thorough root planing. Careful curettage of the pocket wall surface should also be performed to remove granulation tissue and provide better visibility and accessibility to the root surface.

Several substances have been used in attempts to better condition the root surface for attachment of new connective tissue fibers. These include citric acid, fibronectin, and tetracycline.

Citric Acid. Studies by Urist[188] showed that the implantation of demineralized dentin matrix into muscle tissue in animals induced mesenchymal cells to differentiate into osteoblasts and start an osteogenic process. Following up on this concept, Register and Burdick[142] performed a series of studies that showed that citric acid at pH 1, when applied for 2 to 3 minutes on root surfaces, produced a surface demineralization that induced cementogenesis and attachment of collagen fibers.

The following actions of citric acid have been reported:
1. Accelerated healing and new cementum formation occur after surgical detachment of the gingival tissues and demineralization of the root surface by means of citric acid.[142]
2. Topically applied citric acid on periodontally diseased root surfaces has no effect on nonplaned roots, but after root

planing, the acid produces a 4-μm-deep demineralized zone with exposed collagen fibers.[62]
3. Root-planed, non–acid-treated roots are left with a surface smear layer of microcrystalline debris; citric acid application not only removes the smear layer, exposing the dentinal tubules, but also makes the tubules appear wider and with funnel-shaped orifices.[133]
4. Citric acid has also been shown in vitro to eliminate endotoxins[50] and bacteria[35] from the diseased tooth surface.
5. Epithelium does not migrate apically along denuded roots treated with citric acid.[135] This may be due to an early fibrin linkage to collagen fibers exposed by the citric acid treatment.

This technique has been extensively investigated in animals and humans. Studies in dogs have given encouraging results,[142] especially for the treatment of furcation lesions,[33,123] but the results of studies in humans have been contradictory.[144,172]

The recommended technique is as follows:
1. Raise a mucoperiosteal flap.
2. Thoroughly instrument the root surface, removing calculus and underlying cementum.
3. Apply cotton pledgets soaked in a saturated solution of citric acid (pH 1), and leave on for 2 to 5 minutes.
4. Remove pledgets, and irrigate root surface profusely with water.
5. Replace the flap and suture.

The use of citric acid has also been recommended in conjunction with coverage of denuded roots using free gingival grafts (see Chapter 59).

Fibronectin. Fibronectin is the glycoprotein that fibroblasts require to attach to root surfaces. The addition of fibronectin to the root surface may promote new attachment.[22,48,182] However, increasing fibronectin above plasma levels produces no obvious advantages. Adding fibronectin and citric acid to lesions treated with guided tissue regeneration (GTR) in dogs did not improve the results.[20,170]

Tetracycline. In vitro treatment of the dentin surfaces with tetracycline increases binding of fibronectin, which in turn stimulates fibroblast attachment and growth while suppressing epithelial cell attachment and migration.[183] It also removes an amorphous surface layer and exposes the dentin tubules.[194] In vivo studies, however, have not shown favorable results.[195] A human study showed a trend for greater connective tissue attachment after tetracycline treatment of roots; tetracycline alone gave better results than when combined with fibronectin.[2]

Case reports have been presented showing extensive regeneration of the periodontal lesions after antibiotic treatment with penicillin[24] or tetracycline[118] in combination with other forms of therapy.

Growth Factors

Growth factors are polypeptide molecules, released by cells in the inflamed area, that regulate events in wound healing. They can be considered hormones that are not released into the blood stream but have only a local action. Growth substances regulate connective tissue cell migration and proliferation and synthesis of proteins and other components of the extracellular matrix.

These factors, primarily secreted by macrophages, endothelial cells, fibroblasts, and platelets, include platelet-derived growth factor (PDGF), insulin-like growth factor (IGF), basic fibroblastic growth factor (bFGF), and transforming growth factor (TGF)–α and –β. Growth factors could be used to control events during periodontal wound healing (e.g., promoting proliferation of fibroblasts from the periodontal ligament and favoring bone formation).[186] According to Lynch,[98] a combination of PGDF and IGF-1 would be effective in promoting growth of all the components of the periodontium.

For a review of this important topic, see Lynch.[98]

Graft Materials and Procedures

Numerous therapeutic grafting modalities for restoring periodontal osseous defects have been investigated. Periodontal defects as sites for transplantation differ from osseous cavities surrounded by bony walls. Saliva and bacteria may easily penetrate along the root surface, and epithelial cells may proliferate into the defect, resulting in contamination and possible exfoliation of the grafts. Therefore, the principles established to govern transplantation of bone or other materials into closed osseous cavities are not fully applicable to transplantation of bone into periodontal defects.[40]

The considerations that govern the selection of a material have been defined by Schallhorn as follows:[160]

- Biologic acceptability
- Predictability
- Clinical feasibility
- Minimal operative hazards
- Minimal postoperative sequelae
- Patient acceptance

It is difficult to find a material with all of these characteristics, and to date there is no "ideal" material or technique. Once the material is placed in the bony defect, it may act in a number of ways. It may have no effect; it may act only as a scaffolding material for the host to lay down new bone; it may actively induce bone formation; or through its own viability it may deposit new bone in the defect.

Graft materials have been developed and tried in many complex forms. To familiarize the reader with various types of graft material, as defined by either the technique or the material used, a brief discussion of each is provided.

All grafting techniques require presurgical scaling, oc-

clusal adjustment as needed, and exposure of the defect with a full-thickness flap. The flap technique best suited for grafting purposes is the papilla preservation flap,[181] because it provides complete coverage of the interdental area after suturing. (See Chapter 55 for a description of the technique.) The use of antibiotics after the procedure is generally recommended.

Autogenous Bone Grafts

Bone From Intraoral Sites. In 1923, Hegedus attempted to use bone grafts for the reconstruction of bone defects produced by periodontal disease.[74] The method was revived by Nabers and O'Leary[118] in 1965, and numerous efforts have been made since that time to define its indications and technique.

Sources of bone include bone from healing extraction wounds,[76,147] bone from edentulous ridges,[76] bone trephined from within the jaw without damaging the roots, newly formed bone in wounds especially created for the purpose,[71] and bone removed during osteoplasty and ostectomy.

Osseous Coagulum. Robinson described a technique using a mixture of bone dust and blood that he termed osseous coagulum.[146] The technique uses small particles

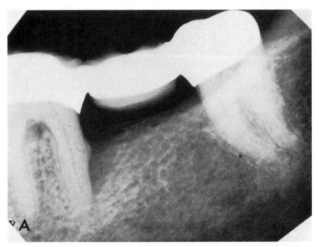

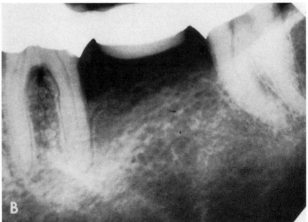

FIGURE 57–14. Bone defect on the distal root of a first molar treated with osseous coagulum implants. *A,* Before treatment. *B,* One year after treatment. (Courtesy of Dr. R. Earl Robinson.)

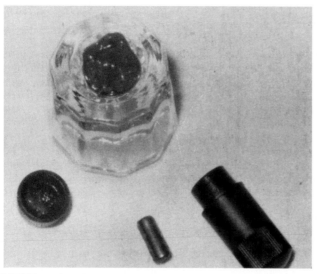

FIGURE 57–15. The sterile capsule shown at the bottom of the photograph is used to produce the soft, pliable osseous mass present in the top of the dappen dish.

ground from cortical bone. The advantage of the particle size is that it provides additional surface area for the interaction of cellular and vascular elements.

Sources of the implant material include the lingual ridge on the mandible, exostoses, edentulous ridges, the bone distal to a terminal tooth, bone removed by osteoplasty or ostectomy, and the lingual surface of the mandible or maxilla at least 5 mm from the roots. Bone is removed with a carbide bur, no. 6 or no. 8, at speeds between 5000 and 30,000 rpm. The coagulum formed by mixing the bone particles and blood is placed in a sterile dappen dish or amalgam cloth.

The coagulum is placed in the defect a little at a time, starting at the bottom and packing and drying with moist gauze until there is a considerable excess. The flap is replaced over the coagulum and sutured (Fig. 57–14). The obvious advantage of this technique is the ease of obtaining bone from already exposed surgical sites. This technique is also very quick to accomplish and can be performed in areas without great preparation. In addition, it complements osseous resective techniques needed in the area (see Chapter 56).

The disadvantages of the technique are centered on its relatively low predictability[54] and on the inability to procure adequate material for large defects. Although notable success has been reported by many individuals, studies documenting the efficacy of the technique are still inconclusive.[32,55,57,146]

Bone Blend. Some of the disadvantages of osseous coagulum derive from the inability to use aspiration during accumulation of the coagulum; another problem is the unknown quantity and quality of the bone fragments in the collected material. To overcome these problems, the so-called bone blend technique has been proposed.[36]

The bone blend technique uses an autoclaved plastic capsule and pestle (Fig. 57–15). Bone is removed from a predetermined site (extraction socket, exostosis, edentulous area, or region of the defect) with chisels or rongeur forceps. The pestle and bone fragments are placed in the cap-

sule, and a few drops of sterile saline are added. The capsule is closed, wrapped in sterile gauze, and placed in the triturator. The bone is triturated for 60 seconds. A dense mass of bone, such as that removed from an exostosis, may require more blending time. After trituration, the bone blend is observed clinging to the walls of the capsule and to the pestle. It is removed from the capsule with a spoon-shaped instrument. Trituration reduces the bone fragments to a workable, plastic-like osseous mass, similar in consistency to slushy amalgam, that can be packed or molded into bony defects (see Fig. 57–15).

Froum and coworkers have found osseous coagulum–bone blend procedures to be at least as effective as iliac autografts and open curettage.[55–57]

Intraoral Cancellous Bone Marrow Transplants. Hiatt and Schallhorn have described the use of cancellous bone obtained from the maxillary tuberosity, edentulous areas, and healing sockets.[76]

The maxillary tuberosity frequently contains a good amount of cancellous bone, particularly if the third molars are not present; also, foci of red marrow are occasionally observed. After a ridge incision is made distally from the last molar, bone is removed with a curved and cutting rongeur. Care should be taken not to extend the incision too far distally, to avoid sectioning the tendons of the palatine muscle; also, the location of the maxillary sinus has to be analyzed on the radiograph to avoid cutting into it.

Edentulous ridges can be approached with a flap, and cancellous bone and marrow are removed with curettes. Healing sockets are allowed to heal for 8 to 12 weeks, and the apical portion is utilized as donor material. The particles are reduced to small pieces (Figs. 57–16 and 57–17).

Bone Swaging.[46,151] This technique requires the existence of an edentulous area adjacent to the defect from which the bone is pushed into contact with the root surface without fracturing the bone at its base (Fig. 57–18). This technique is complicated by varying degrees of elasticity of the bone. Bone with a greater cancellous composition is more flexible. Bone without adequate cancellous material tends to fracture from the alveolus, providing a noncontiguous bone graft. Thus, bone swaging is technically difficult, and its usefulness is limited.

Bone From Extraoral Sites

Iliac Autografts. The use of fresh or preserved iliac cancellous marrow has been extensively investigated. This material has been used by orthopedic surgeons for years. Schallhorn and coworkers[157,158,162] and others[8,17,34,37–39,71] have provided data from human and animal studies to support the use of autogenous iliac grafts. This technique has proved successful in bony defects with various numbers of walls, in furcations, and even supracrestally to some extent (Fig. 57–19). However, problems have also been associated with its use. Schallhorn has observed postoperative sequelae of infection, exfoliation, and sequestration; varying rates of healing; root resorption; and rapid recurrence of the defect.[159] The last two, which of course have the most lasting effects, have been observed by other authors as well[17,39] (Fig. 57–20). For these reasons, in addition to problems of increased patient expense and difficulty in procuring the donor material,[160] the technique is no longer in use.

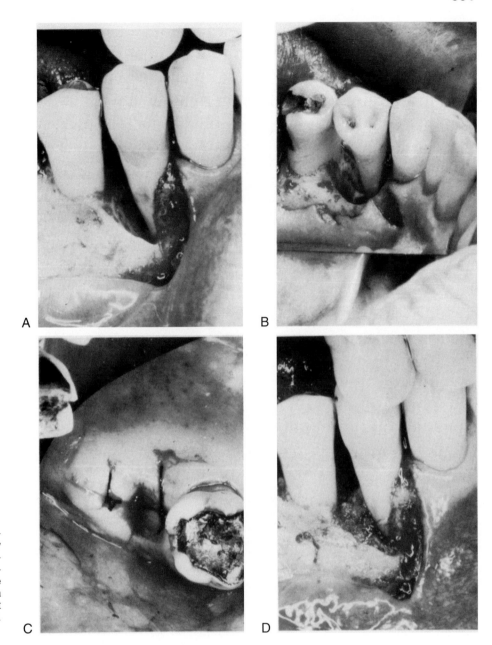

FIGURE 57–16. Autogenous bone transplant from extraction site. *A,* Buccal view of an angular defect on the distal surface of the first premolar. *B,* Elevated lingual mucoperiosteal flap and view of the angular defect. *C,* Bone obtained from a 6-week-old extraction site. *D,* The defect filled with bone implant. (Courtesy of Dr. Edward S. Cohen.)

Allografts

Obtaining donor material for autograft purposes necessitates inflicting surgical trauma on another part of the patient's body. Obviously, it would be to the patient's as well as the therapist's advantage if a suitable substitute could be utilized for grafting purposes that would offer similar potential for repair and not require the additional surgical removal of donor material from the patient. However, both allografts and xenografts are foreign to the organism and therefore have the potential to provoke an immune response.

Attempts have been made to suppress the antigenic potential of allografts and xenografts by radiation, freezing, and chemical treatment.[16]

Bone allografts are commercially available from tissue banks. They are obtained from cortical bone within 12 hours of the death of the donor, defatted, cut in pieces, washed in absolute alcohol, and deep frozen. The material may or may not then be demineralized, and subsequently, it is ground and sieved to a particle size of 250 to 750 μm and freeze-dried. Finally it is vacuum sealed in glass vials.

Numerous steps are also taken to eliminate viral infectivity. These include exclusion of donors from known high-risk groups as well as various tests on the cadaver and the tissues to exclude individuals with any type of infection or malignant disease. The material is then treated with chemical agents or strong acids to effectively inactivate the virus. The risk of human immunodeficiency virus (HIV) infection has been calculated as 1 in 1 to 8 million and characterized as "highly remote."[110]

Undecalcified Freeze-Dried Bone Allograft (FDBA). Several clinical studies by Mellonig, Bowers, and coworkers[109,152,166] reported bone fill exceeding 50% in 67% of the defects grafted with FDBA and in 78% of the defects

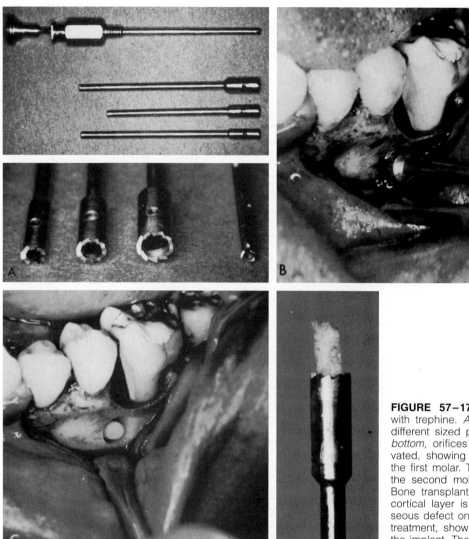

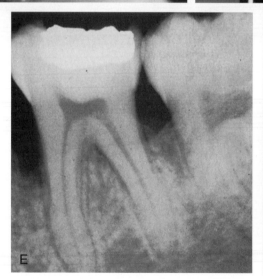

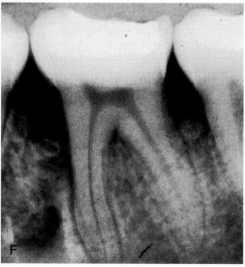

FIGURE 57-17. Autogenous bone transplant obtained with trephine. *A,* Trephines: *top,* manual trephine; *center,* different sized power trephines (no. 2, no. 4, and no. 6); *bottom,* orifices of trephines. *B,* Mucoperiosteal flap elevated, showing osseous defect on the mesial surface of the first molar. The trephine is inserted into bone distal to the second molar. *C,* Bone separated by a trephine. *D,* Bone transplant; the cancellous portion is used, and the cortical layer is removed. *E,* Radiograph showing an osseous defect on mandibular first molar. *F,* Six months after treatment, showing the osseous defect partially filled with the implant. The radiolucent area in the interdental bone is the donor site of the transplant.

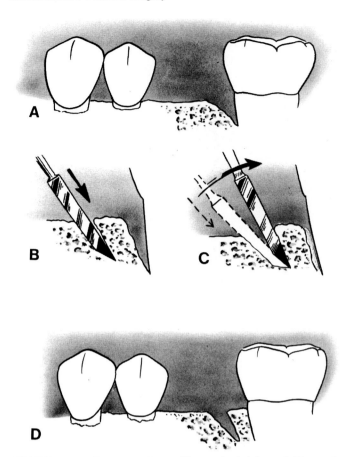

FIGURE 57–18. Bone swaging to fill a vertical defect. *A,* The vertical defect on the mesial aspect of the mandibular molar. *B,* Separate section chiseled. *C,* Bone swaged into the vertical defect *(arrow). D,* The vertical defect filled with bone.

grafted with FDBA plus autogenous bone. FDBA, however, is considered an osteoconductive material, while decalcified FDBA (DFDBA) is considered an osteoinductive graft; laboratory studies[107,108] have found that DFDBA has a higher osteogenic potential than FDBA and is therefore preferred.[106]

Decalcified Freeze-Dried Bone Allografts. Experiments by Urist and coworkers[187–189] have established the osteogenic potential of DFDBAs. Demineralization in cold diluted hydrochloric acid exposes the components of bone matrix, closely associated with collagen fibrils, that have been termed *bone morphogenetic protein.*[189]

In 1975 Libin et al.[95] reported on three patients with 4 to 10 mm of bone regeneration in periodontal osseous defects. Subsequent clinical studies were made with cancellous DFDBA[129] and with cortical DFDBA.[138] The latter resulted in more desirable results (2.4 mm vs. 1.38 mm of bone fill).

Bowers and associates,[14] in a histologic study in humans, showed new attachment (new bone, cementum, and periodontal ligament) in periodontal defects grafted with DFDBA. Mellonig and associates[107,108] tested DFDBA against autogenous materials in the calvaria of guinea pigs and showed it to have similar osteogenic potential.

These studies provide strong evidence that DFDBA in periodontal defects results in significant probing depth reduction, attachment level gain, and osseous regeneration

(Plate XX); the combination of DFDBA and guided tissue regeneration has also proven very successful.[3,176] However, limitations of the use of DFDBA include the possible, albeit remote, potential of disease transfer from the cadaver.

A bone-inductive protein isolated from the extracellular matrix of human bones, termed *osteogenin,* has been tested in human periodontal defects and seems to enhance osseous regeneration.[15]

Xenografts

Calf bone (Boplant), treated by detergent extraction, sterilized, and freeze-dried, has been used for the treatment of osseous defects.[4,163,165] *Kiel bone* is calf or ox bone denatured with 20% hydrogen peroxide, dried with acetone, and sterilized with ethylene oxide. *Anorganic bone* is ox bone from which the organic material has been extracted by means of ethylenediamine; it is then sterilized by autoclaving.[104,105] These materials have been tried and discarded for various reasons; they are mentioned here to provide a historical perspective.

Nonbone Graft Materials

In addition to bone graft materials, many different nonbone graft materials have been tried for restoration of the periodontium. Among them are sclera,[84–86,116,185] dura,[43] cartilage,[153,155] cementum,[154] dentin,[154,164] plaster of Paris,[87,171] plastic materials, calcium phosphate materials,[93,94,122] and coral-derived materials. None of these offers a reliable substitute to bone graft materials, but they are presented here to offer a complete picture of the many attempts that have been made to solve the crucial problem of periodontal regeneration.

Sclera. Sclera was originally utilized in periodontal procedures because it is a dense fibrous connective tissue with poor vascularity and minimal cellularity.[85,86] This affords a low incidence of antigenicity and other untoward reactions.[79] In addition, sclera may provide a barrier to apical migration of the junctional epithelium and serve to protect the blood clot during the initial healing period (Fig. 57–21).

Although some studies show that sclera is well accepted by the host and is sometimes invaded by host cells and capillaries and replaced by dense connective tissue,[47] it does not appear to induce osteogenesis or cementogenesis.[116,127,185] The available scientific research does not warrant the routine use of sclera in periodontal therapy.

Cartilage. Cartilage has been used for repair studies in monkeys and for treatment of periodontal defects in humans.[153,155] It can serve as a scaffolding; when so used, new attachment was obtained in 60 of 70 case studies.[155] However, cartilage has received only limited evaluation.

Plaster of Paris. Plaster of Paris (calcium sulfate) is biocompatible and porous, thereby allowing fluid exchange, which prevents flap necrosis. Plaster of Paris resorbs completely in 1 to 2 weeks. It was found to be useful in one uncontrolled clinical study,[1] but other investigators have reported that it does not induce bone formation.[167] One report[171] suggested its use in combination with DFDBA and

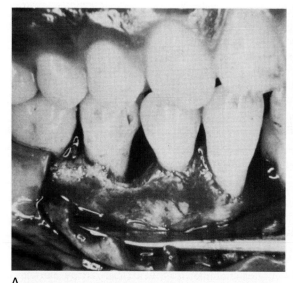
A

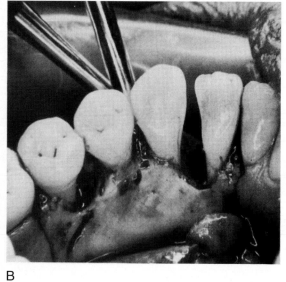
B

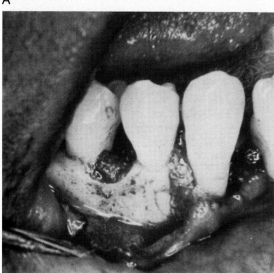
C

FIGURE 57–19. Autogenous hip marrow implant. *A,* Mucoperiosteal flap reveals osseous defect on the second premolar. *B,* Lingual view of infrabony defect revealed by periosteal flap. (Note the defect between the canine and the lateral incisor.) *C,* Hip marrow implant in premolar osseous defect. *D,* Osseous defect before treatment. The gutta-percha point is at the base of the pocket. *E,* Seven months after treatment. The bone is repaired. The gutta-percha point is at the base of the healed sulcus, which is now attached higher on the root. (Courtesy of Dr. Edward S. Cohen.)

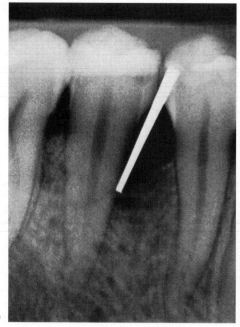
D

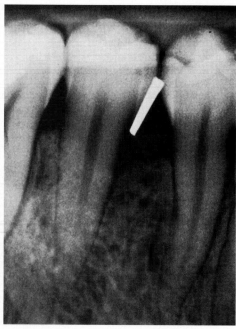
E

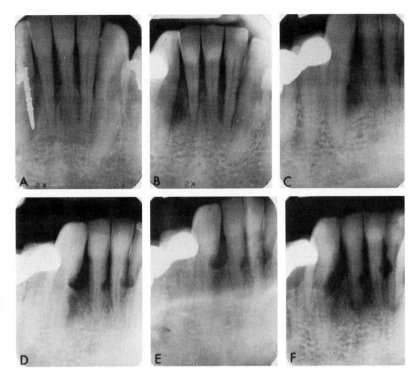

FIGURE 57–20. *A,* November 1973. Radiograph of a patient immediately prior to the placement of a fresh iliac autograft. *B,* Two months later, bone repair is evident. Note the early radiolucent areas on the mesial aspect of the canine. *C,* After 7 months, "bone fill" is occurring, but obvious root resorption is present. *D,* April 1975. Root resorption is apparent on all grafted teeth. Note the obvious degree of fill of the original bone defects. *E,* February 1976. Further involvement. *F,* October 1977. Four years later, root resorption has progressed into the pulp of the lateral incisor, causing a periosteal-endosteal complication.

a Gore-Tex membrane. Its usefulness, however, has not been proven.

Plastic Materials. HTR polymer is a nonresorbable, microporous, biocompatible composite of polymethylmethacrylate and polyhydroxylethylmethacrylate.[199] A clinical 6-month study showed significant defect fill and improved attachment level.[199] Histologically, this material is encapsulated by connective tissue fibers, with no evidence of new attachment.[178]

Calcium Phosphate Biomaterials. Several calcium phosphate biomaterials have been tested since the mid-1970s and are currently available for clinical use. Calcium

phosphate biomaterials have excellent tissue compatibility and do not elicit any inflammation or foreign body response. These materials are *osteoconductive,* and not *osteoinductive,* meaning that they will induce bone formation when placed next to viable bone but not when surrounded by non–bone-forming tissue such as skin.

Two types of calcium phosphate ceramics have been used:

1. Hydroxyapatite (HA), which has a calcium-to-phosphate ratio of 1.67, similar to that found in bone material. HA is generally nonbioresorbable.
2. Tricalcium phosphate (TCP), with a calcium-to-phosphate

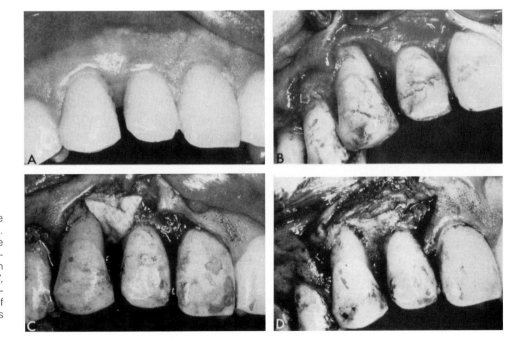

FIGURE 57–21. *A,* Preoperative photograph of a sclera graft area. *B,* An incision is made to conserve gingival tissue, and the area is debrided. Note the vertical defect on the mesial aspect of the canine. *C,* Sclera is placed over defect. *D,* Reentry shows apparent remodeling of defect. (Courtesy of Dr. Jules Klingsberg.)

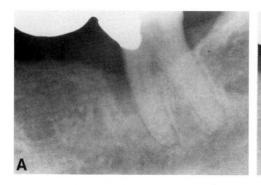
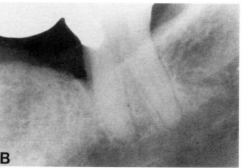

FIGURE 57–22. *A,* Deep angular defect with a 9-mm pocket. *B,* Eleven months after flap surgery and placement of granular porous hydroxyapatite. Note the regeneration of the marginal bone with a remaining shallow area of widened periodontal ligament. Pocket depth is 4 mm.

ratio of 1.5, is mineralogically B-whitlockite. TCP is at least partially bioresorbable.

Case reports and uncontrolled human studies have shown that calcium phosphate bioceramic materials are perfectly tolerated and can result in clinical repair of periodontal lesions. Several controlled studies were conducted on the use of Periograf[139,201] and Calcitite[103]; clinical results were good, but histologically these materials appeared to be encapsulated by collagen.[58]

Coral-Derived Materials. Two different coralline materials have been used in clinical periodontics: natural coral and coral-derived porous hydroxyapatite. Both are biocompatible, but while natural coral is resorbed slowly (several months), porous hydroxyapatite is not resorbed or takes years to do so.

Clinical studies on these materials[77,81,83] showed pocket reduction, attachment gain, and bone level gain (Fig. 57–22 and Plate XX); the materials have also been studied in conjunction with polytetrafluoroethylene membranes, with good results.[89,177] Both materials have demonstrated microscopic cementum and bone formation[25,92,126] (Fig.

57–23), but their slow resorbability or lack thereof has hindered clinical success in practice.

SUMMARY

The subject of new attachment has received a great deal of attention because of its obvious importance in improving the results of therapy. The clinician should make an effort to differentiate between those techniques that have been studied in depth and with acceptable results and others that, although promising, are still experimental. Research papers must be critically evaluated for adequacy of controls, selection of cases, methods of evaluation, and long-range postoperative results.

At present, barrier techniques to prevent epithelial downgrowth, with or without autogenous bone or decalcified freeze-dried bone allograft, are widely used. Coral-derived materials can be used when non–human-derived grafts are preferred.

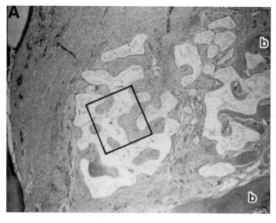
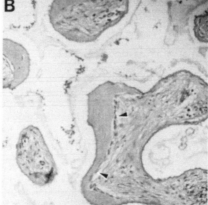
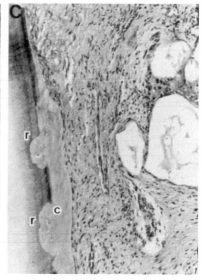

FIGURE 57–23. Microscopic healing, 5½ months after placement of porous hydroxyapatite in an angular osseous defect.[25] *A,* Low-power view of porous hydroxyapatite (clear spaces), lateral and coronal to existing bone (b). Note the lack of inflammatory response to the material and the invasion of the pores by connective tissue. *B,* Higher magnification of area squared in *A*. Note active bone formation within the pores (*arrows*). *C,* Another section of the same case shows formation of new cementum (c) after initial cementum resorption (r).

REFERENCES

1. Alderman NE. Sterile plaster of Paris as an implant in the infrabony environment: A preliminary study. J Periodontol 40:11, 1969.
2. Alger FA, Solt CW, Vuddahanok S, Miles K. The histologic evaluation of new attachment in periodontally diseased human roots treated with tetracycline-hydrochloride and fibronectin. J Periodontol 61:447, 1990.
3. Andereeg CR, Martin SJ, Gray JL, et al. Clinical evaluation of the use of decalcified freeze-dried bone allograft with guided tissue regeneration in the treatment of molar furcation invasions. J Periodontol 62:264, 1991.
4. Arrocha R, Wittwer J, Gargiulo A. Tissue response to heterogenous bone implantation in dogs. J Periodontol 39:162, 1968.
5. Becker W, Becker BE, Berg L, Samsam C. Clinical and volumetric analysis of three-wall intrabony defects following open flap debridement. J Periodontol 57:277, 1986.
6. Becker W, Becker BE, Berg L, et al. New attachment after treatment with root isolation procedures: Report for treated class III and class II furcations and vertical osseous defects. Int J Periodont Restor Dent 8(3):9, 1988.
7. Becker W, Becker BE, Prichard JF, et al. Root isolation for new attachment procedures—a surgical and suturing method: Three case reports. J Periodontol 58:819, 1987.
8. Bierly JA, Sottosanti JS, Costley JM, Cherrick HM. An evaluation of the osteogenic potential of marrow. J Periodontol 46:277, 1975.
9. Bjorn H. Experimental studies on reattachment. Dent Pract 11:351, 1961.
10. Bjorn H, Hollender L, Lindhe J. Tissue regeneration in patients with periodontal disease. Odont Rev 16:317, 1965.
11. Blumenthal NM. The use of collagen materials in bone grafted defects to enhance guided tissue regeneration. Periodont Case Rep 9:16, 1987.
12. Blumenthal NM. The use of collagen membranes to guide regeneration of new connective tissue attachment in dogs. J Periodontol 59:830, 1988.
13. Blumenthal NM, Steinberg J. The use of collagen membrane barriers in conjunction with combined demineralized bone-collagen gel implants in human infrabony defects. J Periodontol 61:319, 1990.
14. Bowers GM, Chadroff B, Carnevale R, et al. Histologic evaluation of new attachment apparatus formation in humans. Part III. J Periodontol 60:683, 1989.
15. Bowers G, Felton F, Middleton F, et al. Histologic comparison of regeneration in human intrabony pockets when osteogenin is combined with demineralized freeze-dried bone allograft and with purified bovine collagen. J Periodontol 62:690, 1991.
16. Buring K, Urist MR. Effects of ionizing radiation on the bone induction principle in the matrix of bone implants. Clin Orthop 55:225, 1967.
17. Burnette WE. Fate of the iliac crest graft. J Periodontol 43:88, 1972.
18. Busschopp J, De Boever J. Clinical and histological characteristics of lyophilized allogenic dura mater in periodontal bony defects in humans. J Clin Periodontol 10:399, 1983.
19. Caffesse RG, Holden MJ, Kon S, Nasjleti C. The effect of citric acid and fibronectin application on healing following surgical treatment of naturally occurring periodontal disease in beagle dogs. J Clin Periodontol 12:578, 1985.
20. Caffesse RG, Nasjleti CE, Anderson GB, et al. Periodontal healing following guided tissue regeneration with citric acid and fibronectin application. J Periodontol 62:21, 1991.
21. Caffesse RG, Smith BA, Castelli WA, Nasjleti CE. New attachment achieved by guided tissue regeneration in beagle dogs. J Periodontol 59:589, 1988.
22. Caffesse RG, Smith BA, Nasjleti CE, Lopatin DE. Cell proliferation after flap surgery, root conditioning and fibronectin application. J Periodontol 58:661, 1987.
23. Card SJ, Caffesse RG, Smith BA, Nasjleti CE. New attachment following the use of a resorbable membrane in the treatment of periodontitis in dogs. Internat J Periodont Restor Dent 9:59, 1989.
24. Carranza FA Sr. A technic for reattachment. J Periodontol 25:272, 1954.
25. Carranza FA Jr, Kenney EB, Lekovic V, et al. Histologic study of healing of human periodontal defects after placement of porous hydroxyapatite implants. J Periodontol 58:682, 1987.
26. Carraro JJ, Sznajder N, Alonso CA. Intraoral cancellous bone autografts in treatment of infrabony pockets. J Clin Periodontol 3:104, 1976.
27. Caton JG, DeFuria EL, Polson AM, Nyman S. Periodontal regeneration via selective cell repopulation. J Periodontol 58:546, 1987.
28. Caton J, Wagener C, Polson A, et al. Guided tissue regeneration in interproximal defects in monkeys. Int J Periodont Restor Dent 12:267, 1992.
29. Caton J, Zander H. Osseous repair of an infrabony pocket without new attachment of connective tissue. J Clin Periodontol 3:54, 1976.
30. Chung KM, Salkin LM, Stein MD, Freedman AL. Clinical evaluation of a biodegradable collagen membrane in guided tissue regeneration. J Periodontol 61:732, 1990.
31. Claffey N, Hahn R, Egelberg J. Effect of placement of occlusive membranes on root resorption and bone regeneration during healing of circumferential periodontal defects in dogs. J Clin Periodontol 16:371, 1989.
32. Coverly L, Toto P, Gargiulo A. Osseous coagulum: A histologic evaluation. J Periodontol 46:596, 1975.
33. Crigger M, Bogle G, Nilveus R, et al. Effect of topical citric acid application in the healing of experimental furcation defects in dogs. J Periodont Res 13:538, 1978.
34. Cushing M. Autogenous red marrow grafts: Potential for induction of osteogenesis. J Periodontol 40:492, 1969.
35. Daly CG. Antibacterial effect of citric acid treatment of periodontally diseased root surface "in vitro." J Clin Periodontol 9:386, 1982.
36. Diem CR, Bowers GM, Moffitt WC. Bone blending: A technique for osseous implants. J Periodontol 43:295, 1972.
37. Dragoo MR, Irwin RK. A method of procuring cancellous iliac bone utilizing a trephine needle. J Periodontol 43:82, 1972.
38. Dragoo MR, Sullivan HC. A clinical and histologic evaluation of autogenous iliac bone grafts in humans. Part I. Wound healing after 2 to 6 months. J Periodontol 44:599, 1973.
39. Dragoo MR, Sullivan HC. A clinical and histologic evaluation of autogenous iliac bone grafts in humans. Part II. External root resorption. J Periodontol 44:614, 1973.
40. Ellegaard B. Bone grafts in periodontal attachment procedures. J Clin Periodontol 3:5, 1976.
41. Ellegaard B, Löe H. New attachment of periodontal tissues after treatment of intrabony lesions. J Periodontol 42:648, 1971.
42. Ellegaard B, Karring T, Löe H. Retardation of epithelial migration in new attachment attempts in intrabony defects in monkeys. J Clin Periodontol 3:23, 1976.
43. Ellegaard B, Nielsen IM, Karring T. Lyodura grafts in new attachment procedures. J Dent Res 55(special issue B):B-304, 1976.
44. Ellegaard B, Karring T, Davies R, Löe H. New attachment after treatment of intrabony defects in monkeys. J Periodontol 45:368, 1974.
45. Ellegaard B, Karring T, Listgarten N, Löe H. New attachment after treatment of interradicular lesions. J Periodontol 44:209, 1973.
46. Ewen SJ. Bone swaging. J Periodontol 36:57, 1965.
47. Feingold JP, Chasens AI, Doyle J, Alfano MC. Preserved scleral allografts on periodontal defects in man. II. Histologic evaluation. J Periodontol 48:4, 1977.
48. Fernyhough W, Page RC. Attachment, growth and synthesis of human gingival fibroblasts on demineralized or fibronectin-treated normal and diseased tooth roots. J Periodontol 54:133, 1983.
49. Fialkoff B, Fry HR. Acid demineralization in periodontal therapy: A review of the literature. J West Soc Periodontol 30:52, 1982.
50. Fine DH, Morris ML, Tabak L, Cole JD. Preliminary characterization of material eluted from the roots of periodontally diseased teeth. J Periodont Res 15:10, 1980.
51. Flanary DB, Twohey SM, Gray JL, et al. The use of a synthetic skin substitute as a physical barrier to enhance healing in human periodontal furcation defects; a follow-up report. J Periodontol 62:684, 1991.
52. Fleisher N, Waal H, Bloom A. Regeneration of lost attachment apparatus in the dog using Vicryl absorbable mesh (Polyglactin 910). Int J Periodont Restor Dent 8(2):45, 1988.
53. Fowler C, Garrett S, Crigger M, Egelberg J. Histologic probe position in treated and untreated human periodontal tissues. J Clin Periodontol 9:373, 1982.
54. Freeman E, Turnbull RS. The value of osseous coagulum as a graft material. J Periodont Res 8:299, 1973.
55. Froum SJ. Comparison of different autograft material for obtaining bone fill in human periodontal defects. J Periodontol 45:240, 1974.
56. Froum SJ, Thaler R, Scoop IW, Stahl SS. Osseous autografts. I. Clinical responses to bone blend or hip marrow grafts. J Periodontol 46:515, 1975.
57. Froum SJ, Thaler R, Scoop IW, Stahl SS. Osseous autografts. II. Histologic responses to osseous coagulum-bone blend grafts. J Periodontol 46:656, 1975.
58. Froum SJ, Kushner L, Scoop IW, Stahl SS. Human clinical and histologic responses to Durapatite implants in intraosseous lesions. J Periodontol 53:719, 1982.
59. Gager AH, Schultz AJ. Treatment of periodontal defects with an absorbable membrane (polyglactin 910) with and without osseous grafting: Case reports. J Periodontol 62:276, 1991.
60. Gantes BG, Garrett S. Coronally displaced flaps in reconstructive periodontal therapy. Reconstruct Periodontics 35(3):495, 1991.
61. Garrett S. Early wound healing stability and its importance in periodontal regeneration. In Polson AM, ed. Periodontal Regeneration; Current Status and Directions. Chicago, Quintessence Books, 1994.
62. Garrett S, Crigger M, Egelberg J. Effects of citric acid on diseased root surfaces. J Periodont Res 13:155, 1978.
63. Glickman I. Clinical Periodontology. 1st ed. Philadelphia, WB Saunders, 1953.
64. Goldman H. A rationale for the treatment of the intrabony pocket. One method of treatment—subgingival curettage. J Periodontol 20:83, 1949.
65. Goldman HM, Cohen DW. The infrabony pocket: Classification and treatment. J Periodontol 29:272, 1958.
66. Gottlow J. Guided tissue regeneration using bioresorbable and non-resorbable devices: Initial healing and long-term results. J Periodontol 64:1157, 1993.
67. Gottlow J, Nyman S, Lindhe J, Karring T. New attachment formation as a result of controlled tissue regeneration. J Clin Periodontol 11:494, 1984.
68. Gottlow J, Nyman S, Lindhe J, et al. New attachment formation in human periodontium by guided tissue regeneration. J Clin Periodontol 13:604, 1986.
69. Greenberg J, Laster L, Listgarten MA. Transgingival probing as a potential estimation of alveolar bone level. J Periodontol 47:514, 1976.
70. Haggerty PC, Maeda L. Autogenous bone grafts: A revolution in the treatment of vertical bone defects. J Periodontol 42:626, 1971.
71. Halliday DG. The grafting of newly formed autogenous bone in the treatment of osseous defects. J Periodontol 40:511, 1969.
72. Han TJ, Carranza FA Jr, Kenney EB. Calcium phosphate ceramics in dentistry: A review of the literature. J West Soc Periodontol 32:88, 1984.
73. Hecker F. Pyorrhea Alveolaris. St Louis, CV Mosby, 1913.

74. Hegedus Z. The rebuilding of the alveolar process by bone transplantation. Dent Cosmos 65:736, 1923.

75. Hiatt WH. Periodontal pocket elimination by combined endodontic-periodontic therapy. J Periodontol 1:153, 1963.

76. Hiatt WH, Schallhorn RG. Intraoral transplants of cancellous bone and marrow in periodontal lesions. J Periodontol 44:194, 1973.

77. Hippolyte MP, Fabre D, Peyrol S. Corail et regeneration tissulaire guidée. Aspects histologiques. J Parodontologie 10:279, 1991.

78. Jarcho M. Biomaterial aspects of calcium phosphates. Dent Clin North Am 30:25, 1986.

79. Johnson W, Parkhill EM, Grindlay JH. Transplantation of homografts of sclera: Experimental study. Am J Ophthalmol 54:1019, 1962.

80. Jones WA, O'Leary TJ. The effectiveness of "in vivo" root planing in removing bacterial endotoxin from the roots of periodontally involved teeth. J Periodontol 49:337, 1978.

81. Kenney EB, Lekovic V, Han T, et al. The use of a porous hydroxylapatite implant in periodontal defects. I. Clinical results after six months. J Periodontol 56:82, 1985.

82. Kenney EB, Lekovic V, Sa Ferreira J, et al. Bone formation within porous hydroxylapatite implants in human periodontal defects. J Periodontol 57:76, 1986.

83. Kenney EB, Lekovic V, Elbaz J-J, et al. The use of a porous hydroxylapatite implant in periodontal defects. II. Treatment of class II furcation lesions in lower molars. J Periodontol 59:67, 1988.

84. Klingsberg J. Preserved sclera in periodontal surgery. J Periodontol 43:634, 1972.

85. Klingsberg J. Scleral allografts in the repair of periodontal osseous defects. NY State Dent J 38:418, 1972.

86. Klingsberg J. Periodontal scleral grafts and combined grafts of sclera and bone: Two year appraisal. J Periodontol 45:262, 1974.

87. Kornbleuth J. Histologic evaluation of plaster as a seal for bone autografts. IADR Abstracts, 1972, p. 184.

88. Lang NP, Hill RW. Radiographs in periodontics. J Clin Periodontol 4:16, 1976.

89. Lekovic V, Kenney EB, Carranza FA Jr, Danilovic B. Treatment of class II furcation defects using porous hydroxyapatite in conjunction with a polytetrafluoroethylene membrane. J Periodontol 61:575, 1990.

90. Lekovic V, Kenney EB, Carranza FA Jr, Martignone M. The use of autogenous periosteal grafts as barriers for the treatment of grade II furcation involvements in lower molars. J Periodontol 62:775, 1991.

91. Lekovic V, Kenney EB, Kovacevic K, Carranza FA Jr. Evaluation of guided tissue regeneration in class II furcation defects. A clinical study. J Periodontol 60:694, 1989.

92. Lekovic V, Ouhayoun JP, Kenney EB, et al. Histologic and histometric evaluation of three implants in periodontal disease (Abstract). J Dent Res 71:624, 1992.

93. Levin MP, Getter L, Cutright DE. A comparison of iliac marrow and biodegradable ceramic in periodontal defects. J Biomed Mater Res 9:183, 1975.

94. Levin MP, Getter L, Adrian J, Cutright DE. Healing of periodontal defects with ceramic implants. J Clin Periodontol 1:197, 1974.

95. Libin BM, Ward HL, Fishman LL. Decalcified lyophilized bone allografts for use in human periodontal defects. J Periodontol 46:51, 1975.

96. Louise F, Borghetti A, Kerebel B. Histologic case reports of coralline hydroxyapatite grafts placed in human intraosseous lesions: Results 6 to 36 months postimplantation. Int J Periodont Restor Dent 12:475, 1992.

97. Louise F, Borghetti A, Simeoni D, Gervasone V. Evaluation clinique a 6 mois du comblement de lesions intra-osseous par un hydroxyapatite poreuse (Interpore 200). J Parodontol 6:203, 1987.

98. Lynch SE. The role of growth factors in periodontal repair and regeneration. In Polson AM, ed. Periodontal Repair and Regeneration. Current Status and Directions. Chicago, Quintessence Books, 1994.

99. Magnusson I, Batich C, Collins BR. New attachment formation following controlled tissue regeneration using biodegradable membranes. J Periodontol 59:1, 1988.

100. Magnusson I, Stenberg WV, Batich C, Egelberg J. Connective tissue repair in circumferential periodontal defects in dogs following use of a biodegradable membrane. J Clin Periodontol 17:243, 1990.

101. Martin M, Gantes B, Garrett S, Egelberg J. Treatment of periodontal furcation defects. (I) Review of the literature and description of a regenerative surgical technique. J Clin Periodontol 15:227, 1988.

102. McClain PK, Schallhorn RG. Long-term assessment of combined osseous composite grafting, root conditioning and guided tissue regeneration. Int J Periodont Restor Dent 13:9, 1993.

103. Meffert RM, Thomas JR, Hamilton KM, Brownstein CN. Hydroxylapatite as an alloplastic graft in the treatment of human periodontal osseous defects. J Periodontol 56:63, 1985.

104. Melcher AH. The use of heterogenous anorganic bone in periodontal bone grafting: A preliminary report. I. Dent Assoc South Afr 13:80, 1958.

105. Melcher A. The use of heterogenous anorganic bone as an implant material in oral procedures. Oral Surg 15:996, 1962.

106. Mellonig JT. Freeze-dried bone allografts in periodontal reconstructive surgery. Dent Clin North Am 35:505, 1991.

107. Mellonig JT, Bowers GM, Bailey RC. Comparison of bone graft materials. Part I: New bone formation with autografts and allografts determined by strontium-85. J Periodontol 52:291, 1981.

108. Mellonig JT, Bowers GM, Bailey RC. Comparison of bone graft materials. Part

II: New bone formation with autografts and allografts; a histological evaluation. J Periodontol 52:297, 1981.

109. Mellonig JT, Bowers GM, Bright RW, Lawrence JL. Clinical evaluation of freeze-dried bone allografts in periodontal osseous defects. J Periodontol 47:125, 1976.

110. Mellonig JT, Prewett AB, Moyer MP. HIV inactivation in a bone allograft. J Periodontol 63:979, 1992.

111. Metzler DG, Seamoons BC, Mellonig JT, et al. Clinical evaluation of guided tissue regeneration in the treatment of maxillary class II molar furcation invasions. J Periodontol 62:353, 1991.

112. Minabe M. A critical review of the biologic rationale for guided tissue regeneration. J Periodontol 62:171, 1991.

113. Moriarty JD, Hutchens LH, Scheitler LE. Histological evaluation of periodontal probe penetration in untreated facial molar furcations. J Periodontol 16:21, 1989.

114. Morris ML. Reattachment of periodontal tissue. A critical study. Oral Surg 2:1194, 1949.

115. Morris ML. Healing of human periodontal tissues following surgical detachment and extirpation of vital pulps. J Periodontol 31:23, 1960.

116. Moskow BS, Gold SI, Gottsegen R. Effects of scleral collagen upon the healing of experimental osseous wounds. J Periodontol 47:596, 1976.

117. Moskow BS, Tannenbaum P. Enhanced repair and regeneration of periodontal lesions in tetracycline-treated patients. Case reports. J Periodontol 62:341, 1991.

118. Nabers CL, O'Leary TJ. Autogenous bone transplants in the treatment of osseous defects. J Periodontol 36:5, 1965.

119. Nabers CL, O'Leary TJ. Autogenous bone grafts: Case report. Periodontics 5:251, 1967.

120. Nabers JM, Meador HL, Nabers CL, O'Leary TJ. Chronology, an important factor in the repair of osseous defects. Periodontics 2:304, 1964.

121. Narang R, Wells H. Bone induction in experimental periodontal bone defects in dogs with decalcified allogenic bone matrix grafts: A preliminary study. Oral Surg 33:306, 1972.

122. Nery EB, Lynch KL. Preliminary clinical studies of bioceramic in periodontal osseous defects. J Periodontol 49:523, 1978.

123. Nilveus R, Bogle G, Crigger M, et al. Effect of topical citric acid application in the healing of experimental furcation defects in dogs. 2. Healing after repeated surgery. J Periodont Res 15:544, 1980.

124. Nyman S, Gottlow J, Karring T, Lindhe J. The regenerative potential of the periodontal ligament. An experimental study in the monkey. J Clin Periodontol 9:257, 1982.

125. Nyman S, Lindhe J, Karring T, Rylander H. New attachment following surgical treatment of human periodontal disease. J Clin Periodontol 9:290, 1982.

126. Ouyahoun JP, Issahakian S, Patat JL, et al. Influence of biomaterials on the healing pattern of bone defects in the miniature pig mandible. Abstract. J Dent Res 68:1022, 1989.

127. Passell MS, Bissada NF. Histomorphologic evaluation of scleral grafts in experimental bony defects. J Periodontol 46:629, 1975.

128. Patur B, Glickman I. Clinical and roentgenographic evaluation of the post-treatment healing of infrabony pockets. J Periodontol 33:164, 1962.

129. Pearson GE, Rosen S, Deporter DA. Preliminary observations on the usefulness of a decalcified freeze-dried cancellous bone allograft material in periodontal surgery. J Periodontol 52:55, 1981.

130. Pitaru S, Tal H, Soldinger M, et al. Collagen membranes prevent the apical migration of epithelium during periodontal wound healing. J Periodont Res 22:331, 1987.

131. Pitaru S, Tal H, Soldinger M, et al. Partial regeneration of periodontal tissues using collagen barriers. Initial observations in the canine. J Periodontol 59:380, 1988.

132. Pitaru S, Tal H, Soldinger M, Noff M. Collagen membranes prevent apical migration of epithelium and support new connective tissue attachment during periodontal wound healing in dogs. J Periodont Res 24:2467, 1989.

133. Polson AM, Frederick GT, Ladenhein S, Hanes PJ. The production of a root surface smear by instrumentation and its removal by citric acid. J Periodontol 55:443, 1984.

134. Polson A, Heijl LC. Osseous repair in infrabony periodontal defects. J Clin Periodontol 5:13, 1978.

135. Polson AM, Proye MP. Fibrin linkage: A precursor for new attachment. J Periodontol 54:141, 1983.

136. Pontoriero R, Lindhe J, Nyman S, et al. Guided tissue regeneration in degree II furcation-involved mandibular molars. A clinical study. J Clin Periodontol 15:247, 1988.

137. Prichard JF. The intrabony technique as a predictable procedure. J Periodontol 28:202, 1957.

138. Quintero G, Mellonig JT, Gambill VM, Pelleu GB Jr. A six-month clinical evaluation of decalcified freeze-dried bone allografts in periodontal osseous defects. J Periodontol 53:726, 1982.

139. Rabalais ML, Yukna RA, Mayer ET. Evaluation of Durapatite ceramic as an alloplastic implant in periodontal osseous defects. J Periodontol 52:680, 1981.

140. Ramfjord SP. Experimental periodontal reattachment in rhesus monkeys. J Periodontol 22:67, 1951.

141. Ramfjord SP, Nissle RR. The modified Widman flap. J Periodontol 45:601, 1974.

142. Register AA, Burdick FA. Accelerated reattachment with cementogenesis to dentin, demineralized in situ. II. Defect repair. J Periodontol 47:497, 1976.

143. Renvert S, Badersten A, Nilveus R, Egelberg J. Healing after treatment of peri-

odontal intraosseous defects. I. Comparative study of clinical methods. J Clin Periodontol 8:387, 1981.

144. Renvert S, Egelberg J. Healing after treatment of periodontal intraosseous defects. II. Effect of citric acid conditioning of the root surface. J Clin Periodontol 8:459, 1981.

145. Rivault AF, Toto PD, Levy S, Gargiulo AW. Autogenous bone grafts: Osseous coagulum and osseous retrograde procedures in primates. J Periodontol 42:787, 1971.

146. Robinson RE. Osseous coagulum for bone induction. J Periodontol 40:503, 1969.

147. Rosenberg MM. Free osseous tissue autografts as a predictable procedure. J Periodontol 42:195, 1971.

148. Rosenberg MM. Reentry of an osseous defect treated by a bone implant after a long duration. J Periodontol 42:360, 1971.

149. Rosling B, Hollender L, Nyman S, Olsson G. A radiographic method for assessing changes in alveolar bone height following periodontal therapy. J Clin Periodontol 2:211, 1975.

150. Ross SE, Cohen DW. The fate of a free osseous tissue autograft: A clinical and histologic case report. Periodontics 6:145, 1968.

151. Ross SE, Malamed EH, Amsterdam M. The contiguous autogenous transplant—its rationale, indications and technique. Periodontics 4:246, 1966.

152. Sanders J, Sepe W, Bowers G, et al. Clinical evaluation of freeze-dried bone allografts in periodontal osseous defects. III. Composite freeze-dried bone allograft with and without autogenous bone. J Periodontol 54:1, 1983.

153. Schaffer EM. Cartilage transplants into periodontium of rhesus monkeys. Oral Surg 11:1233, 1956.

154. Schaffer EM. Cementum and dentine implants in a dog and a rhesus monkey. J Periodontol 28:125, 1957.

155. Schaffer EM. Cartilage grafts in human periodontal pockets. J Periodontol 29:176, 1958.

156. Schaffer EM, Zander HA. Histologic evidence of reattachment of periodontal pockets. Parodontologie 7:101, 1953.

157. Schallhorn RG. The use of autogenous hip marrow biopsy implants for bony crater defects. J Periodontol 39:145, 1968.

158. Schallhorn RG. Postoperative problems associated with iliac transplants. J Periodontol 43:3, 1972.

159. Schallhorn RG. Osseous grafts in the treatment of periodontal osseous defects. In Stahl SS, ed. Periodontal Surgery. Biologic Basis and Technique. Springfield, IL, Charles C Thomas, 1976.

160. Schallhorn RG. Present status of osseous grafting procedures. J Periodontol 48:570, 1977.

161. Schallhorn RG, Hiatt WH. Human allografts of iliac cancellous bone and marrow in periodontal osseous defects. II. Clinical observations. J Periodontol 43:67, 1972.

162. Schallhorn RG, Hiatt WH, Boyce W. Iliac transplants in periodontal therapy. J Periodontol 41:566, 1970.

163. Scoop IW, Kassouny DY, Morgan FH. Bovine bone (Boplant). J Periodontol 37:400, 1966.

164. Scoop IW, Kassouny DY, Register AA. Human bone induction by allogenic dentin matrix. IADR Abstracts, no. 105, 1970, p 100.

165. Scoop IW, Morgan FH, Dooner JJ, et al. Bovine bone (Boplant) implants for infrabony oral lesions (clinical trials in humans). Periodontics 4:169, 1966.

166. Sepe W, Bowers G, Lawrence J, et al. Clinical evaluation of freeze-dried bone allograft in periodontal osseous defects. Part II. J Periodontol 49:9, 1978.

167. Shaffer CD, App GR. The use of plaster of Paris in treating infrabony periodontal defects in humans. J Periodontol 42:685, 1971.

168. Smith B, Caffesse R, Nasjleti C, et al. Effects of citric acid and fibronectin and laminin application in treating periodontitis. J Clin Periodontol 14:396, 1987.

169. Smith BA, Echeverri M. The removal of pocket epithelium. A review. J West Soc Periodontol 32:45, 1984.

170. Smith BA, Smith JS, Caffesse RG, et al. Effect of citric acid and various concentrations of fibronectin on healing following periodontal flap surgery in dogs. J Periodontol 58:667, 1987.

171. Sottosanti J. Calcium phosphate: An aid to periodontal, implant and restorative therapy. J Calif Dent Assoc 20:45, 1992.

172. Stahl SS, Froum SJ. Human clinical and histologic repair responses following the use of citric acid in periodontal therapy. J Periodontol 48:261, 1977.

173. Stahl SS, Froum SJ. Histological and clinical responses to porous hydroxylapatite implants in human periodontal defects three to twelve months post-implantation. J Periodontol 58:689, 1987.

174. Stahl SS, Froum SJ. Healing of human suprabony lesions treated with guided tissue regeneration and coronally anchored flaps. J Clin Periodontol 18:69, 1991.

175. Stahl SS, Froum SJ. Histologic healing responses in human vertical lesions following the use of osseous allografts and barrier membranes. J Clin Periodontol 18:149, 1991.

176. Stahl SS, Froum SJ. Human suprabony healing responses following root demineralization and coronal flap anchorage. J Clin Periodontol 18:685, 1991.

177. Stahl SS, Froum SJ. Human intrabony lesion response to debridement, porous hydroxylapatite implants and Teflon barrier membranes. J Clin Periodontol 18:605, 1991.

178. Stahl SS, Froum SJ, Tarnow D. Human clinical and histologic responses to the placement of HTR polymer particles in 11 intrabony lesions. J Periodontol 61:269, 1990.

179. Stahl SS, Froum SJ, Tarnow D. Human histologic responses to guided tissue regenerative techniques in intrabony lesions. J Clin Periodontol 17:191, 1990.

180. Strub JR, Gaberthal TW, Firstone AR. Comparison of tricalcium phosphate and frozen allogenic bone implants in man. J Periodontol 50:624, 1979.

181. Takei HH, Han TJ, Carranza FA Jr, et al. Flap technique for periodontal bone implants. Papilla preservation technique. J Periodontol 56:204, 1985.

182. Terranova VP, Martin GR. Molecular factors determining gingival tissue interaction with tooth structure. J Periodont Res 17:530, 1982.

183. Terranova VP, Franzetti LC, Hic S, et al. A biochemical approach to periodontal regeneration: Tetracycline treatment of dentin promotes fibroblast adhesion and growth. J Periodont Res 21:330, 1986.

184. Theilade J. An evaluation of the reliability of radiographs in the measurement of bone loss in periodontal disease. J Periodontol 31:143, 1960.

185. Turnbull RS, Freeman E, Melcher AH. Histological evaluation of the osteogenic capacity of sclera. J Dent Res 55:972, 1976.

186. Van Dyke TE, Lester MA, Shapira L. The role of the host response in periodontal disease progression: Implications for future treatment strategies. J Periodontol 64:792, 1993.

187. Urist MR. Bone formation by autoinduction. Science 150:893, 1965.

188. Urist MR. Bone histogenesis and morphogenesis in implants of demineralized enamel and dentin. Oral Surg 29:38, 1971.

189. Urist MR, Strates BS. Bone morphogenetic protein. J Dent Res 50:1392, 1971.

190. Ursell MJ. Relationships between alveolar bone levels measured at surgery, estimated by transgingival probing and clinical attachment level measurements. J Clin Periodontol 16:81, 1989.

191. Wenzel A, Warrer K, Karring T. Digital subtraction radiography in assessing bone changes in periodontal defects following guided tissue regeneration. J Clin Periodontol 19:208, 1992.

192. White E, Shors EC. Biomaterial aspects of Interpore-200 porous hydroxyapatite. Dent Clin North Am 30:49, 1986.

193. Wikesjö UME, Baker PJ, Christersson LA, et al. A biochemical approach to periodontal regeneration: Tetracycline treatment conditions dentin surfaces. J Periodont Res 21:322, 1986.

194. Wikesjö UME, Claffey N, Christersson LA, et al. Repair of periodontal furcation defects in beagle dogs following reconstructive surgery including root surface demineralization with tetracycline hydrochloride and topical fibronectin application. J Clin Periodontol 15:73, 1988.

195. Wikesjö UME, Nilveus R. Periodontal repair in dogs: Effects of wound stabilization in healing. J Periodontol 61:719, 1990.

196. Wikesjö UME, Nilveus RE, Selvig KA. Significance of early healing events on periodontal repair: A review. J Periodontol 63:158, 1992.

197. Younger WJ. Some of the latest phases in implantations and other operations. Dent Cosmos 25:102, 1893.

198. Yukna RA. A clinical and histological study of healing following the excisional new attachment procedure in rhesus monkeys. J Periodontol 47:701, 1976.

199. Yukna RA. HTR polymer graft in human periodontal osseous defects. I. 6-months clinical results. J Periodontol 61:633, 1990.

200. Yukna RA. Clinical human comparison of expanded polytetrafluoroethylene barrier membrane and freeze-dried dura mater allografts for guided tissue regeneration of lost periodontal support. I. Mandibular molar class II furcations. J Periodontol 63:431, 1992.

201. Yukna RA, Mayer ET, Brite DV. Longitudinal evaluation of Durapatite ceramic as an alloplastic implant in periodontal osseous defects after three years. J Periodontol 55:633, 1984.

58

Treatment of Furcation Involvement and Combined Periodontal-Endodontic Therapy

FERMIN A. CARRANZA, JR. and HENRY H. TAKEI

As stated in Chapter 23, the term *furcation involvement* refers to commonly occurring conditions in which the bifurcations and trifurcations of multirooted teeth are invaded by the disease process. The diagnosis, prognosis, and treatment of teeth with furcation involvement (Fig. 58–1) are governed by the general principles applicable to single-rooted teeth. However, in spite of the added stability provided by extra root anchorage, furcated teeth and their surroundings exhibit several anatomic characteristics that make therapy difficult and its results sometimes unpredictable. These anatomic considerations refer to tooth, bone, and gingival interrelationships and are described after the classification of furcation involvements is discussed.

CLASSIFICATION OF FURCATION INVOLVEMENTS

The following classification, introduced by Glickman in 1953,[9] allows a better understanding of patient prognosis and therapy for furcation involvements.

Grade I Involvement. Grade I is the incipient or early lesion. The pocket is suprabony, involving the soft tissue; there is slight bone loss in the furcation area (Fig. 58–2). Radiographic change is not usual, as bone loss is minimal (Fig. 58–3A).

Grade II Involvement. In grade II cases, bone is destroyed on one or more aspects of the furcation, but a portion of the alveolar bone and periodontal ligament remains intact, permitting only partial penetration of the probe into the furcation. The lesion is essentially a cul-de-sac (see Figs. 58–2 and 58–3B).

The depth of the horizontal component of the pocket will vary; this determines whether the furcation involvement is early or advanced. There may also be a vertical or apical component of the pocket that extends into the osseous structure. This vertical bone loss is comparable to an interradicular crater and, when combined with the horizontal component of tissue destruction, can complicate diagnosis, prognosis, and therapy.

The radiograph may or may not reveal the grade II furcation involvement. In the mandibular molars, the close proximity of the roots, thick bone remaining between the roots, or the angulation of the x-ray beam can conceal the furcation involvement. The maxillary molars present additional diagnostic problems because the roots overlap each other radiographically from the facial view. A furcation involvement between the two facial roots may not be seen on the radiograph because the palatal root obscures it.

Grade III Involvement. In this type of furcation involvement, the interradicular bone is completely absent, but the facial and/or lingual orifices of the furcation are occluded by gingival tissue. Therefore, the furcation opening cannot be seen clinically, but it is essentially a through-and-through tunnel (see Fig. 58–2). There may be a crater-like lesion in the interradicular area, creating an apical or vertical component along with the horizontal loss of bone. This type of lesion can be present in both grade III and grade IV lesions.

If the radiograph of the mandibular molars is taken at the proper angle and the roots are divergent, these lesions will appear on the radiograph as a radiolucent area between the roots (Fig. 58–3C,D). The maxillary molars present a diagnostic difficulty similar to that encountered with grade II involvement, owing to the roots overlapping each other.

Grade IV Involvement. As in grade III lesions, the interradicular bone is completely destroyed, but in grade IV involvement, the gingival tissue is also recessed apically so that the furcation opening is clinically visible. Therefore, these involvements also exhibit tunnels, without the orifices being occluded by the gingiva.

The radiographic picture is essentially the same as that of grade III lesions.

Classification of the Vertical Component

The vertical component of furcation involvement is an important feature closely related to resective and regenera-

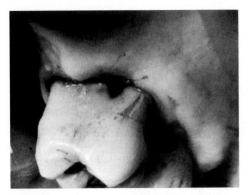

FIGURE 58-1. Typical furcation opening involving the distofacial and palatal roots of a maxillary molar.

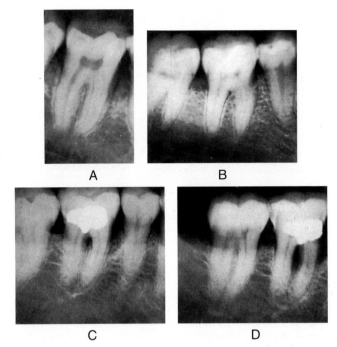

FIGURE 58-3. Radiographs of different degrees of furcation involvement. *A,* Grade I, no marked change. *B,* Grade II, small area of radiolucency. *C,* Distinct triangular area of radiolucency. *D,* Pronounced bone loss. The lesions shown in *C* and *D* would be grade III or grade IV, depending on whether the furcation is clinically visible owing to gingival recession.

tive therapeutic procedures. Tarnow and Fletcher[37] classified each grade of furcation involvement into three subgroups, depending on the distance from the bottom of the defect to the roof of the furcation (on the tooth): subgroup A, 0–3 mm; subgroup B, 4–7 mm; and subgroup C, 7 mm or more. This is a useful addition to the classic classification; however, measuring the subgroups from the imaginary line that joins the two peaks of the remaining bone, rather than from the roof of the furcation, seems to be more advantageous.

Other Classifications

Incorporation of other anatomic features of the furcation (e.g., root proximity, root shape, or root trunk length) into the classification of furcation involvement may help in defining patient prognosis and planning treatment. This would be particularly useful in grade II involvements, but the intricacies and variations of the furcation anatomy would make such a classification too cumbersome. At present, grade II involvements can be subclassified as having good, fair, or poor prognosis for regeneration, depending on the presence or absence of the complex anatomic features described next.

PROBLEMS IN THE TREATMENT OF FURCATIONS

Anatomic and clinical characteristics of tooth, bone, and gingiva are of importance for the clinical management of furcation lesions.

Tooth. The following features should be considered:
1. *Root trunk length.* The root trunk is the portion of the root between the cemento-enamel junction and the separation of the roots. When the root trunk is short, the furcation will become involved early in the disease process. When the root trunk is long, the furcation will be invaded later but will be more difficult to reach and instrument (Fig. 58–4).
2. *Concavity of the inner surface of exposed roots.* All the root surfaces facing the furcation exhibit some degree of concavity or depression in an occluso-apical direction[3,4] (see Chap-

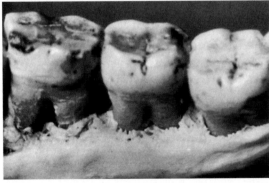

FIGURE 58-2. Teeth in the skull demonstrating the different degrees of furcation involvement. The first molar has a grade III or grade IV involvement; the second molar, a grade II involvement; and the third molar, a grade I, or incipient, involvement.

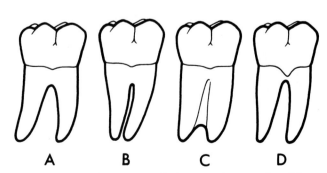

FIGURE 58-4. Different anatomic features that may be of importance in prognosis and treatment of furcation involvement. *A,* Widely separated roots. *B,* Roots are separated but close to one another. *C,* Fused roots (synostosis) separated only in their apical portion. *D,* Presence of enamel projection that may be conducive to an early furcation involvement.

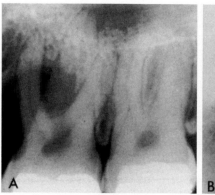
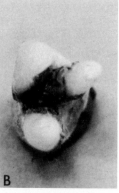

FIGURE 58–5. *A,* Radiograph of furcation involvement of the maxillary first molar. Note the advanced bone loss around the mesiofacial root and the trifurcation area. *B,* Apical view of the first molar shown in *A,* after extraction. Note the heavy calculus deposits in the trifurcation area.

ter 31). This may make instrumentation for calculus removal and root planing almost impossible. After surgical exposure, chances for complete removal improve; in narrow furcations, ultrasonic instrumentation is more effective than hand instrumentation[20] (Fig. 58–5B).

3. *Degree of separation of the roots.* Wide separation of the roots improves access, thereby facilitating instrumentation (see Fig. 58–4A, B).

4. *Enamel projections.* These occur in approximately 15% of molars. They favor plaque accumulation and must be removed to facilitate scaling and root planing.

Bone. Bone shape in the exposed furcation area may be horizontal, or there may be different degrees of vertical bone loss next to the roots or on the furcation side of the facial or lingual bone (Fig. 58–6). Therefore, not only the horizontal depth, but also the vertical or apical depth must be considered.

In addition, a thick buccal or lingual bony ledge—for example, in teeth adjacent to an external oblique ridge or a lingual torus—may favor the formation of trough-like ver-

tical lesions in the furcation area. A thin radicular bone, however, will result in complete loss of the bone, and no vertical lesion will form.

Gingiva. The presence of sufficient attached keratinized gingival tissue and adequate vestibular depth will facilitate the gingival management of the furcation area.

TREATMENT OF FURCATION INVOLVEMENT

Although several decades ago the presence of a furcation involvement was considered an indication for extraction,[22] current techniques have improved prognosis, and these lesions can very often be treated successfully.[8,30,31] Furcation involvement may be confined to a single tooth, but often several teeth are affected. Furcation lesions are treated as they are encountered in the systematic care of the mouth.[7]

Treatment of Grade I Involvement. Grade I furcation involvement usually exhibits suprabony pockets, which are treated by scaling and curettage or by gingivectomy, depending on pocket depth and the fibrosity of the pocket walls. Because the destructive process is in its incipient stages, it is not necessary to enter the furcation during the treatment process. Elimination of the pocket results in resolution of inflammation and repair of the periodontal ligament and adjacent bone margin.

In the treatment of early furcation involvements, the facial groove is sometimes eliminated by reshaping the tooth (*odontoplasty*) to reduce post-treatment accumulation of plaque and debris.[10]

Treatment of Grade II Involvement. Under local anesthesia, each tooth surface is probed down to the bone to determine the pattern of periodontal destruction. One aspect of the furcation is intact in grade II involvement; treatment is performed from the involved side.

Several reports have shown successful osseous repair of grade II furcation lesions with a variety of osseous grafting techniques (i.e., osseous coagulum[29]; autogenous intraoral bone[12]; iliac crest bone[33]; freeze-dried bone with autologous bone[32]; and porous, coral-derived hydroxyapatite[13]), as well as with guided tissue regeneration methods.[2,18,27] However, results with these procedures are not entirely predictable.

Combined techniques using guided tissue regeneration and either porous hydroxyapatite or decalcified freeze-dried bone have been tested in controlled clinical studies in human lower molar furcations,[13,17,27] with very good results.[5] However, further studies are needed to establish precise indications and techniques.

Technique. Practically all clinical research has been conducted in lower molars, but extrapolation of these findings to facial furcations of upper molars seems reasonable. Using this technique in mesiopalatal or distopalatal furcations of upper molars, however, has not given comparable results.

The recommended technique for lower molars uses porous hydroxyapatite or decalcified freeze-dried bone in conjunction with a polytetrafluoroethylene membrane. A full-thickness flap is raised, the area is debrided of granulation tissue, and the root surfaces are carefully scaled and planed with curettes and ultrasonic scalers.[15]

The graft material is placed, filling in the furcation area, particularly the crater area (Fig. 58–7A, B). The entrance to

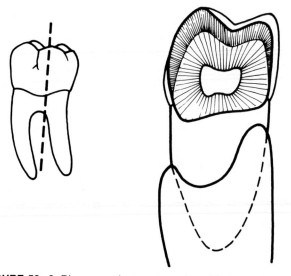

FIGURE 58–6. Diagrammatic representation of faciolingual section of the lower first molar through a furcation area showing crater-like osseous morphology.

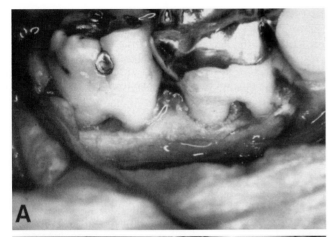

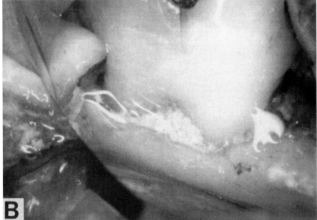

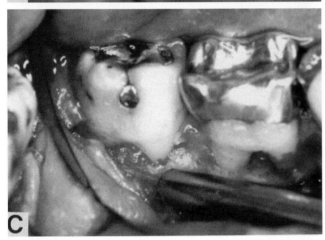

FIGURE 58–7. *A,* After reflection of a mucoperiosteal flap, grade II furcation lesions can be observed in first and second right mandibular molars. *B,* After thorough debridement, porous hydroxyapatite is placed in the second molar defect. The defect in first molar is equally debrided but is left unfilled. *C,* Re-entry after 6 months shows bone fill of the second molar furcation defect. (Patient treated by Dr. J.-J. Elbaz, as part of his clinical research on treatment of furcation defects.[13])

2. Take the suture under the contact point and around the lingual aspect of the tooth to the distal facial papilla, and penetrate from epithelium to connective tissue.
3. Bring the suture back under the contact point to the lingual aspect of the same space and go around the tooth. This will anchor the suture to the tooth.
4. Engage the tissue in front of the furcation in a horizontal mattress suture, starting from the distal surface.
5. Bring the suture back over the distal papilla and around the tooth to the mesial papilla.
6. Tie the suture to the initial thread.

This technique is done independently for each furcation being treated. This type of suture is indicated for grade II furcation involvements in lower molars and for facial furcations in upper molars.

Treatment of Grade III and Grade IV Involvements. In these conditions, interradicular tissue destruction permits a probe to pass freely through the furcation. The gingiva is resected just coronal to the bone or is displaced to the same level to provide visibility and access from all directions so that the involved root surfaces may be thoroughly planed and smoothed without disturbing the bone. The periodontal pack is placed for 1 week, except when patient comfort requires repacking for an additional week.

When infrabony pockets and osseous defects are part of the clinical picture of furcation involvement, the treatment of choice is the flap operation (see Chapters 54 and 55).

Furcation involvements combined with vertical defects require bone contouring as well as instrumentation of the root surface facing the furcation. Success with regenerative procedures in grade III and grade IV furcations, including the use of different graft materials and membranes, has generally been very limited. However, Pontoriero and colleagues[28] reported excellent results in a controlled study of

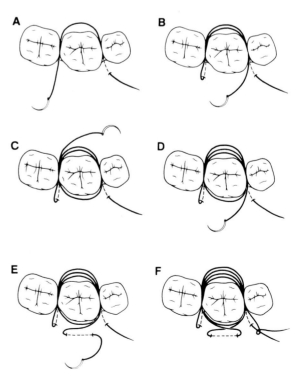

FIGURE 58–8. *A to F,* Suture technique for furcation defects.

the furcation is then covered with a membrane, which is sutured around the tooth.

The flap is sutured back in position. To hold the flap firmly against the tooth in the furcation area, the following suturing technique is recommended (Fig. 58–8):
1. Penetrate the needle from epithelium to connective tissue in the papilla mesial to the furcation.

"incipient" grade III furcation involvements in mandibular molars treated according to the principles of guided tissue regeneration. These furcation defects were not identified as grade III until after surgical exposure, meaning that the "through-and-through" defect was very small and the soft tissue present prevented penetration of the probe until the area was debrided.

The following procedure is recommended:

1. Reflection of a full-thickness flap facially and lingually or palatally; removal of granulation tissue.
2. Bone contouring to adjust angular bone losses to the base of the existing bone.
3. Scaling and planing of exposed root surfaces.
4. Further recontouring of bone to attain a harmonious osseous topography.
5. Suturing of the flap at the level of the bone margin to expose and open the furcation.

The goals of this procedure are to make the furcation accessible for plaque removal by the patient and to eliminate vertical bone loss.

Figure 58–9 shows the post-treatment gingival contour that can be attained with successful treatment of furcation lesions.

Root Conditioning in the Treatment of Furcation Lesions. Several studies[6,23,24] have shown that citric acid conditioning of the root surface increases the rate of success of new attachment procedures on experimentally produced furcation defects in dogs. Clinical human studies, however, have failed to show comparable success rates.[26,36]

Flap Positioning in the Treatment of Furcation Lesions. Adequate postoperative coverage of the furcation by the flap may be critical for successful healing. Klinge and associates[15,16] reported new attachment and complete closure of experimentally created class III furcation defects in the majority of teeth in which the flap had been sutured in a coronal position (see Chapter 57 for a description of the technique).

Coronal positioning of the flap places the marginal epithelium farther from the healing defect and therefore reduces the possibilities of an interfering long junctional epithelium. Cementation of a bracket has been suggested as a

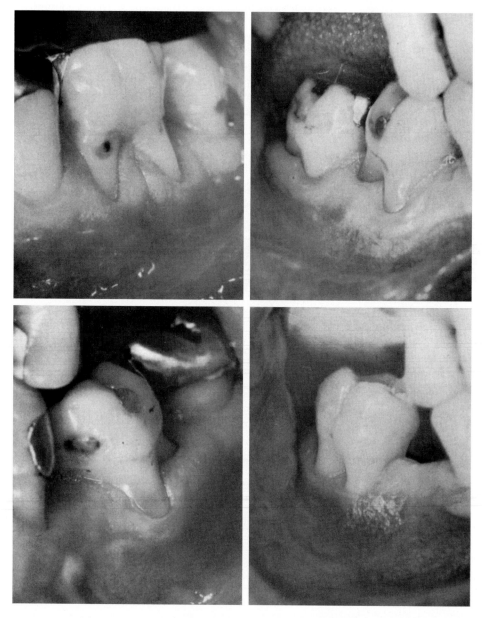

FIGURE 58–9. Optimal gingival contour obtained by treatment of furcation involvements of different severity.

way to raise the flap coronally in humans; the suture would then engage the flap and then go through the bracket.

Occlusal Adjustment in the Treatment of Furcation Lesions. Furcation involvement is not of itself indicative of trauma from occlusion; inflammation may be the only responsible destructive factor. However, of all the areas of the periodontium, the furcation is most susceptible to injury from excessive occlusal forces. When furcation involvement is complicated by infrabony pockets and osseous defects, or if the tooth is excessively mobile, then checking the occlusion and adjusting it, if necessary, are essential.

ROOT RESECTION AND HEMISECTION IN THE MANAGEMENT OF FURCATION INVOLVEMENT

The treatment of advanced grade II and grade III furcation involvements will often require removal or resection of a root.[1,21] This will allow access to the remaining root surfaces for scaling and root planing and for the patient's plaque control regimen. Root resection is the treatment of choice for many of the advanced furcation lesions when positive, definitive results are needed.

The following factors must be considered in the selection of a tooth for root resective therapy:

1. Advanced bone loss around one root with an acceptable level of bone around the remaining root(s).

2. Angulation and position of the tooth in the arch. A molar that is buccally or lingually out of position or mesially or distally tilted cannot be resected.
3. The divergence of the roots. Teeth with divergent roots are easier to resect, whereas teeth with closely approximated or fused roots are poor candidates for root resection.
4. The length and curvature of the roots. Long, straight roots are more favorable for resection than short, conical roots.
5. The feasibility of endodontics and restorative dentistry. If endodontic treatment and/or crown restorations are not possible, the tooth is not a candidate for resective therapy.

Figure 58–10*B*,*C* illustrates the difference between a root resection and a hemisection. The removal of a root without the removal of any portion of the crown is termed a *root resection* or *root amputation* procedure. When one root and its corresponding crown portion are cut and removed, as in Figure 58–10*C*, the procedure is called a *hemisection*. This is often done for the mandibular molars and consists of removal of either the mesial or the distal half, depending on which root is involved. A crown and sometimes a fixed bridge are necessary after a hemisection procedure.

The maxillary first molar usually presents the most favorable anatomic features for resective therapy (Fig. 58–11). If the furcation involvement is between the two buccal roots and there are no interdental furcal lesions, then removal of the distal buccal root is the therapy of choice, as this root is usually the smallest in both diameter and length. When other furcal openings become involved, such

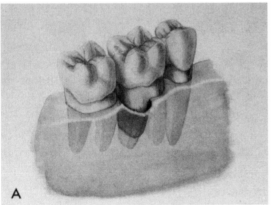
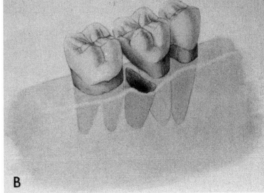
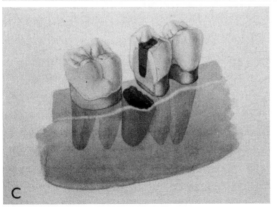

FIGURE 58–10. *A,* Diagrammatic view of furcation involvement in a mandibular first molar, with vertical lesions around the distal root. *B,* After resection of distal root; note the resultant socket. *C,* Another approach using hemisection of the distal half of the tooth (root and crown).

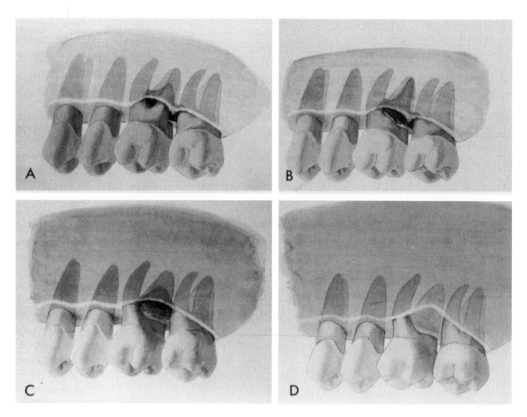

FIGURE 58–11. *A,* Diagrammatic view of furcation involvement around the distofacial root of maxillary first molar; note the bony lesion with a vertical component. *B,* The root has been resected; note the resultant socket and osseous defect. *C,* Partial fill of the socket several months after the resection. *D,* The final osseous contour after osteoplasty of the area.

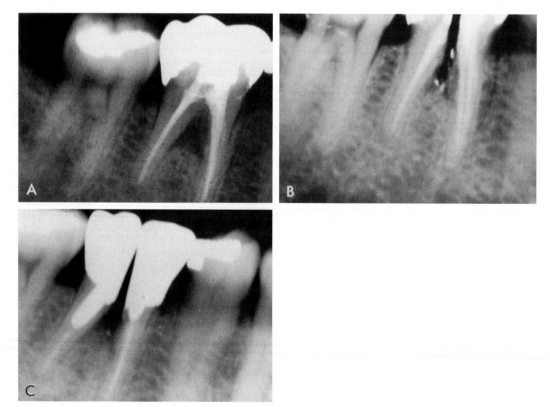

FIGURE 58–12. The bisection technique for treatment of furcation involvements. *A,* Radiograph of a mandibular first molar with a furcation involvement. *B,* Bisection of the molar to eliminate the class III furcation involvement. *C,* The final result of the bisection procedure, with crowns placed on each root.

as the mesial and distal interdental areas of the maxillary molars, the choice of the root to be resected must include a consideration of the numerous factors of tooth and bone anatomy discussed earlier. One clinical study[14] has shown that removal of one of the buccal roots of a maxillary molar does not increase the mobility of the tooth in normal function; splinting is not always necessary.

The treatment of advanced grade II or grade III furcation involvement of a mandibular molar can also be accomplished by a *bisection* (bicuspidization) procedure if the molar exhibits the proper anatomic features and stability. Molars with long, divergent roots and bone loss re-

LEFT   RIGHT

FIGURE 58–13. Apical view of two maxillary molars with different degrees of root proximity. *Left,* Close root proximity. After one root is resected, a defect may form and will require a second intervention. *Right,* Widely separated roots. A second surgical procedure may not be necessary.

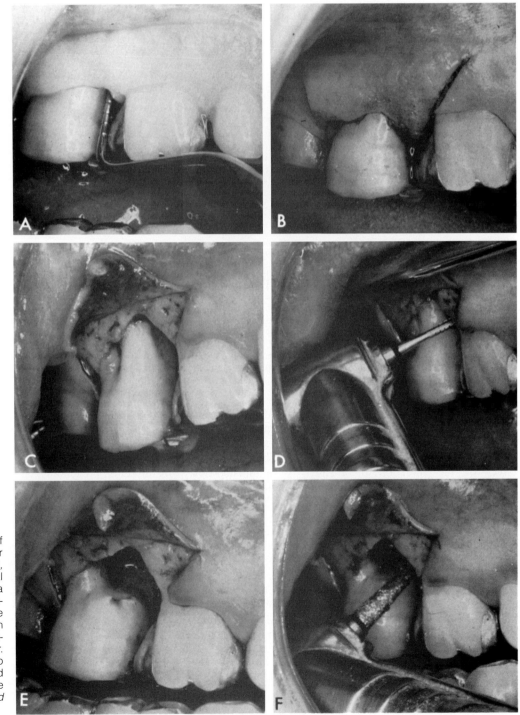

FIGURE 58–14. Resection of the mesiofacial root of a molar with furcation involvement. *A,* Probing the extent of periodontal destruction. *B,* Incisions for a flap. *C,* Mucoperiosteal flap elevated, revealing extensive bone loss and an osseous defect on the mesiofacial root. *D,* Root being resected with cross-cut bur. *E,* Root removed; a sharp stump remains. *F,* Sharp stump planed and tooth contoured to facilitate cleaning. *Illustration continued on following page.*

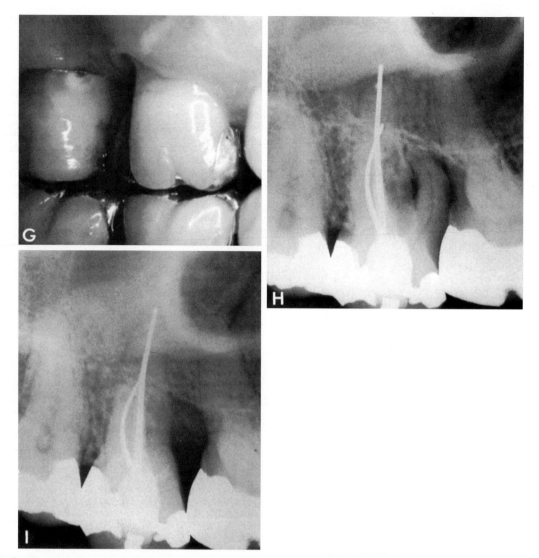

FIGURE 58–14 *Continued G,* Area healed, showing excellent gingival contour where the root was removed. *H,* Radiograph taken before treatment, showing extensive bone loss around the mesiofacial root. *I,* Radiograph taken 9 months after treatment, showing bone repair where the root was removed.

stricted to the furcal area are ideal candidates for this procedure (Fig. 58–12). The molar is simply cut into two separate mesial and distal portions, without the removal of any part of the root or crown. The tunnel-like effect of the furcation involvement is eliminated by creating two separate teeth from the single molar (see Fig. 58–12B). The two portions of the teeth will require crowns.

In most cases of root resection, the endodontic therapy is accomplished first, in which case the procedure is called *nonvital root resection.* However, there are many cases in which the root is resected without endodontic therapy. This is done if the clinician did not anticipate the resection of a root prior to surgery, but the furcation involvement became visible during a periodontal flap procedure. Also, the extent of some furcation involvements is difficult to identify with radiographs and probing alone, and the clinician may not want to commit the patient to an endodontic procedure until the furcation area is examined after the flap is reflected. In these cases, the endodontic therapy can be performed

several days after the periodontal surgical procedure. Root resection without prior endodontic therapy is called *vital resection.*

Endodontic therapy should always be performed prior to hemisection procedures.

Another consideration in root resection procedures is the possibility that a second surgical procedure may be necessary several months after the resective therapy. This may occur in cases of close root proximity in which there are extensive osseous lesions around the resected root. The socket left by the removal of the root requires several months to fill and may leave a residual osseous defect close to the remaining roots. This may result in a vertical bone loss next to the adjacent roots (see Fig. 58–11A). Attempts to recontour the bone at the time of the initial surgery may result in excessive removal of bone. By allowing the bone to fill the socket, the clinician can later reopen the area for a final, definitive osseous correction of the resected area. If the tooth presents widely divergent roots with good interradicular bone, the socket left by the re-

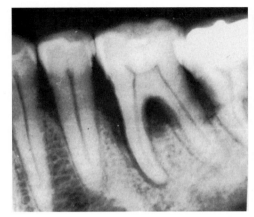
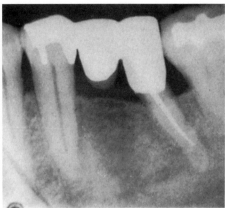

FIGURE 58–15. Hemisection. *Left,* Bifurcation involvement of a first molar. *Right,* Radiograph taken 2 years and 3 months after resection of the mesial half of the first molar. (Courtesy of Dr. John Cane.)

moval of the root may not affect the remaining roots. In these cases, a second surgical procedure may not be necessary (Fig. 58–13).

Technique for Root Resection. The following steps are recommended:

1. Under local anesthesia, probe the area to determine the extent and outline of alveolar bone destruction around the root to be removed (Fig. 58–14*A*).
2. Elevate a mucoperiosteal flap (Fig. 58–14*B,C*).
3. With a contra-angle handpiece and a cross-cut bur, sever the root where it joins the crown (Fig. 58–14*D*). Remove the root (Fig. 58–14*E*).
4. With a stone or diamond point, smooth the resected root

stump and contour the tooth to create an easily cleansable area (Fig. 58–14*F*).
5. Scale and plane the root surfaces, which become visible and more accessible when the root is removed. This is a most critical part of the treatment.
6. Clean the area, replace the flap, suture, and cover with a periodontal pack.

Remove the pack and sutures after 1 week. Physiologic gingival contour is usually restored by 2 months after surgery (Fig. 58–14*G*), and bone repair is detectable radiographically by 9 months (Fig. 58–14*H,I*).

Technique for Hemisection. Hemisection involves the same technique as that used for root resection, except that half the crown is removed along with one of the roots of a mandibular molar. The retained mesial or distal half serves as a useful abutment for a dental restoration (Fig. 58–15). Previous endodontic therapy is mandatory in cases in which the pulp chambers will be opened.

COMBINED PERIODONTAL-ENDODONTIC THERAPY

The periodontium is a continuous unit; pathologic involvement of the periapical area extends into the marginal area, and vice versa. Figure 58–16 diagrams the different ways in which pulpal and periodontal pathologic processes may be interrelated:[34]

1. *A periapical lesion originating in a pulpal infection may have a pathway of fistulization from the apex and along the root to the gingiva* (Fig. 58–16*A*). This can become secondarily complicated into a so-called retrograde periodontitis.[35] Pulpal infection can also extend through an accessory canal directly to the gingiva or to the furcation area, causing bone loss.[25] Differential diagnosis should consider (1) whether the involved area is the only periodontally diseased part of the mouth and (2) the pulpal and periapical status of the tooth. Isolated furcal radiolucencies in pulpally "suspect" teeth with no pockets may point to a pulpal origin of infection. In these cases, endodontic therapy alone or with minimal periodontal treatment may be all that is needed (Fig. 58–17). If a long-standing, primarily endodontic lesion has become periodontally involved, periodontal therapy may be necessary in addition to endodontic treatment. However, it is frequently advisable to perform the endodontic therapy first and wait a few months before proceeding with periodontal treatment, as the remaining lesion may be considerably reduced, if not totally eliminated, after that time (Fig. 58–16*B*).

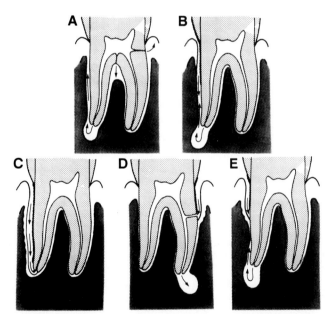

FIGURE 58–16. Diagrammatic representation of different types of endoperiodontal problems. *A,* An originally endodontic problem, with fistulization from the apex and along the root to the gingiva. Pulpal infection can also spread through accessory canals to the gingiva or to the furcation. *B,* A long-standing periapical lesion draining through the periodontal ligament can become secondarily complicated, leading to a "retrograde periodontitis." *C,* A periodontal pocket can deepen to the apex and secondarily involve the pulp. *D,* A periodontal pocket can infect the pulp through a lateral canal, and this in turn can result in a periapical lesion. *E,* Two independent lesions, periapical and marginal, can coexist and eventually fuse with each other. (Redrawn and modified from Simon JHS, Glick DH, Frank AL. The relationship of endodontic-periodontic lesions. J Periodontol *43*:202, 1972.)

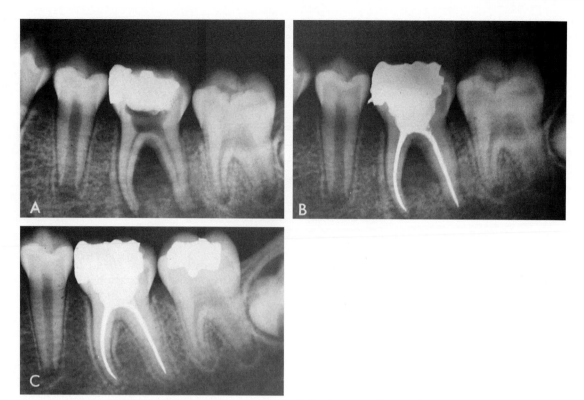

FIGURE 58–17. *A,* Extensive radiolucent area in furcation, apices, and distal aspect of lower first molar. *B,* Immediately after endodontic therapy. *C,* Complete healing of the lesion. No periodontal treatment was performed. (Courtesy of Dr. John I. Ingle and the School of Dentistry, University of Washington.)

2. *Marginal periodontitis can progress to the apex of a root or to the emergence of an accessory canal and induce a secondary pulpal involvement* (Fig. 58–16C,D). Periodontal therapy is necessary in these cases, and the need for endodontic treatment will depend on tooth vitality. If the tooth is nonvital, either as a result of pathologic involvement of the pulp or because the pulp's blood vessels were severed during periodontal treatment, endodontic therapy is indicated.

3. *A true combined lesion is present when two separate lesions of endodontic and periodontal origin coalesce.* In these cases, both periodontal therapy and endodontic therapy are indicated (Fig. 58–16E).

REFERENCES

1. Amen CR. Hemisection and root amputation. Periodontics *4:*197, 1966.
2. Becker W, Becker BE, Berg L, et al. New attachment after treatment with root isolation procedures: Report for treated class III and class II furcations and vertical osseous defects. Int J Periodont Restor Dent *8*(3):9, 1988.
3. Bower RC. Furcation morphology relative to periodontal treatment: Furcation entrance architecture. J Periodontol *50:*23, 1979.
4. Bower RC. Furcation morphology relative to periodontal treatment: Furcation root surface anatomy. J Periodontol *50:*366, 1979.
5. Carranza FA Jr, Jolkovsky DL. Current status of periodontal therapy for furcation involvements. Dent Clin North Am *35:*555, 1991.
6. Crigger M, Bogle G, Nilveus R, et al. The effect of topical citric acid application on the healing of experimental furcation defects in dogs. J Periodont Res *13:*538, 1978.
7. Ericsson I, Nyman S. Treatment of molar furcation involvement. Tandlakart *65:*252, 1973.
8. Farnoush AA, Saadoun AP, Joseph CE. Management of periodontally involved teeth with furcation lesions. J Calif Dent Assoc *14:*11, 1986.
9. Glickman I. Clinical Periodontology. 1st ed. Philadelphia, WB Saunders, 1953.
10. Goldman HM. Therapy of the incipient bifurcation involvement. J Periodontol *29:*112, 1958.
11. Hiatt WH. Periodontic pocket elimination by combined endodontic-periodontic therapy. Periodontics *1:*152, 1963.
12. Hiatt WH, Schallhorn RG. Intraoral transplants of cancellous bone and marrow in periodontal lesions. J Periodontol *44:*194, 1973.
13. Kenney EB, Lekovic V, Elbaz J-J, et al. The use of porous hydroxylapatite implants in periodontal defects. II. Treatment of class II furcation lesions in lower molars. J Periodontol *58:*67, 1988.
14. Klavan N. Clinical observations following root amputations in maxillary molar teeth. J Periodontol *46:*1, 1975.
15. Klinge B, Nilveus R, Kiger RD, Egelberg J. Effect of flap placement and defect size on healing of experimental furcation defects. J Periodont Res *16:*236, 1981.
16. Klinge B, Nilveus R, Egelberg J. Effect of crown attached sutures on healing of experimental furcation defects in dogs. J Clin Periodontol *12:*369, 1985.
17. Lekovic V, Kenney EB, Carranza FA Jr, Danilovic V. Treatment of grade II furcation defects using porous hydroxyapatite in conjunction with a polytetrafluoroethylene membrane. J Periodontol *61:*575, 1991.
18. Lekovic V, Kenney EB, Kovacevic K, Carranza FA Jr. Evaluation of guided tissue regeneration in class II furcation defects. A clinical re-entry study. J Periodontol *60:*694, 1989.
19. Leon LE, Vogel RI. A comparison of the effectiveness of hand scaling and ultrasonic debridement in furcations as evaluated by differential dark-field microscopy. J Periodontol *58:*86, 1987.
20. Matia JB, Bissada NF, Maybury JE, Ricchetti P. Efficiency of scaling of the molar furcation area with and without surgical access. Int J Periodont Restor Dent *6:*25, 1986.
21. Messinger TF, Orban BJ. Elimination of periodontal pockets by root amputation. J Periodontol *25:*213, 1954.
22. Miller SC. Textbook of Periodontia (Oral Medicine). 3rd ed. Philadelphia, Blakiston, 1950.
23. Nilveus R, Bogle G, Crigger M, et al. The effect of topical citric acid application on the healing of experimental furcation defects in dogs. II. Healing after repeated surgery. J Periodont Res *15:*544, 1980.
24. Nilveus R, Egelberg J. The effect of topical citric acid application on the healing of experimental furcation defects in dogs. III. The relative importance of coagulum support, flap design and systemic antibiotics. J Periodont Res *15:*551, 1980.
25. Orban BJ, Johnston H. Interradicular pathology as related to accessory root canals. J Endodont *3:*21, 1948.
26. Parodi RJ, Esper ME. Effect of topical application of citric acid in the treatment of furcation involvement in human lower molars. J Clin Periodontol *11:*644, 1984.
27. Pontoriero R, Lindhe J, Nyman S, et al. Guided tissue regeneration in degree II furcation-involved mandibular molars. A clinical study. J Clin Periodontol *15:*247, 1988.
28. Pontoriero R, Lindhe J, Nyman S, et al. Guided tissue regeneration in the treat-

29. Robinson RE. Osseous coagulum for bone induction. J Periodontol *40*:503, 1969.
30. Ross IF, Thompson RH. A long-term study of root retention in the treatment of maxillary molars with furcation involvement. J Periodontol *49*:238, 1978.
31. Saadoun AP. Management of furcation involvement. J West Soc Periodontol *33*:91, 1985.
32. Sanders JJ, Sepe WW, Bowers GM, et al. Clinical evaluation of freeze-dried bone allografts in periodontal osseous defects. Part III. Composite freeze-dried allografts with and without hip marrow grafts. J Periodontol *54*:1, 1983.
33. Schallhorn RG. Eradication of bifurcation defects utilizing frozen autogenous hip marrow implants. Periodont Abstr *15*:101, 1967.
34. Simon JHS, Glick DH, Frank AL. The relationship of endodontic-periodontic lesions. J Periodontol *43*:202, 1972.
35. Simring M, Goldberg M. The pulpal pocket approach: Retrograde periodontitis. J Periodontol *35*:22, 1964.
36. Stahl SS, Froum S. Human clinical and histologic repair responses following the use of citric acid in periodontal therapy. J Periodontol *48*:261, 1977.
37. Tarnow D, Fletcher P. Classification of the vertical component of furcation involvement. J Periodontol *55*:183, 1984.

59

Mucogingival Surgery

FERMIN A. CARRANZA, JR. and HENRY H. TAKEI

Objectives	Classification
Factors That Affect the Outcome of Mucogingival Surgery	Pedicle Graft: Laterally (Horizontally) Displaced Flap
Irregularity of Teeth	Coronally Displaced Flap
The Mucogingival Line (Junction)	Free Soft Tissue Autograft
Techniques for Increasing Attached Gingiva	Subepithelial Connective Tissue Graft Technique
Free Gingival Autografts	Guided Tissue Regeneration Technique
The Apically Displaced Flap	**Operations for Removal of Frena**
Guided Tissue Regeneration (GTR)	Frenectomy or Frenotomy
Technique for Root Coverage	**Criteria for Selection of Mucogingival Techniques**
Operations for Coverage of Denuded Roots	**Comment**

Mucogingival surgery consists of plastic surgical procedures for the correction of gingiva–mucous membrane relationships that complicate periodontal disease and may interfere with the success of periodontal treatment.

OBJECTIVES

Mucogingival surgery is performed as an adjunct to regular pocket elimination or as an independent procedure for the purpose of widening the zone of attached gingiva when an insufficient amount is present. The width of the attached gingiva varies in different individuals and on different teeth in the same individual (see Chapters 1 and 28). *Attached gingiva* is not synonymous with *keratinized gingiva,* because the latter also includes the free gingival margin. The width of the attached gingiva is determined by subtracting the depth of the sulcus or pocket from the distance from the crest of the margin to the mucogingival junction.

The original rationale for mucogingival surgery was predicated on the assumption that a minimal width of attached gingiva was required for optimal gingival health to be maintained. However, several studies have challenged the view that a wide attached gingiva is more protective against the accumulation of plaque than a thin or a nonexistent zone. No minimal width of attached gingiva has been established as a standard necessary for gingival health. Persons who practice excellent oral hygiene may maintain healthy areas with almost no attached gingiva.

However, those individuals whose oral hygiene practices are less than optimal can be helped by the presence of keratinized gingiva and vestibular depth, which provide room for easier placement of the toothbrush, to avoid brushing on mucosal tissue.

There is also a need for a wider zone of attached gingiva in teeth that serve as abutments for fixed or removable partial dentures, as well as in ridge areas in relation to the dentures. Teeth with subgingival restorations and narrow zones of keratinized gingiva have higher gingival inflammation scores than teeth with similar restorations and wide zones of attached gingiva.[97] Therefore, techniques for widening the attached gingiva are considered preprosthetic periodontal surgical procedures in these cases.

Coverage of denuded roots is another objective of mucogingival surgery. These techniques attempt to solve the aesthetic problem, but also widen the keratinized gingiva.

Still another objective of mucogingival surgery is the creation of some vestibular depth when this is lacking. The amount of keratinized gingiva present may be considered in relation to the depth of the vestibule. Minimal attached keratinized gingiva with good vestibular depth may not require mucogingival surgery, but the same minimal amount of attached keratinized gingiva with no vestibular depth will usually benefit from mucogingival correction.

Reduced or absent attached gingiva may be due to several factors:

1. *The base of the periodontal pocket being apical or close to the mucogingival line* (Fig. 59–1). In these cases, some attached gingiva must be created to separate the healed gingival sulcus from the alveolar mucosa and to prevent pockets from recurring. The functional adequacy of the attached gingiva can be determined by the following tension test: Retract the cheeks and lips laterally with the fingers. If such tension pulls the marginal gingiva from the teeth, widening of the attached gingiva should be considered.
2. *Frenal and muscle attachments that encroach on periodontal pockets and pull them away from the tooth surface.* Tension from such attachments (1) distends the gingival sulcus and fosters the accumulation of irritants that lead to gingivitis and pocket formation and (2) aggravates the progression of periodontal pockets and causes their recurrence after treatment (Fig. 59–2A to C). The problem is more common on the facial surface, but it occasionally occurs on the lingual surface (Fig. 59–2D).
3. *Recession causing denudation of root surfaces* and creating a functional as well as an aesthetic problem (Fig. 59–3A, B). The tension test should also be used in cases of progressive gingival recession to check the effect of soft tissue tension on the gingival margin. Clinical examination and probing will reveal these areas of root denudation.

It should be noted that deepening of the vestibule is not important in relation to periodontal therapy.[5] However, increasing the depth of the vestibule is very important in the surgical preparation of edentulous ridges.

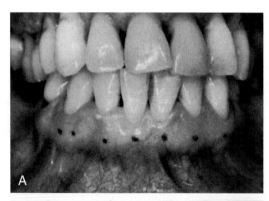
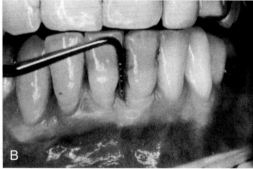

FIGURE 59–1. Periodontal pockets with little or no attached gingiva. *A,* Pockets on mandibular incisors and cuspids extending into the alveolar mucosa. Note the marks inserted to show the location of the base of deep periodontal pockets in relation to the mucogingival line. *B,* Periodontal pockets in the mandibular area, with a probe indicating a 4-mm pocket on the mesial surface of the central incisor, reaching to the mucogingival line.

FACTORS THAT AFFECT THE OUTCOME OF MUCOGINGIVAL SURGERY*

Irregularity of Teeth

Abnormal tooth alignment is an important cause of gingival deformities that require corrective surgery and is an important factor in determining the outcome of treatment. The location of the gingival margin, the width of the attached gingiva, and alveolar bone height and thickness are all affected by tooth alignment. On teeth that are tilted or rotated labially, the labial bony plate is thinner and located farther apically than on the adjacent teeth, and the gingiva is recessed so that the root is exposed.[115] On the lingual surface of such teeth, the gingiva is bulbous and the bone margins are closer to the cemento-enamel junction. The level of gingival attachment on root surfaces and the width of the attached gingiva after mucogingival surgery are affected as much or more by tooth alignment as by variations in treatment procedures.

Orthodontic correction is indicated when mucogingival surgery is performed on malposed teeth in an attempt to widen the attached gingiva or to restore the gingiva over denuded roots. If orthodontic treatment is not feasible, the prominent tooth should be ground to within the borders of the alveolar bone, with special care taken to avoid pulp injury.

Roots covered with thin bony plates present a hazard in mucogingival surgery. Even the most protective type of flap (i.e., a partial-thickness flap) creates the risk of bone resorption on the periosteal surface.[48] Resorption in amounts that ordinarily are not significant may cause loss of bone height when the bony plate is thin or tapered at the crest.

The Mucogingival Line (Junction)

Normally, the mucogingival line in the incisor and canine areas is located approximately 3 mm apical to the crest of the alveolar bone on the radicular surfaces and 5 mm interdentally.[98] In periodontal disease and on malposed, disease-free teeth, the bone margin is located farther apically and may extend beyond the mucogingival line.

The distance between the mucogingival line and the cemento-enamel junction before and after periodontal surgery is not necessarily constant. After inflammation is eliminated, there is a tendency for the tissue to contract and draw the mucogingival line in the direction of the crown.[28]

TECHNIQUES FOR INCREASING ATTACHED GINGIVA

Two types of procedures can widen the zone of attached gingiva: the gingival extension operation and apical displacement of the pocket wall.

Gingival Extension Operation. This consists of surgical deepening of the mucogingival line. To prevent the mucogingival line from creeping back coronally during postoperative healing, a free mucosal or gingival autograft

---

*See also Chapter 51.

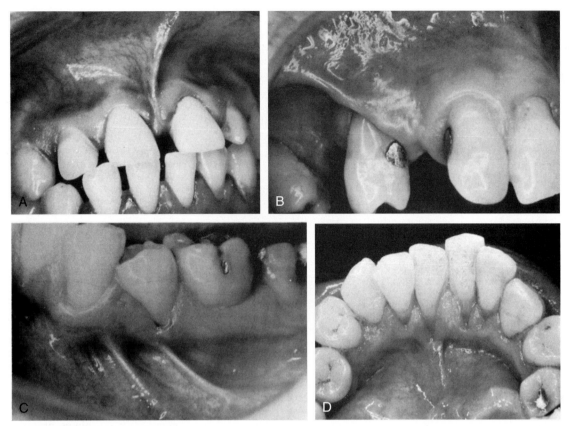

FIGURE 59-2. High frenum attachments. *A,* Frenum between maxillary central incisors. *B,* Frenum on the mesial surface of the maxillary second premolar. *C,* Frenum attached to a pocket wall on a mandibular first premolar. *D,* Frenum attached to a pocket wall on the lingual surface of an incisor.

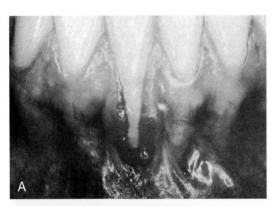

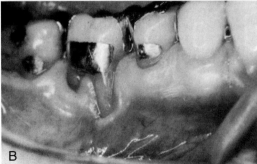

FIGURE 59-3. *A,* Gingival recession and extreme inflammation around a lower central incisor. *B,* Advanced recession of mesiobuccal root of a first lower molar.

is obtained from the palate and placed in the surgical site. Free gingival grafts will also predictably deepen the vestibule.

Apical Displacement of the Pocket Wall. This procedure will eliminate the pocket and transform the pocket wall into attached gingiva. It does not predictably deepen the vestibule.

Free Gingival Autografts

Free gingival grafts are used to create a widened zone of attached gingiva. They were initially described by Bjorn[8] in 1963 and have been extensively investigated since that time.

The Classic Technique

Step 1: Eliminate the Pockets. If pockets are present, resect them with a gingivectomy incision, and scale and plane the root surfaces (Plate XXI). If there are no pockets present in the area, the gingival margin is left intact.

Step 2: Prepare the Recipient Site. The purpose of this step is to prepare a firm connective tissue bed to receive the graft. The recipient site can be prepared by incising at the existing mucogingival junction with a no. 15 Bard-Parker knife to a little more than the desired depth, blending the incision on both ends with the existing mucogingival line (Plate XXI*B*). Periosteum should be left covering the bone.

Another technique consists of outlining the recipient site with two vertical incisions from the cut gingival margin into the alveolar mucosa (Fig. 59–4B). Extend the incisions to approximately twice the desired width of the attached gingiva, allowing for 50% contraction of the graft when healing is complete. The amount of contraction depends on the extent to which the recipient site penetrates the muscle attachments. The deeper the recipient site, the

greater the tendency for the muscles to elevate the graft and reduce the final width of the attached gingiva. The periosteum along the apical border of the graft is sometimes penetrated in an effort to prevent postoperative narrowing of the attached gingiva.

A no. 15 Bard-Parker blade is inserted along the cut gingival margin and used to separate a flap consisting of epithelium and underlying connective tissue without disturb-

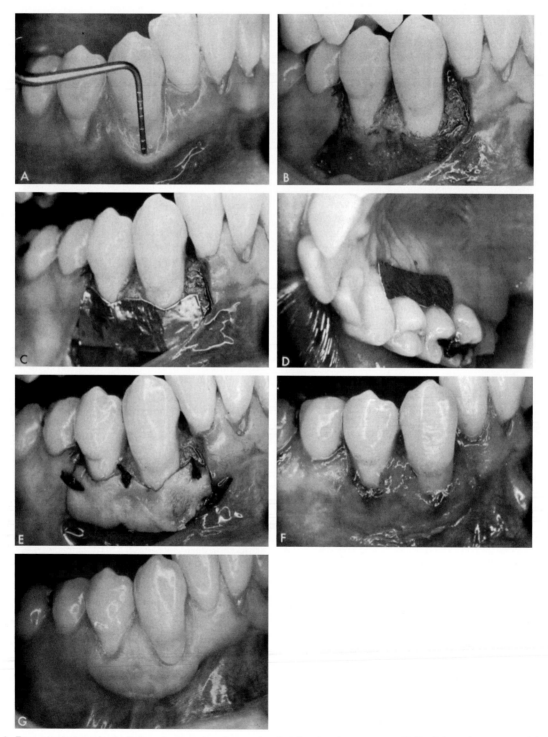

FIGURE 59–4. Free gingival graft. *A*, Before treatment; sulcus extends into alveolar mucosa. *B*, Recipient site prepared for free gingival graft. *C*, Tinfoil template of the desired graft. *D*, Template used to outline the graft in the donor site. *E*, Graft transferred. *F*, After 2 weeks. *G*, After 1 year, showing widened zone of attached gingiva.

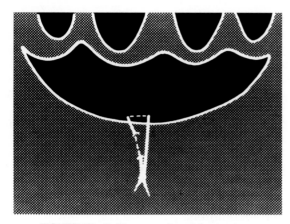

FIGURE 59–5. Diagram of graft bed suture.

ing the periosteum. The flap is extended to the depth of the vertical incisions.

If a narrow band of attached gingiva remains after the pockets are eliminated, it should be left intact and the recipient site started by inserting the blade at the mucogingival junction instead of at the cut gingival margin.

Suture the flap where the apical portion of the free graft will be located. Three to four independent catgut sutures are placed for an average graft. The needle is passed as a superficial mattress suture, first perpendicular to the incision and then on the periosteum parallel to the incision (Figs. 59–5 and 59–6).

Make a tinfoil template of the recipient site to be used as a pattern for the graft (see Fig. 59–4C,D).

Grafts can also be placed directly on bone tissue. For this technique, the flap must be separated by blunt dissection with a periosteal elevator. Reported advantages of this

variant are less postoperative mobility of the graft, less swelling, better hemostasis,[29] and $1\frac{1}{2}$ to 2 times less shrinkage[52,53]; however, a healing lag is observed for the first 2 weeks.[14,15,34]

Step 3: Obtain the Graft From the Donor Site. The classic or conventional free gingival graft technique consists of transferring a piece of keratinized oral mucosa of approximately the size of the recipient site. To avoid the large wound that this procedure sometimes leaves in the donor site, some alternative methods have been proposed. The original technique is described first, followed by several of the most common variants.

For the classic technique (see Fig. 59–4 and Plate XXI), a partial-thickness graft is used; the sites from which it can be obtained are, in order of preference, attached gingiva, masticatory mucosa from an edentulous ridge, and palatal mucosa. The graft should consist of epithelium and a thin layer of underlying connective tissue.

Place the template over the donor site (see Fig. 59–4D), and make a shallow incision around it with a no. 15 Bard-Parker blade. Insert the blade to the desired thickness at one edge of the graft; elevate the edge and hold it with tissue forceps. Continue to separate the graft with the blade, lifting it gently as separation progresses to provide visibility. Placing sutures at the margins of the graft helps control it during separation and transfer and simplifies placement and suturing to the recipient site.[4]

Proper thickness is important for survival of the graft. The graft should be thin enough to permit ready diffusion of nutritive fluid from the recipient site, which is essential in the immediate post-transplant period. A graft that is too thin may shrivel and expose the recipient site.[66,74] If the graft is too thick, its peripheral layer is jeopardized because of the excessive tissue that separates it from new circula-

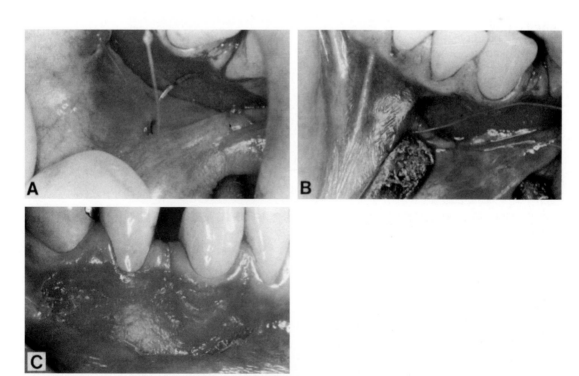

FIGURE 59–6. Graft bed suture. *A,* Suture (vertical mattress) through border of wound. *B,* Suture (horizontal) through periosteum. *C,* Suture completed.

tion and nutrients. Thick grafts may also create a deeper wound at the donor site, with the possibility of injuring major palatal arteries.[108] The ideal thickness of a graft is between 1.0 and 1.5 mm.[44,66] A thick graft can be thinned by holding it between two wet wooden tongue depressors and slicing it longitudinally with a sharp Bard-Parker knife.

After the graft is separated, remove loose tissue tabs from the undersurface. Thin the edge to avoid bulbous marginal and interdental contours. Special precautions must be taken with grafts from the palate. The submucosa in the posterior region is thick and fatty and should be trimmed so that it will not interfere with vascularization. Grafts tend to re-establish their original epithelial structure, so mucous glands may occur in grafts obtained from the palate.

Step 4: Transfer and Immobilize the Graft. Remove the sponge from the recipient site; reapply it, with pressure if necessary, until bleeding is stopped. Clean away excess clot. A thick clot interferes with vascularization of the graft[69]; it is also an excellent medium for bacteria and increases the risk of infection.

Position the graft and adapt it firmly to the recipient site. Space between the graft and the underlying tissue (dead space) will retard vascularization and jeopardize the graft. Suture the graft at the lateral borders and to the periosteum to secure it in position (see Fig. 59–4E and Plate XXIE). Before suturing is completed, elevate the unsutured portion and cleanse the recipient bed beneath it with an aspirator to remove clots or loose tissue fragments. Press the graft back into position and complete the sutures. Be sure that the graft is immobilized, because movement interferes with healing. Avoid excessive tension, which will warp the graft and may pull it away from the underlying surface. Respect for tissue is essential for success. Use every precaution to avoid injury to the graft. Use tissue forceps delicately to

avoid crushing it and a minimal number of sutures to avoid unnecessary tissue penetration. The graft can survive some injury, but abuse may damage it beyond recovery.

Step 5: Protect the Donor Site. Cover the donor site with a periodontal pack for 1 week and repeat if necessary. Retention of the pack on the donor site is sometimes a problem. If facial attached gingiva was used, the pack may be retained by locking it through the interproximal spaces onto the lingual surface. If there are no open interdental spaces, the pack can be covered by a plastic stent wired to the teeth. A modified Hawley retainer is useful to cover the pack on the palate and over edentulous ridges.

Variant Techniques

Four variants to the classic technique are described in this section: the accordion technique, the strip technique, the connective tissue technique, and a combination of the strip and the connective tissue techniques.

The *accordion technique* has been described by Rateitschak and colleagues.[80] It attains expansion of the graft by alternate incisions in opposite sides of the graft (Fig. 59–7).

The *strip technique,* developed by Han and associates,[47] consists of obtaining two or three strips of tissue about 1 mm wide and long enough to cover the entire length of the recipient site (Fig. 59–8). These strips are placed in the base and the center of the recipient site, secured by sutures from the oral mucosa, and wrapped around the tooth. The area is then covered with tinfoil and surgical pack. The donor site usually does not require any protection and heals uneventfully in a few days. Greater shrinkage of the graft results with this technique, and therefore a slightly larger recipient site is required.

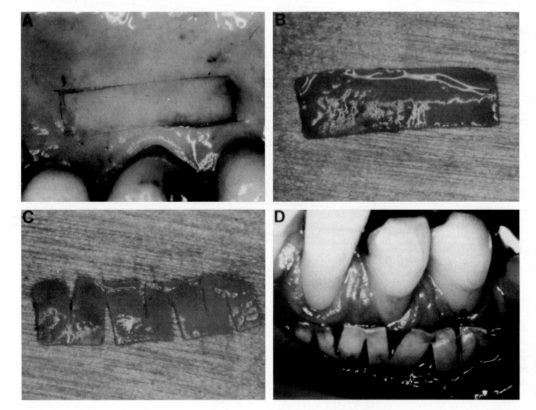

FIGURE 59–7. Free gingival graft: accordion technique. *A,* Donor site with outline of donor tissue. *B,* Donor tissue removed. *C,* Incisions made in donor tissue to obtain expansion. *D,* Expanded donor tissue placed on the recipient site.

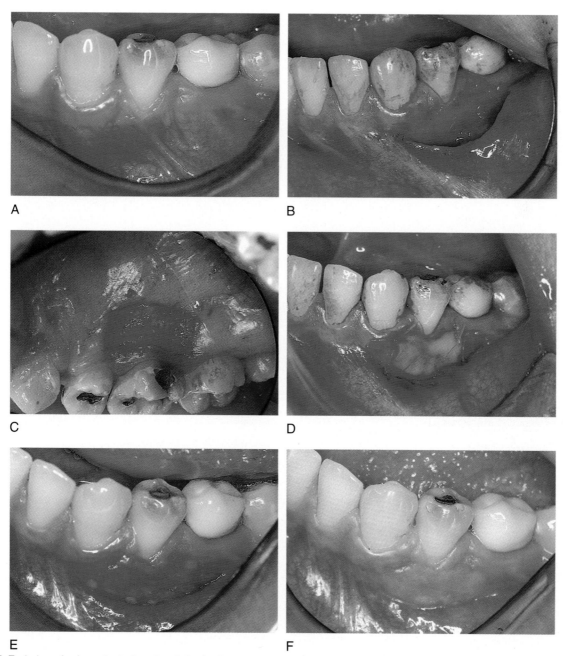

PLATE XXI. Technique for free gingival grafts. *A,* Lack of attached gingiva and the beginning of recession on the lower second premolar. *B,* Surgical bed prepared and the border of the wound sutured to the periosteum. *C,* Donor site in the palatal area immediately after removal of tissue for grafting. Note the presence of periosteum. *D,* Donor tissue placed on the surgical bed and sutured with catgut. *E,* Recipient site 1 month postoperatively. *F,* Recipient site 3 months postoperatively. Compare with *A.* (Courtesy of Dr. Agusti Marfany.)

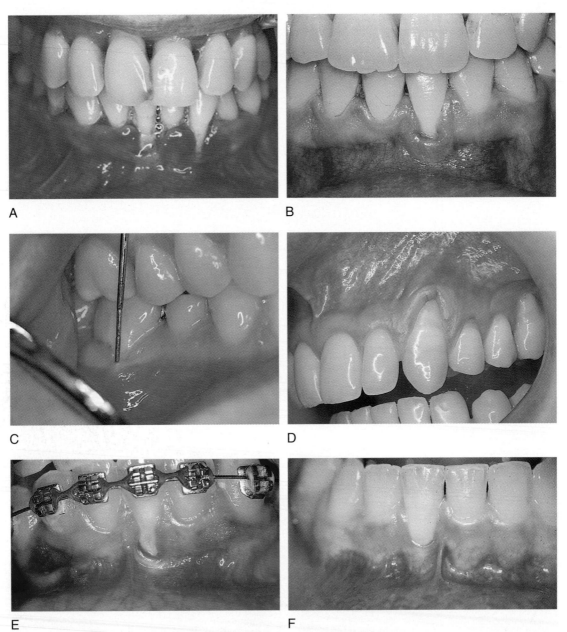

PLATE XXII. Mucogingival defects. *A,* Irregular gingival contours, pocket furcations, and recession with severe gingival inflammation. *B,* Gingival recession and inflammation. Bottom of pocket is beyond mucogingival junction. *C,* Recession on mesiobuccal root of lower first molar. Probe indicates presence of shallow pocket with absence of attached gingiva. *D,* Gingival recession and cleft on upper cuspid. *E,* Advanced gingival recession and inflammation. *F,* After scaling and root planing and adequate plaque control, gingival condition has improved markedly.

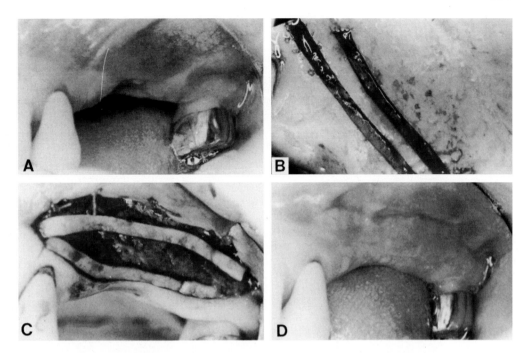

FIGURE 59–8. Free gingival graft: strip technique. *A,* Preoperative view of recipient site. Note the lack of attached tissue in the edentulous area. *B,* Two strips of tissue removed from palatal site. *C,* Strips of tissue placed on the recipient site. *D,* Healing after 4 weeks.

The *connective tissue technique* was originally described by Edel[34] and is based on the fact that the connective tissue carries the genetic message for the overlying epithelium to become keratinized. Therefore, only connective tissue from a keratinized zone can be used as a graft.

This technique has the advantage that the donor material can be obtained from under a palatal flap, which is then sutured back in place so that healing by first intention will take place.[10] Also, the donor site can be from under a flap that is raised for purposes of periodontal treatment of the area.[3] Figure 59–9 shows a case in which the connective tissue graft technique was utilized.

In some cases, a *combination technique* can be performed as follows. Remove a strip of tissue about 3 to 4 mm thick from the palate, place it between two wet tongue depressors, and slice it longitudinally with a sharp Bard-Parker knife. Use as a graft both the superficial portion that contains epithelium and connective tissue and the deeper portion that consists only of connective tissue.

Healing of the Graft

The success of the graft depends on survival of the connective tissue (see Fig. 59–4G and Plate XXI). Sloughing of the epithelium occurs in most cases, but the extent to which the connective tissue withstands the transfer to the new location determines the fate of the graft. Fibrous organization of the interface between the graft and the recipient bed occurs within 2 to several days.[94]

The graft is initially maintained by a diffusion of fluid from the host bed, adjacent gingiva, and alveolar mucosa.[38] The fluid is a transudate from the host vessels and provides nutrition and hydration essential for the initial survival of the transplanted tissues. During the first day, the connective tissue becomes edematous and disorganized and undergoes degeneration and lysis of some of its elements. As healing progresses, the edema is resolved, and degenerated connective tissue is replaced by new granulation tissue.

Revascularization of the graft starts by the second[9] or third day.[54] Capillaries from the recipient bed proliferate into the graft to form a network of new capillaries and anastomose with pre-existing vessels.[54] Many of the graft vessels degenerate and are replaced by new ones, and some participate in the new circulation. The central section of the surface is the last to vascularize, but this is complete by the tenth day.

The epithelium undergoes degeneration and sloughing, with complete necrosis occurring in some areas.[13,72] Necrotic tissue is replaced by new epithelium from the borders of the recipient site. A thin layer of new epithelium is present by the fourth day, with rete pegs developing by the seventh day.

The fact that heterotopically placed grafts maintain their structure (i.e., keratinized epithelium) even after the grafted epithelium has become necrotic and has been replaced by neighboring areas of nonkeratinized epithelium suggests that there exists a genetic predetermination of the specific character of the oral mucosa that is dependent on stimuli that originate in the connective tissue.[55] This is the basis for the technique that uses grafts composed only of connective tissue obtained from areas where it is covered by keratinized epithelium.[10,27,34]

As seen microscopically, healing of a graft of intermediate thickness (0.75 mm) is complete by 10½ weeks; thicker grafts (1.75 mm) may require 16 weeks or longer.[39]

The gross appearance of the graft reflects the tissue changes within it. At the time of transplantation, the graft vessels are empty, and the graft is pale. The pallor changes to an ischemic grayish white during the first 2 days until vascularization begins, after which a pink color appears. The plasmatic circulation accumulates and causes softening and swelling of the graft, which are reduced when the edema is removed from the recipient site by the new blood vessels. Loss of epithelium leaves the graft smooth and shiny. New epithelium creates a thin, gray, veil-like surface that develops normal features as the epithelium matures.

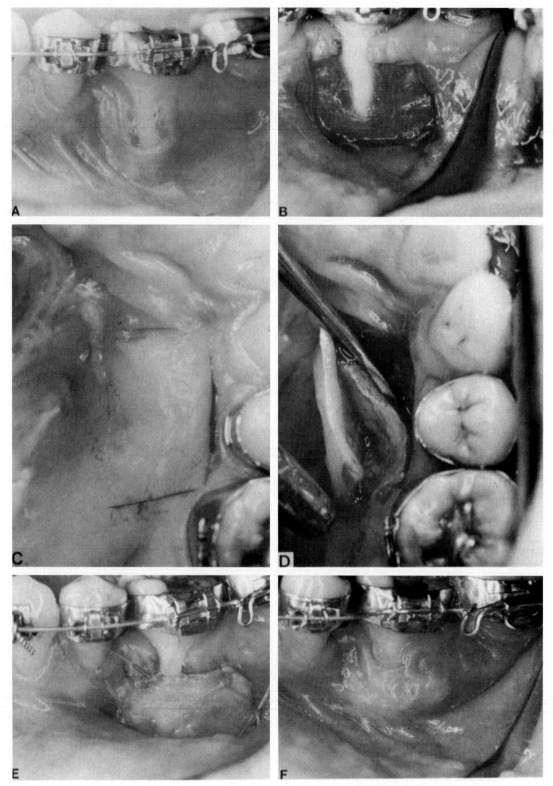

FIGURE 59–9. Connective tissue graft. *A,* Gingival recession and absence of attached gingiva on the facial aspect of the mesial root of the lower left first molar. *B,* Surgical bed prepared; root thoroughly scaled. *C,* Donor tissue outlined on the palatal surface of premolars. *D,* Double flap elevated; the underlying connective tissue is to be used as donor. *E,* Donor tissue sutured with catgut on the recipient site. *F,* Increased band of attached gingiva and partial coverage of the denuded root after 3 months of healing. (Courtesy of Dr. T. J. Han.)

Functional integration of the graft occurs by the 17th day, but the graft will be morphologically distinguishable from the surrounding tissue for months. The graft will eventually blend with adjacent tissues, but sometimes, although pink, firm, and healthy, it will be somewhat bulbous. This ordinarily presents no problem, but if the graft traps plaque or is aesthetically unacceptable, thinning of the graft may be necessary. Thinning of the graft is accomplished by elevating a flap that includes the graft and thinning it from its underside. Paring down the surface will not reduce the thickness of the graft because the surface will proliferate again.

Accomplishments of Free Gingival Grafts

Free gingival grafts effectively widen the attached gingiva. Several biometric studies have analyzed the width of the attached gingiva after the placement of a free gingival graft.[12,48,52] After 24 weeks, grafts placed on denuded bone shrink 25%, whereas grafts placed on periosteum shrink 50%.[59] The greatest amount of shrinkage occurs within the first 6 weeks.

The placement of a gingival graft per se does not improve the status of the gingiva in comparison with that of the gingiva surrounding contralateral teeth with equal degrees of recession where no graft was placed, provided that plaque control is equivalent on both sides.[32,33,106] Therefore, *the indication for a free gingival graft should be based on the presence of progressive gingival recession and inflammation.* When recession continues to progress after a period of a few months with good plaque control, a graft can be placed to prevent further recession and loss of attached gingiva.

Other materials have been used to replace gingival tissue in gingival extension operations. Attempts with lyophilized dura mater[88] and sclera[70] have not been satisfactory; the use of irradiated free gingival allografts showed satisfactory results,[86] but further research is necessary before such grafts can be considered for clinical use.

Free autogenous gingival grafts have been found to be useful for covering nonpathologic dehiscences and fenestrations; ("nonpathologic" refers to openings of the bone through the tooth surface not previously exposed to the oral environment and found in the course of flap surgery).[31]

The use of free mucosal autografts to cover denuded roots is described under "Operations for Coverage of Denuded Roots."

The Apically Displaced Flap

Displaced flaps may be used to correct mucogingival deformities; they avoid some of the limitations of gingival extension operations and require less extensive surgical interference.[2,36,37] This operation utilizes the apically displaced flap (partial-thickness or full-thickness) for the combined purposes of eliminating pockets and widening the zone of attached gingiva. The partial-thickness (mucosal) flap is generally used to avoid exposure of bone and the accompanying risks of bone resorption and aggravation of bone dehiscences and fenestrations.[85,93] The full-thickness (muco-

periosteal) flap is indicated when access to the bone is desired for recontouring purposes.

A step-by-step description of the surgical technique for apically displaced flaps is given in Chapter 55, and the procedure is shown in Figures 59–10 and 59–11.

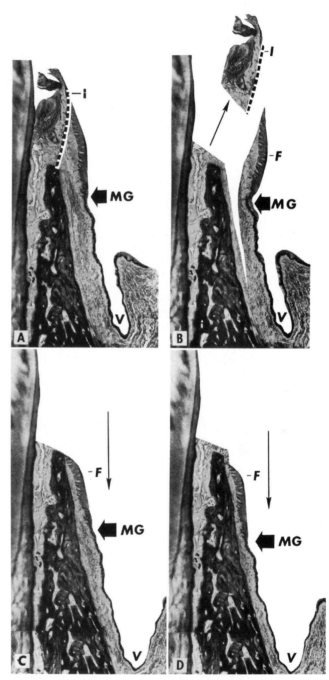

FIGURE 59–10. Apically displaced partial-thickness flap. *A,* Internal incision (I) separates inner wall of periodontal pocket. MG, Mucogingival junction; V, vestibular fornix. *B,* Partial-thickness flap (F) separated, leaving periosteum and a layer of connective tissue on the bone. The inner wall of the periodontal pocket (I) is removed, and the tooth is scaled and planed. *C,* Partial-thickness flap (F) displaced apically with the edge of the flap at the crest of the bone. Note that the vestibular fornix is also moved apically. *D,* Partial-thickness flap (F) displaced apically with the edge of the flap several millimeters below the crest of the bone.

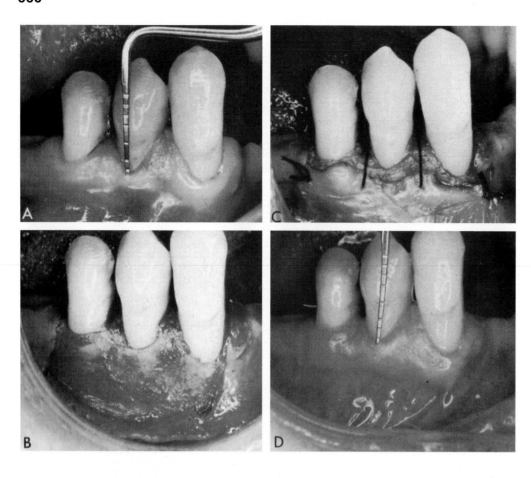

FIGURE 59–11. Apically displaced partial-thickness flap. *A,* Before treatment, the base of pocket extends to the mucogingival line. *B,* Mucosal flap separated from the periosteum; teeth scaled and smoothed. *C,* Flap replaced below the crest of the bone. *D,* Eight months after treatment. Note the shallow sulcus and the widened zone of attached gingiva. Compare with *A.*

Accomplishments

The apically displaced full-thickness flap operation increases the width of the attached gingiva but does not permanently deepen the vestibule. The width of the attached gingiva is increased by approximately half the pretreatment depth of the pockets.[29]

The edge of the flap may be located in any of the three following positions in relation to the bone:

1. *Slightly coronal to the crest of the bone.* This location is chosen to preserve the attachment of supracrestal fibers; however, it may also result in thick gingival margins and interdental papillae with deep sulci and may create the risk of recurrent pockets.
2. *At the level of the crest* (Fig. 59–10C). This results in a satisfactory gingival contour, provided that the flap is adequately thinned.
3. *Two millimeters short of the crest* (Figs. 59–10D and 59–11). This position produces the most desirable gingival contour and the same post-treatment level of gingival attachment as that obtained by placing the flap at the crest of the bone.[37] New tissue will cover the crest of the bone to produce a firm, tapered gingival margin. Placing the flap short of the crest increases the risk of a slight reduction in bone height,[26] but this is compensated for by the advantages of a well-formed gingival margin.

Because the pocket wall contributes to the increase in attached gingiva, the operation is best suited for patients with deep pockets who require additional attached gingiva. The final width of the attached gingiva may be increased by placing the flap farther apically from the crest (see Fig. 59–11).

Other Techniques

Fenestration Operation. The fenestration operation is designed to widen the zone of attached gingiva with a minimal loss of bone height.[82–84] It has also been called *periosteal separation.*[23] It utilizes a partial-thickness flap, except in a rectangular area at the base of the operative field where the periosteum is removed, exposing the bone (Fig. 59–12). This is the area of fenestration. Its purpose is to create a scar that is firmly bound to the bone[19] and will prevent gingival separation from the bone and postsurgical narrowing of the attached zone.

The results obtained with this technique are not as predictable as those obtained with the free gingival graft or the apically displaced flap; therefore, it is not widely performed except for isolated small areas.

Vestibular Extension Operation. The vestibular extension technique, originally described by Edlan and Mejchar,[35] produces statistically significant widening of attached nonkeratinized tissue. This increase in width in the mandibular area reportedly persists in patients observed for periods of up to 5 years.[35,87,107] Currently this technique is of historical interest only; it is presented in Figures 59–13 and 59–14.

OPERATIONS FOR COVERAGE OF DENUDED ROOTS

Denuded roots are covered for two purposes: to solve an aesthetic problem (particularly important in anterior teeth)

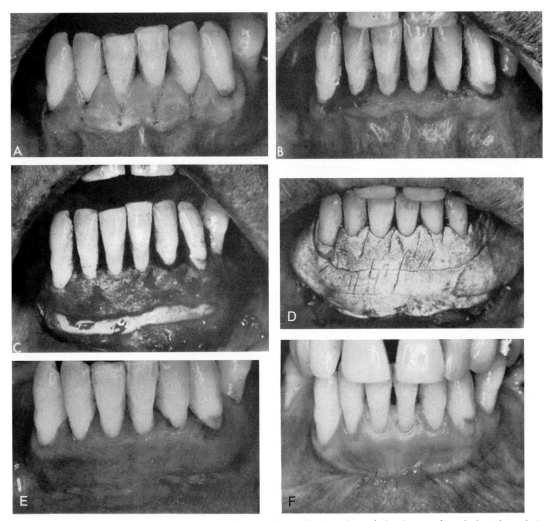

FIGURE 59–12. Fenestration operation. *A,* Pinpoint markings indicate the location of the base of periodontal pockets close to the mucogingival line. *B,* After removal of pockets by gingivectomy. Note the absence of attached gingiva in the lateral incisor and canine area *(left). C,* Flap reflected with periosteum intact. The bone is denuded of periosteum in the horizontal area at the base of the fornix. *D,* Periodontal pack in place. *E,* Three weeks after surgery. *F,* Five months after surgery. Note the wide zone of attached gingiva with a scar at its base.

and to widen the zone of attached gingiva, thereby solving a possible mucogingival problem.

Classification

Several classifications of denuded roots have been proposed. Sullivan and Atkins[101] classified gingival recession into four morphologic categories: (1) shallow-narrow, (2) shallow-wide, (3) deep-narrow, and (4) deep-wide. Miller[61] expanded this classification as follows (Fig. 59–15):

Class I. This includes marginal tissue recession that does not extend to the mucogingival junction. There is no loss of bone or soft tissue in the interdental area. This type of recession can be narrow or wide (groups 1 and 2 in Sullivan and Atkins' classification).

Class II. Class II consists of marginal tissue recession that extends to or beyond the mucogingival junction. There is no loss of bone or soft tissue in the interdental area. This type of recession can be subclassified into wide and narrow (corresponding to groups 3 and 4 of Sullivan and Atkins' classification).

Class III. In Class III, there is marginal tissue recession that extends to or beyond the mucogingival junction; in addition, there is bone and/or soft tissue loss interdentally or malpositioning of the tooth.

Class IV. This is marginal tissue recession that extends to or beyond the mucogingival junction with severe bone loss and soft tissue loss interdentally and/or severe tooth malposition.

Prognosis. In general, the prognosis for class I or II recession is good to excellent, whereas for class III, only partial coverage can be expected. Class IV recession has a very poor prognosis with current techniques.

Several procedures to cover denuded roots are currently being used. These are described in the text that follows.

Pedicle Graft: Laterally (Horizontally) Displaced Flap

This technique, originally described by Grupe and Warren in 1956,[42] was the standard technique for many years and is still indicated in some cases. Other techniques, however, are currently preferred in most cases. The laterally

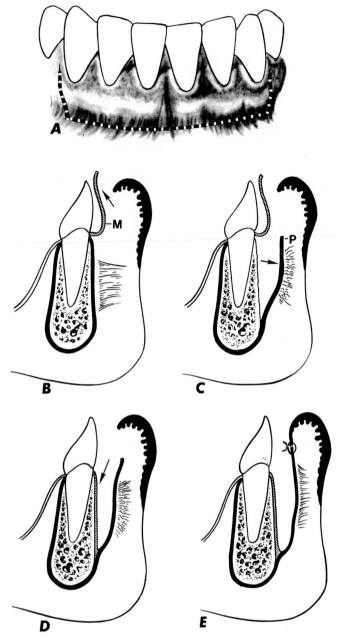

FIGURE 59–13. Edlan-Mejchar operation for vestibular deepening. *A*, The operative field is outlined by two vertical incisions from the junction of the marginal and attached gingivae to approximately 12 mm from the alveolar margin into the vestibule. The vertical incisions are joined by a horizontal incision. *B*, A mucosal flap (M) is elevated, exposing the periosteum on the bone. *C*, The periosteum (P) is separated from the bone, starting from the line of attachment of the mucosal flap; the periosteum, including muscle attachments, is transposed to the lip. *D*, The mucosal flap is folded down over the bone (*arrow*) and is sutured to the inner surface of the periosteum. *E*, The periosteum is transposed to the lip and sutured where the initial horizontal incision was made.

displaced flap can be used to cover isolated denuded roots that have adequate donor tissue laterally.

Step 1: Prepare the Recipient Site. Make an incision, resecting the periodontal pockets or gingival margin around the exposed roots (Figs. 59–16 and 59–17*B*). Remove the resected soft tissue and scale and plane the root surface (Fig. 59–17*C*).

Step 2: Prepare the Flap. The periodontium of the donor site should be healthy, with a satisfactory width of attached gingiva and minimal loss of bone and without dehiscences or fenestrations. A full-thickness or partial-thickness flap may be used, but the latter is preferable because it offers the advantage of more rapid healing in the donor site[6] and reduces the risk of loss of facial bone height, particularly if the bone is thin or the presence of a dehiscence or a fenestration is suspected. However, if the gingiva is thin, partial thickness may not be sufficient for flap survival.

With a no. 15 Bard-Parker blade, make a vertical incision from the gingival margin to outline a flap adjacent to the recipient site. Incise to the periosteum and *extend the incision into the oral mucosa* to the level of the base of the recipient site (Fig. 59–17*D*). The flap should be sufficiently wider than the recipient site to cover the root and provide a broad margin for attachment to the connective tissue border around the root. The interdental papilla at the distal end of the flap, or a major portion of it, should be included to secure the flap in the interproximal space between the donor and the recipient teeth.

Make a vertical incision along the gingival margin and interdental papilla and separate a flap consisting of epithelium and a thin layer of connective tissue, leaving the periosteum on the bone.

It is sometimes necessary to make a releasing incision to avoid tension on the base of the flap that can impair the circulation when the flap is moved (Fig. 59–17*E*). To do this, make a short oblique incision into the alveolar mucosa at the distal corner of the flap, pointing in the direction of the recipient site (Fig. 59–17*F*).

Step 3: Transfer the Flap. Slide the flap laterally onto the adjacent root, making sure that it lies flat and firm, without excess tension on the base. Fix the flap to the adjacent gingiva and alveolar mucosa with interrupted sutures. A suspensory suture may be made around the involved tooth to prevent the flap from slipping apically (Fig. 59–17*G*).

Step 4: Protect the Flap and Donor Site. Cover the operative field with tinfoil and a soft periodontal pack, extending it interdentally and onto the lingual surface to secure it. Remove the pack and sutures after 1 week (Fig. 59–17*H*).

Variations

There are many variations in the incisions for this operation. A common one is the use of converging oblique incisions over the recipient site and a vertical or oblique incision at the distal end of the donor site so that the transposed flap is slightly wider at its base. In another modification, the marginal attachment at the donor site is preserved to reduce the likelihood of recession and marginal bone resorption, but this requires a donor site with a wider zone of attached gingiva.[41]

Sliding partial-thickness grafts from neighboring edentulous areas (pedicle grafts)[24] can be used to restore attached gingiva on teeth adjacent to edentulous spaces with denuded roots and a small vestibular fornix, often complicated by tension from a frenum.

The so-called double papilla flap attempts to cover roots denuded by isolated gingival defects with a flap formed by

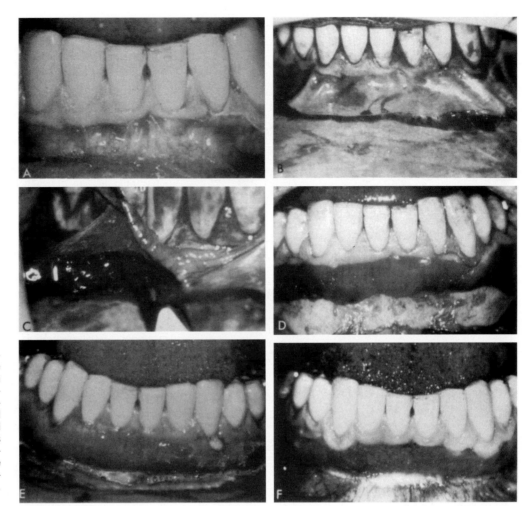

FIGURE 59–14. Vestibular extension operation. *A,* Before surgery. *B,* Horizontal incision in the inner side of the lip. *C,* Dissection of the flap. *D,* After separation of the periosteum and muscle fibers, the flap is folded down over the bone. *E,* Results 1 week after operation. *F,* Results 1 year after operation. Note the nonkeratinized attached tissue. (Courtesy of Dr. Max O. Schmid.)

joining the contiguous halves of the adjacent interdental papillae.[22,49] Results with this technique are frequently poor, because blood supply is impaired by suturing the two flaps over the root surface.

Accomplishments

Coverage of the exposed root surface with the sliding flap operation has been reported to be 60%,[45] 61%,[1] and 72%.[91] Histologic studies in animals have reported 50% coverage.[21,113]

The extent to which the flap establishes a new attachment to the root with the formation of new cementum and the embedding of new connective tissue fibers has not been settled. New attachment on artificially denuded roots in experimental animals[113] and in some clinical studies in humans has been reported,[99,103] but it does not occur consistently enough to be predictable.

In the donor site, there is uneventful repair and restoration of gingival health and contours, with some loss of radicular bone (0.5 mm) and recession (1.5 mm) reported with full-thickness flaps.

Coronally Displaced Flap

The purpose of the coronally displaced flap operation is to create a split-thickness flap in the area apical to the de-

nuded root and displace it coronally to cover the root. Two techniques are available for this purpose.

Procedure I

Step 1. With two vertical incisions, delineate the flap; these incisions should go beyond the mucogingival junction. Make an internal bevel incision from the gingival margin to the bottom of the pocket to eliminate the diseased pocket wall. Elevate a mucoperiosteal flap using careful sharp dissection.

Step 2. Scale and plane the root surface.

Step 3. Return the flap and suture it at a level coronal to the pretreatment position. Cover the area with a periodontal pack, which is removed along with the sutures after 1 week. The pack is replaced for an additional week if necessary.

Variations to Procedure I. Results with the coronally displaced flap technique are not often favorable[46] owing to the presence of insufficient keratinized gingiva. To solve this and increase the chances of success, the following procedure can be performed:

1. *Gingival extension operation with a free autogenous graft.* The technique described earlier in this chapter is performed. This will create several millimeters of attached keratinized gingiva apical to the denuded root.

2. Two months after this operation, a second-stage operation is performed, coronally displacing the flap that will include the

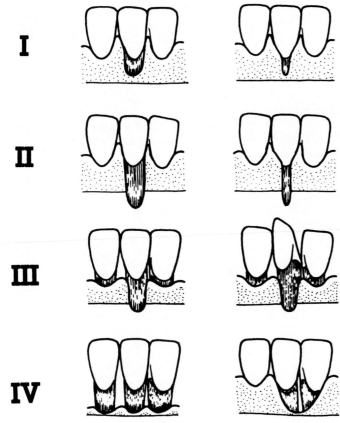

I

II

III

IV

FIGURE 59–15. P. D. Miller's classification of denuded roots.

free autogenous graft. The use of citric acid, pH 1.0, for conditioning the root surface has been suggested[57] (Fig. 59–18).

A significant degree of reduction in recession treated by this double-step operation was reported after 2 years by Bernimoulin and colleagues[6] and confirmed by other authors.[11,58,59]

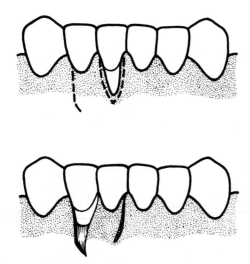

FIGURE 59–16. Laterally displaced flap for coverage of denuded root. *Top,* Incisions removing the gingival margin around the exposed root and outlining flap. *Bottom,* After the gingiva around exposed root is removed, flap is separated, transferred, and sutured.

Procedure II

Tarnow has described the *semilunar coronally repositioned flap* to cover denuded root surfaces.[104] It is performed as follows (Fig. 59–19):

> *Step 1.* A semilunar incision is made following the curvature of the receded gingival margin and ending about 2 to 3 mm short of the tip of the papillae. This is very important, as the flap will derive all its blood supply from the papillary areas. The incision may have to reach the alveolar mucosa if the attached gingiva is narrow.
>
> *Step 2.* Perform a split-thickness dissection coronally from the incision and connect it to an intrasulcular incision.
>
> *Step 3.* The tissue will collapse coronally, covering the denuded root. It is then held in its new position for a few minutes with moist gauze; there is no need to suture or to pack.

This technique is very simple and will predictably provide 2 to 3 mm of root coverage. It can be performed on several adjoining teeth, but even though the incision may be continuous, extreme care should be exercised not to dissect the tissue under the papillae in order to retain an adequate blood supply. The Tarnow technique is successful in upper teeth, particularly in covering the root left exposed by a gingival margin receding from a recently placed crown margin; it is not recommended for mandibular teeth.

Free Soft Tissue Autograft

Successful and predictable root coverage has been reported with free gingival grafts[62,63] and connective tissue grafts, partially covered with a flap.[56]

The *Miller technique*[63] is as follows:

> *Step 1.* Perform root planing and apply saturated citric acid for 5 minutes with a cotton pledget, burnishing it on the root. The usefulness of citric acid application has not been confirmed, however, by other studies.[51]
>
> *Step 2: Prepare the recipient site.* Make a horizontal incision in the interdental papillae at right angles so as to create a margin that the graft may be butted against. Make vertical incisions at the proximal right angles of the adjacent teeth, and totally excise the retracted tissue in the apical area. Maintain an intact periosteum in the apical area.
>
> *Step 3.* Make a pattern of the area with dry foil, and transfer the pattern to the palate to outline the donor tissue. Remove donor tissue by sharp dissection. If glandular or adipose tissue is found on the underside of the graft, remove it.
>
> *Step 4.* Suture the graft in the recipient site with resorbable sutures.

This technique results in adequate coverage of denuded roots, but the tissue covering the root is usually excessively thick and too pale in color.

Subepithelial Connective Tissue Graft Technique

This technique uses a connective tissue graft to cover denuded roots. It was described in 1985 by Langer and Langer,[56] although similar approaches had been previously reported by Perez-Fernandez[75] and Raetzke.[77]

Langer Technique. The Langer technique can be used for coverage of isolated or multiple recessions. Areas to be

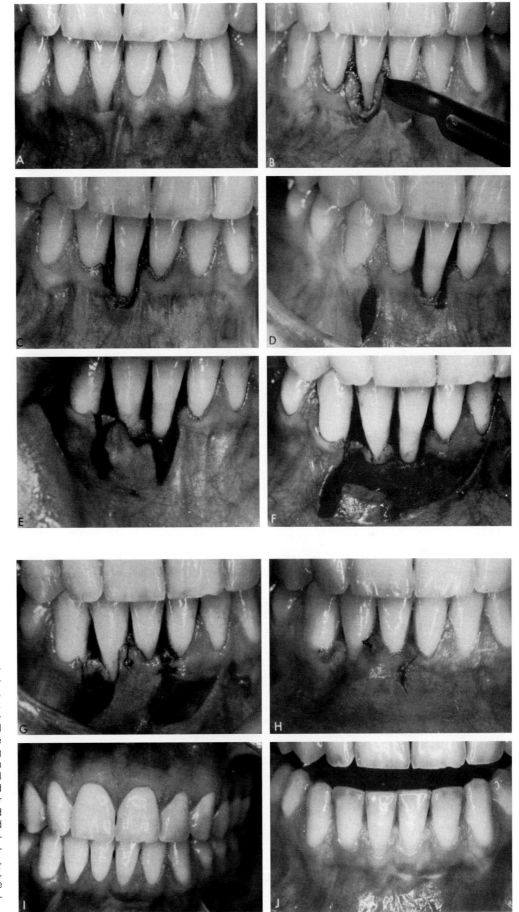

FIGURE 59–17. Horizontally displaced flap combined with relocation of frenum attachment. *A,* Gingival defect of central incisor. *B,* Defect incised. *C,* Gingiva removed and tooth scaled and planed. *D,* Vertical incision on the canine for sliding flap. *E,* Sliding flap detached. Note high frenum attachment between the central incisors. *F,* Frenum detached and resected to level of vestibular fornix. *G,* Sliding flap displaced laterally on central incisor and fixed lateral and suspensory suture. *H,* One week after operation. Sutures to be removed. *I,* Five weeks after operation. *J,* Seven years after treatment. Note the preservation of gingival position and contour.

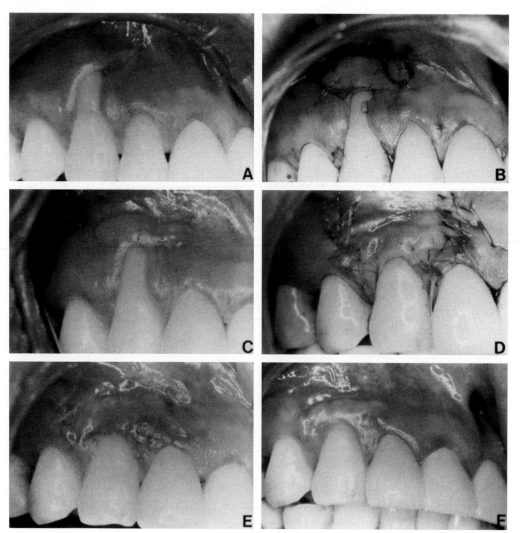

FIGURE 59–18. Coronally displaced flap. *A,* Preoperative view Note the recession and the lack of attached gingiva. *B,* After placement of a free gingival graft. *C,* Three months after placement of the graft. *D,* Flap including the graft, displaced coronally and sutured. *E,* After 2 weeks of healing. *F,* Six months later. Note the root coverage and the presence of attached gingiva. Compare with *A.* (Courtesy of Dr. T. J. Han.)

treated with this technique must be free of inflammation and the patient perfectly trained in plaque control methods. The technique is as follows (Fig. 59–20):

Step 1. Raise a partial-thickness flap with a horizontal incision 2 mm away from the tip of the papilla and two vertical incisions 1 to 2 mm away from the gingival margin of the adjoining teeth (Fig. 59–20*A, B*). These incisions should extend at least one-half to one tooth wider mesiodistally than the area of gingival recession. Extend the flap to the mucobuccal fold without perforations that could affect the blood supply.

Step 2. Thoroughly plane the root, reducing its convexity.

Step 3. Obtain a connective tissue graft from the palate by means of a horizontal incision 5 to 6 mm from the gingival margin of molars and premolars and short vertical incisions on either side (Fig. 59–20*C*). A sheet of connective tissue is carefully removed and freed of all adipose and glandular tissue. The palatal wound is sutured and left completely closed.

Step 4. Place the sheet of connective tissue on the denuded root(s) with its edge about 1 mm apical to the cementoenamel junction. Suture it with removable sutures to the periosteum.

Step 5. Cover the graft with the partial-thickness flap and suture it interdentally with silk sutures going over the connective tissue graft (Fig. 59–20*D*). At least one half to two thirds of the connective tissue graft must be covered

by the flap for the remaining portion to survive over the denuded root.

Step 6. Cover the area with tinfoil and surgical pack.

After 7 days, the dressing and sutures are removed.

This technique has the advantage of covering the receded root with fibrotic tissue that shows excellent tissue tone and texture (Fig. 59–20*E*). The donor site heals by primary intention, with considerably less discomfort than after a free gingival graft.

A variant of the subepithelial connective tissue graft, called a *subpedicle connective tissue graft,* was described by Nelson in 1987.[71] In this technique, a free connective tissue graft is placed under a double papilla flap, which is sutured over it. The author reported 100% coverage in cases of slight denudation (1 to 3 mm), 92% coverage in cases of moderate recession (4 to 6 mm), and 88% coverage in cases of advanced recession (7 to 10 mm).

Guided Tissue Regeneration (GTR) Technique for Root Coverage

Pini-Prato and associates[76] have described a technique based on the principle of guided tissue regeneration (Fig. 59–21). Theoretically this technique results in reconstruction of the attachment apparatus rather than mere coverage

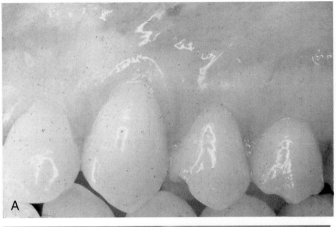
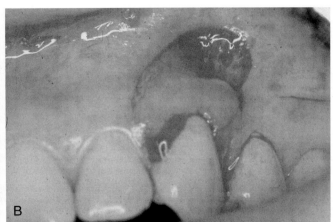
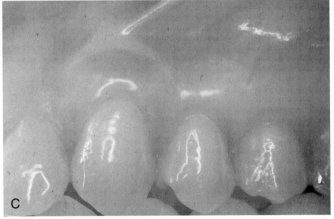

FIGURE 59–19. Semilunar coronally displaced flap. *A,* Slight recession in facial of the upper left canine. *B,* After thorough scaling and root planing of the area, a semilunar incision is made and the tissue separated from the underlying bone. The flap collapses, covering the recession. *C,* Appearance after 7 weeks. Note coverage of the previous root denudation. (Courtesy of Dr. Steven Kwan.)

of the root with gingival tissue attached by a long junctional epithelium; further studies are needed, however, to prove this theory.

The GTR technique consists of the following steps:

Step 1. Create a flap using an intrasulcular incision and oblique releasing incisions carried beyond the mucogingival junction.

Step 2. Elevate a full-thickness flap to the mucogingival junction and a partial-thickness flap beyond it.

Step 3. Perform thorough planing of exposed root surfaces with curettes and burs to create a smooth, concave surface.

Step 4. Trim a Gore-Tex membrane to cover the exposed root and 2 mm of crestal bone.

Step 5. Pass a suture through the apical part of the membrane, tying it in the outside and tightening so as to bend the membrane.

Step 6. Place the membrane on the root so that the bending suture is on bone. This creates a space for the proliferation of tissue.

Step 7. Suture the membrane with sling sutures.

Step 8. Displace the flap as coronally as possible to fully cover the membrane, and place sutures from the corono-proximal edge of the flap, over the contact point and to the palatal gingiva.

Step 9. Place mesial and distal subperiosteal sutures at the base of the flap. Do not apply a periodontal pack.

Four weeks later a small envelope flap is performed, and the membrane is carefully removed. The flap is then again displaced coronally to protect the growing tissue and sutured. One week later these sutures are removed.

Clinical studies comparing this technique with the coronally displaced flap have shown that the GTR technique is better when the recession is more than 4.98 mm apico-coronally.[76] One case analyzed histologically showed 3.66 mm of new connective tissue attachment associated with 2.48 mm of new cementum and 1.84 mm of bone growth.[25]

OPERATIONS FOR REMOVAL OF FRENA

A frenum is a fold of mucous membrane, usually with enclosed muscle fibers, that attaches the lips and cheeks to the alveolar mucosa and/or gingiva and underlying periosteum. *A frenum becomes a problem if its attachment is too close to the marginal gingiva.* It may then pull on healthy gingiva and invite the accumulation of irritants; it may deflect the wall of a periodontal pocket and aggravate its severity; or it may interfere with post-treatment healing, prevent close adaptation of the gingiva, leading to pocket formation, or inhibit proper brushing of the teeth.

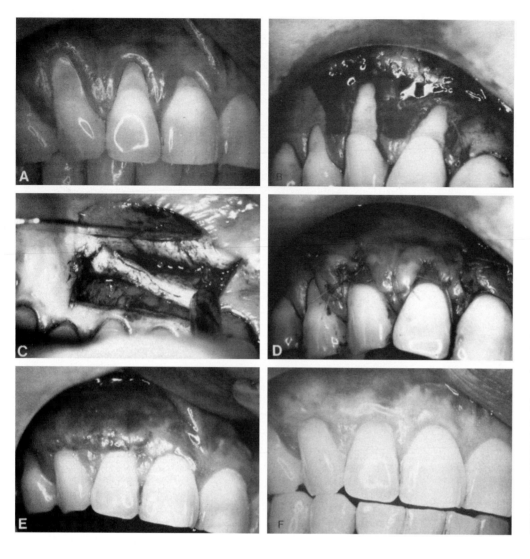

FIGURE 59-20. The Langer technique for root coverage. *A,* Preoperative view. Note the recession on teeth #6-8. *B,* Split-thickness flap elevated on teeth #6 and 7. Note that the interdental papillae are not included in the flap, nor is the gingival margin area of tooth #8, which was treated by means of a coronally positioned flap. *C,* Palatal flap and the removal of the connective tissue graft. *D,* The graft placed under the flap and covering receded areas approximately to the cemento-enamel junction. Sutures in place. *E,* After 1 week of healing. *F,* Roots covered after complete healing. Note the thickness of the tissue in the area covered and excellent color. (Courtesy of Dr. T. J. Han.)

Frenectomy or Frenotomy

The terms *frenectomy* and *frenotomy* signify operations that differ in degree. Frenectomy is complete removal of the frenum, including its attachment to underlying bone, such as may be required in the correction of an abnormal diastema between maxillary central incisors. Frenotomy is the incision of the frenum. Both procedures are used, but frenotomy (i.e., relocating the frenal attachment to create a zone of attached gingiva between the gingival margin and the frenum) generally suffices for periodontal purposes. Frenectomy and frenotomy are usually performed in conjunction with other periodontal treatment procedures but occasionally are done as separate operations.

Frenal problems occur most often on the facial surface between the maxillary and mandibular central incisors and in the canine and premolar areas[111]; they occur less frequently on the lingual surface of the mandible.

Procedure. If the vestibule is deep enough, the operation is confined to the frenum, but it is often necessary to deepen the vestibule to provide space for the repositioned frenum. This is accomplished as follows (Fig. 59-22):

1. After anesthetizing the area, engage the frenum with a hemostat inserted to the depth of the vestibule.

2. Incise along the upper surface of the hemostat, extending beyond the tip.
3. Make a similar incision along the undersurface of the hemostat.
4. Remove the triangular resected portion of the frenum with the hemostat. This exposes the underlying brush-like fibrous attachment to the bone.
5. Make a horizontal incision, separating the fibers, and bluntly dissect to the bone.
6. If necessary, extend the incisions laterally and suture the labial mucosa to the apical periosteum. Sometimes the area is covered with a free gingival graft.
7. Clean the field of operation and pack with gauze sponges until the bleeding stops.
8. Cover the area with dry foil and apply a periodontal pack.
9. Remove the pack after 2 weeks and repack if necessary. One month is usually required for formation of an intact mucosa with the frenum attached in its new position.

High frenal attachments on the lingual surface are uncommon. To correct these without involving the structures in the floor of the mouth, approximately 2 mm of the attachment are separated from the mucosa with a periodontal knife at weekly intervals until the desired level is reached. The area is covered with a periodontal pack during the intervals between treatments.

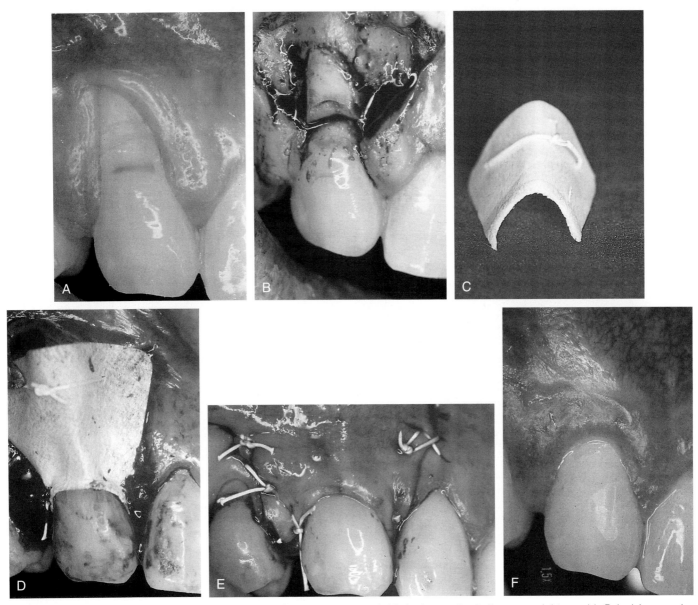

FIGURE 59–21. Guided tissue regeneration technique for root coverage. *A*, Marked recession in the upper right cuspid. *B*, Incisions made and flap elevated. *C*, Membrane trimmed and bent with suture. *D*, Membrane placed on exposed root and covering bone margin. *E*, Sutures in place. *F*, After healing, the root is completely covered. (Courtesy of Dr. Carlo Tinti, Milano, Italy.)

CRITERIA FOR SELECTION OF MUCOGINGIVAL TECHNIQUES

Different techniques are available for solving the mucogingival problems outlined in the first part of this chapter (Plate XXII). The practitioner must know how to choose among them.

Pockets Extending to the Mucogingival Junction. Basically two techniques are available: the apically displaced flap and the free gingival graft. Criteria for selection are based on the character of the gingival pocket wall. *Thick, manageable pocket walls can be used for an apically displaced flap, and this flap should be the first choice.* This technique does not require a second surgical site and offers the added advantage of exposing the bone as needed. *When manageability of the flap is impaired as a result of irregu-*lar contour or soft, friable tissue, the choice is a gingival extension operation with a free gingival graft.

Absence of Attached Gingiva With No Pocket Formation. The need for any type of surgical procedure should be questioned, because many patients' gingival health can be adequately maintained nonsurgically. However, if there is persistent inflammation and plaque control is difficult, *a free gingival graft is the technique of choice.*

Root Coverage. Several techniques are available for this purpose. The techniques recommended are the *Langer technique,* which uses a connective tissue graft under a partial thickness flap, and the *Tarnow technique,* or semilunar coronally displaced flap. Both result in excellent color and tissue thickness in the recipient site. The Langer technique is an excellent solution in most cases, but the Tarnow technique is the first choice in isolated upper teeth.

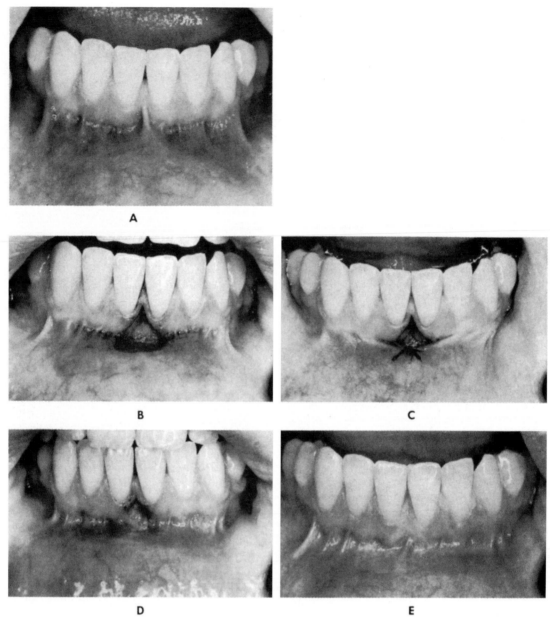

FIGURE 59–22. Relocating the frenum. *A,* Frenum attached close to the gingival margin. *B,* After removal of the frenum. *C,* Mucosa sutured in position. *D,* After 1 week, with periodontal pack and suture removed. *E,* After 6 months, frenum relocated at the mucogingival line.

High Frenum Insertion. Frenectomy is the only technique available; it is usually performed together with other pocket elimination methods. The resulting wound can sometimes be covered with a free gingival graft.

COMMENT

New techniques are constantly being developed and are slowly incorporated into periodontal practice. The practitioner should be aware that new methods are sometimes published without adequate clinical research to ensure the predictability of the results and the extent to which the techniques may benefit the patient. Critical analysis of newly presented techniques should guide our constant evolution toward better clinical methods.

REFERENCES

1. Albano EA, Caffesse RC, Carranza FA Jr. A biometric analysis of laterally displaced pedicle flaps. Rev Asoc Odontol Argent *57:*351, 1969.
2. Ariaudo AA, Tyrrell HA. Elimination of pockets extending to or beyond mucogingival junction. Dent Clin North Am *4:*67, 1960.
3. Becker BE, Becker W. Use of connective tissue autografts for treatment of mucogingival problems. Int J Periodont Restor Dent *6:*89, 1986.
4. Becker NG. A free gingival graft utilizing a pre-suturing technique. Periodontics *5:*194, 1967.
5. Bergenholtz A, Hugoson A. Vestibular sulcus extension surgery in cases with periodontal disease. J Periodont Res *2:*221, 1967.
6. Bernimoulin JP, Loscher B, Muhlemann HR. Coronally repositioned periodontal flap. J Clin Periodontal *2:*1, 1975.
7. Bhaskar SN, Cutright DE, Perez B, Beasley JD III. Full and partial thickness pedicle grafts in miniature swine and man. J Periodontol *42:*66, 1971.
8. Bjorn H. Free transplantation of gingiva propria. Sveriges Tandlak T *22:*684, 1963.
9. Brackett RC, Gargiulo AW. Free gingival grafts in humans. J Periodontol *41:*581, 1970.

10. Broome WC, Taggart EJ Jr. Free autogenous connective tissue grafting. J Periodontol *47:*580, 1976.
11. Caffesse RG, Guinard E. Treatment of localized gingival recessions. Part II. Coronally repositioned flap with a free gingival graft. J Periodontol *49:*358, 1978.
12. Caffesse RG, Albano E, Plot C. Injertos gingivalis libres en perros: Analisis biometrico. Rev Asoc Odontol Argent *60:*517, 1972.
13. Caffesse RG, Carraro JJ, Carranza FA Jr. Injertos gingivales libres en perros: Estudio clinico e histologico. Rev Asoc Odontol Argent *60:*465, 1972.
14. Caffesse RG, Burgett FG, Nasjleti CE, Castelli WA. Healing of free gingival grafts with and without periosteum. Part I. Histologic evaluation. J Periodontol *50:*586, 1979.
15. Caffesse RG, Nasjleti CE, Burgett FG, et al. Healing of free gingival grafts with and without periosteum. Part II. Radioautographic evaluation. J Periodontol *50:*595, 1979.
16. Carranza FA Jr, Carraro JJ. Effect of removal of periosteum on postoperative result of mucogingival surgery. J Periodontol *34:*223, 1963.
17. Carranza FA Jr, Carraro JJ. Mucogingival techniques in periodontal surgery. J Periodontol *41:*294, 1970.
18. Carranza FA Jr, Carraro JJ, Albano EA. Mucogingival surgery. In Stahl SS, ed. Periodontal Surgery: Biologic Basis and Technique. Springfield, IL, Charles C Thomas, 1976.
19. Carranza FA Jr, Carraro JJ, Dotto CA, Cabrini RL. Effect of periosteal fenestration in gingival extension operations. J Periodontol *37:*335, 1966.
20. Carraro JJ, Carranza FA Jr, Albano EA, Joly G. Effect of bone denudation in mucogingival surgery in humans. J Periodontol *35:*463, 1964.
21. Chacker FM, Cohen DW. Regeneration of gingival tissues in non-human primates. J Dent Res *39:*743, 1960.
22. Cohen DW, Ross SE. The double papillae repositioned flap in periodontal therapy. J Periodontol *39:*65, 1968.
23. Corn H. Periosteal separation—its clinical significance. J Periodontol *33:*140, 1962.
24. Corn H. Edentulous area pedicle grafts in mucogingival surgery. Periodontics *2:*229, 1964.
25. Cortellini P, Clauser C, Pini-Prato GP. Histologic assessment of new attachment following the treatment of a human buccal recession by means of a guided tissue regeneration procedure. J Periodontol *64:*387, 1993.
26. Costich ER, Ramfjord SP. Healing after partial denudation of the alveolar process. J Periodontol *39:*127, 1968.
27. Donn BJ Jr. The free connective tissue autograft: A clinical and histologic wound healing study in humans. J Periodontol *49:*253, 1978.
28. Donnenfeld OW, Glickman I. A biometric study of the effects of gingivectomy. J Periodontol *37:*447, 1966.
29. Donnenfeld OW, Marks R, Glickman I. The apically repositioned flap: A clinical study. J Periodontol *35:*381, 1964.
30. Dordick B, Coslet JG, Siebert JS. Clinical evaluation of free autogenous gingival grafts placed on alveolar bone. Part I. Clinical predictability. J Periodontol *47:*559, 1976.
31. Dordick B, Coslet JG, Seibert JS. Clinical evaluation of free autogenous gingival grafts placed on alveolar bone. Part II. Coverage of non-pathologic dehiscences and fenestrations. J Periodontol *47:*568, 1976.
32. Dorfman HS, Kennedy JE, Bird WC. Longitudinal evaluation of free autogenous gingival grafts. J Clin Periodontol *7:*316, 1980.
33. Dorfman HS, Kennedy JE, Bird WC. Longitudinal evaluation of free autogenous gingival grafts. A four-year report. J Periodontol *53:*349, 1982.
34. Edel A. Clinical evaluation of free connective tissue grafts used to increase the width of keratinized gingiva. J Clin Periodontol *1:*185, 1974.
35. Edlan A, Mejchar B. Plastic surgery of the vestibulum in periodontal therapy. Int Dent J *13:*593, 1963.
36. Friedman N. Mucogingival surgery: The apically repositioned flap. J Periodontol *33:*328, 1962.
37. Friedman N, Levine HL. Mucogingival surgery: Current status. J Periodontol *35:*5, 1964.
38. Gargiulo AW, Arrocha R. Histo-clinical evaluation of free gingival grafts. Periodontics *5:*285, 1967.
39. Gordon HP, Sullivan HC, Atkins JH. Free autogenous gingival grafts. II. Supplemental findings—histology of the graft site. Periodontics *6:*130, 1968.
40. Grant DA. Experimental periodontal surgery: Sequestration of alveolar bone. J Periodontol *38:*409, 1967.
41. Grupe HE. Modified technique for the sliding flap operation. J Periodontol *37:*491, 1966.
42. Grupe HE, Warren RF Jr. Repair of gingival defects by a sliding flap operation. J Periodontol *27:*92, 1956.
43. Guinard EA, Caffesse RG. Localized gingival recessions. I. Etiology and prevalence. J West Soc Periodontol *25:*3, 1977.
44. Guinard EA, Caffesse RG. Localized gingival recessions. II. Treatment. J West Soc Periodontol *25:*10, 1977.
45. Guinard EA, Caffesse RG. Treatment of localized gingival recessions. Part I. Lateral sliding flap. J Periodontol *49:*351, 1978.
46. Hall WB. Pure Mucogingival Problems. Etiology, Treatment and Prevention. Chicago, Quintessence Publishing, 1984.
47. Han TJ, Takei HH, Carranza FA Jr. The strip gingival autograft technique. Int J Periodont Restor Dent *13:*181, 1993.
48. Hangorsky V, Bissada NF. Clinical assessment of free gingival graft effectiveness on the maintenance of periodontal health. J Periodontol *51:*274, 1980.
49. Harvey PM. Management of advanced periodontitis. Part I. Preliminary report of a method of surgical reconstruction. NZ Dent J *61:*180, 1965.
50. Hawley CE, Staffileno H. Clinical evaluation of free gingival grafts in periodontal surgery. J Periodontol *41:*105, 1970.
51. Ibbott CG, Oles RD, Laverty WH. Effects of citric acid treatment on autogenous free graft coverage of localized recession. J Periodontol *56:*662, 1985.
52. James WC, McFall WT Jr. Placement of free gingival grafts on denuded alveolar bone. Part I. Clinical evaluations. J Periodontol *49:*283, 1978.
53. James WC, McFall WT Jr, Burkes EJ. Placement of free gingival grafts on denuded alveolar bone. II. Microscopic observations. J Periodontol *49:*291, 1978.
54. Janson WA, Ruben MP, Kramer GM, et al. Development of the blood supply to split-thickness free gingival autografts. J Periodontol *40:*707, 1969.
55. Karring T, Ostergaard E, Löe H. Conservation of tissue specificity after heterotopic transplantation of gingiva and alveolar mucosa. J Periodont Res *6:*282, 1971.
56. Langer B, Langer L. Subepithelial connective tissue graft technique for root coverage. J Periodontol *56:*715, 1985.
57. Liu WJ, Solt CW. A surgical procedure for the treatment of localized gingival recession in conjunction with root surface citric acid conditioning. J Periodontol *51:*505, 1980.
58. Matter J. Free gingival graft and coronally repositioned flap. A 2-year follow-up report. J Clin Periodontol *6:*437, 1979.
59. Matter J, Cimasoni G. Creeping attachment after free gingival grafts. J Periodontol *47:*574, 1976.
60. Maynard JB. Coronal positioning of a previously placed autogenous gingival graft. J Periodontol *48:*151, 1977.
61. Miller PD Jr. A classification of marginal tissue recession. Int J Periodont Restor Dent *5:*9, 1985.
62. Miller PD Jr. Root coverage using a free soft tissue autograft following citric acid application. Part I. Technique. Int J Periodont Restor Dent *2:*65, 1982.
63. Miller PD Jr. Root coverage using a free soft tissue autograft following citric acid application. Part III. A successful and predictable procedure in areas of deep wide recession. Int J Periodont Restor Dent *5:*15, 1985.
64. Miller PD Jr. Root coverage with the free gingival graft. Factors associated with incomplete coverage. J Periodontol *58:*674, 1987.
65. Miyasato M, Crigger M, Egelberg J. Gingival conditions in areas of minimal and appreciable width of keratinized gingiva. J Clin Periodontol *4:*200, 1977.
66. Mormann W, Schaer F, Firestone AC. The relationship between success of free gingival grafts and transplant thickness. J Periodontol *52:*74, 1981.
67. Nabers CL. Repositioning the attached gingiva. J Periodontol *25:*38, 1954.
68. Nabers CL. When is gingival repositioning an indicated procedure? J West Soc Periodontol *5:*4, 1957.
69. Nabers J. Free gingival grafts. Periodontics *4:*243, 1966.
70. Neacy K. The use of allogenic sclera and autogenous gingiva as free gingival grafts. Thesis, University of California, Los Angeles, 1978.
71. Nelson SW. The subpedicle connective tissue graft—a bilaminar reconstructive procedure for the coverage of denuded root surfaces. J Periodontol *58:*95, 1987.
72. Oliver RC, Löe H, Karring T. Microscopic evaluation of the healing and revascularization of free gingival grafts. J Periodontol *3:*84, 1968.
73. Pennel B, King KO, Higgason JD, et al. Retention of periosteum in mucogingival surgery. J Periodontol *36:*39, 1965.
74. Pennel BM, Tabor JC, King KO, et al. Free masticatory mucosa graft. J Periodontol *40:*162, 1969.
75. Perez-Fernandez A. Injerto submucoso libre de encía. Una nueva perspectiva. Bol Inform Dent *42:*63, 1982.
76. Pini-Prato G, Tinti C, Vincenzi G, et al. Guided tissue regeneration versus mucogingival surgery in the treatment of human buccal gingival recession. J Periodontol *63:*919, 1992.
77. Raetzke PB. Covering localized areas of root exposure employing the "envelope" technique. J Periodontol *56:*397, 1985.
78. Ramfjord SP, Costich ER. Healing after exposure of periosteum on the alveolar process. J Periodontol *39:*199, 1968.
79. Rateitschak KH, Egli U, Fingeli G. Recession: A four-year longitudinal study after free gingival graft. J Clin Periodontol *6:*158, 1979.
80. Rateitschak KH, Rateitschak EM, Wolff HF, Hassell TM. Color Atlas of Periodontology. New York, Thieme, 1985.
81. Redondo VF, Bustamante A, Carranza FA Jr. Evaluacion biometrica de la tecnica de extension gingival con fenestracion periostica. Rev Asoc Odontol Argent *56:*346, 1968.
82. Robinson RE. Periosteal fenestration in mucogingival surgery. J West Soc Periodontol *9:*107, 1961.
83. Robinson RE, Agnew RG. Periosteal fenestration at the mucogingival line. J Periodontol *34:*503, 1963.
84. Rosenberg MM. Vestibular alterations in periodontics. J Periodontol *31:*231, 1960.
85. Roth H. Some speculations as to predictable fenestrations prior to mucogingival surgery. Periodontics *3:*29, 1965.
86. Rubenstein HS, Ruben MP, Levy C, Peiser C. Evidence for successful acceptance of irradiated free gingival allografts in dogs. J Periodontol *46:*195, 1975.
87. Schmid MO. The subperiosteal vestibule extension—literature review, rationale and technique. J West Soc Periodontol *24:*89, 1976.
88. Schoo WH, Copes L. Use of palatal mucosa and lyophilized dura mater to create attached gingiva. J Clin Periodontol *3:*166, 1976.
89. Smith RM. A study of the intertransplantation of alveolar mucosa. Oral Surg *29:*328, 1970.

90. Smith RM. A study of the intertransplantation of gingiva. Oral Surg *29:*169, 1970.
91. Smukler H. Laterally positioned mucoperiosteal pedicle grafts in the treatment of denuded roots. J Periodontol *47:*590, 1976.
92. Spengler DE, Hayward JR. Study of sulcus extension wound healing in dogs. J Oral Surg *22:*413, 1964.
93. Staffileno H. Palatal flap surgery: Mucosal flap (split thickness) and its advantages over the mucoperiosteal flap. J Periodontol *40:*547, 1969.
94. Staffileno H, Levy S. Histologic and clinical study of mucosal (gingival) transplants in dogs. J Periodontol *40:*311, 1969.
95. Staffileno H, Levy S, Gargiulo A. Histologic study of cellular mobilization and repair following a periosteal retention operation via split thickness mucogingival flap surgery. J Periodontol *37:*117, 1966.
96. Staffileno H, Wentz F, Orban B. Histologic study of healing of split thickness flap surgery in dogs. J Periodontol *33:*56, 1962.
97. Stetler KJ, Bissada NF. Significance of the width of keratinized gingiva on the periodontal status of teeth with submarginal restorations. J Periodontol *58:*696, 1987.
98. Strahan JD. The relation of the mucogingival junction to the alveolar bone margin. Dent Practit Dent Record *14:*72, 1963.
99. Sugarman EF. A clinical and histological study of the attachment of grafted tissue to bone and teeth. J Periodontol *40:*381, 1969.
100. Sullivan HC, Atkins JH. Free autogenous gingival grafts. I. Principles of successful grafting. Periodontics *6:*5, 1968.
101. Sullivan HC, Atkins JC. Free autogenous gingival grafts. III. Utilization of grafts in the treatment of gingival recession. Periodontics *6:*152, 1968.
102. Sullivan HC, Atkins JH. The role of free gingival grafts in periodontal therapy. Dent Clin North Am *13:*133, 1969.
103. Sullivan HC, Carman D, Dinner D. Histological evaluation of the laterally positioned flap. IADR Abstracts, no. 467, 1971, p 169.
104. Tarnow DP. Semilunar coronally repositioned flap. J Clin Periodontol *13:*182, 1986.
105. Tavtigian R. The height of the facial radicular alveolar crest following apically positioned flap operations. J Periodontol *41:*412, 1970.
106. Trey E, Bernimoulin JP. Influence of free gingival grafts on the health of the marginal gingiva. J Clin Periodontol *7:*381, 1980.
107. Wade AB. Vestibular deepening by the technique of Edlan and Mejchar. J Periodont Res *4:*300, 1969.
108. Ward VJ. A clinical assessment of the use of the free gingival graft for correcting localized recession associated with frenal pull. J Periodontol *45:*78, 1974.
109. Wennstrom J, Lindhe J, Nyman S. Role of keratinized gingiva for gingival health. J Clin Periodontol *8:*311, 1981.
110. Wennstrom J, Lindhe J, Nyman S. The role of keratinized gingiva in plaque-associated gingivitis in dogs. J Clin Periodontol *9:*75, 1982.
111. Whinston GJ. Frenotomy and mucobuccal fold resection utilized in periodontal therapy. NY Dent J *22:*495, 1956.
112. Wilderman MN. Exposure of bone in periodontal surgery. Dent Clin North Am *8:*23, 1964.
113. Wilderman MN, Wentz FM. Repair of a dentogingival defect with a pedicle flap. J Periodontol *36:*218, 1965.
114. Wood DL, Hoag PL, Donnenfeld OW, Rosenfeld LD. Alveolar crest reduction following full and partial thickness flaps. J Periodontol *43:*141, 1972.
115. Woofter C. The prevalence and etiology of gingival recession. Periodont Abstr *17:*45, 1969.

60

Treatment of Gingival Enlargement

FERMIN A. CARRANZA, JR.

Treatment of gingival enlargement is based on an understanding of the cause of enlargement and the underlying pathologic changes (see Chapter 18). Enlargements resulting from inflammation alone can be treated successfully with local procedures, and fastidious oral hygiene prevents recurrence. When systemic or unknown conditions are partially or entirely responsible, surgical removal can eliminate the enlargement, but the persistence of etiologic factors will result in recurrence. Because gingival enlargements differ in cause, treatment of each form is best considered individually.

TREATMENT OF CHRONIC INFLAMMATORY ENLARGEMENT

Scaling and Curettage. Chronic inflammatory enlargements, which are soft and discolored and are caused principally by edema and cellular infiltration, are treated by scaling procedures and curettage, provided the size of the enlargement does not interfere with complete removal of deposits from the involved tooth surfaces.

Surgical Removal. When chronic inflammatory gingival enlargements include a significant fibrotic component that does not undergo shrinkage after scaling and curettage or are of such size that they obscure deposits on the tooth surfaces and interfere with access to them, surgical removal is the treatment of choice. Two techniques are available for this purpose: gingivectomy and flap operation.

Selection of the appropriate technique depends on the size of the enlargement and the character of the tissue. When the enlarged gingiva remains soft and friable even after scaling and root planing, gingivectomy is used to remove it, because a flap requires firmer tissue to adequately perform the incisions and other steps in the

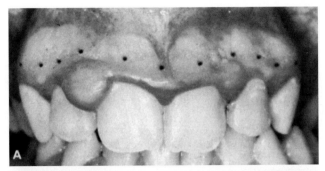

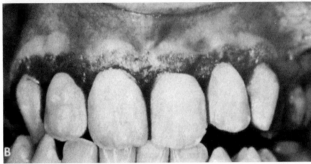

FIGURE 60-1. Gingivectomy incision for gingival enlargement. *A,* Chronic inflammatory gingival enlargement with a tumor-like area. Pinpoint markings outline the extent of the enlargement. *B,* Enlarged gingiva removed. Note the beveled incision.

technique. However, if a gingivectomy incision would remove all of the attached gingiva, thereby creating a mucogingival problem, then a flap operation is indicated.

Gingivectomy Technique. (For a complete description of this technique, see Chapter 53.) For the removal of gingival enlargements, the location and bevel of the gingivectomy incision are particularly critical. The following procedure is used: After the area is anesthetized, the junction of the enlarged gingiva with the adjacent gingiva is probed and outlined with pinpoint markings (Fig. 60–1A). The location of the bleeding points should be at least 1 to 2 mm coronal to the mucogingival line for the gingivectomy technique to be indicated. When indicated, the gingivectomy incision should be placed sufficiently close to the bone to ensure complete removal of the enlarged tissue and complete exposure of all root deposits (Fig. 60–1B).

Tumor-like inflammatory enlargements are treated by gingivectomy as follows: Under local anesthesia the tooth surfaces beneath the mass are scaled to remove calculus and other debris. The lesion is separated from the mucosa at its base with a no. 12 Bard-Parker blade. If the lesion extends interproximally, the interdental gingiva is included in the incision to ensure exposure of irritating root deposits. After the lesion is removed, the involved root surfaces are scaled and planed, and the area is cleansed with warm water. A periodontal pack is applied and removed after 1 week, at which time the patient is instructed in plaque control (Fig. 60–2A,B).

Flap Operation. See Chapters 54 and 55 and the later discussion of the flap technique for fibrotic enlargements.

TREATMENT OF PERIODONTAL AND GINGIVAL ABSCESSES

See Chapter 40.

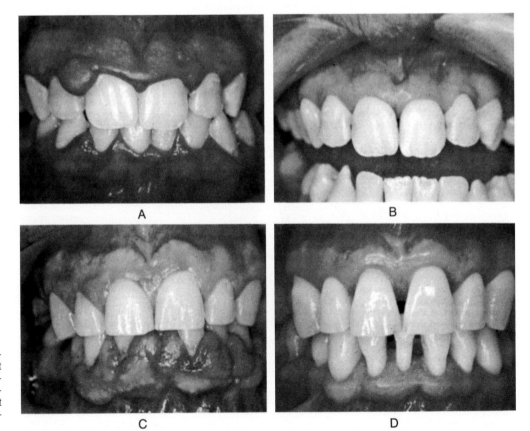

FIGURE 60-2. *A,* Chronic inflammatory gingival enlargement associated with mouth breathing. *B,* Appearance after treatment. *C,* Gingival enlargement associated with phenytoin therapy. *D,* After treatment.

TREATMENT OF DRUG-ASSOCIATED GINGIVAL HYPERPLASIA

Several therapeutic drugs can produce gingival enlargement as a side effect; these include phenytoin, used for treatment of epilepsy; cyclosporine, used as an immune depressant; and nifedipine, used for treatment of hypertension (see Chapter 18). Phenytoin enlargement was initially described in the late 1930s, whereas cyclosporine and nifedipine enlargements have only recently been reported. Therefore, experience with therapy and long-term effects are derived mostly from treatment of phenytoin enlargements. The following description refers mainly to phenytoin hyperplasia, although most of the technical aspects of therapy can be extrapolated to treatment of enlargements caused by the other two drugs.

Gingival enlargement does not occur in all patients receiving phenytoin; when it does occur, it may be of three types:

Type I: Noninflammatory hyperplasia. Discontinuation of phenytoin is the only method of eliminating the hyperplasia. When this is done, the enlargement disappears after a few months. The feasibility of discontinuing the drug should be discussed with the neurologist. Except in cases of severe disfigurement that persists after periodontal treatment and causes psychological problems, the existence of moderate or severe hyperplasia is not sufficient reason to discontinue the use of phenytoin.[8] However, there may be neurologic indications for discontinuing the use of the drug.[8] In most instances, though, the administration of phenytoin must continue, and hyperplasia must be treated by other methods (see discussion of Type III).

Type II: Chronic inflammatory enlargement entirely unrelated to phenytoin. The enlargement is caused entirely by local irritants and resembles inflammatory enlargement in patients not receiving phenytoin. For treatment of this condition, see the preceding discussion of chronic inflammatory enlargements.

Type III: Combined enlargement. This is a combination of hyperplasia caused by phenytoin and inflammation caused

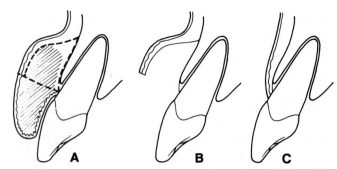

FIGURE 60–4. Diagram showing the flap operation for the removal of gingival enlargements. *A,* Gingivectomy incision at a 90-degree angle to the tooth surface. *B,* After removal of the excised tissue, the hyperplastic tissue is dissected away, maintaining the overlying epithelium and a thin layer of connective tissue. The underlying bone is exposed to ensure complete removal of hyperplasia. *C,* The flap is returned to its original position and sutured.

by local irritation. It is the most common type of enlargement in patients treated with phenytoin. It is treated surgically and by elimination of all sources of local irritation, plus fastidious plaque control by the patient.

Small or even moderate gingival hyperplasias can be removed using a gingivectomy technique (Fig. 60–2*C,D*), described earlier. For voluminous enlargements, however, the gingivectomy technique has the following disadvantages: (1) It does not eliminate the entire hyperplastic tissue (Fig. 60–3). (2) It may result in the loss of all attached gingiva, creating a mucogingival problem. (3) It leaves a wide wound of exposed connective tissue that epithelializes slowly and is painful. For these reasons, whenever possible, the flap technique is preferred.

Flap Technique for Fibrotic Gingival Enlargements

Step 1. Anesthetize the area. Mark depths of pockets with bleeding points on distal, middle, and mesial aspects of each tooth, facially and lingually.

Step 2. With a no. 15 Bard-Parker blade, make a horizontal (nonbeveled) gingivectomy incision following the scalloping of the bleeding points, both facially and lingually (Fig. 60–4).

Step 3. Using an Orban knife, incise the base of each papilla connecting the facial and the lingual incisions.

Step 4. Remove the excised marginal and interdental tissue with a U15/30 scaler.

Step 5. With a no. 11 Bard-Parker knife, thin the remaining gingival tissue, removing the fibrotic component by undermining the tissue. A thin connective tissue layer should remain underlying the epithelium.

Step 6. Remove tissue tabs, and thoroughly scale and plane the roots.

Step 7. Replace the flap, and if necessary, trim it to reach exactly the bone–tooth junction; suture it with a continuous mattress technique and cover with periodontal dressing.

Sutures and pack are removed after 1 week, and the patient is instructed to start plaque control methods. Usually it is convenient to have the patient use chlorhexidine mouthrinses once or twice daily for 2 to 4 weeks.

The initial treatment of combined enlargement presents no difficulty; the problem is recurrence. Recurrence can be kept to a minimum with periodic scaling maneuvers and

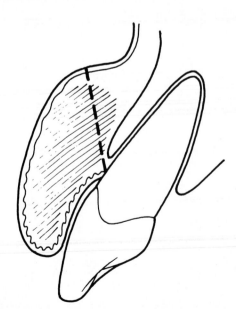

FIGURE 60–3. Gingivectomy incision may not remove the entire hyperplastic tissue (*shaded area*) and may leave a wide wound of exposed connective tissue.

diligent plaque control by the patient[6] (Fig. 60–5). A hard, natural rubber, fitted bite guard worn at night sometimes assists in the control of recurrence.[1,2]

Local treatment is effective; it keeps patients comfortable and without disfigurement for years,[3,5,7] but it does not entirely eliminate enlargement.[9,10] It prevents the return of the inflammatory part of the enlargement (see Fig. 60–3); however, it does not usually prevent recurrence of the phenytoin-induced hyperplastic component of the enlargement, although prevention has been reported in some cases.[4,6] In patients treated with phenytoin whose gingival enlargement is caused by local irritation alone, with no drug-induced hyperplasia, recurrence is totally preventable with local measures.

TREATMENT OF LEUKEMIC GINGIVAL ENLARGEMENT

Leukemic enlargement occurs in acute or subacute leukemia and is uncommon in the chronic leukemic state. The medical care of leukemic patients is often complicated by gingival enlargement with superimposed painful acute necrotizing ulcerative gingivitis, which interferes with eating and creates toxic systemic reactions. The patient's bleeding and clotting times and platelet count should be checked and the hematologist consulted before periodontal treatment is instituted (see Chapter 34).

Treatment of acute gingival involvement is described in Chapter 39. After acute symptoms subside, attention is directed to correction of the gingival enlargement. The rationale is to remove the local irritating factors to control the inflammatory component of the enlargement.

The enlargement is treated with scaling and root planing carried out in stages under topical anesthesia. The initial treatment consists of gently removing all loose accumulations with cotton pellets, superficial scaling, and instructing the patient in oral hygiene for plaque control, which should include, at least initially, daily use of chlorhexidine mouthwashes. Oral hygiene procedures are extremely important in these cases and should be performed by the nurse, if necessary.

Progressively deeper scalings are carried out at subsequent visits. Treatments are confined to a small area of the mouth to facilitate control of bleeding. Antibiotics may be administered systemically the evening before and for 48 hours after each treatment to reduce the risk of infection.

TREATMENT OF GINGIVAL ENLARGEMENT IN PREGNANCY

Treatment requires elimination of all local irritants that are responsible for precipitating the gingival changes in pregnancy. Elimination of local irritants early in pregnancy is a preventive measure against gingival disease, which is preferable to treatment of gingival enlargement after it occurs. Marginal and interdental gingival inflammation and

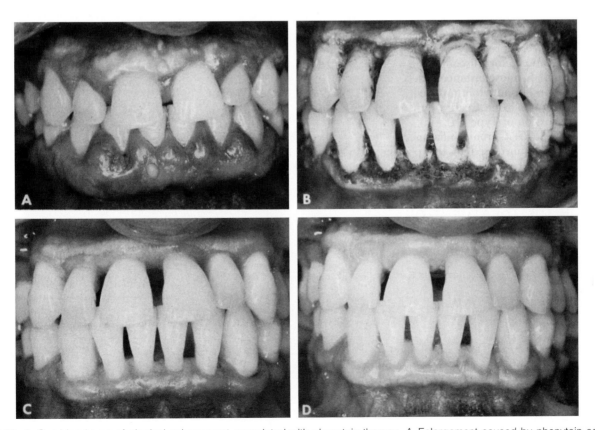

FIGURE 60–5. Combined type of gingival enlargement associated with phenytoin therapy. *A,* Enlargement caused by phenytoin combined with superimposed inflammation. *B,* Appearance at the time of pack removal, 1 week after complete mouth gingivectomy. *C,* After 4 months. *D,* After 5 years. There is some hyperplasia caused by the phenytoin, but gingival size has been kept to a minimum by periodic scalings and diligent plaque control, which prevent inflammation from recurring.

enlargement are treated with scaling and root planing (see Chapters 41 and 52). Treatment of tumor-like gingival enlargements consists of surgical excision and scaling and planing of the tooth surface. The enlargement recurs unless all irritants are removed. Food impaction is frequently an inciting factor.

When to Treat. Gingival lesions in pregnancy should be treated as soon as they are detected, although not necessarily by surgical means. Scaling and root planing procedures and adequate oral hygiene measures may reduce the size of the enlargement. Gingival enlargements do shrink after pregnancy, but they usually do not disappear. After pregnancy the entire mouth should be re-evaluated, a full set of radiographs taken, and the necessary treatment undertaken.

Lesions should be removed surgically during pregnancy only if they interfere with mastication or produce an aesthetic disfigurement that the patient wishes removed.

In pregnancy, the emphasis should be on (1) preventing gingival disease before it occurs and (2) treating existing gingival disease before it becomes worse. All patients should be seen as early as possible in pregnancy. Those without gingival disease should be checked for potential sources of local irritation and should be instructed in plaque control procedures (see Chapter 42). Those with gingival disease should be treated promptly, before the conditioning effect of pregnancy on the gingiva becomes manifest. Precautions necessary for periodontal treatment of pregnant women are presented in Chapter 34.

Every pregnant patient should be scheduled for periodic dental visits, and the importance of such visits in the prevention of serious periodontal disturbances should be stressed.

TREATMENT OF GINGIVAL ENLARGEMENT IN PUBERTY

Gingival enlargement in puberty is treated by scaling and curettage, removal of all sources of irritation, and plaque control. Surgical removal may be required in severe cases. The problem in these patients is recurrence owing to poor oral hygiene.

DRUGS IN THE TREATMENT OF GINGIVAL ENLARGEMENT

Gingival enlargement can be reduced with escharotic drugs, but this is *not* a recommended form of treatment. The destructive action of the drugs is difficult to control; injury to healthy tissue and root surfaces, delayed healing, and excessive postoperative pain are complications that can be avoided when the gingiva is removed with periodontal knives and scalpels or by electrosurgery. Removal of the enlarged gingiva by any method must be accompanied by elimination of local irritants.

RECURRENCE OF GINGIVAL ENLARGEMENT

Recurrence after treatment is the most common problem in the management of gingival enlargement. Residual local irritation and systemic or hereditary conditions that cause noninflammatory gingival hyperplasia are the responsible factors.

Recurrence of chronic inflammatory enlargement immediately after treatment indicates that all irritants have not been removed. Contributory local conditions, such as food impaction and overhanging margins of restorations, are commonly overlooked. If the enlargement recurs after healing is complete and normal contour is attained, inadequate plaque control by the patient is the most common cause.

Recurrence during the healing period is manifested as red, bead-like, granulomatous masses that bleed on slight provocation. This is a proliferative vascular inflammatory response to local irritation, usually a fragment of calculus on the root. The condition is corrected by removing the granulation tissue and scaling and planing the root surface.

Familial, hereditary, or idiopathic gingival enlargement recurs after surgical removal, even if all local irritants have been removed. The enlargement can be maintained at minimal size by preventing secondary inflammatory involvement.

REFERENCES

1. Aiman R. The use of positive pressure mouthpiece as a new therapy for Dilantin gingival hyperplasia. Chron Omaha Dent Soc *131:*244, 1968.
2. Babcock JR. The successful use of a new therapy for Dilantin gingival hyperplasia. Periodontics *3:*196, 1965.
3. Bergmann CL. Dilantin: Its effect on the gingival tissue. Dent Digest *73:*63, 1967.
4. Ciancio SG, Yaffe SJ, Catz CC. Gingival hyperplasia and diphenylhydantoin. J Periodontol *43:*411, 1972.
5. Ginwalla TM, Gomes GC, Nayak RP. Management of gingival hyperplasia in patients receiving Dilantin therapy. J Indian Dent Assoc *39:*124, 1967.
6. Hall WB. Dilantin hyperplasia: A preventable lesion. J Periodont Res *4:*36, 1969.
7. Miller FD. Multipronged attack against Dilantin gingival hyperplasia. Dent Surv *42:*51, 1966.
8. Reynolds NC Jr, Kirkham DB. Therapeutic alternatives in phenytoin-induced gingival hyperplasia. J Periodontol *51:*516, 1980.
9. Russell B, Bay L. The effect of toothbrushing with chlorhexidine gluconate toothpaste on epileptic children. Abstract. J Dent Res *54*(suppl A):L114, 1975.
10. Staple PH, Reed MJ, Mashimo PA, et al. Diphenylhydantoin gingival hyperplasia in *Macaca arctoides.* Prevention by inhibition of dental plaque deposition. J Periodontol *49:*310, 1978.

61

Recent Advances in Surgical Technology

DENNIS A. SHANELEC and LEONARD S. TIBBETTS

Magnification Systems
Magnifying Loupes
The Operating Microscope

Periodontal Microsurgery
Conclusion

The use of magnification in periodontics is not an isolated development but part of a broader trend in medicine and dentistry toward the use of minimally invasive techniques for procedures that previously required extensive surgical incisions.[2,3,8,10] *Microsurgery* may be defined as a refinement in operative technique by which visual acuity is improved through magnification. It has also been described as a methodology through which existing surgical techniques are modified to accommodate the improved vision possible through magnification.[9] In addition to microsurgery, magnification in periodontics may be applied to diagnostic and nonsurgical procedures.

MAGNIFICATION SYSTEMS

A variety of simple and complex magnification systems are available, ranging from simple loupes to prism telescopic loupes and the surgical microscope. Each magnification system has specific advantages and limitations. The assumption that more magnification is always better must be weighed against the decrease in field of view and depth of focus that occurs as magnification increases. Although magnification allows considerable improvement in the accuracy of clinical and diagnostic skills, it also requires increased understanding of the optical principles that govern all magnification systems.

Magnifying Loupes

Surgical loupes are by far the most common system of optical magnification used in periodontics. Loupes are fundamentally two monocular microscopes with side-by-side lenses converged to focus on the operative field. The magnified image formed has stereoscopic properties by virtue of the convergent lenses. A convergent lens system is called a *Keplerian optical system* (Fig. 61–1).

Although loupes are widely used, they have a considerable disadvantage in that the clinician's eyes must converge to view the operative field. This can result in eye strain, fatigue, and even vision changes, especially after prolonged use of poorly fitted loupes.

Three types of Keplerian loupes are commonly employed in periodontics: simple single-element loupes, compound loupes, and prism telescopic loupes. Each type may differ widely in optical sophistication and individual construction.

Simple Loupes. Simple loupes consist of a pair of single-element meniscus lenses (Fig. 61–2). Simple loupes are primitive magnifiers with limited capabilities. Each lens has just two refracting surfaces (Fig. 61–3). Their magnification can be increased only by increasing their lens diameter or thickness. Another disadvantage of simple loupes is that they are highly affected by spherical and chromatic aberration. This distorts both the shape and color of the object being viewed. Size and weight limitations make simple loupes impractical for magnification beyond 1.5 diameters.

Compound Loupes. Compound loupes use multiple-element lenses with intervening air spaces to gain additional refracting surfaces (Fig. 61–4). This allows increased magnification with more favorable working distance and depth of field. Compound loupes can be adjusted to clinical needs without excessive increase in size or weight (Fig. 61–5).

In addition to offering substantially improved optical design, compound lenses can be achromatic. This is a feature that clinicians should choose when selecting magnifying loupes. Achromatic lenses consist of two glass pieces, usually joined together with clear resin. The specific density of each piece counteracts the chromatic aberration of adjacent lenses to produce a color-correct image. Multi-element compound loupes become optically inefficient at magnifications above 3.0 diameters.

Prism Telescopic Loupes. A more advanced type of optical magnification is currently available in the form of prism telescopic loupes. Such loupes contain Schmidt or rooftop prisms that lengthen the light path through a series of mirror reflections within the lens elements (Fig. 61–6). This literally folds the light so the barrel of the telescopic loupe can be shortened. Prism loupes produce better magnification, wider depths of field, longer working distances, and larger fields of view than other types of loupes. The barrels of prism loupes are short enough to be mounted on

677

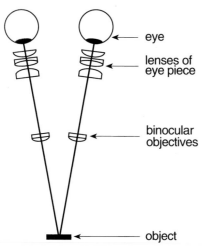

FIGURE 61-1. Keplerian optics.

eye ←

lenses of eye piece ←

binocular objectives ←

object ←

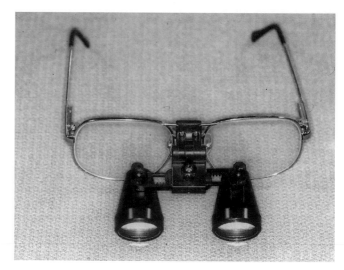

FIGURE 61-4. Compound loupes.

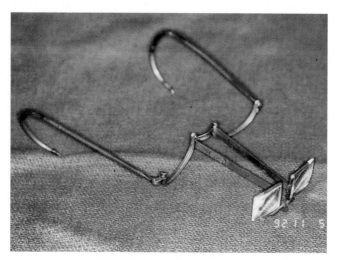

FIGURE 61-2. Simple loupes.

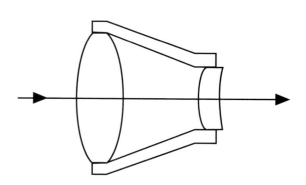

Multiple Lenses
FIGURE 61-5. Compound loupe optical diagram.

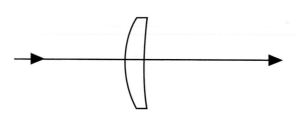

FIGURE 61-3. Simple loupe optical diagram.

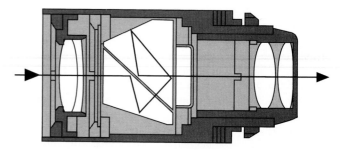

FIGURE 61-6. Prism loupe optical diagram.

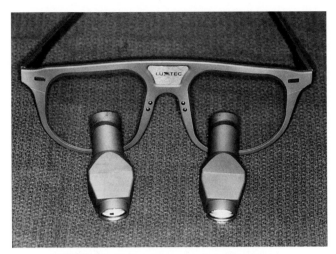

FIGURE 61–7. Eyeglass-mounted prism loupes.

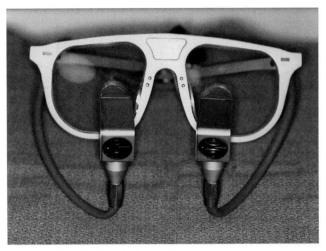

FIGURE 61–9. Coaxial lighted prism loupes.

either eyeglass frames (Fig. 61–7) or headbands (Fig. 61–8). However, the increased weight of prism telescopic loupes with magnification above 3× makes headband mounting more comfortable and stable than eyeglass frame mounting.[6] Recent innovations in prism telescopic loupes include coaxial fiberoptic lighting incorporated in the lens elements to improve illumination (Fig. 61–9).

Magnification Range of Surgical Loupes

Loupes are capable of providing a wide range of magnification (1.5× to 10×). Those delivering less than 2× magnification are usually inadequate for the visual acuity necessary for periodontal microsurgery. Those providing more than 4.5× magnification are awkward to use because of their small field of view and narrow depth of focus and excessive weight.

For most periodontal procedures, prism telescopic loupes of 4× magnification provide an effective combination of magnification, field of view, and depth of focus. Only the surgical operating microscope provides higher magnification and superior optical properties than the prism telescopic loupe does.

The Operating Microscope

The surgical operating microscope offers superior flexibility in magnification and optics compared with magnifying loupes (Fig. 61–10). Although the operating microscope is expensive and requires a long period of adjustment before clinical proficiency is reached, it offers the clinician far better performance and versatility than a loupe. Operating microscopes suitable for use in periodontics utilize Galilean optical principles.[1] They have binocular eyepieces joined by two offset prisms with parallel optical axes (Fig. 61–11). This permits stereoscopic viewing of the operative field without eye convergence. It also permits relaxed viewing of the operative field with the eyes positioned as if focused on infinity without convergence. This reduces eye strain and fatigue. Operating microscopes also incorporate fully coated optics with achromatic lenses to provide the highest resolution and most efficient illumination.

Perhaps the most important advantage of the surgical operating microscope is the ability of the clinician to easily change the working magnification level.[4] Operating microscopes have a rotating variable magnification element that may be changed easily to allow the clinician to quickly

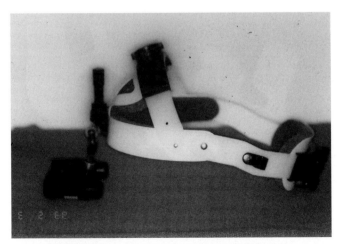

FIGURE 61–8. Headband-mounted prism loupes.

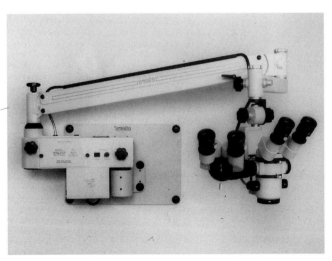

FIGURE 61–10. Surgical operating microscope.

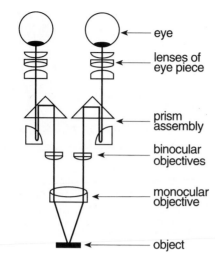

FIGURE 61–11. Galilean optics microscope diagram.

eye

lenses of eye piece

prism assembly

binocular objectives

monocular objective

object

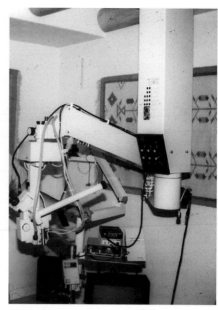

FIGURE 61–13. Ceiling-mounted microscope.

adapt the magnification levels to operative procedure demands (Fig. 61–12). Some operating microscopes incorporate electronic zoom optics for further convenience. Because the optical elements of surgical microscopes are more sophisticated than those found in loupes, depth-of-focus and field-of-view characteristics are enhanced severalfold.

The clinician must establish adequate working distance between the surgical field and the objective lens. This is important to allow the surgical assistant to irrigate and evacuate the surgical field. Such control of hemorrhage is essential for microsurgical visibility. Assistant observer eyepiece attachments are available for most surgical microscopes and greatly aid the progress of microsurgical procedures. Surgical microscopes are available with objective lenses for various working distances. The useful range in dentistry is 200 to 400 mm. Because operating with a mirror adds 100 to 150 mm to the working distance, a ready means of changing working distances is valuable. Quick-change objective lens devices are available for most surgical microscopes.

For practical use in periodontics, a surgical microscope must have both maneuverability and stability. *Microscope mountings* are available for ceiling, wall, or floor (Fig. 61–13). Inclinable eyepieces also lend flexibility to the clinical use of the surgical microscope in periodontics (Fig. 61–14). *Maneuverability* must always be sufficient to meet the requirements of clinicians for increased visual accessibility to the various anatomic structures dealt with in periodontics. Because the optical characteristics of most manufacturers' lenses are comparable, microscope maneuverability is often more important than optical characteristics in determining the appropriate microscope for periodontal procedures.

Illumination of the field is an important consideration. Periodontists are accustomed to lateral illumination from side-mounted dental lights. Clinicians who work with loupes often require a headlamp to compensate for the decreased amount of light passing through the loupes. Until recently, coaxial fiberoptic illumination had been a major

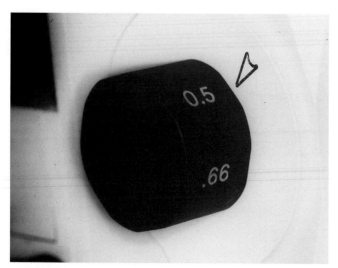

FIGURE 61–12. Microscope variable magnification changer.

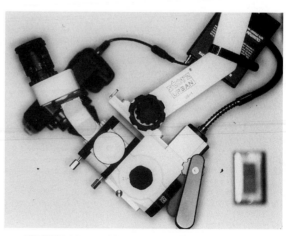

FIGURE 61–14. Microscope inclinable eyepiece.

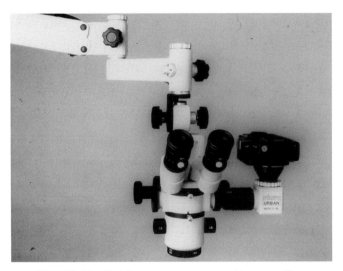

FIGURE 61–15. Microscope camera and beam splitter.

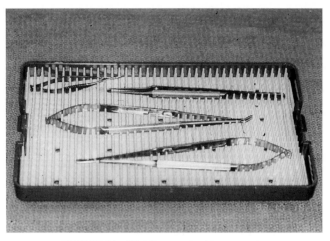

FIGURE 61–17. Microsurgical instruments.

advantage of the operating microscope over surgical loupes. Coaxial lighting places the light source parallel to the optical axis via a prism beam splitter. With coaxial lighting, no shadows are produced, and the clinician can view the farthest reaches of the oral cavity, including deep into subgingival pockets and angular defects. Perfect visualization of root surface irregularities and deposits is possible. The clinician is able to view aspects of normal and abnormal periodontal anatomy never previously accessible. Clinical decisions can be made based on sure knowledge of altered anatomy rather than educated guesses. Coaxial lighting is also available in prism telescopic loupes.

Documentation of periodontal procedures has become increasingly important for dental–legal reasons and for patient and professional education purposes. The surgical operating microscope is ideal for documenting periodontal procedures of all types; 35-mm slides can easily be produced using a beam splitter camera attachment (Fig. 61–15). With a foot-operated shutter control, the surgeon can compose the photographic field as the procedure unfolds without interrupting the surgical process for photography. In addition, the photographic slide represents the surgical field exactly as the surgeon sees it, as opposed to a photographer's view produced while the surgeon works. Excellent video documentation is also available through the operating microscope using a video beam splitter attachment. High-resolution cameras with video and slide printers are currently replacing 35-mm camera photography in many microsurgical disciplines. High-resolution SVHS recorders bring new capabilities for video recording of periodontal procedures for educational purposes.

PERIODONTAL MICROSURGERY

In recent years periodontics has seen increasing refinement of procedures requiring progressively more intricate surgical skills. Regenerative and resective osseous surgery, periodontal plastic surgery, and dental implants demand clinical performance that challenges the technical skills of periodontists beyond the range of ordinary visual acuity.

Periodontal microsurgery introduces the possibility for considerably less invasive surgical procedures in periodon-

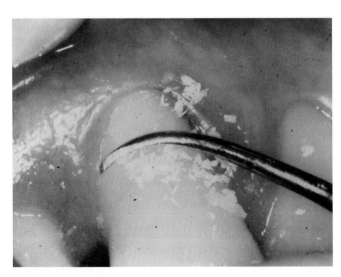

FIGURE 61–16. Magnified root planing.

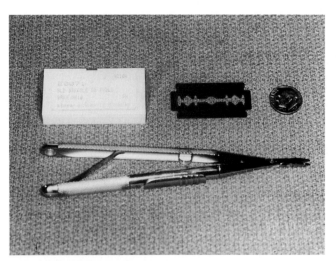

FIGURE 61–18. Castroviejo microsurgical scalpel.

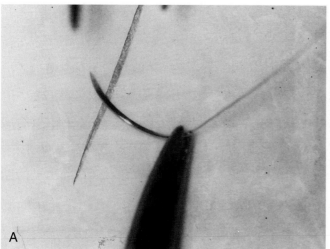

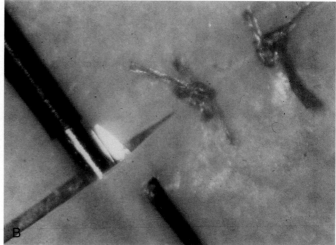

FIGURE 61–19. Microsurgical suturing.

tics, exemplified by a lessened need for vertical releasing incisions and a smaller surgical site. Periodontists, like other microsurgeons, have been surprised by the extent to which reduced incision size is directly related to reduced postoperative patient pain.[12]

Root Preparation. The importance of root debridement is recognized universally, and studies show that the enhanced vision permitted with magnification results in far more complete attainment of the goals of this procedure.

Among the primary goals of periodontal surgery is visual access to the root surface for plaque and calculus removal and for planing of pathologically altered tooth structure. Magnification greatly improves the surgeon's ability to achieve clean, smooth root surfaces (Fig. 61–16). The root surface represents one opposing edge of the microsurgical wound. Root planing is analogous to establishing a clean, right-angled, soft tissue incision. Magnification permits preparation of both hard and soft tissue wound surfaces so they may be joined together according to the microsurgical principle of butt-joint approximation. This encourages primary wound healing with enhanced periodontal regeneration. Wound healing studies have shown epithelialization of microsurgically joined surgical wounds in animals within 48 hours.[5,11]

Surgery Under Magnification. Viewing periodontal surgery under magnification cannot help but impress the clinician with the coarseness of conventional surgical manipulation. What appears to the unaided eye as gentle handling is revealed, under magnification, as gross crushing and tearing of delicate tissues. Periodontists have attempted to treat the surgical site atraumatically to achieve primary wound closure. However, the limits of normal vision dictate the extent to which this goal is possible. Periodontal microsurgery is a natural transition of conventional surgical principles by which magnification is employed to permit accurate and atraumatic handling of soft and hard tissues to enhance wound healing.

Microsurgical Instruments. In addition to the use of magnification and reliance on atraumatic technique, microsurgery entails the use of specially constructed microsurgical instruments specifically designed to minimize trauma

(Fig. 61–17). An important characteristic of microsurgical instruments is their ability to create clean incisions to prepare the wound for healing by primary intention. Such incisions are established at 90-degree angles to the surface using a Castroviejo microsurgical scalpel (Fig. 61–18). Magnification permits easy identification of ragged wound edges for trimming and freshening. To permit primary wound closure, microsutures in the range of 6–0 to 9–0 are required to approximate the wound edges (Fig. 61–19). Microsurgical wound apposition minimizes gaps or voids at the wound edges, which encourages rapid healing with less postoperative inflammation and less pain.

Figures 61-20 through 61-28 illustrate periodontal surgery cases treated using microsurgical techniques.

CONCLUSION

Microsurgery offers new possibilities for periodontics that can improve therapeutic results for a variety of procedures. Its benefits include improved cosmetics, rapid healing, minimal discomfort, and enhanced patient acceptance. Periodontics of the future will see increasing use of magnification in all areas of practice, including implantology.

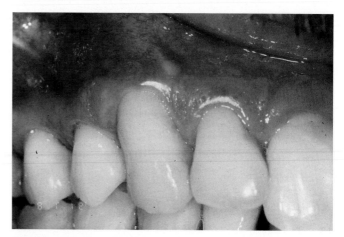

FIGURE 61–20. Subepithelial connective tissue graft, case 1: presurgery.

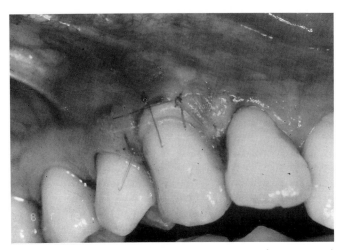

FIGURE 61–21. Subepithelial connective tissue graft, case 1: microsurgical view.

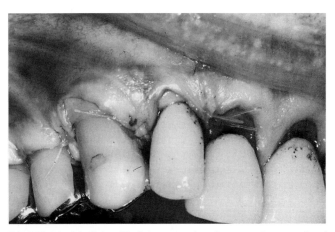

FIGURE 61–24. Subepithelial connective tissue graft, case 2: microsurgical view.

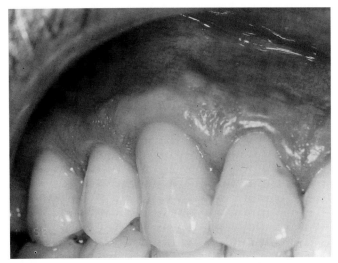

FIGURE 61–22. Subepithelial connective tissue graft, case 1: post-surgery.

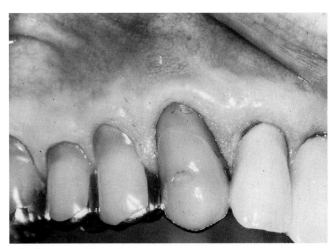

FIGURE 61–25. Subepithelial connective tissue graft, case 2: post-surgery.

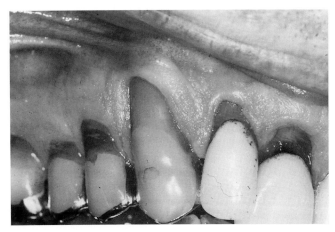

FIGURE 61–23. Subepithelial connective tissue graft, case 2: pre-surgery.

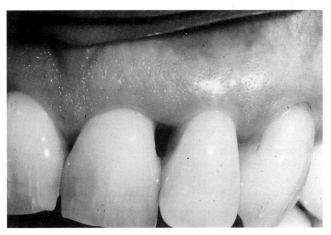

FIGURE 61–26. Papilla reconstruction: presurgery.

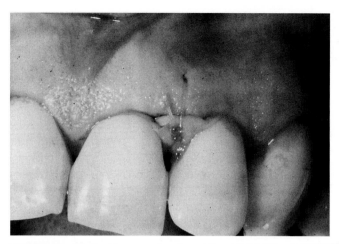

FIGURE 61–27. Papilla reconstruction: microsurgical view.

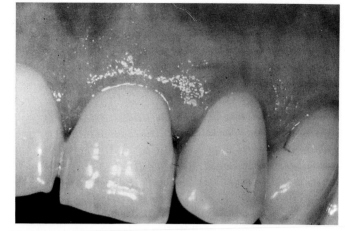

FIGURE 61–28. Papilla reconstruction: postsurgery.

REFERENCES

1. Apotheker H, Jako GJ. A microscope for use in dentistry. J Microsurg *3:*7, 1981.
2. Banowsky LH. Basic microvascular techniques and principles. Urology *23:*495, 1984.
3. Daniel RK. Microsurgery: Through the looking glass. N Engl J Med *300:*1251, 1979.
4. Hoerenz P. The operating microscope. 1. Optical principles, illumination systems and support systems. J Microsurg *1:*367, 1980.
5. Klopper P, Muller JH, Van Hattum AH. Microsurgery and Wound Healing. Amsterdam, Excerpta Medica, 1979, p 280.
6. Labosky DA. Apparatus to relieve nose-bridge pressure from high-power surgical telescopes. J Microsurgery *4:*142, 1983.
7. Owen ER. Practical microsurgery. I. A choice of optical aids. Med Aust *1:*244, 1971.
8. Pecora G, Andreana S. Operating microscope in endodontic surgery. Oral Surg Med Pathol *75:*751, 1993.
9. Serafin D. Microsurgery: Past, present and future. Plast Reconstr Surg *66:*781, 1979.
10. Shanelec DA. Optical principles of loupes. Calif Dent Assoc J *20:*25, 1992.
11. Van Hattum A, James J, Klopper PJ, Muller JH. Epithelial migration in wound healing. Virchows Archiv B Cell Path *30:*221–230, 1979.
12. Way L. Changing therapy for gallstone disease. N Engl J Med *323:*1273, 1990

The periodontist has a well-defined role in the placement of intraoral implants and in their care and maintenance. This part will describe the biologic basis of implantology and its diagnostic and surgical aspects, as well as the diagnosis and treatment of peri-implant disease.

62

Biologic Aspects of Dental Implants

GEORGE W. BERNARD, FERMIN A. CARRANZA, Jr., and
SASCHA A. JOVANOVIC

Biomaterials
The Peri-implant Mucosa
The Implant–Bone Interface

To develop artificial replacements for missing teeth has been an elusive goal for more than 1500 years. A fine, dark stone, shaped like a tooth, was found implanted in a Mayan skull in Central America from 600 AD, and there are reports of implant attempts in ancient Egypt and the Middle East.[31] Interest in developing artificial teeth anchored to the jaws has continued to the present.

The present surge in the use of implants was initiated in 1952 by Brånemark, who conducted extensive experimental and clinical studies.[7-9] Brånemark and associates described the relationship between titanium and bone, for which they coined the term *osseointegration,* defined as the "direct structural and functional connection between ordered, living bone and the surface of a load-carrying implant."[4,7]

BIOMATERIALS

There are many biologically compatible materials that can be used for the manufacturing of implants. Currently, interest is centered on metals and metal alloys, ceramics and carbons, and polymers and composites.

Metals and Metal Alloys. Metallic biomaterials have been extensively used, particularly titanium, tantalum, and alloys of titanium/aluminum/vanadium, cobalt/chromium/molybdenum, and iron/chromium/nickel. Precious metals such as gold and platinum and their alloys are less frequently used. The most widely used material is titanium and its alloy; most available data concern this material.

Ceramics and Carbons. This group includes aluminum oxide (alumina and sapphire) ceramics, carbon, and carbon–silicon compounds. Hydroxyapatite has been proposed as a solid material, and as a surface coating it is also widely used. Because coatings are used on load-bearing metals, there is a need for high interfacial shear strength.[32]

Polymers and Composites. These include cross-linked polymers such as polymethylmethacrylate, silicone rubber, and polyethylene. They are not in general use at present, but technologic developments may bring an increased use of these materials in the future.[32]

THE PERI-IMPLANT MUCOSA

The mucosal tissues around intraosseous implants form a tightly adherent band consisting of a dense collagenous lamina propria covered by stratified squamous keratinizing epithelium (Figs. 62–1 and 62–2).

The implant–epithelium junction is analogous to the junctional epithelium around natural teeth, in that the epithelial cells attach to the titanium implant by means of hemidesmosomes and a basal lamina.[19,20] Evidence for an adhesive junctional epithelium attachment to ceramic implants has also been presented.[30] *This evidence supports the concept that a viable biologic seal can exist between the epithelial cells and the implant.*

A sulcus forms around the implant lined with a sulcular epithelium. The depth of a normal, noninflamed or minimally inflamed sulcus around an intraosseous implant has not yet been accurately determined but is assumed to be between 2.5 and 3.5 mm.[24] Studies on sulcus and pocket depth around normal teeth have determined that the penetration of the probe, particularly if inflammation is present, will be stopped by the first attached collagen fibers (see Chapter 28). Because these are not present around implants, the probe would be expected to attain deeper measurements.[16]

The sulcus around an implant is lined with a sulcular epithelium that is continuous apically with the junctional epithelium. Normal tissues around implants have an intact epithelial lining and about the same number of inflammatory cells as are found around a natural tooth.[1]

Capillary loops in the connective tissue under the junctional and the sulcus epithelia appear to be anatomically similar to those found in the normal periodontium[35] (Fig. 62–3). Some investigators, however, have found reduced vascularity close to the implant surface compared with that around teeth and opined that this may make peri-implant tissues more vulnerable to pathogenic insults.[12,28]

Bleeding on gentle probing rarely occurs in healthy mucosal tissues around implants. The presence of bleeding indicates the presence of plaque-induced inflammation, although false-negative results have been reported.[28]

Although some investigators have suggested that the amount of keratinized tissue around implants is not a factor in the amount of inflammation,[40] others have found an increased chance of peri-implant mucositis in patients without keratinized mucosa.[6,30]

Collagen fibers are nonattached and run parallel to the implant surface owing to the lack of cementum. This is an important difference between peri-implant and periodontal tissues. However, some reports have suggested that microscopic irregularities and porosities, such as would be found

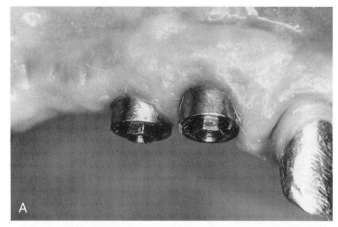
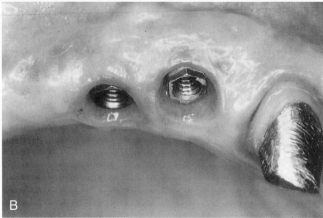

FIGURE 62–1. *A,* Clinically normal gingival mucosa next to two implants. *B,* Normal epithelium lining the implant after removal of the cover screw.

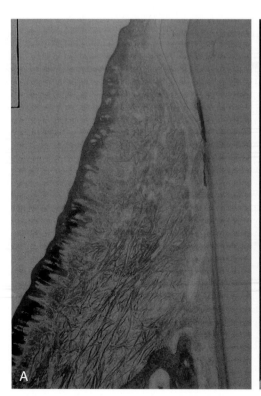
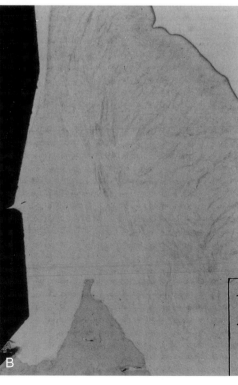

FIGURE 62–2. *A,* Micrograph showing normal periodontium surrounding a tooth. *B,* Micrograph showing normal peri-implant tissues.

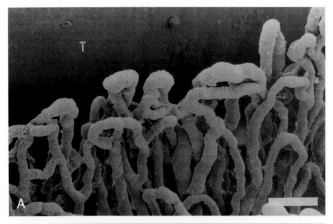

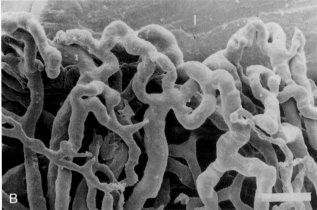

FIGURE 62–3. Microvascular topography surrounding a tooth (*A*) and an implant (*B*). Bar = 5 μm. (Courtesy of Dr. N. Selliseth and Dr. K. Selvig.)

on plasma-sprayed titanium surfaces, may favor the appearance of fibers oriented perpendicularly to the implant surface.[12,23,34]

The marginal portion of the peri-implant mucosa contains significantly more collagen and fewer fibroblasts than the corresponding gingival tissue, which may indicate that tissue turnover in the peri-implant mucosa is less rapid than that in the gingiva.

THE IMPLANT–BONE INTERFACE

The relationship between endosseous implants and bone consists of one of two mechanisms: *osseointegration,* when the bone is in intimate contact with the implant, or *fibro-osseous integration,* in which soft tissues, such as fibers and/or cells, are interposed between the two surfaces.

The proponents of the fibro-osseous system of implant retention opine that the presence of a dense collagenous tissue between implant and bone will act as an osteogenic membrane.[39] There is no wide support, however, for this concept.

The osseointegration concept proposed by Brånemark et al.[7] and called *functional ankylosis* by Schroeder[34] states that there is an absence of connective tissue or any non-bone tissue in the interface between the implant and the bone. A more accurate term, *microinterlock,* is used in orthopedic implantology where tissue and implant are juxtaposed, providing a bioinert fixation with surface porosities, grooves, or beads.[14]

It is important to note that osseointegration refers to the direct contact of bone and implant *at the light microscope level* (Fig. 62–4). Furthermore, osseointegration never occurs on 100% of the implant surface. Successful cases will have between 30% and 95% of the implant

FIGURE 62–4. Peri-implant supporting tissues around an implant at the light microscopy level. *A,* Topographic view. *B,* Higher magnification showing direct apposition of bone and implant.

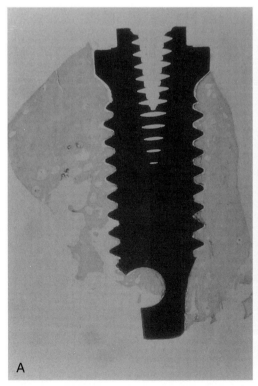

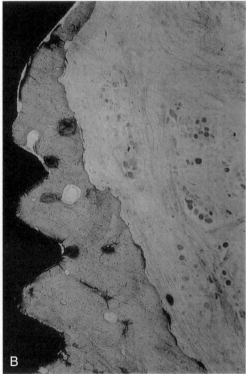

surface, as measured by light microscopy, in contact with bone.

Under the light microscope, bone appears to be in direct contact with the implant. By virtue of its excellent regenerative potential, bone is seen to grow around the ridges and grooves of screw-type implants and through the openings of blade- and hollow cylinder–type implants. Remodeling of bone occurs constantly as part of the normal physiology of bone and continues to occur after the implant has been placed.

Histologic sections of the bone–implant interface, however, are usually thick (20 to 150 μm) and do not permit an accurate view of the interface. These thick sections have been the primary standard of viewing the interface and may have led to the premature definition of the interface as an osteointegrative one.

Although some ultrastructural investigations have reported mineralized matrix in direct contact with titanium without the presence of any amorphous layer,[2,25] others have reported the interposition of connective tissue.[17,32]

Reports using conventional transmission and high-voltage electron microscopy have contradicted the direct bone-to-implant results. These studies suggested a close approximation of calcified tissue to the implant surface but found no conclusive evidence of any molecular bonds between the metal oxide surface of titanium and the adjacent bone.[38] An amorphous cell-free layer, ranging in width from 20 to 1000 nm and composed of glycosaminoglycans and proteoglycans, has been reported to be interposed between bone and titanium.[36] There may also be a lamina limitans–like line,[36] 50 nm thick, and a layer of noncalcified collagen adjacent to the titanium surface. Complete mineralization is seen only 2000 nm (2 μm) from the metal.[36]

An in vitro technique devised by Holden and Bernard[21] has provided a reproducible system to analyze the bone–implant interface. This technique coats Petri dishes

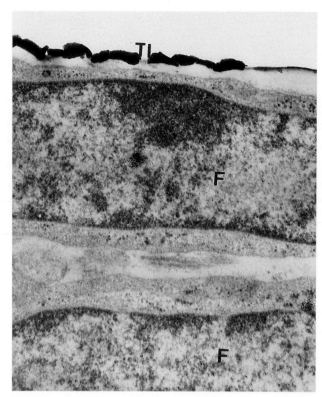

FIGURE 62–6. Transmission electron micrograph of the interface of bone colonies on evaporated titanium (TI). Portions of two fibroblasts (F) are seen with a clear zone between the innermost cells and the titanium. Original magnification ×20,000.

with titanium, titanium alloy, or cobalt/chrome and then grows bone on the thinly coated implant materials. Semithin (2 μm) and thin (80 nm) sections can then be prepared and analyzed using light and transmission electron microscopy.

The compatibility of bone and titanium can be demonstrated by the large number of bone colonies that grow on titanium (Fig. 62–5); a lesser amount grow on titanium alloy, and almost none grow on cobalt/chrome.

Electron microscopy of the bone–titanium interface using this technique shows that there is always connective tissue between the implant and the bone (Fig. 62–6). A carbohydrate-rich adhesive substrate is invariably found on the metal adjoining the fibroblasts in vitro. In vivo, as in vitro, bone is never found in direct contact with titanium.

Plasma-sprayed hydroxyapatite in Petri dishes is even more receptive to bone growth than titanium, forming larger and more numerous colonies. At the interface with hydroxyapatite, fibroblasts and osteoblasts can be demonstrated (Fig. 62–7). Where osteoblasts have developed, collagen is seen in the interface with hydroxyapatite, looking very much like osteoid with matrix vesicles containing hydoxyapatite crystals and growing bone nodules, an indication of woven bone formation. High-resolution electron micrographs show that fine crystals of hydroxyapatite molecularly bond with the implant hydroxyapatite.

The absence of cementum on the implant surface prevents the attachment of collagen fibers to the implant. This lack of cementum is interpreted as being due to the absence of cementum progenitor cells in the area receiving the implant.[27] When these cells are available, cementum can form

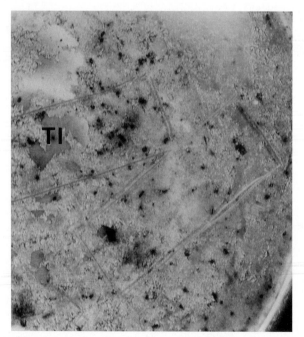

FIGURE 62–5. Petri dish with many dark bone colonies. Evaporated titanium (TI) in areas denuded of cells. Original magnification ×1.

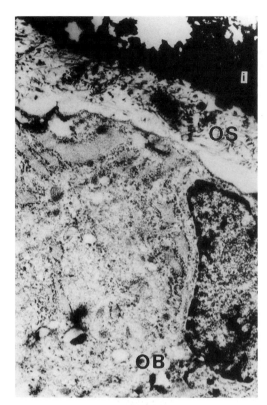

FIGURE 62–7. Transmission electron micrograph showing a portion of an osteoblast (OB) and osteoid with initial calcification (OS) juxtaposed to the hydroxyapatite surface of the implant (i). Original magnification × 18,000.

on the implant surface, and a functional collagen attachment can attach to it. Albrektsson and associates[3] have described the presence of a distinct layer of cementum on the implant surface and a periodontal ligament with fibers oriented perpendicularly when the implant was placed close to retained roots that had a periodontal ligament.

It is important to note that when undecalcified bone interfaces with titanium, whether in vivo or in vitro, electron microscopy has always shown connective tissue interposed between the two surfaces.

This brings up two considerations. In the first place, inflammatory cells are a potential constituent of connective tissue, and improper loading of the implant may trigger an inflammatory response leading to bone resorption. The second is possibly a positive factor in that connective tissue may provide a cushioning structure between the hard surfaces of metal and bone. Furthermore, hydroxyapatite surfaces of implants have true osseointegration but only in a macular fashion with connective tissue in the intervening sites. There is also reason to believe that plasma-sprayed hydroxyapatite with less than optimal crystallinity may not have a long half-life, although long-term studies have not been reported.

REFERENCES

1. Adell R, Lekholm U, Brånemark P-I, et al. Marginal tissue reactions at osseointegrated titanium fixtures. Swed Dent J *28*(suppl):175, 1985.
2. Albrektsson T, Brånemark P-I, Hansson HA, et al. Ultrastructural analysis of the interface zone of titanium and gold implants. Adv Biomater *4:*167, 1982.
3. Albrektsson T, Brånemark P-I, Hansson HA, et al. The interface zone of inorganic implants in-vivo: Titanium implants in bone. Ann Biomed Eng *11:*1, 1983.
4. Albrektsson T, Brånemark P-I, Hansson HA, Lindström J. Osseointegrated titanium implants. Acta Orthop Scand *52:*155, 1981.
5. Albrektsson T, Sennerby L. Direct bone anchorage of oral implants: Clinical and experimental considerations of the concept of osseointegration. Int J Prosthodont *3:*30, 1990.
6. Block M, Kent J. Factors associated with soft and hard tissue compromise of endosseous implants. J Oral Maxillofac Surg *48:*1160, 1990.
7. Brånemark P-I, Adell R, Breine U, et al. Intraosseous anchorage of dental prosthesis. I. Experimental studies. Scand J Plast Reconstr Surg *3:*81, 1969.
8. Brånemark P-I, Hunsson BO, Adell R, et al. Osseointegrated implants in the treatment of the edentulous jaw. Scand J Plast Reconstr Surg *16*(suppl):11, 1977.
9. Brånemark P-I, Zarb GA, Albrektsson T. Tissue-integrated prostheses. In Brånemark P-I, Zarb GA, Albrektsson T, eds. Osseointegration in Clinical Dentistry. Chicago, Quintessence Publishing, 1985.
10. Buser D, Stich H, Krekeler G, Schroeder A. Faserstrukturen der periimplantären Mukosa bei Titanimplantate, Eine Tiereexperimentelle Studie am Beagle-Hund. Zeitschr F Zahnärztliche Implantologie *5:*15, 1989.
11. Buser D, Warre K, Karring T. Formation of a periodontal ligament around titanium implants. J Periodontol *61:*597, 1990.
12. Buser D, Weber HP, Donath K, et al. Soft tissue reactions to non-submerged unloaded titanium implants in beagle dogs. J Periodontol *63:*225, 1992.
13. Buser D, Weber HP, Lang NP. Tissue integration of non-submerged implants. 1 year results of a prospective study with 100 ITI hollow-cylinder and hollow-screw implants. Clin Oral Implant Res *1:*33, 1990.
14. Dienn MG, Maxian SH. Biomaterials used in orthopedic surgery. In Greco RS, ed. Implantation Biology. Boca Raton, FL, CRC Press, 1994, pp 229–252.
15. Elisha J, Bernard GW. The bone/ceramic hydroxyapatite interface following in-vitro bone formation. Unpublished manuscript. University of California, Los Angeles, Los Angeles, CA.
16. Ericsson I, Lindhe J. Probing depths at implants and teeth. J Clin Periodontol *20:*263, 1993.
17. Falez F, Bernard G, Perugia L, Pilloni A. Valutazione quantitativa e qualitativa dell'interfaccia osso-ceramica. Giornale Italiano di Ortop e Traumat 85, 1994.
18. Golijanin L, Bernard GW. Biocompatibility of implant metals in bone tissue culture. J Dent Res *67:*367, 1988.
19. Gould TR, Brunette DM, Westbury C. The attachment mechanism of epithelial cells to titanium in vitro. J Periodont Res *16:*611, 1981.
20. Gould TR, Westbury C, Brunette DM. Ultrastructural study of the attachment of human gingiva to titanium in vivo. J Prosthet Dent *52:*418, 1984.
21. Holden C, Bernard GW. Ultrastructural in-vitro characterization of a porous hydroxyapatite/bone cell interface. J Oral Implantol *16:*86, 1990.
22. Inoue T, Cox JE, Pilliar RM, et al. Effect of the surface geometry of smooth and porous-coated titanium alloy on the orientation of fibroblasts in vivo. J Biomed Mater Res *21:*107, 1987.
23. James RA, Schultz R. Hemidesmosomes and the adhesion of junctional epithelial cells to metal implants. J Oral Implantol *3:*294, 1974.
24. Lekholm U, Ericsson I, Adell R, Slots J. The condition of the soft tissues at tooth and fixture abutment supporting fixed bridges. J Clin Periodontol *13:*558, 1986.
25. Linder L, Albrektsson T, Brånemark P-I, et al. Electron-microscopic analysis of the bone-titanium interface. Acta Orthop Scand *54:*45, 1983.
26. Lindhe J, Berglundh T, Ericsson I, et al. Experimental breakdown of periimplant and periodontal tissues. A study in the beagle dog. Clin Oral Implant Res *3:*9, 1992.
27. Listgarten MA, Buser D, Steinemann SG, et al. Light and transmission electron microscopy of the intact interfaces between non-submerged titanium-coated epoxy resin implants and bone or gingiva. J Dent Res *71:*364, 1992.
28. Listgarten MA, Lang NP, Schroeder HE, et al. Periodontal tissues and their counterparts around endosseous implants. Clin Oral Implant Res *2:*1, 1991.
29. McKinney RV Jr, Steflik DE, Koth DL. The biologic tissue response to dental implants. In McKinney RV Jr., ed. Endosteal Dental Implants. St Louis, CV Mosby, 1991.
30. Meffert R. In the soft tissue interface in dental implantology. Dental Implants NIH Consensus Development Conference, 1988, pp 107–110.
31. Peppas NA, Langer R. New challenges in biomaterials. Science *263:*1715, 1994.
32. Pilloni A, Falez F, Bernard GW. Iddrossiapatite e osteoconduzione: Effetto sulle cellule staminale pluripotenti midollari. Proceedings of the First World Congress on Osseointegration, Venice, September 29–October 2, 1994.
33. Schroeder A, van der Zypen E, Stich H, Sutter F. The reaction of bone, connective tissue and epithelium to endosteal implants with titanium-sprayed surfaces. J Maxillofac Surg *9:*15, 1981.
34. Schroeder A, Sutter F, Krekeler G. Orale Implantologie, Allgemeine Grundlagen und ITI-Hohlzylindersystem. Stuttgart, G Thieme, 1988.
35. Selliseth NJ, Selvig K. Personal communication, June 1994.
36. Sennerby L, Ericsson LE, Thomsen P, et al. Structure of the bone/titanium interface in retrieved clinical oral implants. Clin Oral Implant Res *2:*103, 1992.
37. Steflik MA, McKinney RV Jr. History of Implantology. In McKinney RV Jr., ed. Endosteal Dental Implants. St Louis, CV Mosby, 1991.
38. Steinemann SG, Eulenberg J, Maesuli PA, Schroeder A. Adhesion of bone to titanium. Adv Biomater *6:*409, 1986.
39. Weiss CM. A comparative analysis of fibro-osteal and osteal integration and other variables that affect long term bone maintenance around dental implants. J Oral Implant *13:*467, 1987.
40. Wennstrom J, Bengazi F, Lekholm U. The influence of the masticatory mucosa on the periimplant soft tissue condition. Clin Oral Implant Res *5:*1, 1994.

63

Clinical Aspects
of Dental Implants

SASCHA A. JOVANOVIC

Clinical Management of Dental Implants
Indications and Contraindications
Selection of Cases and Preoperative Diagnosis
Various Implant Systems
Nobelpharma System
ITI System

IMZ System
Integral System
Other Systems
Implant Reconstruction and Aesthetics
Complications
Maintenance Phase

The fundamental work of Brånemark and associates in the 1960s demonstrated that commercially pure titanium implants can be anchored to the jaw bone and used successfully for tooth replacement in edentulous arches. Controlled clinical research showed excellent long-term results achieved after appropriate selection of cases, adequate preparation of biomaterials, and careful handling of patients' soft and hard tissues. The relationship between the bone and the implant was called *osseointegration* (see Chapter 62). Brånemark presented his research for the first time in North America at the conference held in Toronto, Ontario, Canada, in 1982, and his findings were unanimously considered a breakthrough in dental prosthetics and oral rehabilitation and the opening of a new era in clinical dentistry.

Since the mid-1980s, clinical and laboratory research in dental implantology has resulted in the development of numerous implant systems and different techniques for surgical placement and subsequent prosthetic reconstruction. This chapter will present some basic concepts in implant dentistry and will attempt to clarify the indications, advantages, and disadvantages of the various systems.

CLINICAL MANAGEMENT OF DENTAL IMPLANTS

To achieve an osseointegrated dental implant with a high degree of predictability,[7-9] the implant must be (1) sterile; (2) made of a highly biocompatible material such as titanium; (3) inserted with an atraumatic surgical technique that avoids overheating of the bone during preparation of the recipient site; (4) placed with initial stability; and (5) not functionally loaded during the healing period of 4 to 6 months.

When these clinical guidelines are followed, successful osseointegration will occur predictably for submerged[8] and nonsubmerged[24] dental implants. Well-controlled studies of patients with optimal plaque control and appropriate occlusal forces have demonstrated that osseinte-

grated implants show little change in bone height around the implant.[1] After an initial remodeling in the first year that results in 1.0 to 2.0 mm of bone reduction, the bone level around healthy functioning implants remains stable.

Bone quality at the recipient site influences the interface between bone and implant.[14] Compact bone offers a much greater surface area for mineralized tissue–to-implant contact than cancellous bone. Clinical studies have shown that areas of the jaw exhibiting thin layers of cortical bone and large cancellous spaces, such as the posterior maxilla, have significantly lower success rates than areas of denser bone structures. The best results are obtained when contact between bone and implant is most intimate at implant placement.

The surgical preparation of the tissues at the recipient site may also markedly affect healing. Drilling of the bone without proper cooling results in production of temperatures that inflict thermal injury to the tissues.[26]

INDICATIONS AND CONTRAINDICATIONS

The treatment indications for dental implants are broad and can include patients with partially and fully edentulous arches. Many patients can benefit from the osseointegration procedure as long as they fulfill specific requirements for surgical and prosthetic rehabilitation. Patients who are unable to wear removable dentures and have adequate bone for insertion of implants are especially good candidates. However, each patient must be evaluated individually according to clinical parameters such as hygiene, periodontal health (in partially edentulous patients), restorations present, level of decay activity, cause for previous tooth loss, bone quantity and quality, and patient motivation.

Patients must be in good general health. Uncontrolled diabetes, chronic steroid therapy, high-dose irradiation, and abuse of alcohol and smoking[5,11] can increase the occurrence of early and late complications. A thorough physical

690

examination is mandatory if any questions arise about the health status of the patient.[9]

The overall preoperative requirement regarding the local health state is that no pathologic conditions are present in any of the hard or soft tissues of either jaw. All oral lesions, including periodontal inflammation, should be treated in advance and evaluated at a later date for resolution. The presence of nontreated or unsuccessfully treated periodontal disease is a contraindication to implant placement, as the bacterial flora in periodontitis can jeopardize the healing of the implant sites. Only when the periodontitis has been resolved can implant treatment be considered.

Implant placement immediately after extraction has been attempted. Successful immediate placement of implants in extraction sockets of single-rooted maxillary and mandibular teeth has been documented in cases of severe periodontal breakdown, root fractures, or endodontic failures, provided the following conditions are met:

1. After tooth extraction, the socket must have sufficient residual walls.
2. The extraction socket must be free of pathosis.
3. The available soft tissue should allow primary closure.
4. Apical to the socket, a sufficient volume of healthy jawbone must be available to ensure good initial stabilization of the implant.

Covering the implant with a membrane placed under the flap or placing an osseous graft, significantly increases the success rate of implants placed in extraction sockets.[16,25]

SELECTION OF CASES AND PREOPERATIVE DIAGNOSIS

The possibility of implant installation can be determined after studying the jaw structures that are present.[9] Wide variations in jaw anatomy are encountered, and it is therefore important to analyze the anatomy of the maxillofacial and intraoral region via clinical and radiographic examinations before any surgery is started. Chapter 51 describes the anatomic features of interest for implant surgery.

The preoperative diagnosis is necessary to predict the amount of bone available for implant placement and to evaluate presurgically whether the patient is a suitable candidate for implant treatment. Clinical examination of the jawbone consists of palpation and probing through the soft tissue (intraoral bone mapping) to assess the thickness of the soft tissues at the proposed surgical site. Appropriate radiographic procedures, including periapical and panoramic radiographs (Fig. 63–1A), lateral cephalometric views,

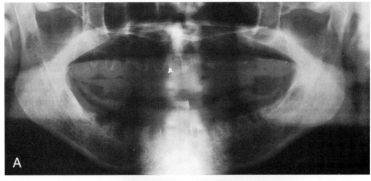

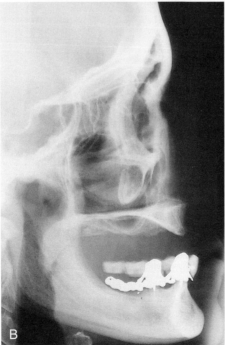

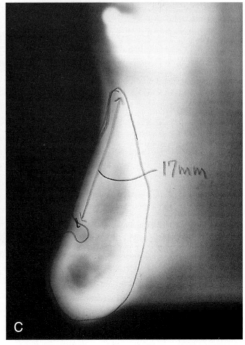

FIGURE 63–1. Different radiographic procedures used in implant dentistry. *A,* Panoramic radiograph. *B,* Lateral cephalometric radiograph. *C,* Tomogram of mandibular premolar area.

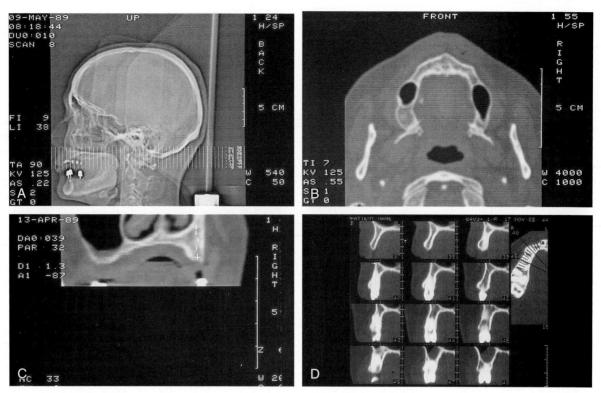

FIGURE 63–2. Computed tomographic scans. *A,* Sagittal view. *B,* Occlusal view. *C,* Cross-sectional view. *D,* Cross-sectional reformatted view.

(Fig. 63–1*B*), and orthopantomograms (Fig. 63–1*C*), can help identify vital structures such as the floor of the nasal cavity, the maxillary sinus, the mandibular canal, and the mental foramen. When only periapical radiographs are used, such findings are severely limited.

The orthopantomogram allows a more comprehensive view of the mandible and maxilla. In the totally edentulous patient, the lateral cephalometric view is very beneficial, especially in the mandible, because it shows angulation, thickness, and vertical bone height. With newer diagnostic techniques such as conventional linear tomograms (see Fig. 63–1) and computed tomographic (CT) scans (Fig. 63–2), it is possible to go beyond the standard two-dimensional radiographs mentioned previously.[22] Exact cross-sectional (three-dimensional) radiographic views of residual bone are possible via specialized software programs. This technology is costly, but it allows a more predictable diagnosis, as it demonstrates whether there is inadequate height and width of bone and the location of vital anatomic structures.

VARIOUS IMPLANT SYSTEMS

Several implant systems are utilized for tooth replacement. These differ mainly in biomaterial, design, and surgical procedure. The three most often used biomaterials are commercially pure titanium, plasma-sprayed titanium surfaces, and plasma-sprayed hydroxyapatite surfaces (Fig. 63–3).

The three main implant designs are the screw-shaped implant form, the cylinder-shaped form, and the hollow basket form.

Surgical procedures can be performed in two interventions (two-stage) or in one stage. In the two-stage procedure, the first operation is for implant insertion and the second operation, several months later, is for uncovering the implant. Implants requiring a one-stage procedure are inserted and left exposed to the oral environment; they are not loaded, however, during the healing period. Chapter 64 describes in detail the surgical procedures for one-stage and two-stage implant placement.

Most implant systems offer a variety of implant lengths

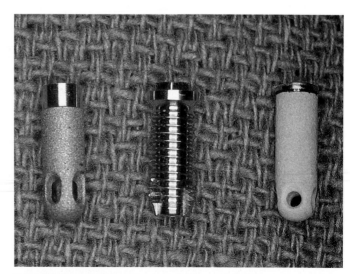

FIGURE 63–3. Different implant designs. *Left,* IMZ. *Center,* Bråne-mark (Nobelpharma). *Right,* Integral-hydroxyapatite.

(7 to 20 mm) and widths (3.25 to 6 mm) to accommodate the available bone quantity. In addition, they include an internally or externally irrigated precision drill set, as well as precisely matched components for surgical and prosthetic needs.

More than 25 different types of implants are available in the United States. Many systems use the term *osseointegration* but lack short- and long-term data to support their claims.[2] For this reason, only implant systems with appropriate clinical and experimental research are presented in the following descriptions (Table 63–1).

Nobelpharma System

The Nobelpharma system[1] consists of a screw-shaped dental implant (Fig. 63–3, *center*), made of commercially pure titanium and applied in a two-stage surgical procedure. The titanium implant surface is machined and forms and maintains an oxide layer without apparent breakdown or corrosion under physiologic conditions. This system was developed by Brånemark in Sweden in the early 1960s, and the term *osseointegration* was coined to designate the relationship of the implant to the bone *at the light microscopy level*.

The Brånemark implant is by far the most extensively researched system, with long-term prospective follow-up studies carried out in fully edentulous and partially edentulous patients. The major advantage of this system is its excellent long-term data (>20 years) and its very meticulous testing in the preclinical stage.

ITI* System

In Switzerland, Schroeder and colleagues initiated clinical and experimental studies evaluating one-stage hollow cylinder implants in the early 1970s.[24] They demonstrated that one-stage implants can also result in direct bone-to-implant contact and in 1976 called this phenomenon *func-*

---

*International Team for Oral Implantology.

tional ankylosis. The ITI implant system[10] has shown good results in long-term retrospective studies in fully edentulous patients and in short-term prospective studies in partially edentulous patients.

This implant system can accommodate several different designs, from the original hollow cylinder (Fig. 63–3, *right*) to a full-body screw design. The surface characteristics—plasma-sprayed titanium coating—have stayed the same since the mid-1970s. Because this implant system protrudes through the mucosa from the day of insertion, it does not require a second intervention, but there is an increased risk of premature loading during the healing period and the danger of titanium showing in the marginal mucosal area.

IMZ System

The intramobile cylinder (IntraMobile Zylinder) implant system[4,18] was developed by Kirsch and Koch in Germany in the early 1970s and has gone through several changes since its early experimental phase. The system includes a commercially pure titanium cylinder with either a plasma-sprayed titanium–coated surface area or a plasma-sprayed hydroxyapatite (HA)–coated surface (Fig. 63–3, *left*), a highly polished titanium transmucosal implant extension for the soft tissue adaptation, and a plastic intramobile element (IME). The theoretical rationale for the IME was to simulate the mobility of the tooth and thereby enable a connection between an osseointegrated implant and a natural tooth. Fracture problems with the plastic IME require replacement of the element at least once a year. The system went into clinical trials in 1978, and several retrospective studies of its longevity have been reported.

Integral System[17]

The first implant system on the market with significant research and clinical studies evaluating cylinder-shaped titanium implants with an HA coating was developed in the

---

Table 63–1. PRINCIPAL FEATURES OF COMMONLY USED IMPLANT SYSTEMS

System	Design	No. of Surgery Stages	Surface	Indication	ADA Accepted	Follow-up Since
Nobelpharma	Screw	Two	Pure Ti machined	Full/partial edentulism	Yes	1965
ITI	Screw, cylinder, hollow basket	One	Ti plasma-sprayed	Full/partial edentulism	Yes	1977*
IMZ	Cylinder	Two	Ti + HA plasma-sprayed	Full/partial edentulism	Yes	1978
Integral	Cylinder, screw	Two	HA plasma-sprayed	Full/partial edentulism	Yes	1985
Dentsply/Core-Vent	Screw, cylinder, hollow basket	Two	Acid-etched Ti + HA plasma-sprayed	Full/partial edentulism	Yes	1984
Steri-Oss	Screw, cylinder	Two	HA plasma-sprayed + acid-etched Ti	Full/partial edentulism	Yes	1988
Astra	Screw	Two	Pure Ti blasted	Full/partial edentulism	No	1990
3i	Screw, cylinder	Two	Ti + HA plasma-sprayed	Full/partial edentulism	No	1990

*Follow-up of the new-generation ITI dental implant since 1986.
ADA, American Dental Association; HA, hydroxyapatite; ITI, International Team for Oral Implantology; 3i, Implant Innovations, Inc.; IMZ, IntraMobile Zylinder; Ti, titanium.

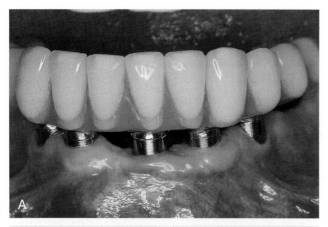

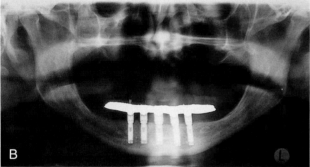

FIGURE 63–4. Fixed bone-anchored bridge retaining a full lower prosthesis. *A*, Clinical view. *B*, Radiographic view.

United States. These HA-coated implants have been recommended for compromised bone sites, because the HA coating accelerates bone apposition to the implant surface in the early healing period and significantly improves the anchorage in bone (see Chapter 62). However, long-term results have reported that the HA coating is biologically unstable over time and shows signs of resorption in histologic studies. This might be one of the factors responsible for controversial data about the increasing rate of complications reported after a 3- to 5-year functional period.

Other Systems

The Dentsply/Core-Vent system, the Steri-Oss system,[23] the Astra Dental Implant System,[13] and the Implant Innovations (3i) system offer a variety of implant designs, from screw-shaped to cylinder type, and implant surface characteristics, from machined pure titanium to HA and plasma-sprayed titanium coatings. These systems have been developed since the early to mid-1980s and resemble some of the previously described systems. Few long-term follow-up data of their clinical results are available.

IMPLANT RECONSTRUCTION AND AESTHETICS

The patients who seem to benefit most from dental implants are those with fully edentulous arches. In these pa-

tients, removable and fixed prosthetic devices can restore almost normal stomatognathic function. The original design of the edentulous arch was a fixed bone-anchored bridge that used five to six implants in the anterior area of the mandible or the maxilla and a cantilever through the premolar area (Fig. 63–4). Most implant bridges currently used are screwed into place and can easily be removed by loosening the fixation screws. This adds a retrievability characteristic to the treatment, which increases the overall comfort and reliability for the patient.

Another treatment option for the rehabilitation of an edentulous arch is the overdenture retained by clips to a bar splinting two to six implants (Fig. 63–5). This treatment results in less prosthesis stability but is still far superior to conventional complete dentures.

Partially edentulous patients with single or multiple missing teeth represent another viable treatment population for osseointegrated implants, but the remaining natural dentition (i.e., its occlusal schemes, periodontal health status, vertical dimension problems, and aesthetics) introduces an additional challenge to achieve a long-lasting, successful rehabilitation.[19] In general, osseointegrated implants can support a freestanding fixed partial denture, and adjacent natural teeth are not necessary for additional support (Fig. 63–6). However, the close proximity of anatomic structures and frequently the limited bone quantity require special attention to diagnosis and treatment planning. The major advantage of implant-supported restorations in partially edentulous patients is that they are less invasive to adjacent teeth (i.e., preparation of abutment teeth becomes unnecessary), and larger edentulous spans can be restored with fixed bridges.[21] Obtaining acceptable aesthetic results, however, poses interesting and difficult challenges for the restorative/surgical team.

The *single-tooth restoration* (Fig. 63–7) requires detailed planning and careful management to achieve perfect harmony among implant position, bone level, soft tissue aesthetics, and tooth form and color.[12] The replacement of single missing teeth with implants has two major advantages over replacement with conventional fixed prostheses. First, there is no need to prepare adjacent teeth, and second, the ridge will be maintained by the implant. The primary candidates for single-tooth implants are all anterior teeth, from central incisor to second premolar, in the maxilla and mandible, provided that no lateral forces are induced by the single standing implant. Molar replacements with single implants are less indicated owing to the high stresses generated in the posterior region of the mouth and the insufficient force distribution over one implant, leading to bone resorption.

Early on, the UCLA abutment[20] was developed by Beumer and coworkers to allow direct connection between the implant-supported restoration and the top of the implant, thereby eliminating the need for the transmucosal abutment cylinder and improving the aesthetic result dramatically, since porcelain rather than titanium emerges from the tissues. Similar techniques have since evolved, and aesthetically pleasing implant restorations are a reality. No significant difference in fully implant-supported bridges or implant-and-tooth–supported bridges have been found in the short term, but the fully implant-supported bridges may have a better long-term outlook.

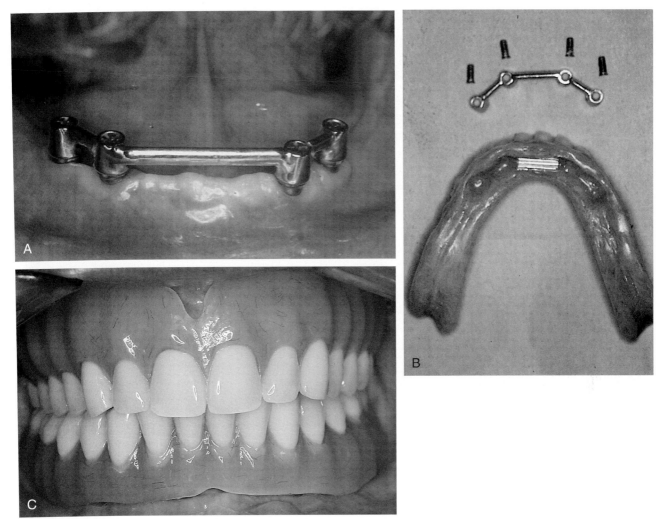

FIGURE 63-5. *A,* Bar over four implants in the mandible. *B,* View of denture with clips and bar. *C,* Upper and lower dentures in place.

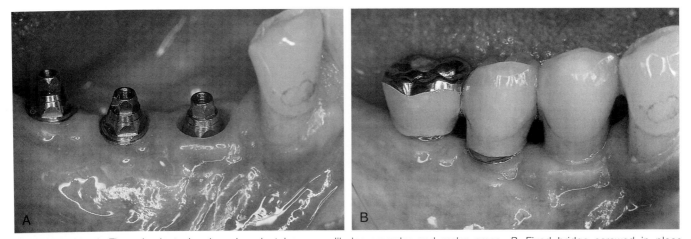

FIGURE 63-6. *A,* Three implants in place in edentulous mandibular premolar and molar areas. *B,* Fixed bridge screwed in place. (Restorative work performed by Dr. S. Lewis, San Antonio, TX.)

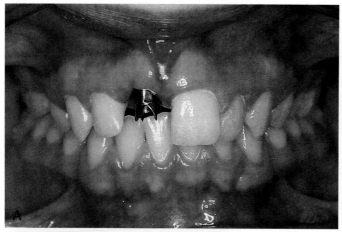
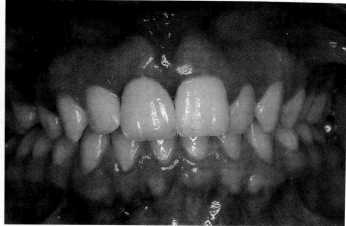
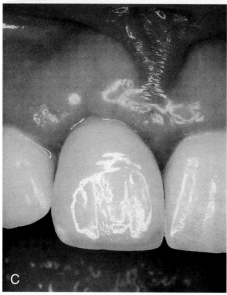

FIGURE 63–7. Single tooth replacement. *A,* Implant in place. *B,* Metalloceramic crown. *C,* Close-up view.

Although long-term data for the partially edentulous patient are still missing, the less invasive dental implant approach is promising and is increasingly preferred by patients and their treatment teams.

COMPLICATIONS

Less than 10% of implants will show some form of complication over the life of the implant.[6] Complications can be detected during the treatment phase (early onset) and/or during the maintenance phase (late onset). When a dental implant demonstrates any degree of mobility *after* the healing period, it is considered a failure. Implant mobility suggests a fibrous connective tissue interface that does not function well over time. When this mobility is detected, the implant with its surrounding fibrous capsule must be removed. After an appropriate healing time it is sometimes possible to place another implant.

During the maintenance phase—once osseointegration is established—complications can be divided into adverse tissue reactions, such as mucosal inflammation and progressive bone loss, and mechanical problems, such as compo-

nent fractures or screw loosenings. These problems are dealt with in detail in Chapter 65.

MAINTENANCE PHASE

Proper oral hygiene and appropriate occlusal forces are critical for long-term function of an implant prosthesis, as poor hygiene and occlusal trauma have been related to marginal bone loss. Plaque control should be started immediately after the implant is exposed to the intraoral environment and monitored over time. Implant superstructures are often bulky and overcontoured, which makes traditional home care procedures more difficult. In addition, implant patients usually have a history of less than ideal home care, which has resulted in their partially or totally edentulous state. Patient recalls should be at 3-month intervals for the first year, and then on a semiannual basis. However, some patients may require more frequent follow-up. Recall visits should include an evaluation of oral hygiene compliance, occlusal harmony, implant and prosthesis stability, overall soft and hard peri-implant tissue health, and radiographic follow-up.

REFERENCES

1. Adell R, Lekholm U, Rockler B, Brånemark P-I. A 15-year study of osseointegrated implants in the treatment of the edentulous jaw. Int J Oral Surg *10:*387, 1981.
2. Albrektsson T, Zarb G, Worthington P, Eriksson AR. The long-term efficacy of currently used dental implants. A review and proposed criteria of success. Int J Oral Maxillofac Implants *1:*11, 1986.
3. Babbush CA, Kent JN, Misiek DJ. Titanium-plasma-sprayed (TPS) screw implants for the reconstruction of the edentulous mandible. J Oral Maxillofac Surg *44:*274, 1986.
4. Babbush CA, Shimura M. Five-year statistical and clinical observations with the IMZ two-stage osteointegrated implant system. Int J Oral Maxillofac Implants *8:*245, 1993.
5. Bain CA, Moy PK. The association between the failure of dental implants and cigarette smoking. Int J Oral Maxillofac Implants *8:*609, 1993.
6. Berman CL. Osseointegration, complications, prevention, recognition, treatment. Dent Clin North Am *33:*635, 1989.
7. Brunski JB. Biomechanics of oral implants: Future research directions. J Dent Educ *52:*775, 1988.
8. Brånemark P-I, Breine U, Adell R, et al. Intraosseous anchorage of dental prostheses. I. Experimental studies. Scand J Plast Reconstr Surg *3:*81, 1969.
9. Brånemark P-I, Zarb GA, Albrektsson T. Tissue-integrated prostheses. Berlin, Quintessence Publishing, 1985.
10. Buser D, Weber HP, Bragger U, Balsiger C. Tissue integration of one stage ITI implants: 3-year results of a longitudinal study with hollow-cylinder and hollow-screw implants. Int J Oral Maxillofac Implants *6:*405, 1991.
11. DeBruyn H, Collaert B. The effect of smoking on early implant failure. Clin Oral Implant Res *5:*260, 1994.
12. Ekfeldt A, Carlsson GE, Börjesson G. Clinical evaluation of single-tooth restorations supported by osseointegrated implants: A retrospective study. Int J Oral Maxillofac Implants *9:*179, 1994.
13. Gotfredsen K, Holm B, Sewerin I, et al. Marginal tissue response adjacent to Astra Dental implants supporting overdentures in the mandible. A 2-year follow-up study. Clin Oral Implant Res *4:*83, 1993.
14. Jaffin RA, Berman CI. The excessive loss of Brånemark implants in type IV bone. A 5-year analysis. J Periodontol *62:*2, 1991.
15. Johnson BW. HA-coated dental implants: Long-term consequences. Calif Dent Assoc J *20:*33, 1992.
16. Jovanovic S, Buser D. Guided bone regeneration in dehiscence defects and delayed extraction sockets. In Buser D, Dahlin C, Schenk RK, eds. Guided Bone Regeneration in Implant Dentistry. Chicago, Quintessence Publishing, 1994.
17. Kent J, Block M. Biointegrated hydroxyapatite coated dental implants: 5 year clinical observations. J Am Dent Assoc *121:*138, 1990.
18. Kirsch A, Ackermann KL. The IMZ osteointegrated implant system. Dent Clin North Am *33:*733, 1989.
19. Lekholm U, van Steenberghe D, Herrmann I, et al. Osseointegrated implants in the treatment of partially edentulous jaws: A prospective 5-year multicenter study. Int J Oral Maxillofac Implants *9:*627, 1994.
20. Lewis SG, Beumer J, Perri GR, et al. The UCLA abutment. J Oral Maxillo-Fac Implants *3:*183, 1989.
21. Pylant T, Triplett RG, Key MC, Brusnvold MA. A retrospective evaluation of endosseous titanium implants in the partially edentulous patient. Internat J Oral Maxillofac Implants *7:*195, 1992.
22. Reddy MS, Mayfield-Donahoo T, Vanderven FJJ, Jeffcoat MK. A comparison of the diagnostic advantages of panoramic radiography and computed tomography scanning for placement of root form dental implants. Clin Oral Implant Res *5:*229, 1994.
23. Saadoun AP, LeGall ML. Clinical results and guidelines on Steri-Oss endosseous implants. Int J Periodont Restor Dent *12:*487, 1992.
24. Schroeder A, van der Zypen E, Stich H, Sutter F. The reactions of bone, connective tissue, and epithelium to endosteal implants with titanium-sprayed surfaces. J Maxillofac Surg *9:*15, 1981.
25. Warrer K, Gotfredsen K, Hjørting-Hansen E, Karring T. Guided tissue regeneration ensures osseointegration of dental implants placed in extraction sockets. Clin Oral Implant Res *2:*166, 1991.
26. Watanabe F, Tawada Y, Komatsu S, Hata Y. Heat distribution in bone during preparation of implant sites: Heat analysis by real-time thermography. Int J Oral Maxillofac Implants *7:*213, 1992.

64

Surgical Aspects of Dental Implants

THOMAS J. HAN

Two-Stage Endosseous Implant Surgery
First-Stage Surgery
Second-Stage Surgery
One-Stage Endosseous Implant Surgery

Surgical Technique
Postoperative Care
Adjunctive Advanced Surgical Techniques

The root form implant surgical techniques are in most part based on research performed on the biologic, physiologic, and mechanical aspects of the Nobelpharma implant system developed by Per-Ingvar Brånemark and colleagues in Sweden.[3]

Nobelpharma implants and other commonly used endosseous implant systems are placed in two surgical stages performed several months apart. The ITI* system, on the other hand, involves only one surgery.[5]

Although treatment planning and evaluation of clinical anatomy of soft and hard tissues are the same, there are some fundamental differences in flap management for both two-stage and one-stage endosseous implant systems; therefore, the two systems will be described separately.

In the two-stage implant system, the first-stage surgery ends by suturing the soft tissues over the implant so that it remains excluded from the oral cavity. *In the mandible the implants are left undisturbed for at least 3 months, while in the maxilla they remain covered for no less than 6 months because of slower healing and less dense bone.* During this period the healing bone makes contact with the implant surface and sometimes grows to its occlusal surface, even covering it.[3]

In the second-stage surgery, the buried implant is uncovered, and a titanium abutment is connected to allow access to the implant from the oral cavity. The restorative dentist

---

*International Team for Oral Implantology.

then proceeds with the prosthodontic aspects of the implant therapy.

In the one-stage implant system, a second intervention is not needed, because the implant is left exposed after the first surgery.

Regardless of the system, to achieve osseointegration the implant must be placed in healthy bone, and an atraumatic and aseptic technique must be followed to avoid damage to vital structures. Generally, implant surgery is done under local anesthesia, and oral or intravenous (IV) sedation can also be used if necessary. The surgical suite should be kept aseptic and the patient appropriately prepared and draped for an intraoral surgical procedure. The patient should rinse with chlorhexidine gluconate for 30 seconds immediately prior to the procedure. Every effort should be made to minimize the risk of contamination of the implant surfaces by such items as gloves, instruments, suction tubing, or saliva.

This chapter presents general considerations and guidance on some of the most commonly used implant systems. The great variety of implant systems with their own specific armamentarium makes it advisable in each case to follow the detailed step-by-step description usually found in the manufacturer's manual.

TWO-STAGE ENDOSSEOUS IMPLANT SURGERY

First-Stage Surgery

Flap Design and Incisions. Two types of incisions—crestal or remote—can be used. In the latter, the incision is made away from the implant site, usually 1 to 2 mm inferior to the mucogingival junction. A back-action chisel or a periosteal elevator is then used to reflect a mucoperiosteal (full-thickness) flap. For the crestal design flap, the incision

is made along the crest of the ridge, bisecting the existing zone of keratinized mucosa (Fig. 64–1A).

The remote incision has the advantage of covering the implant without sutures over its top. The crestal incision, however, is preferred, because it results in less bleeding, easier flap management, less edema, less ecchymosis, less vestibular change postoperatively, faster healing, and easier denture reline.[11] Sutures placed over the implant generally do not interfere with proper healing.

Flap Elevation. A full-thickness flap is raised buccally and lingually to the level of the mucogingival junction, exposing the alveolar ridge of the implant sites (Fig. 64–1B). Elevated flaps may be sutured to the buccal mucosa or the opposing teeth to keep the surgical site open during the surgery.

If a bone augmentation technique, with or without membranes, is anticipated, the flap can be expanded beyond the mucogingival junction with a partial-thickness extension. This will lengthen the flap while providing flexibility to close it without tension after the implantation and ridge augmentation are performed (Fig. 64–1C,D).

When there is a knife-edge alveolar process with sufficient alveolar height and distance from vital structures such as the sinuses or the infraorbital or mental nerves, a suitable round bur is used to recontour the bone to provide a reasonably flat bed for the implant site (see Fig. 64–1B).

Implant Placement. Once the implant site is prepared, a surgical guide or stent is placed intraorally, and a small round bur or spiral drill is used to mark the implant sites. The stent is then removed, and the sites are checked for their appropriate faciolingual location. Slight modifications may be necessary to avoid obvious ridge defects.

The site is then marked to a depth of 1 to 2 mm, breaking through the cortical bone (Fig. 64–2A). A small spiral drill, usually 2 mm in diameter and marked to indicate appropriate depth, is used next to establish the depth and

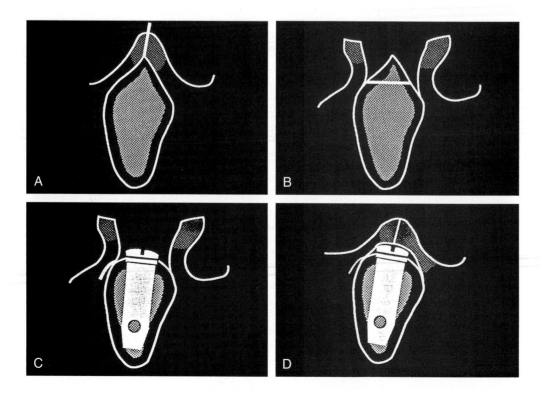

FIGURE 64–1. *A,* Crestal incision made along the crest of the ridge, bisecting the existing zone of keratinized mucosa. *B,* A full-thickness flap is raised buccally and lingually to the level of the mucogingival junction. A sharp ridge can be surgically contoured to provide a reasonably flat bed for the implant. *C,* A partial-thickness flap is raised apically from the mucogingival junction to provide extension of the flap. *D,* Crestal flap closure without tension.

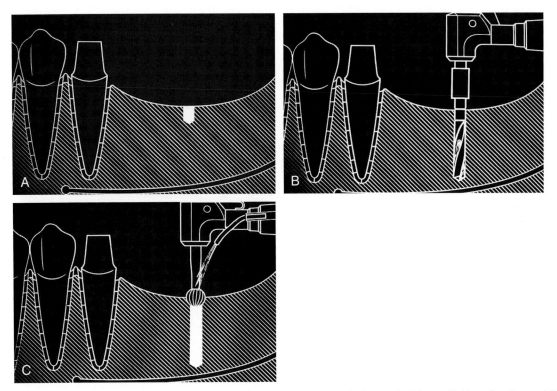

FIGURE 64–2. *A*, Initial site preparation with a small diamond bur to break through the cortical layer. *B*, Use of a 2-mm drill to establish depth and to align the axis of the implant recipient site. *C*, A large round bur is used to create a secure point in the compact bone for the centering of subsequent drills. (Courtesy of IMZ System.)

align the axis of the implant recipient site (Fig. 64–2*B*). This drill may be externally or internally irrigated. In either case, the spiral drill is used at a speed of approximately 800 to 1000 rpm with copious irrigation to prevent overheating the bone.

In press-fit cylindrical implant systems,[1,7] a large round bur is sometimes recommended to create a secure point in the compact bone for the centering of subsequent drills (Fig. 64–2*C*).

If the vertical height of the bone is reduced during the ridge preparation, this must be taken into account when selecting the length of the implant. When multiple implants are used to support a prosthesis, a paralleling or direction-indicating pin should be used to align subsequent implants correctly.

The relationship to neighboring vital structures can be determined by taking a periapical radiograph with a radiographic marker placed at the bottom of the prepared site. Implants should be at least 3 mm apart to ensure sufficient room for adequate oral hygiene once the prosthesis is in place.

The next step is to use a series of drills to systematically widen the site to accommodate the selected size of implant. The shapes of the drills may be slightly different from system to system, but their general purpose is to prepare a recipient site that is accurate in size, both in diameter and in length, for the selected implant without unduly traumatizing the surrounding bone (Fig. 64–3*A–C*).

Regardless of the system used, it is very important that the final diameter drilling be accomplished with a steady hand, without wobbling. There are some techniques that will help accomplish this. If the final drill hits the bottom

of the recipient site before reaching the desired depth, the added hand pressure necessary to achieve the proper depth often causes wobbling and funneling of the recipient site. This is especially true with cannon drills. To minimize this effect, during the preparation of the recipient site with the smaller-diameter drill, the operator should drill to approximately 0.5 mm deeper than needed. This will allow the desired depth to be reached with the final drill without touching the bottom.

In addition, if the final drill is inserted at an inaccurate angle, the result is funneling of the coronal portion of the implant site. To minimize this, when drilling for multiple implant sites, the operator should always keep a direction indicator in adjacent sites. For single implant cases, some type of a direction reference guide should be used. An old set of drills works very well as a direction indicator in multiple implant cases.

Finally, when dealing with very dense bone, a very snugly fitting recipient site can be achieved more predictably when there is minimal diameter change from drill to drill. For example, going from 3.0 to 4.0 mm is far more difficult than going from 3.0 to 3.3 to 3.7 to 4.0 mm.

The placement of screw-type implants[3] is depicted diagrammatically in Figure 64–4*A–G*. For these implants, a tapping procedure may be necessary. With self-tapping implants becoming increasingly popular, there is less need for a tapping procedure, but in very dense bone or when placing very long implants, it is prudent to use a tap (see Fig. 64–4*F*). When dealing with a very soft bone (e.g., in posterior maxillary areas), tapping is not recommended. Also, for screw-type implants with a neck that is wider in diameter than the diameter of the body, it is important to use a

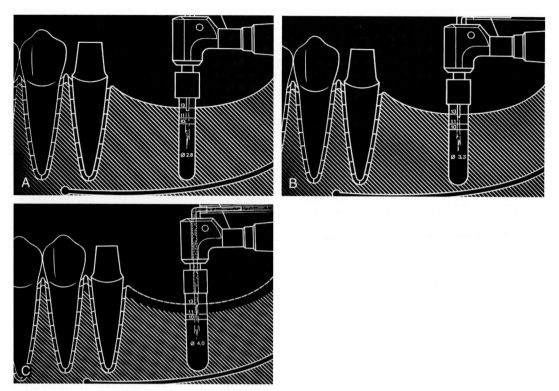

FIGURE 64–3. *A,* A small (2.8-mm) cannon or spade drill is used to increase the diameter of the recipient site to the desired length (10, 11, or 13 mm). *B,* A medium-size (3.3-mm) cannon or spade drill is used to further increase the size of the recipient site. *C,* A large (4.0-mm) cannon or spade drill is used to finalize preparation of the recipient site. (Courtesy of IMZ System.)

countersink drill (see Fig. 64–4*E*). If possible, it is better to stay in cortical bone. However, if the countersinking procedure is done inadequately and the implant cover screw sits too high above the cortical bone, there is a risk of premature exposure. This is especially true when a full or a partial denture is worn over during the integration time, or if there is only thin tissue covering the implant.

It is important to create a recipient site that is accurate in both size and angulation. In partially edentulous cases, a limited opening of the mouth may prevent appropriate positioning of the drills in posterior edentulous areas, so a combination of longer drills or shorter drills, with or without extensions, may be necessary. Anticipating these needs facilitates the procedure and improves the results.

Closure of the Flap. Once the implants are screwed in or tapped in with a mallet and the cover screws are placed (Fig. 64–5; see Fig. 64–4*G*), proper closure of the flap over the implant is very important. One suturing technique that consistently provides the desired result is a combination of inverted mattress and interrupted sutures. The inverted mattress sutures keep the bleeding edges of the flap close together, while the interrupted sutures seal the edges. However, the most important aspect of flap management at this stage is *closure of the flap without tension.* It is better to use a suture that does not require removal during the postoperative visit, such as a 5.0 gut suture.

Postoperative Care. Patients are premedicated with antibiotics (amoxicillin, 500 mg tid) starting immediately before the surgery and continuing for at least 1 week after (see Chapter 50). Swelling is likely to occur, and the patient should apply ice packs extraorally intermittently for the first 24 hours. Chlorhexidine gluconate mouthrinses

should be used twice daily, as oral hygiene and plaque control will be difficult to perform. Adequate pain medication should be prescribed (see Chapter 50). Patients should have a liquid or semisoft diet for the first few days and then gradually return to a normal diet. Patients should also refrain from tobacco and alcohol use on the day of the operation and in the immediate postoperative period.

Plate XXIII shows all steps of Stage 1 implant placement surgery in a clinical case.

Second-Stage Surgery

The objectives of the second-stage surgery are as follows:

1. To expose the submerged implant without damaging the surrounding bone.
2. To control the thickness of the soft tissue surrounding the implant.
3. To preserve or create attached keratinized tissue around the implant.
4. To facilitate oral hygiene.
5. To ensure proper abutment seating.

Thin soft tissue with an adequate amount of keratinized epithelium, along with good oral hygiene, ensures healthier peri-implant soft tissues and better clinical results. The need for keratinized tissue is somewhat controversial depending on the type of implant prosthesis and location of the implant, but one long-term study indicated that, at least in the posterior mandible and in partially edentulous cases, the presence of keratinized tissue is strongly correlated with soft and hard tissue health.[2]

When the two-stage endosseous implant was initially introduced by the manufacturers, the recommended second-

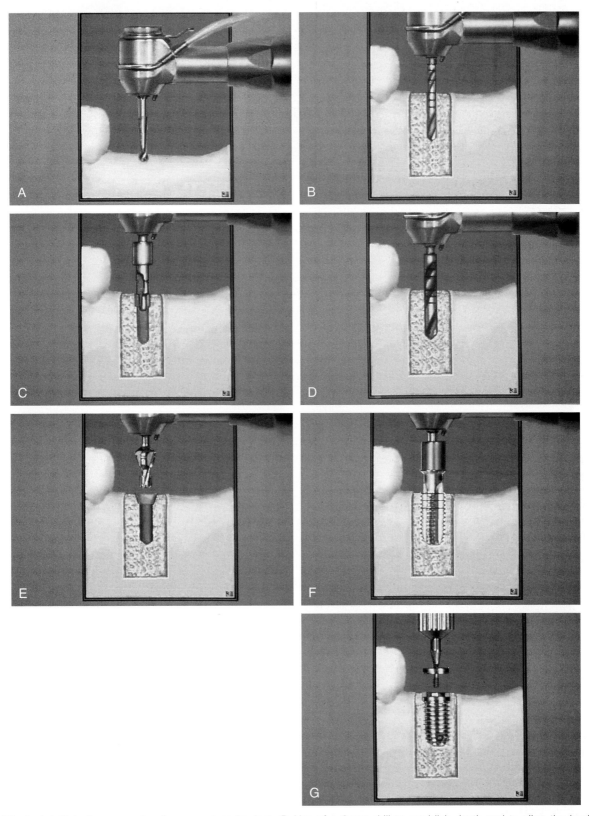

FIGURE 64–4. *A*, Initial site preparation for screw-type implant. *B*, Use of a 2-mm drill to establish depth and to align the implant. *C*, A wider-diameter pilot drill is used to increase the size of the recipient site. *D*, A final size drill is used to finish preparation of the recipient site. *E*, A countersink drill is used to widen the entrance of the recipient site. *F*, A tap is used to create screw threads. *G*, The implant is screwed into the recipient site, and the cover screw is placed. (Courtesy of 3i/Implant Innovations, Inc.)

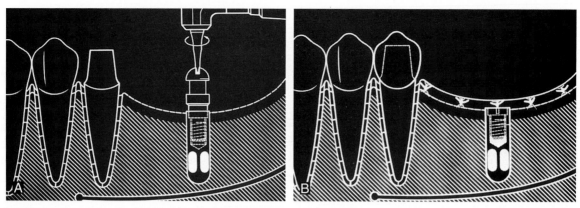

FIGURE 64–5. *A,* The press-fit cylindrical implant is tapped in, flush with the alveolar crest, and the carrier screw is removed. *B,* A cover screw is placed and the flap is closed over the implant without tension. (Courtesy of IMZ System.)

stage surgery consisted of a "punch biopsy" technique. However, very often this technique renders inadequate results because it does not allow any manipulation of the soft or hard tissues to achieve the objectives of the second-stage surgery. To comply with these objectives, a technique was developed that uses a full-thickness flap to place a band of keratinized tissue on one or both sides of the implant and thereby provide some keratinized tissue.[9] However, if there is deficient keratinized tissue to begin with, the resulting amount of keratinized tissue is not predictable, and when multiple implants are involved, denuded alveolar bone may result between the implants. Furthermore, if thin radicular bone is present facial or lingual to the implant, the mere reflection of a full-thickness flap may result in a dehiscence of the implant surface.

Experience with these techniques resulted in the development of a combination technique consisting of a partial-thickness flap and a gingivectomy; this combination technique predictably fulfills all the objectives listed previously. This technique can be used in all posterior areas of the mouth and in the mandibular anteriors. In areas where there is an abundant amount of keratinized tissue, the punch biopsy technique can still be performed; this technique is also used in the maxillary anterior area for aesthetic reasons.

Partial-Thickness Flap–Gingivectomy Technique

Flap Design and Incisions. The initial incision is made approximately 2 mm coronal to the facial mucogingival junction, with vertical incisions both mesially and distally (Plate XXIV*A,B*). When dealing with anterior implants, the flap design should preserve the adjacent papilla.

Flap Elevation and Apical Displacement. A partial-thickness flap is then raised in such a manner that a relatively firm periosteum remains. The flap, containing a band of keratinized tissue, is then placed facial to the emerging head of the implant fixture and fixed to the periosteum with 5.0 gut suture (Fig. 64–6 and Plate XXIV*C*). If initially there is less than 2 mm of keratinized tissue, the flap may be started from the lingual part of the ridge, positioning facially the entire band of keratinized tissue. When a partial-thickness flap is apically displaced in this manner, not exposing the alveolar bone, a band of attached keratinized tissue is maintained or created around the implants.

In the maxillary anterior area, all soft tissue thickness over the implant should be initially maintained, as it is always much easier to later carve out excess tissue than to regenerate it. This technique also allows augmentation of a facial ridge deficiency by harvesting the connective tissue

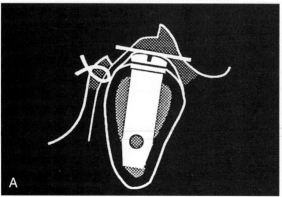
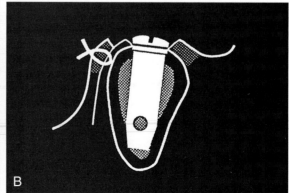

FIGURE 64–6. *A,* A partial-thickness flap is apically sutured to the periosteum, and excess connective tissue coronal to the cover screw is excised by gingivectomy. *B,* A sharp blade is used to eliminate all tissue coronal to the cover screw.

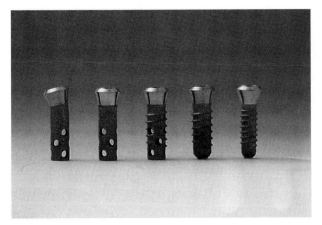

FIGURE 64–7. The most commonly used ITI implants are the solid screw (*left*), the hollow screw (*middle*), and the hollow cylinder (*right*). (Illustration courtesy of The Straumann Company, Cambridge, MA.)

obtained by thinning of the palatal flap and transplanting it onto the facial surface under the flap.

Gingivectomy. Once the flap is positioned facially, the excess tissue coronal to the cover screw is excised, usually using a gingivectomy technique (see Fig. 64–6 and Plate XXIVD). However, if a gingivectomy technique would compromise the lingual keratinized tissue around the implant(s), a similar partial-thickness flap can be made on the lingual side.

Once the excess tissue coronal to the cover screw is removed, the outline of the cover screw is visible. A sharp blade is used to eliminate all tissues coronal to the cover screw (see Fig. 64–6B and Plate XXIVE). The cover screw is then removed, the head of the implant is thoroughly cleaned of any soft or hard tissue overgrowth, and the healing abutments or standard abutments are placed on the fixture (Plate XXIVF). The fit of the implants to the healing abutments can often be visually evaluated.

Postoperative Care. Once the implant is exposed, it is important to remind the patient of the need for good oral hygiene around the implant. A chlorhexidine rinse is highly recommended for at least the initial 2 weeks while the tissues are healing. At this time there should not be any direct pressure to the area from dentures. Fabrication of the suprastructure can begin in about 2 weeks.

Plate XXIVG,H shows the postoperative results in a clinical case after 2 to 3 weeks and 4 months, respectively.

ONE-STAGE ENDOSSEOUS IMPLANT SURGERY

One-stage implants, represented basically by the ITI system, do not remain submerged after being inserted and therefore do not require a second (uncovering) procedure.[4–6] Thus, flap management for this system is fundamentally different from that of the two-stage systems.

In the two-stage technique, the implant is placed flush with the bone crest, and the soft tissue covering it is pur-

posely kept thick to minimize the chances of a premature exposure of the cover screws. In the ITI system, on the other hand, the implant protrudes about 2 to 3 mm from the bone crest, and especially in posterior areas, the flap is thinned and placed apical to the future margin of the prosthesis.

Basically there are three types of ITI implants: the hollow screw, the hollow cylinder, and the solid screw (Fig. 64–7). These come in body diameters of 3.5 mm and 2.8 mm. There are also some differences in placement technique between these three types of ITI implants.

Surgical Technique

Flap Design and Incisions. The flap design for placement of an ITI implant is always a crestal incision bisecting the existing keratinized tissue. Vertical incisions may be needed in one or both ends. Facial and lingual flaps in posterior areas should be carefully thinned before total reflection so that the thickness of the soft tissue does not cover the head of the implant. In anterior or other aesthetic areas of the mouth, the soft tissue is not thinned in order to prevent the metal collar from showing.

Flap Elevation. Full-thickness flaps are elevated facially and lingually.

It is important not to have osseous dehiscences when placing a one-stage implant. For placement of a standard 3.5-mm diameter ITI implant, the ridge should be at least 5.5 to 6 mm wide. It is possible to regenerate deficient ridges using guided bone regeneration techniques, but this implant is designed to stay 2 mm supracrestally, and it is difficult to properly close the flap without oversubmerging the head of the implant.

Placement of the Implant. The implant site is first prepared using a round bur to establish exactly the site(s) where the implant(s) is to be placed. Subsequent steps have slight variations depending on the type of ITI implant to be placed.

With the hollow cylinder (Fig. 64–8A,B) and hollow screw (Fig. 64–8C,D) implants, a predrill is used to prepare the shoulder level, and a trephine with depth markings is then used to the final sink depth.

For the hollow screw implant (see Fig. 64–8C,D), a tapping instrument is used to tap the implant before it is screwed in. For the hollow cylinder system, the tapping procedure is not necessary, and the implant is pushed in with a mallet.

For the solid screw implant (Fig. 64–9A,B), the recipient site is drilled with increasing diameter drills until the final diameter and depth are reached. Again, tapping is necessary if the bone is dense and the implant is screwed in. In this instance a trephine is not used.

Closure of the Flap. In the ITI system, the smooth portion of the implant, approximately 2 to 3 mm in height, remains coronal to the crest of the bone. A healing cover screw is placed, and the keratinized edges of the flap are tied with independent sutures around the implant. When there is an abundant amount of keratinized tissue, scalloping around the implant(s) provides better flap adaptation.

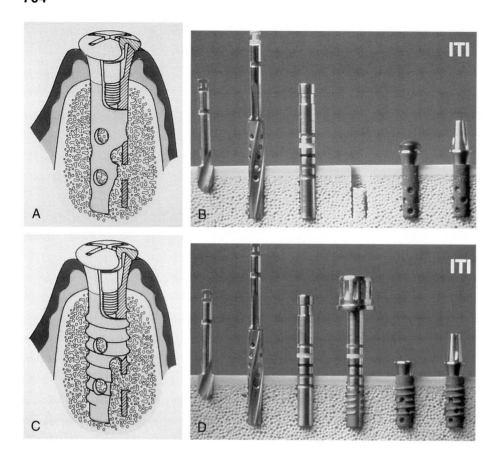

FIGURE 64-8. *A,* Diagram of a hollow cylinder ITI implant. *B,* Drilling sequence of a hollow cylinder ITI implant. *C,* Diagram of a hollow screw ITI implant. *D,* Drilling sequence of a hollow screw ITI implant. (Illustration courtesy of The Straumann Company, Cambridge, MA.)

Postoperative Care

The implants are not loaded for 3 to 4 months, at which time the healing cover screws are removed, and an appropriate abutment installed to begin the prosthetic reconstruction (Fig. 64-10). During the postsurgical period before the prosthetic reconstruction, care includes chlorhexidine mouthrinses twice daily for 2 weeks and, in some cases, oral antibiotics.

ADJUNCTIVE ADVANCED SURGICAL TECHNIQUES

Oral implantology is often made difficult by anatomic limitations of the jaws. There are advanced surgical tech-

niques designed to overcome these difficulties, but often these procedures are very technique sensitive and expensive and have a high degree of postoperative morbidity. It is important to carefully weigh the benefits versus the risks of these procedures. Consider that if the patient has functioned relatively well with a conventional prosthesis before the implants were considered, it may be wise to continue with the traditional type of tooth replacement rather than perform surgical correction of unfavorable anatomic conditions.

One of the most often encountered anatomic limitations in both jaws is *narrow ridges.* Bone augmentation techniques using the principle of guided bone regeneration are indicated.[8] However, the regenerated bone is weaker and requires that the stability of the initial and early loaded stages come from integration with the pre-existing bone. If

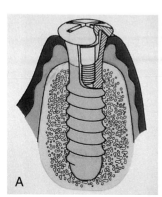

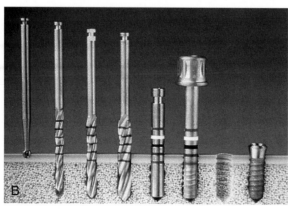

FIGURE 64-9. *A,* Diagram of a solid screw ITI implant. *B,* Drilling sequence of a solid screw ITI implant. (Illustration courtesy of The Straumann Company, Cambridge, MA.)

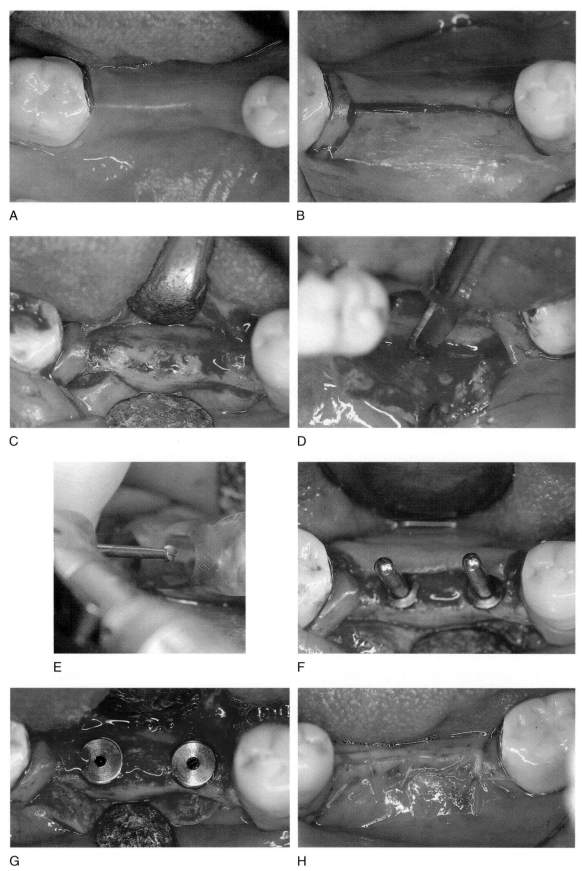

PLATE XXIII. First-stage surgery. *A,* A partial edentulous ridge. A presurgical periodontal and prosthodontic treatment has been completed. *B,* Mesial and vertical incisions are connected by a crestal incision. Notice that bands of gingival collars remain adjacent to teeth. *C,* Minimal flap reflection to expose the alveolar bone. Sometimes a ridge modification is necessary to provide a flat recipient bed. *D,* A buccal flap is partially dissected at the apical portion to provide a flap extension. This is a very critical step to ensure that there is tension-free closure of the flap after the implant placement. *E,* It is important to use the surgical stent to determine the mesial-distal, the buccal-ingual, and the proper angulation of the implant placement. *F,* Frequent use of the guide pins will ensure the parallelism of the implant placement. *G,* After the placement of two Nobelpharma implants, the cover screws are placed. The cover screws should be flush with the crest of the ridge to minimize the chance of their being exposed. This is especially important if a partial denture is to be worn during the healing phase. *H,* Suturing completed. Both regular interrupted and inverted mattress sutures are used intermittently to ensure tension-free, tight closure of the flaps.

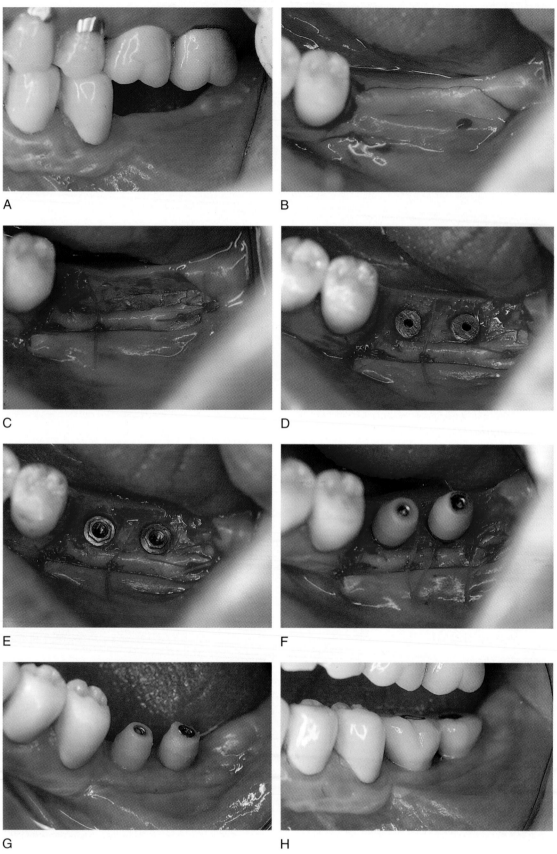

PLATE XXIV. Second-stage surgery. *A,* Two endosseous implants were placed 4 months previously and are ready to be exposed. Notice the narrow band of keratinized tissue. *B,* Two vertical incisions are connected by crestal incision. If there is insufficient facial keratinized tissue, it is necessary to locate the crestal more lingually so that there is a minimum of 2 to 3 mm of keratinized band. *C,* A buccal partial-thickness flap is sutured to the periosteum apical to the emerging implants. *D,* Gingival tissue coronal to the cover screws is excised by utilizing gingivectomy technique. *E,* The cover screws are removed and the heads of the implants are cleared. *F,* Abutments are placed. Visual inspection ensures that there is intimate contact between the abutments and the implants. *G,* Two- to 3-week healing after the second-stage surgery. *H,* Four months after the final restoration. Notice the healthy band of keratinized attached gingiva around the implants.

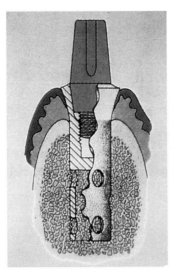

FIGURE 64–10. ITI implant with cement-on abutment in place. (Illustration courtesy of The Straumann Company, Cambridge, MA.)

most of the implant surface is exposed and an extensive amount of bone needs to regenerate to cover the implant, there will be a higher risk of deintegration during the early loaded stage.

Another common anatomic limitation of the maxillary arch is excessive pneumatization of the maxillary sinus leaving a very thin *inferior wall or floor of the maxillary sinus.* There are various techniques for elevating the floor of the sinus and augmenting the bone to accommodate the length of the implants.[6,12] These techniques are generally successful and, if done properly, will benefit the patient.

The sinus lift-augmentation can be done as an initial separate procedure or combined in one intervention with the placement of the implants. The healing period before the second-stage surgery to uncover the implants must be extended to 9 to 12 months.

To perform both objectives in one operation, there must be a sufficient height of bone (usually greater than 5 mm) to provide the initial stability of the implant. In addition, if the existing bone height is sufficient but the bone is very soft, it is better to perform the sinus lift and implantation in separate interventions.

When the sinus lift and the implantation are done in two stages, the bone should be allowed to mature for approximately 9 to 12 months before placing the implants. In addition to this, 6 to 12 months will be required before the second-stage surgery to uncover the implants can be performed.

In the partially edentulous mandibular arch with severely resorbed ridges, a *mandibular nerve repositioning* is an option.[6] This procedure requires extensive manipulation of the mandibular nerve and often results in extended periods of paresthesia and dysesthesia of the lower lip. In most cases, the patient returns to normal sensation in about 6 months. Patients should be carefully selected for these procedures and clearly informed in writing of all the possible side effects.

REFERENCES

1. Babbusch C, Kirsch A, Mentag P, et al. Intramobile cylinder (IMZ) two-stage osteointegrated implant (IME). Part 1: Its rationale and procedures for use. Int J Oral Maxillofac Implants 2:203, 1987.
2. Block MS, Kent JN. Factors associated with soft and hard tissue compromise of endosseous implants. J Oral Maxillofac Implants 48:1153, 1990.
3. Brånemark P-I, Zarb G, Albrektsson I. Tissue-integrated prosthesis. In Osseointegration in Clinical Dentistry. Chicago, Quintessence Publishing, 1987.
4. Buser D, Schroeder A, Sutter F, Lang NP. The new concept of ITI hollow cylinder and hollow-screw implants. Part 2: Clinical aspects, indications and early clinical results. Int J Oral Maxillofac Implants 3:173, 1988.
5. Buser D, Weber HP, Brägger U. The treatment of partially edentulous patients with ITI hollow-screw implants: Presurgical evaluation and surgical procedures. Int J Oral Maxillofac Implants 5:165, 1990.
6. Cranin AN. Atlas of Oral Implantology. New York, Thieme Medical, 1993.
7. Interpore IMZ Technique Manual. Irvine, CA, Interpore International.
8. Jovanovic SA, Giovannoli JL. New bone formation by the principle of guided tissue regeneration for periimplant osseous lesions. J Parodontologie 11:29, 1992.
9. Kenney EB, Weinlander M. Uncovering implants. Calif Dent Assoc J 17:18, 1989.
10. Kent JN, Block MS. Simultaneous maxillary sinus floor bone grafting and placement of hydroxyapatite-coated implant. J Oral Maxillofac Implants 47:238, 1989.
11. Scharf DR, Tarnow DP. The effect of crestal versus mucobuccal incisions on the success rate of implant osseointegration. Int J Oral Maxillofac Implants 8:187, 1993.
12. Wood RM, Moore DI. Grafting of the maxillary sinus with intraorally harvested autogenous bone prior to implant placement. J Oral Maxillofac Implants 3:209, 1988.

65

Diagnosis and Treatment of Peri-implant Disease

SASCHA A. JOVANOVIC

Incidence
Etiology
Diagnosis of Peri-implant Tissue Breakdown
Removal of Failed Implants

Initial Phase of Treatment of Peri-implantitis
Surgical Techniques for Treatment of Peri-implantitis
Maintenance

The long-term predictability of osseointegrated implants for tooth replacement has been documented by several longitudinal studies, resulting in wide use of dental implants.[1,3,11] In spite of these results, however, complications can occur in a small percentage of cases.

Pathologic changes of the peri-implant tissues can be placed in the general category of *peri-implant disease*.[28] Inflammatory changes, which are confined to the soft tissue surrounding an implant, are diagnosed as *peri-implant mucositis*. Progressive peri-implant bone loss in conjunction with a soft tissue inflammatory lesion is termed *peri-implantitis*.[28]

Peri-implantitis begins at the coronal portion of the implant, while the more apical portion of the implant maintains an osseointegrated status.[20,27,31,50] This means that the implant is not clinically mobile until the late stages, when bone loss has progressed to involve the complete implant surface.[17,39]

INCIDENCE

Few studies have reported on the frequency of occurrence of peri-implant disease.[15,18,47,52,53,58,59] Most long-term studies present an average of the marginal bone loss around all reported implants, and therefore statistical means can disguise individual implant sites with peri-implant disease.[1] Depending on the study, mean crestal bone decreases 0.9 to 1.6 mm during the first year of function. In the follow-up period, mean annual rates of bone loss decrease to 0.05 to 0.13 mm.[1,3,11]

Clinical data have shown that after a period of implant function, peri-implant bone loss exceeding 4 mm was seen in 4% to 15% of the implants, and probing depth exceeding 5 mm was seen in 5% to 20% of the implants.[47] Other studies reported that the amount of peri-implant marginal bone loss is influenced by implant design and surface characteristics.[22,43]

A 2-year follow-up study on maxillary overdentures with Brånemark pure titanium implants showed that 6% of the implants had a partial marginal radiolucency, and 28% of the patients showed a peri-implant mucositis or hyperplasia.[52]

A radiographic study of peri-implant bone levels around 80 nonsubmerged titanium plasma-sprayed ITI (International Team for Oral Implantology) implants[59] found a mean bone loss of less than 1.1 mm in the first year of function. However, 7% of implant sites had bone level changes of more than 0.5 mm between year 1 and year 2, and 4% had bone level changes of more than 1 mm.

A significant number of hydroxyapatite-coated implants showed moderate (1 to 3 mm) bone loss, whereas a smaller number of implants demonstrated severe bone loss.[15]

Soft tissue complications such as peri-implant mucositis and hyperplasia were noted[58] in 21% to 28% of the jaws during the first period of clinical experience with osseointegration, but the incidence of these complications has decreased in more recent years. The improvement was attributed to improved oral hygiene methods and the changing of abutments.

Implants with a smooth coronal titanium neck and nonsplinted maxillary implants have shown increased peri-implant bone loss.[43] Under experimental conditions, the character of the implant surface influenced the amount of peri-implant tissue breakdown.[22]

Depending on the severity of the peri-implant bone loss, the morphology of the bone defect, and the implant surface, there is the potential to arrest the progression of the disease process and, in selected cases, to regenerate the lost bone tissue.

ETIOLOGY

The two major etiologic factors associated with resorption of crestal peri-implant bone tissue are bacterial infection and biomechanical factors associated with an overloaded site.[19,39]

Bacterial Infection. If plaque accumulates on the implant surface, the subepithelial connective tissue becomes infiltrated by large number of inflammatory cells and the epithelium appears ulcerated and loosely adherent. When the plaque front continues to migrate apically, clinical and radiographic signs of tissue destruction appear (Fig. 65–1).

Several studies have compared the pathogenesis of experimentally induced periodontitis and peri-implantitis.[20,31,50] The size of the soft tissue inflammatory lesion and the resultant bone loss are greater around implants than around teeth. In addition, the implant lesions extend into the supracrestal connective tissue and approximate or populate the bone marrow (Fig. 65–2), whereas the lesions associated with teeth do not. These studies suggest that plaque-associated soft tissue inflammation around implants may have more serious implications than marginal inflammation around teeth with a periodontal ligament (Fig. 65–3).

Reasons for the increased inflammation around an implant might include the low-vascularity soft tissue band or the difference in the collagen-to-fibroblast ratio of gingival tissue, which affects the defense mechanisms around an implant compared with those seen in tissues around teeth with a periodontal ligament.[20,31,50] In addition, different implant surface characteristics influence the amount of peri-implant tissue breakdown and inflammation; specifically, hydroxy-apatite-coated implants seem to have increased bone loss when compared with titanium implants (Fig. 65–4).[15,18,22]

Subgingival bacterial flora associated with clinically inflamed implant sites is quite different from that seen around "healthy" implants. These microbial shifts are very similar to those occurring around natural teeth, and the bac-

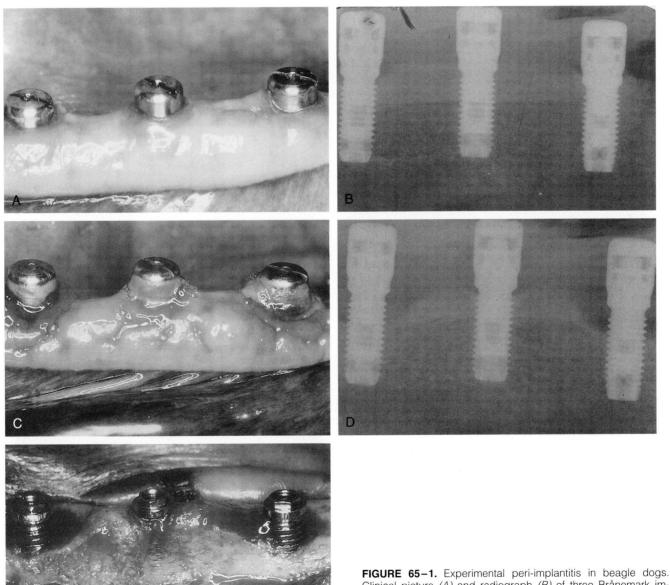

FIGURE 65–1. Experimental peri-implantitis in beagle dogs. Clinical picture *(A)* and radiograph *(B)* of three Brånemark implants in place, 6 months after abutment connection. *C* to *E,* Six months after placement of a ligature to induce plaque accumulation in implants at left and at right; the middle implant represents a nonligated control. *C,* Clinical picture showing inflammatory changes. *D,* Radiograph depicting the resultant bone loss. *E,* Actual bone loss shown after raising a flap.

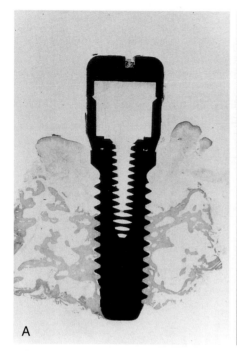 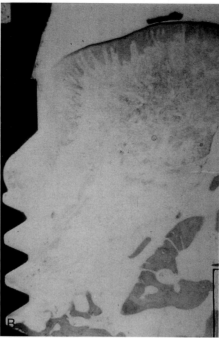 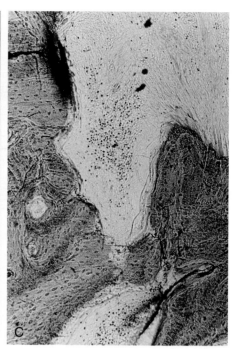

FIGURE 65–2. Microscopic view of experimental peri-implantitis in a beagle dog. *A,* Low-power view of the implant in situ showing vertical bone loss. Note that osseointegration persists in deeper portions of the implant. *B,* Higher power view of the area of bone loss next to the implant. *C,* Higher power view showing extension of inflammation into bone.

florae in adult periodontitis and peri-implantitis seem to have great similarities.[5,21,30,36,37,45]

It is possible that these organisms are the direct cause of the peri-implant breakdown, but proof of such is not available. Nevertheless, a subepithelial inflammatory response occurs, and undoubtedly this plays a role in continuing the inflammatory changes that cause the breakdown to progress.[20,27,31,50] A marked difference has been documented between the bacterial morphotypes of the totally edentulous and the partially edentulous mouth.[4,41] The so-called periodontal pathogens are decreased in the implant sulci of the totally edentulous mouth. This might indicate a higher susceptibility for peri-implantitis in the partially edentulous mouth.

Biomechanical Factors. There is also some experimental and clinical evidence to support the concept that excessive biomechanical forces may lead to high stress or microfractures in the coronal bone-to-implant contact and thereby lead to loss of osseointegration around the neck of the implant.[16,32,43,48,55] The role of loading is likely to have increased influence in four clinical situations:

1. The implant is placed in poor-quality bone.
2. The position of the implant(s) or the total number of implants placed does not favor an ideal load transmission over the implant surface.
3. The patient has a pattern of heavy occlusal function associated with parafunction.
4. The prosthetic superstructure does not fit the implants precisely.

It is important to note that the cause for peri-implant crestal bone loss can be multifactorial, and both bacterial infection and biomechanical factors can be contributing factors. Each factor should be identified and eliminated for treatment of the implant site to be successful.

Other etiologic factors such as traumatic surgical techniques; inadequate amount of host bone, resulting in an exposed implant surface at the time of placement; and a compromised host response can act as cofactors in the development of peri-implant disease.

DIAGNOSIS OF PERI-IMPLANT TISSUE BREAKDOWN

The long-term success of dental implants depends on the continued health of peri-implant hard and soft tissues and an appropriate force distribution to the implants.[39,46] Soft tissue health should be established by obtaining high patient compliance with a plaque removal regimen and having a prosthesis design that follows perioprosthetic guidelines.

The rationale for preferring attached, masticatory mucosa surrounding an implant, especially in the partially edentulous mouth, is based on the difference in microbial composition between the partially and the totally edentulous mouth, the risk for bacterial seeding from adjacent periodontal pockets, the weak soft tissue adherence around the pergingival area of an implant, and the increased inflammatory response around implants with bacterial infection.[4,8,12,20,31,41]

Biomechanical forces on implants are influenced by an adequate number of implants, by favorable implant positions for load distribution, and by establishing an appropriate occlusion.[46,48]

To diagnose a compromised implant site, soft tissue measurements made with manual or automated probes have been suggested. Although some reports say that probing is contraindicated, careful monitoring of probing depth and clinical attachment level over time seems useful in de-

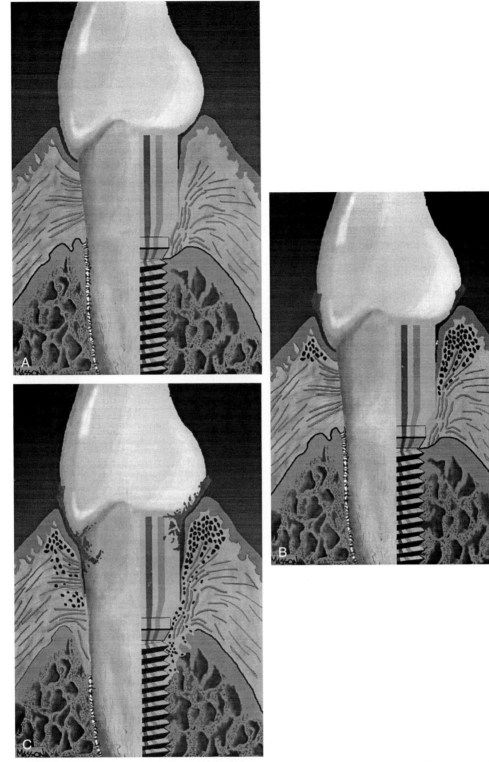

FIGURE 65–3. Diagrammatic representation of periodontitis *(left sides)* and peri-implantitis *(right sides)*. *A,* Normal tissues. *B,* Initial inflammatory involvement of soft tissues representing gingivitis and mucositis stage. *C,* Destruction of supporting structures.

tecting changes in the peri-implant tissue.[11,44,53,54] Radiographs to assess peri-implant bone level are also useful. Standardized radiography, both with and without computerized analysis, has been used to document a number of studies.[1,9,11,20,47]

In addition to pocket formation and radiographic bone destruction, suppuration, calculus buildup (Fig. 65–5),

swelling (Fig. 65–6), color changes, and bleeding on gentle probing have all been documented as signs of peri-implant disease.[36,39]

Mobility has been extensively described in the detection of early and late failures after loading of the implants with the superstructure.[1,39,43] However, mobility should be used only as absolute diagnostic information to determine lack

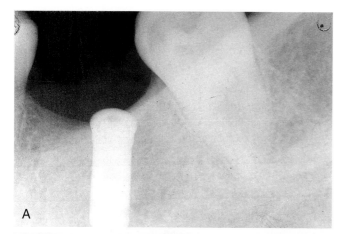

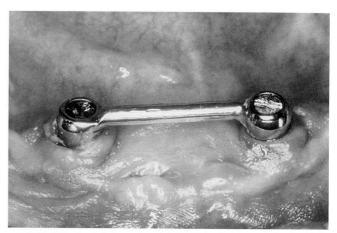

FIGURE 65–6. Peri-implant disease resulting in soft tissue swelling and inflammation.

REMOVAL OF FAILED IMPLANTS

In cases where osseointegration has been reduced severely and bone loss has extended into the apical half of the implant, or if the implant demonstrates mobility, implant removal should be considered (Table 65–1).[3,38] After the implants are removed, the ridge defects can frequently be reconstructed to their original level using bone graft and membrane techniques. This treatment will usually enable the clinician to place new implants in a previously compromised location.

INITIAL PHASE OF TREATMENT OF PERI-IMPLANTITIS

Occlusal Therapy. When excessive forces are considered the main etiologic factor for peri-implant bone loss, treatment involves an analysis of the fit of the prosthesis, the number and position of the implants, and an occlusal evaluation. A change in prosthesis design, an improvement in implant number and position, and occlusal adjustment can all contribute to arresting the progression of peri-implant tissue breakdown.

Anti-infective Therapy. The nonsurgical treatment of peri-implant bacterial infection involves local removal of plaque deposits with plastic instruments and polishing of all accessible surfaces with pumice[54]; subgingival irrigation of all peri-implant pockets with 0.12% chlorhexidine; systemic antimicrobial therapy for 10 consecutive days; and improved patient compliance with oral hygiene procedures until a healthy peri-implant site is established.[35,57] As in treatment of periodontal disease, this initial phase of therapy

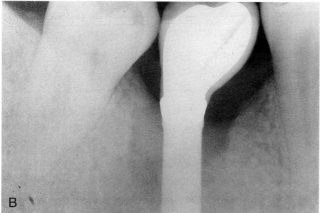

FIGURE 65–4. Rapid destruction of bone after placement of an implant. *A,* Normal supporting tissues after placement of the implant. *B,* Advanced bone loss 12 months later.

of osseointegration. Current electronic diagnostic tools for measuring mobility are not sensitive enough to detect mobility changes in osseointegrated implants undergoing marginal bone loss.

Microbial monitoring is useful in evaluating the peri-implant health condition and the microbial composition of a peri-implantitis site. This information can then potentially be used to determine the etiology of the breakdown and to select a specific antibiotic regimen.[5,35,39]

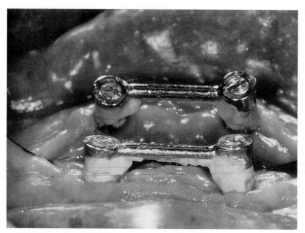

FIGURE 65–5. Plaque and debris accumulation around implants, with resultant inflammation.

Table 65–1. INDICATIONS FOR IMPLANT REMOVAL

- Severe peri-implant bone loss (>50% of implant length)
- Bone loss involving implant vents or holes
- Unfavorable advanced bone defect (one wall)
- Rapid, severe bone destruction (within 1 year of loading)
- Nonsurgical or surgical therapy ineffective

Table 65–2. INDICATIONS FOR NONSURGICAL THERAPY

- Mucosal inflammation detected by clinical signs
- Radiographic bone level stable
- Phase I therapy before surgery

may be sufficient to re-establish gingival health, or it may have to be followed by a surgical approach (Table 65–2).

The implant surface is contaminated with soft tissue cells, bacteria, and bacterial byproducts.[20,26,31] Bacterial adherence is enhanced by the microirregularities of implant surfaces,[42] and as long as the contamination is present, wound healing is compromised. Therefore, if regeneration of new bone and re-osseointegration is to occur, the defect must first be debrided and the contaminated implant surface prepared. Re-osseointegration can be defined as growth of new bone in direct contact with the previously contaminated implant surface without an intervening radiolucent area.[22]

Mechanical devices and chemotherapeutic agents used for implant surface preparation have been evaluated in vitro and in vivo.[14,40,60,61] Conventional hand and ultrasonic instruments are not suitable for preparation and detoxification of the implant surface. *The method of choice involves the use of a high-pressure air spray and a powder abrasive (a mixture of sodium bicarbonate and sterile water).* This method removes microbial deposits completely from titanium surfaces, does not change the surface topography significantly, and has no adverse effect on cell adhesion.[14,40] There have been some warnings regarding the potential for air emphysema when using high-pressure air spray instrumentation in the surgical site.[10] Clinical case reports have shown successful treatment of peri-implant disease with a detoxification protocol utilizing an air–powder abrasive method.[24,33]

Preparation of the implant surface has also been achieved by applying chemotherapeutic agents; several different agents[60,61] have been evaluated for this purpose. The application of a supersaturated solution of citric acid for 30 to 60 seconds has been reported to have the highest potential for removal of endotoxins from hydroxyapatite implant surfaces. Successful treatment of peri-implant disease utilizing only chemotherapeutic agents as a detoxification protocol has been reported.[29,34]

SURGICAL TECHNIQUES FOR TREATMENT OF PERI-IMPLANTITIS

The surgical techniques that are currently advocated to control peri-implant lesions are modified from techniques used to treat bone defects around teeth. The type and size of the bone defect must be determined before deciding on a resective or regenerative treatment modality. This is done by radiographic evaluation and by probing and sounding of the defects under local anesthesia immediately before beginning the procedure. Resective therapy is used to reduce pockets; correct negative osseous architecture and rough implant surfaces; and increase the area of keratinized gingiva, if needed. Regenerative therapy is also used to reduce

pockets, but with the ultimate goal of regeneration of lost bone tissue.

As in the treatment of certain types of periodontitis, systemic antibiotics have been advocated as a supportive regimen during the treatment phase of peri-implant disease.[24,29,35] This may be especially important because of the close proximity of the inflammatory lesion to the implant and the bone marrow (see Fig. 65–2C).[20,31] Antibiotics frequently used without sensitivity testing are doxycycline and metronidazole.[24,29,35] If bacterial sensitivity testing is done, the antibiotic regimen is determined by the laboratory result.

The morphology of osseous defects caused by peri-implant disease will vary and in general will depend on the amount of bone present at the time of implant placement and the length and severity of the pathologic insult. Bone defects can be divided into four main types:

Type I presents moderate horizontal bone loss with a minimal vertical component. These implants are usually covered by a thin buccal and lingual/palatal bone crest at the time of placement and are at an early stage of peri-implant breakdown.

Type II has a moderate to severe horizontal bone loss with a minimal vertical component. This is a more advanced condition than type I.

Type III demonstrates a minimal to moderate horizontal bone loss with an advanced circumferential vertical lesion. These implants are initially covered by a thin coronal bone crest with a wider apical bone base. Frequently the pattern of bone loss has a symmetric feature with a circular trough of uniform width and depth occurring around the circumference of the implant.

Type IV presents more complicated implant defects with moderate horizontal bone loss and with an advanced circumferential vertical lesion; in addition, the buccal and/or lingual plate has been lost (Fig. 65–7). These implants usually demonstrated a thin bone plate at the time of implant placement that resorbed under the pathologic conditions.

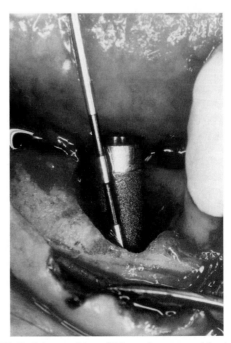

FIGURE 65–7. Advanced type IV bone loss around implants.

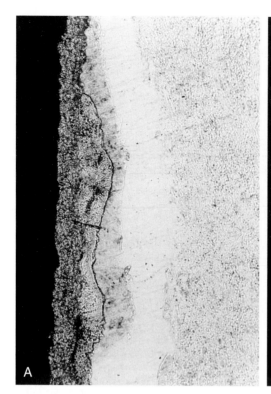
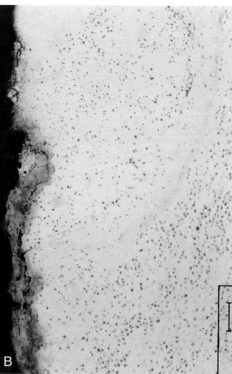

FIGURE 65–8. Light microscopic view of resorption of the surface of a hydroxyapatite-coated implant surrounded by inflammatory cells (Toluidine blue stain). *A.* Early stage of calculus buildup on hydroxyapatite surface showing dense inflammatory infiltrate. *B.* Late stage of inflammation around hydroxyapatite surface resulting in partial resorption.

The implant surface in the defect area is a source of controversy and may play a role in the choice of treatment. There is clinical and histologic evidence that marginal inflammation can cause resorption of the surface of hydroxyapatite-coated implants (Fig. 65–8).[18,22,26] The treated and detoxified peri-implantitis–affected sites show continued phagocytosis of the hydroxyapatite surface.[22] Until further experimental and clinical data are available, a careful and conservative approach should be employed when treating hydroxyapatite-coated implants affected by peri-implant disease.

Titanium implants show little or no resorption of the surface.[20,31] As long as the inflammatory lesion around a titanium implant can be arrested, surgical treatment of selected cases seems indicated.

Peri-implant Resective Therapy. The type of osseous defect should be identified before deciding on the treatment modality (Table 65–3). Apically displaced flap techniques and osseous resective therapy are used to correct horizontal bone loss and moderate (<3 mm) vertical bone defects and to reduce overall pocket depth (Fig. 65–9).[19,33,56,57]

Full-thickness or split-thickness flaps are utilized to access the surgical area. With the flap raised, degranulation of

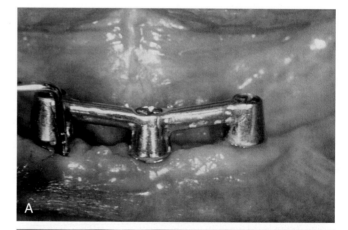
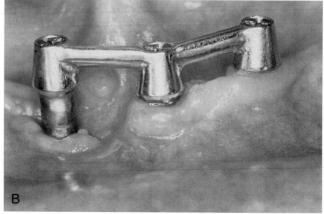

FIGURE 65–9. Treatment of peri-implantitis by resective surgical therapy and implantoplasty. *A,* Before treatment. *B,* After treatment.

Table 65–3. INDICATIONS FOR RESECTIVE THERAPY

- Moderate to advanced horizontal bone loss
- One- and two-wall bone defects
- Implant position in nonaesthetic area

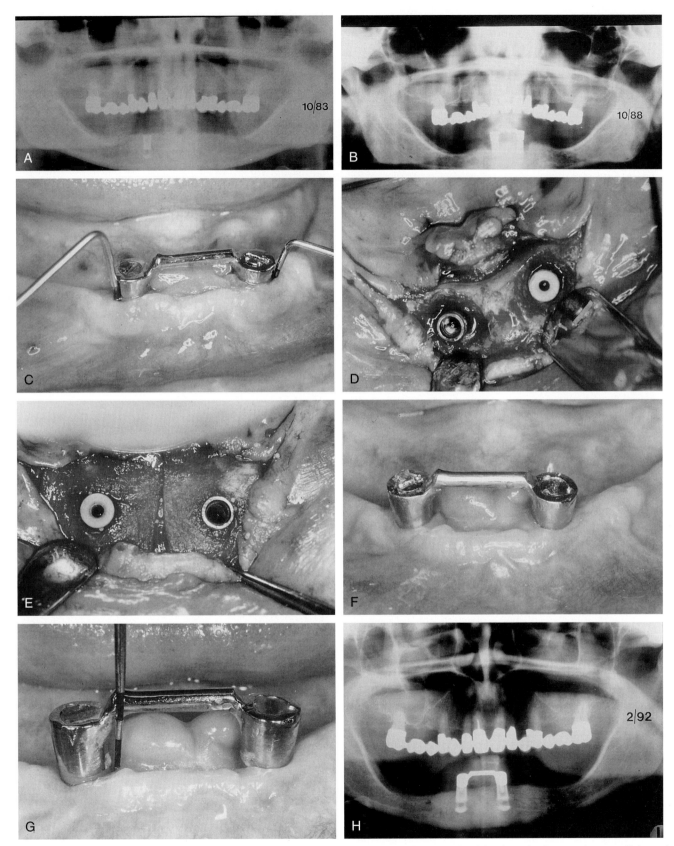

FIGURE 65–10. Treatment of peri-implantitis by regenerative surgical therapy. *A,* Radiograph of implants in the anterior mandible at the time of placement. *B,* Radiograph taken 5 years later shows advanced vertical bone loss around both implants. *C,* Clinical picture with probes showing the presence of very deep peri-implant pockets. *D,* Elevated flaps showing advanced circumferential vertical bone loss around both implants. *E,* After debridement, the area was packed with porous hydroxyapatite covered by a nonresorbable membrane. *F* to *H,* Clinical and tradiographic results after 4 years.

the osseous defect is performed with curettes. This is usually an uncomplicated procedure, as the granulation tissue is loosely adherent to the underlying bone and does not adhere to the implant. Care should be taken to avoid contact between the implant and metal instruments. The implant surface can then be prepared with chemicals and air abrasives. Implant surface preparation is performed by applying the air–powder abrasive spray for a maximum of 60 seconds on the implant surface, followed by copious irrigation with saline solution. Then an antimicrobial solution such as supersaturated citric acid is applied for 30 seconds, followed again by irrigation with saline solution.

Surface Polishing: Implantoplasty. The long-term goal of the surgical treatment of peri-implant breakdown is to arrest the progression of the disease and to achieve a site that is maintainable by the patient. For this purpose, implant surfaces that are smooth and clean coronal to the bone level are preferred. Surfaces with threads or roughened topography (e.g., hydroxyapatite) should be altered with high-speed diamond burs and polishers to produce a smooth continuous surface (Fig. 65–9B).[19,33] The implantoplasty is performed before any osseous resective therapy is initiated and with profuse irrigation.

Surface modifications are performed only when resective surgery is performed and not during regenerative procedures, because the metal particles could interfere with the regeneration of bone. If a rough implant surface or a moderate bone defect still exists after a bone regeneration procedure, a re-entry surgical procedure after a minimum healing time of 6 months may be performed. During this second surgical intervention, resective therapy with modification of the implant surface can be done.

Peri-implant Regenerative Therapy. A few studies have shown successful regenerative treatment of peri-implant bone defects around functioning dental implants (Fig. 65–10).[2,19,24,29,34] The indications for regenerative therapy in submerged and unsubmerged implants are shown in Tables 65–4 and 65–5, respectively.

To accomplish regeneration of lost bone, guided tissue regeneration (GTR) and bone graft techniques have been suggested.[19,34] In several experimental and clinical studies, GTR utilizing membranes has been used for healing of bone defects seen at the time of implant placement[13,23] and around failing implants.[22,24,29]

Regeneration of bone seems to be enhanced if the area is isolated from the oral environment. Therefore, removal of the implant prosthesis is recommended 4 to 8 weeks prior to the regenerative surgical procedure to allow optimal compliance with oral hygiene procedures and to enable the soft tissue to collapse and heal over the implant site with a newly attached cover screw in place. At the time of regenerative surgery a more intact soft tissue flap can be helpful to seal off the peri-implant tissues during the healing period. A crestal incision can then be used to elevate the flap.

If it is not possible to remove the prosthesis beforehand, a sulcular incision can be used to raise a full-thickness flap and to evaluate the surgical site. With the flap raised, degranulation of the osseous defect is performed with curettes, with extreme care taken not to contaminate the implant surface.

Surgical therapy includes implant surface preparation by

Table 65–4. INDICATIONS FOR SUBMERGED REGENERATIVE THERAPY

- Implant allows complete closure with flap
- Moderate to advanced circumferential vertical defects
- Two- and three-wall bone defects
- Detoxification of implant surface possible

---

air–powder abrasive for 30 to 60 seconds, followed by application of an antimicrobial solution such as supersaturated citric acid for 30 to 60 seconds. An elaborate rinse of the surgical area with saline solution is then performed. To achieve increased access of osteogenic cells to the defect, the bone surface is prepared by roughening and penetration with small round burs.

A membrane is then trimmed to extend 3 to 4 mm beyond the margins of the bone defect and is placed over the implant or secured with a cover screw or fixation screws. Care should be taken to position the membrane close to the surrounding bone, but allowing a space for the formation of the blood clot. The flap is closed primarily over the site with mattress and interrupted sutures. Care is taken not to have any tension on the flap; periosteal fenestrations can be used to improve the tension-free suturing of the flap.

Postoperatively patients are instructed to rinse twice daily for 2 weeks with 0.12% chlorhexidine solution, and a systemic antibiotic is prescribed.[25] The sutures are removed after 14 days. If a submerged condition is maintained, the membrane is left undisturbed for at least 4 to 6 months. At that time the membrane is removed and the abutment secured. If the membrane becomes exposed before this time, chlorhexidine application is continued to control infection of the healing tissues over the defect. If exudation is present, immediate removal of the membrane is advised. Otherwise, exposed membranes are usually removed 4 weeks after the perforation occurs.

When one-stage implants are treated or if the prosthesis must be maintained in place, pergingival GTR therapy is applied. The membrane is perforated with a 3-mm hole and slid over the implant. The membrane should ensure complete coverage and isolation of the vertical bone defect. The flap is then sutured closely to the implant neck (Plate XXV).

With a pergingival healing environment, the membranes are removed 6 to 8 weeks after surgery. Removal is necessary because of accumulation of plaque on the membrane and the potential risk of membrane and peri-implant infection. If bioabsorbable membranes are used, no removal procedure is necessary. Postoperative maintenance care is the same as for submerged GTR therapy.

Various bone graft materials can be used in conjunction with GTR therapies, although few studies have looked at

---

Table 65–5. INDICATIONS FOR PERGINGIVAL REGENERATIVE THERAPY

- One-stage implant or nonretrievable prostheses
- Moderate to advanced circumferential vertical defects
- Three-wall bone defects
- Detoxification of implant surface possible

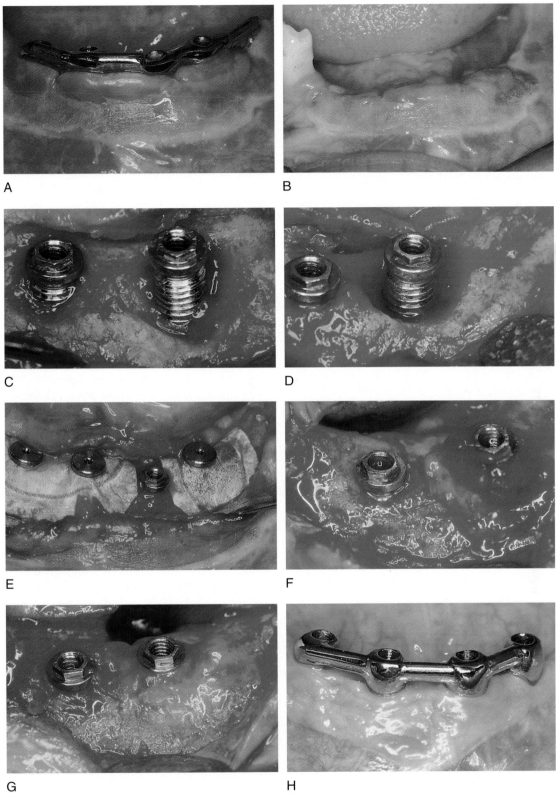

PLATE XXV. Reconstructive treatment of peri-implantitis. *A,* Four osseointegrated implants used for retention of an overdenture in an edentulous lower jaw. Moderate to severe peri-implantitis, with soft tissue hyperplasia and deep pockets around all implants. There was radiographic evidence of progressive bone loss around three of the four implants. *B,* A submerged regenerative therapy was initiated by removal of the abutments 6 months before surgery, and a 1-week period of systemic antibiotic coverage was instituted. Note the improved soft tissue appearance. *C and D,* Elevated flap showing bone loss around three of the four implants. The defects consisted of horizontal bone loss and shallow-to-deep circumferential vertical defects around the implants. The defects were carefully degranulated by hand, and the implant surfaces were detoxified with supersaturated citric acid and an air-abrasive for 30 to 60 seconds and then flushed with sterile water. Bone surfaces were roughened and penetrated with small round burs. *E,* Two membranes placed over the peri-implant bone defects, allowing a blood clot to form underneath. Note the close adaptation of the membranes to the periphery of the bone defects, acting as a tent over the defects. *F and G,* After an uneventful healing period of 4 months, the surgical sites are exposed and the membranes removed. Note the osseous regeneration in the defect area. *H,* Postoperative clinical evaluation 1½ years later. Note healthy peri-implant tissues, minimal probing depth with no bleeding, and minimal soft tissue retraction around all implants.

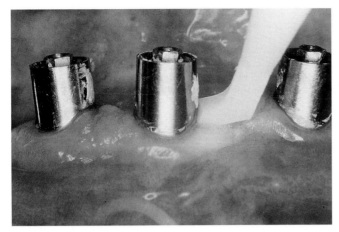

FIGURE 65–11. Professional plaque removal around implants as part of maintenance care.

the value of such combined therapy. Graft materials such as hydroxyapatite, demineralized freeze-dried bone, and autogenous bone have been suggested as support for the membrane.

Hydroxyapatite has an osteoconductive capacity,[34] and it may be more desirable to have a graft completely replaced with the patient's own bone than with a combination of bone and some synthetic material. Demineralized freeze-dried bone has also been utilized as a supporting graft material for the membrane therapy, but with inconclusive results.[51] Demineralized freeze-dried-bone undergoes patterns of incorporation similar to those of autografts, but the incorporation tends to be slower and less complete.[51]

Until more supportive results for allografts or synthetic graft materials are demonstrated, the use of intraoral autogenous bone grafts is preferred.[23] These bone grafts have been extensively evaluated in the surgical literature and have shown potential to be revascularized and eventually replaced by the patient's own bone. Furthermore, the bone grafts stabilize the blood clot, support the membrane, and above all, totally exclude disease transmission. Removal of the bone graft brings minimal morbidity to the intraoral donor site, and the surgical cost is minimal. However, remodeling occurs slowly, and depending on the size and quality of the graft, revascularization may require up to 1 year.

MAINTENANCE

After surgical intervention, all patients are placed on a close recall schedule (Fig. 65–11); maintenance visits every 3 months are advised as a minimum. This allows for monitoring of plaque levels, soft tissue inflammation, and changes in the level of the bone. The importance of maintenance procedures should never be underestimated by either the patient or the therapist.

Acknowledgment

The invaluable help of Dr. Karl Donath with the histologic aspects of this chapter is gratefully acknowledged.

REFERENCES

1. Adell R, Lekholm U, Rockler B, Brånemark P-I. A 15-year study of osseointegrated implants in the treatment of the edentulous jaw. Int J Oral Surg *10:*387, 1981.
2. Adell R, Lekholm U, Brånemark P-I, Lindhe J. Marginal tissue reaction at osseointegrated titanium fixtures. Swed Dent J *28:*175, 1985.
3. Albrektsson T, Zarb G, Worthington P, Eriksson RA. The long-term efficacy of currently used dental implants. A review and prognosis criteria for success. Int J Oral Maxillofac Implants *1:*11, 1986.
4. Apse P, Ellen RP, Overall CM, Zarb GA. Microbiota and crevicular fluid collagenase activity in the osseointegrated dental implant sulcus: A comparison of sites in edentulous and partially edentulous patients. J Periodont Res *24:*96, 1989.
5. Becker W, Becker BE, Newman MG, Nyman S. Clinical and microbiologic findings that may contribute to dental implant failure. Int J Oral Maxillofac Implants *5:*31, 1980.
6. Berglundh T, Lindhe J, Ericsson I, et al. The soft tissue barrier at implants and teeth. Clin Oral Implant Res *2:*81–90, 1991.
7. Berglundh T, Lindhe J, Marinello C, et al. Soft tissue reaction to de novo plaque formation on implants and teeth. Clin Oral Implant Res *3:*1, 1992.
8. Block M, Kent J. Factors associated with soft and hard-tissue compromise of endosseous implants. J Oral Maxillofac Surg *48:*1160, 1990.
9. Bragger U, Burgin W, Fourmousis J, Lang NP. Image processing for the evaluations of dental implants. Dentomaxillofac Radiol *21:*208, 1992.
10. Brown FH, Ogletree RC, Houston GD. Pneumoparotitis associated with the use of an air-powder prophylaxis unit. J Periodontol *63:*642, 1992.
11. Buser D, Weber HP, Bragger U, Balsiger C. Tissue integration of one stage ITI implants: 3-year results of a longitudinal study with hollow-cylinder and hollow-screw implants. Int J Oral Maxillofac Implants *6:*405, 1991.
12. Buser D, Weber HP, Donath K, et al. Soft tissue reactions to nonsubmerged unloaded titanium implants in Beagle dogs. J Periodontol *63:*226, 1992.
13. Dahlin C, Sennerby L, Lekholm U, et al. Generation of new bone around titanium implants using a membrane technique: An experimental study in rabbits. Int J Oral Maxillofac Implants *4:*19, 1989.
14. Dohm GJ, Stender E, Foitzik CH. Die Reinigung von Impllantatoberflachen mit Strahl- und Zahnsteinentfernungsgeraten. Dtsch Z Zahnarztl Implantol *2:*133, 1986.
15. Golec TS, Krauser JT. Long-term retrospective studies on hydroxyapatite-coated endosteal and subperiosteal implants. Dent Clin North Am *36:*39, 1992.
16. Hadeen G, Ismail Y, Garrana H, Pahountis L. Three-dimensional finite element stress analysis of Nobelpharma and Core-Vent implants and their supporting structures. Abstract 1390. J Dent Res *67:*286, 1988.
17. James RA. Periodontal considerations in implant dentistry. J Prosthet Dent *30:*202, 1973.
18. Johnson BW. HA-coated dental implants: Long-term consequences. Calif Dent Assoc J *20:*33, 1992.
19. Jovanovic SA. The management of periimplant breakdown around functioning osseointegrated dental implants. J Periodontol *64:*1176, 1993.
20. Jovanovic SA. Plaque-induced periimplant bone loss in mongrel dogs. A clinical, microbial, radiographic and histological study. Master of Science thesis, University of California, Los Angeles, 1994.
21. Jovanovic SA, James RA, Lessard G. Bacterial morphotypes and PGE2 levels from the perigingival site of dental implants with intact and compromised bone support. Abstract. J Dent Res *67:*28, 1988.
22. Jovanovic SA, Kenney EB, Carranza FA Jr, Donath K. The regenerative potential of plaque-induced periimplant bone defects treated by a submerged membrane technique. An experimental study. Int J Oral Maxillofac Implants *8:*13, 1993.
23. Jovanovic SA, Spiekermann H, Richter EJ. Bone regeneration on titanium dental implants with dehisced defect sites. A clinical study. Int J Oral Maxillofac Implants *7:*233, 1992.
24. Jovanovic SA, Spiekermann H, Richter E-J, Koseoglu M. Guided tissue regeneration around titanium dental Implants. In Laney WR, Tolmen DE, eds. Tissue Integration in Oral, Orthopedic and Maxillofacial Reconstruction. Chicago, Quintessence Publishing, 1992, p 208.
25. Koth DL, McKinney RV, Steflik DE. Microscopic study of hygiene effect on periimplant gingival tissues. J Dent Res *65:*186, 1986.
26. Krauser J, Berthold P, Tamery I, Seckinger R. A SEM study of failed endosseous root formed dental implants. Abstract 65. J Dent Res *70:*274, 1991.
27. Lang NP, Bragger U, Walther D, et al. Ligature-induced periimplant infection in cynomolgus monkeys. I. Clinical and radiographic findings. Clin Oral Implant Res *4:*2–11, 1993.
28. Lang NP, Karring T, eds. Proceedings of the 1st European Workshop on Periodontology. Chicago, Quintessence Publishing, 1994.
29. Lehmann B, Bragger U, Hammerle CHF, et al. Treatment of an early failure according to the principles of guided tissue regeneration. Clin Oral Implant Res *3:*43, 1992.
30. Lekholm U, Ericsson I, Adell R, Slots J. The condition of the soft tissues at tooth and fixture abutments supporting fixed bridges. A microbiological and histological study. J Clin Periodontol *13:*558, 1986.
31. Lindhe J, Berglundh T, Ericsson I, et al. Experimental breakdown of periimplant and periodontal tissues. A study in the beagle dog. Clin Oral Implant Res *3:*9, 1992.

32. Lindquist LW, Rockler B, Carlsson GE. Bone resorption around fixtures in edentulous patients treated with mandibular fixed tissue-integrated prostheses. J Prosthet Dent *59:*59, 1988.
33. Lozada J, James R, Boskovic M, et al. Surgical repair of periimplant defects. J Oral Implant *16:*42, 1990.
34. Meffert RM. Treatment of the ailing, failing implant. J Calif Dent Assoc *20:*42, 1992.
35. Mombelli A, Lang NP. Antimicrobial treatment of periimplant infections. Clin Oral Implant Res *3:*162–168, 1992.
36. Mombelli A, Van Oosten M, Schurch E, et al. The microbiota associated with successful or failing osseointegrated titanium implants. Oral Microbiol Immunol *2:*145, 1987.
37. Nakou M, Mikx FH, Oosterwaal PJM, Kruijsen JCWM. Early microbial colonization of permucosal implants in edentulous patients. J Dent Res *66:*1654, 1987.
38. Nevins M, Mellonig JT. Enhancement of the damaged edentulous ridge to receive dental implants: A combination of allograft and the Gore-Tex membrane. Int J Periodont Restor Dent *12:*97, 1992.
39. Newman M, Flemmig T. Periodontal considerations of implants and implant associated microbiota. J Dent Educ *52:*737, 1988.
40. Parham PL Jr, Cobb CM, French AA, et al. Effects of air–powder abrasive system on plasma-sprayed titanium implant surfaces: An in vitro evaluation. J Oral Implantol *15:*78, 1989.
41. Quirijnen M, Listgarten MA. The distribution of bacterial morphotypes around natural teeth and titanium implants ad modum Brånemark. Clin Oral Implant Res *1:*8, 1990.
42. Quirijnen M, Marechal M, Busscher HJ, et al. The influence of surface free energy and surface roughness on early plaque formation. J Clin Periodontol *17:*138, 1990.
43. Quirijnen M, Naert I, van Steenberghe D. Fixture design and overload influence marginal bone loss and fixture success in the Brånemark system. Clin Oral Implant Res *3:*104, 1992.
44. Quirijnen M, van Steenberghe D, Jacobs R, et al. The reliability of pocket probing around screw-type implants. Clin Oral Implant Res *2:*186, 1991.
45. Rams TE, Link C. Microbiology of failing dental implants in humans: Electron microscopic observations. J Oral Implant *11:*93, 1983.
46. Rangert B, Jemt T, Jorneus L. Forces and moments on Brånemark implants. Int J Oral Maxillofac Implants *4:*241, 1989.
47. Richter EJ, Jansen V, Spiekermann H, Jovanovic SA. Langzeitergebnisse von IMZ-und TPS- Implantaten im interforaminalen Bereich des zahnlosen Unterkiefers. Dtsch Zahnarztl Z *47:*449, 1992.
48. Roberts WE, Garetto LP, de Castro RA. Remodeling of devitalized bone threatens periosteal margin integrity of endosseous titanium implants with treated or smooth surfaces: Indications for provisional loading and axilliary directed occlusion. J Ind Dent Assoc *68:*19, 1989.
49. Sanz M, Newman M, Nachnani S, et al. Characterization of the subgingival microbial flora around endosteal dental implants in partially edentulous patients. Int J Oral Maxillofac Implants *5:*247, 1990.
50. Schou S, Holmstrup P, Stoltze K, et al. Ligature-induced marginal inflammation around osseointegrated implants and ankylosed teeth. Clinical and radiographic observations in cynomolgus monkeys. Clin Oral Implant Res *4:*12, 1993.
51. Simion M, Dahlin C, Trisi P, Piatelli A. Qualitative and quantitative comparative study on different filling materials used in bone regeneration. Int J Periodont Restor Dent *14:*199, 1994.
52. Smedberg J-I, Lothigius E, Bodin I, et al. A clinical and radiological two-year follow-up study of maxillary overdentures on osseointegrated implants. Clin Oral Implant Res *4:*39, 1993.
53. Smithloff M, Fritz M. The use of blade implants in a population of partially edentulous adults. A 15-year report. J Periodontol *58:*589, 1987.
54. Stefani LA. The care and maintenance of the dental implant patient. J Dent Hyg *62:*447, 1988.
55. Strub JR. Langzeitprognose von enossalen oralen Implantaten unter spezieller Beruchsichtigung von periImpllantaren, materialkundlichen und okklusalen Gesichtspunkten. habilitationsschriften der ZMK. Berlin, Quintessenz, 1986, pp 65–91.
56. Strub JR, Gaberthuel TW, Grunder U. The role of attached gingiva in the health of periimplant tissue in dogs. Part I. Clinical findings. Int J Periodont Restor Dent *11:*317, 1991.
57. Thompson-Neal D, Evans G, Meffert R. Effects of various prophylactic treatments on titanium, sapphire, and hydroxylapatite-coated implants: an SEM study. Int J Periodont Restor Dent *9:*301, 1989.
58. Tolman DE, Laney WR. Tissue-integrated prosthesis complications. Int J Oral Maxillofac Implants *7:*477–484, 1992.
59. Weber HP, Buser D, Fiorellini JP, Williams RC. Radiographic evaluation of crestal bone levels adjacent to nonsubmerged titanium implants. Clin Oral Implant Res *3:*181, 1992.
60. Zablotsky M, Diedrich D, Meffert R. Detoxification of endotoxin-contaminated titanium and hydroxyapatite-coated surfaces utilizing various chemotherapeutic and mechanical modalities. Implant Dent *1:*154, 1992.
61. Zablotsky M, Diedrich D, Meffert R, et al. The ability of various chemotherapeutic agents to detoxify the endotoxin infected HA-coated implant surface. Int J Oral Implantol *8:*45, 1991.

66

Preparation of the Periodontium for Restorative Dentistry

FERMIN A. CARRANZA, JR. and HENRY H. TAKEI

Phase I Therapy
Periodontal Surgery
Restorative Considerations in Periodontal Surgery
Preprosthetic Periodontal Surgery

Gingival and periodontal disease must be eliminated before restorative procedures are begun, for the following reasons:

1. Tooth mobility and pain interfere with mastication and function of restored teeth.
2. Inflammation of the periodontium impairs the capacity of abutment teeth to meet the functional demands made on them. Restorations constructed to provide beneficial functional stimulation to a healthy periodontium become a destructive influence when superimposed on existing periodontal disease, shortening the life of the teeth and the restoration.
3. The position of teeth is frequently altered in periodontal disease. Resolution of inflammation and regeneration of periodontal ligament fibers after treatment cause the teeth to move again, often back to their original position. Restorations designed for teeth before the periodontium is treated may produce injurious tensions and pressures on the treated periodontium.
4. Partial prostheses constructed on casts made from impressions of diseased gingiva and edentulous mucosa do not fit properly when periodontal health is restored. When the inflammation is eliminated, the contour of the gingiva and adjacent mucosa is altered (Fig. 66–1). Shrinkage creates spaces beneath the pontics of fixed bridges and the saddle areas of removable prostheses. Resultant plaque accumulation leads to inflammation of the mucosa and gingiva of the abutment teeth.
5. To locate the gingival margin of restorations properly, the position of the healthy gingival sulcus must be established before the tooth is prepared. Margins of restorations hidden behind diseased gingiva are exposed when the inflamed gingiva shrinks after periodontal treatment.

Furthermore, the aims of periodontal treatment are not limited to elimination of periodontal pockets and restoration of gingival health. *Treatment should also create the gingivomucosal environment and osseous topography necessary for the proper function of single-tooth restorations and of fixed and removable partial prostheses.*

In patients with mutilated dentitions and extensive periodontal disease, the sequence of treatment can be modified as follows:

1. "Hopeless" teeth are extracted, followed by construction of a temporary partial denture. Temporary crowns are prepared with provisional margins.
2. Periodontal therapy is performed.
3. Approximately 2 months after periodontal treatment, when gingival health is restored and the location of the gingival sulcus is established, the preparations are modified to relocate the margins in proper relation to the healthy gingival sulcus, and final restorations are constructed.

PHASE I THERAPY

Phase I therapy's specific goal is the control of active dental disease (see Chapters 41 and 42). Therefore, when this phase of therapy is completed, patients should be in a state of dental health with active caries no longer present and active destruction of the periodontium under control. This results in elimination of the acute inflammatory response associated with periodontal destruction. Thus, the status of the gingival tissues should be such that further restorative procedures of a more complex nature can be carried out without detrimental effects from unhealthy gingiva.

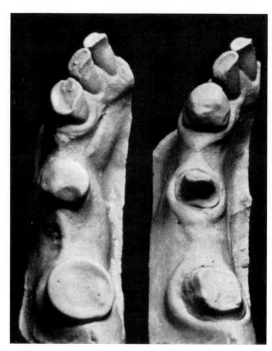

FIGURE 66-1. Change in contour of edentulous mucosa after resolution of inflammation. *Left,* Before treatment. Note the pyramidal contour of the edentulous mucosa. *Right,* After resolution of inflammation. The teeth are in the process of being prepared for a prosthesis.

Obtaining control of periodontal inflammation during Phase I therapy results in restorations of a much higher quality than would be obtained if restoration were carried out in an environment of gingival inflammation. The presence of an acute inflammatory response in the gingiva causes ulceration of the epithelium that lines the gingival pocket and an increase in vascularity and edema of the tissues immediately under this epithelium. There is a possibility of continual bleeding and exudation of inflammatory tissue fluid into the gingival crevice and into the environment of restorative dental procedures. Therefore, it is of utmost importance that all areas of the gingiva that show hemorrhage and significant amounts of inflammatory exudate be brought to an improved state of health before any restorative procedures other than emergency control of dental caries are carried out.

The removal of etiologic factors causing gingival inflammation results in a return to a more healthy gingival state within 1 or 2 weeks. Thus, plaque control, calculus removal, and the removal or correction of any inadequate dental restorations in the gingival environment should be important first-order procedures.

PERIODONTAL SURGERY

Restorative Considerations in Periodontal Surgery

Periodontal surgery is necessary in some patients. These periodontal surgical procedures should be carried out with due regard for the restorative needs of the patient. Therefore, the final level of the periodontium should allow good access to all restorative marginal regions, and any necessary increase in clinical crown length should be obtained by postsurgical positioning of the periodontal tissues. If restorative procedures necessitate the resolution of mucogingival inadequacies, the appropriate surgical procedure should be completed before restorative therapy is begun.

Routine periodontal surgery procedures aimed at the correction of periodontal and mucogingival defects are described in previous chapters. Some of these surgical procedures must be modified because of the restorative or prosthetic needs of the patient. In addition, the goal of some procedures is not treatment of a periodontal condition, but preparation of the mouth for the ensuing restortive or prosthetic therapy. These techniques can be called *preprosthetic periodontal surgery* and include procedures such as crown lengthening, augmentation or reduction of edentulous ridges, and placement of implants. The last procedure has been considered in Part VI; all other preprosthetic surgical techniques are presented in this chapter.

Pockets Adjacent to Edentulous Regions. Periodontal pockets frequently occur on the proximal surface of teeth adjacent to edentulous regions. These periodontal defects should be corrected before any fixed or removable prosthodontic appliance is placed in these areas. The general principles involved in elimination of pockets adjacent to edentulous regions are similar to those used in other areas, but some special procedures are necessary to take into account the special needs of the edentulous space.

Periodontally involved teeth adjacent to edentulous spaces present two problems that must be treated together: elimination of the pockets and management of the edentulous mucosa. Inflammation from the periodontal pockets extends for varying distances into the adjacent edentulous mucosa (Fig. 66-2) and alters its color, consistency, and shape. The edentulous mucosa affected by inflammation may exhibit various degrees of discoloration and edema. It may have a smooth, glistening surface if cellular and fluid exudate predominates. If fibrosis is more prominent, the mucosa is pink, firm, and enlarged, with a lobulated surface.

The contour of the edentulous mucosa and gingiva is affected by mechanical factors, as well as by inflammation from adjacent pockets. The edentulous mucosa may conform to the shape of the underlying bone, it may be swollen and rounded faciolingually, or lateral pressure from the tongue and cheek and food excursion may cause a "pyramiding" of the mucosa to form an elongated triangular ridge (Fig. 66-3). Because of the absence of the normal protective action of the embrasure, the gingiva is often similarly deformed.

The deformed edentulous mucosa reduces the vertical height available for prosthetic replacements. It does not provide a reliable base for the support of saddle areas or for the proper design of pontics. The triangular mucosa is unsatisfactory for the placement of pontics. In an effort to overcome the problem, short pontics with a deep V-shaped base that straddles the ridge are used. These are unsatisfactory, because food wedges between the mucosa and the pontics, and the resultant accumulation of plaque causes inflammation that jeopardizes retention of the bridge (Fig. 66-4).

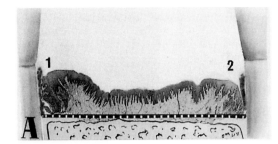

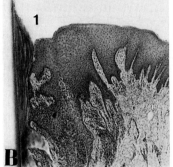 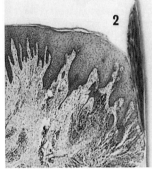

FIGURE 66-2. Preparation of the mouth for prosthesis. *A,* Edentulous mucosa with periodontal pockets (1 and 2) on the adjacent teeth. The location of the necessary incision is indicated by the *dotted line. B,* Inflammation from the periodontal pockets (1 and 2) extends into the edentulous mucosa.

Management of Pockets and Edentulous Mucosa. The area is prepared for the prosthesis, with the following objectives:

1. To establish a healthy gingival sulcus. The pontics adjacent to the natural teeth can be designed to create the gingival embrasure necessary for preservation of gingival health.
2. To eliminate extraneous mucosal tissue to permit adequate vertical space for the replacements.
3. To provide a firm, healthy mucosal base for placement of saddles or pontics.

In some situations, when pockets occur in areas adjacent to edentulous areas, a flap operation may be used to eliminate these pockets and at the same time provide a maintainable contour of the edentulous ridge region (Fig. 66–5). The incisions normally made around the adjacent teeth are

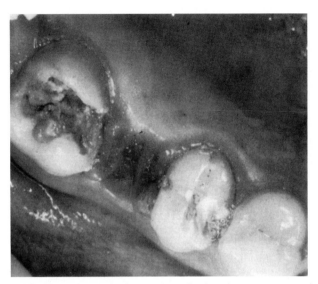

FIGURE 66-4. Chronic inflammation of edentulous mucosa under bridge with ridge-lap pontic.

carried into the edentulous area in the form of parallel buccal and lingual incisions that run across the crest of the ridge so that an adequate band of keratinized gingiva is maintained on both the buccal and lingual portions of the flap. These incisions across the edentulous area are made so that the flap is undermined (Fig. 66–6). The inflamed tissue between the buccal and lingual incisions is removed. The undermining of the buccal and lingual flaps leaves a thin band of tissue that lies close to the underlying bone after the flap is sutured back into position on completion of the operation. The undermining and subsequent repositioning of the flap result in apical positioning of the soft tissue covering the edentulous area.

By means of the parallel incisions over the edentulous area, access is obtained to any osseous defects on the adjacent teeth. These periodontal osseous defects can be recontoured to eliminate angular bone losses and other abnormalities. The flaps provide tissue to cover these corrected osseous defects completely so that subsequent healing is uneventful and of short duration (see Fig. 66–6). The pro-

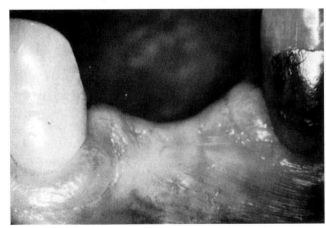

FIGURE 66-3. "Pyramiding" of edentulous mucosa and adjacent gingiva. The gingiva and mucosa are contoured by pressure from the tongue and food excursion.

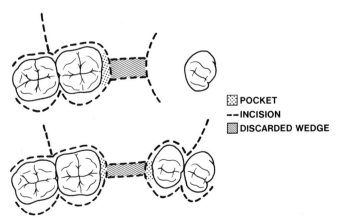

POCKET
--INCISION
DISCARDED WEDGE

FIGURE 66-5. Flap surgery in edentulous areas. Incisions for pockets adjacent to edentulous regions. The *dotted lines* mark the initial incisions. Vertical incisions may be used at the interproximal spaces, or the excision may be continued as an envelope flap design.

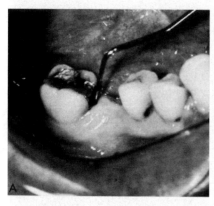
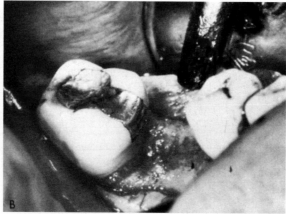
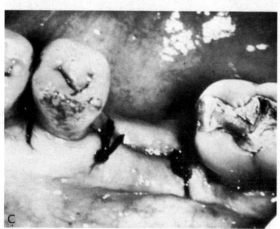
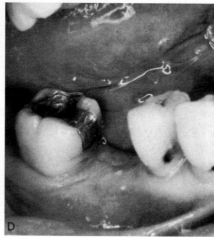

FIGURE 66–6. Flap surgery in edentulous areas. *A,* Pockets adjacent to edentulous region. There is a 6-mm pocket on the mesial aspect of the lower second molar, and additional crown length is required for abutment preparation. *B,* Wedge-shaped tissue removed. The exposed tooth surfaces are root planed, and any necessary osseous recontouring is carried out. *C,* Closure of flaps: lingual view of interrupted sutures used to close the flaps and to hold tissue in an apical position. *D,* Three months after operation. The gingival tissue is established at a more apical level on the tooth. Pocket depth is 2 mm on mesial aspect of second molar. Additional crown length is available for abutment preparation.

cedure also results in the removal of inflamed tissues in the submucosa so that the final tissue has a thin yet dense submucosa bound tightly to the periosteum and covered with an intact keratinized epithelium.

Preprosthetic Periodontal Surgery

Management of Mucogingival Problems. It is often necessary to carry out a free soft tissue autograft in patients who have a mucogingival defect associated with gingival inflammation and require a dental restoration in the immediate environment of the gingiva (Fig. 66–7). The procedure for this free soft tissue autograft is presented in Chapter 59. Mucogingival surgery should be carried out at least 2 months prior to completion of the dental restoration. This allows time for mature tissue to form in the gingival margin so that restorative procedures do not cause a return of clinical inflammation. Augmentation of keratinized gingiva provides stability of the free gingival margin and surrounding gingival tissues so that the dental restoration can be placed in an environment in which gingival health can be maintained.

Crown-Lengthening Procedures. In situations in which a tooth has a short clinical crown that is deemed inadequate for the retention of a required cast restoration, it is necessary to increase the size of the clinical crown using peri-

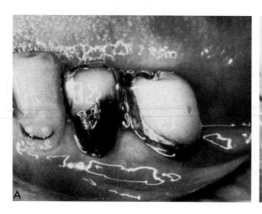
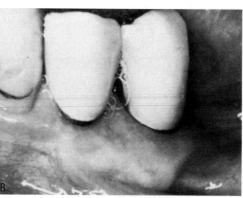

FIGURE 66–7. Mucogingival problems. *A,* Preoperative mucogingival problem. There is inadequate gingiva in the region where a crown margin is to be placed. The presence of a plaque-enhancing margin necessitates the development of an adequate band of gingiva. *B,* Postoperative soft tissue autograft 6 months after mucogingival surgery and placement of restoration. Note the adequate band of gingiva.

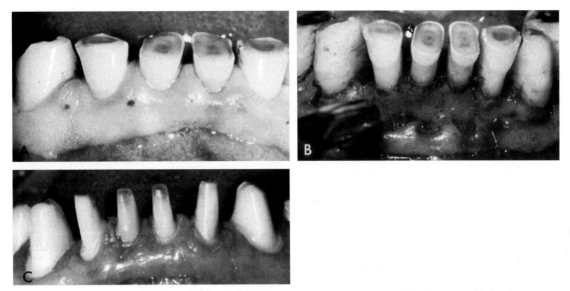

FIGURE 66-8. Crown lengthening using flap surgery. *A,* Before treatment, there are short clinical crowns with inadequate crown length for retention of full crown restorations. *B,* Osseous recontouring has been carried out, with the alveolar crest now positioned apical to original level. *C,* Healing at 6 weeks showing sufficient clinical crowns for preparation of artificial full crowns. (Courtesy of Dr. R. Vandersloot and Dr. I. Logan.)

odontal surgical procedures. These crown-lengthening procedures enable the dentist performing the restoration to develop an adequate area for crown retention without extending the crown margins deep into the periodontal tissues. A gingivectomy technique can be used to eliminate the tissue that forms the pocket or sulcus wall; such tissue may be overgrown (gingival pocket) and may interfere with the intended restorative procedures. This technique will not lengthen the clinical crown, however, except for the minimal area of supracrestal fiber attachment. By definition, the clinical crown is that portion of the tooth that is coronal to the alveolar crest. Therefore, to lengthen it the bone margin has to be remodeled. This is done with an apically displaced flap and osteoectomy (Fig. 66-8), which means that tooth-supporting bone is removed. The removal of bone is usually not necessary all around the tooth but if undertaken should be done with great caution, and no more than what is absolutely necessary should be removed. *It is essential that there be at least 3 mm between the most apical exten-sion of the restoration margin and the alveolar bone crest.* This space allows sufficient room for the supracrestal collagen fibers that are part of the periodontal support mechanism, as well as providing a gingival crevice of 2 to 3 mm. If this guideline is used, the margin of the crown is finally positioned at its correct level, approximately halfway down the gingival crevice. Failure to allow sufficient space between the crown margin and the alveolar crest height means that the finished restoration is positioned deep in the periodontal tissues and results in increased inflammation and pocket formation (Fig. 66-9).

Ridge Augmentation Procedures. These procedures are aimed at correcting the excessive loss of alveolar bone that sometimes occurs in the anterior region as a consequence of advanced periodontal disease, advanced periapical bone loss, traumatic tooth extractions, external trauma, and so forth. This excessive bone loss may create a difficult aesthetic problem and complicate the prosthetic reconstruction. These osseous defects may occur in a coronoapical direc-

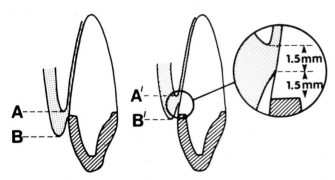

FIGURE 66-9. Guidelines for crown-lengthening procedure. A, Alveolar crest; B, gingival margin; A', level of alveolar crest after surgical crown lengthening; B', level of gingival margin after surgical crown lengthening. Note that crown margins are positioned in the middle of the gingival sulcus. Enlargement shows the crown margin 1.5 mm coronal to the base of the gingival crevice. The alveolar crest is 1.5 mm apical to the base of the gingival crevice.

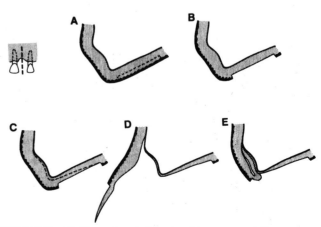

FIGURE 66-10. The roll technique for ridge augmentation.

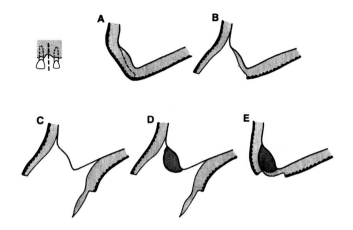

FIGURE 66–11. The double flap for ridge augmentation using hydroxyapatite or a similar material.

tion, in a buccolingual direction, or in both directions simultaneously.[2,7]

Several prosthetic solutions have been proposed for this problem, and the following surgical techniques have been suggested:

1. Placement of a thick mucosal autograft obtained from the palate or the tuberosity.[8,9]
2. Placement of a connective tissue graft beneath a full- or partial-thickness flap[6] or in a "tunnel" created by a lateral incision.[7]
3. The roll technique described by Abrams,[1] which consists of elevating a flap over the deformed area, de-epithelializing its terminal half, and rolling it under the flap, thereby thickening the tissue in the deformed site (Fig. 66–10).
4. Placement of nonporous, dense hydroxyapatite under a split-thickness flap or a pouch created under a full-thickness flap.[3,4]
5. A double flap technique (Fig. 66–11 and Plate XXVI) for use in conjunction with porous hydroxyapatite or other materials to cover the graft while expanding the volume of the area.

Ridge Reduction and Removal of Tori and Exostoses. Sometimes ridges may be too voluminous, or the presence of tori and exostoses may interfere with the prosthetic reconstruction. These areas of excessive osseous tissue are removed with chisels and/or burs after raising a full-thickness flap.

REFERENCES

1. Abrams L. Augmentation of the deformed residual edentulous ridge for fixed prosthesis. Compend Contin Educ Dent *1:*205, 1980.
2. Allen EP, Gainza CS, Farthing GG, Newbold DA. Improved technique for localized ridge augmentation. A report of 21 cases. J Periodontol *56:*195, 1985.
3. Cohen HV. Localized ridge augmentation with hydroxylapatite; report of a case. J Am Dent Assoc *108:*54, 1984.
4. Greenstein GL, Jaffin RA, Hilsen KL, Berman CL. Repair of anterior gingival deformity with Durapatite. A case report. J Periodontol *56:*200, 1985.
5. Kent JL. Reconstruction of the alveolar ridge with hydroxyapatite. Dent Clin North Am *30:*231, 1986.
6. Langer B, Calagna L. The subepithelial connective tissue graft. J Prosthet Dent *44:*363, 1980.
7. Miller PD Jr. Ridge augmentation under existing fixed prosthesis. A simplified technique. J Periodontol *57:*742, 1986.
8. Seibert J. Reconstruction of deformed partially edentulous ridges using full thickness grafts. I. Technique and wound healing. Compend Contin Educ Dent *4:*437, 1983.
9. Seibert J. Reconstruction of deformed partially edentulous ridges using full thickness grafts. II. Prosthodontic/periodontal interrelationships. Compend Contin Educ

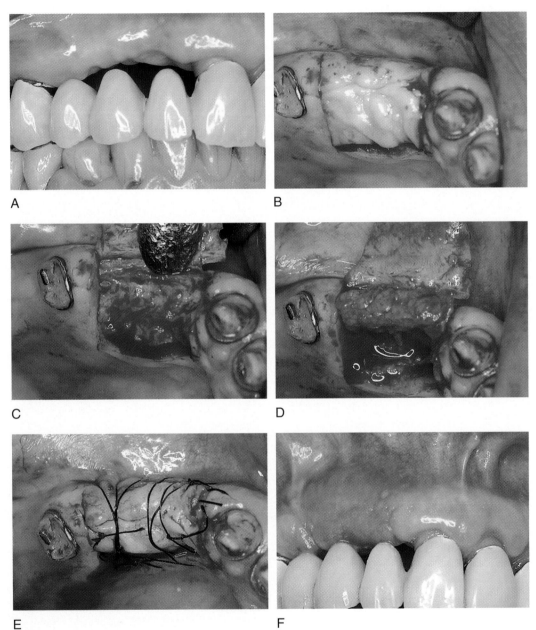

PLATE XXVI. Technique for ridge augmentation. *A,* Temporary bridge over edentulous space. *B,* Flap incision, occlusal view. Note that gingival areas are not involved. *C,* Split-level flap elevated. *D,* Connective tissue obtained from thinning of palatal flap is placed on facial and occlusal areas to augment the ridge. *E,* Flap sutured back in place. Note that there is a gap on the palatal side as a result of the increased tissue volume under the flap. *F,* Healing after 3 months, with temporary bridge in place. Note the improved contour and fuller ridge in comparison with *A.* (Courtesy of Dr. Robert Azzi.)

67

Periodontal-Restorative Interrelationships

MICHAEL K. McGUIRE

Dental restorations and periodontal health are inseparably interrelated. The adaptation of the margins, the contours of the restoration, the proximal relationships, and the surface smoothness have a critical biologic impact on the gingiva and supporting periodontal tissues. Dental restorations therefore play a significant role in maintaining periodontal health.

In addition to cosmetic enhancement, fixed and removable prostheses serve many purposes, including the improvement of masticatory efficiency and speech, the prevention of food impaction, and the prevention of tilting and extrusion of teeth with resultant disruption of the occlusion.

OCCLUSAL ADJUSTMENT BEFORE RESTORATIVE CARE

Traumatic occlusal relationships should be eliminated before restorative procedures are begun, and restorations should be constructed in conformity with the newly established occlusal patterns. If this is not done, the prosthesis will perpetuate occlusal relationships injurious to the periodontium.

The harmful effects of occlusal trauma are not confined to the teeth involved in the restoration and their antagonists. Other areas of the dentition are secondarily affected by an occlusal disharmony created or perpetuated by an inlay or bridge. A delay in occlusal adjustment until the restorations are inserted may interfere with the diagnosis of the perioprosthetic status and result in over- or undertreatment. It may also result in the clinicians grinding through the occlusal surface of the newly created restoration.

The occlusion must be checked at regular intervals after a prosthesis is inserted. Occlusal relationships change with time as the result of micromovement of the natural denti-

tion, wear of restorative materials, and settling of free-end edentulous areas of removable prostheses.

A hard acrylic biteguard should be constructed for all patients with parafunctional habits. The destructive forces created by these parafunctional habits have the potential to destroy restorations, create cervical abrasion, and contribute to the progression of periodontal disease.

Accurate maxillary and mandibular models should be mounted in centric jaw relation. Eccentric jaw records should be utilized to more accurately equilibrate the bite appliance on the articulator. Heat-processed clear acrylic facilitates the fabrication of a durable hygienic and functional appliance. Occlusion should be refined so that bilateral simultaneous contact in centric relation is achieved. Excursive movements should be balanced to allow for dissipation of occlusal forces throughout the appliance. This reduces the untoward effects of the parafunctional habits mentioned earlier. It does not eliminate all of the effects of primary occlusal trauma, however, and behavior modification may be helpful.

FIXED PROSTHODONTICS

Direct Resin Restorations

The combination composite resin and acid etching technique introduced in the 1950s and 1960s by Bowen[6] and Buonocore[8] ushered in a new era for the dental practitioner. Advances in resin manufacturing technology have created third-generation composites with the versatility needed in the demanding field of cosmetic and perioprosthetic dentistry. Direct hybrid resins afford the practitioner a cosmetically and structurally sound way of restoring the dentition to its proper form and function. Composite resin techniques have simplified provisional and long-term alterations of natural tooth surfaces. This allows the practitioner to readily modify embrasure design and interproximal contact/contour, as in diastema closure and occlusal deficiencies. Surface smoothness and durability are important when considering direct resin as a means of therapy. Resins are highly polishable but have deficiencies in strength, porosity, and wear.

Successful tissue response to indirect resin veneers or any composite material depends on many variables. Surface smoothness, an important variable, can be altered significantly if the restorations are finished incorrectly. Also influencing success are the type of composite material, the proximity of the restoration to the soft tissue, whether light curing was complete, and whether air bubbles were incorporated during placement. Soft tissue inflammatory response to resins may not show up initially, because restorations that initially had smooth surfaces may become rough as air bubbles that were incorporated during mixing become exposed.

Organic compounds found in toothpastes, plaque, food, and beverages can soften any composite material or resin cement, resulting in surface roughness and plaque retention. For these and other reasons, clinicians must impress on patients their responsibility in keeping composite restorations free of plaque.

Indirect Resin and Porcelain Restorations

State-of-the-art restorative dentistry realized the long-term inadequacies of many direct-bonded restorations and began research in indirect fabrication of prosthetic solutions to perioprosthetic dilemmas. Cast Rochette resin–bonded restorations provide durable, well-fitting, refined alternatives to "splinting" and full-coverage veneer splinting. Laboratory-prepared porcelain restorations offer a more biocompatible alternative to direct-bonded restorations. They are both aesthetically and marginally superior and provide the integrity that is essential in treating the long-term perioprosthetically compromised patient.

Glass ceramics and porcelain veneers offer a clear advantage over any other type of restorative material in the maintenance of gingival health. Their fine marginal fit results in a thin cement line, which lessens gingival irritation. In addition, the nonporous surface of glass ceramics or porcelain does not allow bacteria to adhere significantly, thus reducing inflammation.

Tooth Preparation in Relation to the Gingival Margin

The first requirement for proper location of the gingival margin of a crown or other restoration close to the gingiva is a healthy gingival sulcus. Periodontal preparation is not complete until the gingiva is healthy and dimensionally stable. Periodontal pockets should not be permitted to remain undisturbed for the ostensible purposes of "keeping the root covered" or "hiding the margins of the restorations." When the periodontal disease is resolved, as it eventually must be, the denuded root and margins of the restoration that were hidden by the inflamed gingiva become visible. In the interim, the patient has suffered unnecessary destruction of

the periodontium, and the longevity of the tooth and the restoration has been jeopardized.

Periodontal therapy, final tooth preparation, and impression-making procedures should not be attempted in one procedure, for this does not allow time for the gingiva to heal, and the location of the margin of the restoration in relation to the healed gingival sulcus can only be estimated.

Dental restorations should be kept away from the gingiva whenever possible. Extension of cavity margins into the gingival sulcus should occur only if there is a definite indication for introduction of restorative materials into the subgingival environment. If the restorative margin is placed subgingivally, it is more difficult for the patient's oral hygiene procedures to control the bacteria that colonize this area.

There are some clinical situations in which the operator must carry the margin of the restoration into the gingival sulcus. These include the existence of a previous restoration extending into the subgingival area, the presence of caries that extend apically into the gingival environment, apical extension to obtain retention of the restoration, and the advantage of subgingival placement on the labial surface of upper anterior teeth in patients for whom aesthetics is of primary importance.

After a decision has been made to place restorative dental materials into the gingival crevice, the level at which the margin should be placed is of critical importance. It is advisable to keep the restorations in the coronal half of the gingival crevice. This allows better access to the margin for oral hygiene procedures and gives better exposure for refining the margin during cavity preparation and impression making.

The dentist should be aware that placing a margin in the gingival crevice at the time of completion of a restoration will not guarantee that the relationship of the gingiva to the margin will be maintained. Movement of the gingival margin over time cannot be reliably predicted.

The position of the gingival margin should be relatively stable in patients who have an adequate amount of keratinized tissue without parafunctional habits and who have an acceptable level of oral hygiene associated with a nontraumatic toothbrushing technique. All clinical signs of gingival inflammation should be resolved before final restorations are initiated, because shrinkage of the gingiva during its resolution results in a more apically positioned gingival margin.

When a subgingival margin is indicated, the operator must be careful to place the margin within the limits of the sulcus. This directive is counter to many restorative concepts promulgated in the past. Even the term *subgingival margin* leads one to believe that placement of the restoration's margin anywhere between the free gingival margin and the alveolar crest is acceptable. Studies have demonstrated that a space of approximately 2 mm is needed for supracrestal connective tissue attachment and for junctional epithelium to attach to the tooth.[34] This 2-mm band is a physiologic dimension that is required around every tooth in the mouth. This constant has been labeled the *biologic width.* If the restoration infringes on or eliminates the biologic width, there is no place for the attachment apparatus to insert. An inflammatory response results, attachment loss with apical migration occurs, and pocket formation ensues.

A crown-lengthening procedure is indicated prior to restoration.

The full crown is extremely useful because it fulfills requirements that can be met by no other type of restoration (Fig. 67–1). However, even when ideally constructed in relation to the gingival sulcus, the full crown introduces the risk of gingival inflammation. Crowns substitute a foreign substance (e.g., gold, resin, or porcelain) for the natural tooth wall of the gingival sulcus. The materials themselves are not irritating, but plaque can accumulate on these surfaces, which can result in gingival inflammation. The junction of the crown and the tooth also presents a problem. Even with a perfect marginal fit, an extremely thin cement line that attracts plaque[49] is unavoidable.

The risk of irritation to the gingiva is reduced by restorations that terminate coronal to the free gingival margin[49,53] (Fig. 67–2). Whenever possible, inlays,[48] pinledges, and three-quarter crowns should be used as individual restorations. This is not a matter of substituting other restorations for purposes that can be fulfilled only by crowns. However, when there is a choice and high caries incidence is not a problem, the gingival third of the tooth should not be involved in the restoration.

Gingival Management for Making Impressions

When using elastic impression materials, it is often necessary to retract the gingiva to gain access to the gingival finish line of the preparation; two methods for accomplishing this are described. These retraction methods should be used only on healthy gingiva. They should not be used for the removal, displacement, or shrinkage of inflamed, swollen gingival tissue. The gingiva must be healthy and its position on the tooth stabilized before the impression is made.

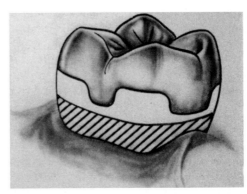

FIGURE 67–2. Avoiding the gingival third. A hypothetical inlay constructed without involving the gingival third of the crown.

Retraction Cord. Cords impregnated with agents are most commonly used for gingival retraction. Among the types of agents used for this purpose are vasoconstrictors (8% racemic epinephrine),[21] which may cause rapid transient elevation in blood pressure and blood glucose concentration and are contraindicated in patients with coronary disease, hyperthyroidism, or diabetes. They also produce local ischemia, which may be injurious to the gingiva. Also used are 8% zinc chloride astringents, 10% tannic acid, and 10% aluminum sulfate. Properly placed cords impregnated with these agents cause lateral displacement and transient dehydration of the gingiva, exposing the finish line of the preparation. The gingiva ordinarily returns to its proper position, provided it was healthy at the outset. Treated retraction cords should be left in the sulcus no longer than suggested by the manufacturer.

Improper placement and removal of retraction cords can result in tissue tearing and inflammation. If the cords are dry,[2] the epithelial lining of the gingival sulcus will adhere to the dry cord and will be torn when the cord is removed prior to taking impressions. The resultant immediate hemorrhage into the area of the gingival sulcus will prevent the operator from making an accurate impression (Fig. 67–3). The operator should moisten retraction cords with saline while they remain in the gingival crevice to limit tearing of the epithelium.

There have been reports of periodontal abscesses associated with impression material and/or retraction cord left in the gingival environment after the making of impressions.[37,42] Immediately after an impression is made, it should be carefully checked for pieces that may have been torn from it and left in the gingival environment. The gingival sulcus should also be inspected carefully for residual impression material.

Electrosurgery. Electrosurgery may be used for gingival management in some situations in which access to finish lines is not available by more conservative methods. It should be carried out so as to minimize tissue damage, and the current should be adapted so that electrosection is used rather than coagulation. The use of equipment that provides a fully rectified current and an undamped waveform results in the least amount of tissue damage.[27] Several studies have shown that careful use of electrosurgery in the superficial part of the gingival crevice results in little, if any, residual damage to the gingiva.[3,11] Reports have emphasized the dangers of electrosurgery when the cutting instrument is al-

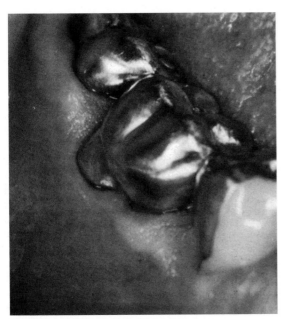

FIGURE 67–1. Tooth contour restored by crown. Note the excellent condition of the gingiva in the furcation area.

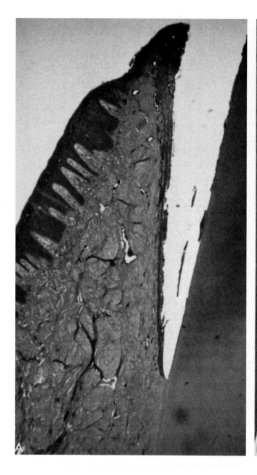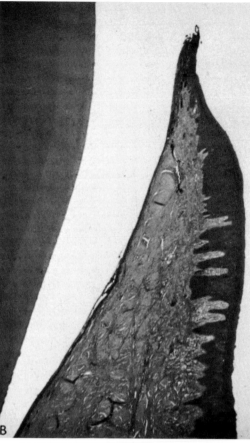

FIGURE 67-3. Gingival response to retraction cords. *A,* Photomicrograph of gingival sulcus region in a dog after removal of a gingival retraction cord that had been placed in the sulcus for 7 minutes. In this case the cord was dried before placement, and the sulcus was air dried during the time the cord was in place and removed dry. Note the tearing of the sulcular epithelium and the initial acute inflammatory reaction in the connective tissue of the gingiva, with dilatation of blood vessels. There is evidence of bleeding into the gingival crevice. *B,* Photomicrograph of gingival sulcus region in a dog after removal of a gingival retraction cord that had been placed in the sulcus for 7 minutes. In this case the cord was moistened with saline before placement, and the gingival sulcus was bathed with saline during the time the cord was in place. Note the intact epithelium, the absence of acute inflammation, and the lack of hemorrhage.

lowed to be in close proximity to the base of the crevice and cementum.[37,59] In patients with a thin covering of gingiva and alveolar bone over the root, electrosurgery should not be used, as the loss of tissue from the internal or crevicular surface can result in gingival recession.[45] In these patients the gingiva should be retracted with retraction cords (Fig. 67–4).

Interim Coverage

Improperly constructed "interim" restorations may cause periodontal inflammation and gingival recession.[15] All interim restorations should be constructed so that they cause no trauma to the gingiva during the time they are in the mouth. The requirements for fit, polish, and contour in the interim restoration should be the same as for the final restoration. The marginal integrity of interim restorations should be as good as is technically possible, and the surfaces of these interim restorations should be highly polished so that plaque accumulation is minimized. The contour of these restorations should also be compatible with the gingival tissues.

Long-term restorations should not be called temporary but should be regarded as provisional or treatment restorations that may remain in place for many months. Provisional or treatment restorations allow the dentist to assess the effect of the final restoration. They can also act as a surgical guide for the periodontist to create proper crown length, and they are important in ridge augmentation procedures. The contour of the restorations, the occlusal pattern, and the patient's oral hygiene procedures may be modified while provisional restorations are in place so that optimal periodontal health is obtained. The final restorations can duplicate the provisional restorations, providing some certainty about the long-term effect of the restorations on the periodontium (Fig. 67–5).

The Embrasures

When teeth are in proximal contact, the spaces that widen out from the contact are known as *embrasures.* Each interdental space has four embrasures: a facial embrasure; a lingual embrasure (Fig. 67–6); an occlusal or incisal embrasure that is coronal to the contact area (Fig. 67–7A); and a gingival embrasure, which is the space between the contact area and the alveolar bone.[7,58] In the healthy state, the gingival embrasure is filled with soft tissue, but periodontal diseases (Fig. 67–7B) may result in attachment loss, creating open gingival embrasures.

The Gingival Embrasure. Embrasures are critical considerations in restorative dentistry. Proximal surfaces of dental restorations are important, because they create the embrasures essential for gingival health (Fig. 67–8). From a periodontal viewpoint, the gingival embrasure is the most significant.

Periodontal diseases cause tissue destruction, which reduces the level of the alveolar bone, increases the size of the gingival embrasure, and creates open interdental space. Restorations may be constructed to preserve the morphologic features of the crown and root and retain the enlarged

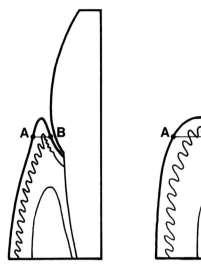

FIGURE 67–4. Electrosurgery for retraction. The use of electrosurgery in patients in whom the gingival tissue is thin buccolingually (i.e., A–B on the left diagram) will result in destruction of almost all the gingival tissue, causing postoperative gingival recession. In these situations retraction cords are the method of choice for obtaining access to the gingival margins. When a thick covering of gingiva is present (i.e., A–B on the right diagram), it is possible to use electrosurgical techniques for gingival retraction.

embrasure and the open interdental space (Fig. 67–9A,B), or, when aesthetic situations dictate, the teeth may be reshaped by the restorations so that the gingival embrasures are relocated close to the new level of the gingiva.

To relocate the gingival embrasure, the dentist changes the contour of the proximal surfaces and broadens the contact areas more apically (Fig. 67–9C). The interdental gingiva assumes its normal shape by filling the new embrasure provided for it, which must be adequate in all dimensions. Although the operator may choose to diminish the gingival embrasure size either because of aesthetic demands or because of requirements for fixed partial denture connectors, this should be done with extreme care.

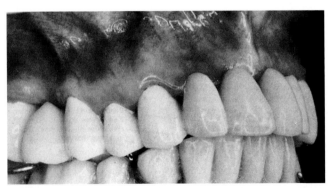

FIGURE 67–5. Provisional restorations. Provisional restorations provide an opportunity to evaluate the patient's response to the final restorations. The aesthetics can be modified, but more importantly, the contour of the restorations can be changed so that the gingival tissues can be kept healthy. When previous restorations have caused gingival inflammation, a provisional restoration provides an environment for the gingiva to return to health. These restorations should be made of resin, have accurate marginal adaptation, and be contoured and polished to duplicate the form of the natural teeth. (Courtesy of Dr. John Flocken.)

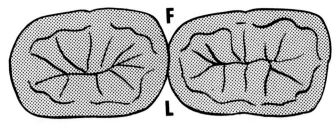

FIGURE 67–6. Occlusal view of mandibular molars showing facial (F) and lingual (L) embrasures.

The following dimensions of the gingival embrasure are important to the preservation of gingival health:

Height: The distance between the contact area and the bone margin (Fig. 67–10A). When the contact area is too close to the cervical line of the tooth, the embrasure is shortened.

Width: The distance mesiodistally between the proximal surfaces (Fig. 67–10B).

Depth: The distance faciolingually from the contact area to a line joining the proximofacial or proximolingual angles (Fig. 67–10C).

The proximal surfaces of crowns should taper away from the contact area facially, lingually, and apically. Excessively broad proximal contact areas and bulky contour in the cervical region crowd out the gingival papillae. This can make oral hygiene difficult, resulting in gingival inflammation and attachment loss (Fig. 67–11).

Restorative dental procedures too often result in the restorative materials taking up space that is normally occupied by the interdental papilla. The problem begins with underpreparation of the tooth, so that the technician is left with no choice except to place an excessive amount of restorative material into the interproximal space. During the preparation of dies for cast restorations, the technician first removes all of the replicated gingival tissue to gain access

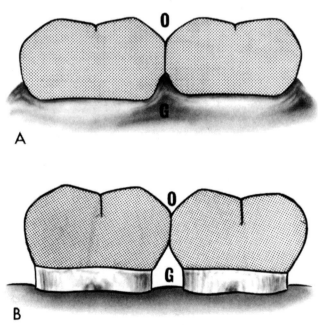

FIGURE 67–7. Occlusal (O) and gingival (G) embrasures. *A,* Interdental gingiva fills gingival embrasure (G). *B,* Open gingival embrasure (G) in patient with periodontal disease.

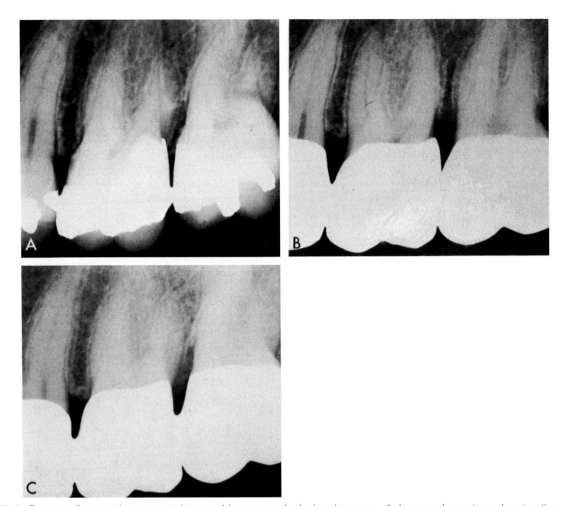

FIGURE 67–8. Contour of restoration corrected to provide proper gingival embrasures. *A,* Improperly contoured restorations on the molars; the gingival embrasure is too narrow. *B,* New restorations; the gingival embrasure between the molars is now wider at its base but too narrow beneath the contact area. *C,* Proper gingival embrasure created by widening the space beneath the molar contact area.

to the finish lines. Thus, it is impossible for him or her to visualize the space available for dental restoration in the interproximal embrasure area. If two models are poured from the same impression and the second one is used as an indi-

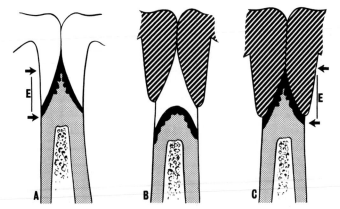

FIGURE 67–9. Relocation of the gingival embrasure. *A,* Normal gingival embrasure (E) filled with gingival tissue. *B,* Space created in gingival embrasure by periodontal disease and restorations constructed to retain the space. *C,* Restorations constructed to move the gingival embrasure (E) close to the gingiva by recontouring the proximal surfaces and locating the contact area further apically.

cator of how much space is currently occupied by the gingival tissues, the technician can have a much better understanding of what the contour of the final restorations should be.

In fixed prostheses and/or multiunit fixed splints, the interproximal connect and/or soldered joint is frequently carried too far apically and so invades the embrasure space from its coronal aspect. This crowding also results in inadequate space for the interdental gingiva and leads to inflammation and destruction of the periodontal tissues (Fig. 67–12).

The responsibility for determining the size of the interproximal connect should rest with the dentist, not the technician. Frequently the technician decides the position and size of the soldered joint without being aware of how much gingival tissue is present in the interproximal embrasure. In patients whose gingival tissue fully occupies the embrasure space, encroachment on this space by restorative materials can be a significant problem.

In patients in whom the interdental papilla has receded, the problem of encroachment into the space is minimized. The principles that determine the size and form of the soldered joint apply equally to the size and form of contact points associated with all interproximal restorations (Fig.

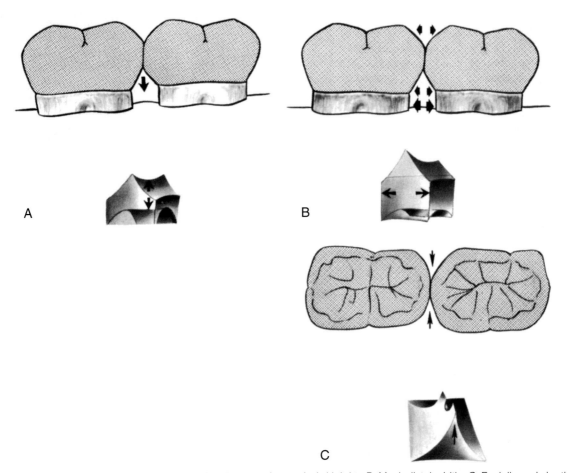

FIGURE 67–10. Dimensions of the gingival embrasure *(arrows)*. *A,* Height. *B,* Mesiodistal width. *C,* Faciolingual depth.

67–13). A tissue transfer model may facilitate correct embrasure design for the technician.

Contours of Restorations

The facial and lingual contours of restorations are also important in the preservation of gingival health. The most common error in re-creating the contours of the tooth in dental restorations is overcontouring of the facial and lingual surfaces. In one study approximately 80% of full gold crowns were wider than the tooth they were replacing, and all porcelain-bonded-to-metal crowns were too wide buccolingually.[39] This overcontouring generally occurs in the gingival third of the crown and results in an area in which oral hygiene procedures are unable to control plaque. Consequently, plaque accumulates, and the gingiva becomes inflamed.

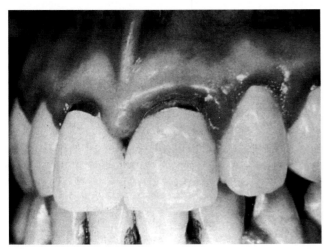

FIGURE 67–11. Inadequate gingival embrasures contribute to periodontal disease.

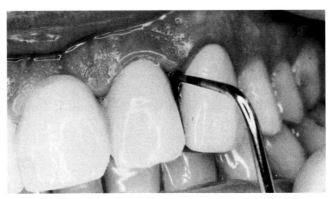

FIGURE 67–12. Excessive contact area. Soldered joint carried too far apically. The periodontal probe is at the apical level of the soldered joint. There is a 7-mm pocket in the adjacent interproximal periodontium.

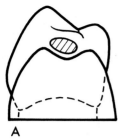 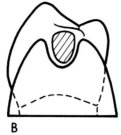

FIGURE 67–13. Size and shape of contact areas. *A,* Correct shape of soldered joint or contact area. *B,* Incorrect shape with excessive apical extension of soldered joint or contact area. The gingival col is disrupted, and the interproximal tissue is forced to take on a structure in which the buccal and lingual portions of the papilla are split. This interproximal tissue is less able to remain healthy because of its form and because of the inaccessibility of the midproximal gingival sulcus region to oral hygiene procedures.

Apparently, undercontouring is not nearly as damaging to the gingiva as overcontouring. Evidence from studies in animals and humans demonstrates that overcontouring is a significant factor in gingival inflammation,[27,29,40,46,61] whereas undercontouring has little, if any, effect on gingival health[25,40] (Fig. 67–14).

Overcontouring on the buccal or labial surfaces frequently occurs in porcelain-bonded-to-metal crowns because of the technician's attempt to obtain a thickness of porcelain adequate to mask the underlying metal and provide the most aesthetic appearance. Frequently the technician has no choice but to put excess porcelain in this area, as tooth preparation has been inadequate. It is important to remove enough tooth material to allow adequate width for the metal and porcelain so that the resulting crowns do not bulge beyond the space normally occupied by the anatomic crown of the tooth. A minimum space of 1.5 mm is required.

In patients in whom periodontal disease causes the gingival margin to be in a much more apical position than it was during health, the facial and lingual contours become even more significant. In these cases, the bulge on the facial contour of the crown, which normally would be subgingival, appears supragingivally.

This makes the portion of the exposed root immediately apical to the bulge less accessible for oral hygiene, with resultant plaque accumulation and gingival inflammation. In

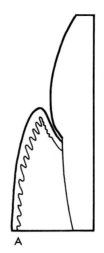 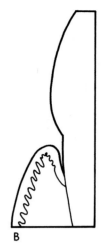 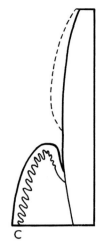

FIGURE 67–15. Facial contour of crowns in relation to gingiva. *A,* The gingival margin is normally coronal to the facial bulge of the anatomic crown. *B,* When the gingiva recedes, it is overprotected by the contour of the crown, and plaque accumulation is thus facilitated. *C,* The crown of the tooth is reshaped so that the gingiva is accessible for proper oral hygiene procedures. This should be carried out in areas where gingival recession is associated with gingival inflammation.

these cases it is frequently necessary to replace existing restorations. This problem is especially important in the area of the facial furcations of maxillary and mandibular molars and in the area of the lingual furcations of mandibular molars (Fig. 67–15).

If the furcation has been exposed by periodontal surgical procedures or by gingival recession, it is important that the restoration be contoured in such a way as to facilitate access for oral hygiene. In these cases, it is important to em-

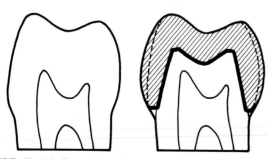

FIGURE 67–14. Buccolingual crown contours. Overcontouring of crowns in the buccolingual dimension is frequently due to inadequate removal of dentin during cavity preparation. The original contour of the tooth in the left diagram cannot be reproduced in the crown (*hatched area in the right diagram*), because there is not enough space for porcelain and metal in the gingival third.

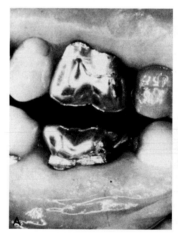 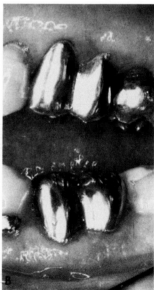

FIGURE 67–16. Recontouring of crowns in periodontally involved teeth. *A,* Preoperative photograph of molar region. There were 6-mm pockets interproximally between the molars and a class I furcation involvement of both upper and lower first molars. *B,* After periodontal surgery, the crowns have been replaced by crowns with accentuated grooves in the furcation region. Note the development of pyramidal gingiva in the mid-facial region.

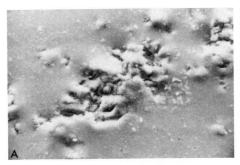 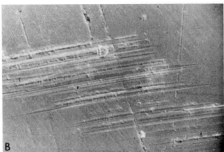 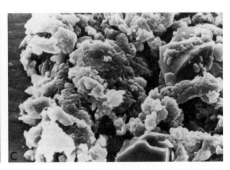

FIGURE 67–17. Surface of restorations. *A,* Scanning electron micrograph of surface of vacuum-fired porcelain (×1100). Note the irregular surface with roughness of approximately 1 microinch. *B,* Scanning electron micrograph of cast gold restoration (×1100). The surface was given a final polish with rouge on a felt wheel. The surface irregularities are approximately 1 microinch. *C,* Scanning electron micrograph of composite restoration (×1100). Note the extreme irregularity of the surface, which would facilitate plaque accumulation.

phasize the mid-facial groove of the crown so that this groove is confluent with the furcation. It is equally important to remove the apical bulge of the restoration, thereby eliminating any plaque traps apical to the cemento-enamel junction (Fig. 67–16).

The Occlusal Surface

Occlusal surfaces should be designed to direct masticatory forces along the long axis of the teeth. They should restore occlusal dimensions and cuspal contours in harmony with the remainder of the natural dentition after occlusal abnormalities have been eliminated by occlusal adjustment. The anatomy of the occlusal surface should provide well-formed marginal ridges and occlusal sluiceways to prevent interproximal food impaction.

The Effect of Surface Finish of Restorative Materials on the Periodontium

The surface of restorations should be as smooth as possible to limit plaque accumulation. Roughened tooth and restoration surfaces in the subgingival region result in increased plaque accumulation and increased gingival inflammation.[26,50,55]

In the clinical situation, porcelain, highly polished gold, and highly polished resin all result in similar plaque accumulation.[9,24,41] There is evidence in dogs that porcelain may accumulate less plaque than gold. This may be due to differences in the inherent properties of these materials, but the surface roughness seems to be the most important factor in humans[9] (Fig. 67–17).

The exact relationship between the degree of surface roughness and plaque accumulation is as yet undetermined. There is evidence that the amount of plaque that accumulates in patients with relatively poor oral hygiene is not affected to a significant degree by minor changes in root surface configuration.[44] In patients with rough dental restorations, however, the surface configuration may play an important role in plaque accumulation.[28,57] Therefore, all restorative materials placed in the gingival environment should have the highest possible polish.

Pontic Design

A pontic should meet the following requirements: it should (1) be aesthetically acceptable; (2) provide occlusal relationships that are favorable to the abutment teeth, opposing teeth, and remainder of the dentition; (3) restore the masticatory effectiveness of the tooth it replaces; (4) be designed to minimize accumulation of irritating dental plaque and food debris and to maximize access for cleansing by the patient; and (5) provide embrasures for the passage of food.

Plaque, which causes inflammation of the mucosa under pontics and the gingiva around abutment teeth, tends to accumulate around fixed prostheses if a special effort is not undertaken to keep them clean. The health of the tissues around fixed prostheses depends primarily on the patient's oral hygiene; the materials with which pontics are constructed appear to make little difference, and pontic design is important only to the extent that it enables the patient to keep the area clean. Plaque accumulates to an equal degree under pontics made of glazed and unglazed porcelain,[21] polished gold, and polished acrylic resin,[42,52] even though the surfaces of the latter two are smoother.[9]

The principles of contours of crowns apply equally to pontics, but with pontics there is an additional concern associated with the contour of the tissue-facing surface. In general, this surface should be kept as convex as possible, and all concavities should be eliminated. The convexity of the tissue surfaces of pontics allows oral hygiene procedures to be effective in keeping the tissue of the edentulous ridge healthy. Concavities in the tissue surfaces of pontics result in plaque trap areas where accumulation of dental bacteria leads to inflammation of the adjacent edentulous tissues (Figs. 67–18 to 67–21).

The *ovate pontic* (Fig. 67–22) is the most hygienic type with the best patient acceptance. The proximal surfaces are tapered to create embrasures between adjoining pontics for self-cleansing passage of food, for stimulation of the edentulous mucosa by food excursion, and for cleansing with toothbrush and dental floss. Tapering should also re-create embrasures adjacent to the abutment teeth that approach the shape and dimension of the natural embrasure to protect the marginal gingiva (see Fig. 67–21). In anterior segments, where aesthetics is a primary consideration, a receptor site can be surgically created in the gingiva for the ovate pontic to rest in. This relatively simple procedure can create the illusion of a free gingival margin and interdental papillae, resulting in the most natural look of all pontics.

Prior to widespread use of the ovate pontic, the *modified ridge-lap design* was considered the most aesthetic (Fig.

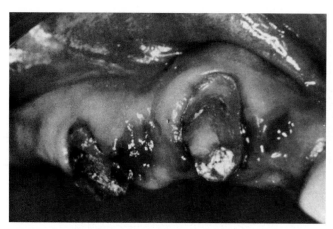

FIGURE 67–18. Consequences of poor pontic design. Chronic inflammation of edentulous mucosa under bridge with ridge-lap type pontic.

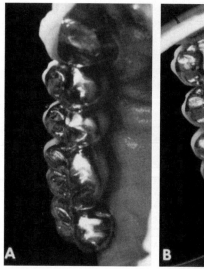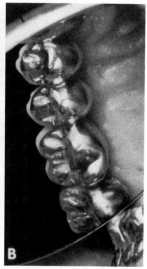

FIGURE 67–20. Replacement of ridge-lap pontics by properly contoured pontics leads to resolution of mucosal inflammation. *A,* Properly shaped pontics inserted in the area previously covered by pontics. Note the inflammation where the ridge-lap pontics had been. *B,* After several months, note the excellent condition of the mucosa under the properly contoured pontics.

67–23). This pontic design has a convex tissue-facing surface, and the tip of the pontic passively contacts the edentulous mucosa. Casts should not be scraped or scored in an attempt to seat the pontic into the mucosa, as this creates a depression around the pontic that makes access for plaque removal difficult. The pontic follows the facial contour of the ridge to the crest, where it joins the lingual surface. The lingual surface of the pontic should follow the normal tooth form for a distance of approximately half its occlusogingival length and should then taper in a convex line to meet the facial portion at the crest of the ridge.[60]

The pontic design with the least effect on the periodontium is the *sanitary* or *hygienic pontic* (Fig. 67–24). This pontic should be designed so that there is at least a 3-mm space between the undersurface of the pontic and the edentulous ridge, allowing the tongue and cheeks to remove any food particles that may lodge in this area. It is often necessary to use a design other than the hygienic pontic for aesthetic reasons.

Ridge-lap pontics, which straddle the ridge and have a concave tissue-facing surface, are the least desirable design and should be avoided. Ridge-lap pontics make it impossible for the patient to control plaque and inevitably result in inflammation of the tissues with which they are in contact.

The natural teeth should guide the design of the occlusal surface of pontics. The width of the occlusal surface should be narrowed to less than that of the tooth being replaced. This reduction in the buccolingual dimension reduces lateral stresses to the bridge and decreases the chances for working/nonworking interferences.

Abnormally shaped spaces between pontics that have been overly narrowed and broad proximal surfaces of adjacent natural teeth may create food impaction problems (Fig. 67–25). An adequate occlusal width is also necessary to shunt the food laterally so that it is not forced into the tissue around the base of the pontic.

The functional relationships of the cusps are the most critical consideration in the design of the occlusal surface of pontics. The cusps should be in harmony with the functional pattern of the entire dentition. Abnormal occlusal re-

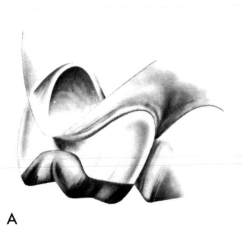

A

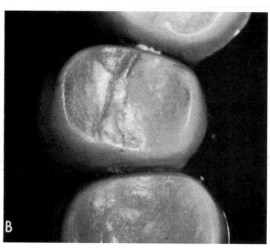

B

FIGURE 67–19. Ridge-lap pontics. *A,* Diagrammatic view of ridge-lap pontic in position. *B,* Undersurface of ridge-lap pontic. Note that the contours that conform to the surface of the underlying mucosa trap food debris.

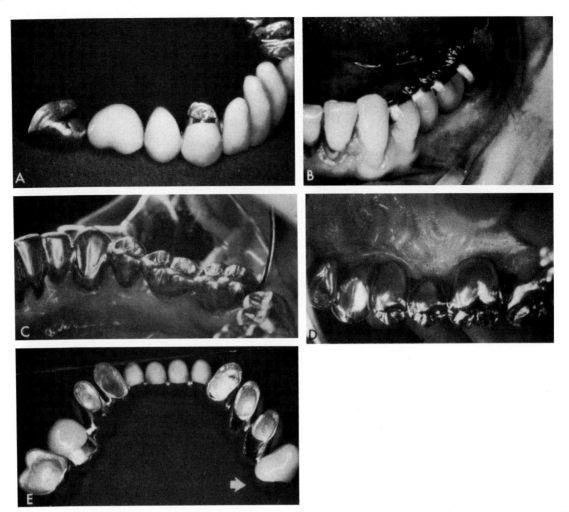

FIGURE 67-21. Proper pontic design. *A,* Ovate anterior and posterior pontics. *B,* Healthy gingiva and edentulous mucosa with ovate pontics. *C,* Lingual view showing spaces required between the pontics and the natural teeth. Note anatomic reconstruction of the occlusal surface of the pontics. *D,* Healthy gingiva and mucosa in relation to properly contoured second premolar pontic. Note the inflammation between the first premolar and canine associated with inadequate gingival embrasure. *E,* Pontics with properly constructed modified ridge-lap design. Note the cantilevered pontic (*arrow*).

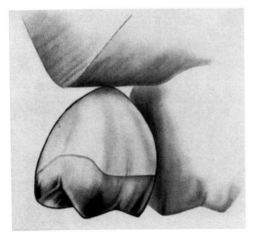

FIGURE 67-22. In the past, ovate pontics were constructed so that they lightly touched the residual ridge, as depicted in the drawing. Currently, ovate pontics resting in gingival receptor sites are often used in anterior regions because of their aesthetic appeal.

lationships jeopardize the opposing teeth and the remainder of the dentition, as well as the periodontium of the abutment teeth.

Cementation

During cementation it is important that the restoration be seated as close to the tooth preparation as possible. A minimal cement line at the margin reduces plaque formation.

It is extremely important that all excess cement be removed from the sulcus after cementation. Retained cement particles can cause gingival inflammation. Removal of cement from the interproximal joints of pontics and abutments can be facilitated by lightly coating the exterior surfaces of the prosthesis with petroleum jelly or disclosing wax prior to cementation.

Restoring the Furcated or Resected Tooth

Mandibular Molars. The most dependable way to restore mandibular molars is to use the hemisection approach,

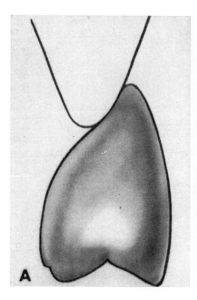

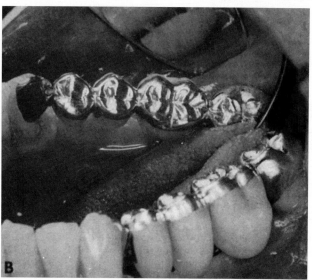

FIGURE 67–23. Modified ridge-lap pontic for aesthetics. *A,* Pontic extended onto the facial aspects of the edentulous ridge. *B,* Modified ridge-lap pontics. Note the excellent condition of the periodontium.

in which the tooth is cut in half through the crown (see Chapter 59). Root canal therapy is necessary on the retained portions of the molar. In some situations it is possible to retain both portions of the hemisected tooth, whereas in other situations half of the tooth will have to be extracted because of advanced periodontal destruction.

If both parts of the tooth are to be retained, it is essential that an adequate embrasure space be created between the two halves of the tooth. All too often, when teeth are hemisected, the resulting restoration is detrimental to periodontal health because the embrasure space is too narrow. The amount of space between the roots should be evaluated preoperatively. An inadequate amount of interradicular bone is a contraindication for hemisection. It is therefore important that when hemisected teeth are prepared for restorative procedures, adequate tooth material is removed in the areas between the roots, so that a wide embrasure space is constructed, which will allow passage of an oral hygiene de-

vice (Fig. 67–26). The two segments of the hemisected mandibular molar should be regarded much the same as two premolar teeth; thus, adequate space must be created between their roots for an interdental papilla and functional periodontal fibers.

When a mandibular molar is hemisected and one portion

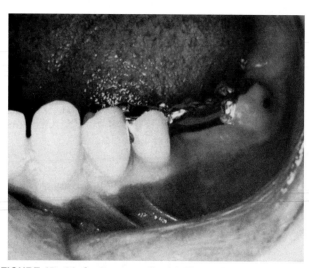

FIGURE 67–24. Sanitary-type fixed bridge with healthy gingiva.

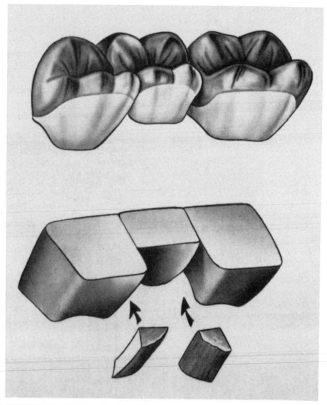

FIGURE 67–25. Occlusal width of pontics. *Top,* Pontic with narrow occlusal width creates food impaction problems. *Bottom,* Occlusal width required to provide proper proximal relations between pontic and adjacent teeth.

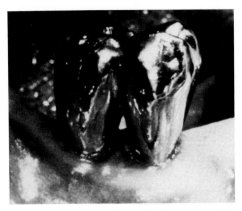

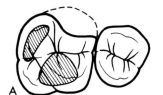
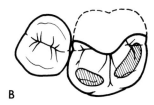

FIGURE 67–28. Crown contours for root-resected maxillary molars. *A,* Mesiobuccal root amputation. Distobuccal and palatal root areas are shaded; original crown contours are shown by *dashed line.* The modified crown contours allow access for oral hygiene while maintaining the contact area. *B,* Palatal root amputation. Note that the contour of the palatal surface is modified to allow adequate plaque control.

FIGURE 67–26. Hemisection of mandibular molar with retention of both roots. Separate full crown preparations have been made on each root. The gold crowns are splinted together with sufficient space between them for interproximal plaque control.

is extracted, the remaining portion often serves as an abutment for a three-unit bridge (Fig. 67–27). It is important when the root is sectioned that care be taken to eliminate any remnants in the furcation areas. The contour of the final restoration should be a smoothly flowing line from the contact area down to the most apical portion of the tooth preparation. Frequently the teeth are sectioned improperly, so that a small amount of the furcation remains on the retained root. This provides a plaque trap, which makes maintenance of periodontal health difficult after the final restoration is placed.

Maxillary Molars. Root-resective techniques in the maxillary molars have applications entirely different from those in the mandibular molars. It is possible for the clinician to temporarily maintain the vitality of many root-resected maxillary molars by placing a pulp-capping medicament over the exposed pulp canal. Root-resected maxillary molars, however, should eventually receive endodontic therapy. (Root canal therapy is generally undertaken 4 to 6 weeks after a vital root resection). The use of endodontic therapy in these teeth provides two major advantages: First, it ensures that there is no pulpal inflammation and patient discomfort subsequent to the resective technique; second, it allows for recontouring of the crown so that plaque control is simplified in the area where the root has been resected. *An improperly contoured crown in the area of the resected root frequently results in accumulation of plaque and a re-*

turn of the periodontal defect because of the patient's inability to cleanse the area.

Crowns that are placed on maxillary molars that have undergone root resection must be contoured in a specific way to ensure that the patient has access for oral hygiene measures (Fig. 67–28). This means that there is a dramatic change from the normal anatomic crowns seen on these teeth. When a mesiobuccal or distobuccal root has been resected, it is necessary to hollow out the crown contours in the area coronal to the area where the root was removed, so that adequate access is available for oral hygiene procedures (Fig. 67–29). When a palatal root has been resected, it is important that the crown be recontoured over the area where the palatal root was previously present. This results in a much thinner crown buccopalatally, with emphasis on a groove running in the mid-palatal surface. In other words, the crown form of this tooth with a palatal root resection would be somewhat similar to that seen in a narrow mandibular molar (Fig. 67–30).

REMOVABLE PARTIAL DENTURE PROSTHESES

Available clinical data show that even with advanced periodontal disease and extensive tooth loss, fixed partial prostheses combined with periodontal therapy, including vigorous maintenance therapy, can result in periodontal health.[36]

From the periodontal viewpoint, fixed prostheses are the

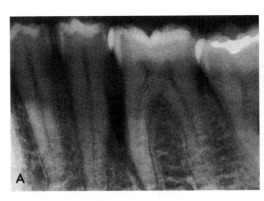
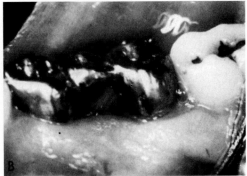

FIGURE 67–27. Hemisection of mandibular molar with retention of one root. *A,* Radiograph showing a localized osseous defect on the mesial root of the first molar. *B,* Lingual view of a fixed prosthesis utilizing the distal root of the first molar; note access for plaque control.

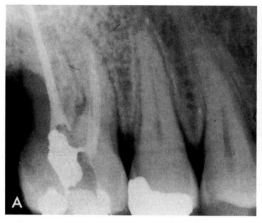
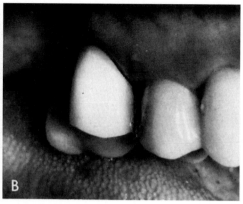

FIGURE 67–29. Root resection of maxillary molar. *A,* Radiograph showing a localized defect on the distobuccal root of maxillary first molar. *B,* After root resection, the molar has been restored, with modifications made to the crown contour to facilitate plaque control.

restorations of choice for replacement of missing teeth, but there are some clinical situations in which removable partial prostheses are the only possible way to restore the lost function of the dentition. The usefulness of removable partial prostheses in the total treatment of periodontal problems should not be minimized.[18] The detrimental effects of caries and periodontal destruction are accentuated in patients with poor oral hygiene; therefore, it is unwise to consider a removable partial denture in patients whose oral hygiene is inadequate. A major part of the treatment plan for patients requiring removable partial prostheses is the establishment of a satisfactory level of oral hygiene.[47] The presence of a partial denture may increase plaque formation around the remaining teeth,[1] so oral hygiene must receive great emphasis in these patients.

Design

To provide maximal stability for removable partial prostheses, every effort should be made to retain posterior teeth for the distal support of the edentulous areas.

When posterior teeth cannot be retained to support edentulous areas, the design for the removable partial prostheses becomes challenging and the relationship of the framework to the distal surface of abutment teeth, especially in bilateral, distal extension partial dentures, becomes an area of controversy. There is some support for the practice of tightly adapting the metal framework to the distal surface and the gingiva of this tooth,[29,30] although some investigators suggest that this area should be relieved of pressure

and that no impingement of the denture framework should occur here.[14]

A clinical study has shown that the I-bar type of removable partial denture can be utilized by many patients with little or no detrimental effect on periodontal health.[5] This particular design utilizes an I-bar infrabulge clasp, mesially positioned occlusal rests, and metal guide planes. The technique emphasizes the need for intraoral adjustment of the denture framework to minimize undue torque on the abutment teeth.[54] This particular design of removable prostheses has also been shown to provide more favorable loading of abutment teeth than that seen with a circumferential clasp design[31] (Fig. 67–31).

Many patients who formerly were treated with removable prosthodontic appliances (e.g., those with bilateral edentulous areas) can now be treated with fixed appliances using dental implants as distal abutments.

Clasps. It has been generally accepted that clasps should be passive and exert no force on the teeth when the partial denture is at rest.[51] Research shows that the use of an improperly designed suprabulge or circumferential clasp exerts a great deal of force on the abutment tooth.[10]

Stress breakers, which connect the retainer and saddle areas with flexible and movable joints, are sometimes used to prevent excessive occlusal forces on abutment teeth. However, comparisons have revealed no advantage of stress breakers over rigid connectors in this respect.[4] With rigid connectors between clasps and saddle areas, the resilience of the mucosa acts as a stress breaker. It permits controlled movement of the prosthesis so that the tissue-borne sections

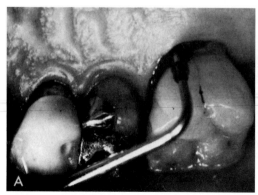
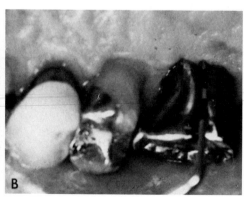

FIGURE 67–30. Palatal root resection. *A,* Preoperative view showing a deep periodontal defect on palatal root. *B,* Postoperative view showing a gold crown narrowed in buccopalatal dimension after resection of palatal root.

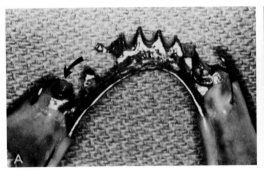
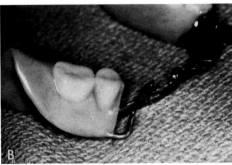

FIGURE 67–31. I-bar design for removable partial denture. *A,* Tissue surface of a removable partial denture for a mandibular bilateral edentulous patient. Note the metal guiding surface that fits tightly against distal surface of distal abutment tooth (*arrow*). *B,* Same removable partial denture showing I-bar clasp and occlusal rest placed in mesial part of abutment tooth.

take the initial occlusal stress and prevent sudden impact on the periodontium of the natural teeth.

Occlusal Rests. Occlusal rests should be designed to direct the forces along the vertical axis of the tooth. To accomplish this, the rest is seated in a spoon-shaped preparation in the abutment tooth with the preparation floor inclined so that the deepest point is toward the vertical axis of the tooth[23] (Fig. 67–32). This purpose is also accomplished if occlusal rests are extended beyond the central zone of the occlusal surface of premolars or if the occlusal surface overlying one of the roots of the molars is covered.

Spreading of anterior teeth can be prevented if a restoration is constructed on the abutment teeth with a horizontal ledge (cingulum rest) on the lingual surface into which the major connector fits (Fig. 67–33). The floor of the ledge should be sloped so as to direct the forces axially. An incisal stop can also prevent settling of clasps (Fig. 67–34). The notch is cut for a slight distance into the tooth substance, at a point approximately one third from the distoincisal angle. The incisal rest fits into the notch and is tapered to terminate in a point on the facial surface.

Removable partial prostheses should always be constructed with occlusal rests. Rests are sometimes omitted for the ostensible purpose of reducing axial load on teeth with weakened periodontal support. Such dentures jeopardize the teeth, because they settle and cause gingival and periodontal disturbances (Fig. 67–35).

Attachments. Attachments are used for aesthetic reasons and to direct occlusal forces axially rather than laterally. There are many types of precision attachments, and advantages have been demonstrated for some.[22] They cause

greater stress and displacement on the abutment teeth of distal extension prostheses than is produced by conventional back-action clasps.[48]

Multiple Abutments. Multiple abutments reduce injurious lateral and torsional stresses on abutment teeth, and their use should be standard procedure in patients with reduced periodontal support and those who are to receive removable partial dentures. The clinician can make multiple abutments by connecting inlays or crowns or by clasping abutment and adjacent teeth in sequence. When the terminal tooth is periodontally weak, more than one adjacent tooth should be used for added support. Joining a weakened tooth to a strong one is as likely to weaken the strong tooth as to strengthen the weak one. It is always advisable to consider whether the long-term interest of the patient would be better served by extracting the prospective weak abutment tooth and making a multiple abutment of two adjacent teeth that are relatively well supported.

Combined Fixed and Removable Partial Prostheses

Isolated teeth with reduced periodontal support are particularly vulnerable to periodontal injury and loosening when used as abutments in removable partial prostheses. They lack mesial and distal buttressing action to assist in withstanding the forces transmitted by the denture. In such cases, fixed and removable prostheses should be combined. The isolated teeth should be joined to their nearest neighbors with a fixed prosthesis (Fig. 67–36) and can then be used as abutments for removable prostheses.

FIGURE 67–32. Occlusal rests in line with vertical axis. *A,* Properly constructed rest in a premolar without a restoration. *B,* Properly constructed rest in a restoration in a premolar. *C,* Clasp in position on a premolar with a rest in a restoration.

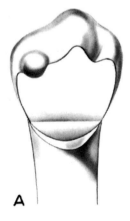
A
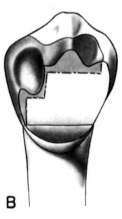
B
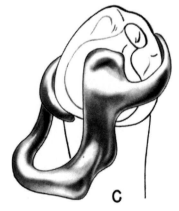
C

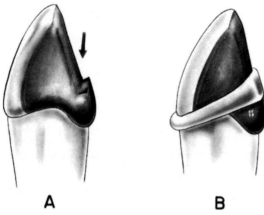

FIGURE 67–33. A method to prevent clasp settling on mandibular cuspid. *A,* Restoration is made for cuspid, including ledge on lingual surface. *B,* Lingual arm of clasp fits into ledge on lingual surface.

Overdentures

The capacity for some teeth to remain in the dental arch for use as abutments for an overdenture has had wide application. This procedure has three obvious advantages for the patient: First, there is increased retention and stability of the denture base. Second, there is evidence that the proprioceptive capacity of a patient with a full denture utilizing some teeth as abutments is dramatically improved over that seen with a conventional full denture design.[33,38] Third, the presence of teeth under a full denture provides a reduced amount of stress on the edentulous ridges, resulting in less bone resorption over time.[13]

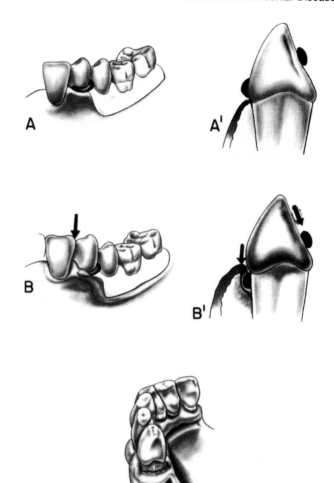

FIGURE 67–35. "Settling" of a lingual bar with no rest on the cuspid. *A,* Lingual bar in position. *A',* Labiolingual view showing cross section of labial and lingual arms of the clasp. (Note there are no rest seals included in the design.) *B,* Lingual bar settles in direction indicated by arrow. *B',* Labial arm digs into gingiva; lingual arm slides down along inclined plane of lingual surface. *C,* View of distal surface of cuspid showing recession of gingiva and marginal gingival disease resulting from settling of partial denture.

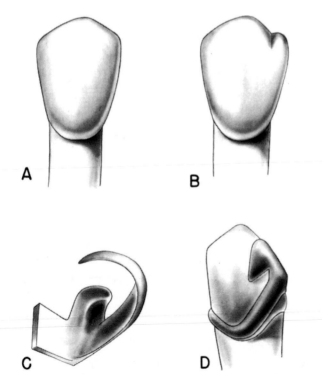

FIGURE 67–34. Incisal rest on anterior tooth. *A,* Mandibular cuspid. *B,* Notch is cut in incisal edge. *C,* View of clasp with incisal rest. *D,* Clasp in position on tooth.

Because many of the teeth utilized for overdenture abutments have had periodontal involvement, it is important that appropriate periodontal considerations be part of the treatment planning process and therapy provided for these areas. In particular, the following are essential:

1. The presence of an adequate zone of attached (keratinized) gingiva around these abutment teeth is of critical importance.
2. Any remaining residual periodontal defects must be treated in the same way as they would be around any periodontally involved tooth prior to the final restoration.

One great advantage that the overdenture concept has for periodontally involved teeth is that it is possible to improve the crown-to-root ratio dramatically. This results in a great diminution in the forces that are applied to the remaining root.

Preparation of the root surface for an overdenture can

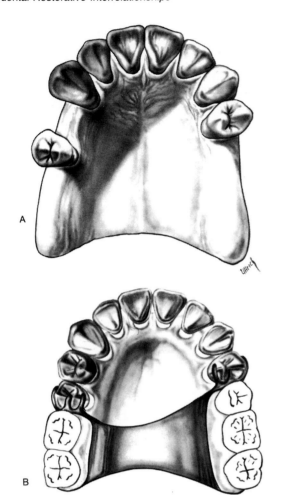

FIGURE 67-36. Combined fixed and removable partial prosthesis. *A,* Prosthesis is required for isolated second premolar. *B,* Isolated second premolar included in fixed prosthesis before the palatal bar is constructed. The first premolar is replaced by a pontic.

utilize any of four different approaches. The simplest is to provide a small, dome-shaped amalgam restoration over the area of the root facing the oral cavity (Fig. 67-37). A cast post and coping can be applied over the root surface. Another alternative is the use of an attachment placed on the root and then mated with an analogous attachment inside the denture. Finally, it is possible to utilize a bar joining two retained roots together to provide a sharing of the load between roots. *It appears that the dome restoration most*

effectively attenuates traumatic forces to the retained roots and therefore should be the method of choice in most cases.[56] The major disadvantage of this doming procedure is that it provides the least amount of retention for the denture compared with other procedures. In cases in which denture retention is of critical importance, the use of a bar or of attachments may be indicated. However, it should be recognized that these bar prostheses complicate the oral hygiene procedures necessary to maintain the periodontal tissues; therefore, they should be used only in patients who have demonstrated an adequate level of and dedication to plaque control. In situations in which recurrent caries is an important consideration, supplemental fluoride therapy should be considered.

Periodontal Splinting

A splint is an appliance for the immobilization or stabilization of injured or diseased parts. Teeth may be splinted as part of Phase I therapy, before periodontal surgery, utilizing temporary or provisional splints. Permanent splints utilizing cast restorations may be placed as part of the restorative phase of therapy.

Splinting of periodontally involved teeth should not be the sole method of obtaining tooth stability. The clinician must always determine the cause of the increased tooth mobility or the pathologic migration of the teeth. Permanent splinting should not be considered until all of the inflammation around the teeth has been resolved. As the inflammation is eliminated, mobility may decrease, making splinting unnecessary. Mobility may also be caused by an abnormal occlusal pattern (e.g., a deflective occlusal contact) resulting in nonaxial forces on teeth and/or excessive occlusal forces associated with parafunctional movement (Fig. 67-38). It is imperative that occlusal stability and control of excessive occlusal forces be obtained first, before splinting is applied. Frequently, the modification of occlusal forces eliminates the need for a splint, as the teeth become less mobile and more stable in their position.

Occlusal forces applied to splints are shared by all teeth within the splint even if the force is applied to only one section of the splint.[19] The rigidity of a splint allows it to act as a lever, so that the forces applied to some teeth in the splint may be much greater than before splinting.[19] Therefore, the inclusion of a mobile tooth in a splint does not completely relieve the tooth of the burden of occlusal forces, nor does it guarantee against injury from excessive

FIGURE 67-37. Preparation of teeth for overdenture. *A,* Preoperative view. Lower cuspid and first premolar have periodontal involvement and unfavorable crown-to-root ratio. *B,* After periodontal flap surgery and endodontic therapy, these teeth have been prepared with dome-shaped contours as abutments for a mandibular complete overdenture. Note the reduced crown-to-root ratio.

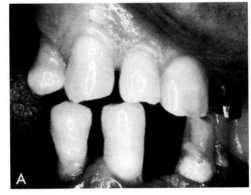
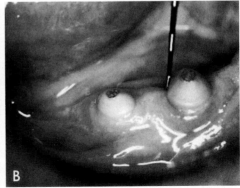

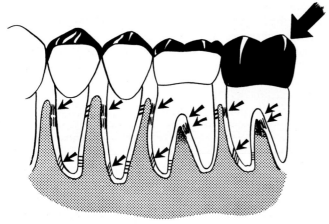

FIGURE 67–38. Transmission of forces in a splint. Excessive occlusal force applied only to the second molar (*large arrow*) injures periodontium of all splinted teeth in comparable locations. *Small arrows* indicate areas of injury. Location of injury depends on the direction of occlusal force.

occlusal forces. If one tooth in a splint is in a traumatic occlusal relationship, the periodontal tissues of the remaining teeth may also be injured. Therefore, it is of primary importance to stabilize the occlusion prior to splinting.

The use of splinting in periodontal therapy is controversial.[32] There is little evidence to support the much-cited rationale that the splinting of mobile teeth enhances resistance to further periodontal breakdown and improves the healing response.[12,35] Therefore, the indications for permanent splinting are more limited than many clinicians believe. Permanent splinting does not necessarily reduce the effect of damaging forces on mobile teeth, nor does it predictably reduce mobility.[43]

The two major indications for periodontal splinting are (1) to immobilize excessively mobile teeth so that the patient can chew more comfortably and (2) to stabilize teeth exhibiting increasing mobility.

The three procedures for provisional stabilization are the following:

1. The reinforced resin splint for use in posterior teeth (Fig. 67–39)
2. The acid etch–resin splint for use in anterior teeth (Fig. 67–40)
3. The resin-bonded metal splint (e.g., Maryland prosthesis)

The introduction of splints into the dental arch generally makes oral hygiene procedures more complicated. Therefore, it is important that patients receive special instruction in the techniques required for control of interproximal plaque (see Chapter 42). When an interdental papilla completely fills the embrasure space, the best method of interdental plaque removal is the use of dental floss via a threader. When the interdental papilla does not fill the embrasure space, the best method for plaque removal is the use of an interdental brush.[17]

Implant-Supported Restorations

The multifaceted field of dental implants is covered in more detail in Part VI, "Oral Implantology" (Chapters 62 to 65). Prosthetic aspects of this subject will be covered here.

Several basic tenets determine the success or failure of the implant-supported restoration. These principles fall into three categories: patient selection, the investing tissues, and force distribution.

Patient selection is one of the most important components of success. Reasonable health is a basic requirement for implant placement, as outlined at the National Institutes of Health Implant Consensus (1988). The patient's psychological profile should also be evaluated.

Investing tissues can be defined as including both hard and soft tissue. Both the bone height and width must be adequate for implant placement. In partially edentulous patients, it has been observed that keratinized tissue around implants seems to offer the greatest resistance to peri-implant infection. An adequate zone of attached gingiva around the abutment also seems to make home care procedures more comfortable for the patient. For these and other reasons, both the hard and soft tissue should be critically evaluated when planning the implant.

Force distribution is the last parameter for discussion. There are a number of general areas of occlusion that must be adhered to in order to avoid disaster:

1. Bilateral simultaneous contact is mandatory. Nothing will destroy an implant restoration faster than an occlusal interference.
2. The occlusal vertical dimension must be in harmony with the patient's neuromuscular system (i.e., free way space must not be violated).
3. The jaw joints should be placed in a retruded, rearmost, reproducible, and unstrained position.
4. All interferences must be eliminated.

Lateral forces, not compressive forces, are the undoing of most dental implant restorations.

A discussion of force distribution limited to describing occlusal load tells only part of the story. The other ingredient relates to the forces (or lack of forces) received by the "healing" implant. The secret of osseointegration lies not with submergibility, but with the concept of implant shielding. Forces that are transmitted to a submerged implant through a transitional prosthesis may generate micromovements to the implant. For successful osseointegration, implant movements should be kept to a minimum; otherwise a fibrous bone–implant interface may result. Therefore, it is critical that clinicians pay close attention to the design of

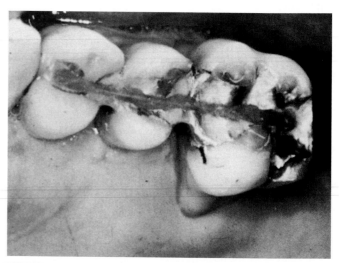

FIGURE 67–39. Posterior splint. Reinforced resin splint. This splint is used for temporary or provisional splinting in posterior teeth.

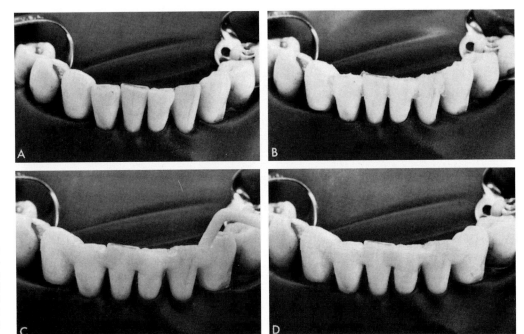

FIGURE 67–40. Anterior splint. Technique for acid etch splint. *A,* Teeth are thoroughly scaled and polished to remove all deposits. *B,* Enamel surface is etched with an acid gel for 2 minutes. *C,* Polymerizing resin restorative material is placed on prepared teeth. *D,* Complete splint.

provisional restorations, especially if the tissue surface sits directly above a submerged endosseous implant.

The long-term success of any dental implant, assuming osseointegration and proper loading of the prosthesis, depends on home care and professional maintenance. It is suggested that implant patients receive professional supportive care every 3 to 4 months, or more frequently if needed. Many implant patients will require extensive oral hygiene instructions and frequent reinforcement.

The profession has watched the evolution of dental implants mature from a crude treatment modality to a predictable and sophisticated entity. Dental implants can no longer be regarded as experimental, and their role in restoring the partially dentate patient is just beginning to be explored.

REFERENCES

1. Addy M, Bates JF. The effect of partial dentures and chlorhexidine on plaque accumulation in the absence of oral hygiene. J Clin Periodontol 4:41, 1977.
2. Al Hamadane KK, Crabb HSM. Marginal adaptation of composite resins. J Oral Rehabil 2:21, 1975.
3. Azzi R, Tsao TF, Carranza FA Jr, Kenney EB. Comparative study of gingival retraction methods. J Prosthet Dent 50:561, 1983.
4. Barkann L. The case for metal ligatures in periodontia. J Sec District D Soc NY 31:341, 1945.
5. Benson D, Spolsky VW. A clinical evaluation of removable partial dentures with I bar retainers. J Prosthet Dent 41:246, 1979.
6. Bowen RL. Adhesive bonding of various materials to hard tissue. V: The effect of a surface active comononer on adhesion to diverse substrates. J Dent Res 44:13–69, 1955.
7. Bryan AW. Some common defects in operative restorations contributing to the injury of the supporting structures. J Am Dent Assoc 14:1486, 1927.
8. Buonocore MD. A simple method of increasing adhesion of acrylic filling materials to enamel surfaces. J Dent Res 50:125, 1955.
9. Clayton JA, Green E. Roughness of pontic materials and dental plaque. J Prosthet Dent 23:407, 1970.
10. Clayton JA, Jaslow C. A measurement of clasp forces on teeth. J Prosthet Dent 25:21, 1971.
11. Coelho DH, Cavallaro J, Rothschild EA. Gingival recession with electrosurgery for impression making. J Prosthet Dent 33:422, 1975.
12. Cross W. The importance of immobilization in periodontology. Paradontologie 8:119, 1954.
13. Crum RJ, Rooney GE. Alveolar bone loss in overdentures: A 5-year study. J Prosthet Dent 40:610, 1978.
14. Derry A, Bertram U. A clinical survey of removable partial dentures after 2 years usage. Acta Odontol Scand 28:581, 1970.
15. Donaldson D. Gingival recession associated with temporary crowns. J Periodontol 44:691, 1973.
16. Fenner W, Gerber A, Muhlemann HR. Tooth mobility changes during treatment with partial denture prosthesis. J Prosthet Dent 6:520, 1956.
17. Gjermo P, Flotra L. The effect of different methods of interdental cleaning. J Periodont Res 5:230, 1970.
18. Glickman I. The periodontal structures and removable partial denture prostheses. J Am Dent Assoc 37:311, 1948.
19. Glickman I, Stein RS, Smulow JB. The effect of increased functional forces upon the periodontium of splinted and nonsplinted teeth. J Periodontol 32:290, 1961.
20. Goransson P, Nyman L. Review of methods for exposing the gingival margin. Sci Educ Bull Int Coll Dent 2:24, 1969.
21. Henry PJ, Johnston JF, Mitchell DF. Tissue changes beneath fixed partial dentures. J Prosthet Dent 16:937, 1966.
22. Homma S, Homma M, Nakamura Y. Dynamic study of attachments. Abstract. J Dent Res 40:228, 1961.
23. Ito H, Inoue Y, Yamada M. Three dimensional photoelastic studies on the clasp-rest and tooth extraction. Abstract. J Dent Res 38:203, 1959.
24. Kaqueler JC, Weiss MB. Plaque accumulation on dental restorative materials. IADR Abstracts 49(615):202, 1970.
25. Karlsen K. Gingival reactions to dental restorations. Acta Odontol Scand 28:895, 1970.
26. Keennan JP, Shillingburg HT, Duncanson MG, Wade CK. Effects of cast gold surface finish on plaque retention. J Prosthet Dent 43:168, 1980.
27. Kelly WJ, Harrison JD. Laboratory experimental evaluation of efficiency of clinical electrosurgical techniques. In Oringer MJ, ed. Electrosurgery in Dentistry. 2nd ed. Philadelphia, WB Saunders, 1975.
28. Knowles JW, Snyder DT. The effect of roughness on supragingival and subgingival plaque formation. IADR Abstracts, no. 345, 1970, p 135.
29. Kratochvil FJ. Influence of occlusal rest position and clasp design on movement of abutment teeth. J Prosthet Dent 13:114, 1963.
30. Kratochvil FJ. Maintaining supporting structures with a removable partial prosthesis. J Prosthet Dent 26:167, 1971.
31. Kratochvil FJ, Caputo AA. Photoelastic analysis of pressure on teeth and bone supporting removable partial dentures. J Prosthet Dent 32:52, 1974.
32. Krogh-Poulsen W. Partial denture design in relation to occlusal trauma and periodontal breakdown. Int Dent J 4:847, 1954.
33. Loiselle RJ, Crum RJ, Rooney GE Jr, Stuever DH Jr. The physiologic basis for the overlay denture. J Prosthet Dent 28:4, 1972.
34. Maynard JD Jr, Wilson RD. Physiologic dimensions of the periodontium significant to the restorative dentist. J Periodontol 50:170, 1979.
35. McCune RJ, Phillips RW, Swartz ML, Mumford G. The effect of occlusal venting and film thickness on the cementation of full cast crowns. J South Cal Dent Assoc 39:36, 1971.
36. Nyman S, Lindhe J, Lunddgren D. The role of occlusion for the stability of fixed

bridges in patients with reduced periodontol support. J Clin Periodontol *2:*53, 1975.

37. O'Leary TN, Standish SM, Coomer RS. Severe periodontal destruction following impression procedures. J Periodontol *44:*43, 1973.

38. Pacer FG, Bowman DC. Occlusal force discrimination by denture patients. J Prosthet Dent *33:*602, 1975.

39. Parkinson CF. Excessive crown contours facilitate endemic plaque niches. J Prosthet Dent *35:*424, 1976.

40. Perel M. Axial crown contours. J Prosthet Dent *25:*642, 1971.

41. Podshadley AG. Gingival response to pontics. J Prosthet Dent *19:*51, 1968.

42. Price C, Whitehead FJH. Impression material as foreign bodies. Br Dent J *133:*9, 1972.

43. Renggli HH. Splinting of teeth. An objective assessment. Helv Odontol Acta *15:*129, 1971.

44. Rosenberg R, Ash MM. The effect of root roughness on plaque accumulation and gingival inflammation. J Periodontol *45:*146, 1974.

45. Ruel J, Schuessler PJ, Malamet K, Morh D. Effect of retraction procedures on the periodontium in humans. J Prosthet Dent *44:*508, 1980.

46. Sacket BP, Gildenhuys RR. The effect of axial crown overcontour on adolescents. J Periodontol *47:*320, 1976.

47. Seemann SK. Study of the relationship between periodontal disease and the wearing of partial dentures. Aust Dent J *8:*206, 1963.

48. Shohet H. Relative magnitudes of stress on abutment teeth and different retainers. J Prosthet Dent *21:*267, 1969.

49. Silness J. Treated with dental bridges. III. The relationship between the location of the crown margin and the periodontal condition. J Periodont Res *5:*225, 1970.

50. Sotres LS, Van Huysen G, Gilmore HW. A histologic study of gingival response to amalgam silicate and resin restorations. J Periodontol *40:*453, 1969.

51. Steffel VL. Clasp partial dentures. J Am Dent Assoc *66:*803, 1963.

52. Stein RS. Pontic-residual ridge relationship: A research report. J Prosthet Dent *16:*251, 1966.

53. Stein RS, Glickman I. Prosthetic considerations essential for gingival health. Dent Clin North Am *4:*177, 1960.

54. Thayer HH, Kratochvil FJ. Periodontal considerations with removable partial dentures. Dent Clin North Am *23:*357, 1980.

55. Waerhaug J. Effect of rough surfaces upon gingival tissues. J Dent Res *35:*323, 1956.

56. Warren AB, Caputo AA. Load transfer to alveolar bone as influenced by abutment designs for tooth supported dentures. J Prosthet Dent *33:*137, 1975.

57. Weitman RT, Eames WB. Plaque accumulation on composite surfaces after various finishing procedures. J Am Dent Assoc *91:*101, 1975.

58. Wheeler RC. A Textbook of Dental Anatomy and Physiology. 3rd ed. Philadelphia, WB Saunders, 1958, pp 64–65.

59. Wilhelmsen NR, Ramfjord SP, Blankenship JR. Effects of electrosurgery on the gingival attachment in rhesus monkeys. J Periodontol *47:*160, 1976.

60. Wing C. Pontic design and construction in fixed bridgework. Dent Pract Dent Rec *12:*390, 1960.

61. Yuodelis RA, Weaver JD, Sapkos S. Facial and lingual contours of artificial complete crowns and their effect on the periodontium. J Prosthet Dent *29:*61, 1973.

68

Supportive Periodontal Treatment

ROBERT L. MERIN

Rationale for Supportive Periodontal Treatment
The Maintenance Program
Classification of Post-treatment Patients

Referring Patients to the Periodontist
Tests for Disease Activity
Maintenance for Implant Patients

Preservation of the periodontal health of the treated patient requires as positive a program as that required for elimination of periodontal disease. After Phase I therapy is completed, patients are placed on a schedule of periodic recall visits for maintenance care to prevent recurrence of the disease (Figs. 68–1 and 68–2).

Transfer of the patient from active treatment status to a maintenance program is a definitive step in total patient care that requires time and effort on the part of the dentist and staff. Patients must be made to understand the purpose of the maintenance program, emphasizing that preservation of the teeth is dependent on it. Patients who are not maintained in a supervised recall program subsequent to active treatment show obvious signs of recurrent periodontitis (e.g., increased pocket depth, bone loss, and tooth loss).[3,6] The more often patients present for recommended supportive periodontal treatment (SPT), the less likely they are to lose teeth.[71] In fact, one study found that tooth loss is three times as common in treated patients who do not return for regular recall visits as in those who do[22]; another showed that patients with inadequate SPT after successful regenerative therapy have a 50-fold increase in risk of probing attachment loss as compared to those with regular recalls.[12] Motivational techniques plus reinforcement of the importance of the maintenance phase of treatment should be considered prior to performing definitive periodontal surgery.[6] Studies have shown that few patients display complete compliance with recommended maintenance schedules[39,69,70] (Fig. 68–3). *It is meaningless simply to inform patients that they are to return for periodic recall visits without clearly explaining the significance of these visits and describing what is expected of patients between visits.*

The maintenance phase of periodontal treatment starts immediately after the completion of Phase I therapy (see Figs. 68–1 and 68–2). While the patient is in the maintenance phase, the necessary surgical and restorative procedures are performed. This ensures that all areas of the mouth retain the degree of health attained after Phase I therapy.

RATIONALE FOR SUPPORTIVE PERIODONTAL TREATMENT

Studies have shown that even with appropriate periodontal therapy, some progression of disease is possible.[15,18,42,51] One likely explanation for the recurrence of periodontal disease is *incomplete subgingival plaque removal.*[68] If subgingival plaque is left behind during scaling, it will regrow within the pocket. The regrowth of subgingival plaque is a slow process compared with that of supragingival plaque. During this period (perhaps months), the subgingival plaque may not induce inflammatory reactions that can be discerned at the gingival margin. The clinical diagnosis may be further confused by the introduction of adequate supragingival plaque control, because the inflammatory reactions caused by the plaque in the soft tissue wall of the pocket are not likely to be manifested clinically as gingivitis. Thus, inadequate subgingival plaque control can lead to continued loss of attachment even without the presence of clinical gingival inflammation.

Bacteria are present in the gingival tissues in adult and juvenile periodontitis cases.[8,11,45,53] Eradication of intragingival microorganisms may be necessary for a stable periodontal result. Scaling, root planing, and even flap surgery may not eliminate intragingival bacteria from some areas.[14] These bacteria may recolonize the pocket and cause recurrent disease.

Bacteria associated with periodontitis can be transmitted between spouses and other family members.[1,66] Patients

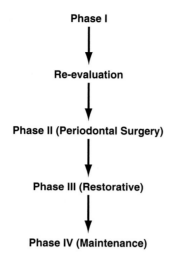

FIGURE 68–1. Incorrect sequence of periodontal treatment phases. Maintenance phase should be started immediately after the re-evaluation of Phase I.

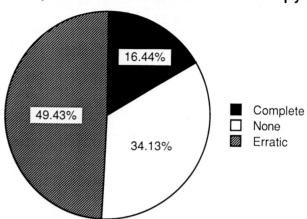

FIGURE 68–3. Compliance with maintenance therapy in 961 patients studied for 1 to 8 years. (Adapted from Wilson TG Jr, Glover ME, Schoen J, et al. J Periodontol *55*:468, 1984.)

who appear to be successfully treated can become infected or reinfected with potential pathogens. This is especially likely in patients with remaining pockets.

Another possible explanation for the recurrence of periodontal disease is the microscopic nature of the dentogingival unit healing after periodontal treatment. Histologic studies have shown that after periodontal procedures, tissues usually do not heal by formation of new connective tissue attachment to root surfaces,[9,58,60] but result in a long junctional epithelium. It has been speculated that this type of dentogingival unit may be weaker and inflammation may rapidly separate the long junctional epithelium from the tooth. Thus, treated periodontal patients may be predisposed to recurrent pocket formation if maintenance care is not optimal.

Subgingival scaling alters the microflora of periodontal pockets.[40,48,56] In one study,[40] a single session of scaling and root planing in patients with chronic periodontitis resulted in significant changes in subgingival microflora. Reported alterations included a decrease in the proportion of motile rods for 1 week, a marked elevation in the proportion of coccoid cells for 21 days, and a marked reduction in the proportion of spirochetes for 7 weeks.

Another study reported that subgingival bacteria had not returned to pretreatment proportions after 3 to 6 months.[56]

However, the rate of return of the pretreatment microbial flora varied from patient to patient. These findings indicate that mechanical debridement produces a relatively long-lasting effect on the microbial flora and that the different groups of microorganisms return to baseline values after varying time periods.

There is reason to believe that both the mechanical debridement performed by the therapist and the motivational environment provided by the appointment are necessary for good maintenance results. Patients tend to reduce their oral hygiene efforts between appointments.[3,69] Knowing that their hygiene will be evaluated causes them to perform better oral hygiene in anticipation of the appointment.

In one study, the proportion of spirochetes obtained in baseline samples of subgingival flora was highly correlated with clinical periodontal deterioration over a period of 1 year.[29] However, subsequent reports in the same longitudinal study concluded that the arbitrary assignment of treated periodontitis patients to 3-month maintenance intervals appears to be as effective in preventing recurrences of periodontitis as assignment of recall intervals based on microscopic monitoring of the subgingival flora.[32,33] Microscopic monitoring was found not to be a reliable predictor of future periodontal destruction in patients on 3-month recall programs, presumably because of the alteration of subgingival flora produced by subgingival instrumentation.

In conclusion, there is a sound scientific basis for recall maintenance, because subgingival scaling alters the pocket microflora for variable but relatively long periods.

THE MAINTENANCE PROGRAM

Periodic recall visits form the foundation of a meaningful long-term prevention program. The interval between visits is initially set at 3 months but may be varied according to the patient's needs.

Periodontal care at each recall visit comprises three parts (Table 68–1). The first part is concerned with examination and evaluation of the patient's current oral health. The second part includes the necessary maintenance treatment and

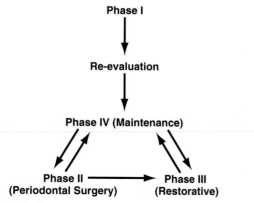

FIGURE 68–2. Correct sequence of periodontal treatment phases.

Table 68–1. MAINTENANCE RECALL PROCEDURES

Part I: Examination (approximate time, 17 minutes)[54]
   Medical history changes
   Oral pathologic examination
   Oral hygiene status
   Gingival changes
   Pocket depth changes
   Mobility changes
   Occlusal changes
   Dental caries
   Restorative and prosthetic status
Part II: Treatment (approximate time, 35 minutes)[54]
   Oral hygiene reinforcement
   Scaling
   Polishing
   Chemical irrigation
Part III: Schedule next procedure (approximate time, 1 minute)[54]
   Schedule next recall visit
   Schedule further periodontal treatment
   Schedule or refer for restorative or prosthetic treatment

oral hygiene reinforcement. The third part involves scheduling the patient for the next recall appointment, additional periodontal treatment, or restorative dental procedures. The time required for a recall visit for patients with multiple teeth in both arches is approximately 1 hour,[54] which includes time for greeting the patient, setting up, and cleaning up.

Examination and Evaluation (Figs. 68–4 to 68–9). The recall examination is similar to the initial evaluation of the patient discussed in Chapter 28. However, because the patient is not new to the office, the dentist will be primarily looking for changes that have occurred since the last evaluation. Analysis of the current oral hygiene status of the patient is essential. Updating of changes in the medical history and evaluation of restorations, caries, prostheses, occlusion, tooth mobility, gingival status, and periodontal pockets are important parts of the recall appointment. The oral mucosa should be carefully inspected for pathologic conditions.

Radiographic examination must be individualized,[35] depending on the initial severity of the case and the findings at the recall visit (Table 68–2). These are compared with findings on previous radiographs to check the bone height and to look for repair of osseous defects, signs of trauma from occlusion, periapical pathologic changes, and caries.

Checking Plaque Control. To assess the effectiveness of their plaque control, patients should perform their hygiene regimen immediately before the recall appointment. Plaque control must be reviewed and corrected until the patient demonstrates the necessary proficiency, even if additional instruction sessions are required. Patients instructed in plaque control have less plaque and gingivitis than uninstructed patients,[3,64,65] and the amount of supragingival plaque affects the number of subgingival anaerobic organisms.[13,57]

Treatment. The required scaling and root planing are performed, followed by an oral prophylaxis (see Chapter 43). Care must be taken not to heavily instrument normal sites with shallow sulci (1 to 3 mm deep), because studies have shown that repeated subgingival scaling and root planing in initially normal periodontal sites result in significant loss of attachment.[28] Irrigation with antimicrobial agents is performed in maintenance patients with remaining pockets.[24,36,54]

Recurrence of Periodontal Disease. Occasionally lesions may recur. This can often be traced to inadequate plaque control on the part of the patient or failure to comply with recommended SPT schedules. It should be understood, however, that it is the dentist's responsibility to teach, motivate, and control the patient's oral hygiene technique, and the patient's failure is the dentist's failure. Surgery should not be undertaken unless the patient has shown proficiency and willingness to cooperate by adequately performing his or her part of therapy.[6,61,70]

Other causes for recurrence are the following:

1. Inadequate or insufficient treatment that has failed to remove all the potential factors favoring plaque accumulation (see Fig. 68–4). Incomplete calculus removal in areas of difficult access is a common source of problems.
2. Inadequate restorations placed after the periodontal treatment was completed.
3. Failure of the patient to return for periodic checkups (see Fig. 68–6). This may be due to the patient's conscious or unconscious decision not to continue treatment or to failure of the dentist and staff to emphasize the need for periodic examinations.
4. Presence of some systemic diseases that may affect host resistance to previously acceptable levels of plaque.

A failing case can be recognized by the following:

1. Recurring inflammation revealed by gingival changes and bleeding of the sulcus on probing.
2. Increasing depth of sulci, leading to the recurrence of pocket formation.
3. Gradual increases in bone loss as determined by radiographs.
4. Gradual increases in tooth mobility as ascertained by clinical examination.

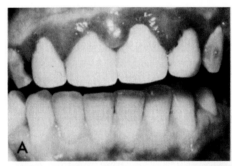
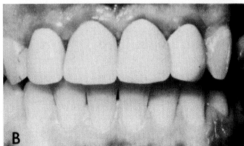

FIGURE 68–4. *A,* Hyperplastic gingivitis related to crown margins and plaque accumulation in a 27-year-old woman. *B,* Four months after treatment, there is significant improvement. However, there is still some inflammation around crown margins, which cannot be resolved without replacing the crowns.

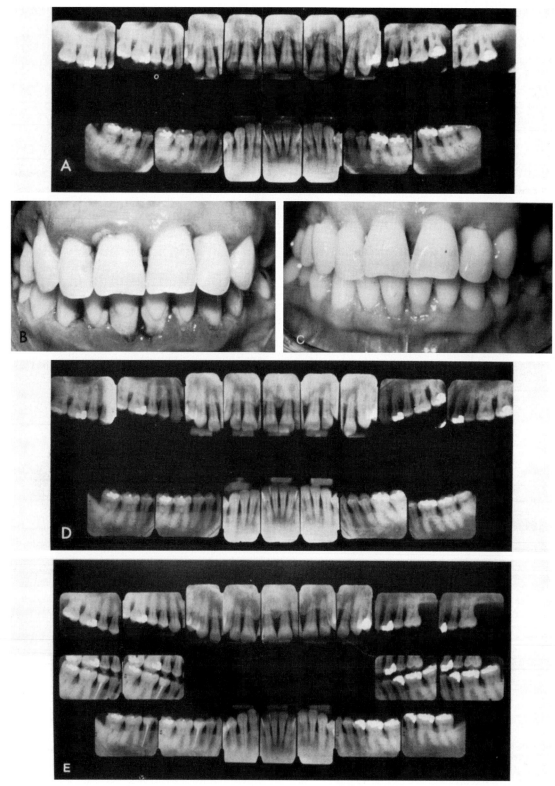

FIGURE 68–5. *A,* The patient was 38 years old when these original radiographs were taken and was treated with a combination of surgical and nonsurgical therapy. This individual is a classic class C maintenance patient. *B,* Pretreatment photographs. Note the inflammation and heavy calculus deposits. *C,* Photograph taken 10 years after treatment. *D,* Radiographs taken 5 years after treatment. *E,* Radiographs taken 10 years after treatment. The radiographic appearance is as good as can be expected in such a severe case. Teeth #15 and #17 were extracted 8 years after treatment.

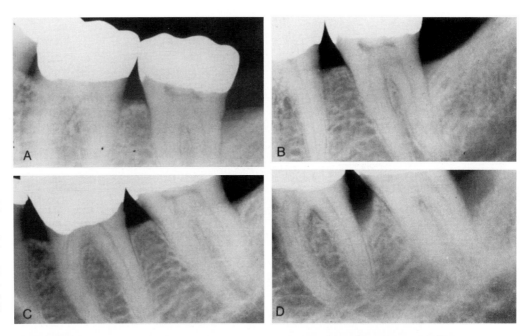

FIGURE 68–6. This series of radiographs clearly shows the importance of maintenance therapy. *A,* Original radiograph of a 58-year-old man. Note the deep distal bone loss on tooth #18 and the moderate distal lesion on tooth #19. Surgical treatment that included osseous grafting was performed. *B,* Radiograph 14 months after surgical therapy. The patient was having recall maintenance performed every 3 to 4 months. *C,* Appearance 3½ years after surgery, with regular recalls every 3 to 4 months. *D,* Appearance after 2 years without recalls (7 years after surgery). The patient retired and traveled around the United States for 2 years. Note the progression of the disease on the distal surfaces of teeth #18 and #19.

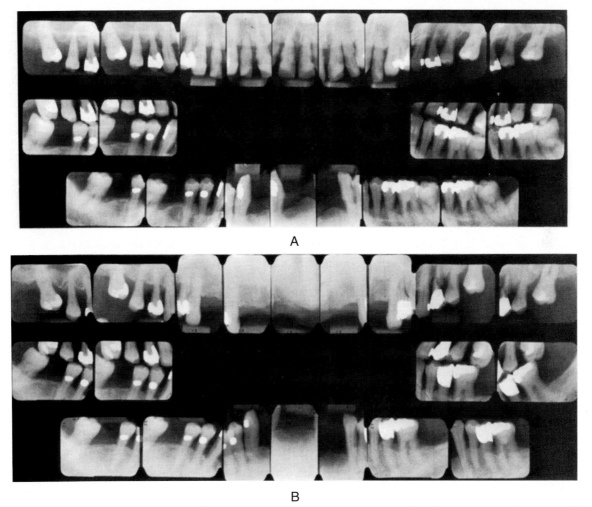

FIGURE 68–7. Advanced cases sometimes do better than expected when the patient complies with maintenance therapy. *A,* Initial radiographs showing a very advanced case. The maxillary arch had extractions and nonsurgical treatment. A plastic treatment partial denture was placed and was expected to grow into a full denture within a few years. The mandibular arch was treated with periodontal surgery, and a permanent metal and plastic removable partial denture was placed. *B,* Radiographs taken 8 years later. The patient performed good oral hygiene and had 3-month recalls. Teeth #12 and #15 required extraction.

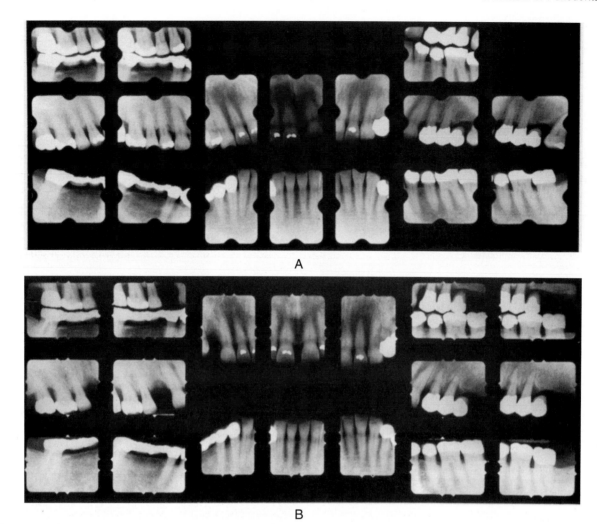

A

B

FIGURE 68–8. *A,* Initial radiographs. The patient was advised to have localized areas of periodontal surgery and periodontal recall every 3 months. However, the patient did not comply and only had dental cleanings once or twice yearly. *B,* Radiographs 4 years later. Note the loss of teeth #5 and #15 and the increased bone loss on several premolars and molars.

Cases that do not respond to adequate therapy or recur for unknown reasons are referred to as refractory periodontitis (see Chapters 26 and 45).

The decision to retreat a periodontal patient should not be made at the preventive maintenance appointment but should be postponed for 1 to 2 weeks.[10] Often the mouth looks a great deal better at that time, owing to the resolution of edema and the resulting improved tone of the gingiva. A summary of the symptoms of recurrence of periodontal disease and their probable causes can be found in Table 68–3.

CLASSIFICATION OF POST-TREATMENT PATIENTS

The first year after periodontal therapy is important in terms of indoctrinating the patient in a recall pattern and reinforcing oral hygiene techniques. In addition, it may take several months to accurately evaluate the results of some periodontal surgical procedures. Consequently, some areas may have to be retreated because the results may not be optimal. Furthermore, the first-year patient often has etio-

logic factors that may have been overlooked and that may be more amenable to treatment at this early stage. For these reasons, *the recall interval for first-year patients should not be longer than 3 months.*

The patients who are on a periodontal recall schedule are a varied group. Table 68–4 lists several categories of maintenance patients and a suggested recall interval for each. Patients can improve or relapse to a different classification with a reduction in or exacerbation of periodontal disease. When one dental arch is more involved than the other, the patient's periodontal disease is classified by the arch that is in worse condition.

In summary, maintenance care is a critical phase of therapy. *The long-term preservation of the dentition is closely associated with the frequency and quality of recall maintenance.*

REFERRING PATIENTS TO THE PERIODONTIST

The majority of periodontal care belongs in the hands of the general dentist. This is because of the overwhelming

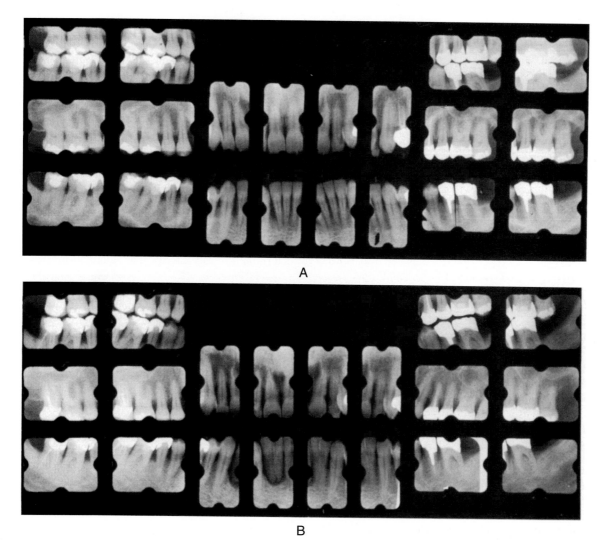

FIGURE 68-9. *A,* Initial radiographs. The patient was advised to have localized areas of periodontal surgery and periodontal recall every 3 months. However, the patient did not comply and had no treatment other than emergency care and occasional dental cleanings. *B,* Radiographs 7 years later. Note the advanced bone loss and caries on many teeth.

number of patients with periodontal disease and the intimate relationship between periodontal disease and restorative dentistry.

For various reasons, an ever greater number of periodontal maintenance patients are expected in future years. The number of caries per capita has dwindled since the mid-1970s by about 50%, and there is some evidence that this decline will continue.[54] As more people retain their teeth throughout their lifetimes and the proportion of older people in the population increases, more teeth will be at risk of periodontal disease. Hence, the prevalence of patients requiring SPT is likely to increase in the future.

This expected increase in the number of periodontal patients will necessitate a greater understanding of periodontal problems and an increased level of expertise for the solution of such problems on the part of the general practitioner of dentistry. However, there will always be a need for specialists to treat particularly difficult cases, patients with systemic health problems, dental implant patients, and situations in which a complex prosthetic construction requires absolute assurance of reliable results.

Where to draw the line between the cases to be treated in the general dental office and those to be referred to a specialist varies for different practitioners and for different patients. The diagnosis indicates the type of periodontal treatment required. If periodontal destruction necessitates surgery on the distal surfaces of second molars, extensive osseous surgery, or complex regenerative procedures, the patient is usually best treated by a specialist. On the other hand, patients who require localized gingivectomy or flap curettage can usually be treated by the general dentist.

It is immediately obvious that some patients should be referred to a specialist, whereas most patients clearly have problems that can be treated by a general dentist. However, there is a third group of patients for whom it will be difficult to decide whether treatment by a specialist is required. Any patient who does not plainly belong in the second of these categories should be considered a candidate for referral to a specialist.[44]

The decision to have the general practitioner treat a patient's periodontal problem should be guided by a consideration of the degree of risk that the patient will lose a tooth or teeth for periodontally related reasons.

The most important factors in the decision are the *extent*

Table 68–2. RADIOGRAPHIC EXAMINATION OF SPT RECALL PATIENTS*[35,63,72]

Patient Condition	Type of Examination
Patients with clinical caries or high-risk factors for caries	Posterior bitewing examination at 12- to 18-month intervals.
Patients with no clinical caries and no high-risk factors for caries	Posterior bitewing examination at 24- to 36-month intervals.
Patients with periodontal disease not under good control	Periapical and/or vertical bitewings of problem areas every 12 to 24 months; full-mouth series every 3 to 5 years.
Patients with history of periodontal treatment with disease under good control	Bitewing examination every 24 to 36 months; full-mouth series every 5 years.
Patients with root form dental implants	Periapical or vertical bitewings at 6, 12, and 36 months after prosthetic placement, then every 36 months unless clinical problems arise.
Transfer periodontal or implant maintenance patients	Full-mouth series if a current set is not available. If a full-mouth series has been taken within 24 months, then radiographs of implants and periodontal problem areas should be taken.

* Radiographs should be taken when they are likely to affect diagnosis and patient treatment. The recommendations in this table are subject to clinical judgment and may not apply to every patient.

and *location of the periodontal deterioration.* Teeth with pockets of 5 mm or more, as measured from the cemento-enamel junction, may have a prognosis of rapid decline. The location of the periodontal deterioration is also an important factor in determining the risk of tooth loss. Teeth with furcation lesions may be at risk even when more than 50% of bone support remains. Therefore, cases in which strategically important teeth fall into these categories are usually best treated by specialists.

An important question remains: *Should the maintenance phase of therapy be performed by the general practitioner or by the specialist?* This should be determined by the amount of periodontal deterioration present. Class A recall patients should be maintained by the general dentist, whereas Class C patients should be maintained by the specialist (see Table 68–4). Class B patients can alternate recall visits between the general practitioner and the specialist (Fig. 68–10). The suggested rule is that *the patient's disease should dictate whether the general practitioner or the specialist should perform the maintenance therapy.*

TESTS FOR DISEASE ACTIVITY

Periodontal patients, even though they have received effective periodontal therapy, are at risk of disease recurrence for the rest of their lives.[17,18] In addition, many pockets in furcation areas may not have been eliminated by surgery.

At present, the best way of determining areas that are losing attachment utilizes a well-organized charting system[52]; some computerized systems offer the possibility of easy retrieval and comparison of past findings.

Comparison of sequential probing measurements gives the most accurate indication of rate of loss of attachment.[2] There are a number of other clinical and laboratory variables that have been correlated with disease activity (see Chapter 30). At present, there is no accurate method of identifying disease activity, and clinicians rely on the information provided by combining probing, bleeding on probing, and sequential attachment measurements.[21,32] Patients whose disease is clearly refractory are candidates for bacterial culturing and antibiotic therapy in conjunction with additional mechanical therapy.

Tests will undoubtedly be developed in the future to help determine disease activity. The clinician must be able to in-

Table 68–3. SYMPTOMS AND CAUSES OF RECURRENCE OF DISEASE

Symptom	Possible Causes
Increased mobility	Increased inflammation Poor oral hygiene Subgingival calculus Inadequate restorations Deteriorating or poorly designed prostheses Systemic disease modifying host response to plaque
Recession	Toothbrush abrasion Inadequate keratinized gingiva Frenum pull Orthodontic therapy
Increased mobility with no change in pocket depth and no radiographic change	Occlusal trauma due to lateral occlusal interference Bruxism High restoration Poorly designed or worn-out prosthesis Poor crown-to-root ratio
Increased pocket depth with no radiographic change	Poor oral hygiene Infrequent recall visits Subgingival calculus Poorly fitting partial denture Mesial inclination into edentulous space Failure of new attachment surgery Cracked teeth Grooves in teeth New periodontal disease
Increased pocket depth with increased radiographic bone loss	Poor oral hygiene Subgingival calculus Infrequent recall visits Inadequate or deteriorating restorations Poorly designed prostheses Inadequate surgery Systemic disease modifying host response to plaque Cracked teeth Grooves in teeth New periodontal disease

Table 68-4. RECALL INTERVALS FOR VARIOUS CLASSES OF RECALL PATIENTS

Merin Classification	Characteristics	Recall interval
First year		
	First-year patient—routine therapy and uneventful healing	3 mo
	or	
	First-year patient—difficult case with complicated prosthesis, furcation involvement, poor crown-to-root ratios, questionable patient cooperation	1 to 2 mo
Class A	Excellent results well maintained for 1 year or more	6 mo to 1 yr
	Patient displays good oral hygiene, minimal calculus, no occlusal problems, no complicated prostheses, no remaining pockets, and no teeth with less than 50% of alveolar bone remaining	
Class B	Generally good results maintained reasonably well for 1 year or more, but patient displays some of the following factors:	3 to 4 mo (decide on recall interval on the basis of the number and severity of negative factors)
	1. Inconsistent or poor oral hygiene	
	2. Heavy calculus formation	
	3. Systemic disease that predisposes to periodontal breakdown	
	4. Some remaining pockets	
	5. Occlusal problems	
	6. Complicated prostheses	
	7. Ongoing orthodontic therapy	
	8. Recurrent dental caries	
	9. Some teeth with less than 50% of alveolar bone support	
Class C	Generally poor results following periodontal therapy and/or several negative factors from the following list:	1 to 3 mo (decide on recall interval on the basis of the number and severity of negative factors; consider retreating some areas or extracting the severely involved teeth)
	1. Inconsistent or poor oral hygiene	
	2. Heavy calculus formation	
	3. Systemic disease that predisposes to periodontal breakdown	
	4. Remaining pockets	
	5. Occlusal problems	
	6. Complicated prostheses	
	7. Recurrent dental caries	
	8. Periodontal surgery indicated but not performed for medical, psychological, or financial reasons	
	9. Many teeth with less than 50% of alveolar bone support	
	10. Condition too far advanced to be improved by periodontal surgery	

terpret whether a test may be useful in determining disease activity and future loss of attachment.[7] Tests should be adopted only when they are based on research that includes a critical analysis of the sensitivity, specificity, disease incidence, and predictive value of the proposed test.

MAINTENANCE FOR IMPLANT PATIENTS

Patients with implants are susceptible to a form of bone loss that has been called *peri-implantitis,* and there is evidence that such patients may be more prone to plaque-induced inflammation with bone loss than are those with natural teeth[5,55,67] (see Chapter 65).

The microflora of implants in partially edentulous patients differs from that in edentulous patients.[4] The implant microflora is similar to tooth microflora in the partially edentulous mouth. Periodontal and implant maintenance are linked, since maintenance of a tooth microflora consistent with periodontal health is necessary to maintain implant microflora consistent with peri-implant health.[4] Because peri-implantitis is difficult to treat,[16] it is extremely important to provide good supportive therapy with implant patients.

In general, procedures for maintenance of patients with implants are similar to those with natural teeth,[38,62] but there are four differences:

1. Plaque control is performed during postsurgical healing periods.
2. No metal instrumention is used for calculus removal on the implants.
3. Acidic fluoride prophylactic agents are avoided.
4. Bacterial monitoring is performed more frequently.

During the phase after uncovering the implants, patients must use ultrasoft brushes, chemotherapeutic rinses, tartar control pastes, irrigation devices, and yarn-like materials to keep the implants and natural teeth clean. Patients will often be afraid to touch the implants but must be encouraged to keep the areas clean.

No metal instruments should be used on the implants during recall appointments.[38] Only plastic instruments should be used for calculus removal, because the implant surfaces can be easily scratched (Fig. 68-11). The rubber cup with flour of pumice provides the smoothest polished abutment surface when used with light intermittent pressure.[37]

Although daily use of topically applied antimicrobials is advised,[38] acidic fluoride agents should not be used because they cause surface damage to titanium abutments.[46]

Because the presence of bacteria associated with peri-

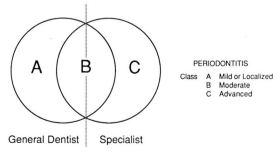

Maintenance Performed by:

PERIODONTITIS
Class A Mild or Localized
       B Moderate
       C Advanced

General Dentist | Specialist

FIGURE 68-10. Scheme for determining which practitioner should perform periodontal maintenance in patients with different degrees of periodontitis.

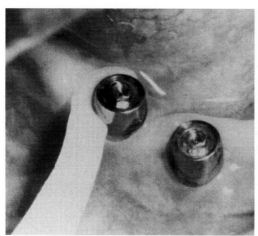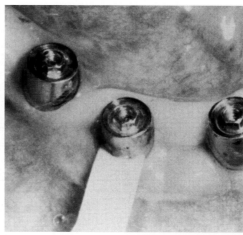

FIGURE 68–11. Plastic instruments used to remove debris from implants.

odontitis and peri-implantitis may play a contributory role in the loss of fixtures, the subgingival plaque of implants with pocketing should be monitored.[5,43]

When prosthetics must be unscrewed and removed for maintenance, it is best done in the office responsible for placing the prosthetics. Each time the prosthetics are re-attached, there will be a slight change in the occlusion. Time must be allowed for occlusal corrections.

REFERENCES

1. Alaluusua S, Asikainen S, Lai CH. Intrafamilial transmission of Actinobacillus actinomycetemcomitans. J Periodontol 62:207, 1991.
2. Armitage GC. Diagnosing periodontal diseases. In Perspectives on Oral Antimicrobial Therapeutics. Littleton, MA, PSG Publishing Co, 1987.
3. Axelson P, Lindhe J. The significance of maintenance care in the treatment of periodontal disease. J Clin Periodontol 8:281, 1981.
4. Bauman GR, Mills M, Rapley JW, et al. Plaque induced inflammation around implants. Int J Oral Maxillofac Implants 7:330, 1992.
5. Bauman GR, Rapley JW, Hallmon WW, et al. The peri-implant sulcus. Int J Oral Maxillofac Implants 8:273, 1993.
6. Becker W, Becker BE, Berg LE. Periodontal treatment without maintenance. A retrospective study in 44 patients. J Periodontol 55:505, 1984.
7. Bennett WI. Screening for bowel cancer. Harvard Med School Health Lett 11:6, 1986.
8. Carranza FA Jr, Saglie FR, Newman MG, Valentin P. Scanning and transmission electron microscope study of tissue invading microorganisms in localized juvenile periodontitis. J Periodontol 54:598, 1983.
9. Caton JG, Zander HA. The attachment between tooth and gingival tissues after periodic root planing and soft tissue curettage. J Periodontol 50:462, 1979.
10. Chace R. Retreatment in periodontal practice. J Periodontol 48:410, 1977.
11. Christersson LA, Albini B, Zambon JJ, et al. Tissue localization of *Actinobacillus actinomycetemcomitans* in human periodontitis. I. Light, immunofluorescence and electron microscopic studies. J Periodontol 58:529, 1987.
12. Cortellimi P, Pini-Prato G, Torretti M. Periodontal regeneration of human infrabony defects. V. Effects of oral hygiene on long-term stability. J Clin Periodontol 21:606, 1994.
13. Dahlen G, Lindhe J, Sato K, et al. The effect of supragingival plaque control on the subgingival microbiota in subjects with periodontal disease. J Clin Periodontol 19:802, 1992.
14. Egloff E, Saglie FR, Newman MG. Intragingival bacteria subsequent to scaling and root planing. Abstract. J Dent Res 65:269, 1986.
15. Greenwell H, Bissada NB, Wittwer JW. Periodontics in general practice: Perspectives on periodontal diagnosis. J Am Dent Assoc 119:537, 1989.
16. Grunder U, Hürzeler MB, Schüpbach P, et al. Treatment of ligature-induced peri-implantitis using guided tissue regeneration: A clinical and histologic study in the beagle dog. Int J Oral Maxillofac Implants 8:282, 1993.
17. Halazonetis TD, Smulow JB, Donnenfeld W, Mejias JE. Pocket formation 3 years after comprehensive periodontal therapy. A retrospective study. J Periodontol 56:515, 1985.
18. Hirschfeld L, Wasserman B. A long-term survey of tooth loss in 600 treated periodontal patients. J Periodontol 49:225, 1978.
19. Kerr NW. Treatment of chronic periodontitis. Br Dent J 150:222, 1981.
20. Krieg AF, Gambino R, Galen RS. Why are clinical laboratory tests performed? JAMA 233:76, 1975.
21. Lang NP, Joss A, Orsanic T, et al. Bleeding on probing. J Clin Periodontol 13:590, 1986.
22. Lietha-Elmer E. Langsfritsgie Ergebnisse reglemassig betreuter und unbetreuter Parodontosepatienten. Schweiz Monatsschr Zahnheilkd 87:613, 1977.
23. Lightner LM, O'Leary TM, Drake RB, et al. Preventive periodontic treatment procedures: Results over 46 months. J Periodontol 42:555, 1971.
24. Lindhe J, Heijl L, Goodson JM, Socransky SS. Local tetracycline delivery using hollow fiber devices in periodontal therapy. J Clin Periodontol 6:141, 1979.
25. Lindhe J, Koch G. The effect of supervised oral hygiene on the gingiva of children. J Periodont Res 1:260, 1966.
26. Lindhe J, Koch G. The effect of supervised oral hygiene on the gingiva of children. Lack of prolonged effect of supervision. J Periodont Res 2:215, 1967.
27. Lindhe J, Nyman S. The effect of plaque control and surgical pocket elimination on the establishment and maintenance of periodontal health. A longitudinal study of periodontal therapy in cases of advanced disease. J Clin Periodontol 2:67, 1975.
28. Lindhe J, Nyman S, Karring T. Scaling and root planing in shallow pockets. J Clin Periodontol 9:415, 1982.
29. Listgarten MA, Hellden L. Relative distribution of bacteria at clinically healthy and periodontally diseased sites in humans. J Clin Periodontol 5:115, 1978.
30. Listgarten MA, Levin S. Positive correlation between the proportions of subgingival spirochetes and motile bacteria and susceptibility of human subjects to periodontal deterioration. J Clin Periodontol 8:122, 1981.
31. Listgarten MA, Lindhe J, Hellden L. Effect of tetracycline and/or scaling on human periodontal disease. Clinical, microbiological and histologic observations. J Clin Periodontol 5:246, 1978.
32. Listgarten MA, Schifter CC, Sullivan P, et al. Failure of a microbiological assay to reliably predict disease recurrence in a treated periodontitis population receiving regularly scheduled prophylaxes. J Clin Periodontol 13:768, 1986.
33. Listgarten MA, Sullivan P, George C, et al. Comparative longitudinal study of 2 methods of scheduling maintenance visit: 4-year data. J Clin Periodontol 16:105, 1989.
34. MacPhee IT, Muir KF. Dark ground microscopy in relation to 3 clinical parameters of chronic inflammatory periodontal disease. J Clin Periodontol 13:900, 1986.
35. Matteson SR, Bottomley W, Finger H, et al. The selection of patients for x-ray examinations: Dental radiographic examinations. DHHS publication no. FDA 88-8273. Washington, DC, Department of Health and Human Services, October 1987.
36. Mazza JE, Newman MG, Sims TN. Clinical and antimicrobial effect of stannous fluoride on periodontitis. J Clin Periodontol 8:213, 1981.
37. McCollum J, O'Neal RB, Brennan WA, et al. The effect of titanium implant abutment surface irregularities on plaque accumulation in vivo. J Periodontol 63:802, 1992.
38. Meffert RM, Langer B, Fritz ME. Dental implants: A review. J Periodontol 63:859, 1992.
39. Mendoza AR, Newcomb GM, Nixon KC. Compliance with supportive periodontal therapy. J Periodontol 62:731, 1991.
40. Mousques T, Listgarten MA, Phillips RW. Effect of scaling and root planing on the composition of human subgingival microflora. J Periodont Res 15:144, 1980.
41. Nyman S, Rosling B, Lindhe J. Effect of professional tooth cleaning on healing after periodontal surgery. J Clin Periodontol 2:80, 1975.
42. Oliver RC. Tooth loss with and without periodontal therapy. Periodont Abstracts 17:8, 1969.
43. Ong ESM, Newman HN, Wilson M, Bulman JS. The occurrence of periodontitis related microorganisms in relation to titanium implants. J Periodontol 63:200, 1992.
44. Parr RW, Pipe P, Watts T. Periodontal Maintenance Therapy. Berkeley, CA, Praxis Publishing, 1974.
45. Pertuiset JH, Saglie FR, Lofthus J, et al. Recurrent periodontal disease and bacterial presence in the gingiva. J Periodontol 58:553, 1987.
46. Probster L, Lin W, Juttemann H. Effect of fluoride prophylactic agents on titanium surfaces. Int J Oral Maxillofac Implants 7:390, 1992.

47. Ramfjord SP, Knowles JW, Nissle RR, et al. Results following three modalities of periodontal therapy. J Periodontol 46:522, 1975.
48. Rosenberg ES, Evian CI, Listgarten MA. The composition of the subgingival microbiota after periodontal therapy. J Periodontol 52:435, 1981.
49. Rosling B, Nyman S, Lindhe J. The effect of systematic plaque control on bone regeneration in infrabony pockets. J Clin Periodontol 3:38, 1976.
50. Rosling B, Nyman S, Lindhe J, Jern B. The healing potential of the periodontal tissues following different techniques of periodontal surgery in plaque-free dentitions. J Clin Periodontol 3:233, 1976.
51. Ross IF, Thompson RH, Galdi M. The results of treatment: A long term study of 180 patients. Parodontologie 25:125, 1971.
52. Ryan RJ. The accuracy of clinical parameters in detecting periodontal disease activity. J Am Dent Assoc 111:753, 1985.
53. Saglie FR, Newman MG, Carranza FA Jr, et al. Immunohistochemical localization of Actinobacillus actinomycetemcomitans in sections of gingival tissue in localized juvenile periodontitis. Acta Odont Lat Am 1:40, 1984.
54. Schallhorn RG, Snider LE. Periodontal maintenance therapy. J Am Dent Assoc 103:227, 1981.
55. Schou S, Holmstrup P, Reibel J, et al. Ligature-induced marginal inflammation around osseointegrated implants and ankylosed teeth: Stereologic and histologic observations on cynomolgus monkeys. J Periodontol 64:529, 1993.
56. Slots J, Mashimo P, Levine MJ, Genco RJ. Periodontal therapy in humans. I. Microbiological and clinical effects of a single course of periodontal scaling and root planing, and of adjunctive tetracycline therapy. J Periodontol 50:495, 1979.
57. Smulow JB, Turesky SS, Hill RG, The effect of supragingival plaque removal on anaerobic bacteria in deep pockets. J Am Dent Assoc 107:737, 1983.
58. Stahl SS. Repair potential of the soft tissue–root interface. J Periodontol 48:545, 1977.
59. Stahl SS, Froum SJ. Human clinical and histologic repair responses following the use of citric acid in periodontal therapy. J Periodontol 48:261, 1977.
60. Stahl SS, Witkin GJ, Heller A, Brown R Jr. Gingival healing. IV. The effects of home care on gingivectomy repair. J Periodontol 40:264, 1969.
61. Sternlich HC. Evaluating long-term periodontal therapy. Tex Dent J 92:4, 1974.
62. Stewart RT. Personal communication. Scripps Clinic, La Jolla, CA.
63. Strid KG. Radiographic procedures. In Brånemark PI, Zarb GA, Albrektsson T, eds. Tissue Integrated Prostheses. Chicago, Quintessence Publishing, 1985.
64. Suomi JD, West JD, Chang JJ, McClendon BJ. The effect of controlled oral hygiene procedures on the progression of periodontal disease in adults: Radiographic findings. J Periodontol 42:562, 1971.
65. Suomi JD, Greene JC, Vermillion JR, et al. The effect of controlled oral hygiene procedures on the progression of periodontal disease in adults: Results after the third and final year. J Periodontol 42:152, 1971.
66. Van Steenbergen TJM, Petit MDA, van der Velden U, de Graaff J. Transmission of Porphyromonas gingivalis between spouses. J Clin Periodontol 20:340, 1993.
67. Van Steenberghe D, Klinge B, Linden U, et al. Periodontal indices around natural and titanium abutments: A longitudinal multicenter study. J Periodontol 64:538, 1993.
68. Waerhaug J. Healing of the dento-epithelial junction following subgingival plaque control. J Periodontol 49:119, 1978.
69. Wilson TG Jr, Glover ME, Schoen J, et al. Compliance with maintenance therapy in a private periodontal practice. J Periodontol 55:468, 1984.
70. Wilson TG Jr. Compliance. A review of the literature. J Periodontol 58:706, 1987.
71. Wilson TG Jr, Glover ME, Malik AK, et al. Tooth loss in maintenance patients in a private periodontal practice. J Periodontol 58:231, 1987.
72. Wilson TG. Maintaining periodontal treatment. J Am Dent Assoc 121:491, 1990.
73. Withers JA, Brunsvold MA, Killoy WJ, Rahe AJ. The relationship of palatogingival grooves to localized periodontal disease. J Periodontol 52:41, 1981.

69

Results of Periodontal Treatment

ROBERT L. MERIN

Prevention and Treatment of Gingivitis
Prevention and Treatment of Loss of Attachment
Prevention of Loss of Attachment

Treatment of Loss of Attachment
Tooth Mortality

The prevalence of periodontal disease and the high tooth mortality rate resulting from it raise an important question: Is periodontal treatment effective in preventing and stopping the progressive destruction of periodontal disease? *Evidence is overwhelming that periodontal therapy is effective in preventing periodontal disease, slowing the destruction of the periodontium, and reducing tooth loss.*

PREVENTION AND TREATMENT OF GINGIVITIS

For many years, the belief that good oral hygiene is necessary for the successful prevention and treatment of gingivitis has been widespread among periodontists. In addition, worldwide epidemiologic studies have confirmed a close relationship between the incidence of gingivitis and lack of oral hygiene.[5,6]

Conclusive evidence on the relation of oral hygiene and gingivitis in healthy dental students was shown by Löe and coworkers.[17,32] After 9 to 21 days without performing oral hygiene measures, experimental subjects with previously excellent oral hygiene and healthy gingiva developed heavy accumulations of plaque and generalized mild gingivitis. When oral hygiene techniques were reinstituted, the plaque in most areas disappeared in 1 or 2 days, and gingival inflammation in these areas disappeared 1 day after the plaque was removed. Thus, gingivitis is reversible and can be resolved by daily effective plaque removal.

A number of long-term studies have shown that gingival health can be maintained by a combination of effective oral hygiene maintenance and scaling procedures.[1,2,8,10,11,19,30,31]

A 3-year study was conducted on 1248 General Telephone workers in California to determine whether progression of gingival inflammation is retarded in an oral environment in which high levels of hygiene are maintained.[30,31] Experimental and control groups were computer matched on the basis of periodontal and oral hygiene status, past caries experience, age, and sex. During the study period, several procedures were instituted to ensure that the oral hygiene status of the experimental group was maintained at a high level. Subjects were given a series of frequent oral prophylaxis treatments, combined with oral hygiene instruction. Subjects in the control group received no attention from the study team except for annual examinations. They were advised to continue their usual daily practices and accustomed visits for professional care. After 3 years, the increase in plaque and debris in the control group was four times as great as that in the experimental group. Similarly, gingivitis scores were much higher in control subjects than in the matching experimental group. Therefore, *chronic marginal gingivitis can be controlled with good oral hygiene and dental prophylaxis.*

PREVENTION AND TREATMENT OF LOSS OF ATTACHMENT

Although periodontal therapy has been used for more than 100 years, it is only since the mid-1970s that a number of studies have been conducted to determine the effect of treatment on reducing the progressive loss of periodontal support for the natural dentition.

Prevention of Loss of Attachment

A longitudinal investigation to study the natural development and progression of periodontal disease was conducted by Löe and coworkers.[15,18] The first group, established in Oslo, Norway, in 1969, consisted of 565 healthy male nondental students and academicians between 17 and 40 years of age. The principal reason for selecting Oslo as a study site was that this city had had a preschool, school, and postschool dental program offering systematic preventive, restorative, endodontic, orthodontic, and surgical therapy on an annual recall basis for all children and adolescents, complete with a documented attendance record, for the previous 40 years. Members of the study population had had maximum exposure to conventional dental care throughout their lives. A second group, established in Sri Lanka in 1970, consisted of 480 male tea laborers between 15 and 40 years of age. They were healthy and well built by local standards, and their nutritional condition was clinically fair. The workers had never been exposed to any programs relative to the prevention or treatment of dental diseases. Toothbrushing was unknown, and dental caries was virtually nonexistent.

The results of this study are quite interesting. The Norwegian group, as the members approached 40 years of age, had a mean individual loss of attachment of slightly above 1.5 mm, and the mean annual rate of attachment loss was 0.08 mm for interproximal surfaces and 0.10 mm for buccal surfaces. As the Sri Lankans approached 40 years of age, the mean individual loss of attachment was 4.50 mm, and the mean annual rate of progression of the lesion was 0.30 mm for interproximal surfaces and 0.20 mm for buccal surfaces. Figure 69-1 shows a graphic interpretation of the difference between the two groups. This study suggests that without interference, periodontal lesions progress at a relatively even pace, and this progress is continuous.

Further analysis of the Sri Lankan laborers[15] showed that they were not all losing attachment at the same rate (Figs. 69-2 and 69-3). Virtually all gingival areas showed inflammation, but attachment loss varied tremendously. Based on interproximal loss of attachment and tooth mortality, three subpopulations were identified: individuals with rapid progression (RP) of periodontal disease (8%), individuals with moderate progression (MP) (81%), and individuals who exhibited no progression (NP) of periodontal disease beyond gingivitis (11%). At age 35, the mean loss of attachment in the RP group was 9 mm; in the MP group, 4 mm; and in the NP group, less than 1 mm. At the age of 45, the mean loss of attachment in the RP group was 13 mm and in the MP group, 7 mm. It is obvious that under natural conditions and in the absence of any therapy, 89% of the Sri Lankan laborers had severe periodontitis that progressed at much greater rates than in the Norwegian group.

In the previously discussed study of General Telephone workers in California, loss of attachment was measured clinically and alveolar bone loss was measured radiographically.[30,31] After 3 years, the control group showed loss of attachment at a rate more than 3½ times that of the matching experimental group during the same period (Fig. 69-4). In addition, subjects who received frequent oral

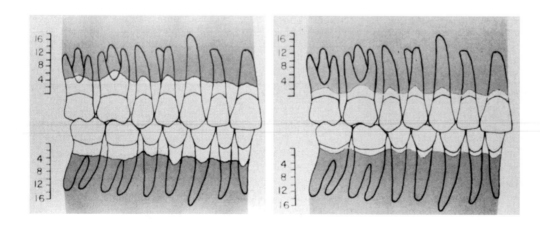

FIGURE 69-1. *Left,* Mean periodontal support of teeth of Sri Lankan tea laborers at approximately 40 years of age. *Right,* Mean periodontal support of teeth of Norwegian academicians at approximately 40 years of age. (From Löe H, et al. J Periodontol *49*:607, 1978.)

Classification of 480 Sri Lanka Laborers According to Progression of Periodontal Disease

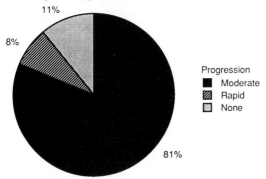

Progression
■ Moderate
▨ Rapid
▢ None

FIGURE 69–2. Progression of periodontal disease in an untreated population. (Data from Löe H, Anerud A, Boysen H, Morrison E. Natural history of periodontal disease in man. J Clin Periodontol *13*:431, 1986.)

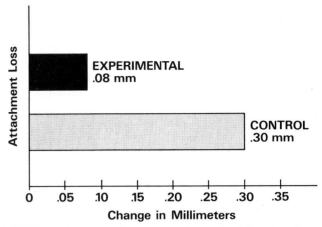

FIGURE 69–4. Change in mean attachment level from baseline to third-year examination for experimental and control groups. (From Suomi JD, West JD, Chang JJ, McClendon BJ. The effect of controlled hygiene procedures on the progression of periodontal disease in adults: Radiographic findings. J Periodontol *42*:152, 1971.)

prophylaxis and were instructed in good oral hygiene practices showed less bone loss radiographically after 3 years than did control subjects. It is clear that *loss of attachment can be reduced by good oral hygiene and frequent dental prophylaxis.*

Treatment of Loss of Attachment

A longitudinal study of patients with moderate to advanced periodontal disease conducted at the University of Michigan showed that the progression of periodontal disease can be stopped for a period of 3 years postoperatively regardless of the modality of treatment.[23–26] With long-term observations, the average loss of attachment was only 0.3 mm over 7 years.[26] These results indicated a more favorable prognosis for treatment of advanced periodontal lesions than previously assumed.

Another study was conducted in 75 patients with advanced periodontal disease to determine the effect of plaque control and surgical pocket elimination on the establishment and maintenance of periodontal health.[13] This study showed that no further alveolar bone loss occurred during the 5-year observation period. The meticulous plaque control practiced by the patients in this study was considered a major factor in the excellent results produced.

Mean Loss of Attachment at Various Ages (mm)

Progression Group	AGE	
	35	45
• Rapid	9	13
• Moderate	4	7

FIGURE 69–3. Loss of attachment in untreated Sri Lankan laborers. (Data from Löe H, Anerud A, Boysen H, Morrison E. Natural history of periodontal disease in man. J Clin Periodontol *13*:431, 1986.)

After 14 years, results for 61 of the initial 75 individuals were reported.[14] Repeated examinations demonstrated that treatment of advanced forms of periodontal disease resulted in clinically healthy periodontal conditions and that this state of health was maintained in most patients and sites during the 14-year period. A more detailed analysis of the data revealed, however, that a small number of sites in a few patients lost a substantial amount of attachment. Forty-three surfaces in 15 different patients were exposed to recurrent periodontal disease of significant magnitude. The frequency of sites that lost more than 2 mm of attachment during the 14 years of maintenance was 0.8% to 0.1% per year.

Neither of these studies used a control group, because failing to treat advanced periodontal patients cannot be justified for ethical reasons. However, in a study in private practice, an effort was made to find and evaluate patients with diagnosed moderate to advanced periodontitis who had not followed through with recommended periodontal therapy.[3] Thirty patients ranging in age from 25 to 71 years were evaluated after periods ranging from 18 to 115 months. All of these untreated patients had progressive increases in pocket depth and radiographic evidence of progressive bone resorption.

In a study of the progression of periodontal disease in the absence of therapy, two different populations were monitored.[12] One group of 64 Swedish adults with mild to moderate periodontal disease and one group of 36 Americans with advanced destructive disease were monitored, but not treated, for 6 years and 1 year, respectively. During the course of 6 years, 11.6% of all sites in the Swedish population (1.9% per year) showed attachment loss of greater than 2 mm, and the corresponding figure for the American population was 3.2% per year. Thus, the frequency of sites with disease progression was 20 to 30 times higher in untreated groups of patients than in the treated and well-maintained groups described in the preceding discussion.[14] *Thus, treatment is effective in reducing loss of attachment.*

Table 69–1. AVERAGE LOSS OF TEETH DURING A 5-YEAR PERIOD AS COMPARED WITH "NORMAL" LOSS OF TEETH IN 1428 MEN AND WOMEN AGES 20 THROUGH 59

	Grade of Oral Hygiene		
	Good	*Fairly Good*	*Not Good*
"Normal" loss of teeth (estimate based on data recorded at initiation of study period)	1.1	1.4	1.8
Actual loss of teeth during 5-year period	0.4	0.6	0.9

From Lovdal A, Arno A, Schei O, Waerhaug J. Combined effect of subgingival scaling and controlled oral hygiene on the incidence of gingivitis. Acta Odontol Scand *19:*537, 1961.

TOOTH MORTALITY

The ultimate test for the effectiveness of periodontal treatment is whether the loss of teeth can be prevented. There are now enough studies from both private practice and research institutions to document that loss of teeth is retarded or prevented by therapy.

The combined effect of subgingival scaling every 3 to 6 months and controlled oral hygiene was evaluated over a 5-year period in 1428 factory workers in Oslo, Norway.[19] Tooth loss was significantly reduced in all patients. This study showed that frequent subgingival scalings reduce tooth loss even when oral hygiene is not good (Table 69–1).

In the previously mentioned longitudinal study conducted at the University of Michigan, 104 patients with a total of 2604 teeth were included.[23–26] After 1 to 7 years of treatment, 53 teeth were lost for various reasons (Table 69–2). Thirty-two teeth were lost during the first and second years after initiation of treatment. The remaining 21 teeth were lost in a random pattern over the next 6 years. Therefore, the loss of teeth owing to advanced periodontal disease following treatment was minimal (1.15%).

Another study was undertaken to test the effect of periodontal therapy in cases of advanced disease.[13,14] The subjects were 75 patients who had lost 50% or more of their periodontal support (Fig. 69–5). Treatment consisted of

Table 69–2. TOOTH MORTALITY FOLLOWING TREATMENT OF ADVANCED PERIODONTITIS IN 104 PATIENTS WITH 2604 TEETH TREATED OVER A 10-YEAR PERIOD

Teeth Lost*	Reason
2	Pulpal disease
3	Accidents
4	Prosthetic considerations
14	One patient wanted a maxillary denture for cosmetic reasons
30	Periodontal
53	All reasons

* Two percent of the teeth were lost during the study period.
Adapted from data in Ramfjord SP, Knowles JW, Nissle RR, et al. Longitudinal study of periodontal therapy. J Periodontol *44:*66, 1973.

oral hygiene measures, scaling procedures, extraction of untreatable teeth, periodontal surgery, and prosthetics if indicated. After completion of periodontal treatment, there followed a 5-year period during which none of the patients showed any further loss of periodontal support. No teeth were extracted in the 5-year post-treatment period. It should be pointed out that the patients in this study were selected because of their capacity to meet high requirements of plaque control after repeated instruction in oral hygiene techniques. This fact does not detract from the validity of the study but tends to show the etiologic importance of bacterial plaque. The results indicate that periodontal surgery coupled with a detailed plaque control program not only temporarily cures the disease, but also reduces further progression of periodontal breakdown, even in patients with severely reduced periodontal support. After 14 years, 61 of the original patients were still in the study.[14] Recurrence of destructive periodontal disease in isolated sites of the dentition resulted in loss of a certain number of teeth during the observation period (Fig. 69–6). In the 6 to 10 years after active therapy, one tooth in each of three different patients was lost, and during the final observation period (11 to 14 years), three teeth in one patient, two teeth in each of three patients, and one tooth in each of four patients had to be extracted because of recurrent periodontal disease. In addition, three teeth in each of three different patients and one tooth in each of five patients were extracted owing to the development of extensive caries, periapical lesions, or other endodontic complications. During the entire course of the study, there was a total loss of 30

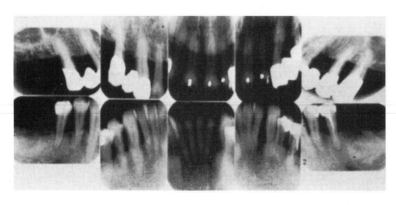

FIGURE 69–5. Radiographs taken 5 years after typical periodontal treatment. Note the advanced bone loss, in spite of which teeth were retained in a healthy condition for the duration of the study. (From Lindhe J, Nyman S. The effect of plaque control and surgical pocket elimination on the establishment and maintenance of periodontal health. A longitudinal study of periodontal therapy in cases of advanced disease. J Clin Periodontol *2:*67, 1975. ©1975 Munksgaard International Publishers Ltd., Copenhagen, Denmark.)

Cumulative Tooth Loss After 10-14 Years of Therapy in 61 Patients

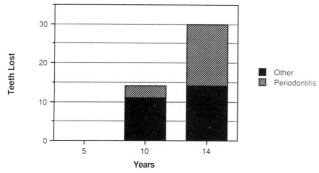

FIGURE 69–6. Tooth loss in treated patients with very advanced periodontal disease. (Data from Lindhe J, Nyman S. Long-term maintenance of patients treated for advanced periodontal disease. J Clin Periodontol *11*:504, 1984.)

teeth (for all reasons) out of 1330 teeth. The tooth mortality rate was therefore 2.3%.

There have been several studies in private practice that have attempted to measure frequency of tooth loss after periodontal therapy. In one study, 180 patients who had been treated for chronic destructive periodontal disease were evaluated.[27] The average age of the patients before treatment was 43.7 years. A total of 141 teeth were lost. From the beginning of treatment to the time of the survey, the majority of patients lost no teeth (Fig. 69–7). Three patients out of 180 (1.7%) lost 35 teeth, approximately 25% of the teeth lost. Twelve additional patients lost 46 teeth, or 32.6% of the teeth lost. Many patients in the study had advanced alveolar bone loss, including extensive furcation involvements. However, only a relatively small number (141) of the teeth were lost in the study group of 180 patients between the beginning of periodontal treatment and the time of the study.

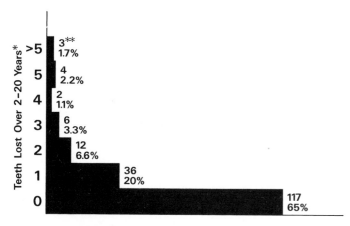

Number of Patients (n=180) with Percentage of Total

*Average of 8.6 years.
**3 patients lost 35 teeth.

The average tooth loss per patient was 0.9 per 10 years.

FIGURE 69–7. Tooth mortality. (Adapted from Ross IF, Thompson RH, Galdi M. The results of treatment. A long term study of one hundred and eighty patients. Parodontologie *25*:125, 1971.)

% of Patients (n=211) with Teeth Lost Over 15-34 Years

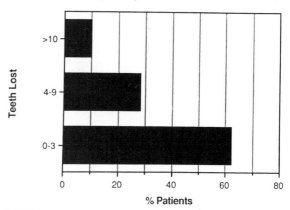

FIGURE 69–8. Tooth mortality 15 to 34 years after initiation of therapy (average, 22.2 years). Average tooth loss is 1.6 teeth per 10 years. Compare with the same study population in Figure 69–7. As the treated population ages, the rate of bone loss appears to increase. (Adapted from Goldman MJ, Ross IF, Goteiner D. Effect of periodontal therapy on patients maintained for 15 years or longer. J Periodontol *57*:347, 1986.)

The teeth were lost for several reasons, including periodontal disease as well as caries and other nonperiodontal causes.* The length of time after treatment varied from 2 to 20 years, with an average of 8.6 years. Of considerable significance is the large number of teeth (81 teeth, or 57.5%) lost by a few patients (15 patients, or 8.4%). Even when this group is considered with the remaining 165 patients, it may be seen that the periodontal care provided helped to retain most teeth, as the average tooth loss was slightly less than one tooth (0.9) over the 10 years following treatment.

In a follow-up study, the long-term results of periodontal therapy were evaluated after 15 to 34 years (average, 22.2 years).[4] The average tooth loss at this time was 1.6 teeth per 10 years. Patients were classified into three groups according to tooth loss. Sixty-two percent had an average tooth loss of 0.45 per 10 years and were considered "well maintained." Twenty-eight percent lost an average of 2.6 teeth per 10 years and were considered "downhill." Ten percent lost an average of 6.4 teeth per 10 years and were considered "extreme downhill" (Fig. 69–8).

---

*U.S. Public Health Surveys conducted in the 1960s indicated that an average of 4.3 teeth were lost after age 35 in the general population.[9]

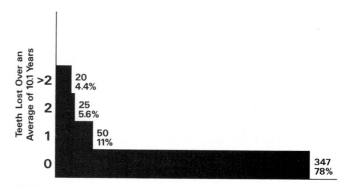

FIGURE 69–9. Tooth mortality in 442 periodontal patients treated over a period of 10 years. (Courtesy of Dr. R. G. Oliver.)

Another study included all patients in a practice who had been treated 5 or more years previously and had received regular preventive periodontal care since that time.[22] There were 442 patients, with an average length of time since treatment of 10.1 years. Two thirds of the patients were older than 40 at the time of treatment. These patients had been seen every 4.6 months, on average, for their preventive periodontal care, which consisted of oral hygiene instruction and prophylaxis (Figs. 69–9 and 69–10).

The total tooth loss owing to periodontal disease was 178 of just over 11,000 teeth available for treatment. More important, 78% of the patients did not lose a single tooth following periodontal therapy, and 11% lost only one tooth. When one considers that more than 600 teeth had furcation involvements at the time of the original treatment and that well over 1000 teeth had less than half of the alveolar bone support remaining, the tooth loss was low. During the same average 10-year period following periodontal therapy, only

Table 69–3. TOOTH MORTALITY IN TREATED PERIODONTITIS PATIENTS

Study	Average Number of Teeth Lost per 10 Years With Periodontal Treatment
Hirschfeld and Wasserman[7]	1.0
McFall[21]	1.4
Oliver[22]	0.72
Ross et al.[27]	0.9
Goldman et al.[4]	1.6

45 teeth were lost through caries or pulpal involvement. Even more surprising are the statistics over an average 10-year period for teeth with a less than optimal prognosis. Only 85 (14%) of a total of 601 teeth with furcation involvement were lost, and 117 (11%) of 1039 teeth with half or less of the bone remaining were lost. Of the 1043 teeth listed as having a guarded prognosis for any reason by the clinician performing the initial examination, only 126 (12%) were lost over this 10-year average period. The average tooth mortality rate was 0.72 tooth lost per patient per 10 years.

In a third study in private practice, 600 patients were followed for a period of between 15 and 53 years after periodontal therapy[7] (Table 69–3; Figs. 69–11 and 69–12). The majority (76.5%) had advanced periodontal disease at the start of treatment. There were 15,666 teeth present, for an average of 26 teeth per patient. During the follow-up period (average, 22 years), a total of 1312 teeth were lost owing to all causes. Of this number, 1110 were lost for periodontal reasons. The average tooth mortality rate per patient was 2.2 teeth; when this is converted to a 10-year rate, an average of one tooth was lost per 10 years in each patient. During this period of observation, 666 teeth with a questionable prognosis were lost out of a total of 2141. This means that 31% of the teeth with a questionable prognosis were lost over 22 years of treatment. A total of 1464 teeth with furcation involvement were treated, and 31.6% were lost during the period of study. Eighty-three percent of the patients lost fewer than three teeth over the 22-year average treatment period and were classified as "well maintained." The remaining 17 percent of the patients were di-

Furcation Involvement

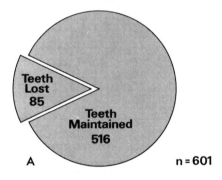

A   n = 601

One-half Bone Lost

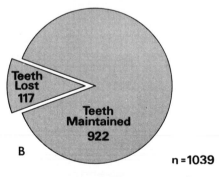

B   n = 1039

Guarded Prognosis

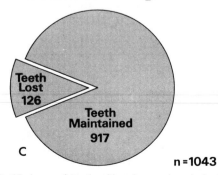

C   n = 1043

FIGURE 69–10. Loss of teeth with advanced periodontal disease over a period of 10 years. (Courtesy of Dr. R. G. Oliver.)

Status at Start

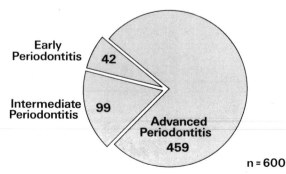

n = 600

FIGURE 69–11. Status at start of study of 600 patients reported by Hirschfeld and Wasserman. (Data from Hirschfeld L, Wasserman B. A long-term survey of tooth loss in 600 treated periodontal patients. J Periodontol 49:225, 1978.)

Tooth Mortality

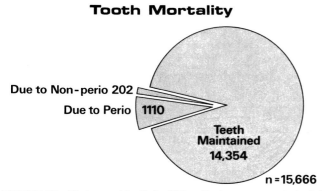

Due to Non-perio 202

Due to Perio 1110

Teeth Maintained 14,354

n=15,666

FIGURE 69-12. Loss of teeth in 600 patients over a period of 15 to 53 years. (Data from Hirschfeld L, Wasserman B. A long-term survey of tooth loss in 600 treated periodontal patients. J Periodontol 49:225, 1978.)

vided into two groups: "downhill" (four to nine teeth lost) or "extreme downhill" (10 to 23 teeth lost). Thus, 17% of the patients studied accounted for 69% of the teeth lost owing to periodontal causes. This study also showed that relatively few teeth are lost following periodontal therapy. In addition, relatively few of the teeth with guarded prognosis, including those with furcation involvement, are lost, and a small percentage of patients lose most of the teeth.

There are two studies that give insight into tooth mortality in untreated patients. The studies of Löe and coworkers in Sri Lankan laborers[15] showed that after the age of 35, an average of 5 and 16 teeth were lost per 10 years in the moderate progression and rapid progression groups, respectively (Fig. 69-13). In a previously discussed study in private practice,[3] an effort was made to find and evaluate patients with diagnosed moderate to advanced periodontitis who did not follow through with recommended periodontal therapy. Patients with untreated periodontal disease were losing teeth at a rate greater than 0.61 tooth per year (6.1 teeth per 10 years). A total of 83 teeth were lost in 30 patients, but the investigators excluded one patient who had lost 25 teeth. Including this patient would have increased the tooth loss in untreated patients to an even higher rate.

Table 69-4. TOOTH MORTALITY IN UNTREATED PERIODONTITIS PATIENTS

Study	Average Number of Teeth Lost per 10 Years Without Periodontal Treatment
Becker et al.[3]	6
Löe et al.[15] (moderate progression)	5
Löe et al.[15] (rapid progression)	16

When one compares Tables 69-3 and 69-4, it is obvious that tooth mortality is much greater in untreated groups.

In summary, the prevalence of periodontal disease and the high tooth mortality rate resulting from the disease have raised the need for effective treatment. Treatment is now available that is effective in preventing the disease and in stopping the progression of bone destruction after periodontitis is present. In addition, there is overwhelming evidence that periodontal therapy greatly reduces tooth mortality. Every dental practitioner should be familiar with the philosophy and techniques of periodontal therapy. Failure to diagnose and treat periodontal disease or to make periodontal treatment available to patients causes unnecessary dental problems and tooth loss.

REFERENCES

1. Axelsson P, Lindhe J. Effect of controlled oral hygiene procedures on caries and periodontal disease in adults. Results after 6 years. J Clin Periodontol 8:239, 1981.
2. Bay I, Moller IJ. The effect of a sodium monofluorophosphate dentifrice on the gingiva. J Periodont Res 3:103, 1968.
3. Becker W, Berg L, Becker EB. Untreated periodontal disease: A longitudinal study. J Periodontol 50:234, 1979.
4. Goldman MJ, Ross IF, Goteiner D. Effect of periodontal therapy on patients maintained for 15 years or longer. J Periodontol 57:347, 1986.
5. Greene JC. Periodontal disease in India: Report of an epidemiological study. J Dent Res 39:302, 1960.
6. Greville TNE. United States life tables by dentulous or edentulous condition, 1971, and 1957-58. Publication no. (HRA) 75-1338. Washington, DC, U.S. Department of Health, Education and Welfare, August 1974.
7. Hirschfeld L, Wasserman B. A long-term survey of tooth loss in 600 treated periodontal patients. J Periodontol 49:225, 1978.
8. Hoover DR, Lefkowitz W. Reduction of gingivitis by toothbrushing. J Periodontol 36:193, 1955.
9. Kelly JE, Van Kirk LE Jr, Garst CC. Decayed, missing and filled teeth in adults. United States 1960-1962. Public Health Service Publication no. 1000, Series 11, No. 23. Washington, DC, February 1967.
10. Ladavalya MRN, Harris R. A study of the gingival and periodontal conditions of a group of people in Chieng Mai povince. J. Periodontol 30:219,1959.
11. Lightner LM, O'Leary JT, Drake RB, et al. Preventive periodontic treatment procedures: Results over 46 months. J Periodontol 42:555, 1971
12. Lindhe J, Haffajee AD, Socransky SS. Progression of periodontal disease in adult subjects in the absence of periodontal therapy. J Clin Periodontol 10:433, 1983.
13. Lindhe J, Nyman S. The effect of plaque control and surgical pocket elimination on the establishment and maintenance of periodontal health. A longitudinal study of periodontal therapy in cases of advanced disease. J Clin Periodontol 2:67, 1975.
14. Lindhe J, Nyman S. Long-term maintenance of patients treated for advanced periodontal disease. J Clin Periodontol 11:504, 1984.
15. Löe H, Anerud A, Boysen H, Morrison E. Natural history of periodontal disease in man. J Clin Periodontol 13:431, 1986.
16. Löe H, Silness J. Periodontal disease in pregnancy. I. Prevalence and severity. Acta Odontol Scand 21:533, 1976.
17. Löe H, Theilade E, Jensen SB. Experimental gingivitis in man. J Periodontol 36:177, 1965.
18. Löe H, Anerud A, Boysen H, Smith M. The natural history of periodontal disease in man. J Periodontol 49:607, 1978.
19. Lovdal A, Arno A, Schei O, Waerhaug J. Combined effect of subgingival scaling and controlled oral hygiene on the incidence of gingivitis. Acta Odontol Scand 19:537, 1961.

Tooth Loss in Sri Lankan Laborers

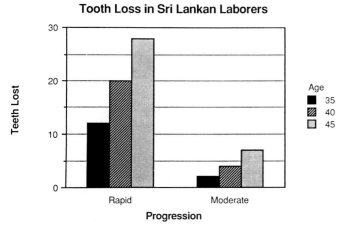

Teeth Lost

30

20

10

0

Rapid   Moderate

Progression

Age
■ 35
▨ 40
□ 45

FIGURE 69-13. Tooth loss in a population with untreated periodontal disease. (Data from Löe H, Anerud A, Boysen H, Morrison E. Natural history of periodontal disease in man. J Clin Periodontol 13:431, 1986.)

20. Marshall-Day CD, Stephens RG, Quigley LF. Periodontal disease: Prevalence and incidence. J Periodontol *26:*185, 1955.
21. McFall WT Jr. Tooth loss with and without periodontal therapy. Periodont Abstracts *17:*8, 1969.
22. Oliver RC. Personal communication, 1977.
23. Ramfjord SP, Nissle RR. The modified Widman flap. J Periodontol *45:*601, 1974.
24. Ramfjord SP, Nissle RR, Shick RA, Cooper H. Subgingival curettage versus surgical elimination of periodontal pockets. J Periodontol *39:*167, 1968.
25. Ramfjord SP, Knowles JW, Nissle RR, et al. Results following three modalities of periodontal therapy. J Periodontol *46:*522, 1975.
26. Ramfjord SP, Knowles JW, Nissle RR, et al. Longitudinal study of periodontal therapy. J Periodontol *44:*66, 1973.
27. Ross IF, Thompson RH. A long-term study of root retention in the treatment of maxillary molars with furcation involvement. J Periodontol *49:*238, 1978.
28. Ross IF, Thompson RH, Galdi M. The results of treatment. A long term study of one hundred and eighty patients. Parodontologie *25:*125, 1971.
29. Russell AL. Some epidemiological characteristics of periodontal diseases in a series of urban populations. J Periodontol *28:*286, 1957.
30. Suomi JD, West JD, Chang JJ, McClendon BJ. The effect of controlled oral hygiene procedures on the progression of periodontal disease in adults: Radiographic findings. J Periodontol *42:*152, 1971.
31. Suomi JD, Greene JC, Vermillion JR, et al. The effect of controlled oral hygiene on the progression of periodontal disease in adults: Results after the third and final year. J Periodontol *42:*152, 1971.
32. Theilade E, Wright WH, Jensen SB, Löe H. Experimental gingivitis in man. II. J Periodont Res *1:*1, 1966.

Index

Note: Page numbers in *italics* refer to illustrations; roman numerals refer to color plates. Page numbers followed by t refer to tables.

ISBN 0-7216-6728-7

90071

9 780721 667287